Respiratory Emergencies

Respiratory Emergencies

Edited by

Alan M. Fein
Clinical Professor of Medicine at the New York University School of Medicine and Chief of Pulmonary, Critical Care and Sleep Medicine, ProHealth Care Associates, LLP. He is an attending physician at North Shore University Hospital and Long Island Jewish Medical Center, New York, USA

Stephan Kamholz
David J. Greene Professor of Medicine at the New York University School of Medicine, and Chairman of the Department of Medicine at North Shore University Hospital and Long Island Jewish Medical Center, New York, USA

David Ost
Associate Professor of Medicine at the New York University School of Medicine and Director of Interventional Pulmonology at New York University Medical Center, New York, USA

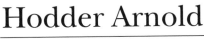

Hodder Arnold
A MEMBER OF THE HODDER HEADLINE GROUP

First published in Great Britain in 2006 by
Hodder Arnold, an imprint of Hodder Education, a member of the
Hodder Headline Group,
338 Euston Road, London NW1 3BH

http://www.hoddereducation.com

Distributed in the United States of America by
Oxford University Press Inc.,
198 Madison Avenue, New York, NY10016
Oxford is a registered trademark of Oxford University Press

Whilst the advice and information in this book are believed to be true and
accurate at the date of going to press, neither the author[s] nor the
publisher can accept any legal responsibility or liability for any errors or
omissions that may be made. In particular, (but without limiting the
generality of the preceding disclaimer) every effort has been made to check
drug dosages; however it is still possible that errors have been missed.
Furthermore, dosage schedules are constantly being revised and new side-
effects recognized. For these reasons the reader is strongly urged to consult
the drug companies' printed instructions before administering any of the
drugs recommended in this book.

British Library Cataloguing in Publication Data
A catalogue record for this book is available from the British Library

Library of Congress Cataloging-in-Publication Data
A catalog record for this book is available from the Library of Congress

ISBN-10   0 340 81195 1
ISBN-13   978 0 340 81195 5

1 2 3 4 5 6 7 8 9 10

Commissioning Editor: Philip Shaw
Project Editor: Heather Fyfe
Production Controller: Karen Tate
Cover Design: Tim Pattinson

Typeset in 10/12pt Minion by Phoenix Photosetting, Chatham, Kent
Printed and bound in Great Britain by CPI Bath

What do you think about this book? Or any other Arnold title?
Please send your comments to **www.hoddereducation.com**

Contents

Contributors

Alexandre R Abreu MD
Chief Fellow, Division of Pulmonary and Critical Care Medicine
Miller School of Medicine
University of Miami
Miami Beach, FL
USA

Sandra G Adams MD
Assistant Professor, Department of Medicine
Division of Pulmonary Diseases/Critical Care Medicine
University of Texas Health Science Center at San Antonio
and
South Texas Veterans Health Care System
Audie L Murphy Memorial Veterans Hospital Division,
San Antonio, TX
USA

Gautam Ahluwalia MD
Associate Professor, Department of Medicine
Dayanand Medical College and Hospital
Ludhiana
India

Shoaib Alam MD
Assistant Professor of Medicine
Division of Pulmonary, Allergy and Critical Care
Penn State University-Hershey Medical Center
Hershey, PA
USA

Nicolino Ambrosino MD
Head, Pulmonary Unit
Cardio-Thoracic Department
Azienda Ospedaliera-Universitaria Pisana
Pisa
Italy

Antonio Anzueto MD
Professor of Medicine
Division of Pulmonary Diseases/Critical Care Medicine
University of Texas Health Science Center at San Antonio
and
South Texas Veterans Health Care System
Audie L Murphy Memorial Veterans Hospital Division,
San Antonio, TX
USA

Anup Banerjee MD
Pulmonary and Critical Care Medicine
Indiana University Hospital
Indianapolis, IN
USA

Nicolas Baudouin
Department of Pulmonary and Intensive Care University Hospital
Dijon
France

Philippe Bonniaud
Department of Pulmonary and Intensive Care University Hospital
Dijon
France

Clio Camus
Department of Pulmonary and Intensive Care University Hospital
Dijon
France

Philippe Camus
Department of Pulmonary and Intensive Care University Hospital
Dijon
France

Matthew D Cham MD
Assistant Professor of Radiology
Department of Radiology
Weill Medical College of Cornell University
New York, NY
USA

Mildred Chen MD
Assistant Professor of Radiology
Department of Radiology
Weill Medical College of Cornell University
New York, NY
USA

Brian M Cuneo MD, FCCP
Director, Medical Intensive Care Unit and Respiratory Care Services
Pulmonary and Critical Care Medicine Service
Walter Reed Army Medical Center
Washington DC
USA

Steven Deitelzweig MD
Section Head, Hospital-Based Internal Medicine
Ochsner Clinic Foundation
New Orleans, LA
USA

Asha Devereaux MD, MPH, FCCP
Attending Physician
Pulmonary/Critical Care Medicine
Sharp-Coronado Hospital
Cornado, CA
USA

Sean T Devine
Attending Physician
Geisinger Health System
Danville, PA
USA

George A Eapen MD
Associate Professor of Medicine,
MD Anderson Cancer Center
Houston, TX
USA

Ali A El Solh MD, MPH
Associate Professor of Medicine
Department of Medicine, Division of Pulmonary, Critical Care, and
Sleep Medicine
University at Buffalo School of Medicine and Biomedical Sciences
Buffalo, NY
USA

Marcia Epstein MD, FACP, FIDSA
Assistant Professor
NYU School of Medicine
Infectious Disease Attending at
North Shore University Hospital
Manhasset, NY
USA

Armin Ernst MD
Director, Interventional Pulmonology
Beth Israel Deaconess Medical Center and Harvard Medical School
Boston, MA
USA

John E Fitzgerald MD
Associate Professor of Medicine
Pulmonary/Critical Care Division
UT Southwestern Medical Center
Dallas, TX
USA

Pascal Foucher
Department of Pulmonary and Intensive Care University Hospital
Dijon
France

Wolfgang Frank MD
Medical Director
Klinik Amsee
Malchiner Landstrasse
Waren (Müritz)
Germany

James A Geiling MD, FACP, FCCP
Chief, Medical Service, Department of Veterans Affairs Medical
Center
and
Associate Professor of Medicine, Dartmouth Medical School
White River Junction, VT
USA

Liziamma George MD, FCCP, FACP
Director, Medical Intensive Care Unit and Respiratory Care Unit
New York Methodist Hospital
Brooklyn, New York
USA

Colin K Grissom MD, FCCP
Assistant Professor of Medicine
Pulmonary and Critical Care Division
Department of Medicine
LDS Hospital and the University of Utah
Salt Lake City, UT
USA

Jay T Heidecker MD
Senior Pulmonary Fellow
Division of Pulmonary and Critical Care Medicine
Medical University of South Carolina
Charleston, SC
USA

John E Heffner MD
Professor of Medicine
Executive Medical Director
Medical University of South Carolina
Charleston, SC
USA

Claudia I Henschke PhD, MD
Professor of Radiology and Chief of Chest Imaging
Department of Radiology
Weill Medical College of Cornell University
New York, NY
USA

Nicholas S Hill MD
Chief, Division of Pulmonary, Critical Care and Sleep Medicine
Tufts-New England Medical Center
Boston, MA
USA

John T Huggins MD
Senior Fellow
Medical University of South Carolina
Charleston, SC
USA

Hemwattie Shantie Jaimangal DO
Infectious Disease Fellow at
North Shore University Hospital
Manhasset, HY
USA

Ahmad Jibbaoui
Department of Pulmonary and Intensive Care University Hospital
Dijon
France

Jill P Karpel MD
Department of Pulmonary and Critical Care Medicine
North Shore University Hospital
Manhasset, NY
USA

Kabeya Kazambu
Department of Pulmonary and Intensive Care University Hospital
Dijon
France

Felix Khusid RRT–NPS, RPFT
Administrative Director, Respiratory Therapy
New York Methodist Hospital
Brooklyn, New York
USA

Angela Kim MD
Instructor in Medicine
NYU School of Medicine
Infectious Disease Attending at
North Shore University Hospital
Manhasset, NY
USA

Antonia Koutsoukou MD
Associate Professor of Critical Care Medicine
Department of Critical Care and Pulmonary Services
University of Athens Medical School
Evangelismos Hospital
Athens
Greece

Kevin L Kovitz MD, MBA
Professor of Medicine and Pediatrics
and
Director, Interventional Pulmonology and Medical Critical Care
Medical Director and Associate Dean for Medical Affairs
Section of Pulmonary Diseases, Critical Care and Environmental
Medicine
Tulane University Health Sciences Center
New Orleans, LA
USA

Bruce P Krieger MD, FACP, FCCP
Professor of Medicine (Vol.)
Miller School of Medicine
University of Miami
Associate Medical Director, Critical Care Center
Memorial Hospital Jacksonville
USA

Deepa G Lazarous MD
Fellow, Division of Pulmonary, Critical Care and Sleep Medicine
Georgetown University Hospital
Washington DC
USA

Michael Lippmann MD
Head, Pulmonary/Critical Care
Albert Einstein Medical Center
Philadelphia, PA
USA

Robert Loddenkemper MD
Professor of Medicine
Charité–Universitäts–Medizin Berlin
and former Medical Director of Dept of Pneumology
Lungenklinik
Heckeshorn
Helios Klinikum
Emil von Behring
Berlin
Germany

Mark E Lund MD
Director, Regional Center for Complex Airways Disease Management
Lewiston, ME
USA

Vinay Maheshwari MD
Fellow, Pulmonary and Critical Care
Tufts-New England Medical Center
Boston, MA
USA

Praveen N Mathur MB BS
Professor of Clinical Medicine
Indiana University Hospital
Pulmonary and Critical Care Medicine
Indianapolis, IN
USA

Nuala J Meyer MD
Fellow
Pulmonary and Critical Care Medicine
University of Chicago
Chicago, IL
USA

Dorothy I McCauley MD
Professor of Radiology
Department of Radiology
Weill Medical College of Cornell University
New York, NY
USA

James E Mojica MD
Pulmonary Critical Care Unit
Harvard Medical School
Massachusetts General Hospital
Boston, MA
USA

Lisa K Moores MD, FACP, FCCP
Associate Professor of Medicine
Uniformed Services University of the Health Sciences
Pulmonary and Critical Care Medicine Service
Walter Reed Army Medical Center
Washington, DC
USA

Ali M Nadroo MD
Assistant Professor of Clinical Pediatrics
Weill Medical College of Cornell University
Attending Neonatologist, Department of Pediatrics
New York Methodist Hospital
Brooklyn, NY
USA

Pramod Narula MD
Associate Professor of Clinical Pediatrics
Weill Medical College of Cornell University
Chairman Department of Pediatrics
New York Methodist Hospital
Brooklyn, NY
USA

Anne E O'Donnell MD
Chief, Division of Pulmonary, Critical Care and Sleep Medicine
Georgetown University Hospital
Washington DC
USA

Jonathan B Orens MD
Associate Professor of Medicine, Medical Director Lung
Transplantation Program
Associate Director, Division of Pulmonary and Critical Care Medicine
Johns Hopkins University
Division of Pulmonary and Critical Care Medicine
Baltimore, MD
USA

Harold I Palevsky MD
Professor of Medicine
University of Pennsylvania School of Medicine
Chief, Pulmonary, Allergy and Critical Care
Penn Presbyterian Medical Center
Director, Pulmonary Vascular Disease Program
USA

Suhail Raoof MD, FCCP, FACP, FCCM
Professor of Clinical Medicine
Weill Medical College of Cornell University
Chief, Division of Pulmonary and Critical Care Medicine
Medical Director, Respiratory Therapy
New York Methodist Hospital
Brooklyn, New York
USA

Nitin P Ron MD
Assistant Professor of Clinical Pediatrics
Weill Medical College of Cornell University
Attending Neonatologist, Department of Pediatrics
New York Methodist Hospital
Brooklyn, NY
USA

Charis Roussos MD, MSc, PhD, MRS, FRCP(C)
Professor of Critical Care Medicine
Department of Critical Care and Pulmonary Services
University of Athens Medical School
Evangelismos Hospital
Athens
Greece

Steven A Sahn MD, FCCP, FACP, FCCM
Professor of Medicine and Director
Division of Pulmonary and Critical Care Medicine
Medical University of South Carolina
Charleston, SC
USA

Jonathan Sackner–Bernstein MD
Former Clinical Scholars Program
Heart Failure and Cardiomyopathy Center
Division of Cardiology
North Shore University Hospital
Manhasset, NY
USA

Massimiliano Serradori MD
Cardio-Thoracic Department
Azienda Ospedaliera-Universitaria Pisana
Pisa
Italy

Marvin I Schwarz MD
The James C Campbell Professor of Pulmonary Medicine
Division of Pulmonary Sciences and Critical Care Medicine
University of Colorado Health Sciences Center
Denver, CO
USA

Gregory A Schmidt MD
Professor, Division of Pulmonary Diseases, Critical Care and
Occupational Medicine
University of Iowa
Iowa City, IA
USA

Lawrence Shulman DO
Department of Pulmonary and Critical Care Medicine
North Shore University Hospital
Manhasset, NY
USA

Hal A Skopicki MD, PhD, FACC
Assistant Professor of Medicine
Director, Heart Failure and Cardiomyopathy Program
SUNY – Stony Brook School of Medicine
Stony Brook, NY
USA

Vickie R Shannon MD
Associate Professor of Medicine,
MD Anderson Cancer Center
Houston, TX
USA

Mario Solomita DO
Department of Internal Medicine
North Shore University Hospital
Manhasset, NY
USA

Sean Studer MD
Assistant Professor of Medicine
Divisions of Pulmonary and Critical Care Medicine
Departments of Medicine
University of Pittsburgh Medical Center
Pittsburgh, PA
USA

Arthur Sung MD
Instructor in Medicine
and
Fellow, Interventional Pulmonology
Section of Pulmonary Diseases, Critical Care and Environmental
Medicine
Tulane University Health Sciences Center
New Orleans, LA
USA

Arunabh Talwar MD, FCCP
Attending, Division of Pulmonary and Critical Care Medicine
Department of Internal Medicine
North Shore University Hospital Manhasset
and
Assistant Professor, Medicine
New York University School of Medicine
New York
USA

Victor F Tapson MD
Professor of Medicine, Director, Pulmonary Hypertension Center
Director, Center for Pulmonary Vascular Disease
Division of Pulmonary, Allergy, and Critical Care Medicine
Duke University Medical Center
Durham, NC
USA

Antoni Torres
Chief of Pulmonology Department
Institut Clinic de Pneumologia I Cirurgia Toràcica
Hospital Clínic de Barcelona
Barcelona
Spain

Mauricio Valencia
Clinical Researcher
Respiratory Intensive Care Medicine
Hospital Clínic de Barcelona
Barcelona
Spain

Aaron B Waxman MD, PhD
Director, Pulmonary Disease Program
Pulmonary Critical Care Unit
Harvard Medical School
Massachusetts General Hospital
Boston, MA
USA

Kathleen Williams DO
Past Fellow, Interventional Pulmonology
Section of Pulmonary Diseases, Critical Care and Environmental
Medicine
Tulane University Health Sciences Center
New Orleans, LA
and
Interventional Pulmonologist
Portland, OR
USA

David F Yankelevitz MD
Professor of Radiology
Department of Radiology
Weill Medical College of Cornell University
New York, NY
USA

Abbreviations

2PAMCl	pralidoxime chloride	CPR	cardiopulmonary resuscitation
AAP	American Academy of Pediatrics	CRDQ	Chronic Respiratory Disease Questionnaire
ACCP	American College of Chest Physicians	CT	computed tomography
ACE	angiotensin-converting enzyme	CTPA	CT pulmonary angiography
ACEI	angiotensin-converting enzyme inhibitor	CTV	CT venography
ACh	acetylcholine	CVC	central venous catheter
AChE	acetylcholinesterase	DAH	diffuse alveolar hemorrhage
ACR	American College of Radiology	DCI	decompression illness
ACTH	adrenocorticotropic hormone	DCS	decompression sickness
AECC	American–European Consensus Conference	DHS	dengue hemorrhagic fever
AECOPD	acute exacerbations of chronic obstructive pulmonary disease	D_LCO	diffusion capacity for carbon monoxide
		DSS	dengue shock syndrome
AEP	acute eosinophilic pneumonia	DVT	deep vein thrombosis
AGE	arterial gas embolus	EBRT	external beam radiation therapy
ALI	acute lung injury	$ECCO_2R$	extracorporeal carbon dioxide removal
AMP	adenosine monophosphate	ECMO	extracorporeal membrane oxygenation
AMS	acute mountain sickness	EELV	end-expiratory lung volume
APC	argon plasma coagulation	EKG	electrocardiogram
APT	amiodarone pulmonary toxicity	EPAP	expiratory positive airway pressure
aPTT	activated partial thromboplastin time	ERS	European Respiratory Society
ARDS	acute respiratory distress syndrome	ETC	esophageal tracheal combitube
ATA	atmosphere absolute units	ETT	endotracheal tube
ATRA	all *trans*-retinoic acid	FBI	fiberoptic endotracheal intubation
ATS	American Thoracic Society	FDA	Food and Drug Administration
AV	arteriovenous	FEV_1	forced expiratory volume in 1 second
BAE	bronchial arterial embolization	Fio_2	fractional inspired oxygen
BAL	bronchoalveolar lavage	FIVC	forced inspiratory vital capacity
BDI	Baseline Dyspnea Index	FRC	functional residual capacity
BiPAP	bilevel positive airway pressure	FVC	forced vital capacity
BNP	B-type natriuretic peptide	GMP	guanosine monophosphate
BOOP	bronchiolitis obliterans organizing pneumonia	GVHD	graft-versus-host disease
BPD	bronchopulmonary dysplasia	HAART	highly active antiretroviral therapy
BUN	blood urea nitrogen	HACE	high-altitude cerebral edema
CABG	coronary artery bypass graft surgery	HAP	hospital-acquired pneumonia
CAO	central airway obstruction	HAPE	high-altitude pulmonary edema
CAP	community-acquired pneumonia	HCAP	healthcare-associated pneumonia
CCB	calcium-channel blocker	HDR	high dose rate
CDC	Centers for Disease Control and Prevention	HIT	heparin-induced thrombocytopenia
CDH	congenital diaphragmatic hernia	HPA	hypothalamic–pituitary–adrenal (axis)
CMV	cytomegalovirus	HRCT	high-resolution computed tomography
CNS	central nervous system	HRQoL	health-related quality of life
COP	cryptogenic organizing pneumonia	HSCT	hematopoietic stem cell transplant
COPD	chronic obstructive pulmonary disease	IABP	intraaortic balloon pump
CPAP	continuous positive airway pressure	IC	inspiratory capacity

ICP	intracranial pressure		PCP	*Pneumocystis carinii* pneumonia
ICU	intensive care unit		PCR	polymerase chain reaction
IL	interleukin		PCT	portable computed tomography
ILD	interstitial lung disease		PDT	percutaneous dilatational tracheostomy
iLMA	intubated laryngeal mask airway		PDT	photodynamic therapy
iNO	inhaled nitric oxide		PE	pulmonary embolism
IPAH	idiopathic pulmonary arterial hypertension		$P_E co_2$	expired partial pressure of carbon dioxide
IPAP	inspiratory positive airway pressure		PEF	peak expiratory flow (sometimes given as PEFR)
IPF	idiopathic pulmonary fibrosis		PEFR	peak expiratory flow rate
IPS	idiopathic pneumonia syndrome		PERDS	peri-engraftment respiratory distress syndrome
IRS	immune reconstitution syndrome		PH	pulmonary hypertension
IRV	inverse ratio ventilation		PIF	PIF, peak inspiratory flow
ISHLT	International Society for Heart and Lung Transplantation		PLV	partial liquid ventilation
			PPE	personal protective equipment
IVCF	inferior vena caval filter		PPH	primary pulmonary hypertension
IVOX	intravenous oxygenator		PPHN	persistent pulmonary hypertension of the new born
LDH	lactate dehydrogenase		P_{pl}	pleural pressure
LMA	laryngeal mask airway		P_{plat}	plateau pressure
LMWH	low-molecular-weight heparin		P_{pw}	pulmonary capillary wedge pressure
LTOT	long-term oxygen therapy		PSI	Pneumonia Severity Index
LVS	live vaccine strain		PSP	primary spontaneous pneumothorax
Mch	methacholine		PSV	pressure support ventilation
MDI	metered-dose inhaler		RAR	rapidly adapting receptor
MEB	middle ear barotrauma		R_{aw}	airways resistance
MODS	multiple organ dysfunction syndrome		RBC	red blood cell
MRC	Medical Research Council		RDS	respiratory distress syndrome
MSAF	meconium-stained amniotic fluid		RV	residual volume
MSOF	multisystem organ failure		$Sa\sco_2$	arterial oxygen saturation
Nd:YAG	neodymium:yttrium aluminum garnet		SARS	severe acute respiratory syndrome
NFA	near-fatal asthma		SASR	slowly adapting stretch receptor
NGT	nasogastric tube		SCBA	self-contained breathing apparatus
NICU	neonatal intensive care unit		SEMS	self-expandable metallic airway stents
NIPPV	noninvasive positive pressure ventilation		SIDS	sudden infant death syndrome
NIV	noninvasive ventilation		SSP	secondary spontaneous pneumothorax
NVD	neuro-ventilatory dissociation		TDI	Transition Dyspnea Index
NYHA	New York Heart Association		TEF	tracheoesophageal fistula
OHS	obesity hypoventilation syndrome		TLC	total lung capacity
$Pa co_2$	alveolar carbon dioxide tension (or pressure)		TNF	tumor necrosis factor
Pco_2	partial pressure of carbon dioxide		TRALI	transfusion-related acute lung injury
Po_2	partial pressure of oxygen		TTI	tension time index
PA	pulmonary artery		UFH	unfractionated heparin
$Paco_2$	arterial carbon dioxide tension (or pressure)		VAS	visual analog scale
Pao_2	arterial oxygen tension (or pressure)		VATS	video-assisted thoracoscopic surgery
PAC	pulmonary artery catheter		VB	virtual bronchoscopy
PACS	picture archiving and communications system		$\dot{V}_E$	minute ventilation
PAF	platelet activating factor		$\dot{V}/Q$	ventilation–perfusion
PAH	pulmonary arterial hypertension		VTE	venous thromboembolism
PAI	plasminogen activator inhibitor		WBC	white blood cell

Reference annotation

The reference lists are annotated, where appropriate, to guide readers to primary articles, key review papers, and management guidelines, as follows:

- ●   Seminal primary article
- ◆   Key review paper
- ✳   First formal publication of a management guideline

We hope that this feature will render extensive lists of references more useful to the reader and will help to encourage self-directed learning among both trainees and practicing physicians.

Pathophysiology

Dyspnea: pathophysiology, diagnosis, and quantitation

NICOLINO AMBROSINO, MASSIMILIANO SERRADORI

INTRODUCTION

The most common symptom in patients with respiratory diseases is dyspnea – 'difficult, labored, uncomfortable breathing'.[1] The American Thoracic Society (ATS) defines dyspnea as:[2]

> a term used to characterize a subjective experience of breathing discomfort that consists of qualitatively distinct sensations that vary in intensity. The experience derives from interactions among multiple physiological, psychological, social and environmental factors, and may induce secondary physiological and behavioral responses.

Dyspnea is characterized by a measurable intensity and qualitative dimensions, which may vary depending on the individual, the underlying disease, and other circumstances.[3]

NEUROPHYSIOLOGIC BASIS OF DYSPNEA

Receptors in the airways, lung parenchyma, respiratory muscles, and chemoreceptors provide sensory feedback via the vagal, phrenic, and intercostal nerves to the spinal cord, medulla, and higher centers[4] (Fig. 1.1).

Chemoreceptors

Both peripheral and central chemoreceptors can sense changes in arterial oxygen (Pa_{O_2}) and carbon dioxide

(Pa_{CO_2}) tension and pH to ensure that alveolar ventilation can adapt to changes in metabolic needs. Hypercapnia stimulates ventilation, therefore it must influence the perception of breathing. At a given level of ventilation, dyspnea is greater during hypercapnic than exercise hyperpnea.[5] The urge to breathe at a constant level of ventilation increases with increasing P_{CO_2}, but the sense of

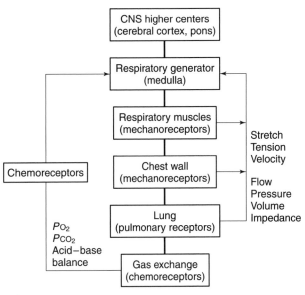

Figure 1.1 *Neurophysiological basis of dyspnoea. CNS, central nervous system. (Redrawn with permission from Voduc N, Webb K, O'Donnell D. Physiological basis of dyspnea. In: Donner CF, Ambrosino N, Goldstein RS, eds.* Pulmonary Rehabilitation: Efficacy and Scientific Basis. *London: Hodder Arnold.[4])*

effort to breathe actually decreases.[6] An independent role for carbon dioxide in the pathogenesis of dyspnea and, in particular, the perception of 'air hunger' is suggested by several observations: subjects paralyzed with curare do not complain of 'air hunger' after carbon dioxide inhalation;[7] high-level quadriplegic patients report 'air hunger' with increasing levels of carbon dioxide, without any increase in ventilation;[8] and pharmacologically paralyzed healthy subjects still report severe dyspnea in response to relatively mild hypercapnia.[9] One study found that in patients with chronic obstructive pulmonary disease (COPD) during exercise central chemoresponsiveness explained about 28 percent of peak breathlessness variance,[10] no mechanical factor being involved. These results conflict with previous reports.[11]

The effects of arterial hypoxia on dyspnea are still under discussion.[12] Hypoxia may act both indirectly by increasing ventilation and directly, independent of change in ventilation. The response to induced hypoxemia in health is quite variable, and the response to supplemental oxygen in patients with pulmonary diseases, even with severe resting hypoxemia, is unpredictable.[13] Arterial hypoxia acutely stimulates the peripheral chemoreceptors, whose afferent activity may directly reach consciousness. The resultant increased central motor output and respiratory muscle activation may contribute to breathing discomfort. The possible sensory consequences of hypoxic effects on the heart and pulmonary vessels are still poorly understood. Hypoxia may cause ventilatory muscle fatigue, which requires greater motor activation and effort for a given muscle contraction, leading to respiratory discomfort. In patients with airflow limitation, hypoxic hyperventilation will result in air trapping and dynamic lung hyperinflation, which may *per se* contribute to dyspnea.[14,15] Nevertheless although one study showed that oxygen reduced the degree of dynamic lung hyperinflation during recovery from exercise, it did not make patients feel less breathless than breathing air.[16] The relative contribution of each of the multiple sensory inputs arising from hypoxia is still to be clarified.

Pulmonary receptors

Different types of pulmonary receptor have been identified.[17] Slowly adapting stretch receptors (SASRs), which are located principally in large airways, respond to increases in lung volume. Rapidly adapting receptors (RARs) in the airway epithelium respond to different stimuli, such as particulate irritants, direct stimulation of the airways, and pulmonary congestion. Juxtapulmonary (J) receptors are nonmyelinated fibers (C fibers) located near pulmonary capillaries and in the bronchial and laryngeal mucosa. These fibers are stimulated by mechanical and chemical stimuli which result in apnea, rapid shallow breathing, bronchoconstriction, and mucus hypersecretion. Almost all

of the afferent signals from pulmonary receptors are ultimately carried to the central nervous system (CNS) via the vagus nerve.

Pulmonary receptors, in particular the J receptors, might be implicated in the sensation of dyspnea.[18] Vagal blocking has resulted in inconsistent effects on dyspnea associated with pulmonary diseases such as emphysema, interstitial lung disease (ILD) or in patients with heart-lung transplants.[19–21] In contrast, the vagus nerve may have an important role in conveying sensory information related to bronchoconstriction.[22] As a whole, these results suggest that, although peripheral receptors contribute to dyspnea in some situations, they are not the exclusive source of the sensation.

Mechanoreceptors

Mechanical receptors for volume, flow, muscle shortening, muscle tension, and chest wall displacement provide peripheral sensory feedback modulating the intensity of central motor output at central sensory level (see Fig. 1.1). The feedback is negative because its inhibition increases the perception of breathlessness.[23] Several studies have suggested that stimulation of chest wall afferents reduces rather than increases dyspnea. Inspiratory chest wall vibration decreases the breathlessness induced by a combination of hypercapnia and resistive load.[24] Compared with no vibration, inspiratory vibration over the parasternal intercostals significantly reduces dyspnea whereas expiratory vibration (out of phase) has an opposite effect, both in healthy subjects and in patients with chronic respiratory disease.[25]

Respiratory muscle effort

Dyspnea may reflect greater respiratory muscle activity or 'effort'. Perception of effort is the awareness of the efferent motor command from the CNS to the respiratory muscles. Sense of effort is a central sensation that increases whenever the central motor command or muscle load increases, or when the muscles are weakened, fatigued, or paralyzed. During voluntary increase in ventilation, the increased motor command is sent to the ventilatory muscles, and the motor cortex transmits a copy signal to the sensory cortex through receptors spread out in the cortex. This copy signal is called 'central corollary discharge'. A corollary discharge is also sent to the sensory cortex by the brainstem. However, this signal is weaker and probably associated with either the perception of 'air hunger' or a lesser sense of effort.[3,6]

The sense of muscle 'effort' reflects the magnitude of this corollary discharge and is dependent not only on the absolute magnitude of the load and its duration, but also on the relative magnitude of the load compared with the maximum capacity of the muscle. With regard to the respiratory muscles, inspiratory effort is proportional to the intrathoracic pressures generated during tidal breathing, related to the peak pressures generated during a maximum inspiratory effort.[26–28] Increased contractile muscle effort may explain the presence of dyspnea in a variety of clinical settings. Chronic obstructive pulmonary disease and ILD as well as pulmonary vascular diseases are all associated, in varying degrees, with increased ventilatory demand, excessive mechanical loading, and functional weakness of the ventilatory muscles. All of these derangements are ultimately associated with increased breathing effort. However, the perception of respiratory muscle effort is not always synonymous with dyspnea. Studies in asthmatic patients during acute bronchoconstriction have shown that some patients on mechanical ventilation may continue to experience severe dyspnea despite effective reduction in tidal esophageal (pleural) pressure swings, i.e. a reduced respiratory effort.[29] In such patients ventilatory muscle unloading is not enough to reduce dyspnea, which thus also must have other causes.

Neuro–ventilatory dissociation

Dyspnea may occur when a greater than expected respiratory muscle activity is required to produce a given amount of ventilation. This was formerly described as 'length–tension inappropriateness'.[30] With regard to the respiratory system 'length' actually corresponds to the change in lung volume whereas 'tension' corresponds to the respiratory pressures produced. It has been suggested that dyspnea is the result of a 'dissociation' or discrepancy between the ventilatory drive and the amount of produced ventilation.[31] That is, dyspnea may be the result of an interaction between efferent and afferent signals (neuro-ventilatory dissociation [NVD]).[32,33] The afferent signal might be the sum of sensory information related to respiratory pressures, airflow, and lung and chest wall motion. In health there is an appropriate matching between efferent motor signals and afferent feedback during rest and exercise. Dyspnea may result from a dissociation between the amplitude of the central efferent discharge and afferent sensory inputs (feedback).

These findings suggest that dyspnea results from multiple and simultaneous sensory inputs, thus highlighting the crucial importance of the CNS in the final integration of this complex sensation. A functional brain imaging study[34] showed that high loaded breathing was associated with neural activation in three distinct brain regions: the right anterior insula, the cerebellar vermis, and the medial pons. This suggests that conscious perception of acutely induced respiratory discomfort during loaded breathing results from two distinct, parallel integration processes. The first may be involved in sensorimotor integration of loaded breathing and thus in the perception of the predominant part of perceived intensity of respiratory discomfort, whereas the second may be involved in the modulation of perceived intensity, which presumably includes emotional processing of this sensory experience.

THE LANGUAGE OF DYSPNEA

Different pathophysiologic abnormalities result in different qualities of respiratory discomfort. Therefore verbal descriptors could help to define one or more of the responsible abnormalities and contribute to a specific diagnosis. In one study,[35] dyspnea descriptors were obtained from normal volunteers able to distinguish between sensations induced by different stimuli such as breath holding, carbon dioxide inhalation, exercise, resistive and elastic respiratory loads, constrained tidal volume (V_T) and from symptomatic patients with different cardiorespiratory diseases. Standardized descriptors were grouped in discrete clusters with high discriminating value among diseases: the pathologic conditions characterized by many clusters suggests that:

- dyspnea comprises more than one sensation
- each condition is characterized by a unique set of clusters
- some clusters are shared by more than one condition, suggesting that similar pathways or receptors modify dyspnea.

There was no obvious relation between the qualitative descriptors of dyspnea and the quantitative intensity among the patient groups: different diseases may be distinguished by the quality of the sensation and not by the intensity.[35]

Dyspnea descriptors can help in understanding the language of dyspnea.[8,36–38] Nevertheless differences in language and among races, cultures, and in the manner in which concepts or symptoms are held can all influence the idea of dyspnea.[39,40] Indeed, in a study in COPD patients[41] the relation between breathlessness and exercise performance was different between men and women: at any given level of exercise, women were more breathless than men.

Chest tightness

Vagal activity contributes to the sensation of 'chest tightness', a term frequently reported by asthmatic patients. The sensation of 'chest tightness' induced by acute bronchoconstriction receded after vagal blockade.[42] Airway anesthesia reduces the sensation of 'chest tightness' associated with histamine-induced bronchoconstriction.[43] During acute bronchospasm, 'chest tightness' may arise from the stimulation of sensory receptors within the lungs mediated through vagal and autonomic pathways. Contraction of airway smooth muscle stimulates SASRs whereas RARs (irritant) and J receptors may respond to local inflammation of the airways.[44]

Work/effort

Several clinical conditions are characterized by descriptors comprised in the cluster 'work/effort'.[35] The respiratory muscles are important to the experience of dyspnea. The intensity of the motor command to ventilatory muscles relayed to the sensory cortex (corollary discharge), alone or in combination with force generation and respiratory muscle contraction, can be perceived as a sensation of 'effort' and considered as difficult breathing.[45,46] Indeed during methacholine (Mch)-induced bronchoconstriction, unloading of respiratory muscles by means of assisted ventilation is associated with decrease in the effort score compared with spontaneous breathing.[47]

Unrewarded inspiration

The central motor command output to the sensory cortex (the corollary discharge) is modulated by peripheral feedback from several respiratory mechanoreceptors including muscle spindles, Golgi tendon organs, vagal lung and airway mechanoreceptors.[46] In patients with low cervical quadriplegia the quality and intensity of dyspnea during Mch-induced bronchoconstriction leading to dynamic lung hyperinflation were similar to the quality and intensity in asthma at maximal response and not altered by extensive chest wall deafferentation.[22] The mismatch between respiratory motor output and the mechanical response of the system may play a major role in the increased perception of exercise dyspnea in patients with COPD[32,33,48] and ILD.[49]

Rapid breathing

Healthy subjects exercising with external thoracic restriction, and patients with ILD frequently use terms such as 'rapid' and 'shallow' to describe their respiratory discomfort.[35,36,38,49,50] Due to inadequate lung distensibility, the increased respiratory drive results in increased respiratory frequency, potentially through vagal afferents.

Air hunger

Qualitatively different sensations can result from voluntary (cortical) versus reflex (brainstem) drives to breathe, consistent with the possibility that corollary discharge from medullary respiratory centers gives rise to 'air hunger', whereas corollary discharge from cortical motor centre gives rise to a sense of breathing 'effort'.[8] When respiratory rate is voluntarily increased or decreased with reciprocal changes in V_T from the spontaneous adopted level, dyspnea at any given level of ventilation worsens.[51] This indicates that breathing responses to change in chemical drive may be regulated, partially to minimize sensations of respiratory effort and discomfort.[51,52]

CLINICAL APPLICATIONS OF THE LANGUAGE OF DYSPNEA

Chronic obstructive pulmonary disease

Pathophysiologic factors known to contribute to dyspnea in patients with COPD include increased intrinsic mechanical loading of inspiratory muscles, the inspiratory threshold load (that is the dynamic intrinsic positive end-expiratory pressure [iPEEP][53]), increased mechanical restriction of the thorax, inspiratory muscle weakness, increased ventilatory demand relative to capacity, gas exchange abnormalities, dynamic airway compression, cardiovascular factors, and any combination of the above.[54]

DYNAMIC HYPERINFLATION

Expiratory flow limitation is the pathophysiologic condition in COPD. It is due to difficulty exhaling during forced and quiet expiration with related alveolar air retention and lung hyperinflation. Reduced lung recoil in emphysema alters the balance of forces between the lung and chest wall to a higher end-expiratory lung volume (EELV): inspiration begins before tidal expiration is complete and lung hyperinflation results. When respiratory rate acutely increases (and expiratory time diminishes), as during exercise, hyperventilation or exacerbations, there is further dynamic lung hyperinflation as a result of air trapping, with related mechanical and sensory consequences. Dynamic lung hyperinflation results in increased elastic and inspiratory threshold loading of inspiratory muscles (the iPEEP)[53] already burdened with increased resistive work. Moreover, acute-on-chronic hyperinflation compromises the ability of the ventilatory muscles, particularly the diaphragm, to increase pressure generation in response to the increased ventilatory drive during exercise.

Neither the forced expiratory volume at 1 second (FEV_1) nor the FEV_1 to vital capacity ratio (FEV_1/VC) is a good predictor of dyspnea in patients with severe chronic airflow obstruction. There is a close correlation between hyperinflation (as demonstrated by reduction of inspiratory capacity [IC]) during exercise and the intensity of exercise dyspnea.[32,33] Indeed long-acting β_2-agonists significantly reduced the transdiaphragmatic pressure–time product, an index of respiratory muscle activity, dynamic lung hyperinflation, and dyspnea during endurance treadmill walk. It has been shown that improvements in dyspnea scores correlate significantly with changes in the V_T to esophageal pressure swings ratio, EELV, and IC.[55] Furthermore, breathing heliox–oxygen mixture during cycle ergometer high-intensity constant work rate exercise has been shown to be associated with a reduction in dynamic lung hyperinflation, as reflected by an increase in IC correlated to the decrease in dyspnea.[56]

DIFFUSION CAPACITY

Patients with COPD, who have a reduced diffusion capacity for carbon monoxide ($D_L CO$), often experience more severe dyspnea and disability than those with a preserved $D_L CO$.[35]

WORK OF BREATHING

To the extent that intrinsic mechanical loading and functional inspiratory muscle weakness in COPD contribute to dyspnea, assisted ventilation should provide symptomatic benefit by unloading and assisting such overburdened ventilatory muscles. Several studies have examined the acute effects of different modalities of ventilatory assistance on dyspnea and exercise tolerance in advanced COPD.[57] The message of these physiologic studies could be summarized as follows: assisted ventilation during exercise reduces dyspnea and work of breathing and enhances exercise tolerance in COPD patients.

LANGUAGE

The effect of the physiologic derangement of COPD increases both corollary discharge and central output to skeletal muscles, and likely reduces the peripheral instantaneous feedback from the lung and chest wall receptors.[3] In contrast with healthy subjects, who report a perception of increased effort/work at the end of exhaustive exercise, patients with COPD select descriptors of inspiratory difficulty and unsatisfied inspiration (i.e. 'Can't get enough air in').[33] Neuro-ventilatory dissociation may form the basis for these discrete qualitative dimensions of dyspnea (Fig. 1.2). Patients with COPD also report qualitative perceptions of 'unsatisfied' or 'unrewarded' inspiration, 'shallow breathing' and 'inspiratory difficulty' during exercise. These distinct sensations are associated with dynamic lung hyperinflation and its negative mechanical effects, i.e. the iPEEP and the uncoupling of the normal association between respiratory effort and ventilatory output.[33,49,58,59]

Asthma

Patients use similar terms to describe spontaneous and induced asthma.[47,60] In induced asthma, the initial sensation of 'chest tightness' reflects the breathing discomfort resulting from mild bronchoconstriction; with more severe decrease in FEV_1 and hyperinflation, the sensation of 'work' or 'effort' of breathing takes place.[61] This may be due to the related inflammatory component of asthma, and associated mechanical load on the ventilatory muscles.[62] There may be, therefore, two distinct sensations of dyspnea; the first sensation is 'chest tightness' which probably arises from stimulation of pulmonary receptors secondary to bronchospasm and is relieved with bronchodilators. The second, 'work/effort' is likely to be associated with both

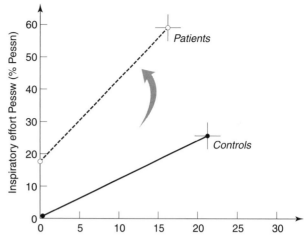

Figure 1.2 *Schematic representation of neuro-ventilatory dissociation of the respiratory pump. The figure is a plot of inspiratory effort to inspiratory tidal volume. In normal subjects (controls) a linear regression line starts from between inspiratory effort and the concurrent volume or flow. In patients with respiratory load and muscle weakness the slope increases, indicating the need for a greater effort for any given volume or flow. Furthermore, the intercept shifts to a greater effort, indicating an inspiratory threshold load. Pessw: esophageal pressure swings; Pessn, esophageal pressure during sniff maneuver. (Redrawn from Lung 180, 2002; 131–48, Pathophysiology of dyspnea, Scano G, Ambrosino N, Fig. 2, with kind permission of Springer Science and Business Media.[3])*

dynamic lung hyperinflation and more severe airway obstruction.

Like patients with asthma, patients with cystic fibrosis select the cluster 'tight'.[38] Because airway reactivity/bronchoconstriction is a common feature of these diseases, it is possible that the descriptor 'My chest feels tight' originates from airway receptors and reflects airway tone. Because of the underlying mechanism, the score of 'chest tightness' does not decrease with assisted ventilation compared with spontaneous breathing during Mch-induced bronchoconstriction. For the same reason, the 'chest tightness' score is higher with bronchospasm and hyperinflation than with ventilatory-induced hyperinflation and PEEP.[47]

Many descriptors that characterize bronchial asthma indicate that different pathophysiologic mechanisms are potentially in play.[39] A discrimination analysis showed that symptoms that can be reliably discriminated ('chest tightness' and 'chest pain') imply different neural processes, whereas symptoms that cannot be reliably discriminated ('breathlessness' and 'air hunger') imply a similar neural process. The study[39] also showed that dyspnea is more intense with bronchoconstriction, baseline pulmonary impairment, weight and female sex; dyspnea is less intense with age, bronchial hyperresponsiveness, low level of fear, coping, and adaptation.[39] Thus, attention to the language of dyspnea is useful in monitoring the response to bronchodilator therapy in patients with acute asthma. For instance rating of 'work/effort' may reflect the persistence of obstruction/inflammation of the airways more clearly than ratings of overall intensity of dyspnea alone.[63,64]

Perception and descriptors of dyspnea are also and more remarkably important for defining the severity of asthma. It has been shown that patients experiencing near-fatal asthma (NFA) attacks have a blunted perception of dyspnea.[65] Among patients with a low perception of dyspnea significantly more hospitalizations, NFA attacks, and deaths have been reported during the follow-up period.[66] It has been also found that perception of dyspnea is blunted in patients who have had an NFA at both rest and the end point of various exercises.[67] In addition, the mechanisms involved in the exercise limitation observed in NFA patients were different from those found in non-NFA subjects: the former stop exercising mainly because of leg discomfort, whereas the latter stop predominantly because of dyspnea.[67] Barreiros et al. propose that early detection of NFA candidates and assessment of their asthma status should be based on both subjective (dyspnea scales under different conditions) and objective (lung function) measurements. Existence of a dichotomy between these two types of evaluation would suggest an NFA risk.[67]

Interstitial/restrictive lung disease

Patients with restrictive lung disease frequently complain of 'work/effort', 'unsatisfied inspiration', 'inspiratory difficulty', 'rapid' and 'shallow'.[35,36,38,49] To avoid dyspnea, they adopt a tightly constrained breathing pattern.[52] These sensations have their physiologic basis partially in an impaired ability to increase lung volume and displace the thorax appropriately in the setting of an increased ventilatory drive. A slight variation in the patient's average tidal volume at rest provokes considerable dyspnea and this vulnerability to dyspnea probably explains why the resting respiratory cycle is so tightly controlled in patients with restrictive lung disease.[52] 'Air hunger' rating changes more deeply when $PaCO_2$ is altered and ventilation ($\dot{V}_E$) is constant, whereas the 'work/effort' rating changes more deeply when minute ventilation increases and $PaCO_2$ is constant.[68]

In patients with neuromuscular diseases a normal inspiratory motor output per unit change in PCO_2 results in a shallower breathing pattern.[69,70] The consequent impairment of neuro-ventilatory coupling underlies the high scoring of dyspnea in these patients. In turn, the association of muscle weakness and elastic load in neuromuscular disease is responsible for the modulation of a normal central respiratory output into a shallow breathing pattern. Neuromuscular disease,[69] COPD,[33,58] ILD,[49] and airway involvement in multisystem disease[71] share common mechanisms underlying the discomfort of breathing, explaining the similarity of clusters selected in different disorders.[39]

Congestive heart disease

Patients with chronic heart failure may stop exercising because of intolerable exercise dyspnea or leg fatigue or both at a point where there is apparent cardiopulmonary reserve.[72] During exercise these patients describe their dyspnea using the cluster 'suffocating at rest', 'rapid breathing', 'air hunger',[35] a 'need to sight'[36] or 'work/effort'.[38] There is no clear pathophysiologic explanation for that. Assisted ventilation decreases leg effort, probably by reducing the left ventricular afterload, increasing peripheral blood flow, and improving local acid–base equilibrium which reduces muscular afferents associated with the perception of 'effort'.[73] Nonetheless, the observation of no evident effect on dyspnea during the constant load exercise test suggests that factors other than mechanical loading contribute predominantly to dyspnea.

Hamilton et al.[74] and Killian[75] found that among patients with angina, pulmonary impairment, ischemic heart disease or cardiopulmonary disease the proportion of patients limited by dyspnea, leg effort, or a combination of both was similar for all disease types. Only the angina group selected 'chest pain'. Verbal descriptors may help to differentiate between patients with chronic heart failure and patients deconditioned who describe 'heavy breathing'.[76] In a study that aimed to determine whether differences existed between reports of dyspnea in stable COPD and chronic heart failure the most common terms given by COPD patients were 'scary', 'hard to breath', 'shortness of breath', and 'cannot get enough air', whereas chronic heart failure subjects used the terms 'shortness of breath', 'gasping', and 'cannot get enough air'.[77]

Despite the attention given by practitioners to different descriptors of dyspnea, often it can still be difficult to distinguish the underlying pathology. This may be the case in patients with chronic heart failure and patients with dyspnea from other causes. Therefore there is a need of objective markers, such as assessment of B-type natriuretic peptide levels, which are higher in patients with chronic heart failure than in other patients. Used together with other clinical information, Meuller et al. showed that rapid measurement of B-type natriuretic peptide in the emergency department improved the evaluation and treatment of patients with acute dyspnea, thereby reducing the time to discharge and total costs of treatment.[78] Also in a setting of primary care patients complaining of dyspnea N-terminal pro-brain peptide has been shown to be promising for disproval of heart failure.[79]

MEASUREMENT OF DYSPNEA

Both healthy subjects and patients with heart and lung disease use descriptors of dyspnea.[38,80] Several variables influence the patient's perception of intensity and/or descriptors of physical symptoms, including age, sex, socioeconomic status, medical history, and interaction with other patients.[40,41] These interactions become more complex with multiple comorbidities, such as depression, anxiety, and distress. Therefore there is the need to quantify, i.e. to measure, dyspnea. The two major purposes for measuring dyspnea are:

- to discriminate the severity of a symptom between individuals
- to evaluate changes in dyspnea within an individual patient.[81]

Both psychophysical methods and clinical scales have been used to assess breathlessness.[82] Although dyspnea is a subjective sensation, the principles of psychophysics (the study of the relation between a stimulus and the response) can be applied to quantify the severity of breathing discomfort.[83] Psychophysical testing usually involves the measurement of perception of breathing changes in response to externally added loads.[84] This approach has led to greater understanding of respiratory sensations but several factors, including technical aspects and time requirements, limit its application in the routine setting.

Visual analog scale

During an exercise test, dyspnea is usually measured by means of a visual analog scale (VAS) or a category ratio scale (see next section).[82,85–87] The VAS consists of a horizontal or vertical line, usually 100 mm in length, with or without descriptors or significant images positioned as anchors.[88] The descriptors at the two extremes may be 'no breathlessness' and 'intolerable breathlessness'. The subject is instructed to place a mark on the line, thus quantifying their dyspnea (Fig. 1.3).

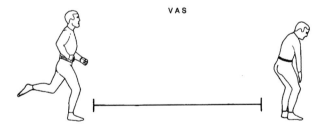

VAS

Figure 1.3 *A visual analog scale (VAS). The VAS consists of a horizontal or vertical line, usually 100 mm in length, with or without descriptors or significant images positioned as anchors.[89] Descriptors at the two extremes may be 'no breathlessness' and 'greatest breathlessness'. The subject is instructed to place a mark on the line with a pen. The location of the mark provides a quantification of the dyspnea.*

Category ratio scale

The most widely used scale to rate dyspnea during exercise testing is the modified 0–10 category ratio Borg scale.[90] This

scale consists of a vertical line labeled 0–10 with nonlinear spacing of verbal descriptors of severity corresponding to specific numbers that can be chosen by the subject to reflect presumed ratio properties of sensation or symptom intensity (Box 1.1). The VAS and the Borg scale provide similar scores during incremental cardiopulmonary exercise testing in healthy subjects[91] and in COPD patients.[92] Nevertheless it has been suggested that Borg scale is more correlated with pulmonary function tests values than VAS.[89]

Box 1.1 Borg scale

0 = Nothing at all
0.5 = Extremely weak (just noticeable)
1 = Very weak
2 = Weak (light)
3 = Moderate
4 = Somewhat strong
5 = Strong (heavy)
6
7 = Very strong
8
9
10 = Extremely strong (almost maximal)
Maximal score = 11

Initially, investigators were interested in peak values of dyspnea on the VAS or the Borg scale during exercise testing. The descriptors on the Borg scale permit comparisons among individuals based on the assumption that the verbal descriptors on the scale describe the same intensity for different subjects. Two subjects may select the same number on the Borg scale as the proper indication of their subjective peak breathlessness despite different levels of peak workload. For example, although a wide range of values have been reported, both healthy individuals and patients with cardiorespiratory disease usually stop exercise (at ratings between 5 and 8 on the Borg scale) at submaximal intensities of dyspnea and/or leg discomfort.[82] Killian *et al.*[93] reported that despite peak power output on the cycle ergometer being almost twice as high in their healthy subjects compared with the patients with varying grades of severity of COPD, the healthy subjects and patients had similar ratings for peak values for dyspnea.

Patients can also give ratings at specific times (iso-time) or work load (iso-workload) increment during the exercise test.[82] The subject is instructed to provide ratings at each power output increment (typically at 1-minute intervals) 'on cue' during the exercise test. A series of discrete dyspnea ratings can be obtained over the course of 1-minute intervals of time. Based on these data the slope and intercept of the workload to Borg score relation can be calculated over a range of stimulus (workload) values. In general, the slope of the regression between power production and dyspnea is higher in patients with respiratory disease compared with healthy individuals.[82,94] A numerical value or descriptor on the Borg scale may be used as a dyspnea 'target' (as opposed to a measured length in millimeters on the VAS) for prescribing and monitoring exercise training.[95,96] A recent study[97] suggests that elderly individuals, both healthy as well as patients with COPD, can successfully use a computer system to provide spontaneous and continuous ratings of breathlessness during exercise. The continuous method illustrates clearly how the perception of breathlessness changes throughout the entire course of an exercise test rather than only at arbitrary 1-minute time intervals. Thus, the standard discrete approach of obtaining ratings each minute may not accurately reflect the individual's perceptual changes in dyspnea.[97]

Recalling dyspnea

In all the approaches discussed above, validity depends on the accuracy of patient reports. People may overestimate or underestimate their capacity to exercise.

MRC SCALE

To assess symptoms more directly, dyspnea has been evaluated during performance of supervised tasks. Since 1959, the Medical Research Council (MRC) scale[98] has been used extensively as a discriminative instrument based on a single dimension (i.e. magnitude of task) that provokes dyspnea (Box 1.2). The MRC scale is simple to administer and correlates with other dyspnea scales and with scores of health status.[99,100] It has been recently included in a global index able to predict the risk of death from any cause and from respiratory causes among patients with COPD.[101] Although MRC and other similar scales are appropriate discriminative instruments, they are limited by two factors. The scales focus only on one dimension that affects breathlessness; furthermore the grades are quite broad so that it may be difficult to detect small but important changes with particular interventions.[82]

Box 1.2 The MRC scale

Five statements about perceived breathlessness:

1 – I only get breathless with strenuous exercise
2 – I get short of breath when hurrying on the level or up a slight hill
3 – I walk slower than people of the same age on the level because of breathlessness or have to stop for breath when walking at my own pace on the level
4 – I stop for breath after walking 0.1 km (100 yards) or after a few minutes on the level
5 – I am too breathless to leave the house

BASELINE AND TRANSITION DYSPNEA INDEXES

To enhance the ability to measure changes in dyspnea, multidimensional instruments have been developed that consider additional factors influencing patients' dyspnea. The Baseline Dyspnea Index (BDI) and Transition Dyspnea Index (TDI) include two components – functional impairment and magnitude of effort – in addition to magnitude of task that provoked breathing difficulty.[82,99] The BDI was developed as a discriminative instrument to measure dyspnea at a single point in time, whereas the TDI was developed as an evaluative instrument to measure changes in dyspnea from the baseline state. Ratings or scores for dyspnea are obtained from an interviewer who selects a score for each of the three components based on the patient's answers using specific criteria for the grades as described for the instruments. Translations in different languages are available.[82]

CHRONIC RESPIRATORY DISEASE QUESTIONNAIRE

The Chronic Respiratory Disease Questionnaire (CRDQ) includes dyspnea as one of four components of a quality-of-life instrument in patients with respiratory disease.[102] The individual patient is asked to select the five most important activities that caused breathlessness over the past 2 weeks by recall and by then reading from a list of 26 activities. The severity of dyspnea is graded by the patient selecting a score on a scale (range 1–7) for each of the five activities. The overall score can then be divided by the number of activities (usually five) selected by the patient. There is no correlation between the effort dyspnea evaluated by Borg scale and the dyspnea category of the CRDQ.[82,100]

OTHER QUESTIONNAIRES

Other multidimensional questionnaires include the UCSD Shortness of Breath Questionnaire,[103] the Pulmonary Functional Status and Dyspnea Questionnaire,[104] and the oxygen-cost diagram.[82] The UCSD questionnaire asks patients to indicate how frequently they experience shortness of breath on a seven-point scale during 21 activities of daily living. There are three additional questions about limitations due to shortness of breath, fear of harm from overexertion, and fear of shortness of breath for a total of 24 items. Although the St George's Respiratory Questionnaire includes questions about dyspnea as part of the symptoms component for measuring health status, there is no specific score or grade for dyspnea.[105]

Why should we measure dyspnea?

Several studies have shown that the VAS as well as BDI/TDI and CRDQ are valid, reliable, and responsive instruments for measuring breathlessness in chronic respiratory diseases. A cross-sectional study found that the BDI/TDI and the UCSD Shortness of Breath questionnaire demonstrated the highest levels of reliability and validity among six different measures of dyspnea (including the ATS dyspnea scale, oxygen-cost diagram, VAS, and the Borg scale).[106] In this study the BDI exhibited consistently higher correlations than the UCSD questionnaire with the 6-minute walking distance test, quality of wellbeing score, lung function, depression score, and anxiety score.[106] In patients with chronic airflow obstruction, breathlessness measured with VAS and BDI correlated with measures of exercise capacity but the proportion of shared variance with exercise loaded to the greatest with breathlessness measured with the BDI. Borg scores for dyspnea, whether at rest or at maximum work rate, did not correlate with any of the measures of exercise capacity.[41] In a factor analysis of clinical methods used to evaluate dyspnea in patients with COPD, the MRC, the BDI, the oxygen-cost diagram, the activity component of St George's Respiratory Questionnaire, and dyspnea of the CRDQ were all grouped into the same factor, and the frequency distribution histograms of these measurements showed virtually the same distribution.[100] The Borg scale at the end of maximum exercise was found to be a different factor. These measurements demonstrated the same pattern of correlation with physiologic data. In a prospective clinical study in healthy subjects, Grant et al.[107] found that subjective scales such as VAS, the Borg scale or the Likert scale could reproducibly measure symptoms during steady-state exercise and could detect the effect of drug intervention. The VAS and Borg scales appeared to be the best subjective scales for this purpose. VAS peak exercise, BDI/TDI, and CRDQ adequately reflect the beneficial effects of pulmonary rehabilitation.[108] In a factor analysis study in asthmatic patients, airway obstruction appeared as an independent dimension or factor. Dyspnea independently characterized the condition of asthma. Submaximal exercise tolerance could not be associated with the symptom of breathlessness.[109] Furthermore it is well known that the FEV_1, the degree of dyspnea and exercise performance provide independent information regarding the degree of disability in patients with COPD.[110–112]

From the above and other evidence, we can argue that it is not possible to predict a patient's intensity of dyspnea and related disability from the physiologic data. This is especially true for COPD patients who may have relatively mild airflow obstruction but severe dyspnea. Borg dyspnea score at peak exercise appears to be the best NFA indicator.[67] Therefore there is the need to specifically measure dyspnea with a specific tool according to the desired purpose. Indeed the Global Initiative for Chronic Obstructive Lung Disease[113] and ATS[114] recommend that a patient's perception of breathlessness should be included in any new staging system for COPD.

CONCLUSION

Dyspnea should be related to pathophysiology rather than to a specific disease.[2] Standard tools to measure dyspnea are available. In addition, there are tools to relate the severity of symptoms with observed levels of cardiac and pulmonary responses during performance of supervised tasks. Inventories that involve aspects of dyspnea related to quality of life are not yet a routine part of the history and physical examination, but have demonstrated a useful role in the clinic. Measurement instruments may involve a cost for use, may be self-administered or require an interviewer, and will vary in the time required for completion and scoring.

Key learning points

- Dyspnea is the sensation of breathing discomfort, which can be described in different terms depending on the different pathophysiologic mechanisms, and varies in intensity.

- The mechanisms of dyspnea are complex.

- The neuro-ventilatory dissociation theory of dyspnea involves a mismatch between the central reflex drive to breathe and the simultaneous afferent feedback from peripheral sensory receptors throughout the respiratory system. This feedback system provides information about the extent and appropriateness of the mechanical response to central drive.

- In COPD, the intensity and quality of dyspnea during activity correlates with the magnitude of lung hyperinflation and inspiratory events; it correlates poorly with FEV_1.

- Valid, reliable, and responsive instruments are available to measure the severity of breathlessness in patients with respiratory disease.

REFERENCES

1. Comroe JH. Some theories of the mechanism of dyspnea. In: Howell JB, Campbell EJM, eds. *Breathlessness*. Boston: Blackwell Scientific Publications, 1966: 1–7.

2. American Thoracic Society. Dyspnea. Mechanisms, assessment and management: a consensus statement. *Am J Respir Crit Care Med* 1999; **159**: 321–40.

3. Scano G, Ambrosino N. Pathophysiology of dyspnea. *Lung* 2002; **180**: 131–48.

4. Voduc N, Webb K, O'Donnell D. Physiological basis of dyspnea. In: Donner CF, Ambrosino N, Goldstein RS, eds. *Pulmonary Rehabilitation: Efficacy and Scientific Basis*. London: Arnold, 2005: 124–35.

5. Chonan T, Mulholland MB, Leitner J, et al. Sensation of dyspnoea during hypercapnia, exercise and voluntary hyperventilation. *J Appl Physiol* 1990; **68**: 2100–6.

6. Demediuk BH, Manning H, Lilly J, *et al.* Dissociation between dyspnoea and respiratory effort. *Am Rev Respir Dis* 1992; 146: 1222–5.

7. Campbell EJM, Godfrey S, Clark TJH, *et al.* The effect of muscular paralysis induced by tubocurarine on the duration and sensation of breath-holding during hypercapnia. *Clin Sci* 1969; 36: 323–8.

8. Banzett RB, Lansing RW, Reid MB, Brown R. 'Air hunger' arising from increasing PCO_2 in mechanically ventilated quadriplegics. *Respir Physiol* 1989; 76: 53–68.

9. Gandevia SC, Killian K, McKenzie DK, *et al.* Respiratory sensations, cardiovascular control, kinaesthesia and transcranial stimulation during paralysis in humans. *J Physiol* 1993; 470: 85–107.

10. Marin JM, Montes de Oca M, Rassulo J, Celli BR. Ventilatory drive at rest and perception of exertional dyspnea in severe COPD. *Chest* 1999; 115: 1293–300.

11. Montes de Oca M, Rassulo J, Celli BR. Respiratory and cardiopulmonary function during exercise in very severe COPD. *Am J Respir Crit Care Med* 1996; 154: 1284–8.

12. Lane R, Cockcroft A, Adams L, Guz A. Arterial oxygen saturation and breathlessness in patients with chronic obstructive airways disease. *Clin Sci* 1987; 72: 693–8.

13. Mak VHF, Bugler JR, Roberts CM, Spiro SG. Effect of arterial oxygen desaturation on six-minute walk distance, perceived effort and perceived breathlessness in patients with airflow limitation. *Thorax* 1993; 48: 33–48.

14. O'Donnell DE, Bain DJ, Webb KA. Factors contributing to relief of exertional breathlessness during hyperoxia in chronic airflow limitation. *Am J Respir Crit Care Med* 1997; 155: 530–5.

15. Somfay A, Porszasz J, Lee SM, Casaburi R. Dose-response effect of oxygen on hyperinflation and exercise endurance in nonhypoxaemic COPD patients. *Eur Respir J* 2001; 18: 77–84.

16. Stevenson NJ, Calverley PMA. Effect of oxygen on recovery from maximal exercise in patients with chronic obstructive pulmonary disease. *Thorax* 2004; 59: 668–72.

17. Coleridge HM, Coleridge JCG. Reflexes evoked from tracheobronchial tree and lungs. In: Cherniak NS, Widdicombe JG, eds. *Handbook of Physiology*. Section 3: the respiratory system, volume 2: control of breathing, part 1. Bethesda, MD: American Physiological Society, 1986: 395–429.

18. Raj H, Singh VK, Anand A, Paintal AS. Sensory origin of lobeline-induced sensations: a correlative study in man and cat. *J Physiol* 1995; 482: 235–46.

19. Bradley GW, Hale T, Pimble J, *et al.* Effect of vagotomy on the breathing pattern and exercise ability in emphysematous patients. *Clin Sci* 1982; 62: 311–19.

20. Winning AJ, Hamilton RD, Guz A. Ventilation and breathlessness on maximal exercise in patients with interstitial lung disease after local anesthetic aerosol inhalation. *Clin Sci* 1988; 74: 275–81.

21. Kimoff RJ, Cheong TH, Cosio MG, *et al.* Pulmonary denervation in humans: Effects on dyspnea and ventilatory pattern during exercise. *Am Rev Respir Dis* 1990; 142: 1034–40.

22. Lougheed MD, Flannery J, Webb KA, O'Donnell DE. Respiratory sensation and ventilatory mechanics during induced bronchoconstriction in spontaneously breathing low cervical quadriplegia. *Am J Respir Crit Care Med* 2002; 166: 370–6.

23. Shannon R. Reflexes from respiratory muscles and costovertebral joints. In: Cherniak NS, Widdcombe JG, eds. *Handbook of Physiology*. Section 3: the respiratory system, volume 2: control of breathing, part 1. Bethesda, MD: American Physiological Society, 1986: 431–47.

24. Edo H, Rimura H, NiiJima M, *et al.* Effects of chest wall vibration on breathlessness durino hypercapnic ventilatory response. *J Appl Physiol* 1998; 84: 1487–91.

25. Manning HL. Effect of chest wall vibration on breathlessness during hypercapnic ventilatory response. *J Appl Physiol* 1998; 1485–6.

26. McCloskey DI. Corollary discharges: motor commands and perception. In: Brookahrt, JM, Mountcastle VB, eds. *Handbook of Physiology*. Section 1, the nervous system, vol 2. Bethesda MD: American Physiological Society, 1981: 1415–47.

27. Chen Z, Eldridge FL, Wagner PG. Respiratory-associated firing of midbrain neurones in cats: relation to level of respiratory drive. *J Physiol* 1991; 437: 305–25.

28. Redline S, Gottfried SB, Altose MD. Effect of changes in inspiratory muscle strength on the sensation of respiratory force. *J Appl Physiol* 1991; 70: 240–5.

29. Lougheed MD, Webb KA, O'Donnell DE. Breathlessness during induced lung hyperinflation in asthma: the role of the inspiratory threshold load. *Am J Respir Crit Care Med* 1995; 152: 911–20.

30. Campbell EJM, Howell JBL. The sensation of breathlessness. *Br Med Bull* 1963; 18: 36–40.

31. Schwartzstein RM, Simon PM, Weiss JW, *et al.* Breathlessness induced by dissociation between ventilation and chemical drive. *Am Rev Respir Dis* 1989; **139**: 1231–7.

32. O'Donnell DE, Webb KA. Exertional breathlessness in patients with chronic airflow limitation: the role of hyperinflation. *Am Rev Respir Dis* 1993; **148**: 1351–7.

33. O'Donnell DE, Bertley JC, Chau LKL, Webb KA. Qualitative aspects of exertional breathlessness in chronic airflow limitation: pathophysiologic mechanisms. *Am J Respir Crit Care Med* 1997; **155**: 109–15.

34. Pfeiffer C, Poline JB, Thivard L, *et al.* Neural substrate for the perception of acutely induced dyspnoea. *Am J Respir Crit Care Med* 2001; **163**: 951–7.

35. Simon PM, Schwartzstein RM, Woodrow Weiss J, *et al.* Distinguishable types of dyspnoea in patients with shortness of breath. *Am Rev Respir Dis* 1990; **142**: 1009–14.

36. Elliot MW, Adams L, Cockcroft A, *et al.* The language of breathlessness: use of verbal descriptors by patients with cardiorespiratory disease. *Am Rev Respir Dis* 1991; **144**: 826–32.

37. Banzett RB, Lansing RW, Brown R, *et al.* 'Air hunger' arising from increased PCO_2 persists after complete neuromuscular block in humans. *Respir Physiol* 1990; **81**: 1–17.

38. Mahler DA, Harver A, Lentine T, *et al.* Descriptors of breathlessness in cardiorespiratory diseases. *Am J Respir Crit Care Med* 1996; **154**: 1357–63.

39. Killian KJ, Watson R, Otis J, *et al.* Symptom perception during acute bronchoconstriction. *Am J Respir Crit Care Med* 2000; **162**: 490–6.

40. Hardie GE, Jonson S, Gold WM, *et al.* Ethnic differences: word descriptors used by African American and white asthma patients during induced bronchoconstriction. *Chest* 2000; **117**: 928–9.

41. Foglio K, Carone M, Pagani M, *et al.* Physiological and symptom determinants of exercise performance in patients with chronic airway obstruction (CAO). *Respir Med* 2000; **94**: 256–63.

42. Petit JM. Afferent pathways. In: Porter R, ed. *Breathing: Hering-Breuer Centenary Symposium.* London: J & A Churchill, 1970: 111–24.

43. Taguchi O, Kikuchi Y, Hida W, *et al.* Effects of bronchoconstriction and external resistive loading on the sensation of dyspnoea. *J Appl Physiol* 1991; **71**: 2183–90.

44. Paintal AS. Vagal receptors and their reflex effects. *Physiol Rev* 1973; **53**: 15–27.

45. Manning HL, Schwartzstein RM. Pathophysiology of dyspnoea. *New Engl J Med* 1995; **33**: 1547–52.

46. Killian KJ, Campbell EJM. Dyspnoea. In: Roussos C, ed. *The Thorax Part B.* New York: Marcel Dekker 1995: 1709–47.

47. Binks AP, Moosavi SH, Banzett RB, *et al.* 'Tightness' sensation of asthma does not arise from the work of breathing. *Am J Respir Crit Care Med* 2002; **165**: 78–82.

48. O'Donnell DE. Breathlessness in patients with chronic airflow limitation: mechanisms and management. *Chest* 1994; **106**: 904–12.

49. O'Donnell DE, Chau LKL, Webb AK. Qualitative aspects of exertional dyspnoea in patients with interstitial lung disease. *J Appl Physiol* 1998; **84**: 2000–9.

50. Harty ER, Corfield DR, Schwartzstein RM, Adams L. External thoracic restriction, respiratory sensation, and ventilation during exercise in men. *J Appl Physiol* 1999; **86**: 1142–50.

51. Chonan T, Mulholland MB, Altose MD, Cherniack NS. Effects of changes in level and pattern of breathing on the sensation of dyspnoea. *J Appl Physiol* 1990; **69**: 1290–5.

52. Brack T, Jubran A, Tobin M. Dyspnoea and decreased variability of breathing in patients with restrictive lung disease. *Am J Crit Care Med* 2002; **165**: 1260–4.

53. Rossi A, Polese G, Brandi G, Conti G. Intrinsic positive end-expiratory pressure (PEEPi). *Intensive Care Med* 1995; **21**: 522–36.

54. O' Donnell DE. Exertional breathlessness in chronic respiratory disease. In: DA Mahler, ed. *Dyspnea.* New York: Marcel Dekker, 1998: 97–14.

55. Man WDC, Mustfa N, Nikoletou D, *et al.* Effect of salmeterol on respiratory muscle activity during exercise in poorly reversible COPD. *Thorax* 2004; **59**: 471–6.

56. Palange P, Valli G, Onorati P, *et al.* Effect of heliox on lung dynamic hyperinflation, dyspnea and exercise endurance capacity in COPD patients. *J Appl Physiol* 2004; **97**: 1637–42.

57. Ambrosino N, Strambi S. New strategies to improve exercise tolerance in chronic obstructive pulmonary disease. *Eur Respir J* 2004; **23**: 313–22.

58. O'Donnell DE, Revill SM, Webb KA. Dynamic hyperinflation and exercise intolerance in COPD. *Am J Respir Crit Care Med* 2001; **164**: 770–7.

◆ 59. Pride NB, Macklem PT. Lung mechanics in disease. In: Fishman AP, ed. *Handbook of Physiology*. Section 3 Vol 3, part 2: the respiratory system. Bethesda, MD: Am Physiology Society, 1986: 659–92.

● 60. Lougheed MD, Lam M, Forkert L, Webb KA. O'Donnell DE. Breathlessness during acute bronchoconstriction in asthma. *Am Rev Respir Dis* 1993; **148**: 452–9.

● 61. Moy ML, Woodrow Weiss J, Sparrow D, *et al.* Quality of dyspnoea in bronchoconstriction differs from external resistive loads. *Am J Respir Crit Care Med* 2000; **162**: 451–5.

● 62. Gorini M, Iandelli I, Misuri G, *et al.* Chest wall hyperinflation during acute bronchoconstriction in asthma. *Am J Respir Crit Care Med* 1999; **160**: 808–16.

● 63. Moy ML, Latin ML, Harver A, *et al.* Language of dyspnoea in assessment of patients with acute asthma treated with nebulized albuterol. *Am J Respir Crit Care Med* 1998; **158**: 749–53.

◆ 64. Scano G, Grazzini M, Stendardi L, Ambrosino N. Dyspnoea and asthma. *Monaldi Arch Chest Dis* 1998; **53**: 672–6.

● 65. Kikuchi Y, Okabe S, Tamura G, *et al.* Chemosensitivity and perception of dyspnea in patients with a history of near-fatal asthma. *N Engl J Med* 1994; **330**: 1329–34.

● 66. Magadle R, Berar-Yanay N, Weiner P. The risk of hospitalization and near-fatal and fatal asthma in relation to the perception of dyspnea. *Chest* 2002; **121**: 329–33.

● 67. Barreiro E, Gea J, Sanjuas C, Marcos R, *et al.* Dyspnoea at rest and at the end of different exercises in patients with near-fatal asthma. *Eur Respir J* 2004; **124**: 219–25.

● 68. Lansing RW, Im BS-H, Thwing JI, *et al.* The perception of respiratory work and effort can be independent of the perception of air hunger. *Am J Respir Crit Care Med* 2000; **162**: 1690–6.

● 69. Lanini B, Misuri G, Gigliotti F, *et al.* Perception of dyspnoea in patients with neuromuscular disease. *Chest* 2001; **120**: 402–8.

● 70. Lanini B, Gigliotti F, Coli C, *et al.* Dissociation between respiratory effort and dyspnoea in a subset of patients with stroke. *Clin Sci* 2002; **103**: 467–73.

● 71. Scano G, Seghieri G, Mancini M, *et al.* Dyspnoea, peripheral airway involvement and respiratory muscle effort in patients with Type I diabetes mellitus under good metabolic control. *Clin Sci* 1999; **96**: 499–506.

● 72. Clark AL, Sparrow JL, Coates AJS. Muscle fatigue and dyspnoea in chronic heart failure; two sides of the same coin? *Eur Heart J* 1995; **16**: 49–52.

● 73. O'Donnell DE, D'Arsigny C, Raj S, *et al.* Ventilatory assistance improves exercise endurance in stable congestive heart failure. *Am J Respir Crit Care Med* 1999; **160**: 1804–11.

● 74. Hamilton AL, Killian KJ, Summers E, Jones NL. Muscle strength, symptom intensity, and exercise capacity in patients with cardiorespiratory disorders. *Am J Respir Crit Care Med* 1995; **152**: 2021–31.

◆ 75. Killian KJ. The mechanisms of dyspnoea. *Eur Respir Rev* 2002; **82**: 31–3.

◆ 76. Schwartzstein RM. The language of dyspnoea. *Eur Respir Rev* 2002; 12; **82**: 28–30.

● 77. Caroci Ade S, Lareau SC. Descriptors of dyspnea by patients with chronic obstructive pulmonary disease versus congestive heart failure. *Heart Lung* 2004; **33**: 102–10.

● 78. Mueller C, Scholer A, Laule-Kilian K, *et al.* Use of B-type natriuretic peptide in the evaluation and management of acute dyspnea. *N Engl J Med* 2004; **350**: 647–54.

● 79. Nielsen LS, Svanegaard J, Klitgaard NA, Egeblad H. N-terminal pro-brain natriuretic peptide for discriminating between cardiac and non-cardiac dyspnoea. *Eur J Heart Fail* 2004; **6**: 63–70.

● 80. Harver A, Mahler DA, Schwartzstein RM, Baird JC. Descriptors of breathlessness in healthy individuals. Distinct and separate constructs. *Chest* 2000; **118**: 679–90.

◆ 81. Mahler DA. Measurement of dyspnea. In: Donner CF, Ambrosino N, Goldstein RS, eds. *Pulmonary Rehabilitation: Efficacy and Scientific Basis.* London: Arnold, 2005: 136–42.

◆ 82. Mahler DA, Jones PW, Guyatt GH. Clinical measurement of dyspnea. In: Mahler DA, ed. *Dyspnea.* New York: Marcel Dekker, **199**: 149–98.

◆ 83. Baird JC, Noma E. *Fundamentals of Scaling and Psychophysics.* New York: Wiley Interscience, 1978.

◆ 84. Gandevia SC. Neural mechanisms underlying the sensation of breathlessness: kinesthetic parallels between respiratory and limb muscles. *Aust N Z J Med* 1988; **18**: 83–91.

◆ 85. Ambrosino N, Stendardi L, Scano G. Measurement of dyspnoea. *Monaldi Arch Chest Dis* 1998; **53**: 661–3.

◆ 86. Ambrosino N, Porta R. Measurement of dyspnoea. *Monaldi Arch Chest Dis* 2001; **56**: 39–42.

◆ 87. Ambrosino N, Scano G. Measurement and treatment of dyspnoea. *Respir Med* 2001; **95**: 539–47.

◆ 88. Gift AG. Visual analogue scales: measurement of subjective phenomena. *Nurs Res* 1989; **38**: 286–8.

● 89. Rampulla C, Baiocchi S, Dacosto E, Ambrosino N. Dyspnea on exercise. *Chest* 1992; **101**: 248s–252s.

● 90. Borg GAV. Psychological bases of perceived exertion. *Med Sci Sports Exerc* 1982; **14**: 377–81.

● 91. Wilson RC, Jones PW. A comparison of the visual analogue scale and modified Borg scale for the measurement of dyspnea during exercise. *Clin Sci* 1989; **76**: 277–82.

● 92. Muza SR, Silverman MT, Gilmore GC, et al. Comparison of scales used to quantitate the sense of effort to breathe in patients with chronic obstructive pulmonary disease. *Am Rev Respir Dis* 1990; **141**: 909–13.

● 93. Killian KJ, LeBlanc P, Martin DH, et al. Exercise capacity and ventilatory, circulatory, and symptom limitation in patients with chronic airflow limitation. *Am Rev Respir Dis* 1992; **146**: 935–40.

● 94. Hamilton AL, Killian KJ, Summers E, Jones NL. Symptom intensity and subjective limitation to exercise in patients with cardiorespiratory disorders. *Chest* 1996; **110**: 1255–63.

● 95. Mejia R, Ward J, Lentine T, Mahler DA. Target dyspnea ratings predict expected oxygen consumption as well as target heart rate values. *Am J Respir Crit Care Med* 1999; **159**: 1485–9.

● 96. Mahler DA, Ward J, Mejia-Alfaro R. Stability of dyspnea ratings after exercise training in patients with COPD. *Med Sci Sports Exerc* 2003; **35**: 1083–7.

● 97. Fierro-Carrion G, Mahler DA, Ward J, Baird JC. Comparison of continuous and discrete measurements of dyspnea during exercise in patients with COPD and normal subjects. *Chest* 2004; **125**: 77–84.

● 98. Fletcher CM, Elmes PC, Wood CH. The significance of respiratory symptoms and the diagnosis of chronic bronchitis in a working population. *Br Med J* 1959; **1**: 257–66.

● 99. Mahler DA, Weinberg DH, Wells CK, Feinstein AR. The measurement of dyspnea: contents, interobserver agreement, and physiologic correlates of two new clinical indexes. *Chest* 1984; **85**: 751–8.

● 100. Hajiro T, Nishimura K, Tsukino M, et al. Analysis of clinical methods used to evaluate dyspnea in patients with chronic obstructive pulmonary disease. *Am J Respir Crit Care Med* 1998; **158**: 1185–9.

● 101. Celli BR, Cote CG, Marin JM, et al. The body-mass index, airflow obstruction, dyspnea, and exercise capacity index in chronic obstructive pulmonary disease. *N Engl J Med* 2004; **350**: 1005–12.

● 102. Guyatt GH, Berman LB, Townshend M, et al. A measure of quality of life for clinical trials in chronic lung disease. *Thorax* 1987; **42**: 773–8.

● 103. Eakin EG, Resnikoff PM, Prewitt LM, et al. Validation of a new dyspnea measure: the UCSD shortness of breath questionnaire. *Chest* 1998; **113**: 619–24.

● 104. Lareau SC, Carrieri-Kohlman V, Janson-Bjerklie, Ross PJ. Development and testing of the pulmonary functional status and dyspnea questionnaire. *Heart Lung* 1994; **23**: 242–50.

● 105. Jones PW, Quirk FH, Baveystock CM, Littlejohns P. A self-complete measure of health status for chronic airflow limitation: the St. George's Respiratory Questionnaire. *Am Rev Respir Dis* 1992; **145**: 1321–7.

● 106. Eakin EG, Sassi-Dambron DE, Ries AL, Kaplan RM. Reliability and validity of dyspnea measures in patients with obstructive lung disease. *Int J Behavioral Med* 1995; **2**: 118–34.

● 107. Grant S, Aitchison T, Henderson E, et al. A comparison of the reproducibility and the sensitivity to change of visual analogue scales, Borg scales, and Likert scales in normal subjects during submaximal exercise. *Chest* 1999; **116**: 1208–17.

● 108. de Torres JP, Pinto-Plata V, Ingenito E, et al. Power of outcome measurements to detect clinically significant changes in pulmonary rehabilitation of patients with COPD. *Chest* 2002; **121**: 1092–8.

● 109. Grazzini M, Scano G, Foglio K, et al. Relevance of dyspnoea and respiratory function measurements in monitoring of asthma: a factor analysis. *Respir Med* 2001; **95**: 246–50.

● 110. Ries AL, Kaplan RM, Blumberg E. Use of factor analysis to consolidate multiple outcome measures in chronic obstructive pulmonary disease. *J Clin Epidemiol* 1991; **44**: 497–503.

● 111. Mahler DA, Harver A. A factor analysis of dyspnea ratings, respiratory muscle strength, and lung function in patients with chronic obstructive pulmonary disease. *Am Rev Respir Dis* 1992; **145**: 467–70.

● 112. Wegner RB, Jorres RA, Kirsten DK, Magnussen H. Factor analysis of exercise capacity, dyspnoea ratings and lung function in patients with severe COPD. *Eur Respir J* 1994; **7**: 725–9.

✴ 113. Pauwels RA, Buist AS, Calverley PMA, *et al.* Global strategy for the diagnosis, management and prevention of chronic obstructive lung disease. NHLBI/WHO global initiative for chronic obstructive lung disease (GOLD) workshop summary. *Am J Respir Crit Care Med* 2001; **163**: 1256–76.

✴ 114. ATS statement. Standards for the diagnosis and care of patients with chronic obstructive pulmonary disease. *Am J Respir Crit Care Med* 1995; **152**: S77–120.

2

Acute and chronic respiratory failure: pathophysiology and mechanics

ANTONIA KOUTSOUKOU, CHARIS ROUSSOS

INTRODUCTION

Respiratory failure is a condition in which the respiratory system fails in one or both of its gas-exchanging functions, i.e. oxygenation of mixed venous blood and/or elimination of carbon dioxide from it. Respiratory failure is conventionally defined as the condition in which the arterial P_{O2} (PaO_2) is less than 60 mm Hg, the arterial P_{CO2} ($PaCO_2$) is higher than 45 mm Hg or both. Therefore, the diagnosis of respiratory failure is a laboratory one but it is important to emphasize that these cut-off values are not rigid; they simply serve as a general guide in combination with the history and clinical assessment of the patient. Respiratory failure may be acute, chronic, or acute on chronic. The clinical presentation of patients with acute and chronic respiratory failure is usually quite different. While acute respiratory failure is characterized by life-threatening derangements in arterial blood gases and acid–base status, the manifestations of chronic respiratory failure are more indolent and may be clinically inapparent. Although the causes of respiratory failure are diverse, common underlying pathophysiologic mechanisms exist.[1]

The respiratory system can be said to consist of two parts: the lung that is the gas-exchanging organ and the pump that ventilates the lungs.[2] The pump consists of the chest wall, including the respiratory muscles, the respiratory controllers in the central nervous system and the pathways that connect the central controllers with the respiratory muscles (spinal and peripheral nerves). Failure of each part of the system will lead to a distinct entity (Fig. 2.1). In general, failure of the lung caused by a variety of lung diseases (e.g. pneumonia, emphysema, interstitial lung disease) leads to hypoxemia with normocapnia or hypocapnia (hypoxemic or type I respiratory failure). Failure of the pump (e.g. drug overdose) results in alveolar hypoventilation and hypercapnia (hypercapnic or type II respiratory failure); although hypoxemia coexists, the hallmark of ventilatory failure is the increase in $PaCO_2$. Undoubtedly, both types of respiratory failure may coexist in the same patient as, for example, in patients with chronic obstructive pulmonary disease (COPD) and carbon dioxide retention, or in patients with severe pulmonary edema or asthmatic crisis who first develop hypoxemia and as the disease persists or progresses, hypercapnia appears.

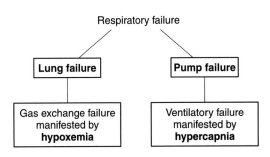

Figure 2.1 *The respiratory system is depicted as consisting of two parts: (i) the lung, the gas-exchanging organ, the failure of which is manifested as hypoxemia; and (ii) the pump, which ventilates the lung, the failure of which is manifested as hypercapnia. (Redrawn with permission from Roussos C, Koutsoukou A. Respiratory failure. Eur Respir J 2003; 21 (Suppl 47): 3s–14s.[1])*

PATHOPHYSIOLOGY OF RESPIRATORY FAILURE

Hypoxemic (type I) respiratory failure

Four principal pathophysiologic mechanisms account for the hypoxemia seen in a wide variety of diseases: ventilation/perfusion inequality ($\dot{V}/Q$), increased shunt (Q_s/Q_t), diffusion impairment, and alveolar hypoventilation.[3] Abnormal desaturation of mixed venous blood in the face of extensive lung disease is an important mechanism of hypoxemia.

Abnormal ventilation/perfusion ratio is the most common mechanism of hypoxemia. The P_{O_2} and P_{CO_2} values in any alveolar unit and, hence, the end-capillary P_{O_2} and P_{CO_2} of each lung, are basically determined by the composition of the inspired gas, the composition of mixed venous blood and the proper matching of ventilation with blood flow. In an ideal situation, all alveolar–capillary units should have equal matching of ventilation and perfusion, i.e. a ratio of 1. However, even in the normal lungs some $\dot{V}/Q$ inequality is present. This is because there is normally a gradient of blood flow from the apex to the base of a lung, which is much greater than the similar gradient of ventilation, thus leading to higher $\dot{V}/Q$ ratios in the lung apex than at the lung base.[4] It should be kept in mind that blood coming from regions of the lung with high $\dot{V}/Q$ ratio and a high P_{O_2} cannot compensate for blood coming from regions with a low $\dot{V}/Q$ ratio and a low P_{O_2}. This is due to the fact that the net P_{O_2} and P_{CO_2} of the arterial blood depends on the average of individual values of oxygen content of the blood coming from all areas of the lung. Given that the shape of the oxyhemoglobin dissociation curve is nonlinear (sigmoidal), and that hemoglobin is almost fully (~90 percent) saturated at a P_{aO_2} of 60 mm Hg, the oxygen content is not significantly augmented even with a substantial elevation of P_{O_2} above 60 mm Hg. Hypoxemia due to $\dot{V}/Q$ mismatch develops when there is decreased ventilation to normally perfused regions or when there are lung regions with greater reduction in ventilation than in perfusion. Hypoxemia resulting from pure $\dot{V}/Q$ mismatching can be easily corrected by supplementing inspired oxygen.

A shunt is a blood pathway that does not allow any contact between alveolar gas and red cells, so that no gas exchange occurs in the affected region and the blood passing through the shunt maintains a mixed venous composition. This blood mixes with other blood that has undergone alveolar gas exchange resulting in a fall in arterial P_{O_2}. In the normal lung, a 2–3 percent shunt normally occurs because of drainage of venous blood through the thebesian veins into the left ventricle. This is called extrapulmonary shunting and can be increased in pathologic conditions such as cyanotic right-to-left congenital heart disease or in the presence of abnormal arteriovenous vascular channels in the lungs. However, intrapulmonary shunting is the most common cause of

venous admixture and occurs when deoxygenated mixed venous blood traverses alveoli that are nonaerated either because they are completely collapsed or because they are filled with edema fluid or inflammatory cells, such as in patients with pulmonary edema (cardiogenic or noncardiogenic), atelectasis, or pneumonia. Shunting can be differentiated from $\dot{V}/Q$ mismatching on the basis of the different response to inhalation of 100 percent oxygen. In patients with pure shunt, hypoxemia cannot be corrected even with high concentrations of inspired oxygen.[5]

Impaired oxygen diffusion prevents complete equilibration of alveolar oxygen with pulmonary capillary blood. Diseases that increase the distance between alveolus and erythrocyte because of a thickening of the alveolar–capillary membrane, decrease capillary surface area, or shorten transit time of the blood through the pulmonary capillaries, may lead to impaired diffusion of oxygen through the alveolar wall and pulmonary capillary endothelium. However, a diffusion abnormality is rarely severe enough to result in arterial hypoxemia at rest.[6] Exercise testing can often demonstrate physiologically significant abnormalities due to impaired diffusion. Oxygen supplementation improves the hypoxemia caused by diffusion impairment.

Hypoventilation leads to hypoxemia because oxygen uptake by the blood crossing the gas-exchange units is faster than the rate of oxygen replenishment by the inspired air, while at the same time blood and consequently alveolar carbon dioxide rises, resulting in a reduction of the concentration of oxygen in the alveoli. In the absence of underlying pulmonary disease, hypoxemia accompanying hypoventilation is characterized by normal alveolar–arterial oxygen difference (DA–aO2). In contradistinction, disorders in which any of the other three mechanisms are operative are characterized by a widening of the alveolar–arterial gradient.

Hypercapnic (type II) respiratory failure

Ventilatory failure resulting in carbon dioxide retention implies alveolar hypoventilation for a given level of carbon dioxide production ($\dot{V}_{CO_2}$). The respiratory equation relates the arterial P_{CO_2} to alveolar ventilation ($\dot{V}_A$):

$$P_{aCO_2} = k \times \left(\frac{\dot{V}_{CO_2}}{\dot{V}_A} \right) \quad [1]$$

where k denotes the constant of proportionality.

Since $\dot{V}_A = \dot{V}_E - \dot{V}_D$, where $\dot{V}_E$ denotes minute ventilation and $\dot{V}_D$ dead space ventilation, this relation may be expressed as follows:

$$P_{aCO_2} = k \times \frac{\dot{V}_{CO_2}}{\dot{V}_E - \dot{V}_D}$$

$$= k \times \dot{V}_{CO_2}/\dot{V}_E \left(1 - \frac{\dot{V}_D}{\dot{V}_E} \right)$$

$$= k \times \dot{V}co_2/\dot{V}E \left(1 - \frac{fVD}{fVT} \right)$$

$$= k \times \dot{V}co_2/\dot{V}E \left(1 - \frac{VD}{VT} \right) \quad [2]$$

$$= k \times \dot{V}co_2/\dot{V}T \, f \left(1 - \frac{VD}{VT} \right) \quad [3]$$

where V_T is tidal volume and f is the frequency of breathing.

Equation [1] states that the $Paco_2$ rises if carbon dioxide production increases (e.g. hyperthermia) at constant alveolar ventilation or when at a constant $\dot{V}co_2$, $\dot{V}_A$ decreases. For a young adult carbon dioxide production is about 200 mL/min. Carbon dioxide production increases during hyperthermia (by ~14 percent per each degree Celsius rise in temperature), during muscular activity (~700–800 mL/min during resistive breathing), during shivering, or increase in muscular tone, such as in tetanus. Under normal conditions, an increase in carbon dioxide production will be detected promptly by the central nervous system (CNS) and then easily compensated by increasing minute ventilation to maintain a normal $Paco_2$. However, if a patient's ventilatory capacity is impaired, an increase in $\dot{V}co_2$ will greatly stress the ventilatory system and lead to an increase of arterial Pco_2.

Alveolar ventilation decreases on the basis of a rise in the V_D/V_T ratio (either by increasing V_D or decreasing V_T) at a constant minute ventilation, of a decrease in minute ventilation or of both an increase in V_D/V_T and a decrease in minute ventilation.[7,8] Under conditions of unchanged minute ventilation any increase in frequency will be accompanied by a decrease in V_T. This will result in an increased V_D/V_T ratio thus leading to hypercapnia. $\dot{V}_E$ in equation [2] may be further separated to its two components, namely inspiratory flow and duty cycle:

$$\dot{V}_E = VT \times f = VT \times \frac{1}{T_{TOT}} = \frac{V_T}{T_I} \times \frac{T_I}{T_{TOT}}$$

where T_{TOT} is the total respiratory cycle and T_I the inspiratory time.

Thus, a reduction in mean inspiratory flow (V_T/T_I), in duty cycle (T_I/T_{TOT}), or in both will cause increase on $Paco_2$. In daily clinical practice, as a patient becomes hypercapnic generally more than one factor contributes to the rise of $Paco_2$.

PATHOPHYSIOLOGY OF VENTILATORY PUMP FAILURE

Three major causes of pump failure lead to hypercapnia:[9]

- inadequate output of the respiratory centers
- mechanical or functional defect of the chest wall
- fatigue of the inspiratory muscles, that is, they become unable to continue to generate an adequate pleural

pressure despite an appropriate central respiratory drive and an intact chest wall.

It is obvious that if the activation from the CNS is insufficient, the respiratory efforts will be inadequate for the demands and hypoventilation will ensue. Conditions characterized by impaired respiratory drive may be either temporal (e.g. anesthesia, overdose, CNS infections, head trauma) or permanent (e.g. diseases of the medulla). Besides that, the output of the respiratory centers may be reflexively modified to prevent respiratory muscles injury and avoid or postpone fatigue (see below).

Motor output emanating from the CNS should be transferred to the respiratory muscles, a process requiring anatomic and functional adequacy of the spinal cord, peripheral nerves, and neuromuscular junction. Any disorder along this pathway (Guillain–Barré syndrome, poliomyelitis, myopathies) will result in an insufficient inflation of the chest cavity inadequate to reduce intrathoracic pressure, which is essential for the air to flow into the lungs. Mechanical defects of the chest wall (flail chest, kyphoscoliosis, and hyperinflation) are entities that predispose to alveolar hypoventilation since they impose additional work on the inspiratory muscles which have to displace the noncompliant chest wall and lungs.

Severe hyperinflation is one of the most common causes of impaired mechanical performance of the inspiratory muscles. In normal subjects at rest, the end-expiratory lung volume (functional residual capacity [FRC]) corresponds to the relaxation volume (V_r) of the respiratory system, i.e. the lung volume at which the elastic recoil pressure of the total respiratory system is zero. Pulmonary hyperinflation, which is defined as an increase in FRC above predicted normal range, may be due to increased V_r as a result of loss of elastic recoil of the lung (e.g. emphysema), and/or dynamic pulmonary hyperinflation, which is said to be present when the FRC exceeds V_r.[10] Hyperinflation imposes significant constraints on inspiratory muscles. As lung volume increases, their effectiveness as pressure generators is decreased because their fibers become shorter (force–length relation) and their geometrical arrangement changes.[9]

When working under excessive inspiratory load (elastic or resistive) the inspiratory muscles may become fatigued. Fatigue must be distinguished from weakness, which is reduction in force generation fixed and not reversible by rest, although muscle weakness may be a predisposition to muscle fatigue. Fatigue occurs when the energy supply to the respiratory muscles does not meet the demands. Factors predisposing to respiratory muscle fatigue are those that increase inspiratory muscle energy demands and/or those that decrease energy supplies.[11] Energy demands are determined by the work of breathing, and the strength and efficiency of the inspiratory muscles (Fig. 2.2).

The work of breathing increases proportionally with the mean pressure developed by the inspiratory muscles per breath (mean tidal pressure – P_i), expressed as a fraction of

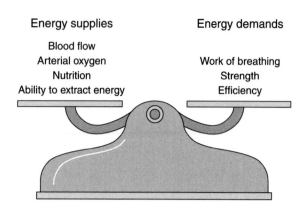

Energy supplies

Blood flow
Arterial oxygen
Nutrition
Ability to extract energy

Energy demands

Work of breathing
Strength
Efficiency

Figure 2.2 *Respiratory muscle endurance is determined by the balance between energy supplies and demands. Normally, the supplies meet the demands and a large reserve exists. Whenever this balance weighs in favor of demands, the respiratory muscles ultimately become fatigued, leading to inability to sustain spontaneous breathing. (Redrawn with permission from Roussos C, Koutsoukou A. Respiratory failure. Eur Respir J 2003; 21 (Suppl 47): 3s–14s.[1])*

maximum inspiratory pressure that inspiratory muscles can perform [P_i/P_{imax}]), with $\dot{V}_E$, with duty cycle, and the mean inspiratory flow rate.[9]

Mean tidal pressure is increased if elastic (stiff lungs – pulmonary edema) or resistive load (airways obstruction – asthma) imposed on the inspiratory muscles is increased. Roussos et al.[12] have directly related P_i/P_{imax} with the time that the diaphragm can sustain the load imposed on it (endurance time). The critical value of P_i/P_{imax} that could be generated indefinitely at FRC was around 0.60. Greater values of P_i/P_{imax} ratio were inversely related to the endurance time. The critical value of P_i/P_{imax} increases when end-expiratory lung volume increases. Bellemare and Grassino[13] found that the maximum pressure which can be sustained indefinitely decreases when duty cycle increases, and suggested that the product of P_i/P_{imax} and T_I/T_{TOT} defines a useful 'tension time index' (TTI) that is related to the endurance time. Whenever TTI is smaller than a critical value (0.15 for the diaphragm) the load can be sustained indefinitely.

The force developed by a skeletal muscle that is sufficient to produce fatigue is a function of the maximum force the muscle can develop. Any condition that decreases the maximum force decreases the muscle's strength and predisposes to fatigue. Such conditions include atrophy (a likely result of prolonged mechanical ventilation), immaturity, neuromuscular diseases and performance on an inefficient part of the muscle's length–tension characteristics.[14]

Finally, muscle efficiency, the ratio of external work performed to energy consumed, is an important factor in energy demands. Inspiratory muscle efficiency is known to fall in patients with hyperinflation. It has been shown that for the same work of breathing the oxygen cost is markedly higher in patients with emphysema than in normal subjects.[15] This happens either because in emphysematous patients some inspiratory muscles may contract isometrically (they consume energy but do not perform work), or because the inspiratory muscles are operating on an inefficient part of their force–length relation: a more forceful contraction is required to produce a given pressure change, and an even greater degree of excitation is required to develop a given force. Thus both conditions lead to increased energy consumption for a given pressure development.[16] Factors determining inspiratory muscle energy available are the muscle blood flow, the oxygen content of the arterial blood, the blood substrate concentration as well as the ability of the muscles to extract energy (see Fig. 2.2).

Diaphragmatic blood flow is essentially determined by the perfusion pressure which is a function of cardiac output and peripheral vascular resistance, and by the vascular resistance of the muscle, which is a function of the intensity and duration of contraction.[17] As it has been described in animal models, a reduction of cardiac output accompanying cardiogenic or septic shock is a cause of respiratory muscle fatigue leading to severe alveolar hypoventilation, bradypnea, and respiratory arrest.[18,19] Energy supply to inspiratory muscles also depends on the ability of the muscle to increase blood flow parallel to the increased work. The diaphragm has a greater capacity to increase blood flow than other skeletal muscles.[20] However, the amount that the inspiratory muscle blood flow can be increased may be affected by the intensity and duration of muscle contraction. If the respiratory muscles remain contracted throughout the respiratory cycle, as occurs in asthma,[21] the overall blood flow to the muscles may be less than required. In addition, the hemoglobin concentration and oxyhemoglobin saturation will influence the aerobic energy supply to the muscle and, hence, its endurance. Conditions characterized by inability of the muscles to extract and use energy, such as sepsis or cyanide poisoning or diminished energy stores and glycogen depletion as in extreme inanition, may potentially lead to respiratory muscle fatigue.

It is clear from the above discussion that fatigue may occur in a variety of clinical entities that either alone or in combination result in an imbalance between respiratory muscle's energy supplies and demands. No matter what the causes are, it is well known that fatigue is characterized by loss of force output[22] leading to inability of the respiratory muscles to develop adequate P_i during tidal breathing with consequent decrease in tidal volume and minute ventilation and hypercapnia.

Patients in acute and chronic respiratory failure as well as normal subjects and animals subjected to fatiguing respiratory loads tend to adapt rapid shallow breathing, consisting of a decrease in tidal volume and increased breathing frequency. Although this pattern may not be efficient in terms of gas exchange, it may reduce the load on the muscles, thereby preventing fatigue from occurring.[23–26]

Reduction of tidal volume by means of shortening inspiratory time for the P_i to be diminished, is accompanied by reduction of the energy demands per breath (TTI per breath). The reduction in tidal volume is compensated for at least in the beginning by increasing breathing frequency so that minute ventilation is maintained or increased. Such a situation leads to increased V_D/V_T and hypercapnia. This frequency of breathing, however, is no longer optimal and, for the same alveolar ventilation, the energy demands will increase. Thus, although shortening of inspiratory time seems to be a better option in terms of energy demands, if coupled with high frequency and possibly inadequate energy supply, as it occurs during strenuous contractions, may lead to muscle fatigue. In such a situation pressure generated by the inspiratory muscles will decrease with a consequent decrease in tidal volume, minute ventilation, and a further increase in V_D/V_T,[27] with a following reduction of $\dot{V}_A$ that is accompanied by an increase in $P\text{CO}_2$. At a later stage, inspiratory time increases again and the respiratory frequency gradually decreases resulting in a further drop of minute ventilation.[28] In extreme fatigue, the CNS reduces the output signals per breath leading to respiratory arrest.[18]

When the respiratory muscles are extensively loaded, however, it is likely that feedback mechanisms modify central drive. The central drive alters the ventilatory pattern and serves in reducing the load and alleviating fatigue by exerting a 'central wisdom'. Thus it protects the ventilatory pump from exhaustion, which undoubtedly is a very terminal event. Although there are no data from patients to substantiate the existence of 'central wisdom' in ventilatory failure, there is enough evidence supporting this notion. In animals, it has been shown that the reduction of tidal volume that followed resistive breathing could be restored promptly to normal by administration of naloxone[29] or by bilateral cervical vagotomy.[30] Furthermore, the fact that most hypercapnic patients with COPD can achieve normocapnia by voluntarily increasing their ventilation implies that although these patients could increase their ventilation they choose not to do so. Thus, alveolar hypoventilation with consequent hypercapnia is the result of reduced TTI, which may be due to muscle fatigue or possibly to adaptation of the central nervous system before the development of overt fatigue.

The neurophysiologic mechanisms that cause an altered pattern of breathing are not well elucidated. Rapid shallow breathing may be produced by activation of vagal irritant receptors in the airways,[31] or may represent a behavioral response to minimize the sense of dyspnea.[32] Activation of endogenous opioid pathways has also been postulated to alter the pattern of breathing, perhaps as a mechanism by which the sense of dyspnea might be reduced.[29] Small fiber afferents have been implicated widely in the response of central respiratory output to prolonged stresses such as shock, hypoxia, acidosis, and vigorous exercise.[19,33,34] It is possible that, during loaded breathing, afferents through the small fibers modulate endogenous opioids as an adaptive response to minimize

breathlessness and to avoid or delay the onset of respiratory muscle fatigue.[35] In fact, strenuous inspiratory resistive breathing has been found to produce β-endorphin[36,37] not only in animals but also in human beings. However, the source of these substances remains elusive, and both central sites, such as the hypothalamic–pituitary–adrenal (HPA) axis, and peripheral sites, such as the spinal cord and peripheral nerves, have been implicated.[38] It has been shown that in normal human volunteers strenuous resistive breathing leads to a significant rise of the proinflammatory cytokines interleukin (IL)-1β, IL-6, adrenocorticotropic hormone (ACTH), and β-endorphin.[39] The strong relation between the rise in the β-endorphin and ACTH and the preceding increase in circulating IL-6 allowed the authors to suggest that proinflammatory cytokines, and especially IL-6, are responsible for the activation of the HPA axis, leading eventually to an increase in plasma β-endorphin and ACTH, given that both are derived from posttranslational modification of the same molecule, namely propiomelanocortin,[40] and are concomitantly secreted by the pituitary gland.[41,42] It is tempting to suggest that the mechanism accounting for the increase of β-endorphin and ACTH could be the stimulation of small afferent nerve fibers by the cytokines that are produced during resistive breathing. In fact, global depletion of small afferent fibers inhibits the plasma ACTH response to intravenous IL-1β.[43]

Whatever the mechanisms however, the limit of this strategy is that, with rapid shallow breathing V_D/V_T will be increased (see respiratory equation above) with worsening of hypercapnia.

COMMON CLINICAL CONDITIONS ASSOCIATED WITH RESPIRATORY FAILURE

Although failure of the lungs leads mainly to hypoxemia and failure of the ventilatory pump causes hypercapnia, these two entities share mechanisms leading to altered respiratory system mechanics, respiratory muscle dysfunction, and eventually fatigue. Furthermore, these two types of respiratory failure may coexist in the same patient or failure of one part may be followed by failure of the other.

Respiratory diseases that cause hypoxemia are usually characterized by abnormal lung mechanics, a situation accompanied by increased work of breathing (resistive or elastic), and therefore energy demands. Taking into account that the amount of energy available is reduced due to hypoxemia, it becomes obvious that these lung diseases may result in muscle fatigue and ventilatory failure through the imbalance between demands and supplies. Similarly, diseases that involve the ventilatory pump (myopathies) and present with hypercapnia are usually characterized by the patient's inability to cough, which leads to accumulation of secretions and possibly atelectasis, situations eventually aggravating $\dot{V}/\dot{Q}$ inequality with the result of hypoxemia.

Acute hypoxemic respiratory failure

Acute hypoxemic respiratory failure is characterized by severe hypoxemia that is relatively refractory to oxygen therapy; it usually results from processes that cause collapse or filling of the alveoli. Common clinical examples in this category are diffuse lesions, such as pulmonary edema or pulmonary hemorrhage, or focal lesions, such as lobar pneumonia or pulmonary contusion (Box 2.1). Hypoxemia may also develop acutely in a few other nosologic entities that are not encompassed in the above categories.

Box 2.1 Most common causes of acute hypoxemic respiratory failure

- Cardiogenic pulmonary edema
- Acute respiratory distress syndrome (ARDS)
- Alveolar hemorrhage
- Lobar pneumonia
- Atelectasis

Pulmonary edema is characterized by excessive lung liquid accumulation arising either from increased hydrostatic pressure (high pressure or cardiogenic pulmonary edema) or from increased alveolar–capillary membrane permeability (increased permeability pulmonary edema or ARDS). The exit of fluid into the interstitial and alveolar spaces floods alveoli and inhibits surfactant, contributing to widespread atelectasis. A major component of the gas-exchange abnormalities in such patients is shunt due to the presence of a large number of collapsed and flooded alveoli. Shunt fraction appears to relate to the degree of pulmonary edema, as long as other factors remain unchanged.[44] Ventilation/perfusion abnormalities may also occur and coexisting interstitial edema may impair diffusion across the alveolar–capillary membrane, thus further impairing oxygenation of mixed venous blood.

The effects of hydrostatic pulmonary edema and acute lung injury on respiratory system mechanics have been the subject of many investigations. Generally, it has been acknowledged that either form of pulmonary edema may result in decreased lung volume, decreased static compliance, and increased resistance of the respiratory system.[45] The reduction in lung compliance has been attributed to decreased lung volume or to intrinsic modifications of the mechanical properties of lung tissues, and has been used as a good indicator of the amount of liquid in the airspaces.[44] The high values of respiratory system resistance are due to airway flooding, airway hyperactivity, and reduced lung volume. Finally, apart from altered lung mechanics, a marked decrease in chest wall compliance has been reported as a result of intrinsic alterations of the chest wall due to abdominal distension, edema, or pleural effusions.[45] High resistance and low compliance impose a marked increase in the resistive and elastic loads. This in conjunction with heightened ventilatory demand due to hypoxia results in a substantial increase in the work of breathing.

The prototype of focal acute hypoxemic respiratory failure is lobar pneumonia. Hypoxemia is principally caused by persistence of pulmonary artery blood flow to the consolidated lung, resulting in an intrapulmonary shunt fraction amounting up to 40 percent of total cardiac output despite consolidation involving a smaller anatomic part of the lung. This is probably due to failure of pulmonary hypoxic vasoconstriction to reduce pulmonary arterial blood flow to consolidated lung segments and/or to consumption of oxygen by the aerobically active leukocytes and bacteria within the consolidated lobe.[44] Yet shunt is not the only cause of hypoxemia, since it has been found that areas of low $\dot{V}/Q$ ratio develop either as a result of mechanical interaction of the consolidated lobe with the adjacent lung or due to peripheral airways obstruction with secretions and cellular debris.

Respiratory system mechanics have been found to be abnormal in pneumonia.[46] Inflammatory exudate fills alveoli, causing a volume loss roughly proportional to the extent of the pulmonary infiltrate. The loss in volume reduces total lung compliance. There is also evidence that the dynamic compliance of the remaining ventilated lung is reduced, possibly by reduction in surfactant activity. The work of breathing is increased and ventilatory failure may ensue.

Blunt chest trauma, particularly when it is sufficient to cause rib fractures, often contuses the underlying lung. The central region of the contused lung often manifests significant hemorrhage and interruption of the pulmonary arterial circulation, therefore intrapulmonary shunt is minimal. However, hypoxemia can be quite profound due to mechanical interdependence of the contused regions with the surrounding lung, which leads to large number of low $\dot{V}/Q$ units. Other clinical entities that may be accompanied by acute hypoxemia are acute asthmatic crisis, acute exacerbation of COPD, massive pulmonary embolism as well as perioperatively in selected groups of patients. Since shunt is minimal in these conditions, enrichment of inspired oxygen usually alleviates this gas exchange abnormality.

In a severe asthmatic crisis, airways obstruction results in maldistribution of alveolar ventilation relative to perfusion, thus leading to considerable $\dot{V}/Q$ inequalities but to minimal shunt, which implies the importance of collateral ventilation in keeping obstructed areas protected from atelectasis. The poor relation between gas-exchange and spirometric abnormalities indicate different origins of each abnormality, bronchoconstriction of large airways dominating spirometric indices, and mucus secretion and edema in peripheral airways determining gas exchange. Dead space ventilation increases substantially, presumably due to hypoperfusion of regions of the hyperinflated lung.[47] Despite this increase, most patients present with low $PaCO_2$. When the airways obstruction is severe or nonresponding to therapy, acute asthmatic attack may result in respiratory muscle fatigue and ventilatory failure (see below).

In patients with angiographically proved pulmonary embolism, hypoxemia is mainly due to $\dot{V}/Q$ inequalities which may consist of several different patterns: low $\dot{V}/Q$ areas, because of overperfusion of nonembolized regions, or bronchoconstriction and reduced ventilation near areas of infarct; high $\dot{V}/Q$ areas presumably reflect the hypoperfused embolized regions, whereas shunt is the result of alveolar collapse, edema, or open arterial foramen ovale. Furthermore, reduced mixed venous PO_2 is a significant additional factor in depressing PaO_2.[44,48]

In the postoperative period, many patients develop hypoxemic respiratory failure, which has atelectasis as the primary causative mechanism.[49] In these patients, abnormal abdominal mechanics reduce the end-expiratory lung volume below the closing volume leading to progressive collapse of dependent lung units. This is usually the case in morbidly obese patients during anesthesia and supine position.

The characteristic pulmonary function abnormalities in obese people consist of decreased expiratory reserve volume and FRC, reduced total respiratory system compliance (the decrease being more pronounced in the supine position), and increased airway and respiratory system resistances. In nonsmokers, the FRC has been found to be below the closing volume, implying that peripheral airway closure can occur during tidal breathing thus leading to maldistribution of ventilation and impaired gas exchange.[50,51] Obese people are at greater risk of developing further respiratory impairment when exposed to factors associated with increased respiratory morbidity, such as thoracic or intraabdominal operations, and anesthesia and mechanical ventilation. In anesthetized morbidly obese patients, substantial impairment of oxygenation has been reported both in the preoperative and postoperative period.[50,52–55] Hypoxemia has been attributed to ventilation/perfusion mismatch given that the lung bases are well perfused but hypoventilated because of airway closure and alveolar collapse.[50] In contrast, the $PaCO_2$ has been reported to be normal, indicating that hypoventilation does not contribute to impaired oxygenation under these conditions.

Hypercapnia of acute onset

Pathologic entities resulting in acute carbon dioxide retention are anatomic and functional defects of the CNS, impairment of the neuromuscular transmission, and mechanical defect of the rib cage as well as conditions leading to fatigue of the respiratory muscles (Box 2.2). Mechanisms responsible for carbon dioxide retention decrease minute ventilation as well as increase V_D/V_T.

Box 2.2 Causes of acute hypercapnia

Decreased central drive
- Drugs (sedatives)
- Central nervous system diseases (encephalitis, stroke, trauma)

Altered neural and neuromuscular transmission
- Spinal cord trauma
- Transverse myelitis
- Tetanus
- Amyotrophic lateral sclerosis
- Poliomyelitis
- Guillain–Barré syndrome
- Myasthenia gravis
- Organophosphate poisoning
- Botulism

Muscle abnormalities
- Muscular dystrophy
- Disuse atrophy
- Prematurity

Chest wall and pleural abnormalities
- Acute hyperinflation
- Chest wall trauma (flail chest, diaphragmatic rupture)

Lung and airways diseases
- Acute asthma
- Acute exacerbation of COPD
- Cardiogenic and noncardiogenic pulmonary edema
- Pneumonia
- Upper airways obstruction
- Bronchiectasis

Other causes
- Sepsis
- Circulatory shock

Depression of the CNS due to pharmacologic agents, infections or head trauma leads to hypoventilation because of impaired respiratory drive. Mechanical defects of the chest wall (flail chest, acute hyperinflation), neuromuscular diseases (bilateral diaphragmatic paralysis, myasthenia gravis, botulism, Guillain–Barré syndrome) and pharmacologic agents, such as curare, may acutely result in hypercapnia. Acute hypercapnia may occur in every clinical condition that is characterized by increase in mechanical load of breathing and, consequently, in the energy demands that cannot be met by the energy supplies.

In an acute asthmatic attack characterized by severe airways obstruction, the rapid shallow breathing associated with increased elastic and resistive inspiratory loads increase the work of breathing and, consequently, the energy demands. Air trapping and lung hyperinflation with consequent diaphragmatic flattening and worsening of inspiratory muscles mechanics result in reduced strength and efficiency of the respiratory muscles as well as impaired blood supply to the muscles due to strong contractions. This will probably lead to decreased P_{imax}, while at the same time, P_i is increased. Increased P_i/P_{imax} leads to dyspnea[30] and, potentially, if a critical value is crossed, to fatigue. Such a situation forces alveolar hypoventilation by reducing tidal volume, either as a protective mechanism for the muscles, since there is enough evidence that strenuous breathing causes muscle injury,[56,57] or as a consequence of fatigue of the muscles. In noncardiogenic (ARDS) and cardiogenic pulmonary edema, energy demands are increased due to increased elastic and resistive work as well as hyperventilation, whereas energy supply is diminished due to hypoxemia in the former, and hypoxemia as well as low cardiac output in the latter. In such situations, the respiratory muscles may fail.

Acute hypercapnic respiratory failure may also develop in patients with acute respiratory failure and mechanical ventilation during the weaning trial. Early research regarding this issue showed that most patients who failed the weaning trial presented with tachypnea, acidosis, and fatigue of the respiratory muscles.[28] Latter studies have shown that rapid shallow breathing (with the consequent rise in V_D/V_T) as well as a significant increase in the elastic and resistive load of the respiratory muscles, are the major causes of carbon dioxide retention in these patients.[24,58] Disuse atrophy of the respiratory muscles, a well documented condition after short- and long-term mechanical ventilation,[59] malnutrition, decreased perfusion that is often seen in these patients, and also decreased strength and efficiency of the muscles due to hyperinflation, are conditions that decrease respiratory muscles capacity. These, coupled with increased mechanical load, are situations that may lead to respiratory muscle fatigue.

In most neuromuscular diseases with acute onset (e.g. diaphragmatic paralysis or poisons such as organophosphates), weakness of the respiratory muscles is a common feature that leads to ventilatory failure. Weakness could be also the result of muscle atrophy, malnutrition, electrolytic disorders or immature respiratory muscles as in newborn babies. In these situations, the remaining normal muscle cells cannot develop sufficient force to maintain adequate alveolar ventilation, and they eventually become fatigued.

Hypercapnia of insidious onset

Patients with chronic hypercapnia have to breathe against increased forces imposed either by the lung (as in bronchitis, emphysema) or by the chest wall (as in kyphoscoliosis, extreme obesity or neuromuscular disorders), or by both, as in scleroderma and polymyositis (Box 2.3).

Box 2.3 Causes of chronic hypercapnia

Lung and airways diseases
- Chronic obstructive airway disease (bronchitis, emphysema, bronchiectasis)

Chest wall abnormalities
- Kyphoscoliosis
- Thoracoplasty
- Obesity
- Pleural effusion
- Neuromuscular disorders

Lung and chest wall diseases
- Scleroderma
- Polymyositis
- Systemic lupus erythematosus

Central nervous system abnormalities
- Primary alveolar hypoventilation
- Ondine curse

Other
- Electrolyte abnormalities
- Malnutrition, endocrine disorders

Although chronic hypercapnia is most frequently seen in COPD, where it is associated with an ominous prognosis,[60] the mechanisms leading to its occurrence are not completely understood. The relation between Pa_{CO_2} and indices of airways obstruction or $\dot{V}/Q$ mismatch is weak,[61] suggesting that factors other than lung pathology may be operative.

Given the increase in V_D/V_T ratio that occurs in COPD, Pa_{CO_2} could be maintained normal, or near normal, provided that minute ventilation could be preserved at a sufficient high level. The fact that in patients with steady-state COPD deep breathing brings the respiratory muscles near to fatigue and cannot be tolerated for more than a few minutes[62] suggests that hypercapnic COPD patients choose to act as 'wise fighters', who instead of increasing their ventilation (an option that could potentially lead to muscle fatigue) choose to hypoventilate.

The problem with maintaining minute ventilation above normal is associated with significant mechanical impediments to breathing. Since COPD patients have increased airflow resistance and reduced dynamic compliance, the resistive and elastic loads are increased and, hence, the inspiratory muscles have to generate higher forces to inflate the lung. The emphysematous changes in the lung cause hyperinflation, which forces the inspiratory muscles to operate at shorter than normal lengths and altered geometry, thus reducing their ability to lower the intrathoracic pressure. More importantly, dynamic hyperinflation that develops in these patients due to expiratory flow limitation imposes a severe strain on the respiratory muscles because of the additional load that is placed on them (the intrinsic positive end-expiratory pressure [$PEEP_i$]).

Subsequently, the balance between the mechanical impediments to breathing and the capacity of the inspiratory muscles to cope with them, expressed by P_i/P_{imax}, is shifted to an unfavorable direction (more work–less muscle reserve). Under such conditions COPD patients choose to reduce P_i by reducing tidal volume. Reduced tidal volume may reflect reduced central respiratory drive or, alternatively, mechanical limitation and/or inspiratory muscle dysfunction.

A subnormal respiratory output has long been postulated as a mechanism for hypercapnia in patients with COPD. However, neural drive has been found to be higher in these patients than in normal subjects, although no significant differences were found between normocapnic and hypercapnic patients.[63,64] Furthermore, the voluntary drive to breathe[65] has been shown not to be decreased in hypercapnic COPD patients. Consequently, although in these patients the respiratory drive to breath is increased, they are better off terminating inspiratory time early, a process that results in lower tidal volume.

The reduction in tidal volume is largely offset by an increase in the respiratory rate, so that minute ventilation is well preserved. However, rapid shallow breathing aggravates dynamic hyperinflation and increases V_D/V_T. The pattern of breathing in COPD patients has been examined by Sorli *et al.*, who compared normal people with hypercapnic and normocapnic stable COPD patients[63] and found that hypercapnic patients were breathing faster and more shallowly than either the normal persons or their normocapnic co-subjects and so, at equal minute ventilation, V_D/V_T was higher in the carbon dioxide retainers. Decreased tidal volume and increased V_D/V_T were also found by Begin and Grassino,[66] who suggested that chronic alveolar hypoventilation is likely to develop in COPD patients who have a combination of high inspiratory loads (resistive and elastic) and greater hyperinflation, factors that effectively reduce P_{imax}, thus increasing the fraction of force developed/force available to breathe (less efficient muscles). These data were subsequently confirmed by the finding that tidal volume was related directly to inspiratory time, indicating that a small tidal volume was primarily the consequence of alteration in respiratory timing.[67]

The mechanisms leading to alteration in respiratory timing in patients with COPD have not yet been clearly defined. Changes in the pattern of breathing may represent a behavioral response to minimize the sense of dyspnea. Studies indicate that the sense of breathlessness increases with an increase in the intrathoracic pressure required to maintain airflow and tidal volume, with the duration of inspiration (relative to total breath cycle) and with respiratory rate.[32] Thus, at a given level of minute ventilation and set of respiratory mechanics, the pattern of breathing determines the intensity of breathlessness.

Given that in the COPD patients who presented with gross hyperinflation and hypercapnia, P_i/P_{imax} was markedly increased compared with normals,[66] it could be suggested that, as the disease progresses the critical level of power output for muscle fatigue will be exceeded to permit the patient to maintain adequate alveolar ventilation. Therefore, it seems probable that when the muscles become unable to develop enough force, the activation system comes into play and may alter the pattern of breathing in an attempt to optimize the performance of the muscles and possibly to postpone or prevent severe fatigue. Although the underlying mechanisms are not known, it is speculated that afferents from the small fibers stimulated by the heavy work (ergoreceptors, type III) or by noxious substances (nociceptors, type IV) modify the CNS output.

Acute-on-chronic respiratory failure

Acute deterioration in a patient with chronic respiratory failure is termed acute-on-chronic respiratory failure. Patients may present with worsening dyspnea, deteriorating mental status, or respiratory arrest after relatively minor, although often multiple, insults. Patients with severe but stable COPD live on a subtle equilibrium between their increased demands and limited reserves. Any factor that potentially interferes with this equilibrium (either increase in demands or decrease in reserves) will lead to breakdown of this balance with consequent acute respiratory failure.

Patients with COPD exacerbation face a further increase in respiratory system load due to abnormal airway resistance and respiratory system elastance. The increased resistance is caused by bronchospasm, airway inflammation, or physical obstruction by mucus and scarring. The most significant contributor to the elastic load is dynamic hyperinflation that develops whenever the duration of expiration is insufficient to allow the lungs to deflate to relaxation volume (V_r) prior to the next inspiration. This tends to occur under conditions in which expiratory flow is impeded (increased airway resistance) or when the expiratory time is shortened (increased breathing frequency).[10,68] Expiratory flow may also be retarded by other mechanisms such as persistent constriction of the respiratory muscles during expiration. Most commonly however, dynamic pulmonary hyperinflation is observed in COPD patients who exhibit expiratory flow limitation during resting breathing and plays a paramount role in causing respiratory failure.

When breathing takes place at lung volumes higher than V_r, positive elastic recoil pressure that remains at end expiration ($PEEP_i$) acts as an inspiratory threshold load which increases the static elastic work of breathing. On average it has been found that the inspiratory work due to $PEEP_i$ represented 57 percent of the overall increase in the

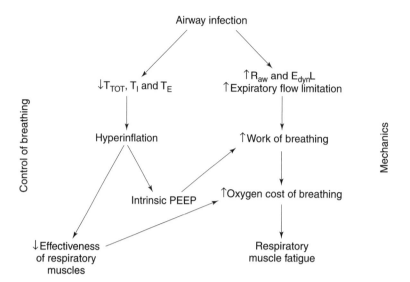

Figure 2.3   *Schematic representation of the sequence and the responsible mechanisms that lead to acute on chronic respiratory failure in patients with COPD. T_{TOT}, total respiratory cycle; T_I, inspiratory time; T_E, expiratory time; R_{aw}, airways resistance; E_{dyn}, dynamic elastance of the lung; PEEP, positive end-expiratory pressure. (Redrawn with permission from Roussos C, Koutsoukou A. Respiratory failure. Eur Respir J 2003; 21(Suppl 47): 3s–14s.[1])*

work of breathing exhibited by the COPD patients, relative to normal subjects.[69]

Due to hyperinflation, tidal breathing occurs at a steeper portion of the pressure–volume curve of the lung (increased elastance), increasing the inspiratory load. Apart from increasing elastic loads, dynamic hyperinflation is accompanied by a concomitant decrease in the effectiveness of the inspiratory muscles as pressure generators because the inspiratory muscle fibers become shorter and their geometrical arrangement changes. Still patients presenting with acute-on-chronic respiratory failure may not only have worsening hyperinflation, but also other conditions (protein–calorie malnutrition, steroid myopathy) that cause muscle weakness. Figure 2.3 shows a schematic representation of the sequence and the responsible mechanisms that lead to acute-on-chronic respiratory failure in COPD patients.

Acute ventilatory failure in these patients is usually triggered by airway infection. The increased respiratory frequency, which is invariably present in acutely ill COPD patients due to shortened expiration time,[10,70] further exacerbates dynamic hyperinflation, which promotes an increase in the static elastic work of breathing (due to both iPEEP and decreased lung compliance). At the same time, acute increase in airway resistance (bronchoconstriction, copious secretions) cause an increase in the resistive work of breathing. The increased work of breathing associated with the impaired muscle effectiveness will lead to an increase of energy requirements, which at a critical point will exceed the diminished energy available (hypoxemia, impaired diaphragmatic blood flow due to forceful contractions), and respiratory muscle fatigue will ensue with a further increase in P_{CO_2}.

Key learning points

- Respiratory failure is mainly due either to lung failure resulting in hypoxemia or pump failure resulting in alveolar hypoventilation and hypercapnia.

- Four pathophysiologic mechanisms are responsible for hypoxemic respiratory failure: ventilation/perfusion inequalities, shunt, diffusion impairment and hypoventilation.

- Hypoxemia accompanying hypoventilation is characterized by normal alveolar–arterial oxygen difference, whereas the disorders in which any of the other three mechanisms are operative are characterized by a widening of the alveolar–arterial gradient.

- Abnormal desaturation of systemic venous blood in the face of extensive lung disease is an important mechanism of hypoxemia.

- Hypercapnic respiratory failure may be the result of central nervous system depression, functional or mechanical defect of the chest wall, imbalance of energy demands and supplies of the respiratory muscles, and/or adaptation of central controllers in order to prevent respiratory muscles injury and avoid or postpone fatigue.

- Hypercapnic respiratory failure may occur either acutely, insidiously, or acutely upon a chronic carbon dioxide retention. In all these conditions, pathophysiologically, the common denominator is reduced alveolar ventilation for a given carbon dioxide production.

ACKNOWLEDGMENT

Supported by THORAX Foundation.

REFERENCES

1. Roussos C, Koutsoukou A. Respiratory failure. *Eur Respir J* 2003; **21**(Suppl 47): 3s–14s.

2. Roussos C. Ventilatory failure and respiratory muscles. In: Roussos C, Macklem PT., eds. *The Thorax*. New York: Marcel Dekker, 1985: 884–8.

3. Hall JB, Schmidt GA, Wood LD. Acute hypoxemic respiratory failure. In: Murray JF, Nadel JA, eds. *Textbook of Respiratory Medicine*. Philadelphia: WB Saunders, 2000: 2413–42.

4. Wagner P, Laravuso RB, Uhl RR, West JB. Continuous distribution of ventilation/perfusion ratios in normal subjects breathing air and 100% O$_2$. *J Clin Invest* 1974; **54**: 54–68.

5. Wagner P. Ventilation, pulmonary blood flow and ventilation/perfusion relationships. In: Fishman AP, Elias JA, Fishman JA, et al, eds. *Fishman's Pulmonary Diseases and Disorders*. New York: McGraw-Hill, 1998: 177–92.

6. Wagner P. Diffusion and chemical reaction in pulmonary gas exchange. *Physiol Rev* 1977; **57**: 257–312.

7. Roussos C. The failing ventilatory pump. *Lung* 1985; **160**: 59–84.

8. Roussos C. Function and fatigue of respiratory muscles. *Chest* 1985; **88**: 124S–132S.

9. Roussos C, Macklem PR. The respiratory muscles. *N Engl J Med* 1982; **307**: 786–97.

10. Gottfried SB, Rossi A, Higgs BD. Non-invasive determination of respiratory system mechanics during mechanical ventilation for acute respiratory failure. *Am Rev Respir Dis* 1985; **131**: 414–20.

◆ 11. Vasilakopoulos T, Zakynthinos S, Roussos C. Respiratory muscles and weaning failure. *Eur Respir J* 1996; **9**: 2383–400.

● 12. Roussos C, Fixley D, Gross D, Macklem PT. Fatigue of the respiratory muscles and their synergistic behavior. *J Appl Physiol* 1979; **46**: 897–904.

13. Bellemare F, Grassino A. Effects of pressure and timing of contraction on human diaphragm fatigue. *J Appl Physiol* 1982; **53**: 1190–5.

● 14. Farkas G, Roussos C. Acute diaphragmatic shortening: in vitro mechanics and fatigue. *Am Rev Respir Dis* 1984; **130**: 434–8.

15. McGregor M, Beklake MR. The relationship of oxygen cost of breathing to respiratory mechanical work and respiratory force. *J Clin Invest* 1961; **40**: 971–80.

● 16. Macklem PT, Gross D, Grassino A, Roussos C. Partitioning of the inspiratory pressure swings between diaphragm and intercostal/accessory muscles. *J Appl Physiol* 1978; **44**: 200–8.

17. Humphreys PS, Lind AR. Blood flow through active and inactive muscle of the forearm during isolated hand grip contractions. *J Physiol (Lond)* 1963; **166**: 120–35.

● 18. Aubier M, Trippenbach T, Roussos C. Respiratory muscle fatigue during cardiogenic shock. *J Appl Physiol* 1981; **51**: 449–508.

● 19. Hussain SNA, Simkus G, Roussos C. Respiratory muscle fatigue: a cause of ventilatory failure in septic shock. *J Appl Physiol* 1985; **58**: 2033–40.

20. Robertson CH, Eschenbacher JW, Johnson RL. Respiratory muscle blood flow distribution during expiratory resistance. *J Clin Invest* 1977; **60**: 473–80.

21. Muller N, Bryan A, Zamel N. Tonic inspiratory muscle activity as a cause of hyperinflation in histamine-induced asthma. *J Appl Physiol* 1980; **49**: 869–74.

22. Roussos C, Moxham J, Bellemare F. Respiratory muscle fatigue. In: Roussos C, ed. *The Thorax*. New York: Marcel Dekker, 1995: 1405–61.

23. Roussos C. Ventilatory muscle fatigue governs breathing frequency. *Clin Respir Physiol* 1984; **20**: 445–51.

24. Tobin MJ, Perez W, Guenther SM, Semmes BJ. The pattern of breathing during successful and unsuccessful trials of weaning from mechanical ventilation. *Am Rev Respir Dis* 1986; **143**: 1111–18.

25. Milic-Emili J. Is weaning an art or a science? *Am Rev Respir Dis* 1986; **134**: 1107–8.

26. Bellemare F. Respiratory muscle function. In: Kelley WN, ed. *Textbook of Internal Medicine*. Philadelphia: JP Lippincott, 1989: 1843.

27. Gallacher CG, Im Hof V, Younes M. Effect of inspiratory muscle fatigue on breathing pattern. *J Appl Physiol* 1985; **59**: 1152–8.

● 28. Cohen C, Zagelbaum G, Gross D, *et al.* Clinical manifestations of inspiratory muscle fatigue. *Am J Med* 1982; **73**: 308–16.

29. Scardella AT, Parisi RA, Phair DK, et al. The role of endogenous opioids in the ventilatory response to acute flow–resistive loads. *Am Rev Respir Dis* 1986; **133**: 26–31.

30. Adams JM, Farkas GA, Rochester DF. Vagal afferents, diaphragm fatigue and inspiratory resistance in the anesthetized dog. *J Appl Physiol* 1988; **64**: 2279–86.

31. Coleridge HM, Coleridge JCG. Reflexes evoked from tracheobronchial tree and lungs. In: Cherniac NS, Widdicombe JG, eds. *Handbook of Physiology*. Section 3: The Respiratory System Vol 2. Control of breathing, part 1. Bethesda MD: American Physiological Society, 1986: 395–429.

32. Killian KJ, Summers E, Basalygo M, Campbell EJ. Effect of frequency on perceived magnitude of added loads to breathing. *J Appl Physiol* 1985; **58**: 1616–21.

33. Jammes Y, Buchler B, Delpierre S, et al. Phrenic afferents and their role in inspiratory control. *J Appl Physiol* 1986; **60**: 854–60.

34. Hussain SNA, Magder S, Chatillon A, Roussos C. Chemical activation of thin fiber phrenic afferents: respiratory responses. *J Appl Physiol* 1990; **69**: 1002–11.

35. Petrozzino JJ, Scardella AT, Santiago TV, Edelman NH. Dichloroacetate blocks endogenous opioid effects during inspiratory flow–resistive loading. *J Appl Physiol* 1992; **72**: 590–6.

36. Santiago TV, Edelman NH. Opioid and breathing. *J Appl Physiol* 1985; **59**: 1675–85.

37. Wanke T, Lahrmann H, Auinger M, et al. Endogenous opioid system during inspiratory loading in patients with type I diabetes. *Am Rev Respir Dis* 1993; **148**: 1335–40.

38. Petrozzino JJ, Scardella AT, Edelman NH, Santiago TV. Respiratory muscle acidosis stimulates endogenous opioids during inspiratory loading. *Am Rev Respir Dis* 1993; **144**: 607–15.

39. Vasilakopoulos T, Zakynthinos S, Roussos C. Strenuous resistive breathing induces proinflammatory cytokines and stimulates the HPA axis in humans. *Am J Physiol* 1999; **277**: 1013–19.

40. Kjoer A, Knigge U, Bach FG, Warberg J. Stress-induced secretion of pro-opiomelanocortin-derived peptides in rats: relative importance of anterior and intermediate pituitary lobes. *Neuroendocrinology* 1995; **61**: 167–72.

41. Drenth JP, Van Uum SH, Van Deuren M, et al. Endurance run increases circulating IL-6 and IL-1ra but downregulates ex vivo TNF-a and IL-1b production. *J Appl Physiol* 1995; **79**: 1497–503.

42. Guillemin R, Vargo T, Rossier J. β-endorphin and adrenocorticotropin are secreted concomitantly by the pituitary gland. *Science* 1977; **197**: 1367–9.

43. Watanabe TA, Morimoto A, Tan N, et al. ACTH response induced in capsaicin-desensitized rats by interleukin-1 or prostaglandin E. *J Physiol (Lond)* 1994; **457**: 139–45.

44. Wagner P, Rodriguez-Roisin R. Clinical advances in pulmonary gas exchange. *Am Rev Respir Dis* 1991; **143**: 883–8.

45. Polese G, Rossi A, Appendini L, et al. Partitioning of respiratory mechanics in mechanically ventilated patients. *J Appl Physiol* 1991; **71**: 2425–33.

46. Bruce Light R. Pulmonary pathophysiology of pneumococcal pneumonia. *Semin Respir Infect* 1999; **14**: 218–26.

47. Rodriguez-Roisin R, Ballester E, Roca J, et al. Mechanisms of hypoxemia in patients with status asthmaticus requiring mechanical ventilation. *Am Rev Respir Dis* 1989; **139**: 732–9.

48. Santolicandro A, Pediletto R, Fornal E, et al. Mechanisms of hypoxemia and hypocapnia in pulmonary embolism. *Am J Respir Crit Care Med* 1995; **152**: 336–47.

49. Hedenstierna J. Mechanisms of postoperative pulmonary dysfunction. *Acta Chir Scand* 1989; **550**: 152–8.

50. Bae J, Ting EY, Giuffrida JG. The effect of changes in the body position of obese patients on pulmonary volume and ventilatory function. *Bull N Y Acad Med* 1976; **52**: 830–7.

51. Hedenstierna G, Santesson J, Norlander O. Airway closure and distribution of inspired gas in the extreme obese, breathing spontaneously and during anesthesia with intermittent positive pressure ventilation. *Acta Anaesthesiol Scand* 1976; **20**: 334–42.

52. Koutsoukou A, Koulouris N, Bekos B, et al. Expiratory flow limitation in morbidly obese postoperative mechanically ventilated subjects. *Acta Anaesthesiol Scand* 2004; **48**: 1080–8.

53. Holley H, Milic-Emili J, Becklake M, Bates D. Regional distribution of pulmonary ventilation and perfusion in obesity. *J Clin Invest* 1967; **46**: 475–81.

54. Farebrother MJB, McHardy GJR, Munro JF. Relation between pulmonary gas exchange and volume before and after substantial weight loss in obese subjects. *Br Med J* 1974; **3**: 391–3.

55. Ferretti A, Giampiccollo P, Cavalli A, et al. Expiratory flow limitation and orthopnea in massively obese subjects. *Chest* 2001; **119**: 1401–8.

56. Zhu E, Petrof BJ, Gea J, *et al.* Diaphragm muscle fiber injury after inspiratory resistive breathing. *Am J Resp Crit Care Med* 1997; **155**: 1110–16.

57. Jiang T-X, Reid WD, Road JD. Delayed diaphragm injury and diaphragm force production. *Am J Resp Crit Care Med* 1998; **157**: 736–42.

● 58. Zakynthinos S Vasilakopoulos T, Roussos C. The load of inspiratory muscles in patients needing mechanical ventilation. *Am J Respir Crit Care Med* 1995; **152**: 1248–55.

59. Le Bourdelles G, Viires N, Boczkowski J, *et al.* Effects of mechanical ventilation on diaphragmatic contractile properties in rats. *Am J Respir Crit Care Med* 1994; **149**: 1539–44.

60. Burrows B, Earle RH. Course and prognosis of chronic obstructive lung disease. A prospective study of 200 patients. *N Engl J Med* 1969; **280**: 397–404.

61. Lane DJ, Howel JBL, Giblin B. Relation between airways obstruction and carbon dioxide tension in chronic obstructive pulmonary disease. *Br Med J* 1968; **3**: 707–9.

62. Bellemare F, Grassino A. Force reserve of the diaphragm in patients with chronic obstructive pulmonary disease. *J Appl Physiol* 1983; **55**: 8–15.

● 63. Sorli J, Grassino A, Lorange G, Milic-Emili J. Control of breathing in patients with chronic obstructive pulmonary disease. *Clin Sci Mol Med* 1978; **54**: 295–304.

64. Gorini M, Spinelli A, Ginnani R, *et al.* Neural respiratory drive and neuromuscular coupling in patients with chronic obstructive pulmonary disease. *Chest* 1990; **98**: 1179–86.

65. Topeli A, Laghi F, Tobin MJ. The voluntary drive to breath is not decreased in hypercapnic patients with severe COPD. *Eur Respir J* 2001; **18**: 53–60.

● 66. Begin P, Grassino A. Inspiratory muscle dysfunction and chronic hypercapnia in chronic obstructive pulmonary disease. *Am Rev Respir Dis* 1991; **143**: 905–12.

67. Gorini M, Misuri J, Corrado A. Breathing pattern and carbon dioxide retention in severe chronic obstructive pulmonary disease. *Thorax* 1996; **51**: 677–83.

68. Rossi A, Gottfried SP, Zocchi L. Measurement of static compliance of the total respiratory system in patients with acute respiratory failure during mechanical ventilation. *Am Rev Respir Dis* 1985; **131**: 672–7.

● 69. Coussa ML, Guerin C, Eissa NT, *et al.* Partitioning of work of breathing in mechanically ventilated COPD patients. *J Appl Physiol* 1993; **75**: 1711–19.

70. Sharp JT. The chest wall and respiratory muscles in airflow limitation. In: Roussos C, Macklem PT, eds. *The Thorax*. New York: Marcel Dekker, 1985: 1155–202.

3

Pulmonary vascular physiology

JAMES E MOJICA, AARON B WAXMAN

INTRODUCTION

A thorough understanding of the pulmonary circulation is a prerequisite for the prompt recognition and successful management of a variety of respiratory emergencies. Previously the domain of pediatricians and cardiologists, various practitioners are now expected to manage derailments of the pulmonary circulation in emergency departments, inpatient wards, and intensive care units. This chapter reviews some of the fundamental principles of the physiology of the adult pulmonary circulation that serve as a foundation for clinical practice.

OVERVIEW OF HEMODYNAMICS

The pulmonary circulation is a circuit within the body's circulatory system. Its cardinal function, as implied by the term circulation, is transport. Flow through this circuit delivers systemic venous blood to adequately ventilated alveoli for gas exchange. This circuit stands in series with the larger systemic circulation and, despite differences in structure and function, is governed by the same hemodynamic principles.

Pressure

The contraction of the heart's ventricles imparts energy to the blood that it pumps. Blood vessels are therefore filled under pressure, defined as the force applied by the circulating blood over the surface of a vessel. Since blood vessels are elastic, they readily accommodate the ejected blood volume and store the kinetic energy in the form of elastic potential energy. The distension of a vessel filled under pressure is analogous to stretching a spring with a weight.

Arterial pressures in the pulmonary circulation are lower than in the systemic circulation. Normal pulmonary artery pressures are approximately 25 mm Hg during systole and 8 mm Hg during diastole with a mean pressure of 15 mm Hg.[1] These pressures, as will be discussed below, are subject to the effects of gravity and vary between the apex and the base of the lungs.

Flow

Fluids flow across pressure gradients. As flow occurs through a tube, the natural properties of the fluid and the tube will generate resistance and impede flow. Ohm's law[2] simplifies these basic tenets of hemodynamics, whereby flow (Q) is equal to the pressure difference (ΔP) across a cylinder (or vessel) divided by its resistance (R):

$$Q = \Delta \frac{P}{R}$$

In the circulation, flow (Q) varies directly with the perfusion pressure (ΔP) and inversely with vascular resistance (R). The variables in Ohm's equation can be replaced with measurements obtained from the right and left heart. So cardiac output (CO):

(i) for the left heart:

$$CO = \frac{(Mean\ arterial\ pressure - right\ atrial\ pressure)}{Systemic\ vascular\ resistance}$$

(ii) for the right heart:

$$CO = \frac{(Mean\ pulmonary\ artery\ pressure - left\ atrial\ pressure)}{Pulmonary\ vascular\ resistance}$$

The flow through blood vessels is equal to cardiac output in the steady state. The perfusion pressure driving cardiac output is the difference between the aortic (i.e. mean arterial pressure [MAP]) and the right atrial pressures (RAP). The total frictional resistance to flow offered to by the blood vessels is the systemic vascular resistance.

Cardiac output is defined as the volume of blood ejected from the heart per unit time. The amount of blood ejected by a ventricular contraction is known as the stroke volume (i.e. the difference between end-diastolic and end-systolic volumes). Cardiac output (CO) can be obtained by multiplying the stroke volume (SV) by the heart rate (HR):

$$CO = SV \times HR$$

Therefore, a normal stroke volume of ~70 mL at a resting heart rate of 70 beats per minute results in a normal cardiac output of 5 L/min.[3]

The stroke volume is dependent on the end-diastolic volume of the ventricle, which in turn determines the force of ventricular contraction. In the face of varying venous return, the stroke volume is determined by the degree of ventricular stretch (preload). This regulatory mechanism is known as the Frank–Starling relation and refers to the length/tension relation of the muscle.[3] Therefore, venous return is the primary determinant of cardiac output under normal conditions. Any process that increases venous return will increase cardiac output (e.g. changes in blood volume, vascular resistance, or inotropic effects).

Since the pulmonary circulation accommodates the entire stroke volume of the right ventricle with each heartbeat, flow through this circuit is equal to the cardiac output. Determinants of the cardiac output vary flow through the systemic circulation and, therefore, also flow through the lungs.

Resistance

The Poiseuille–Hagen equation[2] describes the variables that affect resistance met by fluid flowing through a tube (i.e. radius [r], viscosity [η], and length [l]).

$$R = \frac{(8 \times \eta \times l)}{p \times r^4}$$

Ohm's law can now be expanded to:

$$Q = \frac{p \times \Delta P \times r^4}{8 \times \eta \times l}$$

By this equation, the most important determinants of blood flow are pressure gradients (ΔP) and the caliber of the vessels (r^4). Since, under normal conditions, pressures in the cardiovascular system are maintained constant, the vessels are the gatekeepers to flow through the circulation.[4]

This idealized description of blood flow is simplified and makes assumptions that are likely incorrect *in vivo* and certainly incorrect in pathologic states:

- Blood vessels are not the rigid tubes of constant diameter studied and described by Poiseuille.[5]
- Blood viscosity can be variable, rather than a constant, with changes in hematocrit or protein concentration.
- Flow through vessels is not laminar, but instead susceptible to turbulence with changes in vessel diameter and blood viscosity.[6]

With these caveats in mind, one can begin to apply these idealized principles to the circulatory system.

In addition to pressure, pulmonary vascular resistance (PVR) is much lower than systemic (SVR) values. This can be illustrated by calculating right- and left-sided values using the described formulas (i.e. variants of Ohm's Law):

$$SVR = \frac{(MAP - RAP)}{CO}$$

$$= \frac{(80 - 5)}{5} = 15\ mm\ Hg/L/min$$

$$PVR = \frac{(mean\ pulmonary\ arterial\ pressure - left\ atrial\ pressure)}{CO}$$

$$= \frac{(15 - 8)}{5} = 1.4\ mm\ Hg/L/min$$

The low vascular resistance is an important characteristic of the pulmonary circulation (approximately one-tenth systemic resistance). Although the calculated values are helpful in illustrating this point, they are static measurements that can be misleading. Mechanical factors, such as lung volume and recruitment of new blood vessels, have direct effects on vascular resistance and confound this simple calculation. But, under controlled conditions, the calculated pulmonary vascular resistance likely represents pulmonary vasomotor tone.

DISTRIBUTION OF BLOOD FLOW IN THE LUNGS

Unlike the systemic circulation, the pulmonary circulation needs to selectively distribute blood flow. The goal is to deliver deoxygenated blood to alveoli with adequate ventilation for gas exchange, avoiding shunt physiology. Several factors have clear effects on pulmonary vascular resistance and, therefore, blood flow.

Effect of hypoxia

An alveolar oxygen tension of <60 mm Hg causes vasoconstriction of small arteries in the pulmonary vasculature within seconds.[7] This is the complete *opposite* of the systemic circulation's vasodilatory response to hypoxia (although both, respectively, attempt to enhance systemic delivery of oxygen). The vasoconstriction of the pulmonary circulation is thought to autoregulate perfusion to match ventilation and can be focal or diffuse within the lung.[8]

The most dramatic example of this effect is seen *in utero*. As the lungs develop and mature during gestation, the placenta fulfills the future role of the pulmonary circulation. Deoxygenated blood in the fetus is delivered to the placenta via the umbilical arteries. Fetal blood is oxygenated by the placenta and enters fetal systemic circulation via the umbilical vein. With a PO_2 near 20 mm Hg, oxygenated placental blood is diverted from the airless, fluid-filled lungs through hypoxic vasoconstriction.[9] Less than 10 percent of the cardiac output will flow through the pulmonary circulation as most of the oxygenated blood is diverted via the foramen ovale to the left heart for systemic distribution.[10] Flow to the lungs is further minimized by the presence of the ductus arteriosus, which shunts blood from the pulmonary arteries to the aorta.

Hypoxia inhibits voltage-gated potassium channels in pulmonary artery smooth muscle cells.[11] This inhibition causes membrane depolarization and an influx of calcium via voltage-dependent calcium channels. The increase in cytosolic calcium stimulates smooth muscle contraction and, therefore, vasoconstriction.[12,13] Despite our current understanding of the vascular response to hypoxia, since its original description in humans,[14] the sensing mechanism of hypoxic pulmonary vasoconstriction remains elusive. Regardless of the mechanism, the hypoxia sensor appears particularly sensitive to changes in alveolar rather than vascular oxygen tension.[15] The identification of the process that induces vasoconstriction may have significant therapeutic promise and is an area of active research.

Lung volumes

In a collapsed lung, small pulmonary arteries are closed and allow no flow (resistance is infinite).[16] With progressive lung inflation, vascular recruitment occurs, resistance drops, and flow is generated even at low pressures. As the lung inflates, lung recoil increases with a resultant increase in transmural pressure and, therefore, vessel diameter. This effect plateaus at the lung's functional residual capacity (FRC). Lung inflation beyond FRC is notable for a rise in pulmonary vascular resistance peaking at the other extreme, total lung capacity. As maximal lung inflation nears, vascular resistance rises as the changes in transmural pressure decrease and mechanical strain on capillaries limit flow. Extreme lung volumes have opposite effects on pulmonary vascular resistance. This is graphically represented by a U-shaped curve.[17]

Furthermore, changes in intrapleural pressure have direct effects on systemic venous return and cardiac output.[18] Pleural pressure (P_{pl}) is subatmospheric throughout most of the respiratory cycle. Pleural pressure oscillates between −4 and −7 cm H_2O during tidal volume breathing, favoring venous return. However, at total lung capacity, pleural pressures can drop to a level of −20 cm H_2O.[19] At these subatmospheric pressures, the great veins collapse and alveolar inflation can compress pulmonary vessels. The net effect is an increase in total vascular resistance, with a resultant drop in venous return. A concomitant rise in afterload from increased arterial pressures explains the drop in cardiac output. At this new steady state (equilibrium point), venous return and cardiac output are both reduced.

Positive pressure ventilation raises intrapleural pressures into the atmospheric range. The positive intrapleural pressure will promptly decrease the gradients for venous return to the right atrium and the ejection pressure of the left ventricle.[20,21] This effect may be theoretically augmented by the external compression of the expanding lungs and the descent of the diaphragm creating increased venous resistance.[22]

Hydrostatic pressure gradients (the zones)

The weight of circulating blood creates a gradient of flow across the lung in the upright position. Three theoretical zones have been described to characterize this model.[23,24] In the uppermost portion of the lung, the perfusion pressure is lower than the intraalveolar pressure, resulting in little to no flow (zone 1). In contrast, in the lung bases, high perfusion pressures maintain constant flow that is not impeded by alveolar pressures (zone 3). In normal individuals, the majority of the lung functions under zone 3 conditions. The apex of the lung probably experiences zone 2 physiology. Therefore, given prevailing intravascular pressures, there is no zone 1 in the lung under normal conditions. Marked intravascular depletion or high intraalveolar pressures are required to create zone 1 areas.[25]

Positive pressure ventilation will theoretically impair oxygenation by creating areas of zone 1 blood flow. By increasing lung volume and airway pressure, intraalveolar pressures surpass the perfusion pressure (converting zone 2 blood flow to zone 1).[25,26] Exercise, on the other hand, increases zone 3 blood flow. Exercise produces substantial increases in blood flow. High flow and pulmonary vascular pressures recruit the entire pulmonary vasculature, thereby enhancing blood flow to the upper areas of the lung.[27] In addition to improving the efficiency of gas exchange, this vascular recruitment prevents abrupt rises in capillary pressures (which could result in pulmonary edema and right ventricular strain/failure).

Vasoactive mediators

The vascular endothelium plays a critical role in the regulation of the function of smooth muscle cells. Studies in patients with endothelial dysfunction (e.g. pulmonary arterial hypertension) have allowed the description of a number of biologic mediators with direct effects on vasomotor tone. Under normal physiologic conditions, these mediators are homeostatic, maintaining vascular tone and preventing proliferation of smooth muscle cells.[28,29]

EICOSANOIDS

Lipids from the cell membranes of endothelial cells play an important role in regulation of vascular tone, platelet aggregation, and inflammation. Under certain conditions, phospholipids on the cell membrane are degraded by phospholipase A_2, yielding arachidonic acid. The latter is the precursor for the eicosanoids, a family of fatty acid derivates with potent hormonelike effects. Prostaglandins, thromboxanes, and leukotrienes are all members of the eicosanoid family and share the characteristic 20-carbon backbone provided by their common precursor (*eikosi* is Greek for 20). But, despite structural similarities, their effects are varied and, at times, dichotomous.[30]

Prostaglandins are known to act on a variety of tissues by regulating the synthesis of cyclic adenosine monophosphate (AMP), an intracellular messenger molecule. These fatty acid derivatives can stimulate strong contractions of smooth muscle (e.g. uterine contractions during labor). In the pulmonary vascular bed, prostacyclin causes relaxation of smooth muscle by stimulating production of cyclic AMP. In addition to its function as a potent vasodilator, the increase in cyclic AMP also inhibits smooth muscle cell proliferation.[31]

The metabolites of arachidonic acid also have important effects on thrombosis. Thromboxanes promote clotting by enhancing platelet aggregation. They are also potent vasoconstrictors and further enhance thrombosis by reducing blood flow to the site of a clot. Prostacyclins, in addition to their vasodilatory properties, inhibit platelet aggregation. An imbalance in the circulating concentration of these two molecules is believed to be a key component in the pathogenesis of pulmonary arterial hypertension.[32]

NITRIC OXIDE

The endothelium is also capable of regulating vascular tone by breaking down the amino acid L-arginine to produce nitric oxide gas. Formerly known as endothelium-derived relaxing factor, nitric oxide is a potent vasodilator. As the gas diffuses into the surrounding smooth muscle, it induces smooth muscle relaxation by increasing intracellular cyclic guanosine monophosphate (GMP).[33] Cyclic GMP activates potassium channels via protein kinases that result in the loss of intracellular potassium. This ion flux hyperpolarizes the cell membrane, decreasing calcium influx, and thereby causing vasodilatation.[34] The endothelium produces nitric oxide at a basal rate but can also release it in response to an agonist (e.g. acetylcholine) or physical forces (e.g. shear stress). Impairment in the endothelium's production of nitric oxide has been associated with pulmonary hypertension.[35]

ENDOTHELIN

The endothelins are a family of three peptides produced by a wide variety of cells. These peptides have mitogenic and vasoactive properties. Endothelial cells and vascular smooth muscle cells produce one of its members, endothelin-1, in response to various stimuli. Endothelin-1 has paracrine effects on neighboring cells, via binding to endothelin receptors, resulting in vasoconstriction and smooth muscle cell proliferation. Two endothelin receptors have been characterized and cloned. Type A receptors show a vascular smooth muscle cell predominance and mediate vasoconstriction. Type B receptors are found in endothelial cells and mediate vasodilation. The role of endothelin-1 in homeostasis and/or disease remains unclear and is also active area of investigation.[36]

OTHER MEDIATORS

The list of biologic mediators with effects in the pulmonary vasculature is extensive and continues to grow. Angiotensin II, serotonin, histamine, platelet-activating factor, vasoactive intestinal peptide, and bradykinin are among the prominent agents currently under investigation. Furthermore, the integrity of the endothelium appears to also play a role in the effect these mediators have on the vessels. Bradykinin and acetylcholine stimulate vasodilation of an intact endothelium, but cause vasoconstriction in the presence of endothelial dysfunction.[37,38] Homeostasis appears to depend on the balance of these mediators, but their interactions and physiologic significance remain in the penumbra of our current understanding.

COMPARING THE CIRCUITS

As previously mentioned, the pulmonary circulation lies in series with the systemic circulation. An anatomic survey of the pulmonary vascular bed reveals key differences from systemic beds. This section will review these teleologic differences that appear to optimize respiratory and nonrespiratory functions of the pulmonary circulation.

The right ventricle

Despite a common origin, the ventricles begin to differ upon folding of the heart tube early in gestation. Once remodeling of this tube is completed, the right ventricle leads a low-key existence, eclipsed by its left-sided sibling. Physicians disregarded the right-sided chamber for centuries, labeling it as passive and prone to failure under stress. Its retrosternal location has continued to plague attempts at noninvasive assessments of its function.

The mature right ventricle is a thin-walled chamber. In cross-section, it has a crescent shape as a result of the encroachment by the muscular intraventricular septum. Thin walls also limit the ventricle's ability to increase the force of its contractions. In the face of rising pulmonary vascular resistance, the ventricle dilates in an effort to maintain stroke volume.[39] However, the fibrous pericardium that encases the heart limits the extent to which the right ventricle can dilate.

Blood flow to the right ventricle from the coronary circulation also differs. Whereas the left ventricle is nourished by oxygenated blood during diastole, coronary blood flow to the right ventricle occurs during systole. Flow occurs as a result of the systolic pressure gradients between the right and left ventricles under normal conditions. Pathologic increases in pulmonary vascular resistance (afterload) will lead to right, and eventually left, ventricular failure. As mentioned above, as the ventricle dilates to maintain stroke volume, increases in end-diastolic volume result in a concomitant rise in pressure within the chamber. Increase in wall stress and peak systolic pressures jeopardize coronary blood flow to the right ventricle with resultant ischemia. The dilated ventricle also pushes back on the intraventricular septum, impairing the compliance of the left ventricle and, eventually, its contractility.[40,41]

The arterial system

Pulmonary arteries are thin and distensible with a large capacitance. They are compliant, with the ability to expand when receiving blood under pressure. Compliance is the physical property that describes how volume changes in response to changes in distending or transmural pressure ($C=\Delta V/\Delta P$).[2] Transmural pressure (ΔP), in turn, is calculated by subtracting the pressure inside a vessel from the pressure outside the vessel.[3] A vessel's ability to stretch is, therefore, determined by change in volume and transmural pressure.

Dynamic flow through the pulmonary vessels is accompanied by changes in intravascular volume and intravascular pressure. Pulmonary vessels are surrounded by air-filled lung that is highly compliant, resulting in a low transmural pressure. The net effect is the dilatation of these arteries, rather than a rise in arterial pressure, thereby maintaining a low-pressure system.[6]

The extensive vasculature of the lung with high compliance and large capacitance allows the lung to act as a blood reservoir. This represents a second, nonrespiratory, function of this circulation. The lungs hold approximately 9 percent (~450 mL) the total body blood volume (which in turn is ~6–8 percent total body weight).[42] This volume of stored blood can be mobilized in response to changes in sympathetic nerve activity, lung inflation, or total body blood volume.

Pulmonary arteries are shorter and have branches with large diameters than their systemic counterparts.[1] As demonstrated by the Poiseuille–Hagen equation, vessels with shorter lengths (l) and larger diameters ($2r$), allow for greater flow. Enhancing flow, in turn, permits the pulmonary circulation to accommodate the entire cardiac output of the right ventricle and deliver deoxygenated blood to the extensive capillary meshwork.

The pulmonary capillaries

The structure of the pulmonary capillaries also differs from their systemic bed counterparts. Rather than being distinct vessels, pulmonary capillaries run in sheets within alveolar septa. The capillary sheets create a lattice resembling a spider's web with a large surface area for the blood–gas interface.

The low resistance of the entire pulmonary circulation stems from this lattice. In the systemic circulation, arterioles play a major role in the control of blood flow. Dynamic changes in the caliber of these vessels can delay or expedite flow through the entire system. Though these muscular arterioles are present in the lungs, their relative collapsibility and distensibility make them less effective than their systemic counterparts in regulating flow.[5] Most of the resistance in the pulmonary circulation therefore originates in the capillary beds and, as previously mentioned, is quite low (approximately one-sixth that of the systemic vascular resistance).[43]

The endothelium of the capillary network provides several pathways for fluid and solute exchange. Oxygen and carbon dioxide use diffusion to cross the endothelium. Water and lipid-soluble substances travel between cells and across channels. Solutes are sieved by the capillary's extracellular matrix in a size-selective manner. The filtration of fluid across the capillary wall is described by the Starling equation:[3]

$$J_v = L_p \times S \left[(P_c - P_i) - \sigma_d (\pi_c - \pi_i) \right]$$

The flow or net filtration across the capillary (J_v) is related to the membrane conductivity (L_p), surface area (S), a reflection coefficient (σ), and the hydrostatic (P) and oncotic (π) pressure gradients between capillary and interstitium. In the normal lung, the filtration across the pulmonary vessels is greater than the rate of absorption. Using the Starling equation with measure values, the net filtration pressure is approximated at +7 mm Hg.[4]

As with vascular tone, vasoactive mediators can alter the permeability of the endothelium. Histamine and thrombin, for example, can rapidly increase vascular endothelial permeability through intracellular signaling and even cytoskeletal alterations. Direct injury of endothelial cells can result in a marked increase in capillary filtration.[44]

CONCLUSION

The remaining chapters of this book will present and discuss various direct and indirect challenges to the pulmonary circulation. Trauma, infections, extreme environments, and intrinsic diseases push compensatory mechanisms beyond their limit while requiring clinicians to tailor their therapies and driving researchers to improve our armamentarium.

Key learning points

- The primary role of the pulmonary circulation is the delivery of deoxygenated blood to ventilated alveoli for gas exchange. The pulmonary circulation is unique in that it accommodates the entire cardiac output every cardiac cycle. Flow through this circulation is therefore equivalent to the cardiac output and dependent on venous return.

- The hemodynamic principles that describe the circulatory system apply to the systemic and pulmonary circuits. These are idealized and summarized by Ohm's law and the Poiseuille–Hagen equation. Flow occurs across pressure gradients, limited by the natural properties of the fluid and the channel through which it occurs.

- The pulmonary vascular bed is extensive, and normally has a large capacitance and high compliance. Blood flow through the lungs is tailored to match perfusion with ventilation such that changes in the alveolar Pa_{O_2}, lung volumes, and gravity have direct effects on flow. Resistance to flow through the pulmonary circulation can be dramatically increased or decreased by changes in the diameter of the pulmonary blood vessels. Most of the resistance originates in the pulmonary capillaries.

- The endothelium of the pulmonary vessels regulates the tone (and therefore resistance) of the pulmonary vascular bed under normal conditions. Pathologic states, extrinsic and intrinsic to the endothelium, can result in pulmonary hypertension through vasoactive mediators.

- Coronary blood flow to the right ventricle differs from the left ventricle in that it occurs during systole. Dilatation of the right ventricle may contribute to ischemia on the basis of decreased coronary perfusion with increases in wall stress. Dilatation of the right ventricle, in response to pulmonary hypertension, is limited by the pericardium.

REFERENCES

1. Fishman AP, ed. *The Pulmonary Circulation: Normal and Abnormal*. Philadelphia: University of Philadelphia Press, 1990.

2. Halliday D, Resnick R, Walker J. *Fundamentals of Physics*, 4th ed. New York: John Wiley, 1993.

3. Guyton AC, Hall JE. *Textbook of Medical Physiology*, 9th ed. Philadelphia: WB Saunders, 1996.

4. West JB. *Respiratory Physiology – The Essentials*, 6th ed. Baltimore: Williams & Wilkins, 2000.

5. Krenz GS, Dawson CA. Flow and pressure distributions in vascular networks consisting of distensible vessels. *Am J Physiol* 2003; **284**: 2192–203.

6. Nichols WW, O'Rourke MF. *McDonald's Blood Flow in Arteries: Theoretical, Experimental, and Clinical Principles*, 4th ed. New York: Oxford University Press, 1998.

7. Hales CA, Ahluwalia B, Kazemi H. Strength of pulmonary vascular response to regional alveolar hypoxia. *J Appl Physiol* 1975; **38**: 1083–7.

8. Marshall BE, Marshall C, Magno M, *et al*. Influence of bronchial arterial PO_2 on pulmonary vascular resistance. *J Appl Physiol* 1991; **70**: 405–15.

9. Morin F, Eagan E, Norfleet W. Development of pulmonary vascular response to oxygen. *Am J Physiol* 1988; **254**: H542–6.

10. Coceani F, Olley PM. The control of cardiovascular shunts in the fetal and neonatal period. *Can J Physiol Pharmacol* 1988; **66**: 1129–34.

11. Madden JA, Vadula MS, Kurup VP. Effects of hypoxia and other vasoactive agents on pulmonary and cerebral artery smooth muscle cells. *Am J Physiol* 1992; **263**: L384–93.

12. Post JM, Hume JR, Archer SL, Weir EK. Direct role for potassium channel inhibition in hypoxic pulmonary vasoconstriction. *Am J Physiol* 1992; **262**: C882–90.

13. Coppock EA, Martens JR, Tamkun MM. Molecular basis of hypoxia-induced pulmonary vasoconstriction: role of voltage-gated K channels. *Am J Physiol Lung Cell Mol Physiol* 2001; **281**: L1–12.

14. Motley HL, Cournand A, Werko L, *et al*. The influence of short periods of induced acute anoxia upon pulmonary artery pressures in man. *Am J Physiol* 1947; **150**: 315–20.

15. Sylvester JT. Hypoxic pulmonary vasoconstriction. *Circ Res* 2001; **88**: 1228–30.

16. Benumof, JL. Mechanism of decreased blood flow to atelectatic lung. *J Appl Physiol* 1979; **46**: 1047–8.

17. Strieder, Denise J. Physical factors in lung function. In: Kazemi H, ed. *Disorders of the Respiratory System.* New York: Grune & Stratton, 1976: 12–40.

18. Mead, J, Whittenberger JL. Lung inflation and hemodynamics. In: Fenn WO, Rahn H, eds. *Handbook of Physiology. Section 3: Respiration. Volume I.* Washington DC: American Physiological Society, 1964: 477–87.

19. Lai-Fook SJ, Rodarte JR. Pleural pressure distribution and its relationship to lung volume and interstitial pressure. *J Appl Physiol* 1991; **70**: 967–78.

20. Pinsky MR. The hemodynamic consequences of mechanical ventilation: an evolving story. *Intensive Care Med* 1997; **23**: 493–503.

21. Fessler HE, Brower RG, Wise RA, *et al.* Effects of positive end-expiratory pressure on the gradient for venous return. *Am Rev Respir Dis* 1991; **143**: 19–24.

22. Mead J. Mechanical properties of the lungs. *Physiol Rev* 1961; **41**: 281–330.

23. Hughes JMB, Glazier JB, Maloney JE, West JB. Effect of lung volume on distribution of pulmonary blood flow in man. *Respir Physiol* 1968; **4**: 58–72.

24. West JB, Dollery CT. Distribution of blood flow and ventilation-perfusion ratio in the lung, measured with radioactive CO_2. *J Appl Phys* 1960; **15**: 405–10.

25. Jellinek H, Krenn H, Oczenski W, *et al.* Influence of positive airway pressure on the pressure gradient for venous return in humans. *J Appl Phys* 2000; **88**: 926–32.

26. Haney MF, Johansson G, Haggmark S, Biber B. Heart-lung interactions during positive pressure ventilation: left ventricular pressure-volume momentary response to airway pressure elevation. *Acta Anaesthesiol Scand* 2001; **45**: 702–9.

27. West JB. Blood flow to the lung and gas exchange. *Anesthesiology* 1974; **41**: 124–38.

28. Barnes PJ, Liu SF. Regulation of pulmonary vascular tone. *Pharmacol Rev* 1995; **47**: 87–131.

29. Bergofsky EH. Humoral control of the pulmonary circulation. *Annu Rev Physiol* 1980; **42**: 221–33.

30. Sprague RS, Stephenson AH, Olearczyk JJ, Lonigro AJ. COX and the control of the pulmonary circulation. *Thromb Res* 2003; **110**: 335–8.

31. Clapp LH, Finney P, Turcato S, *et al.* Differential effects of stable prostacyclin analogues on smooth muscle proliferation and cyclic AMP generation in human pulmonary artery. *Am J Respir Cell Mol Biol* 2002; **26**: 194–201.

32. Christman BW, McPherson CD, Newman JH, *et al.* An imbalance between the excretion of thromboxane and prostacyclin metabolites in pulmonary hypertension. *N Engl J Med* 1992; **327**: 70–5.

33. Palmer RMJ, Ferrige AG, Moncada S. Nitric oxide release accounts for the biological activity of endothelium-derived relaxing factor. *Nature* 1987; **327**: 524–6.

34. Nelson MT, Quayle JM. Physiological roles and properties of potassium channels in arterial smooth muscle. *Am J Physiol* 1995; **254**: H542–6.

35. Giaid A, Saleh D. Reduced expression of endothelial nitric oxide synthase in the lungs of patients with pulmonary hypertension. *N Engl J Med* 1995; **333**: 214–21.

36. Giaid A, Yanagisawa M, Langleben D, *et al.* Expression of endothelin-1 in the lungs of patients with pulmonary hypertension. *N Engl J Med* 1993; **328**: 1732–9.

37. Chen YF, Oparil S. Endothelial dysfunction in the pulmonary vascular bed. *Am J Med Sci* 2000; **320**: 2123–32.

38. Downing SE, Lee JC. Nervous control of the pulmonary circulation. *Annu Rev Physiol* 1980; **42**: 199–210.

39. Wauthy P, Pagnamenta A, Vassalli F, *et al.* Right ventricular adaptation to pulmonary hypertension: an interspecies comparison. *Am J Physiol Heart Circ Physiol* 2004; **286**: H1441–7.

40. McNeil K, Dunning J, Morrell NW, *et al.* The pulmonary circulation and right ventricular failure in the ITU. *Thorax* 2003; **58**: 157–62.

41. Vlahakes GJ, Turley K, Hoffman JI. The pathophysiology of failure in acute right ventricular hypertension: hemodynamic and biochemical correlations *Circulation* 1981; **63**: 87–95.

42. Harris P, Heath D. *The Human Pulmonary Circulation*, 2nd ed. New York: Churchill Livingstone, 1977.

43. Takala J. Pulmonary capillary pressure. *Intensive Care Med* 2003; **29**: 890–3.

44. Lakshminarayan S, Bernard S, Polissar NL, Glenny RW. Pulmonary and bronchial circulatory responses to segmental lung injury. *J Appl Physiol* 1999; **87**: 1931–6.

Diagnostics and Interventions

4

Airway management: endotracheal intubation and tracheostomy

ARTHUR SUNG, KATHLEEN WILLIAMS, KEVIN L KOVITZ

INTRODUCTION

It is essential to have the skills to assess and to establish a stable airway when managing patients with respiratory failure. Endotracheal intubation is a life-saving procedure commonly performed in the critical care setting. Even under emergent circumstances, proper planning is crucial to ensure optimal outcomes. Poor understanding of anatomy, and a lack of alternative methods or tools when intubating – especially in patients with difficult airways – may prove catastrophic and increase complication rates. The purpose of this chapter is to familiarize the reader with various techniques used in endotracheal intubation and tracheostomies in the intensive care setting.

The indications for endotracheal intubation include: hypoxic or hypercapneic respiratory failure; loss of airway protective mechanisms due to neurologic insults such as strokes or drug overdoses; airway obstructions from malignancies or benign causes; and inability to clear secretions, blood, or foreign materials. Regardless of the underlying cause, restoring adequate oxygenation and ventilation is of utmost importance. Noninvasive positive pressure ventilation (NIPPV), such as continuous or bi-level devices, is used increasingly in the setting of respiratory failure in order to avoid ETI. In specific clinical settings, such as acute exacerbations of obstructive diseases, randomized trials have shown its benefits.[1,2] However, the use of NIPPV in other clinical scenarios such as cardiogenic pulmonary edema and noncardiogenic respiratory failures is still under active investigation.[3,4] In addition, NIPPV is contraindicated in various conditions that often occur concomitantly in patients with respiratory failure, such as inability to cooperate due to change in mentation, copious secretions, and comorbidities such as active myocardial infarction. Therefore, ETI remains the mainstay of mechanical ventilatory support, particularly in the intensive care setting.

AIRWAY ANATOMY

Good understanding of the anatomy of the airway is a prerequisite to successful intubation. The airway is divided into the upper (nares to glottis) and lower (trachea and conducting bronchi) segments.

Upper airway

The oral cavity is where initial airway assessment and manipulations take place: tongue size, tooth integrity, and temporomandibular joint mobility are important anatomic factors affecting the outcome of difficulty of the intubation process. The oropharynx is bordered superiorly by the soft palate and extends to the tip of the epiglottis. The hypopharynx contains three major structures: the piriform recess, postcricoid region, and the posterior pharyngeal wall. Complex musculature in this area is responsible for swallowing. The pharynx consists of three outer circular muscles (the superior, middle, and inferior constrictors) and three inner longitudinal muscles (stylopharyngeus, palatopharyngeus, and salpingopharyngeus).[5] During swallowing, the constrictors sequentially propel the food bolus into the esophagus, while the inner longitudinal muscles raise the pharynx.

The larynx is composed of muscles, cartilage, ligaments, and fibrous membranes. Its major structures are the epiglottis, thyroid cartilage, arytenoid cartilages, cricoid cartilage, and the upper trachea.[5] It lies at the level of the third through sixth cervical vertebrae and is higher in women and children. The space between the base of the tongue and the anterior surface of the epiglottis on either side is called the vallecula. The valleculae are separated by the median glossoepiglottic fold and bordered laterally on either side by the lateral glossoepiglottic folds.[6] The vallecula is a potential site of foreign body entrapment, such as food, in upper airway obstruction. The thyroid cartilage connects to the cricoid by the cricothyroid membrane, which is relatively avascular[7,8] and is easily palpated. The cartilage serves as the landmark for emergent cricothyroidotomy (discussed below). The tracheal rings connect to the cricoid cartilage by ligaments and muscles.

The vocal cord apparatus is surrounded by the laryngeal structures. In standard intubation position, the larynx is viewed from above, the epiglottis is seen at the anterior border and the interarytenoid notch posteriorly. Leading from the interarytenoid notch anterolaterally, there are several structures (corniculate and cuneiform tubercles) before the aryepiglottic folds meet at the posterolateral aspects of the epiglottis to form the vestibule. Here the ventricular folds (false cords) are seen before the true vocal cords are observed medially.

The glossopharyngeal nerve and the vagus nerve supply the motor and sensory pathways for the larynx. Stimulation of the external layer of pharyngeal muscles that is innervated by motor and sensory branches of the vagus and glossopharyngeal nerves, such as by blunt trauma to the posterior pharynx during direct laryngoscopy, can result in vagally mediated hypotension.[8] Stimulation of the superior laryngeal nerve, which provides sensory innervation to the epiglottis, the arytenoids and the vocal cords, can induce protective closure of the glottis. Furthermore, nerve endings in the piriform recess in the hypopharynx are exquisitely sensitive to touch, heat, and chemical stimulation. Manipulations can also cause glottic closure.[7] Therefore, careful topical anesthesia should be considered in this region before awake intubation.

Lower airway

The lower airway (tracheal to conductive bronchi) begins at the cricoid cartilage (at about the level of the sixth cervical vertebra). The adult trachea is at least 1.2 cm in diameter and has 16–20 cartilage rings.[8] The trachea divides at the carina, at the level of fifth thoracic spine, into the left and right main stem bronchi.[8] The horseshoe-shaped tracheal cartilage shapes the anterior part of the trachea, whereas the posterior part of the trachea consists of smooth muscle that joins the ends of the tracheal cartilage.[8]

ENDOTRACHEAL INTUBATION

Pre-intubation assessment

The patient's environment influences decision making. For example, a hemodynamically unstable patient should not be intubated in a room lacking equipment for adequate monitoring during the procedure. Any history of adverse events with regard to medications, especially anesthetics including topical anesthetic agents such as lidocaine, should be noted. History of craniofacial or head trauma, neck trauma, or surgery should alert one to the possibility of anatomic abnormalities. Patients with history of surgical procedures of their cervical spine may have limited neck flexion or atlanto-occipital extension.

The history immediately prior to onset of respiratory failure may suggest obstruction as the cause. Upper airway obstruction can be caused by aspiration of gastric contents, blood, or foreign body. In addition, laryngeal edema or spasm may lead to inspiratory stridor and paradoxical breathing. When an obstruction occurs at the level of the epiglottis, vocal cords, or trachea, tracheal intubation or a surgical airway is necessary.

Assessment of a difficult airway

The American Society of Anesthesiologists (ASA) Task Force on Management of the Difficult Airway published guidelines for management of the difficult airway in 2002.[9] It defined a difficult airway as 'the clinical situation in which a conventionally trained anesthesiologist experiences difficulty with face mask ventilation of the upper airway, difficulty with tracheal intubation, or both'. The key to airway management is the recognition of patient characteristics strongly suggestive of difficult mask ventilation, difficult endotracheal intubation, or both.

Difficult intubation, commonly viewed as greater than three attempts by an unassisted anesthesiologist, is associated with increased morbidity. Complications include oxygen desaturation,[10] dental damage,[10,11] hypertension,[11] cardiac arrest, and aspiration.[11] Furthermore, previous experience of difficult bag valve mask ventilation is important to note as adequate pre-oxygenation before intubation is essential. Previous history of failed repeated direct laryngoscopy should prompt the consideration of other modalities, such as fiberoptic laryngoscopy or laryngeal mask airway.

Anatomic assessment

Various scoring systems have been developed to predict and assess the risk of endotracheal intubation. In 1983,

Mallampati published a classification system based on viewing the oropharyngeal cavity.[12] The patient is seated with head in neutral position, mouth open wide, and the tongue protruded. The examiner rates the distance between the base of the tongue to the uvula, soft palate, and pharyngeal pillars:

- Class I – uvula, soft palate, and pharyngeal pillars are clearly visible.
- Class II – soft palate and the pharyngeal pillars only are visible.
- Class III – only the soft palate is visible.

Sampson and Young added class IV – where only the hard palate is visible.[13] The Mallampati classification is improved with phonation, whereas a supine position has a negative effect.

Laryngoscopic views as defined by the Cormack–Lehane (C-L) scale range from grade 1 (easiest, full view) to grade 4 (most difficult, glottis not visualized). There is good correlation between the Mallampati classification and the C-L scale but neither method necessarily predicts difficult intubations,[14] particularly in the emergent setting.[15] Other parameters used include the thyromental distance, mentohyoid distance, mouth opening, and interincisor gap. In adults, adequate mouth opening should ideally be 2.5–3 finger breadths between the upper and lower incisors to allow enough room for the laryngoscope to sweep the tongue to the left and visualize the larynx.[16] The thyromental distance is reduced in patients with micrognathia. The distance from the mandibular symphysis to the hyoid bone should be three finger breadths. If lesser, the angles between the mouth, the oropharynx, and larynx become more acute and difficult to visualize.[14]

Many studies have been published on physical predictors of a difficult intubation using the Mallampati or C-L scale, however, as discussed earlier, no one predictor has proved to be accurate. A history of difficult intubation, systemic or congenital disease, and trauma suggests difficult intubation.[17] Decreased mandibular opening has been found to have a relative risk of 10.3 for difficult intubation[18] and is defined as less than two finger breadths opening between the upper and lower incisors. Mallampati class III or IV is only able to predict a difficult airway about 50 percent of the time, due in part to patient phonation during evaluation and lack of consistency among observers.[19]

PRE-INTUBATION VENTILATION TECHNIQUES

Basic maneuvers

With the patient supine, elevation of the upper thoracic vertebrae by several centimeters by placing a towel roll or blanket between the shoulders helps to align the trachea, larynx, and oropharynx. Simple maneuvers, such as the head tilt/chin lift and jaw thrust can immediately improve airway patency, keeping in mind that hyperextension or flexion of the neck should be avoided in patients with head and neck injuries. To perform head tilt/chin lift, tilt the head backward by placing one hand on the patient's forehead and the other behind the neck. The chin lift maneuver is performed by pulling the chin anteriorly and superiorly by putting several fingers under the mandibular symphysis while using the thumb to depress the lower lip, keeping the mouth opened. The jaw thrust is an effective technique to clear obstruction by the tongue. With both hands on the angle of the jaw, the mandible is displaced forward.

Oral airways

Oral and nasal airways are additional tools that are valuable when relieving tongue obstruction or to prevent the patient from biting down. Most oral airways are curved and are intended to fit the curvature of the tongue and palate and end just above the epiglottis. The device can be inserted either in the same orientation in which it will lie in the mouth or initially at 180° with the tip facing upward. If the latter method is used, the airway is advanced about half of the length and then rotated 180° and advanced into position. If ventilation is ineffective despite an oral airway, one must ensure that the tongue is not pushed back into the oropharynx by grasping the tip of the tongue and pulling it forward while simultaneously pushing the oral airway posteriorly. Complications include aspiration and laryngeal spasm.[20] Therefore, patients who are awake or semiconscious, with full stomachs, friable oral lesions, poor dentition, or active laryngospasm may be poor candidates for oral airways.

A nasopharyngeal airway is indicated when a patient cannot tolerate oral insertion due to oral trauma or significant gag reflex in a conscious or semi-conscious state. In addition, this airway should be preferentially used in situations such as in the presence of tongue abnormalities or oral cavity or dental pathologies. On the other hand, patients with bleeding disorders, nasal deformities, and basilar skull fractures should be considered for an oral airway instead. Various sizes are available, ranging from 6 mm to 9 mm inner diameter for adults. Most nasopharyngeal airways are soft and pliable with a bevel at the distal end to facilitate insertion and a flared proximal end to limit the depth of insertion. During insertion, the leading tip of the bevel should be against the nasal septum and perpendicular to the face. Once the tip of the nasopharynx is reached, the nasal airway should be turned 90° counterclockwise, aligning the bevel against the posterior pharyngeal wall. Adequate lubricant, gentle insertion, and a tube with a diameter no larger than the nasal opening should be used. Complications include bleeding due to nasal mucosal trauma during insertion and esophageal intubation if the device is too long.

Bag valve mask

During the pre-intubation period, adequate oxygenation can be achieved with proper facemask ventilation by a bag valve mask. The device can correct both oxygenation and ventilation problems, and can be maintained until more definite artificial airways are established. Problems encountered during facemask ventilation include insufficient seal (such as in edentulous patients) and excessive air leak. Causal factors include age, weight, male sex, history of snoring, and Mallampati class IV.[21] The presence of a beard may prevent optimal seal the mask and patient's skin. Furthermore, it can hide anatomic abnormalities such as micrognathia. When shaving the beard is impractical, placing wide tape on the beard and placing the mask over the tape can improve the seal.

With bag valve mask ventilation, the airway is not protected and high airway pressures and tidal volumes increase the risk of gastric insufflation. The air may preferentially go down the esophagus if the patient has redundant tissue over the larynx or in the setting of laryngeal spasm and glottic closure. Gastric insufflation is also likely when there is reduced pulmonary compliance with pulmonary fibrosis, mucus plugs in the airways, bronchospasm, pulmonary edema, obesity, or the supine position. A number of studies in both apneic volunteers and preoperative settings have compared different tidal volumes with bag valve mask ventilation. These studies have shown that smaller tidal volumes (ranges from 365 mL to 500 mL) with supplemental oxygen achieved adequate oxygenation without significant gastric insufflation.[22,23] Current guidelines by the American Heart Association revised in 2000 recommend that bag valve mask ventilation for resuscitations with $FiO_2 > 40$ percent should be performed with tidal volumes of 6–7 mL/kg with delivery time over 1–2 s/breath.[24,25]

TECHNICAL ASPECTS OF ENDOTRACHEAL INTUBATION

Proficiency in endotracheal intubation requires experience and practice. Although there are useful tools available to aid in gaining skills, such as models or even full-scale simulators, they do not fully duplicate the real-life situations physicians, residents, and allied health providers encounter. In addition, although not uncommon, there is a lack of policies and guidelines regarding consent from family members with respect to the practice of cadaver intubations in the recently deceased, and there are inherent ethical concerns.[26,27] This section describes the fundamental techniques of endotracheal intubation in an intensive care setting.

Laryngoscopes

Standard laryngoscopy blades are of two types: the curved Macintosh blade and the straight Miller blade. Both blades have a flange on the left side of the blade to keep the tongue out of the line of sight. The tip of the curved blade is placed in the vallecula. The tip of the straight blade should be passed just beyond the epiglottis, on its posterior surface, and then a forward and upward movement of the clinician's hand should bring the arytenoid cartilages and glottic opening into view. Insertion of the curved blade too far into the vallecula may push the epiglottis posteriorly and cover the glottic opening. Curved blades are thought to be less traumatic because when properly positioned, they should not come into contact with the epiglottis. Straight blades provide a better view of the glottis in patients with a long epiglottis or anterior larynx, and they are preferred in children due to their floppy epiglottis.

The endotracheal tube

Endotracheal intubation with a single lumen tube is the gold standard for providing emergency airway. The standard single-lumen endotracheal tube is sterile and made of polyvinyl chloride or silicone; some have a continuous metal coil embedded in the plastic to limit kinking. The tube may or may not have a distal cuff; if it does, the distal cuff is connected to a pilot balloon and is inflated once the tube is in position to prevent leaking of air between the tube and the trachea, thus minimizing aspiration of pharyngeal content. In general, the endotracheal tube should be 7.0–7.5 mm in diameter for an average adult female and 7.5–8.0 mm for an average adult male. Larger diameter tubes can lead to vocal cord trauma, as the glottis is the narrowest portion of the adult larynx. A small endotracheal tube increases the resistance of airflow, which is inversely related to the fourth power of luminal radius. The high-volume, low-pressure cuff should not be inflated to a pressure above 30 cm H_2O. High pressures can lead to tracheal mucosa necrosis,[27] malacia, stenosis,[28] and fistula formation.[29] Disastrous complications with overzealous inflation include tracheal ruptures and erosions into carotid arteries.[30] Insufficient cuff pressure predisposes to aspiration of pharyngeal contents, and it is recommended that at least 20–25 cm H_2O should be used.[31] Manometry measurements are recommended routinely with intubated patients as there are considerable cuff pressure variations outside the recommended range.[32,33]

Orotracheal intubation

In preparation for oral endotracheal intubation, the patient should be supine and the patient's head should be at the level of the physician's midchest. In the absence of trauma or neck injury, the sniff position, which is achieved by lifting up the head and extending the atlanto-occipital joint, allows maximal visualization of the vocal cords. A small rolled towel can be placed underneath the patient's neck for facilitation. The oropharynx should be suctioned just prior to intubation, and the laryngoscope light should be tested for illumination. The patient should be pre-oxygenated with 100 percent oxygen for 4–5 minutes by bag valve mask ventilation. Once adequate oxygenation is achieved, the blade is held in the left hand and placed in the right side of the patient's mouth while the left fifth finger pushes the patient's chin downward, opening the mouth. Alternatively, the mouth is gently opened by the left thumb and index finger in a scissorlike fashion. The blade is advanced toward the base of the tongue on the right side of the patient's mouth while simultaneously sweeping the tongue to the left by bringing the blade into the center of the mouth. Once the tip of the blade is at the vallecula anterior to the epiglottis (if using Macintosh blade), the laryngoscope handle is lifted in a 45° angle to the axis of the spine, anterior and caudad. Care is taken to avoid using the teeth as the fulcrum or rotation of the blade. Anterior and caudad movement of the laryngoscope stretches the hyoepiglottic ligament, moving the epiglottis anteriorly and exposing the aryepiglottic folds and the glottis anteriorly. When the epiglottis is visualized, the endotracheal tube with or without stylet (which assists the curvature of the endotracheal tube to align with the airway) is inserted, with visualization of the tube passing through the glottis. Adult endotracheal tubes are generally advanced to 20–24 cm from the distal tip of the tube to the teeth. If advanced further, the right mainstem bronchus can be intubated with occlusion of the left mainstem. Cricoid pressure, or the Sellick maneuver, is routinely applied during emergent intubation to avoid aspiration of gastric contents. This maneuver may alter laryngoscopic view,[34,35] but has not been proved to increase the difficulty of intubations.[36] Once the endotracheal tube is observed to pass through the vocal cords, and felt to be positioned correctly in the upper trachea, the cuff is inflated to create an adequate seal.

Nasotracheal intubation

Nasotracheal intubation provides another route to obtain a secure airway, particularly in the setting of oral trauma. Similar to placing a nasopharyngeal airway, a nasotracheal tube is placed against the nasal septum perpendicular to the face and inserted with the curvature of the tube along the larynx. Once the tube is advanced to the posterior oropharynx, a direct laryngoscope can be used to further visualize the advancement of the tube into the glottis. Magill forceps can also be used to aid the intubation. Complications include significant epistaxis, tube contamination, and infection.[37]

Blind nasal intubation is accomplished by advancing an endotracheal tube through the nares and posteriorly through the inferior nasal meatus into the pharynx. The patient may be supine or sitting in the sniffing position. The leading edge of the tube is placed along the nasal septum of the nostril and the tube is directed parallel to the hard palate in a posterior direction, with the concave curve of the tube facing superiorly. Once in the nasopharynx, the tube is rotated 180°, aligning the curve of the endotracheal tube with the curvature of the patient's airway. The tube is advanced 2–5 cm until air is felt to flow through the tube. During patient inhalation, the tube is advanced through the vocal cords.

Confirmation of tube placement

The patient is observed for symmetric chest rise and auscultation is done to check for equal bilateral breath sounds immediately after intubation to confirm tracheal intubation. In obese patients or in the setting of poor chest wall compliance, these signs may not be reliable. Although fogging of the endotracheal tube after intubation is often felt to be a sign of tracheal intubation, water condensation in the endotracheal tube was demonstrated in 85 percent of esophageal intubations in one study and in 28 percent in another.[38,39] The detection of carbon dioxide is felt to be reliable enough to merit the ASA statement: 'when an endotracheal tube is inserted, its correct positioning in the trachea must be verified by clinical assessment and by identification of carbon dioxide in the expired gas'.[40] Capnography and colorimetric detection of carbon dioxide are the most commonly used methods.

Calorimetric end-tidal carbon dioxide detection is a readily available tool in which the device is attached between the endotracheal tube and the ventilator or bag and mask assembly. The device contains a pH-sensitive paper filter that reversibly turns from purple to yellow – carbon dioxide levels are less than 0.5 percent when the paper is purple and greater than 2 percent when it is yellow. In patients who have not had a cardiac or pulmonary arrest, this has been shown to be a reliable tool.[41–43] The capnograph measures the exhaled carbon dioxide on a breath-to-breath basis and displays the exhaled carbon dioxide level on a continuous monitor. False-negative results (absent waveform and tube in the trachea, as in severe bronchospasm) and false-positive results (present waveform with the tube in the esophagus, due to ventilating the stomach) have been reported.[44]

Esophageal intubation with reservoir bag breaths can cause expansion of the chest wall, simulating endotracheal intubation. An esophageal detector bulb is a 75–90 mL self-inflating bulb with a standard 15 mm endotracheal adapter. The esophagus collapses when negative pressure is applied in its lumen but the trachea does not due to its stiffness. After intubation, the bulb is attached to the end of the endotracheal tube and compressed and then quickly released. If the tube is in the esophagus, air may be heard moving through the esophagus and the bulb will not inflate, as the negative pressure pulls the esophageal mucosa up to occlude the tube. In one study, the sensitivity and specificity of the esophageal detector bulb were evaluated in 2140 consecutively anesthetized adult patients. The proportion of false-negative results was 3.6 percent. Most of the false-negative results (85 percent) were in morbidly obese patients (body mass index [BMI] >35 kg/m^2).[45] Tracheal occlusion with an esophageal bulb has been reported.[46]

ALTERNATIVE ARTIFICIAL AIRWAYS FOR DIFFICULT INTUBATIONS

In the case of a recognized difficult airway, an awake intubation should be considered. A planned strategy with a back-up plan may lead to an improved outcome.[47] Local anesthetic to the upper airway, pre-oxygenation, and sufficient sedation are essential so that the patient is awake and relaxed. Awake tracheal intubation can be performed by direct laryngoscopy, blind nasal or oral routes, stylet, fiberoptic, or retrograde. The preference for an awake intubation takes into account the desire to preserve the natural airway, airway patency, spontaneous respirations, the patient's ability to protect the airway, and laryngeal position (it moves anteriorly after paralysis).

Alternative methods to bag valve mask ventilation and direct laryngoscopy include supraglottic ventilatory devices (the laryngeal mask airway [LMA], esophageal-tracheal Combitube™), blind intubation, indirect and fiberoptic laryngoscopes (Bullard™, WuScope™, Shikani Seeing Optical Stylet™). All these will be discussed below.

Laryngeal mask airway

The LMA (LMA Company Limited, UK), developed in 1981 in the United Kingdom by Dr Archie Brain, is made of silicone and is latex free. There is a variety of sizes able to accommodate both pediatric and adult patients. It is often used in patients undergoing general anesthesia and can be used as a rescue device after failed attempts to intubate by direct laryngoscopy. In the setting of a difficult airway, it can be used for awake intubation, blind intubation, or combined with fiberoptic bronchoscopy. Furthermore, endotracheal intubation can be accomplished by placing an endotracheal tube through an LMA (Fastrach™, discussed later in the chapter). Another distinct advantage of the LMA is its reliable ease of placement by an inexperienced operator in an emergent situation. A 94 percent success rate has been reported for positioning on the first attempt of an LMA by paramedical personnel and students attempting to access known difficult airways.[48–50]

To place the LMA, lubricate it and place the deflated cuff of the LMA facing the patient's tongue and advance it posterior along the palate. Once past the tongue, the LMA will move easily into position. When resistance is felt, the LMA is at the upper esophageal sphincter. The cuff is then inflated, and its leading edge should pass between the tip of the epiglottis and the posterior pharyngeal wall. The positioned LMA sits at the opening of the larynx and rests in the oropharynx at an oblique angle. The cuff of the LMA abuts the firm posterior pharyngeal wall and forms a seal. The anterior margin of the LMA lies at the base of the hypopharynx, with the tip at the level of upper esophageal sphincter. Pathologies at or above the vocal cords are contraindications to its use, including laryngeal obstruction, tumor, bleeding of the oropharynx, epiglottitis, and laryngeal abscess.

Complications include higher frequency of gastric insufflation due to the lower sealing pressure of the cuff as compared with endotracheal tubes.[50] Therefore, use of LMA is contraindicated in patients with full stomachs, history of significant esophageal reflux, and near-term gestation pregnancies. Coughing or laryngospasm are also seen if the LMA makes contact with the vocal cords. In addition, epiglottic downward folding may occur in the event of glottic insertion.

The Proseal™ LMA is a newer version of Classic LMA™ designed with a different cuff to improve insertion and a gastric conduit for access to the gastrointestinal tract. Airway obstruction occurs in between 2 percent and 10 percent of cases.[51,52] The Fastrach™ LMA, or intubating LMA (iLMA), is a modified standard LMA with addition of a metallic handle and tunnel for endotracheal tube insertion. During emergent and initial failed attempt intubations, it can be used to establish supraglottic airway and, subsequently, endotracheal tube intubation can be accomplished through its metallic channel. Standard endotracheal tubes can be used. Furthermore, insertion of an iLMA can be facilitated by fiberoptic bronchoscope or lightwand.[53] In a study using manikins, both experienced and nonexperienced operators were able to achieve high success rates for intubation on the first attempt after having a less than 60 second demonstration.[54]

Blind intubation

ESOPHAGEAL–TRACHEAL COMBITUBE®

The esophageal-tracheal Combitube™ (ETC, Kendall-Sheridan Corporation, Argyle, NY) is a disposable polyvinyl chloride double lumen artificial airway. It is designed for emergent intubations and can be placed blindly, laryngoscopically, or over a bronchoscope. The device contains two cuffs with the distal one designed to occlude either the trachea or the esophagus while the proximal oropharyngeal balloon is situated the patient's hypopharynx, sealing the oral and nasal cavities.

A wall separates the two lumens, and the tube is opened at the distal end resembling a standard endotracheal tube. The other lumen, blocked at its distal end, is similar to an esophageal obturator airway with perforations at the pharyngeal level.[55] Ventilatory outlets are positioned between the two cuffs. If the distal end is placed in the esophagus, which is more than 95 percent of the time, the longer blue inlet is used for connection to a bag valve or a ventilator and air comes out of the pharyngeal outlets between the two sealed cuffs. On the other hand, if the trachea is intubated, then the shorter clear inlet is used and air comes out of the distal end opening, similar to conventional endotracheal tubes.

The sniff position should be avoided, since esophageal intubation is intended. After insertion to the ring mark at the level of teeth, the proximal (pharyngeal) balloon is inflated with air (85 mL of air for the 37 Fr and 100 mL for the 41 Fr) followed by the distal balloon (10–12 mL of air for the 37 Fr and 10–15 mL for the 41 Fr). Correct positioning is attained when the ventral part of the proximal balloon reaches the posterior part of the hard palate. If the patient is difficult to ventilate, the ETC may be too deep. Both balloons should then be deflated; the ETC is withdrawn 1–2 cm and the balloons inflated with ventilation reinitiated. Complications of ETC include esophageal injury, subcutaneous emphysema, pneumomediastinum,[56] and tongue engorgement.[57]

Other supraglottic devices include the Pharyngeal Airway Xpress™, which is a latex-free, single-use artificial airway and is intended for routine procedures. It is curved, and has a large or pharyngeal cuff and a 3.5 cm hooded window that is designed to lift the epiglottis forward and allow ventilation. However, there are no studies showing its benefit over alternative airway devices.[58]

Blind nasal intubation

Nasal intubation (discussed earlier) causes less discomfort (less gag response) but a higher possibility of bleeding than oral intubation. It is also simpler than the oral approach because the tube is aimed at the epiglottis when it emerges into the hypopharynx. Nasotracheal intubation is indicated if the patient cannot tolerate the supine position or the oral cavity is not accessible (seizures, temporomandibular joint trismus, oral pathology). Turbinate trauma, necrosis, and sinusitis are associated with long-term nasal intubation. Contraindications to nasotracheal intubation include bleeding disorders (including uremia, nasal hematoma, or hemorrhage), facial trauma, nasopharyngeal obstruction, and acute epiglottis.

Tracheal introducer

Sir Robert R Macintosh introduced the original tracheal introducer, or gum elastic bougie, in 1949. It was a urethral dilator used as a directional guide for intubating difficult airways with an endotracheal tube. Currently, an Eschmann tracheal introducer, which is modified from the original and still called the gum elastic bougie,[59] can be used to guide an endotracheal tube or an LMA into the trachea by the Seldinger technique.[60] It is a 60 cm long, 15 Fr catheter with a curved tip, and made of a polyester tube core and is resin coated.[59]

The gum elastic bougie is useful when grade 3 (C-L scale) laryngoscopic view is encountered (visualization of the tip of epiglottis). With patient in standard sniff position, a laryngoscope is used to achieve the best view possible. The introducer is advanced blindly into the glottis while the

operator notes the length and advances to approximately 20–24 cm at the teeth. Furthermore, the operator or/and assistant can feel the sensation when the stiff tip runs against the tracheal ring, causing clicking sensation as the tube is advanced through the trachea. The endotracheal tube, which is placed over the proximal end of the catheter, is advanced into the glottis by Seldinger technique, also called 'railroading'. Other signs of airway (versus esophageal) intubation include resistance felt when advancing into the bronchial tree at maximal insertion distance of 45 cm, and induction of cough when the catheter is being advanced if the patient is not paralyzed.[61] The bougie tracheal introducer technique is highly successful, given practice and experience.[62]

Indirect intubation devices

FIBEROPTIC LARYNGOSCOPE

Rigid fiberoptic laryngoscopes include the WuScope™ (Achi Corporation, San Jose, CA) and the Bullard laryngoscope™ (ACMI Circon, Santa Barbara, CA), both intended for use in difficult intubations for patients in neutral position, such as in cervical spine immobilizations.[63] The WuScope™ consists of the rigid laryngoscope and the fiberoptic flexible scope portion. It has been used for exchange of endotracheal tubes, as well as postsurgical complications in neck surgery.[64,65] The Bullard laryngoscope is similar to the WuScope™ and is also reported to have improved airway access in trauma patients.[66] Real-time fluoroscopic studies have demonstrated that fiberoptic laryngoscopic intubation reduces cervical vertebral movement compared with direct laryngoscopy.[67] As in all intubating techniques, familiarity with these devices is essential before attempting difficult intubations.

LIGHTED STYLETS

A lighted stylet, Trachlight™ (Laerdal Medical Corp., Wappingers Falls, New York), uses a strong light source to transilluminate the neck when it is positioned in the upper airway, but light is not seen if it is placed in the esophagus. The technique has been described by Hung and colleagues.[68,69] The unit consists of a lightwand with a light bulb at its distal end; the proximal end is attached to a handle. The endotracheal tube is placed over the lightwand shaped with a detachable stylet in a 'hockey stick' configuration.[68] The tip is advanced toward the laryngeal prominence, using the glow of the light as a guide. Once the lightwand enters the glottis, a bright yellow glow should be seen in the anterior neck, just below the thyroid prominence. The stiff inner stylet is retracted and the endotracheal tube is advanced into the trachea. Hung et al. published their experience of using the lightwand in patients who were difficult to intubate.[70] In 206 patients with known or anticipated difficult airways, 204 were successfully intubated. In another study Weiss and Hatton successfully intubated

250 of 253 patients in emergency room, operating room, and intensive care units. The three failed intubations were due to obesity with poor transillumination.[71] Possible contraindications include epiglottitis, retropharyngeal hematoma or abscess, tracheal stenosis, laryngeal pathology, foreign bodies, or airway compromise of unknown etiology.[68] The Shikani Optical Seeing™ (SOS) stylet (Clarus Medical, Minneapolis, MN) incorporates the properties of the transilluminating lightwand and the fiberoptic bronchoscope.[72,73] The advantage of the system include its portability and reusability.[72] Recent literature has described its use in children.[74]

Many new types of intubating fiberoptic stylet have been introduced recently for difficult intubations. They differ in size, angle of view, light source, and rigidity. Liem *et al.* have published a summary.[73]

Flexible bronchoscopic intubation

Flexible bronchoscopes have assisted in oral and nasal intubations since Stiles *et al.* published results of 100 fiberoptic endotracheal intubations (FBI) in 1972.[75] In experienced hands, a flexible fiberoptic bronchoscope is a valuable tool for difficult airway intubations. It is particularly useful in situations where oral–pharyngeal–laryngeal alignment is not possible, such as in cervical spine injuries. Another advantage of FBI is the ability to perform awake intubations with adequate topical anesthesia. This option is often considered in obstetrics where general anesthesia patients may present with 'cannot intubate, cannot ventilate' situations.[76]

The major indication for FBI is known or suspected difficult intubation. Secretions or blood can usually be suctioned, washed, or cleared by injecting air or sterile normal saline through the fiberoptic scope. Preferably, the posterior pharynx should be topically anesthetized with benzocaine (Cetacaine®) or lidocaine. The endotracheal tube is placed over the bronchoscope. The bronchoscope is advanced beyond the vocal cords into the trachea. The patient is then asked to inhale and the endotracheal tube is gently advanced over the bronchoscope, through the vocal cords, and into the trachea. Contact of the endoscope or the endotracheal tube with the carina will induce intense coughing and should be avoided. The passage of the endotracheal tube can be difficult due to the gap between the inside of the tube and the bronchoscope.[77] Fiberoptic tracheal intubation skills are considered critical in airway management. Mastering the technique requires practice and it should be undertaken by any clinician responsible for airway management.

Fiberoptic compatible oral airways (FCOAs) are also available for assisting fiberoptic-guided intubations. Several FCOAs are commercially available, but all have channels for fiberoptic cables to pass through. Depending on the design, the channel is positioned at either the anterior or the posterior aspect of the body. Those with anterior channels, such as Patil-Syracuse™ (Keomed, Inc., Minnetonka, MN) and Williams Intubating Airway™ (Mainline Medical, Inc. Norcross, GA), allow more direct access to the glottis, whereas Ovassapian™ (Kendall Healthcare Products Co., Mansfield, MA) and Luomanen™ (Luomanen Medical Products, Sparta, NJ) FCOAs have posterior channels with less immediate access to glottis but are easier to remove after intubation.[78]

Emergent cricothyroidotomy

The ASA Task Force on Management of the Difficult Airway published the guidelines for management of the difficult airway, which suggested that equipment for cricothyrotomy should be available to all personnel managing airways.[9] In the ASA closed claims study, adverse outcomes due to respiratory-related events accounted for the largest class of injury with brain damage or death in 85 percent of cases.[79] Approximately 0.01–2.0 percent of 10 000 patients were difficult to mask ventilate and intubate; 0.05–0.35 percent were unable to be intubated.[80] This underscores the need for any clinician who manages airways to have the equipment readily available and be knowledgeable about the technique of cricothyroidotomy.

When confronted with 'cannot intubate, cannot ventilate' situations, such as unrelieved glottic or supraglottic obstructions, cricothyroidotomy is the most important approach to establish an emergent airway. It is also a life-saving procedure when equipment for endotracheal intubation is lacking. Cricothyroidotomy may be performed by one of two methods: needle and surgical, both of which require good knowledge of clinical anatomy of the neck. The anterior structures of the neck pertinent to cricothyroidotomy are described below.

The anterior structures of the neck include the hyoid bone, hyoid–thyroid membrane, thyroid cartilage, cricothyroid membrane, and the cricoid cartilage. The cricothyroid membrane is a fibroelastic membrane surrounded by cricothyroid muscles below the thyroid cartilage and is devoid of major blood supplies or nerves.[81] The larynx is supplied by the superior laryngeal artery, which is a branch of the superior thyroid artery, and the inferior laryngeal artery from the inferior thyroid artery. The cricothyroid artery, a branch of the superior laryngeal artery, courses through the superior portion of the cricothyroid membrane.[81] Therefore, it is recommended that the incision during cricothyroidotomy should be aimed at the inferior portion of the membrane, rather than immediately below the thyroid cartilage.[81]

Needle method

Standing on the left side of the patient, with the left thumb and index finger stabilizing the trachea, the operator inserts a 12 or 14 G needle catheter attached to a 5 mL syringe inferiorly at 45° through the cricothyroid membrane so not to damage the vocal cords. With constant aspiration during insertion, advancement is stopped once air is seen in syringe, indicating location in the lumen of the trachea. Then the needle is withdrawn and the catheter is connected to oxygen supply or a jet ventilator. Specific kits are also available.

Transtracheal jet ventilation

After successful cannulation of the cricothyroid membrane with needle catheter assembly, high-pressure oxygen (344.74 kPa) can be connected from wall outlet via a Luer-lock connector. It has been shown that TJV is useful in supplying adequate oxygenation after unsuccessful bag valve mask ventilation, and perhaps improving glottic view for laryngoscopy with high pressure opening the glottis.[82] Complications result from barotrauma, including pneumothorax, pneumomediastinum, and subcutaneous emphysema.

Surgical method

The location of surgical cricothyroidotomy is the same level as the needle method, except a 1 cm transverse incision is made. Care is taken not to extend the incision laterally beyond 1 cm as the common carotid artery and the internal jugular vein lie posterolaterally.[81] Once the incision is made, the scalpel handle is used to insert into the opening and is turned 90° to open the airway. Subsequently, an appropriate-size cuffed endotracheal tube or tracheostomy tube is inserted and secured with sutures and tied around the neck.

Complications include esophageal rupture due to forceful entry through the lumen, laryngeal damage due to oversized cuff used to insert into the small cricothyroid space, and tracheal ring fracture.[83,84]

The complication rate for an elective cricothyroidotomy is 6–8 percent and for an emergent cricothyrotomy is 10–40 percent.[83,84] There is a 25 percent overall complication rate, with a 15 percent incidence of persistent voice dysfunction and a 4 percent risk of subglottic stenosis.[80,81] The early complications of a cricothyroidotomy include: asphyxia, hemorrhage, improper tube placement, subcutaneous emphysema, mediastinal emphysema, pneumothorax, airway obstruction, esophageal perforation, mediastinal perforation, vocal cord injury, aspiration, and laryngeal disruption. Late complications include: tracheal stenosis, subglottic stenosis, aspiration, swallowing dysfunction, tube obstruction, tracheoesophageal fistula, voice changes, infection, hemorrhage, persistent stoma, tracheomalacia.[83,84]

Retrograde tracheal intubation

Retrograde intubation is an invasive technique involving cricothyroid membrane puncture and passage of a guidewire 'retrogradely' into the oropharynx. It is considered a nonsurgical airway access that can be performed in the hospital or prehospital setting. It can be used in the management of the difficult airway and as a rescue technique after failed intubation using conventional methods. It was originally described in 1960 and is relatively simple to perform and has been successfully used in adults and children.[85]

Ideally, the patient's neck should be extended and local anesthesia and aseptic technique used. Commercial kits are available. An 18 G or larger needle attached to a 20 mL syringe and partially filled with saline is advanced in the midline through the cricothyroid membrane. When a large volume of air is aspirated, entrance into the trachea is likely. The needle is aimed superiorly, and the syringe is removed. A guidewire is then threaded through the needle into the oropharynx. The patient's tongue should be pulled anteriorly to prevent coiling of the wire in the mouth. The wire tip is retrieved with Magill forceps under direct visualization. The wire is placed through the Murphy eye of the endotracheal tube and the proximal portion of the wire held with one hand while the endotracheal tube is slid down into the trachea. The guidewire is removed in a retrograde fashion (through the mouth) once the endotracheal tube is in the trachea and the endotracheal tube advanced into place. Cases have been reported in which retrograde intubation has been effective in patients with abnormal anatomic or pathologic conditions of the upper airway.[86] It can be performed in patients with an immobilized neck and in the prehospital setting. Contraindications include patients who require immediate intubation (retrograde intubation can take 5–10 minutes), complete upper airway obstruction, laryngeal trauma, severe infections, or inability to open the mouth to retrieve the wire.

TRACHEOSTOMY (PERCUTANEOUS VERSUS SURGICAL)

Tracheostomy is a commonly performed procedure for relief of airway obstruction, pulmonary hygiene, and prolonged mechanical ventilatory support.[87] However, due to its inherent complications which include stoma infections, bleeding, and even death,[88,89] the ideal timing for performing a tracheostomy has not been established.[90] It has not been clearly established that laryngeal injury from endotracheal intubation is time dependent.[91] Because patients may benefit from tracheostomy to different degrees and at different times during their clinical course, factors unique to the individual patient must be considered.[92] The individualization of tracheotomy timing has been termed the 'anticipatory approach' – the patient's likelihood of benefiting from tracheostomy and anticipated duration of continued ventilatory support. Recent literature suggests that tracheostomy as early as 48 hours after intubation in patients who are expected to need long-term mechanical ventilation improves survival and decreases ventilator days.[93] Furthermore, a recent systemic review and metaanalysis suggests shortened stay in the intensive care unit and artificial ventilation with an early approach.[94] These conclusions needs to be confirmed by additional studies.

Tracheostomy can be performed by the open surgical technique or by several percutaneous dilation techniques. The classic open surgical tracheotomy was standardized by Chevalier Jackson in 1909.[95,96] In 1985, Ciaglia and colleagues performed a modified Seldinger serial percutaneous dilatational tracheostomy (PDT).[97]

Surgical tracheostomy

Surgical tracheostomy is an operation typically performed by general surgeons, cardiothoracic surgeons, otolaryngologists, and other surgeons. Some centers create a surgical environment and it is done at the bedside in the intensive care unit, but the operating room with adequate equipment is the usual setting. The operation is done under general anesthesia, and the anesthesiologist is responsible for the security and removal of the endotracheal tube. The standard surgical technique involves a 2 cm transverse incision about 2 cm above the suprasternal notch.[98] After dissection and division of cervical fascia and underlying neck muscles with lateral retraction, the midline is developed with exposure of the thyroid gland.[98] Lateral retraction sutures are placed around the second or third tracheal ring. A vertical tracheostomy at midline is created ideally between the second and fourth tracheal ring and is subsequently dilated.[98] The tracheostomy tube is placed, secured and connected to the ventilation source. The endotracheal tube is then removed.

Percutaneous dilatational tracheostomy

The first or second tracheal interspace is the preferred site for PDT. The patient begins with an endotracheal tube in place and should have continuous pulse oximetry and vital signs monitored throughout the procedure. An amnesic such as a benzodiazepine and an analgesic such as an opioid are administered intravenously to produce moderate to deep sedation. A neuromuscular blocker is given, and 100 percent oxygen is administered throughout the procedure. The neck is extended to open the tracheal cartilage interspaces, and the surgical field is prepped and draped, with aseptic technique. Local anesthesia is injected subcutaneously at the incision site. A 2 cm skin incision is made over the first or second tracheal interspaces and hemostats or curved forceps are used to bluntly dissect down to the anterior tracheal wall. The bronchoscope is inserted through the endotracheal tube and maintained just proximal to the end of the tube to protect it. The endotracheal tube cuff is deflated and the tube is withdrawn to just above the first tracheal ring. The

endotracheal tube cuff is reinflated and the introducer needle with the bevel facing downward is inserted in the midline through the skin incision under bronchoscopic visualization. Saline or lidocaine in the syringe shows bubbling when aspiration is performed and the needle is in the trachea. Bronchoscopic visualization is preferred and bubbling can be seen if the needle is in the esophagus. When the needle bevel is seen in the trachea, the syringe is disconnected and the J-tipped guidewire is advanced through the needle, into the trachea and down to the carina. Keeping the wire in place, the needle is removed. Plastic dilators are advanced over the wire, each sequentially larger (Cook Critical Care, Indianapolis, IN and Simms Portex, Keene, NH). Alternatively, a single progressive dilator may be used (Blue Rhino™, Cook Critical Care, Indianapolis, IN). When the incision is dilated, a tracheostomy tube, with a dilator inside it serving as an obturator, is advanced over the wire and into the trachea. The wire and obturator are removed and the patient's tracheostomy tube is connected to the ventilator and the cuff inflated. The endotracheal tube and bronchoscope are withdrawn after visual confirmation of the tracheostomy tube is in the trachea. Care should be taken during the procedure not to puncture the cuff of the endotracheal tube.

Complications of PDT include stoma infections, bleeding, accidental extubation, pneumothorax, tracheal ring fracture, and tracheal stenosis.[99,100] The rate of complication is as follows: 1–4 percent rate of bleeding,[100,101] 0.8–3.7 percent rate of tracheal stenosis,[100,101] and mortality less than 1 percent.[102]

Many studies have compared surgical and percutaneous tracheostomy. One metaanalysis concluded that the percutaneous technique was easier to perform and had a lower incidence of peristomal infection and bleeding.[103] Another metaanalysis concluded that an increase in complication rates accompanied the percutaneous tracheostomy.[104] Theoretically, because the dilatational technique has less tissue trauma, it should result in less bleeding, infection, and deformity. It is better suited for the critically ill patient, as the patient does not need to be transported to the operating room, and theoretically is less costly. Both surgical and percutaneous dilatational tracheostomy can be performed quickly with little significant difference in procedure time.[105] There is also no statistically significant difference in mortality attributed to the two techniques.[106] Friedman and colleagues found that the time from intubation to tracheostomy was 28.5 hours in PDT and 100.4 hours in surgical tracheostomy.[107] Certainly, there is an inherent logistical bias toward a shorter time period for PDT due to the ease of performing the procedure at the bedside versus procuring a time slot for the operating room. Concurrently, the cost of performing PDT versus surgical tracheostomy is markedly reduced. As an example, total patient cost at one hospital was reduced by about 50 percent (US$3000 vs. $1600) in 2001.[108]

Key learning points

- Endotracheal intubation is a procedure to establish an airway for delivery of oxygen and assisted ventilation. In the setting of acute respiratory failure, knowledge of indications and alternative treatment modalities is essential.

- Understanding of airway anatomy is a prerequisite to proper intubation techniques, prevention of complications, and guidance in choosing appropriate procedures.

- Pre-intubation set-ups, proper positioning of patients, and knowledge of available equipment and resources assure optimal outcome for endotracheal intubation.

- There are a variety of methods for endotracheal intubation, including direct, indirect or blind procedures. Familiarity with the different modalities is a major requirement for those being trained in advanced airway management.

- Tracheostomy provides long-term airway security. Options include surgical and percutaneous tracheostomy. Due to the technical differences and potential complications of each, the decision to opt for one over the other needs to be individualized and risks and benefits weighed.

- Percutaneous tracheostomy should only be performed by trained personnel who are familiar with the procedure and possess good knowledge of neck anatomy.

REFERENCES

1. Brochard L, Mancebo J, Wysocki M, *et al.* Noninvasive ventilation for acute exacerbations of chronic obstructive pulmonary disease. *N Engl J Med* 1995; **333**: 817–22.

2. Khilnani GC, Saikia N, Sharma SK, *et al.* Efficacy of non-invasive positive pressure ventilation for management of COPD with acute or acute on chronic respiratory failure: A randomized controlled trial. *Am J Respir Crit Care* 2002; **165**: A387.

3. Nava S, Carbone G, DiBattista N, *et al.* Noninvasive ventilation in cardiogenic pulmonary edema: a multicenter randomized trial. *Am J Respir Crit Care Med* 2003; **168**: 1432–7.

4. Keenan SP, Sinuff T, Cook DJ, Hill NS. Does noninvasive positive pressure ventilation improve outcome in acute hypoxemic respiratory failure? A systematic review. *Crit Care Med* 2004; **32**: 2516–23.

5. Emory University.Pharynx and larynx [updated August 19, 1997]. Available at: www.emory.edu/ ANATOMY/AnatomyManual/pharynx.ht mL (accessed July 15, 2005).

6. Hanafee WN, Ward PH. Anatomy and physiology. In: Hanafee WN, Ward PH, eds. *The Larynx: Radiology, Surgery, Pathology.* New York: Thieme, 1990.

7. Thach BT, Neuromuscular control of upper airway patency. *Clin Perinatol* 1992; **42**: 941.

8. Boerner TF, Ramanathan S. Functional anatomy of the airway. In: Benumof JL, ed. *Airway Management: Principles and Practice*, 1st ed. St Louis, MO: Mosby-Year Book 1996: 15.

9. American Society of Anesthesiologists Task Force on Management of the Difficult Airway. Practice guidelines for the management of the difficult airway. 1993, amended 2002. *Anesthesiology* 2003; **98**: 1269–77.

10. Rose DK, Cohen MM., The airway: problems and predictions in 18,500 patients. *J Anaesth* 1994;41(5 Pt 1):372–83.

11. Burkle CM, Walsh MR, Harrison BA, *et al.* Airway management after failure to intubate by direct laryngoscopy: outcomes in a large teaching hospital. *Can J Anaesth* 2005; **52**: 634–40.

12. Mallampati SR. Clinical signs to predict difficult tracheal intubation. *Can J Anaesth* 1983; **30**: 316.

13. Sampson GLT, Young JRB. Difficult tracheal intubation: a retrospective study. *Anesthesia* 1987; **42**: 487.

14. Cattano D, Panicucci E, Paolicchi A, *et al.* Risk factors assessment of the difficult airway: an Italian survey of 1956 patients. *Anesth Analg* 2004; **99**: 1774–9.

15. Levitan RM, Everett WW, Ochroch EA. Limitations of difficult airway prediction in patients intubated in the emergency department. *Ann Emerg Med* 2004; **44**: 307–13.

16. Behringer E. Approaches to managing the upper airway. *Anesthesiol Clin North Am* 2002; **20**: 813–32.

17. Rose DK, Cohen MM. The airway: problems and predictions in 18500 patients. *Can J Anaesth* 1994; **41**: 361.

18. Rosin P, Barkin R eds. *Emergency Medicine: Concepts in Clinical Practice*, 4th ed. St Louis, MO: Mosby-Year Book, 1998.

19. Reed MJ, Dunn MJ, Mckeown DW. Can an airway assessment score predict difficulty at intubation in the emergency department? *Emerg Med J* 2005; **22**: 99–102.

20. Soliz J, Sinha A, Thakar D. Airway management: a review and update. *Internet Journal of Anesthesiology* 2002; 6 [online]. Available at: www.ispub.com/ostia/index.php?xmlFilePath=journ als/ija/vol6n1/airway.xml (accessed April 12, 2006).

21. Yildiz TS, Solak M, Toker K. The incidence and risk factors of difficult mask ventilation. *J Anesth* 2005; **19**: 7–11.

22. Wenzel V, Keller C, Idris AH, *et al.* Effects of smaller tidal volumes during basic life support ventilation in patients with respiratory arrest: good ventilation, less risk? *Resuscitation* 1999; **43**: 25–9.

23. Dorges V, Ocker H, Hagelberg S, *et al.* Smaller tidal volumes with room-air are not sufficient to ensure adequate oxygenation during bag-valve-mask ventilation. *Resuscitation* 2000; **44**: 37–41.

◆ 24. Idris AH, Gabrielli A. Advances in airway management. *Emerg Med Clin North Am* 2002; **20**: 843–57.

✳ 25. The American Heart Association in collaboration with the International Liaison Committee on Resuscitation. Guidelines 2000 for cardiopulmonary resuscitation and emergency cardiovascular care. Part 3: adult basic life support. *Circulation* 2000; **102**(8 Suppl): I22–59.

26. Fourre MW. The performance of procedures on the recently deceased. *Acad Emerg Med* 2002; **9**: 595–8.

◆ 27. Hudson TS. Is it ethical to practice intubations on the deceased? *JONAS Healthc Law Ethics Regul* 2000; **2**: 22–8.

28. Liu H, Chen JC, Holinger LD, Gonzalez-Crussi F. Histopathologic fundamentals of acquired laryngeal stenosis. *Pediatr Pathol Lab Med* 1995; **15**: 655–77.

29. Reed MF, Mathisen DJ. Tracheoesophageal fistula. *Chest Surg Clin North Am* 2003; **13**: 271–89.

30. Locicero J, 3rd. Tracheo-carotid artery erosion following endotracheal intubation. *J Trauma* 1984; **24**: 907–9.

31. Lomholt N. A device for measuring the lateral wall cuff pressure of endotracheal tubes. *Acta Anaesthesiol Scand* 1992; **36**: 775–8.

32. Sengupta P, Sessler DI, Maglinger P, *et al.* Endotracheal tube cuff pressure in three hospitals, and the volume required to produce an appropriate cuff pressure. *BMC Anesthesiol* 2004; **4**: 8.

● 33. Vyas D, Inweregbu K, Pittard A. Measurement of tracheal tube cuff pressure in critical care. *Anaesthesia* 2002; **57**: 275–7.

● 34. Brimacombe J, White A, Berry A. Effect of cricoid pressure on the ease of insertion of the laryngeal mask airway. *Br J Anaesth* 1993; **71**: 800–2.

35. Snider DD, Clarke D, Finucane BT. The 'BURP' maneuver worsens the glottic view when applied in combination with cricoid pressure. *Can J Anaesth* 2005; **52**: 100–4.

36. Turgeon AF, Nicole PC, Trepanier CA, *et al.* Cricoid pressure does not increase the rate of failed intubation by direct laryngoscopy in adults. *Anesthesiology* 2005; **102**: 315–19.

37. Piepho T, Thierbach A, Werner C. Nasotracheal intubation: look before you leap. *Br J Anaesth* 2005; **94**: 859–60.

38. Andersen K, Hald A. Assessing the position of the tracheal tube: the reliability of different methods. *Anaesthesia* 1989; **44**: 984.

39. Gillespie JH, Knight RG, Middaugh RE, *et al.* Efficacy of endotracheal tube cuff palpation and humidity in distinguishing endotracheal from esophageal intubation [abstract]. *Anesthesiology* 1988; **69**: A265.

✳ 40. *Standards for Basic Intraoperative Monitoring. 1994 Directory of Members.* Park Ridge, IL: American Society of Anesthesiologists, 1994: 736.

41. O'Flaherty D, Adams AP. The end-tidal CO_2 detector: assessment of a new method to distinguish esophageal from tracheal intubation. *Anaesthesia* 1990; **45**: 653.

42. Goldberg JS, Rawle PP, Zehnder IL, *et al.* Colormetric end-tidal CO_2 monitoring for tracheal intubation. *Anesth Analg* 1990; **70**: 191.

43. MacLeod GJ, Heller MB, Gerard J, *et al.* Verification of endotracheal tube placement with colorimetric end-tidal CO_2 detection. *Ann Emerg Med* 1991; **20**: 267.

44. Dunn SM, Mushlin PS, Lind LJ, *et al.* Tracheal intubation is not invariably confirmed by capnography. *Anesthesiology* 1990; **73**: 1285.

45. Wafai Y, Salem MR, Joseph NJ, *et al.* The self-inflating bulb for confirmation of tracheal intubation: incidence and demography of false negatives. *Anesthesiology* 1994; **81**: A1303.

46. Write RS, Burdumy TJ. Acute endotracheal tube occlusion caused by use of an esophageal detector device: report of a case and a discussion of its utility. *Ann Emerg Med* 2004; **43**: 626–9.

47. American Society of Anesthesiologists Task Force on Management of Difficult Airway. Practice guidelines for management of the difficult airway: an updated report by the American Society of Anesthesiologists

Task Force on Management of the Difficult Airway *Anesthesiology* 2003; **98**: 1269–77.

48. Verghese C, Brimacombe JR. Survey of laryngeal mask airway usage in 11,910 patients: safety and efficacy for conventional and non-conventional usage. *Anesth Analg* 1996; **82**: 129–33.

49. Pennant JH, Walker MB. Comparison of the endotracheal tube and the laryngeal mask in airway management by paramedical personnel. *Anesth Analg* 1992; **74**: 531–4.

50. Brimacombe J. The advantages of the LMA over the tracheal tube or facemask: a meta-analysis. *Can J Anaesth* 1995; **42**: 1017–23.

51. Brimacombe J, Keller C, Fullekrug B, *et al.* A multicenter study comparing the ProSeal with the Classic laryngeal mask airway in anesthetized, nonparalyzed patients. *Anesthesiology* 2002; **96**: 289–95.

52. Keller C, Brimacombe J, Kleinsasser A, Brimacombe L. The laryngeal mask airway ProSeal™ as a temporary ventilatory device in grossly and morbidly obese patients before laryngoscope-guided tracheal intubation. *Anesth Analg* 2002; **94**: 737–40.

53. Joo HS, Rose DK. The intubating laryngeal mask airway with and without fiberoptic guidance. *Anesth Analg* 1999; **88**: 662–6.

54. Levitan RM, Ochroch EA, Stuart S, Hollander JE. Use of the intubating laryngeal mask airway by medical and nonmedical personnel. *Am J Emerg Med* 2000; **18**: 12–16.

55. Agro F, Frass M, Benumof JL, Krafft P. Current status of the Combitube: a review of the literature. *J Clin Anesth* 2002; **14**: 307–14.

56. Vezina D, Lessard MR, Bussieres J, *et al.* Complications associated with the use of the esophageal-tracheal Combitube. *Can J Anaesth* 1998; **45**: 76–80.

57. McGlinch BP, Martin DP, Volcheck GW, Carmichael SW. Tongue engorgement with prolonged use of the esophageal-tracheal Combitube. *Ann Emerg Med* 2004; **44**: 320–2.

58. Cook TM, McCormick B, Gupta K, *et al.* An evaluation of the PA(Xpress) pharyngeal airway – a new single use airway device. *Resuscitation* 2003; **58**: 139–43.

59. El-Orbany MI, Salem MR, Joseph NJ. The Eschmann tracheal tube introducer is not gum, elastic, or a bougie. *Anesthesiology* 2004; **101**: 1240.

60. Brimacombe J, Keller C, Judd DV. Gum elastic bougie-guided insertion of the ProSeal laryngeal mask airway is superior to the digital and introducer tool techniques. *Anesthesiology* 2004; **100**: 25–9.

61. Henderson JJ, Popat MT, Latto IP, Pearce AC; Difficult Airway Society. Difficult Airway Society guidelines for management of the unanticipated difficult intubation. *Anaesthesia* 2004; **59**: 675–94.

62. Latto IP, Stacey M, Mecklenburgh J, Vaughan RS. Survey of the use of the gum elastic bougie in clinical practice. *Anaesthesia* 2002; **57**: 379–84.

63. Smith CE, Pinchak AB, Sidhu TS, *et al.* Evaluation of tracheal intubation difficulty in patients with cervical spine immobilization: fiberoptic (WuScope) versus conventional laryngoscopy. *Anesthesiology* 1999; **91**: 1253–9.

64. Sprung J, Wright LC, Dilger J. Use of WuScope for exchange of endotracheal tube in a patient with difficult airway. *Laryngoscope* 2003; **113**: 1082–4.

65. Sprung J, Weingarten T, Dilger J. The use of WuScope fiberoptic laryngoscopy for tracheal intubation in complex clinical situations. *Anesthesiology* 2003; **98**: 263–5.

66. Rodricks MB, Deutschman CS. Emergent airway management: indications and methods in the face of confounding conditions. *Crit Care Clin* 2000; **16**: 389–409.

67. Sahin A, Salman MA, Erden IA, Aypar U. Upper cervical vertebrae movement during intubating laryngeal mask, fibreoptic and direct laryngoscopy: a video-fluoroscopic study. *Eur J Anaesthesiol* 2004; **21**: 819–23.

68. Hung OR. Stewart R. Illuminating stylets (Lightwand). In: Benumof JL, ed. *Airway Management: Principles and Practice*, 1st ed. St Louis MO: Mosby-Year Book, 1996: 342–52.

69. Agro F, Hung OR, Cataldo R, *et al.* Lightwand intubation using the Trachlight: a brief review of current knowledge. *Can J Anaesth* 2001; **48**: 592–9.

70. Hung O, Pytka S, Morris I, *et al.* Lightwand intubations: I. Clinical trial of a new lightwand for tracheal intubation in patients with difficult airway equipment. *Can J Anaesth* 1995; **42**: 826–30.

71. Weiss FR, Hattin MN. Intubation by use of the lightwand: experience in 253 patients. *J Oral Maxillofac Surg* 1989; **47**: 577–80.

72. Shikani AH. New 'seeing' stylet-scope and method for the management of the difficult airway. *Otolaryngol Head Neck Surg* 1999; **120**: 113–16.

73. Liem EB, Bjoraker DG, Gravenstein D. New options for airway management: intubating fibreoptic stylets. *Br J Anaesth* 2003; **91**: 408–18.

74. Pfitzner L, Cooper MG, Ho D. The Shikani Seeing Stylet for difficult intubation in children: initial experience. *Anaesth Intensive Care* 2002; **30**: 462–6.

75. Stiles CM, Stiles QR, Denson JS. A flexible fiberoptic laryngoscope. *JAMA* 1972; **221**: 1246.

76. Trevisan P. Fiber-optic awake intubation for caesarean section in a parturient with predicted difficult airway. *Minerva Anesthesiol* 2002; **68**: 775–81.

77. Jones HE, Pearce AC, Moore P. Fiberoptic intubation: Influence of tracheal tube tip design. *Anaesthesia* 1993; **48**: 672–4.

78. Glen M. Atlas. A comparison of fiberoptic-compatible oral airways. *J Clin Anesth* 2004; **16**: 66–73.

79. Caplan RA, Vistica MF, Posner KL, Cheney FW. Adverse respiratory events in anesthesia: a closed claims analysis. *Anesthesiology* 1990; **72**: 828.

80. Bellhouse CP, Dore C. Criteria for estimating the likelihood of difficulty of endotracheal intubation with Macintosh laryngoscope. *Anaesth Intensive Care* 1998; **16**: 329.

81. Boon JM, Abrahams PH, Meiring JH, Welch T. Cricothyroidotomy: a clinical anatomy review. *Clin Anat* 2004; **17**: 478–86.

82. Patel RG. Percutaneous transtracheal jet ventilation. *Chest* 1999; **116**: 1689–94.

83. Walls RM. Cricothyroidotomy. *Emerg Med Clin North Am* 1998; **6**: 725–36.

84. Melker RJ, Florete OG. Cricothyrotomy: a review and debate. *Anesthesiol Clin North Am* 1995; **13**: 565.

85. Sanchez TF. Retrograde intubation. *Anesthesiol Clin North Am* 1995; **13**: 439.

86. Blanda M, Gallo U. Emergency airway management. *Emerg Med Clin North Am* 2003; **21**: 1.

87. Freeman BD, Isabella K, Cobb JP, *et al.* A prospective, randomized study comparing percutaneous with surgical tracheostomy in critically ill patients. *Crit Care Med* 2001; **29**: 926–30.

88. Skaggs JA, Cogbill CL. Tracheostomy: management, mortality, complications. *Am Surg* 1969; **35**: 393–6.

89. Ryan DW, Kilner AJ. Another death after percutaneous dilational tracheostomy. *Br J Anaesth* 2003; **91**: 925–6.

90. Heffner JE. Tracheostomy application and timing. *Clin Chest Med* 2003; 389–90.

91. Colice GL, Stukel TA, Dain B. Laryngeal complications of prolonged intubation. *Chest* 1989; **96**: 877–84.

92. Pelosi P, Severgnini P. Tracheostomy must be individualized!. *Crit Care* 2004; **8**: 322–4.

93. Rumbak MJ, Newton M, Truncale T, *et al.* A prospective, randomized, study comparing early percutaneous dilational tracheotomy to prolonged translaryngeal intubation (delayed tracheotomy) in critically ill medical patients. *Crit Care Med* 2004; **32**: 1689–94.

94. Griffiths J, Barber VS, Morgan L, Young JD. Systematic review and meta-analysis of studies of the timing of tracheostomy in adult patients undergoing artificial ventilation. *BMJ* 2005; **330**: 1243.

95. Jackson C. Tracheostomy. *Laryngoscope* 1909; **19**: 285–90.

96. Toye FJ, Weinstein JD. A percutaneous tracheostomy device. *Surgery* 1969; **65**: 384.

97. Ciaglia P, Firshing R, Syniec C. Elective percutaneous dilatational tracheostomy: a new simple bedside procedure. *Chest* 1985; **87**: 715–19.

98. Walts PA, Murthy SC, Decamp MM. Techniques of surgical tracheostomy. *Clin Chest Med* 2003; **24**: 413–22.

99. Sue RD, Susanto I. Long-term complications of artificial airways. *Clin Chest Med* 2003; **24**: 457–71.

100. Marx WH, Ciaglia P, Graniero KD. Some important details in the technique of percutaneous dilatational tracheostomy via the modified Seldinger technique. *Chest* 1996; **110**: 762–6.

101. Hill BB, Zweng TN, Maley RH, *et al.* Percutaneous dilational tracheostomy: report of 356 cases. *J Trauma* 1996; **41**: 238–43.

102. Goldenberg D, Ari EG, Golz A, *et al.* Tracheotomy complications: a retrospective study of 1130 cases. *Otolaryngol Head Neck Surg* 2000; **123**: 495–500.

103. Freedman BD, Isabella K, Lin N, Buchman TG. A meta-analysis of prospective trials comparing percutaneous and surgical tracheostomy in critically ill patients. *Chest* 2000; **118**: 1412–18.

104. Dulguerov P, Gysin C, Perneger TV, Chevrolet JC. Percutaneous or surgical tracheostomy: a meta-analysis. *Crit Care Med* 1999; **27**: 1617–25.

105. Heikkinen M, Aarnio P, Hannukainen J. Percutaneous dilatational tracheostomy or conventional surgical tracheostomy? *Crit Care Med* 2000; **28**: 1399–402.

106. Angel LF, Simpson CB, Comparison of surgical and percutaneous dilatational tracheostomy. *Clin Chest Med* 2003; **24**: 423–9.

◆ 107. Friedman Y, Fildes J, Mizock B, *et al.* Comparison of percutaneous and surgical tracheostomies. *Chest* 1996; **110**: 480–5.

108. Massick DD, Yao S, Powell DM, *et al.* Bedside tracheostomy in the intensive care unit: a prospective randomized trial comparing open surgical tracheostomy with endoscopically guided percutaneous dilatational tracheostomy. *Laryngoscope* 2001; **111**: 494–500.

5

Basic and advanced mechanical ventilation modalities

LIZIAMMA GEORGE, FELIX KHUSID, SUHAIL RAOOF

INTRODUCTION

Ventilators are mechanical devices that assist in the breathing of an individual when the breathing apparatus fails to provide adequate ventilation or oxygenation. Ventilators deliver gases at the alveolar level and artificially support the respiratory system.

Mechanical ventilators have evolved over the years into complicated machines. A detailed discussion of the evolution of mechanical ventilators is beyond the scope of this chapter.[1-3]

BASIC CONCEPTS

Mechanical ventilators generate force or use pressure to carry out the work of breathing. To accomplish this, the machine needs a power input, conversion of power into a drive mechanism, a control scheme, and an output to simulate breathing (Fig. 5.1).

In patients who assist the ventilator, the force generated by the muscle contraction is added to the force generated by the ventilator. The pressure, volume, and flow vary with time; therefore they are the variables. On the other hand,

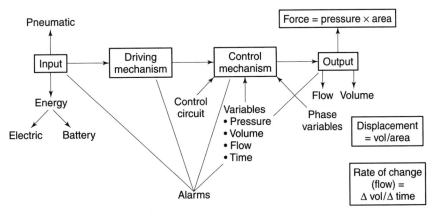

Figure 5.1 *Mechanism of operation of mechanical ventilators.*

compliance and resistance are constant and are called the parameters. The relation between these variables and parameters can be expressed using the following formula:

$$\text{Muscle pressure} + \text{ventilator pressure} = \frac{\text{Volume}}{\text{compliance}} + \text{resistance} \times \text{flow} \quad (1)$$

The variables are measured in relation to end-expiratory values. The parameters are assumed to be constant and in combination with variables, they constitute the load. Elastic load (volume/compliance) is the load needed to expand the lungs and chest wall and resistive load (flow × resistance) is the pressure required to deliver the gas at a particular flow rate.[4,5] Muscle pressure and ventilator pressure is the force required to overcome the elastic load and resistive load. Equation 1 can also be written as:

$$P = \text{Elastic load} + \text{resistive load} \quad (2)$$

where P = total pressure applied.

If the respiratory system is compared to a piston attached to a straight tube, which in turn, is attached to a balloon, the pressure generated by the piston is equal to the pressure required to expand the balloon. The tube will provide the resistive load and the balloon will provide the elastic load. If the flow is maintained constant in this apparatus, the initial pressure is used to overcome the resistive load of the tube. It then rises linearly over time to overcome the elastic load of the balloon. The maximal pressure attained at the end of inspiration is the peak pressure (P_{peak}) of the system and the amount of gas released into the balloon is called the tidal volume (V_T).[6]

When the flow ceases at the end of inspiration, the resistive load is abolished since it is flow dependent. At this time, the pressure becomes equal to the elastic load (P_{el}) of the system. The P_{el} is otherwise known as the end-inspiratory plateau pressure and is used to calculate the static compliance of the respiratory system. The pressure returns to zero at end exhalation. It is important to remember that the P_{el} can be increased if there is dynamic hyperinflation of the system, in which case the end-expiratory P_{el} is positive.[7]

Using the tidal volume and plateau pressure, compliance can be calculated using following formula:

$$\text{Static compliance} = \frac{VT}{Pplat} - PEEP \quad (3)$$

$$\text{Dynamic compliance} = \frac{VT}{PIP} - PEEP \quad (4)$$

where PIP = peak inspiratory pressure, P_{plat} = plateau pressure, and PEEP = positive end-expiratory pressure. Static compliance may be used as an indicator to assess severity of acute respiratory distress syndrome (ARDS) and to follow the course of the disease process in patients being ventilated.

Mean airway pressure (P_{aw}) is the average pressure measured at the airway opening throughout the respiratory cycle. It is equal to the average pressure the ventilator applies to the patient.[8,9] The average pressure that distends the alveolus is called the mean alveolar pressure (P_A), and it can vary with mean airway pressure, minute ventilation, positive end-expiratory pressure (PEEP), or with the flow pattern. The relation between the mean airway pressure and the mean alveolar pressure is given by the formula:

$$P_A = P_{aw} + \left(\frac{\dot{V}_E}{60}\right)(RE - RI)$$

where P_A= mean alveolar pressure, P_{aw} = mean airway pressure, $\dot{V}_E$ = minute ventilation, RE = expiratory resistance, and RI= inspiratory resistance. Thus, P_A approximates P_{aw} except in conditions of increased minute ventilation and expiratory resistance.

INDICATIONS FOR MECHANICAL VENTILATION

The primary indication for mechanical ventilation is respiratory failure which could be hypoxemic, hypercapnic, or combined. The failure can be due to abnormalities of the gas exchange units, the ventilatory pump, decreased central drive, or a combination of any one of these.[10–13] The failure occurs when the patient's ventilatory load exceeds the ventilatory muscle strength and endurance. Bellemare and Grassino were able to show the relation between load, strength, endurance, and duration of the inspiratory muscle contraction. They were able to calculate the pressure time index from transdiaphragmatic pressure and the average time of inspiration as a fraction of the duty cycle. Breathing pattern associated with pressure time index above 0.18 may indicate impending respiratory failure if the condition is not improved.[14] Patients with respiratory failure present with dyspnea except patients with a central cause, who can present with apnea or respiratory arrest. The usual indications for mechanical ventilation include:

- apnea or unstable respiratory drive from head trauma, drug overdose, anesthesia or a stroke
- impending ventilatory failure with rising Pa_{CO_2} (usually 10 mm Hg above baseline; pH <7.30) as in status asthmaticus, chronic obstructive pulmonary disease (COPD) exacerbation, flail chest, etc.
- severe hypoxemic respiratory failure (Pa_{CO_2} <60 mm Hg or an Sa_{O_2} <90 percent on an Fi_{O_2} >0.6) as seen in severe pneumonia, ARDS, pulmonary edema, lung contusion, etc.

CLASSIFICATION OF MECHANICAL VENTILATORS

There is no universal classification of mechanical ventilators at this time.[15] As the ventilators become more sophisticated, the classification of ventilators become more complex.[16] A clinical system of classifying ventilators is based upon the application of negative or positive pressure (Box 5.1).

Box 5.1 Clinical classification of ventilators

(A) Positive pressure ventilation

Invasive ventilation

Conventional modes of ventilation:
- Continuous mandatory
- Assist-control, synchronized intermittent mandatory, pressure control, pressure support

Nonconventional modes of ventilation:
- Inverse ratio
- High frequency
- Closed loop systems
- Volume assured pressure support/pressure augmentation
- Volume support/variable pressure support
- Pressure regulated volume control/adaptive pressure ventilation
- Automode/variable pressure support/variable pressure control
- Adaptive support ventilation
- Mandatory minute volume
- Proportional assist ventilation

Non-invasive

Acute respiratory failure

Chronic respiratory failure

(B) Negative pressure ventilation

Cyclical negative pressure

Negative positive pressure

Continuous negative extrathoracic pressure

Box 5.2 Components of a mechanical ventilator

Input
- Pneumatic
- Electric – alternating current, direct current

Power conversion and transmission
- External compressor
- Internal compressor
- Output control valves

Control scheme
- Control circuit
- Control variables and wave forms
- Phase variables
- Conditional variables

Output
- Pressure
- Volume
- Flow
- Effects of patient circuit

Alarm systems
- Input power alarms
- Control circuit alarms
- Output alarms
- Inspired gas alarms

information.[18–20] The pneumatic system delivers a gas mixture (varying from 100 percent oxygen to room air) to the patient. Before delivery, the gas mixture is filtered, warmed, and humidified (Fig. 5.2).

Control variables

These are variables that the ventilator manipulates to cause inspiration. The particular variable is held constant as ventilatory load changes. The four control variables are pressure, volume, flow, and time.

- *Pressure control ventilator.* The pressure waveform remains constant irrespective of the change in the compliance and resistance of the respiratory system.
- *Volume control ventilator.* The waveform is constant with varying load (resistance and compliance) and measured volume is used to control the volume waveform.
- *Flow control ventilator.* A constant volume curve in the face of changing compliance and resistance, where volume is not used for feedback control.
- *Time control ventilator.* The inspiratory and expiratory time is the only variable controlled.

Mechanical ventilators may be classified using power input, power conversion, control scheme, output, and alarm systems (Box 5.2).[17]

Power input

The energy to drive the ventilator comes from either an electric/battery source or from compressed gas (pneumatic system). First generation ventilators were pneumatically powered and used compressed gas to power the ventilator and also to ventilate the patient. Current generation ventilators are electronically controlled with a microprocessor and use both a pneumatic system and an electronic system. The microprocessor controls the opening and closure of inspiratory and exhalation valves, integrates the monitoring system of ventilator (pressure, flow, and volume), controls alarms, and displays monitored

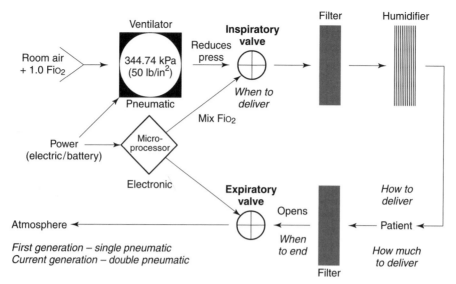

Figure 5.2 *A simplified diagrammatic representation of the ventilatory system. The newer generation ventilators are equipped with microprocessors that regulate the opening and closure of inspiratory and exhalation values, integrate with the monitoring systems, control alarms and display monitored information. The pneumatic system mixes air and oxygen to provide the requisite oxygen concentration to the patient. The gases are filtered, warmed, and humidified.*

Phase variables

These variables denote how specific components of respiration are initiated or terminated. The phase variables are trigger, limit, and cycle (Fig. 5.3).

- *Trigger* allows inspiration to commence. It can be preset for pressure, volume, flow, and time. An example of preset pressure change is sensitivity. When the patient effort drops the airway pressure by a preset level or the expiratory flow reaches a certain preset level, inspiratory phase starts.[21,22]
- *Limit variable*: during the inspiratory phase, the pressure, volume, or flow cannot exceed the preset upper limit. Inspiratory phase may still continue when the limit is reached. All new generation ventilators will alarm when the limit variable is exceeded.
- *Cycle variable* is one that terminates the inspiratory phase. The inspiratory flow can be terminated when a preset pressure, volume, flow or time interval is reached. Modern ventilators employ complex algorithms of these variables for feedback and control. In volume-cycled ventilation, inspiration is terminated after a preset tidal volume is delivered. In pressure-cycled ventilation, inspiration is terminated after a preset pressure is reached. In flow cycled, the termination of inspiration occurs when the flow falls to a particular level, as seen with pressure support, or in time cycled after a particular duration of time, as seen with pressure assist-control.

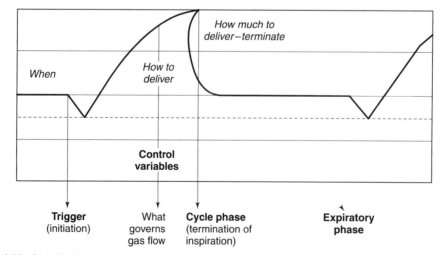

Figure 5.3 *Phase variables include trigger, which allows inspiration to begin, limit variables (pressure, volume, or flow) that define the upper limit of the variable during inspiration, and the cycle variable that terminates inspiration.*

Conditional variables

Conditional variables allow the ventilators to synchronize the delivery of a breath with patient's intrinsic efforts, to deliver sigh breaths as well as to allow the patient to breathe spontaneously during ventilatory support. These variables help the patient to have mandatory (ventilator starts or ends the breath), assisted, supported, or spontaneous (patient starts and ends) breaths.

Take the example of a ventilator delivering a flow triggered, flow limited and volume cycled breath (tidal volume set to 500 mL). In addition, the ventilator is programmed to deliver eight sighs per hour at a tidal volume of 1000 mL (or two sighs every 15 minutes). Before delivering each breath, the ventilator scrutinizes the values of these conditional variables and decides when it should deliver the sighs. In this example, the conditional variable is the time that has to elapse before the sigh is delivered.

TYPES AND MODES OF MECHANICAL VENTILATION

Positive pressure ventilation

Positive pressure ventilation generates supra-atmospheric pressures in the upper airway. The pressure gradient between upper airway and pleura will drive the gas mixture in the lungs. Positive pressure ventilation can be provided using a mask (noninvasive) or through an endotracheal tube (invasive). Positive pressure ventilation uses different modes to provide appropriate settings to the patient.

Negative pressure ventilation

Mechanical ventilatory support can be given using negative pressure as well as positive pressure ventilators.[23] Negative pressure ventilators apply a subatmospheric pressure to the chest wall during inspiration. This in turn will create negative pleural pressure, which will allow the air to move into the lungs. Exhalation can be either passive or active by applying positive pressure to the chest wall.

Modes of ventilation

Modes of ventilation are defined as a particular set of control, phase, and conditional variables that determine how the patient will receive a tidal breath. In a simplistic form, modes of the ventilation can be grouped as *pressure targeted* or *volume targeted*.[24,25]

In volume-targeted modes, the primary target is a predetermined tidal volume. The peak inspiratory pressures vary from breath to breath. The clinician sets the flow rates, frequency (inspiratory time), and the flow waveform pattern.

In the pressure-targeted ventilatory mode, the peak pressure and inspiratory time (pressure assist control) is set and the tidal volume and flow rates vary from breath to breath.[26] A comparison between volume- and pressure-targeted ventilation is shown in Table 5.1.

Table 5.1 *Comparison of volume- and pressure- targeted ventilation*

	Volume-targeted	Pressure targeted
Rate	Minimum rate set	Minimum rate set
Tidal volume	Set	Variable
Peak alveolar pressure	Variable	Set
Peak inspiratory flow	Set	Variable
Pattern of flow wave	Set	Decelerating (variable pattern)
Inspiratory time	Set, may be determined by inspiratory flow rate	Variable pressure support
Set pressure control

Modified with permission from *Mechanical Ventilation Manual.* American College of Physicians, 1998.

CONVENTIONAL MODES OF VENTILATION

Table 5.2 presents a summary of the common modes of mechanical ventilation with their indications and some of the precautions that should be observed with their use.

Controlled mechanical ventilation (CMV)

This could be either volume or pressure targeted. It does not allow triggering by the patient and the cycle variables are time, pressure, volume, or flow. Controlled ventilation provides maximal ventilatory support with reduction in the oxygen cost of breathing. The minute ventilation is guaranteed to the patient. Most of the patients who receive controlled ventilation need deep sedation or paralysis or do not have a ventilatory drive. This mode also allows the clinician to provide nonphysiologic ventilatory support to patients with severe cardiopulmonary disease. Modern ventilators do not prevent patients from triggering the ventilator. This mode has been replaced by assist-control mode.

Assist–control mechanical ventilation

Assist-control ventilation differs from CMV as it responds to patient's effort in triggering the inspiratory phase. Thus, the ventilator senses that the patient wants to breathe and delivers a clinician-determined volume or pressure to the patient. A minimum rate is set to ensure that ventilation occurs even if the patient does not trigger the ventilator. Ideally, the pleural or tracheal pressure changes should initiate the breath but due to mechanical difficulties, the pressure changes are measured from the ventilatory circuit. The magnitude of the triggering effort as well as the delay to trigger response is important.[27]

Table 5.2 *Common modes of mechanical ventilation*

Mode	Description	Indications	Initial setup	Precautions
Controlled mechanical ventilation (CMV)	Targeted volume or pressure will be delivered to the patient independent of patient's effort or demand	In rare neurologic cases where sedation might affect hemodynamic stability	Set volume/pressure, mandatory respiratory rate, flow rate/inspiratory time and Fio$_2$ if desired.	Patient will not be able to trigger machine breaths, since every breath is going to be time controlled. Attempt to breathe between mandatory breaths will result in patient fighting the ventilator, which may result intrinsic PEEP, air trapping and hemodynamic instability
Assist/control (A–C)	Combines the ability to deliver targeted volume or pressure breath at a prescribed rate as well as responding to patient's demand by delivering volume/ pressure targeted breath	Considered to be the mode of choice when full ventilatory support is indicated	Set volume/pressure, mandatory respiratory rate, Fio$_2$ and flow rate. For pressure assist, inspiratory time and for volume assist, flow rate may have to be set	In the presence of excessive patient triggering activity, patient may develop: respiratory alkalosis, air trapping, increased peak pressures, and intrinsic PEEP
Synchronized intermittent mandatory ventilation with pressure support (SIMV + PSV)	Allows patient to take pressure supported breaths during the time interval between mandatory breaths	SIMV + PSV is occasionally utilized as a weaning mode. As patient's own ventilation increases, the SIMV rate is decreased. PSV breaths will take place between mandatory SIMV breaths. PSV is added to eliminate or decrease inspiratory resistance within the endotracheal/tracheal tube during spontaneous breathing	Set volume/pressure, mandatory respiratory rate, and flow rate for volume targeted ventilation. PSV level is also set	May not provide adequate ventilatory support; Fio$_2$ may result in prolonged weaning process
Continuous positive airway pressure + PSV (CPAP + PSV)	Permits patient to breathe with the help of PSV while maintaining a constant level of airway pressure within the lungs. Every PSV breath is initiated by the patient and terminated by flow or time. V$_T$, respiratory rate, and inspiratory time are patient determined	Every spontaneous breath is inhaled from CPAP level and exhaled to the same CPAP level. Pressure support will be applied to every spontaneously initiated breath, to eliminate inspiratory resistance of an endotracheal or tracheal tube. In patients who are difficult to wean, PSV$_{max}$ or high levels of pressure support may be applied in order to augment patient's spontaneous breathing. Primary indication for CPAP + PSV is weaning from mechanical ventilation	Set necessary level of CPAP, select appropriate level of pressure support. Newer ventilators give the ability to fine tune flow for pressure support. Apply necessary level of Fio$_2$	Inappropriately low levels of pressure support may result in patient fatigue, underventilation, and increased work of breathing leading to respiratory acidosis. Inappropriately high level of pressure support may result in overventilation, respiratory alkalosis, and development of volutrauma and barotrauma

Table 5.2 *Continued*

Pressure regulated volume control (PRVC)	Is time cycled and pressure limited. V_T and respiratory rate are constant while flow is variable. Flow will vary based on lung compliance and airway resistance	PRVC is applicable when use of control mode is indicated. The main advantage of this mode is delivery of preset V_T with decelerating flow at a prescribed rate. The ventilator adjusts on a breath to breath basis, constant inspiratory pressure to deliver the breath at the lowest possible peak pressure	Set V_T, respiratory rate, inspiratory time, inspiratory rise time (%) and FiO_2	If lung compliance and airway resistance changes, peak pressures will change accordingly. Common factors that may affect peak pressures are: presence of secretions, bronchospasm, presence of tracheoesophageal fistula, pneumothorax, etc.
PRVC (automode)	If patient is capable of triggering ventilator for 2 breaths every 7–12 seconds (depending on the ventilator used), patient will be switched to volume support where patient's V_T would be supported by variable pressure support levels based on lung compliance and airway resistance	Primary indication for this mode is to facilitate the weaning process. As lung compliance and airway resistance changes, level of pressure support necessary to maintain targeted volume will be automatically adjusted	Set V_T, respiratory rate, inspiratory time, inspiratory rise time (%), FiO_2, engage automode	Assure that patient has steady respiratory drive; otherwise the ventilator will keep switching back to PRVC
Volume control automode	The same as PRVC automode, only in A–C format with square waveform	Primary indication for this mode is to facilitate weaning. As lung compliance and airway resistance changes, level of pressure support necessary to maintain targeted volume will be automatically adjusted	Set V_T, respiratory rate, inspiratory time, inspiratory rise time (%), FiO_2, engage automode	Assure that patient has a steady respiratory drive; otherwise the ventilator will keep switching back to volume control
Pressure control	Pressure control is time cycled. A pressure limited breath is delivered at a preset rate. This mode offers ability to have constant peak pressures with decelerating flow pattern. The following factors affect the pressure control: pressure limit, respiratory rate, inspiratory time, lung compliance, and airways resistance. (The same as A–C pressure targeted strategy)	Pressure control is used to control patient's peak pressures as well as peak intraalveolar pressures. Utilization of pressure control might also help to satisfy patient's high inspiratory demand	Set pressure control level, respiratory rate, inspiratory time and FiO_2. When selecting starting point for pressure control level, choose necessary level of pressure that will result in adequate minute ventilation. One formula that might be useful as a starting point is: Peak pressure–PEEP/2	Monitoring minute volume V_T, and in pressure control is paramount, since volumes are variable and pressure is constant. If clinical conditions affecting lung compliance and airway resistance deteriorate, V_T and minute volume will decrease. If lung compliance and airway resistance improve, ensure that lungs are not overinflated and overventilated, otherwise it might result in volutrauma and respiratory alkalosis

Table 5.2   Continued

Pressure control automode	In this mode, if the patient is triggering the ventilator 2 breaths every 7–12 seconds (depending on the ventilator utilized), patient will be switched to preset level of pressure support	The main indication for use of automode pressure control is to facilitate comfort and control of patient's spontaneously triggered breaths. For example, patient recovering from sedation and beginning to trigger the ventilator might respond much more favorably to ability to control their own inspiratory time than with fixed inspiratory time in pressure control	Set pressure control level, respiratory rate, inspiratory time, PSV level, Fio_2 and activate automode. When selecting starting point for pressure control and pressure support level, choose necessary level of pressure that will result in adequate minute ventilation	Ensure that patient has steady respiratory drive; otherwise the ventilator will keep switching back to pressure control. Close monitoring of minute and V_T volume is paramount, since it will be variable. A patient who has high mandatory respiratory rate in pressure control must have minute volumes monitored closely, because in automode the only requirement is to maintain 2 triggered breaths every 7–12 seconds pressure control
Inversed I:E ratio pressure control	The same as pressure control ventilation, but the inspiratory time will exceed expiratory time	Primarily indicated in patients with ARDS to improve oxygenation	Set pressure control level, respiratory rate, inspiratory time and Fio_2. Inspiratory time will be longer than exhalation. When selecting starting point for pressure control level, choose necessary level of pressure that will result in adequate minute ventilation.	Inversed I:E ratio pressure control may result in development of intrinsic PEEP, increased intrathoracic volume and decreased venous return to the heart, resulting in compromised hemodynamic stability
Pressure augmentation A–C (PA A-C)	PA A–C is a pressure initiated volume guaranteed breath. Patient will initialize the breath within PSV format where flows will be matched to patient's demand, but if target V_T is not reachable, the ventilator will increase the flow over time in order to guarantee the V_T	Primary indication for using pressure augmentation A–C is to enhance patient–ventilator synchrony by offering pressure supported volume guaranteed breath. If patient–ventilator synchrony is improved, it may help in lowering work of breathing and decreasing intrinsic PEEP, if it is present	Set inspiratory pressure level, targeted minimum V_T minimum necessary peak flow, select appropriate pressure slope, and Fio_2, activate pressure augmentation	Inappropriately low-set targeted V_T may result in inadequate ventilation which may result in respiratory acidosis. If targeted V_T volume is too high, ventilator will continuously interfere by attempting to guarantee the volume and supplying additional flow
Mandatory minute ventilation (MMV)	This mode offers machine breaths at preset rate and preset V_T in case of inadequate or absent spontaneous breathing. If spontaneous pressure supported breathing is sufficient and meets the goal of preset minimum minute ventilation, no machine breaths will be delivered	The main goal of MMV is to allow the patient to take spontaneous pressure supported breaths as soon as possible instead of being ventilated in the controlled mode. MMV might be useful in postoperative patients or patients requiring short-term ventilatory support	Set V_T, respiratory rate, pressure support level, and Fio_2	Monitoring of respiratory rates is critical, since ventilator is targeting minimum minute volumes, which can be achieved not only through sufficient V_T levels but also through increased respiratory rates

Table 5.2 *Continued*

Volume support	Volume support mode offers constant inspiratory pressure with decelerating flow pattern. Level of pressure support necessary will vary as lung compliance and airway resistance change	The goal of this mode is to automate weaning process by achieving targeted volume with lowest level of pressure necessary	Set initial expected V_T respiratory rate, inspiratory time and FiO_2	If patient develops apnea, volume support will be reverted to PRVC until apnea alarm is reset. The high pressure limit must be set appropriately since it serves an important role of limiting level of pressure necessary to deliver V_T should sudden changes in lung compliance and airway resistance occur
Airway pressure release ventilation (APRV)	Offers patient an ability to breathe spontaneously with periodic release of pressure from higher to the lower level of CPAP. Mandatory time interval is set for both levels of CPAP. APRV could be utilized in conjunction with automatic tube compensation (ATC). The purpose of ATC is to overcome inspiratory airway resistance	Main goal of APRV is to improve oxygenation while offering patient an ability to breathe spontaneously at both levels of CPAP. Weaning of APRV is achieved by gradually decreasing high pressure (P-high) until it is equal to low pressure (P-low); at that point it simply turns into CPAP	Set P-high inspiratory pressure P-low PEEP, T-high inspiratory time, T-low expiratory time, FiO_2, and ATC if desired. Typically when setting up T-low try to maintain it between 0.8 and 1.2 seconds. Prolonged T-low interval may cause alveolar derecruitment	Should not be used in patients with COPD. Might not provide adequate ventilatory support. Patients being managed with APRV should not be heavily sedated. Prior to placement on APRV ensure patient's hemodynamic stability

PEEP, positive end-expiratory pressure; VT, tidal volume.; ARDS, acute respiratory distress syndrome; COPD, chronic obstrutive pulmonary disease.

The triggers could be either pressure change or flow change. The pressure changes are detected from the inhalation port or exhalation port or from the patient. The phase changes occur when the machine detects the pressure change of 1–2 cm below the end-expiratory pressure. The disadvantages of these triggering points are that moisture accumulation can dampen or overestimate the pressure changes. The flow triggering occurs either using a bias flow or by actually measuring the flow in the airway. In the flow-by mode, a continuous flow of gas 5–20 L/min is presented to the patient and is measured at the expiratory limb. With the patient's effort, some of this gas is diverted to the patient's lung and the resultant change in the flow triggers the ventilator breath. Weak respiratory efforts do not trigger the ventilators by both of these triggering mechanisms. If there is any system leak, the ventilator will recognize this as patient effort and autocycling of the ventilator will occur. If the patient is ventilated using a noncuffed tube and is breathing around the tube, the triggering mechanism will not work. Assisted ventilation does not abolish work of breathing for the patient. The disadvantages of assist-control mode ventilation are excessive work of breathing by the patient if the sensitivity and flow rate are not adequately set, worsening air trapping in patients with COPD and dyssynchrony in awake patients.[28] However, it is the preferred mode in most clinical settings, at least initially.

Intermittent mandatory ventilation (IMV) and synchronized intermittent mandatory ventilation (SIMV)

The major disadvantage of assist-control mode of ventilation was that it does not allow the patient to take spontaneous breaths.[29] The SIMV mode allows the patient to take spontaneous breaths but only with mandatory breaths. The mandatory breaths are given at a preset frequency. If the machine detects patient's effort during preset intervals, the mandatory breath is synchronized with patient's effort. Between the preset intervals, the patient can breathe spontaneously at a rate and tidal volume chosen by the patient.[30] The IMV mode does not affect the respiratory timing but decreases the frequency of mandated breaths, increasing the respiratory drive. The spontaneous breaths are taken through a demand valve or a continuous flow of gases. This mode is associated with increased work of breathing especially in the presence of PEEP.[31] Continuous flow system has only minimal pressure fluctuations during spontaneous breathing.[32] The mandatory breaths can be either volume targeted or pressure targeted. In the synchronized form, the machine breath is synchronized with patient's inspiratory effort.[33] The spontaneous breaths can be augmented with pressure support in most modern ventilators.

Pressure assist-control ventilation

Positive pressure mechanical ventilation has been associated with the development of barotrauma in patients with severe lung disease. High peak inspiratory pressure, mean airway pressure, and PEEP have been reported as contributory factors for this complication.[34] In addition atelectasis,

hypoxemia, and decreased compliance have also been seen in animals ventilated with high peak pressures.[35] Pressure assist-control ventilation allows the clinician to set the peak inspiratory pressure at the desired level. In addition to the pressure, the minimum frequency and inspiratory time or fraction of duty cycle is also set. The newer ventilators allow the clinician to choose from different options to regulate the rise time (the time required by the ventilator to reach the peak inspiratory pressure). The shorter the rise time, the greater the initial flow. This may be advantageous to the patient who is severely dyspneic and has a high intrinsic inspiratory flow (air hunger).[36] Alveolar ventilation varies with the compliance, resistance, breathing pattern, and development of intrinsic PEEP. The inspiratory flow during the pressure-controlled ventilation is of a decelerating nature. When the frequency of respiration is increased, both inspiratory and expiratory time is decreased. This may lead to development of intrinsic PEEP, thus decreasing effective driving pressure, decreasing tidal volume and resulting in hypercapnia. With higher frequencies, the minute ventilation reaches a plateau depending on the resistance and duty cycle.[37] Spontaneous breathing is allowed during pressure assist-control ventilation, giving the patient some control on regulation of minute ventilation.

Pressure support ventilation

Pressure support ventilation gives greater flexibility to patient to trigger, determine the flow rate, inspiratory time and tidal volume and indicate when the breath should be terminated.[38] The ventilator recognizes the patient's effort to inspire. Triggering of the breath is either by using a pressure sensor or by using 'flow by' method. The ventilator quickly delivers an inspiratory pressure to a preset level. The inspiratory rise time may be regulated by the clinician in some modern ventilators. Once the clinician-determined pressure is achieved, it is maintained during the inspiratory phase. The ventilator continuously alters the inspiratory flow to ensure that the peak inspiratory pressure (clinician determined) is not exceeded. This mode of ventilation is flow cycled, i.e. inspiration is terminated when the inspiratory flow decreases to a particular level.[39] This level of flow is usually specific to the ventilator. Inspiration may cease when the flows drop to 5 L/min or 25 percent of the peak inspiratory flow.

Pressure support ventilation may be used as an independent mode for ventilation or can be added to SIMV. The workload of respiratory muscles decreases as the pressure support increases.[40] This mode does not guarantee the tidal volume as in assist-control mode, but the patient can regulate flow and tidal volume as they wish, which improves the patient–ventilator synchrony. Ventilators vary in their mechanisms to deliver pressure support ventilation, and the measurement of pulmonary mechanics is difficult with this mode. The estimation of appropriate level of pressure support for ventilation is determined by a stable and comfortable breathing pattern,[41] adequate tidal volume,[42] or assessment of accessory muscle activity in the neck. Pressure support is also used as a weaning mode for patients and in this instance pressure support is used to overcome the resistance generated by the endotracheal and ventilator tubes. Pressure support ventilation should not be used in patients with an unstable respiratory drive.

NONCONVENTIONAL MODES OF VENTILATION

Inverse ratio ventilation

Extended inspiratory time has been shown to improve oxygenation in infants with respiratory distress syndrome.[43] In patients with ARDS, similar extension of the inspiratory time to reverse I:E ratio was shown to improve oxygenation. The extended inspiratory time will allow lung recruitment utilizing high mean airway pressure and low tidal volume.[44] The mean airway pressure is high; however the peak inspiratory pressure is lower. Decreased expiratory time may generate intrinsic PEEP, which in turn will increase alveolar pressure in volume-targeted ventilation or decrease the tidal volume in pressure-targeted ventilation. It is for this reason that we do not recommend prolonging the ratio by greater than 2:1 in most clinical settings. Inverse ratio ventilation is applied either through pressure-controlled ventilation by increasing the inspiratory time, or by decreasing the flow rate (with or without an inspiratory pause) in volume-controlled ventilation.[45–47]

Familiarity with ventilators should help one determine which mode to use to deliver inverse ratio ventilation. The complications of inverse ratio ventilation include development of intrinsic PEEP, barotrauma with high mean airway pressure, the need for sedation and paralysis, and decreased cardiac output secondary to the intrinsic PEEP. The patient should be carefully evaluated for the benefits of inverse ratio ventilation. It should be promptly discontinued if the desired benefit has not occurred.

High-frequency ventilation

Conventional modes of mechanical ventilation try to emulate normal breathing parameters as much as possible. Delivery of high tidal volumes by these modes can damage the lung by overdistension or by generating high peak airway pressures. High-frequency ventilation, developed in the 1960s, uses rapid respiratory rates and small tidal volumes. Depending on the frequency of breaths, high-frequency ventilation is classified into: high-frequency positive pressure ventilation (HFPPV), high-frequency jet ventilation (HFJV), and high-frequency oscillation (HFO)[48] (Table 5.3).

High-frequency ventilators were developed to prevent ventilator-associated lung injury, ventilate patients during rigid bronchoscopy and laryngeal surgery, in the presence of bronchopleural fistula and in cases of ARDS.[49,50] In high-frequency jet ventilation, placement of an endotracheal tube is not required. Gas is delivered either under high flow or high pressure through a small bore cannula placed in the middle or upper part of the endotracheal tube. The gas mixture is humidified using aerosolized saline solution. The operator sets the frequency, driving pressure, I:E ratio, and mean airway pressure.

The exact mechanism of gas exchange in high-frequency ventilation is not clear. The proximal alveoli are probably ventilated by direct bulk flow of gas as in conventional ventilation. The second mechanism proposed is longitudinal (Taylor) dispersion. In this form the turbulent flow will superimpose on diffusion to improve the gas exchange. Pendelluft or movement of gas within the lung secondary to regional differences in ventilation also may have a role in gas exchange in high-frequency ventilation. The laminar flow pattern in the airway is associated with different flow rates in the center and periphery of the airway. The gas in the center of the airway moves faster and flows toward the alveoli. In the periphery, flow of gases is slower and moves in the opposite direction especially during expiratory effort. Cardiogenic mixing and molecular diffusion are the other mechanisms of gas exchange in this form of ventilation.

The most common adverse effects of this type of ventilation are air trapping and drying of secretions.[51] High-frequency oscillation with volume recruitment maneuvers was shown to improve gas exchange without hemodynamic compromise in patients with severe ARDS.[52,53]

NEWER MODES OF VENTILATION

Positive pressure mechanical ventilation plays an important role in the management of patients with respiratory failure. Different forms of positive pressure ventilation as described above have several disadvantages. The mechanical breath may not match the patient's needs; it may control only one aspect of ventilation at one time. As the new generation of ventilators emerge, they use closed loop systems which allow

Table 5.3 *Comparison of types of high frequency ventilation*

Ventilator modes	Breaths freq/min	Tidal volume (mL/kg)	Flow rate (L/min)	Inspiration	Exhalation
Conventional	2–40	4–10	up to 120	Active	Passive
High-frequency positive pressure ventilation	60–100	3–4	175–250	Active	Passive
High-frequency jet ventilation	100–200	2–5	Depends on pressure	Active	Passive
High-frequency oscillation	up to 2400	1–3	Depends on pressure	Active	Active

the ventilator to adjust for leaks, changing compliance or resistance, and patient needs.[54] Some ventilator modes are able to analyze each breath and appropriately control the volume and pressures of that breath (*intra-breath*). Others analyze a series of breaths and make volume and pressure changes to fit the clinician's description for subsequent breaths (*inter-breath*). These ventilators have the capability for dual mode control. Dual modes can operate during mandatory and spontaneous breaths. The machine will give a series of test breaths to the patient to measure different variables used for control of the system. The feedback loop allows either pressure or volume (one variable at a time) to be altered or regulated.

Volume assured pressure support or pressure augmentation

Volume assured pressure support or pressure augmentation use dual control within a single breath. The breath usually starts as a pressure control breath, reaching the preset pressure rapidly. The flow is variable as in pressure-targeted ventilation. The ventilator determines the tidal volume delivered to the patient. If the volume delivered is equal to the preset volume, the breath is pressure controlled or pressure supported. If the tidal volume delivered is below the preset value, the pressure control mode will change into a volume control mode assuring the volume delivery to the patient. This is achieved either by increasing the inspiratory time or increasing the pressure limit.[55,56]

Volume support or variable pressure support ventilation

In volume support or variable pressure support ventilation, all breaths are patient triggered. The breaths are pressure limited and flow cycled.[57] The machine will attempt to maintain the tidal volume by adjusting the pressure support and the breaths are terminated when the flow falls below 25 percent of peak value. The theoretical advantage of these modes is that the level of pressure support is automatically reduced as the patient's capacity to carry out the work of breathing improves. The disadvantage is that in patients with obstructive airway disease this may contribute to the development of intrinsic PEEP.

Pressure regulated volume control

Pressure regulated volume control uses tidal volume as the feedback control mechanism to adjust the pressure. The breaths are ventilator or patient triggered, pressure controlled, and flow cycled. The pressure limit is calculated by the ventilator and is influenced by the compliance of the respiratory system. The first few breaths are delivered at a pressure limit that is 75 percent of what is required to achieve the desired tidal volume. Based on the measured tidal volume of these breaths, the pressure limit is adjusted to achieve the desired tidal volume. The pressure fluctuation between breaths does not vary more than 3 cm H_2O per breath. The ventilator can also adjust flow according to the patient's demand making this mode more comfortable for the patient. The downside of this type of ventilation is alveolar overdistension due to the fixed minute ventilation in the face of varying compliance of the lung.[58]

Adaptive support ventilation

Adaptive support ventilation adjusts both spontaneous and ventilator delivered breaths to the patient's needs by adjusting different variables.[59] Adaptive support ventilation analyzes the mechanical properties of the respiratory system and the patient's breathing effort to deliver the clinician-set minute ventilation, while at the same time minimizing the work of breathing.[60,61] The ventilator can provide 100 mL/min/kg minute ventilation to the adults and 200 mL/min/kg ventilation to children. The physician can determine what percentage of the minute ventilation is to be supported by the ventilator. Initially, the machine delivers a series of test breaths to calculate variables like dead space, compliance, resistance, and intrinsic PEEP. With this information, it then determines the frequency, pressure limit, inspiratory time, and I:E ratio. The lung mechanics are measured and adjusted breath to breath to meet prescribed targets. Patient triggered breaths are recognized and appropriate reduction in mandatory breaths is made, always assuring that the targets are met.

Automode and variable pressure support/variable pressure control

Automode ventilator combines volume support for spontaneously breathing patients and pressure-regulated volume-controlled (PRVC) mode for mandatory breaths. It was originally designed for automated weaning (changing pressure control to pressure support) with the escalation of support if a patient's effort diminishes below a threshold. When the machine recognizes two consecutive patient breaths it switches from either pressure control to pressure support or volume control to volume support. The volume support ventilation changes to mandatory breaths when the patient becomes apneic for a predetermined time.[62]

Proportional assist ventilation

Unlike the conventional modes of mechanical ventilation where the ventilator support diminishes with patient effort and cycle changes depend on the preset ventilator values (rather than the patient needs), proportional assist ventilation supports the patient effort without imposing predetermined targets.[63,64] The ventilator support increases proportionately to the patient demand with better neuro-ventilatory coupling. The proportion of assist is determined from continuous calculation of the elastance and the airway pressure and is amplified to assist the patient. The degree of assist can be half or two-thirds of the patient's effort. In certain conditions, the ventilator can oversupport the patient resulting in continuous inspiratory flow even when the patient's inspiratory effort stops. This results in increased volume or pressure delivery to the patient and is called a runaway condition. The runaway condition occurs when there is an overestimation of airway pressures, presence of leak, or rapid change in the lung conditions. The tidal volume, inspiratory time, and flow pattern is determined by the patient. This may cause hypercapnia or respiratory acidosis in patients with decreased central drive.

Automatic tube compensation

The endotracheal tube imposes significant resistance to flow during the initial part of inspiration. In spontaneously breathing patients, pressure support is added to overcome the increased work of breathing related to the endotracheal tubes. The constant pressure applied will not adjust for the additional narrowing of the tube caused by secretions or kinking. Automatic tube compensation continuously calculates the tube resistance from tracheal pressure, tube coefficient, and flow rate. It is based on the premise that tracheal pressure change can be calculated by knowing the inspiratory and expiratory flow and the flow dependent resistive properties of the endotracheal tube. With the usage of automatic tube compensation (ATC), it is essential to put in the caliber of the airway for the ventilator to calculate pressure change needed to generate the requisite flow. In several respects, ATC is similar to pressure support ventilation. The basic difference is that the inspiratory pressure support provided in ATC is continuously being calculated and changed. In contrast, the level of inspiratory pressure support provided in pressure support ventilation is constant unless manually changed by the operator. Also, ATC serves to obviate the effects on airways resistance (and hence increased work of breathing) imposed by the artificial airways.[65,66]

Mandatory minute ventilation

Mandatory minute ventilation mode is used during weaning to support patients who failed to meet the set minute ventilation.[67] The ventilator adjusts the output according to the patient's performance. If the minute ventilation exceeds the goal, there will be no support from the ventilator and if the patient fails to meet the set goal the ventilator compensates either by increasing tidal volume or by increasing rate. The disadvantages of this mode include measurement of exhaled volume to calculate minute ventilation. The patient can have rapid shallow breathing, but may have reached the desired minute ventilation. Thus, muscle fatigue may be developing (as indicated by the rapid-shallow breathing) and the ventilator may not provide any support in such a situation.[68]

Airway pressure release ventilation

Airway pressure release ventilation was designed to augment alveolar ventilation for patient receiving continuous positive airway pressure (CPAP) and at the same time minimizes the development of alveolar overdistension and high airway pressures.[69,70] The patient receives ventilation using CPAP and the pressure is released by opening the expiratory valve. This allows for a rapid decrease in lung volume. The pressure is reestablished immediately and the lungs are reinflated. The advantages of this type of ventilation are decrease in peak airway and thoracic pressures and it may improve ventilation/perfusion matching with more uniform distribution of ventilation. This mode of ventilation may interfere with spontaneous breathing, decreasing tidal volumes in noncompliant lungs, and difficulty providing optimal release time for patients with unequal lung involvement.

Negative pressure ventilation

Mechanical ventilatory support can be given using negative pressure as well as positive pressure ventilators. Negative pressure ventilators apply a subatmospheric pressure to the chest wall during inspiration. This in turn will create negative pleural pressure, which will allow the air to move to the lungs. Exhalation phase can be either passive or active by applying positive pressure to the chest wall.

The first negative pressure ventilator used a tight fitting body box and bellows and was developed in 1832 by Dalziel and was modified later by Woillez, Emerson, and Drinker. The patient's body rested in the ventilator and a tight collar was applied around the neck. A negative pressure was created in the tank using either manually operated bellows or by an electric pump. Negative pressure ventilators like 'poncho wrap', or 'pneumo wrap' consist of water impermeable and air proof nylon parkas. This apparatus is suspended over rigid metallic or plastic shields, which are applied to the anterior part of the abdomen to provide negative pressure. These ventilators are not as effective as the iron lung, but have the advantage of portability and ease of application. The chest 'cuirass' consists of a rigid shell applied to the anterior chest wall and is probably the least effective of the negative pressure ventilators.[71]

Negative pressure ventilation can be delivered in five different modes: cyclical negative pressure; negative/positive pressure; continuous negative extrathoracic pressure; negative pressure/continuous negative extrathoracic pressure and external high frequency ventilation.

CYCLICAL NEGATIVE PRESSURE

The machine generates a preset subatmospheric pressure during inspiration. This allows air to flow into the lungs. The pressure returns to atmospheric pressure during exhalation. This mode of ventilation can increase the tidal volume in patients with chest wall disorders.[72]

NEGATIVE/POSITIVE PRESSURE

The machine generates negative pressure during inspiration and positive pressure during exhalation.

CONTINUOUS NEGATIVE EXTRATHORACIC PRESSURE

This type of mechanical ventilation provides continuous subatmospheric pressure to the chest wall while the patient breathes spontaneously. It augments the tidal volume.

NEGATIVE PRESSURE/CONTINUOUS NEGATIVE EXTRATHORACIC PRESSURE

Besides applying continuous negative extrathoracic pressure for ventilatory support, additional negative pressure is applied to augment the tidal volume to the patient.

EXTERNAL HIGH–FREQUENCY VENTILATION

A high frequency ventilator connected to a chest or abdominal cuirass was approved for secretion clearance in COPD patients, but can augment the minute volume in normal subjects and COPD patients with improvement in gas exchange. The frequencies range from 60 to 140 cycles per minute and pressure changes are from $-26\,cm\,H_2O$ to $+10\,cm\,H_2O$. These modalities can provide short-term ventilation for COPD patients and relieve muscle fatigue.[73,74]

CLINICAL USE OF NEGATIVE PRESSURE VENTILATION

In COPD patients with acute respiratory failure, negative pressure ventilation can be as beneficial as controlled ventilation. Duration of ventilation was shorter in patients with negative pressure ventilation.[75]

Negative pressure ventilators were extensively used for patients with acute respiratory failure during the polio epidemic in 1930s until 1950. Since the invention of positive pressure ventilation, negative pressure ventilators have been mainly used in patients with slowly progressive respiratory failure secondary to neuromuscular disorders, chest wall disorders, and central hypoventilation. Some patients with chest wall deformities require special fitting for cuirass ventilators. Nocturnal ventilation using negative pressure ventilation improves gas exchange and survival in these patients.[76]

ADJUNCTS TO MECHANICAL VENTILATION

POSITIVE END-EXPIRATORY PRESSURE

Positive end-expiratory pressure is applied to a patient on mechanical ventilatory support to improve oxygenation. Ashbaugh and coworkers applied PEEP to patients who had acute respiratory failure secondary to diffuse lung injury to improve oxygenation.[77] Since then PEEP has become the cornerstone for management of patients with acute hypoxemic respiratory failure. Under static conditions, functional residual capacity (FRC) is determined by the opposing elastic properties of the chest wall and the lungs. In patients with acute respiratory failure secondary to pulmonary edema, the FRC is decreased markedly causing reduction of the number of alveoli for gas exchange. Gas dilution and computed tomographic studies have confirmed decreased FRC in patients with acute respiratory failure.[78–80]

Application of PEEP to patients with acute respiratory failure increases the FRC by recruitment of collapsed alveoli or by overdistension of the normal alveoli. The PEEP keeps the alveoli open during the expiratory phase in the dependent portions of the lungs.[81] In patients with pulmonary edema, PEEP redistributes the water from alveolar space to perivascular interstitial space without decreasing the overall lung edema.[82] PEEP with low lung volumes decreases formation of lung edema compared with large volume lung inflation.[83] Applied PEEP can increase, decrease, or cause no change in the respiratory system compliance. Increasing compliance denotes alveolar recruitment whereas decreasing compliance usually points to alveolar over distension.[84,85] When the compliance is unchanged, it usually indicates underlying fibrosis of lung. Effect of PEEP on the cardiovascular system depends on:

- compliance of the respiratory system
- right and left ventricular contractility
- compensatory mechanisms.

Transmission of PEEP to the pleural space is decreased in patients with low lung compliance (ARDS) and/or increased chest wall compliance (rib fractures). In contrast there will be increased transmission of the pressures in lungs with high compliance (as seen in COPD). The primary effect of increased pleural pressure is decreased cardiac output and subsequent reduction in oxygen delivery.[86] The net cardiac output depends on the effect of PEEP on preload, afterload, and the volume status of the patient.

SIGHS

In the past, deliberate increases in the tidal volume at predetermined intervals were given regularly to patients being mechanically ventilated. This may prevent microatelectasis and also recruit the dependent lung. Presently, it is rarely used and the value of this intervention is to be determined. The addition of sigh breaths in recently weaned patients on pressure support ventilation has not been shown to improve the oxygenation.[87] On the other hand, sigh breaths improved the oxygenation in patients with early ARDS on pressure support ventilation.[88]

PERMISSIVE HYPERCAPNIA

One of the strategies to decrease the ventilator induced lung injury is to decrease the tidal volume and distending pressure. In patients with severe lung injury or severe obstructive airway disease, retention of carbon dioxide and respiratory acidosis may ensue.[89,90] Increased carbon dioxide produces certain physiologic effects through the sympathomimetic stimulation – elevation of intracranial pressure; stimulation and depression of the cardiovascular system; ventilatory stimulation; hypoxemia; and depression of the central nervous system.[91] The safe level of hypercapnia is unknown. In patients with no contraindication – acute neurologic and cardiac events – cautious use of permissive hypercapnia may be inevitable to prevent ventilator-induced lung injury.[92,93]

PRONE VENTILATION

There is significant regional variation in the disease distribution and hence distribution of ventilation in patients with ARDS. This has been demonstrated by computed tomography of patients with ARDS.[94] Supine position is associated with decreased ventilation in the dependent and in the topmost part of the lung. Improvement in oxygenation after a patient with respiratory failure has been put in the prone position has been known since the 1970s.[95] The mechanism of improvement includes: increase in lung volume, improvement of ventilation/perfusion matching, and more homogeneous distribution of ventilation.[96,97] Not all patients benefit from prone ventilation. Some patients maintain oxygenation after returning to supine position; in others the improvement is seen only in prone position, and a third group comprises nonresponders.[98] Improvement in oxygenation is seen more commonly in early ARDS from extrapulmonary causes. Prone positioning is associated with some mechanical complications. These are accidental dislodgment of endotracheal tubes, central venous lines, drains, and development of pressure ulcers. None of the studies so far has shown a survival benefit in ARDS from prone positioning.[99]

INITIATION OF MECHANICAL VENTILATION

It is important to set specific goals in relation to individual patient's needs at the onset of mechanical ventilatory support. Patient comfort and avoidance of patient–ventilator dyssynchrony is also of paramount importance. The initial settings include selection of mode of ventilation, fractional concentration of inspired oxygen, tidal volume, respiratory frequency, I:E ratio, sensitivity, and flow rates.

Fractional concentration of inspired oxygen

For patients with hypoxemic respiratory failure, most physicians start with fractional concentration of inspired oxygen (Fio_2) of 1.0 and titrate it down to the lowest Fio_2 required to keep the arterial oxygen tension more than 60 mm Hg and/or oxygen saturation above 90 percent. Pulse oximetry or arterial blood gases can be used to titrate oxygen down to the lowest possible concentration required for the patient. If the patient's Fio_2 cannot be titrated below 60 percent, other modalities to improve oxygenation should be considered. High oxygen concentration can damage the lungs and the changes are often indistinguishable from acute lung injury.[100,101] Concomitant administration of bleomycin, amiodarone, and radiation can potentiate the toxic effects of these medications.

Tidal volume

Depending on the mode of ventilation used, the tidal volume can be preset or depends on the inflation pressure and the compliance of the respiratory system. The deleterious effects of high tidal volumes have been demonstrated both in animals and humans and are indistinguishable from acute lung injury.[102] In patients with acute lung injury and ARDS, a tidal volume of 4–6 mL/kg ideal body weight (IBW) is recommended to prevent ventilator-associated lung injury.[103] This may be modified to some extent by observing the plateau pressures. If the plateau pressure is <25 cm H_2O, a tidal volume of 8–10 mL/kg IBW may be used, especially if the patient demonstrates 'air hunger'. If the plateau pressure is between 25 cm H_2O and 30 cm H_2O, a tidal volume of 6–8 mL/kg IBW may be used for the patient with a strong intrinsic inspiratory drive. For those whose plateau pressure is >30 cm H_2O, the tidal volume may have to be dropped to 4–6 mL/kg IBW. Patients with obstructive airway disease should usually also be ventilated in the range of 6–8 mL/kg IBW, ensuring that the plateau pressures are less than 30 cm H_2O.

The gas in the circuit is compressed during inspiration resulting in expansion of the tubing. So part of the volume delivered to the patient does not reach the patient.[104] During expiration the volume that is stored in the tubing is released and measured tidal volume will be higher than the set tidal volume. The compression volume varies with the characteristics of the tubing (length, diameter, compliance) and the inflation pressure. The compression volume is expressed as the compression factor which is the ratio of compression volume to plateau pressure. The actual tidal volume can be calculated subtracting compression volume (compression factor × peak inspiratory pressure) from exhaled tidal volume. Measurement of compression volume is important for calculation of the compliance, intrinsic PEEP, oxygen consumption and carbon dioxide production.[105,106]

Inflation pressures

In volume-controlled ventilation, inflation pressure is a dependent variable and is affected by the delivered tidal volume. The alarms are set to alert the clinician when the pressure exceeds the set limit. In pressure-controlled setting, the inflation pressure is the control variable and is usually set to give the appropriate tidal volume for that patient but should not usually exceed 30 cm H_2O. The one exception to keeping plateau pressures below 30 cm H_2O is an individual with morbid obesity and chest burns (increased chest wall stiffness) or abdominal compartment syndrome (increased pleural pressures resulting in lower transpulmonary pressures).

Respiratory rate

The rate setting depends on the demand of the patient and should be close to the patient's actual rate. Patients who assist the ventilator can exceed the back-up rate. In volume preset ventilators, when the respiratory rate increases, the ventilator does not adjust the inspiratory time or the flow rate. This may cause reversal of I:E ratio, which may result in patient–ventilator dyssynchrony.

When ARDSNet trial guidelines are implemented for ARDS patients, it is important to remember that permissive hypercapnia is not recommended. Since low tidal volumes were used, respiratory rates were kept at about 30 breaths per minute.[103]

Inspiratory flow rate

Even though inspiratory flows are not a necessary physician order for the ventilator setting, most of the ventilators require either a flow rate or inspiratory time (Ti). The flow rate affects the tidal volume and the Ti. The common practice is to start with a flow rate of 60 L/min and to adjust it according to the patient's needs.[107]

Expiratory flow rate is the ratio of tidal volume and expiratory time and is determined by the patient's actual respiratory rate, not the set rate. High actual rates are associated with short expiratory time and high flow rates. In patients with obstructive airway disease, the shortened expiratory time will cause dynamic hyperinflation. In these conditions, it is prudent to begin with an inspiratory flow rate of 80 L/min if volume-targeted ventilation is used.

Inspiratory time

In modes of mechanical ventilation in which inspiratory time has to be set (such as pressure assist-control), it is important to determine what the patient's intrinsic inspiratory time is. A reasonable idea may be obtained by looking at the waveform of the respiratory cycle. The usual range is 0.6–1.0 seconds. Some patients who are breathing rapidly may require short inspiratory times (0.6 seconds).

Sensitivity

Sensitivity should be set to as sensitive as possible without auto-triggering occurring. In most clinical settings, flow-triggering is preferred over pressure triggering.

VENTILATORY MANAGEMENT IN SPECIFIC CLINICAL CONDITIONS

Acute lung injury and acute respiratory distress syndrome

Acute lung injury (ALI) and ARDS are manifestations of lung injury associated with various disease processes. The lung involvement is nonuniform, and the initial exudative phase may progress to fibrotic phase in 3–10 days. Due to the

heterogeneity of the disease process, ARDS patients are more prone to develop ventilator-associated lung injury.

Besides improving oxygenation and decreasing work of breathing, the ventilator mode must gear toward decreasing ventilator-induced lung injury. ARDSNet trial, a multicenter, randomized study comparing high versus low tidal volumes showed absolute survival benefit in the low tidal volume group. The guidelines for the ventilator strategy are given in Box 5.3.[103,108–110]

Chronic obstructive pulmonary disease

Patients with COPD have significantly altered pulmonary mechanics due to airflow limitation, structural lung damage, and respiratory muscle dysfunction secondary to hyperinflation. These patients also develop PEEP as a result of altered mechanics and different time constants of different lung units.

Noninvasive mechanical ventilation must be considered in all patients admitted to a hospital with COPD exacerbation, who are demonstrating rising $PaCO_2$ or muscle fatigue.[111–114] Noninvasive positive pressure ventilation (NIPPV) is preferable for COPD patients if they are alert, hemodynamically stable, able to clear secretions, and experienced personnel are available to institute ventilatory support.

If the patient needs invasive mechanical ventilation, either pressure control or volume control mode can be used successfully. The most important point to remember in ventilating these patients is to prevent the development of intrinsic PEEP. The ventilator is initially set to tidal volume of 6–8 mL/kg IBW, rate 10–14/min, flow rate ≥80 L/min, FiO_2 to maintain O_2 saturation >90 percent, and P_{plat} <30 cm H_2O. Adding small PEEP (5 cm H_2O) to the initial ventilator setting is advisable. If pressure control mode of ventilation is used the inspiratory time is set for 0.6–1.0 seconds. The ventilator settings are adjusted according to arterial blood gases, which must be maintained close to the baseline arterial blood gases of the patient. Development of intrinsic PEEP must be monitored carefully and ventilator settings must be adjusted accordingly. Application of external PEEP up to 80 percent in intrinsic PEEP will decrease the work of breathing and usually not result in further hyperinflation[115] (Fig. 5.4).

There are some important differences between mechanical ventilation of asthmatic patients and COPD patients as it pertains to mechanical ventilation. There is an abundance of data for the use of NIPPV in COPD patients. In COPD patients, dynamic hyperinflation develops due to loss of lung elasticity. The PEEP (intrinsic) results in increased work of breathing and dyssynchrony. Giving extrinsic PEEP up to 80 percent of intrinsic PEEP is appropriate. These patients have problems mainly in exhalation (exhalation is a passive process that requires lung elasticity which is reduced in emphysema). The airway pressure proximal to the airway narrowing (equal pressure point) is relatively normal. Since these patients may have a

Box 5.3 ARDSNet protocol for ventilation of patients with severe ARDS[103]

Goals (decreasing order of importance)

- Pa_{O_2}: 55–80 mm Hg
- Tidal volumes: 6 mL/kg IBW
- Plateau pressures: <30 cm H_2O in patients with normal chest wall compliance
- PEEP: appropriate to maintain alveolar recruitment (5–24 cm H_2O), determined by Fi_{O_2} used
- Pa_{CO_2}: 40 mm Hg ideally, permissive hypercapnia if plateau pressure >30 cm H_2O

Initiating mechanical ventilation

A – calculate ideal body weight (IBW)
(male = 50 + 2.3 [ht (in) – 60] kg;
female = 45.5 + 2.3 [ht (in) – 60] kg)

B – select volume assist-control mode

C – set initial tidal volume 8 mL/kg IBW,
decrease to 7 mL/kg IBW after 1 hour,
then 6 mL/kg IBW in 1–2 hours

D – Set respiratory rate to maintain baseline minute
ventilation of the patient, but not >35 breaths/min

E – I:E ratio 1:2

F – Fi_{O_2} and PEEP according to the table below

Fi_{O_2} 0.3 0.4 0.5 0.6 0.7 0.8 0.9. 1.0

PEEP 5 5–8 8–10 10 10–14 14 14–18 20–24

Subsequent adjustments

Plateau pressure – goal <30 cm H_2O

- Check plateau pressure every 4 hours and after each PEEP and tidal volume changes
- If P_{plat} >30 cm H_2O, decrease the tidal volume by 1 mL/kg to a minimum of 4 mL/kg IBW
- If P_{plat} <25 cm H_2O , and tidal volume is 4 mL/kg, increase the tidal volume to a maximum of 6 mL/kg
- If patient develops dyspnea tidal volume may be increased to 7–8 mL/kg, provided the P_{plat} remains <30 cm H_2O

Arterial pH, Pa_{CO_2}, and respiratory rate

Goal:

- pH 7.30–7.45

Respiratory rate – maximum 35 breaths/min

- pH 7.15–7.30

(i) increase the set rate until pH >7.30 or Pa_{CO_2} <25 mm Hg
(ii) if set rate >35/min and pH <7.30, sodium bicarbonate may be given intravenously

- pH <7.15

(i) increase the set rate to maximum
(ii) consider intravenous sodium bicarbonate after maximum respiratory rate failed to correct the pH
(iii) may increase the tidal volume 1 mL/kg and occasionally and the tidal volume limit may be exceeded

- pH >7.45

(i) determine the cause of alkalosis respiratory versus metabolic
(ii) if respiratory, decrease the set rate until the patient's rate is more than the set rate, but not under 6 breaths/min

high inspiratory drive, pressure assist-control may best meet their needs. In contrast, there are few data on using NIPPV in the setting of status asthmaticus.[116] There are more data on the usage of helium–oxygen mixture in the setting of asthma than COPD.[119–122] Permissive hypercapnia is almost always required in the first 24–48 hours when mechanically ventilating an acute asthmatic patient. Intrinsic PEEP measurements in such patients may be an underestimation of the degree of intrinsic PEEP (due to complete obstruction of alveolar ducts and bronchi).

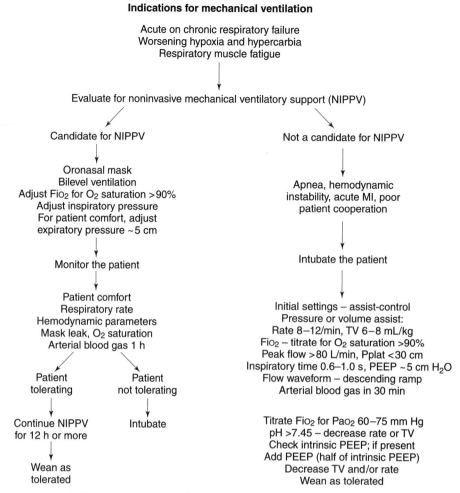

Figure 5.4 *Algorithm for treatment of chronic obstructive pulmonary disease. MI, myocardial infarction; PEEP, positive end-expiratory pressure; TV, tidal volume.*

High driving pressures in the range of 60–80 cm H_2O may be needed to overcome proximal airways resistance. However, in both conditions, plateau pressures should be maintained below 30 cm H_2O.

Table 5.4 summarizes the ventilatory management of some of the other common causes of respiratory failure.

WEANING

Recent guidelines from the American College of Chest Physicians make the following recommendations:

- Daily assessments should be made for weaning patients beginning from the first day of mechanical ventilation.
- Each hospital should develop its own guidelines or protocols for weaning patients.
- Certain prerequisites should be fulfilled prior to conducting a spontaneous breathing trial (SBT). These include:
  — partial or complete reversal of conditions that lead to respiratory failure

  — oxygenation parameters support SBT: (i) P/F ≥150 with PEEP <8 cm H_2O (ii) FiO_2 <0.5 (P/F stands for PaO_2/FiO_2 ratio)
  — absence of severe acidosis usually assessed by a pH of >7.25
  — hemodynamic stability
  — spontaneous respiratory drive is present
  — absence of copious secretions that may prevent successful extubation.

Patients fulfilling these prerequisites should be given a daily SBT. This may be given as CPAP (up to a pressure of 5 cm H_2O or pressure support ventilation of 5–7 cm H_2O or a T-piece breathing trial). They should be observed for about 5 minutes at the bedside. If the patients appear to be tolerating the SBT, a total duration of 30–120 minutes is given. Patients should be assessed at the end of the SBT. Simple parameters are used to indicate failure of the SBT. These include:

- Respiratory instability
  — tachypnea (respiratory rate >35/min)

Table 5.4 *Ventilatory management in specific conditions*

Disease	Main problems	Special vent settings	Precautions
Head trauma	Raised intracranial pressure Unstable respiratory drive	RR to keep Pa_{CO_2} between 25 and 30 mm Hg if raised intracranial pressure	Prevent hypercapnia and hypoxemia (keep Pa_{O_2} >70 mm Hg) Keep PEEP usually below 5–8 cm H_2O to prevent further rise in intracranial pressure
Chest trauma	Flail chest Lung contusion ARDS Rupture of large airways	Avoid mechanical vent if possible A-C mode of vent	Pain relief is important If a large air leak is present, bronchoscopic evaluation of the airways may be useful
Cardiogenic pulmonary edema	Excessive work of breathing Hypoxemia (especially in cardiac ischemia or MI) Pulmonary congestion	Try CPAP approx 10 cm H_2O first and Fi_{O_2} of 1.0 If hypercapnia is developing, use NIPPV (PSV 10 H_2O and PEEP 5 cm H_2O) Use pressure or volume assist if mechanical ventilation is required V_T 8–10 cm H_2O Consider PEEP of 5–10 cm H_2O	Venous return may be augmented when these patients are given spontaneous breathing trials. Observe carefully for development of pulmonary edema on extubation Ensure adequate oxygenation (Pa_{O_2} >70–80 mm Hg)
Postoperative patient	Atelectasis Hypoxemia Pain and splinting Nausea and vomiting	A-C control (pressure or volume) Larger tidal volumes up to 10 mL/kg are acceptable 5–10 cm H_2O PEEP	Patients may be given a rapid spontaneous breathing trial with PSV PCA pumps usually ensure adequate analgesia without respiratory drive suppression

ARDs, acute respiratory distress syndrome; MI, myocardial infarction; A-C, assist-control; RR, respiratory rate; CPAP, continuous positive airway pressure; NIPPV, noninvasive positive pressure ventilation; PSV, pressure support ventilation; PEEP, positive end-expiratory pressure; V_T, tidal volume; PCA, patient-controlled analgisia.

— Sa_{O_2} <90 percent
— obvious respiratory distress (diaphoresis, significant anxiety, etc.)
- Hemodynamic instability
  — systolic blood pressure >180 mm Hg
  — heart rate >140/min or sustained increase in the heart rate of >20 percent from baseline.

Remove artificial airway if patient demonstrates successful SBT. Consideration needs to be made for the following prior to extubation:

- airway patency
- ability to protect airway
- copious respiratory secretions.

If the patient fails SBT, the respiratory muscles should be rested, usually for 24 hours. An effort to determine the reason for failure of the SBT is made[121–125] (Fig. 5.5).

COMPLICATIONS OF MECHANICAL VENTILATION

Even though mechanical ventilatory support is life saving in many situations, it is commonly associated with many complications. The complications can occur as a result of mechanical ventilation itself or as a complication of underlying disease process.

- Reversal of underlying problem
- Prerequisites fulfille d
  (Fi_{O_2}, PEEP, P/F, BP, respiratory drive)

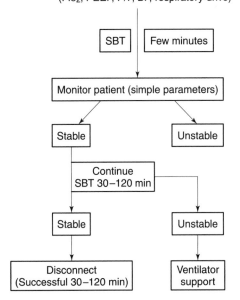

Figure 5.5 *Algorithm for weaning. PEEP, positive end-expiratory pressure; BP, blood pressure; P/F, PaO_2/Fi_{O_2}; SBT, spontaneous breathing trial.*

Ventilators are complex and sophisticated machines and malfunction can occur due to defective machines as well as human error.[126] Common machine associated problems are circuit leaks, disconnections, and mechanical failure of ventilator components.

Tracheal intubations cause immediate and late complications for the patient. Immediate complications include trauma to the upper airway, trachea, right main stem intubations and aspiration to the lung. Common delayed complications are ulcerations of mouth, pharynx, larynx, and trachea. Patients can also develop tracheal granulations, tracheomalacia, destruction of tracheal cartilages, tracheoesophageal and tracheoinnominate fistulas. Mechanical problems from the endotracheal tube include obstruction of the tube with secretions and malfunction of the tracheal tube cuff.

Pulmonary barotrauma includes pneumomediastinum, subcutaneous emphysema, pneumopericardium, pneumoperitoneum, and pneumothorax. Presence of extraalveolar air in patients receiving positive pressure ventilation may be due to factors other than mechanical ventilation. In the early days of mechanical ventilation, barotrauma was solely attributed to high peak pressures.[127–129] Increased peak pressure is not synonymous with alveolar overdistension. Factors contributing to high peak pressure include increased resistance to the ventilator circuit and patient airways, patient ventilator asynchrony, extrathoracic causes such as morbid obesity, tense ascites or abdominal packing, and alveolar overdistension. In patients with alveolar overdistension, asymmetric pressure differences between the alveoli and bronchovascular bundle result in alveolar rupture and escape of air into the subcutaneous tissues.[130,131] Barotrauma is rare in normal lungs but the incidence is increased in patients with underlying lung diseases such as ARDS, obstructive lung diseases, and *Pneumocystis carinii* pneumonia.

Ventilator-associated lung injury was known from the inception of mechanical ventilatory support. Animals ventilated with high peak pressures developed atelectasis, severe congestion, and pulmonary edema.[132–134] Alterations of alveolar and arterial permeability contributed to these changes in the mechanically ventilated lung. Microscopic studies of the lungs showed destruction of the epithelial cells, denudation of basement membranes, gaps in capillary endothelium, and hyaline membrane formation.[135] High peak pressures are associated with high volumes in normal lung. Subsequent animal studies showed that high volume inflation of the lung, not the high pressure caused the lung damage.[102] Alveolar overdistension can be avoided using low tidal volumes, limiting peak and plateau pressure (<30 cm H_2O) and use of optimal PEEP.

Nosocomial infections are common in patients being ventilated due to disruption of the normal defense mechanisms, contamination of the ventilator circuit, adherence of microorganisms to the endotracheal tubes, and increased susceptibility of the patient to infections. The incidence nosocomial pneumonia varies widely among different studies (9–41 percent) and mortality exceeds 50 percent. Gram-negative bacilli including *Pseudomonas aeruginosa*, *Staphylococcus aureus*, and polymicrobial pneumonia are the common etiological agents. Diagnosis of nosocomial infections is difficult due to the contamination of the specimens with colonized bacteria in the endotracheal tubes. Meticulous attention to infection control measures, oral care, elevation of head of bed >30°, judicious use of H_2 blockers and proton pump inhibitors, early extubation, and use of antimicrobial coated endotracheal tube may decrease the incidence of nosocomial pneumonia in patients being ventilated.[136]

Positive pressure ventilation decreases the venous return to the heart, which may decrease the cardiac output. This commonly occurs in patients with hypovolemia and in patients who develop intrinsic PEEP.[137] Overdistension of the lung is associated with increase in pulmonary vascular resistance and increased right ventricular afterload. In patients with severe left ventricular dysfunction, increased intrathoracic pressure can augment cardiac output by decreasing the afterload. Patients on mechanical ventilation have decreased excretion of sodium and water. Possible mechanisms implicated are decreased cardiac output, atrial natriuretic peptide, and increased antidiuretic hormone. Of these, decrease in atrial natriuretic hormone definitely has been shown to decrease urine output in patients on positive pressure ventilation and PEEP.[138]

Gastrointestinal complications of mechanical ventilation include development of pneumoperitoneum. Pneumoperitoneum occurs in patients with barotrauma as well as in rupture of viscera and must be evaluated urgently. Gastrointestinal bleeding secondary to stress ulceration occurs in severely ill patients on mechanical ventilation.[139] Prophylactic use of antacids, H_2 blockers and proton pump inhibitors decrease the incidence of bleeding in these patients. Nutritional support in patients being mechanically ventilated is often a big challenge. Undernutrition leads to muscular atrophy and decreased immune function, and overfeeding may increase metabolism and ventilator requirements. In patients with raised intracranial pressure, positive pressure ventilation, especially the application of PEEP, may decrease the cerebral venous return and increase the intracranial pressure further.[140]

In summary, mechanical ventilation is associated with multiple pulmonary and extrapulmonary complications. Awareness and attention to preventive measures may prevent some of these complications in patients being ventilated.

Key learning points

- Most of the recent advancements in the field of mechanical ventilation pertain to the development of ventilator-induced lung injury and the concept of lung protection strategy.

- The ARDSNet guidelines should be adhered to in the setting of ARDS and mechanical ventilation. For most clinical diagnoses, tidal volumes in the range of 6–10 mL/kg IBW are appropriate.

- Newer modes of mechanical ventilation are now commercially available. Although they have theoretical advantages, none has shown to decrease the mortality in different clinical settings.

- The use of pressure-targeted ventilation is able to better match the patient's intrinsic drive and has some definite advantages, although reduction in mortality has not been demonstrated.

- NIPPV has been shown to reduce the mortality and complications in patients presenting with moderate to severe COPD exacerbation. It should be considered in all patients prior to initiating invasive mechanical ventilation.

- Weaning should be considered on a daily basis. The importance lies not in how the patient is weaned (pressure support ventilation, CPAP, T-piece) but how frequently weaning trials are initiated. The involvement of respiratory therapists and nurses to carry out weaning trials according to predetermined guidelines and protocols should be strongly advocated.

REFERENCES

1. Snider GL. Historical perspective on mechanical ventilation. From a simple life support system to ethical dilemma. *Am Rev Respir Dis* 1989; **140**: S2–S7.

2. Colice GL. Historical perspective on the development of mechanical ventilation. In: Tobin M, ed. *Principles and Practice of Mechanical Ventilation*. New York: McGraw-Hill, 1994: 1–35.

3. Bach JR. A historical perspective on the use of noninvasive ventilatory support alternatives. *Respir Care Clin North Am* 1996; **2**: 161–81.

4. Bone RC, Eubanks DHJ. A clinician's guide to ventilators: how they work and why they can fail. A classification system to make sense of available options. *J Crit Illn* 1992; **7**: 379–82, 387–94.

5. Guttmann J. Analysis of respiratory mechanics during artificial ventilation. *Biomed Tech (Berl)* 1998; **43**: 107–15.

6. Maggiore SM, Brochard L. Pressure-volume curve: methods and meaning. *Minerva Anesthesiol* 2001; **67**: 228–37.

7. Rossi A, Ganassini A, Polese G, Grassi V. Pulmonary hyperinflation and ventilator-dependent patients. *Eur Respir J* 1997; **10**: 1663–74.

8. Marini J, Ravencraft S. Mean airway pressure: physiologic determinants and clinical importance: Part 1. Physiologic determinants and measurements; Part 2 clinical implications. *Crit Care Med* 1992; **20**: 1461–72, 1604–16.

9. Kacmarek R, Hess D. Basic principles of ventilator machinery. In: Tobin M, ed. *Principles and Practice of Mechanical Ventilation*. New York: McGraw-Hill, 1994: 65–110.

10. Hanley ME, Bone RC. Acute respiratory failure. Pathophysiology, causes, and clinical manifestations. *Postgrad Med* 1986; **79**: 166–9, 172–6.

11. Seriff NS, Khan F, Lazo BJ. Acute respiratory failure. Current concepts of pathophysiology and management. *Med Clin North Am* 1973; **57**: 1539–50.

12. Poggi R, Masotti A, Rossi A. Acute respiratory failure. *Monaldi Arch Chest Dis* 1994; **49**: 488–92.

13. Roussos C, Koutsoukou A. Respiratory failure. *Eur Respir J Suppl* 2003; **47**: 3s–14s.

14. Bellemare F, Grassino A. Effect of pressure and timing of contraction on human diaphragm fatigue. *J Appl Physiol* 1982; **53**: 1190–5.

15. Smallwood R. Ventilators – reported classifications and their usefulness. *Anaesth Intensive Care* 1986; **14**: 251–7.

16. Bone RC, Eubanks DH. Second- and third-generation ventilators: sorting through available options. When, and for which patients, are special functions needed? *J Crit Illn* 1992; **7**: 399–416.

17. Chatburn RL. Classification of mechanical ventilators. *Respir Care* 1992; **37**: 1009–25.

18. Chatburn RL. Computer control of mechanical ventilation. *Respir Care* 2004; **49**: 507–17.

19. Branson R. Understanding and implementing advances in ventilator capabilities. *Curr Opin Crit Care* 2004; **10**: 23–32.

20. Bone RC, Eubanks DH, Gluck E. Beyond the basics: operating the new generation of ventilator. A look at the features and functions of these units. *J Crit Illn* 1992; **7**: 770–82.

21. Aslanian P, El Atrous S, Isabey D, *et al.* Effects of flow triggering on breathing effort during partial ventilatory support. *Am J Respir Crit Care Med* 1998; **157**: 135–43.

22. Leung P, Jubran A, Tobin MJ. Comparison of assisted ventilator modes on triggering, patient effort, and

dyspnea. *Am J Respir Crit Care Med* 1997; **155**: 1940–8.

23. Corrado A, Gorini M. Negative-pressure ventilation: is there still a role? *Eur Respir J* 2002; **20**: 187–97.

24. Botz GH, Sladen RN. Conventional modes of mechanical ventilation. *Int Anesthesiol Clin* 1997; **35**: 19–27.

25. Popovich J, Jr. Mechanical ventilation. Physiology, equipment design, and management. *Postgrad Med* 1986; **79**: 217–20.

26. Campbell RS, Davis BR. Pressure-controlled versus volume-controlled ventilation: does it matter? *Respir Care* 2002; **47**: 416–24.

27. Sassoon CSH. Mechanical ventilator design and function: the trigger variable. *Respir Care* 1992; **37**: 1056–69.

28. Chiumello D, Pelosi P, Calvi E, *et al.* Different modes of assisted ventilation in patients with acute respiratory failure. *Eur Respir J* 2002; **20**: 925–33.

29. Willatts SM. Alternative modes of ventilation. Part I. Disadvantages of controlled mechanical ventilation: intermittent mandatory ventilation. *Intensive Care Med* 1985; **11**: 51–5.

30. Weiss JW, Rossing TH, Ingram RH Jr. Effect of intermittent mandatory ventilation on respiratory drive and timing. *Am Rev Respir Dis* 1983; **127**: 705–8.

31. Sassoon CS, Del Rosario N, Fei R, *et al.* Influence of pressure- and flow-triggered synchronous intermittent mandatory ventilation on inspiratory muscle work. *Crit Care Med* 1994; **22**: 1933–41.

32. Mecklenburgh JS, Latto IP, Al-Obaidi TA, *et al.* Excessive work of breathing during intermittent mandatory ventilation. *Br J Anaesth* 1986; **58**: 1048–5.

33. Kacmarek RM, Wilson RS. IMV systems: Do they make a difference? *Chest* 1985; **87**: 557.

34. Tuxen DV, Lane S. The effects of ventilatory pattern on hyperinflation, airway pressures, and circulation in mechanical ventilation of patients with severe air-flow obstruction. *Am Rev Respir Dis* 1987; **136**: 872–9.

35. Tsuno K, Sakanashi Y, Kishi Y, *et al.* Acute respiratory failure induced by mechanical pulmonary ventilation at peak pressure of 40 cm of H_2O. *J Anesth* 1988; **2**: 176–83.

36. MacIntyre NR, McConnell R, Cheng KC, Sane A. Patient-ventilator flow dyssynchrony: flow-limited versus pressure-limited breaths. *Crit Care Med* 1997; **25**: 1671–7.

37. Marini J. Pressure controlled ventilation. In: Tobin M, ed. *Principles and Practice of Mechanical Ventilation* New York: McGraw-Hill 1994: 305–17.

38. Dekel B, Segal E, Perel A. Pressure support ventilation. *Arch Intern Med* 1996; **156**: 369–7.

39. Williams P, Kratohvil J, Ritz R, Hess DR, *et al.* Pressure support and pressure assist/control: are there differences? An evaluation of the newest intensive care unit ventilators. *Respir Care* 2000; **45**: 1169–81.

40. Yamada Y, Shigeta M, Suwa K, Hanaoka K. Respiratory muscle pressure analysis in pressure-support ventilation. *J Appl Physiol* 1994; **77**: 2237–43.

41. MacIntyre N. Respiratory function during pressure support ventilation. *Chest* 1986; **89**: 677–83.

42. Hurst JM, Branson RD, Davis K, Barrette RR. Cardiopulmonary effects of pressure support ventilation. *Arch Surg* 1989; **124**: 1067–70.

43. Reynolds E. Effect of alterations in mechanical ventilator settings on pulmonary gas exchange in hyaline membrane disease. *Arch Dis Child* 1971; **46**: 152–9.

44. Zavala E, Ferrer M, Polese G, *et al.* Effect of inverse I:E ratio ventilation on pulmonary gas exchange in acute respiratory distress syndrome. *Anesthesiology* 1998; **88**: 35–42.

45. Armstrong BW Jr, MacIntyre NR. Pressure-controlled, inverse ratio ventilation that avoids air trapping in the adult respiratory distress syndrome. *Crit Care Med* 1995; **823**: 279–85.

46. Mancebo J, Vallverdu I, Bak E, *et al.* Volume-controlled ventilation and pressure-controlled inverse ratio ventilation: a comparison of their effects in ARDS patients. *Monaldi Arch Chest Dis* 1994; **49**: 201–7.

47. Marcy TW, Marini JJ. Inverse ratio ventilation in ARDS. Rationale and implementation. *Chest* 1991; **100**: 494–504.

48. Gillespie DJ. High-frequency ventilation. A new concept in mechanical ventilation. *Mayo Clin Proc* 1983; **58**: 187–96.

49. el-Baz NM, Caldarelli DD, Holinger LD, *et al.* High frequency ventilation through a small catheter for laser surgery of laryngotracheal and bronchial disorders. *Ann Otol Rhinol Laryngol* 1985; **94**(5 Pt 1): 483–8.

50. Fort P, Farmer C, Westerman J, *et al.* High-frequency oscillatory ventilation for adult respiratory distress syndrome – a pilot study. *Crit Care Med* 1997; **25**: 937–47.

51. Delafosse C, Chevrolet JC, Suter P, Cox JN Necrotizing tracheobronchitis: a complication of high frequency jet ventilation. *Virchows Arch A Pathol Anat Histopathol* 1988; **413**: 257–64.

52. Mehta S, Lapinsky SE, Hallett DC, *et al.* Prospective trial of high-frequency oscillation in adults with acute respiratory distress syndrome. *Crit Care Med.* 2001; **29**: 1360–9.

53. Derdak S, Mehta S, Stewart TE, *et al.* Multicenter Oscillatory Ventilation For Acute Respiratory Distress Syndrome Trial (MOAT) Study Investigators High-frequency oscillatory ventilation for acute respiratory distress syndrome in adults: a randomized, controlled trial. *Am J Respir Crit Care Med* 2002; **166**(6): 801–8.

54. Branson RD, Johannigman JA, Campbell RS, Davis K Jr. Closed-loop mechanical ventilation. *Respir Care* 2002; **47**: 427–51.

55. Branson RD, Davis K, Jr. Dual control modes: combining volume and pressure breaths. *Respir Care Clin North Am* 2001; **7**: 397–408.

56. Amato MB, Barbas CS, Bonassa J, *et al.* Volume-assured pressure support ventilation (VAPSV). A new approach for reducing muscle workload during acute respiratory failure. *Chest* 1992; **102**: 1225–34.

57. MacIntyre NR, Gropper C, Westfall T. Combining pressure-limiting and volume-cycling features in a patient-interactive mechanical breath. *Crit Care Med* 1994; **22**: 353–7.

58. Guldager H, Nielsen SL, Carl P, Soerensen MB. A comparison of volume control and pressure-regulated volume control ventilation in acute respiratory failure. *Crit Care* 1997; **1**: 75–7.

59. Brunner JX, Iotti GA. Adaptive Support Ventilation (ASV). *Minerva Anesthesiol* 2002; **68**: 365–8.

60. Tassaux D, Dalmas E, Gratadour P, Jolliet P. Patient-ventilator interactions during partial ventilatory support: a preliminary study comparing the effects of adaptive support ventilation with synchronized intermittent mandatory ventilation plus inspiratory pressure support. *Crit Care Med* 2002; **30**: 801–7.

61. Petter AH, Chiolero RL, Cassina T, *et al.* Automatic 'respirator/weaning' with adaptive support ventilation: the effect on duration of endotracheal intubation and patient management. *Anesth Analg* 2003; **97**: 1743–50.

62. Holt SJ, Sanders RC, Thurman TL, Heulitt MJ. An evaluation of Automode, a computer-controlled ventilator mode, with the Siemens Servo 300A ventilator, using a porcine model. *Respir Care* 2001; **46**: 26–36.

63. Grasso S, Ranieri VM. Proportional assist ventilation. *Respir Care Clin North Am* 2001; 465–73.

64. Ambrosino N, Rossi A. Proportional assist ventilation (PAV): a significant advance or a futile struggle between logic and practice? *Thorax* 2002; **57**: 272–6.

65. Fabry B, Haberthur C, Zappe D, *et al.* Breathing pattern and additional work of breathing in spontaneously breathing patients with different ventilatory demands during inspiratory pressure support and automatic tube compensation. *Intensive Care Med* 1997; **23**: 545–52.

66. Sasaki C, Hoshi K, Wagatsuma T, *et al.* Comparison between tube compensation and pressure support ventilation techniques on respiratory mechanics. *Anaesth Intensive Care* 2003; **31**: 371–5.

67. Hewlett AM, Platt AS, Terry VG. Mandatory minute volume. A new concept in weaning from mechanical ventilation. *Anaesthesia* 1977; **32**: 163–9.

68. Quan SF, Parides GC, Knoper SR Mandatory minute volume (MMV) ventilation: an overview. *Respir Care* 1990; **35**: 898–905.

69. Stock MC, Downs JB, Frolicher DA. Airway pressure release ventilation. *Crit Care Med* 1987; **15**: 462–6

70. Frawley PM, Habashi NM. Airway pressure release ventilation: theory and practice. *AACN Clin Issues* 2001; **12**: 234–46.

71. Hill NS. Clinical applications of body ventilators. *Chest* 1986; **90**: 897–905.

72. Kinnear W, Petch M, Taylor G, Shneerson J. Assisted ventilation using cuirass respirators. *Eur Respir J* 1988; **1**: 198–203.

73. Spitzer SA, Fink G, Mittelman M. External high frequency ventilation in severe chronic obstructive pulmonary disease. *Chest* 1993; **104**: 1698–701.

74. Hardinge FM, Davies RJ, Stradling JR. Effect of short-term high frequency negative pressure ventilation on gas exchange using the Hayek oscillator in normal subjects *Thorax* 1995; **50**: 44–9.

75. Corrado A, Gorini M, Ginnani R, *et al.* Negative pressure ventilation versus controlled mechanical ventilation in the treatment of acute respiratory failure in COPD patients. *Eur Respir J* 1998; **12**: 519–25.

76. Mehta S, Hill NS. Noninvasive ventilation. *Am J Respir Crit Care Med* 2001; **163**: 540–77.

77. Ashbaugh DG, Bigelow DB, Petty TL, Levine BE. Acute respiratory failure in adults. *Lancet* 1967; **2**: 319–23.

78. Suter PM, Scholobom RM. Determination of functional residual capacity during mechanical ventilation. *Anaesthesiology* 1974; **41**: 605–7.

79. Stokke DB. Review: artificial ventilation with positive end expiratory pressure. Historical background, terminology and pathophysiology. *Eur J Intensive Care Med* 1976: **2**: 77–85.

80. Gattinoni L, Pesanti A, Avalli L, *et al.* Pressure volume curve of total respiratory system in acute respiratory failure: Computed tomographic scan study. *Am Rev Respir Dis* 1987; **136**: 730–6.

81. Gattinoni L, D'Andrea L, Pelosi P *et al.* Regional effects and mechanisms of positive end expiratory pressure in early adult respiratory distress syndrome. *JAMA* 1993; **16**: 2122–7.

82. Malo J, Ali J, Wood LDH. How does positive end expiratory pressure reduce intrapulmonary shunt in canine pulmonary edema? *J Appl Physiol* 1984; **57**: 1002–10.

83. Corbridge TC, Wood LDH, Crawford GP *et al.* Adverse effects of large tidal volumes and low PEEP in canine acid aspiration. *Am Rev Respir Dis* 1990; **142**: 311–15.

84. Gottfried SB, Rossi A, Calverly PM, *et al.* Interrupter technique for measurement of respiratory mechanics anaesthetized cats. *J Appl Physiol* 1984; **56**: 681–90.

85. Bates HT, Rossi A, Milic EJ. Analysis of the behavior of the respiratory system with constant inspiratory flow. *J Appl Physiol,* 1985; **58**: 1840–8.

86. O'Quinn RJ, Marini JJ, Culver BH, *et al.* Transmission of airway pressure to pleural space during lung edema and chest wall restriction. *J Appl Physiol* 1985; **59**: 1171–7.

87. Davis K Jr, Branson RD, Campbell RS, *et al.* The addition of sighs during pressure support ventilation. Is there a benefit? *Chest* 1993; **104**: 867–70.

88. Patroniti N, Foti G, Cortinovis B, *et al.* Sigh improves gas exchange and lung volume in patients with acute respiratory distress syndrome undergoing pressure support ventilation *Anesthesiology* 2002; **96**: 788–94.

89. Hickling KG, Walsh J, Henderson S, Jackson R. Low mortality rate in adult respiratory distress syndrome using low-volume, pressure-limited ventilation with permissive hypercapnia: a prospective study. *Crit Care Med* 1994; **22**: 1568–78.

90. Mutlu GM, Factor P, Schwartz DE, Sznajder J. Severe status asthmaticus: management with permissive hypercapnia and inhalation anesthesia. *Crit Care Med* 2002; **30**: 477–80.

91. Bigatello LM, Patroniti N, Sangalli F. Permissive hypercapnia. *Curr Opin Crit Care* 2001; **1**: 34–40.

92. Burchardi H. New strategies in mechanical ventilation for acute lung injury. *Eur Respir J* 1996; **9**: 1063–7.

93. O'Croinin D, Ni Chonghaile M, Higgins B, Laffey JG. Bench-to-bedside review: Permissive hypercapnia. *Crit Care* 2005; **9**: 51–9.

94. Pelosi P, D'Andrea L, Vitale G, *et al.* Vertical gradient of regional lung inflation in adult respiratory distress syndrome. *Am J Respir Crit Care Med* 1994; **149**: 8–13.

95. Douglas WW, Rehder K, Beynen FM, *et al.* Improved oxygenation in patients with acute respiratory failure: the prone position. *Am Rev Respir Dis* 1977; **115**: 559–66.

96. Guerin C, Badet M, Rosselli S, *et al.* Effects of prone position on alveolar recruitment and oxygenation in acute lung injury. *Intensive Care Med* 1999; **25**: 1222–30.

97. Lamm WJE, Graham MM, Albert RK. Mechanism by which the prone position improves oxygenation in acute lung injury. *Am J Respir Crit Care Med* 1994; **150**: 184–93.

98. Chatte G, Sab J, Dubois J, *et al.* Prone position in mechanically ventilated patients with severe acute respiratory failure. *Am J Respir Crit Care Med* 1997; **155**: 473–8.

99. Albert RK. Prone ventilation. *Clin Chest Med* 2000; **21**: 511–17.

100. Jackson RM. Pulmonary oxygen toxicity. *Chest* 1985; **88**: 900–5.

101. Capellier G, Maupoil V, Boussat S, *et al.* Oxygen toxicity and tolerance. *Minerva Anesthesiol* 1999; **65**: 388–92.

102. Dreyfuss D, Soler P, Bassett G, Saumon G. High inflation pressure pulmonary edema: respective effects of high airway pressure, high tidal volume, and positive end expiratory pressure. *Am Rev Respir Dis* 1988; **137**: 1159–64.

103. ARDS Network (The Acute Respiratory Distress Syndrome Network). Ventilation with lower tidal volumes as compared with traditional tidal volumes for acute lung injury and the acute respiratory distress syndrome. *N Engl J Med* 2000; **342**: 1301–8.

104. McGough EK, Banner MJ, Melker RJ. Variations in tidal volume with portable transport ventilators. *Respir Care* 1992; **37**: 233–9.

105. Bartel LP, Bazik JR, Powner DJ. Compression volume during mechanical ventilation: comparison of ventilators and tubing circuits. *Crit Care Med* 1985; **13**: 851–4.

106. Hess D, McCurdy S, Simmons M. Compression volume in adult ventilator circuits: a comparison of five disposable circuits and a nondisposable circuit. *Respir Care* 1991; **36**: 1113–18.

107. Sassoon CS, Foster GT. Patient ventilator asynchrony. *Curr Opin Crit Care* 2001; 7: 28–33.

108. Brower RG, Lanken PN, MacIntyre N, *et al*. National Heart, Lung, and Blood Institute ARDS Clinical Trials Network. Higher versus lower positive end-expiratory pressures in patients with the acute respiratory distress syndrome. *N Engl J Med* 2004; **351**: 327–36.

109. Parsons PE, Eisner MD, Thompson BT, *et al*. NHLBI Acute Respiratory Distress Syndrome Clinical Trials Network. Lower tidal volume ventilation and plasma cytokine markers of inflammation in patients with acute lung injury. *Crit Care Med* 2005; **33**: 1–6.

110. Ferguson ND, Frutos-Vivar F, Esteban A, *et al*. Mechanical Ventilation International Study Group. Airway pressures, tidal volumes, and mortality in patients with acute respiratory distress syndrome. *Crit Care Med* 2005; **33**: 21–30.

111. Conti G, Antonelli M, Navalesi P, *et al*. Noninvasive vs. conventional mechanical ventilation in patients with chronic obstructive pulmonary disease after failure of medical treatment in the ward: a randomized trial. *Intensive Care Med* 2002; **28**: 1701–7.

112. Brochard L, Mancebo J, Wysocki M, *et al*. Noninvasive ventilation for acute exacerbations of chronic obstructive pulmonary disease. *N Engl J Med* 1995; **333**: 817–22.

113. Lightowler JV, Wedzicha JA, Elliott MW, Ram FS. Non-invasive positive pressure ventilation to treat respiratory failure resulting from exacerbations of chronic obstructive pulmonary disease: Cochrane systematic review and meta-analysis. *BMJ* 2003; **326**: 185.

114. Vitacca M, Lanini B, Nava S, *et al*. Inspiratory muscle workload due to dynamic intrinsic PEEP in stable COPD patients: effects of two different settings of non-invasive pressure-support ventilation. *Monaldi Arch Chest Dis* 2004; **61**: 81–5.

115. Guerin C, Milic-Emili J, Fournier G. Effect of PEEP on work of breathing in mechanically ventilated COPD patients. *Intensive Care Med* 2000; **26**: 1207–14.

116. Fernandez MM, Villagra A, Blanch L, Fernandez R Non-invasive mechanical ventilation in status asthmaticus. *Intensive Care Med* 2001; **27**: 486–92.

117. Tassaux D, Jolliet P, Roeseler J, Chevrolet JC. Effects of helium-oxygen on intrinsic positive end-expiratory pressure in intubated and mechanically ventilated patients with severe chronic obstructive pulmonary disease. *Crit Care Med* 2000; **28**: 2721–8.

118. Georgopoulos D, Kondili E, Prinianakis G. How to set the ventilator in asthma. *Monaldi Arch Chest Dis* 2000; **55**: 74–83.

119. Jain S, Hanania NA, Guntupalli KK. Ventilation of patients with asthma and obstructive lung disease. *Crit Care Clin* 1998; **14**: 685–705.

120. Schaeffer EM, Pohlman A, Morgan S, Hall JB. Oxygenation in status asthmaticus improves during ventilation with helium-oxygen. *Crit Care Med* 1999; 27: 2666–70.

121. Esteban A, Frutos F, Tobin MJ, *et al*. A comparison of four methods of weaning patients from mechanical ventilation. Spanish Lung Failure Collaborative Group. *N Engl J Med* 1995; **332**: 345–50.

122. Jounieaux V, Duran A, Levi-Valensi P Synchronized intermittent mandatory ventilation with and without pressure support ventilation in weaning patients with COPD from mechanical ventilation. *Chest* 1994; **105**: 1204–10.

123. Alia I, Esteban A. Weaning from mechanical ventilation. *Crit Care* 2000; **4**: 72–80.

124. Ely EW, Baker AM, Dunagan DP, *et al*. Effect on the duration of mechanical ventilation of identifying patients capable of breathing spontaneously. *N Engl J Med* 1996; **335**: 1864–9.

125. Perren A, Domenighetti G, Mauri S, *et al*. Protocol-directed weaning from mechanical ventilation: clinical outcome in patients randomized for a 30-min or 120-min trial with pressure support ventilation. *Intensive Care Med* 2002; **28**: 1058–63.

126. Abramson NS, Wald KS, Grenvik ANA, *et al*. Adverse occurrences in intensive care units. *JAMA* 1980; **244**: 1582–4.

127. Peterson HP, Baier H. Incidence of pulmonary barotraumas in a medical ICU. *Crit Care Med* 1983; **11**: 67–9.

128. Anzueto A, Frutos-Vivar F, Esteban A, *et al*. Incidence, risk factors and outcome of barotrauma in mechanically ventilated patients. *Intensive Care Med* 2004; **30**: 612–9.

129. Sandur S, Stoller JK. Pulmonary complications of mechanical ventilation. *Clin Chest Med* 1999; **20**: 223–47.

130. Maunder RJ, Pierson DJ, Hudson LD. Subcutaneous and mediastinal emphysema: pathophysiology, diagnosis, and management. *Arch Intern Med* 1984; **144**: 1447–53.

131. Woodside KJ, van Sonnenberg E, Chon KS, *et al.* Pneumothorax in patients with acute respiratory distress syndrome: pathophysiology, detection, and treatment. *J Intensive Care Med* 2003; **18**: 9–20.

132. Webb HH, Tierny DF. Experimental pulmonary edema due to intermittent positive pressure ventilation with high inflation pressures: protection by positive end expiratory pressure *Am Rev Respir Dis* 1974; **110**: 556–65.

133. Kolobow T, Morretti MP, Fumagalli R, *et al.* Severe impairment in lung function induced by high peak airway pressure during mechanical ventilation *Am Rev Respir Dis* 1987; **135**: 312–15.

134. Tsuno K, Prato P, Kolobow T. Acute lung injury from mechanical ventilation at moderately high pressure. *J Appl Physiol* 1990; **69**: 577–83.

135. Dreyfuss D, Saumon G. Ventilator induced lung injury Lessons from experimental studies. *Am J Respir Crit Care Med* 1998; **157**: 294–323.

136. American Thoracic Society; Infectious Diseases Society of America. Guidelines for the management of adults with hospital-acquired, ventilator-associated, and healthcare-associated pneumonia. *Am J Respir Crit Care Med* 2005; **171**: 388–416.

137. Dambrosio M, Cinnella G, Brienza N, *et al.* Effects of positive end-expiratory pressure on right ventricular function in COPD patients during acute ventilatory failure. *Intensive Care Med* 1996; **22**: 923–32.

138. Andrivet P, Adnot S, Brun-Buisson C, *et al.* Involvement of ANF in the acute antidiuresis during PEEP ventilation. *J Appl Physiol* 1988; **65**: 1967–74.

139. Pingleton SK. Complications of acute respiratory failure. *Med Clin North Am* 1983; **67**: 725–46.

140. Burchiel KJ, Steege TD, Wyler AR. Intracranial pressure changes in brain-injured patients requiring positive end-expiratory pressure ventilation. *Neurosurgery* 1981;8:443–9.

6

Emergency applications of noninvasive ventilation

VINAY MAHESHWARI, NICHOLAS S HILL

INTRODUCTION

Noninvasive ventilation (NIV) refers to techniques that assist ventilation without requiring an invasive airway. The most commonly used noninvasive technique is noninvasive positive pressure ventilation (NIPPV), which provides intermittent positive pressure to the upper airway via a mask or similar interface. In the early twentieth century, NIV was provided mainly by negative pressure ventilators (so called 'body ventilators'). In the 1960s, NPPV delivered via mouthpieces was used at some centers for patients with neuromuscular conditions but did not gain widespread acceptance. With the introduction of nasal masks to deliver continuous positive airway pressure (CPAP) to patients with obstructive sleep apnea, NIPPV delivered nocturnally via nasal masks was developed and used to treat hypoventilation related to neuromuscular disease.[1,2] This has been shown to be effective and is widely accepted as a standard therapy for chronic hypercapnic respiratory failure due to neuromuscular disease, chest wall deformity, or disorders of respiratory drive.[3]

More recently, NIPPV via nasal or oronasal masks has been extensively studied for treatment of acute respiratory failure in various settings. Randomized controlled trials have shown that this method of ventilation is efficacious in acute exacerbations of chronic obstructive pulmonary disease (COPD),[4–7] cardiogenic pulmonary edema,[8,9] hypoxemic respiratory failure in immunocompromised patients,[10,11] and persistent weaning failure.[12,13] Results of these studies have shown that NIV decreases the need for invasive mechanical ventilation, reduces mortality, and shortens the length of hospital stay, particularly in COPD exacerbations.[14,15]

For the purposes of this chapter, NIV refers to the delivery of positive pressure via noninvasive techniques using nasal or facial masks. Ventilatory support is offered by providing higher inspiratory and lower expiratory pressures, similar to invasive ventilation. Portable ventilators, known as 'bilevel' ventilators, can be set to provide inspiratory positive airway pressure (IPAP) and expiratory positive airway pressure (EPAP). These settings are akin to pressure support and positive end-expiratory pressure (PEEP) found in critical care ventilators, except that IPAP is the total inspiratory pressure and is equal to the pressure support plus PEEP. Continuous positive airway pressure delivers positive airway pressure that is maintained steadily throughout the respiratory cycle in a spontaneously breathing patient and does not actively assist ventilation. However, we discuss both NIV and CPAP here because the two modalities are administered in essentially the same manner, and CPAP has important applications in certain forms of respiratory failure.

Our focus will be on the use of NIV in emergency settings, including the selection of appropriate patients for NIV as well as some practical suggestions for selection of ventilator modes and mask interfaces, initiation of NIV, techniques of monitoring, and management of complications.

RATIONALE FOR NONINVASIVE VENTILATION

The rationale for using NIV as opposed to invasive methods is to avoid complications associated with invasive mechanical ventilation. Endotracheal intubation can be complicated by aspiration, trauma to upper airway structures, arrhythmias, and hypotension. Tracheostomy placement carries the risk of hemorrhage, stomal infections, and intubation of a false lumen. Furthermore, endotracheal invasion provides a direct conduit to the lower airways, thereby increasing the risk of nosocomial pneumonia. In comparison with NIV, invasive mechanical ventilation is associated with higher rates of pneumonia, sinusitis, and sepsis (see Table 6.1).[16–18] Persistent intubation can lead to difficulties with upper airway obstruction and speech by causing tracheal stenosis, tracheomalacia, or damage to the vocal cords and larynx. In properly selected patients, NIV is preferred over invasive mechanical ventilation because it avoids these complications while better preserving speech, eating by mouth, and expectoration.

Table 6.1 *Relative advantages of noninvasive and invasive mechanical ventilation*

Noninvasive ventilation	Invasive ventilation
Lower incidence of pneumonia and aspiration	Ability to provide higher inspired oxygen concentration
Minimal risk for barotrauma	Higher inspiratory pressures achieved
Reduced trauma to larynx, trachea and vocal cords	Requires less initial time investment by staff
Less sedation required	
Improved speech capability	Less trouble with air leaking
Able to receive oral nutrition	Better suited for patients with copious secretions
More comfortable for most patients	No conjunctival irritation
Easier expectoration	No risk of nasal bridge ulceration
	More assured ventilation and oxygenation

MECHANISMS OF ACTION IN ACUTE RESPIRATORY FAILURE

Noninvasive ventilation reverses gas exchange abnormalities without the need for airway invasion by reducing the work of breathing, improving alveolar ventilation, and avoiding respiratory muscle fatigue.[19] By intermittently applying positive airway pressure during inspiration, pressure support ventilation (PSV) administered noninvasively reduces esophageal pressure swings and diaphragmatic electromyographic (EMG) signals during spontaneous breathing, providing clear evidence that it reduces inspiratory muscle work. It also augments spontaneous tidal volumes, improving the efficiency of breathing.[19,20] Positive end-expiratory pressure applied noninvasively further reduces work of breathing in hyperinflated patients by counterbalancing intrinsic PEEP and lowering the inspiratory threshold load and, in patients with pulmonary edema, by improving respiratory system compliance.[19] When combined in patients with COPD, pressure support and

PEEP have an additive effect on the reduction in work of breathing.[21]

Gas exchange improvements with pressure support alone are mostly due to improvements in alveolar ventilation and not changes in ventilation/perfusion ($\dot{V}/Q$) matching.[22] However, the application of PEEP or CPAP opens collapsed airways, thereby improving $\dot{V}/Q$ mismatch and shunt.[23] Also, by increasing intrathoracic pressure and thus lowering preload and afterload, CPAP can have either beneficial or deleterious hemodynamic effects. Those with high pulmonary capillary wedge pressures and impaired left ventricular systolic function benefit from the reductions in preload and afterload, whereas those with diminished intravascular volume and normal systolic function may experience a decline of cardiac output due to reduced ventricular filling.[24] Thus, the combination of pressure support and PEEP offers advantages over either modality alone, but CPAP alone (with attention paid to volume status) has beneficial actions, particularly in patients with cardiogenic pulmonary edema.

INDICATIONS OF NONINVASIVE VENTILATION

Obstructive disorders

CHRONIC OBSTRUCTIVE PULMONARY DISEASE

The strongest evidence for the use of NIV in the emergency setting is for exacerbations of COPD. Several prospective, randomized controlled trials have established that, compared with conventional therapy, NIV improves gas exchange, relieves dyspnea, reduces intubation rates, decreases mortality, and shortens intensive care unit (ICU) and length of hospital stay.[5,6,14,15,25,26] Although NIV is commonly initiated in the emergency ward with patients then transferred to an ICU, one study showed that patients with arterial pH values between 7.25 and 7.35 managed using NIV on general respiratory wards had lower rates of intubation (15 vs. 27 percent) and mortality (10 vs. 20 percent) compared with patients treated conventionally.[7] However, more acidemic patients (pH <7.30) did not manifest significant reductions in intubation or mortality rates, leading the authors to suggest that such patients might have benefited from an ICU admission.

Recent metaanalyses have combined the results of selected randomized controlled studies that compared effects of NIV with conventional therapy in COPD patients exclusively. Endotracheal intubation rates (relative risk reduction of 42 percent), hospital length of stay (mean reduction 3.24 days) and inhospital mortality (relative risk reduction of 41 percent) were significantly reduced with NIV.[15] Subgroup analysis showed that these beneficial effects occurred only in patients with severe exacerbations (pH <7.30), and not in those with milder exacerbations.[27] Although these studies assessing the efficacy of NIV for treatment of COPD exacerbations are heterogeneous with regard to the severity of illness, techniques and equipment used, location of use, and experience of the caregiver team, the benefit of NIV for these patients has been demonstrated repeatedly. Thus, NIV should be considered the ventilatory mode of first choice and a standard of care for selected patients with respiratory insufficiency due to COPD exacerbations.

ASTHMA EXACERBATIONS

Few studies have evaluated the use of NIV for asthma exacerbations partly because most patients respond promptly to medical therapy. In a small study, NIV was successful in improving gas exchange abnormalities and associated with a low rate of intubation in patients presenting with severe respiratory acidosis (mean pH 7.25).[28] A more recent study comparing NIV versus conventional medical therapy in severe acute asthma found that NIV more rapidly improved forced expiratory volume in 1 second (FEV_1) (53.5 vs. 28.5 percent increase in FEV_1 in the first hour) and reduced the rate of hospitalization (17.6 vs. 63.5 percent).[29] These results are promising but there is insufficient evidence to recommend NIV for routine treatment of acute asthma. In patients not responding promptly to medical therapy who manifest evidence of impending respiratory muscle fatigue, however, a cautious trial of NIV should be considered.

CYSTIC FIBROSIS AND BRONCHIECTASIS

The physiologic defects of these diseases resemble those of COPD in a number of ways, but an important difference is that both are characterized by thick, copious secretions that may be difficult to expectorate. Nonetheless, success with NIV has been reported during acute exacerbations in cystic fibrosis patients with end-stage lung disease and the modality may be useful as a bridge to lung transplantation.[30,31] If NIV is to be used in these patients, particular attention should be paid to assisting with secretion removal.

Hypoxemic respiratory failure

Treatment of hypoxemic respiratory failure (PaO_2/ FiO_2 ratio <200, severe tachypnea with respiratory rate >35/min, and respiratory distress) with NIV has been studied extensively with conflicting results. This category comprises a heterogeneous group of etiologies including pneumonia, cardiogenic pulmonary edema, acute respiratory distress syndrome (ARDS), aspiration pneumonia, atelectasis, and trauma. An early randomized trial showed benefit of NIV only in a hypercapnic subgroup of patients.[6] Subsequently, other studies have observed favorable effects in nonhypercapnic patients as well. One randomized trial demonstrated that NIV improved oxygenation as rapidly as intubation, reduced the need for intubation to a third of patients, and showed trends toward a decreased mortality and ICU length of stay.[18] In addition, complications such as pneumonia and sinusitis were more frequent in the conventionally ventilated group.

Most recently, Ferrer et al. compared NIV with conventional oxygen therapy in patients with severe hypoxemic respiratory failure and observed a lower incidence of septic shock, ICU mortality, and 90-day mortality in the NIV group.[32] This effect was most pronounced in patients with pneumonia but was insignificant in those with ARDS. Thus, NIV improves gas exchange and avoids intubation in some patients with hypoxemic respiratory failure, but the category is so broad, it is difficult to apply the results to individual patients. Therefore, the individual diagnostic categories will be considered below.

Cardiogenic pulmonary edema

The use of CPAP alone to treat acute pulmonary edema was first described many decades ago. Three randomized controlled trials have demonstrated that CPAP (10–12.5 cm H_2O) more rapidly improves oxygenation and reduces the need for intubation among patients with pulmonary edema compared with conventional medical treatment.[8,23,33] A metaanalysis of these studies derived an absolute 26 percent reduction in the need for intubation and a trend toward reduced hospital mortality among patients treated with CPAP.[34]

Based on the rationale that it would more rapidly reduce work of breathing and dyspnea than CPAP alone, a number of studies have evaluated the use of pressure support plus PEEP (or 'bilevel' ventilation) to treat acute pulmonary edema. In a randomized trial comparing NIV with conventional medical management in 40 patients, NIV lowered intubation rates and more rapidly improved oxygenation, but had no effect on inhospital mortality and length of stay.[9] In a randomized trial comparing CPAP to bilevel airway positive pressure ventilation, bilevel ventilation more rapidly improved oxygenation and lowered $PaCO_2$, but again there was no difference in mortality or intubation rates.[35] This study was terminated early, however, due to an increased incidence of myocardial infarction in the bilevel ventilation group, although a subsequent trial reported in preliminary form has shown no such increase. More recently, it has been shown that patients presenting to the emergency ward with pulmonary edema and treated with NIV had no improvement in overall clinical outcomes, although patients in the hypercapnic subgroup had significantly lower intubation rates.[36] Thus, CPAP or 'bilevel' ventilation is indicated for the initial management of selected patients with acute cardiogenic pulmonary edema. Either may be used with the expectation that outcomes will be similar, but adding inspiratory pressure support may be advantageous in patients with hypercapnia or persistent dyspnea.[19]

Pneumonia

One randomized trial has compared NIV with conventional management in the treatment of hypoxemic respiratory failure due to severe community-acquired pneumonia. Patients treated with NIV had lower rates of intubation and shorter ICU lengths of stay but the benefit was restricted to the COPD subgroup of patients.[37] In another randomized trial with CPAP (10 cm H_2O) alone compared with conventional oxygen therapy in patients with hypoxemic, nonhypercapnic respiratory failure, Delclaux et al. found no benefit of CPAP other than an earlier improvement in oxygenation.[38] Subsequently, Ferrer et al. found that NIV reduced intubation rates in a subgroup of 34 patients with pneumonia compared with conventional oxygen therapy.[32] These studies suggest that NIV may be superior to CPAP alone in the therapy of patients with hypoxemic respiratory failure, but no trials have yet directly compared them. Also, intubation rates are still high in patients with respiratory failure due to severe community-acquired pneumonia, even when treated with NIV (two-thirds of patients).[39] Thus, NIV can be recommended for patients with pneumonia who have underlying COPD, but should be used only with great caution in patients with severe pneumonia without underlying COPD.

Acute respiratory distress syndrome

A brief report examined the effects of NIV on patients with ARDS/acute lung injury. Intubation was avoided in 6 of 12 episodes of ARDS in 10 patients when NIV was used as the initial mode to assist ventilation.[40] However, the more recent Ferrer study showed no benefit of NIV in the cohort of ARDS patients.[32] Based on this, NIV cannot be recommended routinely to treat ARDS patients. However, a cautious trial might be considered in otherwise stable patients with single organ system involvement without very severe oxygenation defects (PaO_2/FiO_2 >100) and with the proviso that they are intubated without delay if they show any signs of deterioration.

Restrictive/neuromuscular disease

Treatment of chronic respiratory failure in patients with neuromuscular disorders and thoracic cage abnormalities with NIV is well accepted. However, few studies have examined the use of NIV in this population in the setting of acute respiratory failure. In one small study, four kyphoscoliotic patients with acute respiratory decompensation were treated with nasal NIV and experienced significant improvements in PaO_2, $PaCO_2$ and pulmonary function.[41] With the success of NIV for these patients in the chronic setting, it is considered the treatment of first choice when decompensation occurs.[3]

Bach et al. have described an approach to treating patients using long-term NIV for restrictive thoracic disorders at home who develop acute respiratory infections.[42] They use NIV 24 hours daily to assist ventilation, with a cough assist device to facilitate clearance of secretions as often as necessary and if the oxygen saturation drops below 90 percent. This approach avoids the need for intubation or even hospitalization in most cases, but requires well-trained patients and caregivers.[43] However, bulbar dysfunction, as occurs with amyotrophic lateral sclerosis, limits the success of this approach.

There is little information regarding NIV use for deteriorations of idiopathic pulmonary fibrosis (IPF). In a small retrospective study of patients with IPF admitted to an ICU with acute respiratory failure, only 5 of 15 were deemed candidates for NIV. Three of these died and the others required invasive mechanical ventilation.[44] Thus, NIV appears to offer little or no benefit to this subgroup of patients.

Immunocompromised patients

Avoidance of intubation is of particular importance in immunocompromised patients. Invasive mechanical ventilation is associated with poor outcomes in this population because of the associated increase in infectious complications.[45,46] When compared with invasive mechanical ventilation for respiratory failure due to Pneumocystis carinii pneumonia, NIV improved survival.[47] In a study of neutropenic patients with hypoxemia and pulmonary infiltrates, most of whom had hematologic malignancies, the intermittent use of NIV reduced the need for intubation, serious complications, and ICU and hospital mortality.[48] Similar results have been noted in patients with acute respiratory failure following solid-organ transplantation.[10] In immunocompromised patients who do not require emergent intubation or have other contraindications (see section on Patient selection), NIV is now considered the ventilatory mode of first choice to treat respiratory failure. However, it is important not to delay intubation if there is deterioration or a lack of improvement despite initiation of NIV.

Weaning and extubation

Complications increase as intubation becomes prolonged, so strategies that shorten its duration would be expected to lower complication rates. In difficult-to-wean patients NIV has been used as a way to facilitate extubation. In one series, trauma patients were extubated before meeting standard extubation criteria and supported using NIV with 59 percent avoiding reintubation.[49] Patients with COPD intubated for 48 hours, who failed a T-piece weaning trial were randomized to either extubation followed by facemask NIV or continued invasive pressure support ventilation. Early extubation to NIV in these patients increased the percentage of patients weaned at 28 days, reduced the duration of mechanical ventilation and ICU stay, improved survival, and was associated with a trend for fewer pneumonias. Another study confirmed that early extubation to NIV shortened the duration of invasive mechanical ventilation but other outcomes were not improved.[50] A more recent prospective trial of 43 patients with 'persistent' weaning failure, who had failed weaning trials on three consecutive days, randomized patients to either early extubation to NIV or continued invasive mechanical ventilation and conventional weaning.[13] The NIV group had shorter durations of invasive mechanical ventilation, decreased lengths of stay and need for tracheostomies, lower incidence of complications, and improved survival. Thus, evidence supports the use of NIV to expedite extubation, mainly in COPD patients, but evidence to support this approach in patients with other diagnoses is lacking.

Noninvasive ventilation has also been used in respiratory failure occurring after extubation in patients who meet standard extubation criteria.[51] Although it may be effective in COPD patients,[52] a recent trial examining this approach in patients with various causes for their respiratory failure (only 13 percent COPD patients) found that NIV failed to lower extubation rates and was associated with a higher ICU mortality.[53] Intubations were delayed longer, perhaps excessively, in the NIV supported group than in the conventional treatment group, possibly explaining the higher mortality. Thus, NIV to treat extubation failure cannot be recommended as a routine therapy except in COPD patients.

Other applications

CHEST TRAUMA

Chest trauma patients have been successfully supported with CPAP. In a trial of 69 patients with multiple rib fractures and hypoxemia, those randomized to CPAP had shorter ICU and hospital lengths of stay and fewer infectious complications than patients intubated immediately.[54] However, patients requiring FiO_2 >40 percent were excluded and the intubated group had a greater injury severity on presentation. Some anecdotal reports indicate that NIV can also be used to assist patients with chest trauma, but those with burns fare less well.[55] Given the lack of evidence, however, it is difficult to make recommendations.

POSTOPERATIVE PATIENTS

In an uncontrolled study, patients who received surgery for various reasons and developed respiratory failure postoperatively were treated with bilevel positive pressure ventilation via facemask and had low reintubation rates.[56] Controlled trials have demonstrated that NIV improves oxygenation and survival after lung resection[57,58] and better sustains lung function after gastroplasty.[59] Thus, accumulating evidence supports the use of NIV to treat postoperative respiratory insufficiency after certain types of surgery, particularly lung resection. More work, however, is needed to establish the role of NIV after other types of surgery.

'DO NOT INTUBATE' PATIENTS

The use of NIV to treat patients who refuse intubation has aroused controversy. Some have argued that NIV can reduce dyspnea and even reverse respiratory failure in patients who would otherwise die, whereas others opine that it merely prolongs the dying process and contributes to discomfort in terminally ill patients.[60] Observational studies on the use of NIV in patients who refuse intubation indicate that survival to discharge may be as high as 60 percent, with the best survival in patients with COPD or congestive heart failure.[61] For this reason, NIV may be tried in such patients as long as they and their families are informed that it is being used as a form of life support and given the option to decline.

PRACTICAL APPLICATION OF NONINVASIVE VENTILATION

Patient selection

Noninvasive ventilation avoids the need for intubation by serving as a 'crutch', providing the critical time needed to allow medical therapy to reverse the underlying cause of the respiratory failure. Therefore, the likelihood of success is greater if NIV is used as soon as the need for ventilatory assistance arises. It may be ineffective if the patient severely decompensates, and undue delay of needed intubation by a futile trial of NIV may even be harmful. Patients with elevated $PaCO_2$ (>90 mm Hg) and severely reduced pH levels (<7.10), as well as higher acuity of illness (APACHE II >20), have lower rates of success with NIV, consistent with the idea that early use of NIV enhances success.[62] In addition, patients who manifest no improvements in gas exchange and vital signs within the first 2 hours of NIV initiation are more likely not to respond.[63]

Based on these predictors of success and entry criteria used by previous studies, patient selection criteria for the application of NIV in acute respiratory failure can be distilled into a simple two-step process. Using clinical markers of respiratory distress such as moderate to severe dyspnea, tachypnea, accessory muscle use, and paradoxical breathing, the first step identifies patients who require ventilatory assistance and are at risk for intubation. The level of tachypnea used as a criterion depends on the cause of respiratory failure; patients with hypoxemic respiratory failure usually having higher respiratory rates (>30/min) for a given level of distress than those with COPD exacerbations (>24/min).[19] Blood gas criteria are also used for patients with hypercapnic respiratory failure, either acute or acute-on-chronic (pH <7.35, $PaCO_2$ >45 mm Hg), as well as hypoxemic respiratory failure (PaO_2/FiO_2 <200). Noninvasive ventilation is not indicated for patients with only mild respiratory distress or minimal gas exchange abnormalities who are likely to succeed with medical management alone.

The second step in selecting patients for NIV is to screen out those with a low likelihood of success who should be promptly intubated. Noninvasive ventilation requires time for initiation and is inappropriate for those with cardiac or respiratory arrest who should be intubated immediately. Other contraindications include hemodynamic instability, acute severe cardiac ischemia, uncontrolled arrhythmias, or upper gastrointestinal bleeding (Box 6.1).[3,63] Other reasons to withhold NIV include an inability to cooperate, protect the airway, or fit a mask. Excessive secretions and mental obtundation are relative contraindications, and judgment must be exercised when deciding on individual cases.[19]

Box 6.1 Relative contraindications to NIV use

- Cardiac/respiratory arrest
- Hemodynamically unstable (i.e. systolic blood pressure <90 mm Hg resistant to fluids)
- Uncontrolled arrhythmias
- Severe uncontrolled upper gastrointestinal bleeding
- Undrained pneumothorax
- Multiorgan system failure
- High risk for aspiration
- Unable to clear respiratory secretions
- Agitation
- Unable to cooperate
- Unable to fit mask
- Facial surgery, trauma, or deformity
- Upper airway or esophageal surgery

The etiology of respiratory failure is another important consideration in patient selection and predicts success. The potential to reverse the predisposing factors within hours to days with the use of treatments such as diuretics, bronchodilators, and/or steroids, is important. Acting as a 'crutch', NIV provides support and allows time for medical management to be effective. However, the need for prolonged (more than a few days) continuous ventilatory assistance, particularly when coupled with the need for nutritional support and multiple diagnostic procedures, is a challenge for NIV. Figure 6.1 outlines an approach to NIV application in the setting of acute respiratory failure.

Modes and ventilators

Both 'critical care' and portable pressure-limited 'bilevel' ventilators have been used to deliver NIV in the emergency setting but there are no studies directly comparing efficacies. Gas exchange and work of breathing improvements appear to be equivalent with both types of ventilators as long as expiratory pressure is applied along with inspiratory pressure during 'bilevel' ventilation.[64] 'Bilevel' devices are pressure generators that deliver adjustable inspiratory and expiratory pressures (IPAP and EPAP) and have the ability to compensate for leaking.[65] Some of these devices have features that may enhance patient comfort and synchrony, including an adjustable 'rise time' (i.e. the rapidity of reaching target inspiratory pressure) and the ability to limit inspiratory duration. Critical care ventilators, on the other hand, offer greater pressure and flow delivery capabilities, oxygen blenders, and better alarm and monitoring features, but have less capability to compensate for leaks. Newer 'bilevel' devices include graphic display screens and oxygen blenders, thus narrowing the differences between the two types. Lacking studies directly comparing the efficacy of both types, the selection of a ventilator usually depends on equipment availability and practitioner preferences and experience.

Most clinicians use pressure-limited as opposed to volume-limited modes for NIV, based on studies showing greater compliance or tolerance with pressure-limited modes.[66,67] However, other outcomes comparing the use of pressure-cycled and volume-cycled ventilators in patients with COPD are similar.[67]

Interfaces

The 'interface', or device used to direct pressurized gas into the upper airway during NIV, is usually a nasal or oronasal mask. Mouthpieces and nasal 'prongs' or 'pillows' (pledgets that insert directly into the nostrils) are sometimes used. Proper mask fit is of the utmost importance to enhance comfort and minimize air leaks, thus optimizing synchrony and maximizing the likelihood of success. Care should be taken to avoid excessive tightening of the mask straps as this may increase pressure on the skin over the bridge of the nose and promote the development of nasal ulcers. Routine use of artificial skin over the nasal bridge reduces the risk of this complication.

Nasal masks have the advantages of facilitating speech, oral intake, and expectoration compared with oronasal masks, and are rated as more comfortable by patients with stable hypercapnia.[68] However, they require patent nasal passages and mouth closure to prevent leaks and are less effective in edentulous patients.[69] Compared with full facial masks, they leak more, deliver lower tidal volumes and eliminate $PaCO_2$ less effectively (see Table 6.2).[68] In the setting of acute respiratory failure, nasal masks are more prone to excessive air leakage through the mouth. Consequently, although efficacy to prevent intubation is similar between both nasal and oronasal masks, initial patient tolerance is better with oronasal masks.[70] For this reason, we recommend oronasal masks for initiating NIV in acute respiratory failure. Because they may cause initial apprehension, discomfort and occasional claustrophobic reactions, however, experienced practitioners who can reassure patients, make adjustments, minimize the adverse reactions and enhance patient comfort should apply oronasal masks.

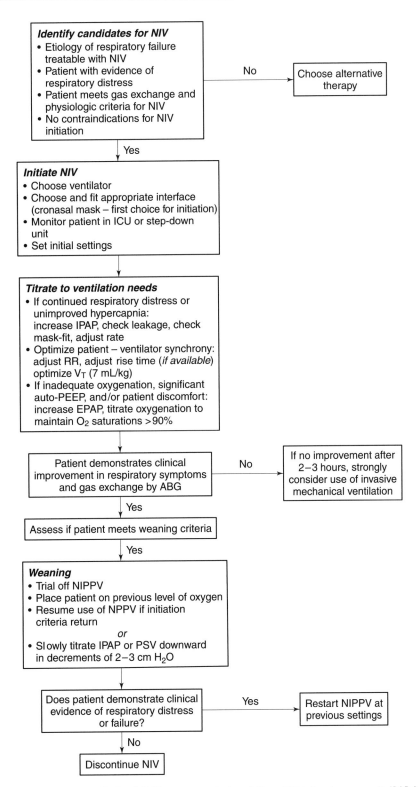

Figure 6.1 *Algorithm for use of noninvasive ventilation (NIV) in acute respiratory failure. ICU, intensive care unit; IPAP, inspiratory positive airway pressure; RR, respiratory rate; V_T, tidal volume, PEEP, positive end expiratory pressure; EPAP, expiratory positive airway pressure; ABG, arterial blood gases; NIPPV, noninvasive positive pressure ventilation; PSV, pressure support ventilation.*

Table 6.2   *Relative advantages of nasal masks and oronasal masks*

Nasal mask	Oronasal mask
Greater comfort	Lowers Pa_{CO_2} more effectively
Less claustrophobia	Delivers higher tidal volumes
Allows easier speech	Reduces air leaking through mouth
Allows oral intake	More effective for mouth breathers
Less gastric distention	Recommended as first line for acute respiratory failure
Expectoration easier	

Newer interfaces include a helmet device that is like a clear inverted bucket fitting over the head and fastening under the axillae. Compared with a conventional facemask, the helmet has lower rates of intolerance, fewer complications, and similar efficacy for preventing intubation.[71] In addition, the helmet may offers an effective way to deliver CPAP to treat cardiogenic pulmonary edema.[72] A mask that covers the entire face (Total Facemask, Respironics, Murraysville, PA) resembling a goalie mask, has also shown promise for enhancing comfort without increasing claustrophobia.[73]

Initiation and settings

INSPIRATORY PRESSURE OR TIDAL VOLUME

Little evidence is available to guide NIV settings, so clinician skill and experience are important. We advocate initiation with a relatively low inspiratory pressure (8–10 cm H_2O) and then increasing over subsequent minutes to hours to 12–20 cm H_2O as tolerated to alleviate respiratory distress. Pressure-limited ventilation delivers preset inspiratory and expiratory pressures that are time cycled. Some investigators have advocated the initial use of higher initial inspiratory pressures (20 cm H_2O), but patients may have difficulty tolerating these high pressures initially. Regardless of the initial pressures chosen, inspiratory pressures should be titrated as tolerated with the following goals in mind: a comfortable patient, alleviation of respiratory distress, decreased respiratory rate, good patient–ventilator synchrony, and enhanced gas exchange. These goals are not always entirely compatible, and it is often necessary to arrive at the best compromise.

EXPIRATORY PRESSURES

Expiratory pressures are set at 3–5 cm H_2O initially, partly to minimize rebreathing in the single ventilator circuit of 'bilevel' ventilators. Higher levels may be necessary, however, to counterbalance intrinsic PEEP in obstructive patients, as well as to improve oxygenation in patients with hypoxemic respiratory failure.

OTHER ADJUSTMENTS

A back-up rate is often used in the acute setting to prevent apneas and assure ventilator cycling in the presence of air leaks. Other adjustments to enhance comfort and synchrony include features to limit inspiratory duration and adjust the 'rise time' required to reach the targeted inspiratory pressure. A shorter inspiratory duration (0.7–1.0 seconds) helps to minimize expiratory asynchrony in COPD patients (who may start exhaling before the ventilator cycles to expiratory pressure), and dyspneic patients usually prefer a short 'rise time' (0.05–0.1 seconds).

OXYGEN SUPPLEMENTATION AND HUMIDIFICATION

Supplemental oxygen is titrated during NIV to maintain oxygen saturation between 90 percent and 92 percent. 'Critical care' ventilators provide the desired Fi_{O_2} via oxygen blenders. With older 'bilevel' ventilators, oxygen is provided directly via a connector in the mask or tubing itself. It is important to recognize, though, that this set-up fails to achieve high levels of oxygenation (maximum Fi_{O_2} 40–50 percent, even at oxygen flow rates of 15 L/min, the maximum recommended). As mentioned previously, newer models, such as the Vision® (Respironics), are now equipped with oxygen blenders. Humidification is usually unnecessary for brief applications (<12 h), but may enhance comfort and is usually recommended for longer applications. If there is significant air leaking, a heated humidifier may maintain a lower nasal resistance.

Monitoring

Prospective randomized trials have shown that NIV can be initiated successfully and safely in many different settings.[3] These include the emergency ward, ICU, step-down units, and general medical wards. Acutely ill patients receiving NIV should be closely monitored to ensure that goals are met. This requires an experienced staff, high-level monitoring capabilities, and the ability to convert to invasive mechanical ventilation if necessary. Current recommendations are that following initiation in an emergency ward, acutely ill patients receiving NIV should be transferred to an ICU setting or a specialized step-down unit until stabilized.[63] COPD patients with milder exacerbations may be managed on general wards if local expertise is adequate.[63] However, such patients should be promptly transferred to an ICU with any sign of deterioration.

Monitoring should consist of frequent assessments of patient comfort and vital signs, particularly respiratory rate. A reduction in respiratory rate within the first 2 hours predicts success.[69] Patient–ventilator synchrony, accessory muscle use, and mask fit should also be assessed frequently. Early improvements in gas exchange are also indicators of success. Pulse oximetry should be monitored continuously, at least during the acute phase, and arterial blood gases obtained intermittently.[67,69,74] If stabilization has not occurred within the first 2–3 hours, then failure of NIV should be declared and the patient intubated if they have not declined. Delay in intubation may lead to increased morbidity and mortality and should be avoided.[75]

COMPLICATIONS

When properly applied in selected patients, NIV is associated with few adverse events and is generally well tolerated. The majority of events that do occur are related to pressure effects of the mask and straps (see Table 6.3).[19] Excessive pressure from the mask seal predisposes to nasal bridge erythema and/or ulceration. With proper mask fitting, use of artificial skin over the nose, newer mask designs with softer silicone, and avoidance of overtightening of straps, this complication can be minimized.

Table 6.3 *Side effects and complications of noninvasive ventilation*

Effect	Remedy
Mask-related	
Discomfort	Readjust, loosen straps, try new mask
Facial erythema	Artificial skin
Nasal bridge ulceration	Nasal instead of oronasal
Claustrophobia	
Air pressure/flow-related	
Air leaks	Re-seat mask, adjust strap tension
Conjunctival irritation	Humidify, nasal saline, steroids
Oronasal dryness congestion	Reduce inspiratory pressure as tolerated
Sinus/ear pain	
Gastric distention	
Patient–ventilator asynchrony	
Major complications	Reduce air leaks, adjust rise time
Barotrauma	and/or inspiratory duration
Hypotension	Unusual; lower pressures
Aspiration pneumonia	Adequate hydration
	Exclude patients at high aspiration risk

Ventilator airflow and pressure can cause air leakage into the eyes, leading to conjunctival dryness and irritation. Excessive inspiratory pressure may cause sinus and ear pain and necessitate a lower pressure. Oral and nasal dryness are frequent problems with excessive air leaks through the mouth and may be relieved with mask adjustments or chin straps to minimize leakage, or nasal saline and/or humidification, particularly if NIV is used for a prolonged period of time. Nasal congestion and discharge frequently occur and may require treatment with decongestants and/or topical steroids. Gastric distension is common but rarely interferes with efficacy and may be ameliorated with agents such as simethicone.

More serious adverse events are rare and occur in less than five percent of applications.[19] Because insufflation pressures are low compared with invasive mechanical ventilation, barotrauma, hypotension, reduced cardiac output or arrhythmias are uncommon.[76] The incidence of pneumonia, including aspiration, is also low with NIV and is decreased compared with invasive mechanical ventilation.[12,77]

SUMMARY

Noninvasive ventilation, long used for chronic respiratory failure and sleep-related hypoventilation, has more recently been applied in the setting of acute respiratory failure. Both portable and critical care ventilators can be used to deliver NIV via a variety of interfaces, usually either nasal or oronasal masks, the latter being preferred initially for acute applications. NIV has proved efficacy in reducing intubation rates, mortality, and ICU lengths of stay in patients with respiratory failure due to exacerbations of COPD. It is thus considered the ventilatory mode of first choice for these patients. Also, both noninvasive CPAP alone and NIV rapidly improve gas exchange and reduce the need for intubation in patients with cardiogenic pulmonary edema, and either may be chosen to treat these patients. NIV also appears to be effective in avoiding intubation and lowering mortality in immunocompromised patients with acute respiratory failure and facilitating extubation in COPD patients. The indications for NIV in other conditions causing acute respiratory failure are less clear. NIV may be used to avoid intubation in hypoxemic respiratory failure due to a number of causes, but the evidence supporting these applications is less clear, and such patients must be monitored closely.

Important considerations for the successful application of NIV include careful patient selection, early initiation, proper and comfortable mask fitting and close monitoring. NIV should be used to avoid intubation, but not to replace or delay needed intubation. When used properly, NIV enhances patient comfort and improves clinical outcomes and is associated with few adverse events. Success is greatest when an experienced, skilled team applies NIV, but failure rates up to 33–40 percent are still reported, and some centers even now use NIV very little, if at all. As improvements in ventilator and interface technology continue and more practitioners become knowledgeable about NIV, we can expect enhanced success rates and more consistent use among centers in the future.

Key learning points

- Noninvasive ventilation refers to techniques that assist ventilation without requiring an invasive airway. It reduces breathing effort and improves ventilation and/or oxygenation and thereby may avoid the need for intubation and its attendant risks. In this sense it serves as a 'crutch', providing the critical time needed to allow medical therapy to reverse the underlying cause of the respiratory failure.

- The strongest evidence for support of use of NIV is in: COPD exacerbations with pH <7.35; acute cardiogenic pulmonary edema; hypoxemic respiratory failure in immunocompromised patients; and persistent weaning failure in COPD patients.

- Results of randomized controlled trials demonstrate that NIV decreases the need for invasive mechanical ventilation, reduces mortality and shortens the length of hospital stay in COPD exacerbations.

- The success of NIV in the setting of acute respiratory failure is largely based on proper patient selection. This involves consideration of the etiology of failure, clinical and physiologic parameters, and recognition of the limits of NIV application.

- Noninvasive ventilation should not be used as a substitute for invasive mechanical ventilation if the latter is clearly indicated.

- The application of NIV requires proper mask fit to ensure patient tolerance and comfort, appropriate initial and subsequent ventilator settings and adjustments to achieve goals, and experienced and well-trained staff.

REFERENCES

1. Rideau Y, Gatin G, Bach J, Gines G. Prolongation of life in Duchenne's muscular dystrophy. *Acta Neurol* 1983; **5**: 118–24.

2. Sullivan CE, Berthon-Jones M, Issa FG. Nocturnal nasal-airway pressure for sleep apnea. *N Engl J Med* 1983; **309**: 112.

3. British Thoracic Society Standards of Care C. Non-invasive ventilation in acute respiratory failure [see comment]. *Thorax* 2002; **57**: 192–211.

4. Bott J, Carroll MP, Conway JH, *et al.* Randomised controlled trial of nasal ventilation in acute ventilatory failure due to chronic obstructive airways disease [see comment]. *Lancet* 1993; **341**: 1555–7.

5. Brochard L, Mancebo J, Wysocki M, *et al.* Noninvasive ventilation for acute exacerbations of chronic obstructive pulmonary disease [see comment]. *N Engl J Med* 1995; **333**: 817–22.

6. Wysocki M, Tric L, Wolff MA, *et al.* Noninvasive pressure support ventilation in patients with acute respiratory failure. A randomized comparison with conventional therapy. *Chest* 1995; **107**: 761–8.

7. Plant PK, Owen JL, Elliott MW. Early use of non-invasive ventilation for acute exacerbations of chronic obstructive pulmonary disease on general respiratory wards: a multicentre randomised controlled trial [see comment]. *Lancet* 2000; **355**: 1931–5.

8. Bersten AD, Holt AW, Vedig AE, *et al.* Treatment of severe cardiogenic pulmonary edema with continuous positive airway pressure delivered by face mask. *N Engl J Med* 1991; **325**: 1825–30.

9. Masip J, Betbese AJ, Paez J, *et al.* Non-invasive pressure support ventilation versus conventional oxygen therapy in acute cardiogenic pulmonary oedema: a randomised trial [see comment]. *Lancet.* 2000; **356**: 2126–32.

10. Antonelli M, Conti G, Bufi M, *et al.* Noninvasive ventilation for treatment of acute respiratory failure in patients undergoing solid organ transplantation: a randomized trial [see comment]. *JAMA* 2000; **283**: 235–41.

11. Hilbert G, Gruson D, Vargas F, *et al.* Noninvasive ventilation in immunosuppressed patients with pulmonary infiltrates, fever, and acute respiratory failure [see comment]. *N Engl J Med* 2001; **344**: 481–7.

12. Nava S, Ambrosino N, Clini E, *et al.* Noninvasive mechanical ventilation in the weaning of patients with respiratory failure due to chronic obstructive pulmonary disease. A randomized, controlled trial. *Ann Intern Med* 1998; **128**: 721–8.

13. Ferrer M, Esquinas A, Arancibia F, *et al.* Noninvasive ventilation during persistent weaning failure: a randomized controlled trial [see comment]. *Am J Respir Crit Care Med* 2003; **168**: 70–6.

14. Peter JV, Moran JL, Phillips-Hughes J, Warn D. Noninvasive ventilation in acute respiratory failure – a meta-analysis update [see comment]. *Crit Care Med* 2002; **30**: 555–62.

15. Lightowler JV, Wedzicha JA, Elliott MW, Ram FS. Non-invasive positive pressure ventilation to treat respiratory failure resulting from exacerbations of chronic obstructive pulmonary disease: Cochrane systematic review and meta-analysis [see comment]. *BMJ* 2003; **326**: 185.

16. Girou E, Schortgen F, Delclaux C, *et al.* Association of noninvasive ventilation with nosocomial infections and survival in critically ill patients [see comment]. *JAMA* 2000; **284**: 2361–7.

17. Girou E, Brun-Buisson C, Taille S, *et al.* Secular trends in nosocomial infections and mortality associated with noninvasive ventilation in patients with exacerbation of COPD and pulmonary edema. *JAMA* 2003; **290**: 2985–91.

● 18. Antonelli M, Conti G, Rocco M, *et al.* A comparison of noninvasive positive-pressure ventilation and conventional mechanical ventilation in patients with acute respiratory failure [see comment]. *N Engl J Med* 1998; **339**: 429–35.

◆ 19. Mehta S, Hill NS. Noninvasive ventilation. *Am J Respir Crit Care Med* 2001; **163**: 540–77.

20. Brochard L, Isabey D, Piquet J, *et al.* Reversal of acute exacerbations of chronic obstructive lung disease by inspiratory assistance with a face mask. *N Engl J Med* 1990; **323**: 1523–30.

21. Appendini L, Patessio A, Zanaboni S, *et al.* Physiologic effects of positive end-expiratory pressure and mask pressure support during exacerbations of chronic obstructive pulmonary disease [see comment]. *Am J Respir Crit Care Med* 1994; **149**: 1069–76.

22. Diaz O, Iglesia R, Ferrer M, *et al.* Effects of noninvasive ventilation on pulmonary gas exchange and hemodynamics during acute hypercapnic exacerbations of chronic obstructive pulmonary disease. *Am J Respir Crit Care Med* 1997; **156**: 1840–5.

23. Lin M, Yang YF, Chiang HT, *et al.* Reappraisal of continuous positive airway pressure therapy in acute cardiogenic pulmonary edema. Short-term results and long-term follow-up. *Chest* 1995; **107**: 1379–86.

24. Bradley TD, Holloway RM, McLaughlin PR, *et al.* Cardiac output response to continuous positive airway pressure in congestive heart failure. *Am Rev Respir Dis* 1992; **145**(2 Pt 1): 377–82.

25. Kramer N, Meyer TJ, Meharg J, *et al.* Randomized, prospective trial of noninvasive positive pressure ventilation in acute respiratory failure [see comment]. *Am J Respir Crit Care Med* 1995; **151**: 1799–806.

◆ 26. Keenan SP, Sinuff T, Cook DJ, Hill NS. Which patients with acute exacerbation of chronic obstructive pulmonary disease benefit from noninvasive positive-pressure ventilation? A systematic review of the literature [summary for patients in *Ann Intern Med* 2003; **138**: 861–70.

27. Keenan SP, Kernerman PD, Cook DJ, *et al.* Effect of noninvasive positive pressure ventilation on mortality in patients admitted with acute respiratory failure: a meta-analysis [see comment]. *Crit Care Med* 1997; **25**: 1685–92.

28. Meduri GU, Cook TR, Turner RE, *et al.* Noninvasive positive pressure ventilation in status asthmaticus. *Chest* 1996; **110**: 767–74.

29. Soroksky A, Stav D, Shpirer I. A pilot prospective, randomized, placebo-controlled trial of bilevel positive airway pressure in acute asthmatic attack. *Chest* 2003; **123**: 1018–25.

30. Madden BP, Kariyawasam H, Siddiqi AJ, *et al.* Noninvasive ventilation in cystic fibrosis patients with acute or chronic respiratory failure. *Eur Respir J* 2002; **19**: 310–13. [Erratum appears in *Eur Respir J* 2002; **20**: 790.]

31. Hodson ME, Madden BP, Steven MH, *et al.* Non-invasive mechanical ventilation for cystic fibrosis patients – a potential bridge to transplantation. *Eur Respir J* 1991; **4**: 524–7.

32. Ferrer M, Esquinas A, Leon M, *et al.* Noninvasive ventilation in severe hypoxemic respiratory failure: a randomized clinical trial. *Am J Respir Crit Care Med* 2003; **168**: 1438–44.

33. Rasanen J, Heikkila J, Downs J, *et al.* Continuous positive airway pressure by face mask in acute cardiogenic pulmonary edema. *Am J Cardiol* 1985; **55**: 296–300.

34. Pang D, Keenan SP, Cook DJ, Sibbald WJ. The effect of positive pressure airway support on mortality and the need for intubation in cardiogenic pulmonary edema: a systematic review [see comment]. *Chest* 1998; **114**: 1185–92.

● 35. Mehta S, Jay GD, Woolard RH, *et al.* Randomized, prospective trial of bilevel versus continuous positive airway pressure in acute pulmonary edema [see comment]. *Crit Care Med* 1997; **25**: 620–8.

36. Nava S, Carbone G, DiBattista N, *et al.* Noninvasive ventilation in cardiogenic pulmonary edema: a multicenter randomized trial [see comment]. *Am J Respir Crit Care Med* 2003; **168**: 1432–7.

● 37. Confalonieri M, Potena A, Carbone G, *et al.* Acute respiratory failure in patients with severe community-acquired pneumonia. A prospective randomized evaluation of noninvasive ventilation [see comment]. *Am J Respir Crit Care Med.* 1999; **160**(5 Pt 1): 1585–91.

38. Delclaux C, L'Her E, Alberti C, *et al.* Treatment of acute hypoxemic nonhypercapnic respiratory insufficiency with continuous positive airway pressure delivered by a face mask: A randomized controlled trial [see comment]. *JAMA* 2000; **284**: 2352–60.

39. Jolliet P, Abajo B, Pasquina P, Chevrolet JC. Non-invasive pressure support ventilation in severe community-acquired pneumonia [see comment]. *Intensive Care Med* 2001; **27**: 812–21.

40. Rocker GM, Mackenzie MG, Williams B, Logan PM. Noninvasive positive pressure ventilation: successful outcome in patients with acute lung injury/ARDS. *Chest* 1999; **115**: 173–7.

41. Finlay G, Concannon D, McDonnell TJ. Treatment of respiratory failure due to kyphoscoliosis with nasal intermittent positive pressure ventilation (NIPPV). *Irish J Med Sci* 1995; **164**: 28–30.

42. Bach JR, Ishikawa Y, Kim H. Prevention of pulmonary morbidity for patients with Duchenne muscular dystrophy. *Chest* 1997; **112**: 1024–8.

43. Tzeng AC, Bach JR. Prevention of pulmonary morbidity for patients with neuromuscular disease. *Chest* 2000; **118**: 1390–6.

44. Blivet S, Philit F, Sab JM, *et al.* Outcome of patients with idiopathic pulmonary fibrosis admitted to the ICU for respiratory failure [see comment]. *Chest* 2001; **120**: 209–12.

45. Afessa B, Tefferi A, Hoagland HC, *et al.* Outcome of recipients of bone marrow transplant who require intensive-care unit support [see comment]. *Mayo Clinic Proc* 1992; **67**: 117–22.

46. Rubenfeld GD, Crawford SW. Withdrawing life support from mechanically ventilated recipients of bone marrow transplants: a case for evidence-based guidelines [see comment]. *Ann Intern Med* 1996; **125**: 625–33.

47. Confalonieri M, Calderini E, Terraciano S, *et al.* Noninvasive ventilation for treating acute respiratory failure in AIDS patients with *Pneumocystis carinii* pneumonia. *Intensive Care Med* 2002; **28**: 1233–8.

48. Hilbert G, Gruson D, Vargas F, *et al.* Noninvasive ventilation in immunosuppressed patients with pulmonary infiltrates, fever, and acute respiratory failure [see comment]. *N Engl J Med* 2001; **344**: 481–7.

49. Gregoretti C, Beltrame F, Lucangelo U, *et al.* Physiologic evaluation of non-invasive pressure support ventilation in trauma patients with acute respiratory failure. *Intensive Care Med* 1998; **24**: 785–90.

50. Girault C, Daudenthun I, Chevron V, *et al.* Noninvasive ventilation as a systematic extubation and weaning technique in acute-on-chronic respiratory failure: a prospective, randomized controlled study. *Am J Respir Crit Care Med* 1999; **160**: 86–92.

51. Keenan SP, Powers C, McCormack DG, Block G. Noninvasive positive-pressure ventilation for postextubation respiratory distress: a randomized controlled trial [see comment]. *JAMA* 2002; **287**: 3238–44.

52. Hilbert G, Gruson D, Portel L, *et al.* Noninvasive pressure support ventilation in COPD patients with postextubation hypercapnic respiratory insufficiency. *Eur Respir J* 1998; **11**: 1349–53.

● 53. Esteban A, Frutos-Vivar F, Ferguson ND, *et al.* Noninvasive positive-pressure ventilation for respiratory failure after extubation [see comment]. *N Engl J Med* 2004; **350**: 2452–60.

54. Bolliger CT, Van Eeden SF. Treatment of multiple rib fractures. Randomized controlled trial comparing ventilatory with nonventilatory management. *Chest* 1990; **97**: 943–8.

55. Beltrame F, Lucangelo U, Gregori D, Gregoretti C. Noninvasive positive pressure ventilation in trauma patients with acute respiratory failure. *Monaldi Arch Chest Dis* 1999; **54**: 109–14.

56. Pennock BE, Crawshaw L, Kaplan PD. Noninvasive nasal mask ventilation for acute respiratory failure. Institution of a new therapeutic technology for routine use. *Chest* 1994; **105**: 441–4.

57. Aguilo R, Togores B, Pons S, *et al.* Noninvasive ventilatory support after lung resectional surgery. *Chest* 1997; **112**: 117–21.

58. Auriant I, Jallot A, Herve P, *et al.* Noninvasive ventilation reduces mortality in acute respiratory failure following lung resection. *Am J Respir Crit Care Med* 2001; **164**: 1231–5.

59. Joris JL, Sottiaux TM, Chiche JD, *et al.* Effect of bi-level positive airway pressure (BiPAP) nasal ventilation on the postoperative pulmonary restrictive syndrome in obese patients undergoing gastroplasty. *Chest* 1997; **111**: 665–70.

60. Benhamou D, Muir JF, Melen B. Mechanical ventilation in elderly patients. *Monaldi Arch Chest Dis* 1998; **53**: 547–51.

61. Meduri GU, Fox RC, Abou-Shala N, *et al.* Noninvasive mechanical ventilation via face mask in patients with acute respiratory failure who refused endotracheal intubation. *Crit Care Med* 1994; **22**: 1584–90.

62. Ambrosino N, Foglio K, Rubini F, *et al.* Non-invasive mechanical ventilation in acute respiratory failure due to chronic obstructive pulmonary disease: correlates for success [see comment]. *Thorax* 1995; **50**: 755–7.

✷ 63. International Consensus Conferences in Intensive Care Medicine: Noninvasive Positive Pressure Ventilation in Acute Respiratory Failure. Organized Jointly by the American Thoracic Society, the European Respiratory Society, the European Society of Intensive Care Medicine, and the Societe de Reanimation de Langue Francaise, and approved by the ATS Board of Directors, December 2000. *Am J Respir Crit Care Med* 2001; **163**: 283–91.

64. Patel RG, Petrini MF. Respiratory muscle performance, pulmonary mechanics, and gas exchange between the BiPAP S/T-D system and the Servo Ventilator 900C with bilevel positive airway pressure ventilation following gradual pressure support weaning. *Chest* 1998; **114**: 1390–6.

65. Liesching T, Kwok H, Hill NS. Acute applications of noninvasive positive pressure ventilation [see comment]. *Chest* 2003; **124**: 699–713.

66. Girault C, Richard JC, Chevron V, *et al.* Comparative physiologic effects of noninvasive assist-control and pressure support ventilation in acute hypercapnic respiratory failure [see comment]. *Chest* 1997; **111**: 1639–48.

67. Vitacca M, Rubini F, Foglio K, *et al.* Non-invasive modalities of positive pressure ventilation improve the outcome of acute exacerbations in COLD patients [see comment]. *Intensive Care Med* 1993; **19**: 450–5.

68. Navalesi P, Fanfulla F, Frigerio P, *et al.* Physiologic evaluation of noninvasive mechanical ventilation delivered with three types of masks in patients with chronic hypercapnic respiratory failure [see comment]. *Crit Care Med* 2000; **28**: 1785–90.

69. Soo Hoo GW, Santiago S, Williams AJ. Nasal mechanical ventilation for hypercapnic respiratory failure in chronic obstructive pulmonary disease: determinants of success and failure. *Crit Care Med* 1994; **22**: 1253–61.

70. Kwok H, McCormack J, Cece R, *et al.* Controlled trial of oronasal versus nasal mask ventilation in the treatment of acute respiratory failure. *Crit Care Med* 2003; **31**: 468–73.

71. Antonelli M, Pennisi MA, Pelosi P, *et al.* Noninvasive positive pressure ventilation using a helmet in patients with acute exacerbation of chronic obstructive pulmonary disease: a feasibility study. *Anesthesiology* 2004; **100**: 16–24.

72. Tonnelier JM, Prat G, Nowak E, *et al.* Noninvasive continuous positive airway pressure ventilation using a new helmet interface: a case-control prospective pilot study. *Intensive Care Med* 2003; **29**: 2077–80.

73. Criner GJ, Travaline JM, Brennan KJ, Kreimer DT. Efficacy of a new full face mask for noninvasive positive pressure ventilation. *Chest* 1994; **106**: 1109–15.

74. Meduri GU, Turner RE, Abou-Shala N, *et al.* Noninvasive positive pressure ventilation via face mask. First-line intervention in patients with acute hypercapnic and hypoxemic respiratory failure. *Chest* 1996; **109**: 179–93.

75. Wood KA, Lewis L, Von Harz B, Kollef MH. The use of noninvasive positive pressure ventilation in the emergency department: results of a randomized clinical trial [see comment]. *Chest* 1998; **113**: 1339–46.

76. Confalonieri M, Gazzaniga P, Gandola L, *et al.* Haemodynamic response during initiation of non-invasive positive pressure ventilation in COPD patients with acute ventilatory failure. *Respir Med* 1998; **92**: 331–7.

77. Guerin C, Girard R, Chemorin C, *et al.* Facial mask noninvasive mechanical ventilation reduces the incidence of nosocomial pneumonia. A prospective epidemiological survey from a single ICU. *Intensive Care Med* 1997; **23**: 1024–32. [Erratum appears in *Intensive Care Med* 1998; **24**: 27.

7

Imaging of adult respiratory emergencies

MATTHEW D CHAM, DOROTHY I McCAULEY, MILDRED CHEN, DAVID F YANKELEVITZ, CLAUDIA I HENSCHKE

INTRODUCTION

Respiratory emergencies represent a spectrum of cardiopulmonary conditions that are commonly encountered in the emergency room and intensive care unit (ICU) settings. Due to the tremendous overlap of conditions between the emergency room and the ICU, this chapter will focus primarily on adult respiratory emergencies in the ICU.

Radiology of the ICU patient has become increasingly complex due to our deeper understanding of pathology and our consequent vigilance. Clinical management of patients in the ICU requires constant radiologic monitoring. Up to 65 percent of routine chest radiographs from the ICU have been shown to reveal unsuspected abnormalities that could affect patient management.[1] The objective of this chapter is to provide an overview of the imaging modalities used during respiratory emergencies and the common cardiopulmonary diseases and complications they help identify.

IMAGING MODALITIES IN THE INTENSIVE CARE UNIT

Imaging of critically ill patients is particularly challenging due to the several key factors. Critically ill patients are often imaged in suboptimal conditions due to their fixed supine positioning and inability to hold their breath. Patients are often clinically unstable, require constant monitoring, and are unable to spend more than a few minutes outside of the ICU. Over the past decades, imaging modalities have been developed and refined to cater to the special needs of these patients.

Portable chest radiography

Portable chest radiography allows for the imaging of supine patients in the ICU setting. Despite the decreased image quality of this test compared with the standard posteroanterior chest radiograph, the convenience afforded by portable chest radiography has made it the most commonly ordered radiologic test in the ICU. With the introduction of the picture archiving and communications system (PACS), the chest radiograph has become an even more powerful imaging tool, as the images are rapidly and readily accessible. Not only are the radiographs less prone to physical loss, but they can also be simultaneously viewed by multiple clinicians and radiologists at remote locations as well as in the ICU itself.

Portable chest radiography in the ICU can be acquired either routinely or nonroutinely. Routine portable chest radiographs are acquired to monitor the progress of a patient's acute cardiopulmonary disease. Nonroutine radiographs are acquired to determine the cause of a new clinical abnormality or to determine the outcome of recent instrumentation. Numerous studies have debated the merits of performing routine radiographs in all ICU patients. One large prospective study, comprising over 1132 consecutive medical and surgical ICU radiographs, found a 65 percent increase in incidence of unsuspected abnormal findings after a chest radiograph of both stable and nonstable ICU patients.[1] However, other smaller studies have shown only a 3 percent increase in unsuspected findings from routine chest radiographs of stable ICU patients.[2] In a recent comprehensive metaanalysis encompassing 15 large prospective studies, Graat *et al.* concluded that the ongoing debate over usefulness of daily routine chest radiographs is still not settled.[3] From a medicolegal standpoint, the American College of Radiology (ACR) Appropriateness Criteria consensus panel supports the use of daily chest radiographs in patients with acute cardiopulmonary disease; with clinical decompensation; on mechanical ventilation; and with recent instrumentation.[4] The ACR does not recommend routine chest radiographs in stable cardiac patients after the initial admission radiograph.[4]

Computed tomography

Computed tomography (CT) is commonly used in evaluation of critically ill patients. With the advent of multidetector-row CT scanners, CT has become a more powerful tool as the short scan times reduce motion artifacts in mechanically ventilated patients. One of the major obstacles to CT imaging is the inconvenience associated with transporting potentially unstable patients. Over the past 10 years, portable CT (PCT) scanners have been developed to address this concern, allowing unstable ICU patients to be safely scanned within the confines of the ICU.[5] Despite this technologic advancement, PCT is plagued by several disadvantages: it is more costly to operate than fixed CT scanners; the quality of PCT produced images is inferior to those of fixed CT scanners; it can be impossible to navigate through the tight spaces of some ICUs; it requires an impractical 4.8 m (16 ft) minimum clearance between scanner and ICU staff to abide by radiation safety standards.[6,7] Thus, it has been increasingly common for hospitals to strategically place fixed CT scanners in close proximity to the ICU.

The most common indications for CT imaging in ICU patients are sepsis of unknown etiology, thromboembolic disease, and CT-guided drainage of abscess.

Ultrasound and Doppler imaging

Ultrasound is frequently employed in the ICU for its portability and lack of ionizing radiation. Ultrasound is an excellent modality for imaging patients who are too unstable for transport to the CT scanner. The most common indications for ultrasound imaging of ICU patients include ultrasound-guided central venous catheter placement, deep vein thrombosis, and ultrasound-guided thoracentesis or abscess drainage.

In the surgical ICU, Doppler ultrasound also provides flow information that is highly useful for posttransplant vascular evaluation.

RADIATION DOSE IN INTENSIVE CARE UNIT IMAGING

Critically ill patients undergo dozens of radiologic studies during their hospital stay. Each ICU patient typically has one to two portable chest radiographs each day in addition to CT and fluoroscopic imaging.[8] In a retrospective study involving 46 patients who spent at least 30 days in the surgical ICU, Kim *et al.* found that the average patient had a total of 70.1 chest radiographs, 7.8 CT scans, and 2.5 fluoroscopic imaging studies.[9] Kim *et al.* also found that CT imaging constituted less than 10 percent of the total number of radiologic studies performed but accounted for two-thirds of the total radiation dose.[9] Kim *et al.* estimated that the mean cumulative effective dose of radiation resulting from these studies is 106 mSv per patient, which is 30 times higher than the mean yearly radiation dose from all sources for individuals in the United States, and translates to a theoretical additional morbidity attributable to radiologic studies of 0.78 percent.[9]

Several new technologies have been developed to further reduce the radiation dose during CT imaging, while potentially maintaining diagnostic efficacy. Most multidetector-row CT scanners are now equipped with dose-reducing applications that automatically modulate the tube current in the z axis and/or the x and y axes. Depending on patient's anatomy, radiation dose may decrease by up to 60 percent using these applications.[10] One of the limitations of this technology is that radiation dose may not be reduced in markedly obese patients.

RESPIRATORY EMERGENCIES AND COMPLICATIONS IN THE INTENSIVE CARE UNIT

Respiratory emergencies can result from a myriad of causes, few of which can be determined by clinical examination alone. Portable radiographs or CT of the chest is often necessary to identify the underlying cause of a patient's respiratory distress. Several complications also arise from malpositioned ICU support devices, which are discussed in the last section of this chapter.

Pulmonary edema and acute respiratory distress syndrome

Pulmonary edema can be classified into four categories based on pathophysiology:

- increased hydrostatic pressure edema
- permeability edema with diffuse alveolar damage or acute respiratory distress syndrome (ARDS)
- permeability edema without diffuse alveolar damage
- mixed edema due to simultaneous increase in hydrostatic pressure and pulmonary vascular permeability.

These four categories share many common findings, making it difficult at times to distinguish one category from another.[11]

Increased hydrostatic pressure edema is seen with increased pulmonary capillary wedge pressures of 15–25 mm Hg. This is the most common form of pulmonary edema in the ICU setting, often occurring during left-sided heart failure, also known as cardiogenic pulmonary edema, and during fluid overload. Initially, extravascular fluid accumulates within the interlobular septa, seen as Kerley B lines on the chest radiograph and CT. When elevated pulmonary vascular pressures persist, this interstitial fluid migrates centrally towards the hila, seen as perihilar peribronchial cuffing on the chest radiograph (Fig. 7.1). Above a pulmonary capillary wedge pressure of 25 mm Hg, fluid fills the alveolar spaces, seen as nodular areas that can coalesce into frank consolidation on the chest radiograph and CT.[12] In the most patients, this form of pulmonary edema is characterized by a gravitational or dependent distribution that affects both lungs symmetrically. Less commonly, an asymmetric and nondependent distribution can occur as a result of numerous entities including chronic obstructive pulmonary disease, mitral regurgitation, upper airway obstruction, chronic pulmonary embolism, pulmonary venoocclusive disease, and near-drowning episodes.[13] Other commonly associated findings include dilatation of the azygos vein, pleural effusions, and cardiomegaly. The mainstay of treatment for cardiogenic pulmonary edema includes the use of diuretics, supplemental oxygen, opioids, nitrates, and occasionally ventilatory support. Portable chest radiographs are often useful to monitor the patient's condition and to determine the efficacy of a particular treatment regimen.

Permeability edema with diffuse alveolar damage, most commonly seen with ARDS, affects between 50 000 and 100 000 ICU patients annually in the United States.[14] The underlying mechanism involves both a direct insult to lung tissue, such as a pneumonia, and an indirect insult from an acute systemic inflammatory response, resulting in rapid accumulation of proteinaceous fluid within alveolar spaces. Radiographically, ARDS has a variable appearance that commonly includes progressive symmetric ground glass opacification, small- to moderate-sized pleural effusions, and air bronchograms.[15] Interlobular septal thickening or Kerley B lines are only rarely seen in ARDS (Fig. 7.2). Due to the nonspecific radiographic findings in ARDS, the diagnosis is

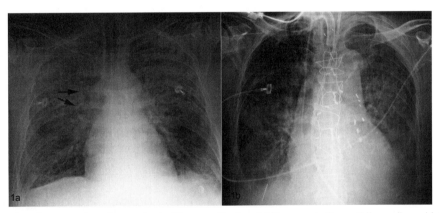

Figure 7.1   *(a) Hydrostatic pulmonary edema in a patient with congestive heart failure – note the perihilar peribronchial cuffing on this chest radiograph (arrows). (b) With increasing hydrostatic pressure, fluid fills the alveolar spaces and pleural spaces, seen as frank consolidation and pleural effusions in this second patient with congestive heart failure.*

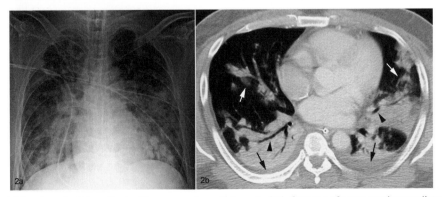

Figure 7.2   *(a) Permeability edema in this patient with pneumonia and characteristic features of acute respiratory distress syndrome (ARDS), demonstrating bilateral pulmonary infiltrates on the chest radiograph. (b) Chest computed tomography scan of the same patient shows symmetric ground-glass opacification (white arrows), small-to-moderate-sized pleural effusions (black arrows), and air bronchograms (arrowheads). Note the absence of interlobular septal thickening – which is not a typical finding in ARDS.*

traditionally made clinically. Thus, ARDS is defined as a clinical syndrome of acute persistent respiratory failure characterized by severe hypoxia and bilateral pulmonary infiltrates in the absence of congestive heart failure.[16] With advancements in the treatment and diagnosis of ARDS, the associated mortality has steadily decreased from 70 percent in the 1980s to less than 30 percent in recent literature.[17]

Permeability edema without diffuse alveolar damage is distinguished from ARDS by its rapid resolution after reversal of the predisposing factor. This form of pulmonary edema is often drug induced. It can be seen in 2 percent of patients with heroin overdose and about 20 percent of patients undergoing interleukin-2 cytokine treatment.[18,19] It has also been frequently reported in mountain climbers who ascend rapidly to heights of 2500 m above sea level over a 24–48-hour period, referred to as high-altitude pulmonary edema.[20] As with ARDS, the diagnosis of this form of pulmonary edema is also made clinically, supported by radiographic findings.

Mixed edema, as its name implies, occurs as a result of both increased hydrostatic pressure and increased pulmonary vascular permeability. The most common form of mixed edema is neurogenic pulmonary edema, seen during cerebral and cerebrovascular injury.[21] The exact pathophysiology of neurogenic edema is poorly understood. Chest radiographs typically demonstrate bilateral homogeneous airspace consolidations that are difficult to distinguish from simple fluid overload, thus requiring clinical correlation. Other causes of mixed edema include pulmonary thromboendarterectomy (reperfusion pulmonary edema), lung transplantation, hydrothorax or hemothorax evacuation (reexpansion pulmonary edema), and pneumonectomy.[13] Mixed edema typically resolves over time in patients who survive the initial acute event.

Barotrauma: pneumothorax and pneumomediastinum

Ventilator-associated barotrauma is defined as extraalveolar air resulting from overdistension of alveoli and rupture of their walls into their bronchovascular bundle. In the ICU, barotrauma occurs as the result of mechanical ventilation in patients with predisposing factors such as ARDS, chronic obstructive pulmonary disease, and pneumonia.[22] Due to our improved understanding of its pathophysiology, barotrauma has become much less common in the modern ICU. In recent literature, barotrauma was found to occur in only 6.5 percent of ventilated patients with ARDS compared with 40–60 percent of ventilated patients 15 years ago.[23,24] Radiographically, barotrauma is seen in the form of pneumothorax, pneumomediastinum, pneumatocele, and in neonates, pulmonary interstitial emphysema.

The risk of pneumothorax and pneumomediastinum increases with the duration of mechanical ventilation and presence of underlying lung disease.[25] During mechanical

ventilation, pneumothoraces tend to expand rapidly and can progress to tension if untreated.[26,27] In patients standing upright, the displaced pleural line from a pneumothorax is usually evident along the lung apex (Fig. 7.3). In critically ill patients undergoing supine or semi-erect chest radiographs, images should be carefully reviewed for evidence of a deep sulcus sign, a continuous diaphragm sign, or subcutaneous emphysema (Fig. 7.4). The deep sulcus sign refers to the lucency of the lateral costophrenic angle produced by pneumothorax within the nondependent pleural space of supine patients.[28] The continuous diaphragm sign refers to a pneumomediastinum that is trapped posterior to the pericardium, which gives the appearance of a continuous collection of supradiaphragmatic air on portable chest radiography.[29,30] When the radiographic findings are equivocal, a chest CT should be performed due to its increased sensitivity for small pneumothoraces that can be missed in up to 38 percent of supine radiographs.[31] The high mortality of ventilator-associated barotrauma is high, ranging between 50 percent and 71 percent, thus necessitating prompt radiologic diagnosis, appropriate ventilator adjustment, and chest tube placement.[32,33]

Thromboembolic disease

Pulmonary embolism (PE) and deep vein thrombosis (DVT) are different manifestations of the same disease spectrum that affects between 10 percent and 13 percent of ICU patients.[34–36] Predisposing factors such as immobility,

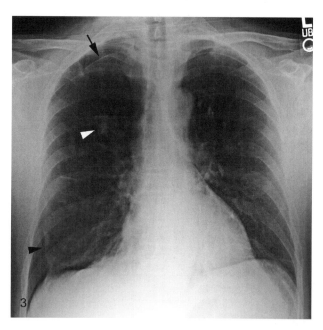

Figure 7.3 *Pneumothorax in this upright patient demonstrates a displaced pleural line along the lung apex (arrow) and the right lung base (black arrowhead). This patient's pneumothorax occurred after biopsy of a right upper lobe pulmonary nodule (white arrowhead).*

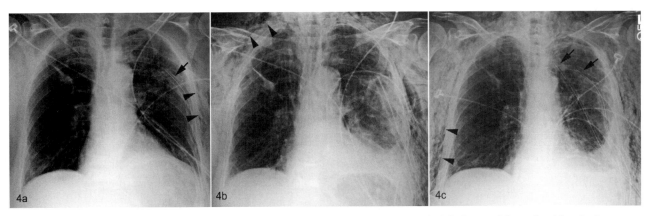

Figure 7.4 *(a) A small pneumothorax in this patient led to subcutaneous emphysema along the left chest wall (arrowheads) and subsequent left chest tube placement (arrow). (b) Radiograph of the same patient obtained 8 hours later demonstrates interval worsening of subcutaneous emphysema, now extending to the contralateral neck (arrowheads), despite of the chest tube. (c) Radiograph of the same patient obtained 8 days later demonstrates persistent worsening of subcutaneous emphysema, now extending to the contralateral chest wall, and consequent placement of a second chest tube (arrows).*

myocardial infarction, sepsis, malignancy, prior surgery, burn, trauma, and malignancy, place ICU patients at high risk for thromboembolic disease. Although conventional pulmonary angiography is traditionally regarded as the gold standard for the diagnosis of PE, major advances in multidetector-row CT has made CT pulmonary angiography (CTPA) the initial imaging study for suspected PE at many institutions.[37–41] On CTPA, acute PE appears as an intravascular filling defect in a pulmonary artery that partially or completely occludes the vessel and may be associated with increased diameter of the affected vessel (Fig. 7.5a). Several prospective studies have found that it is safe to withhold anticoagulation in patients with no thromboembolic disease identified on CT imaging. [42–44]

Although conventional lower extremity venography is traditionally regarded as the gold standard for the diagnosis of DVT, the noninvasive nature, lower cost, and high accuracy of lower extremity Doppler sonography has made it the most commonly ordered test for suspected DVT. On Doppler ultrasound, DVT appears as a segment of venous noncompressibility that may be associated with a flow void.

The prevalence of DVT in suspected PE is approximately 18 percent, and 36–45 percent in proved PE.[45] Because of this strong association between PE and DVT, pelvic and lower extremity CT venography (CTV) has been frequently employed to concurrently evaluate the deep venous system of patients undergoing CTPA.[46,47] Several studies comparing CTV and sonography have found high concordance rates and similar accuracy between these two modalities.[48–50] In addition, CTV has the advantage of detecting pelvic deep venous thrombi, which are difficult to detect on ultrasound imaging.[51] On CTV, acute DVT appears as an intravascular filling defect in the deep venous system that partially or completely occludes the vein and may be associated with

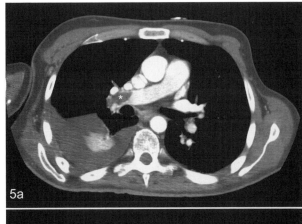
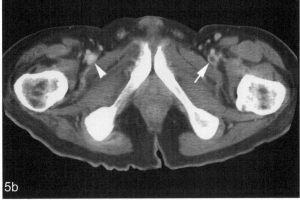

Figure 7.5 *(a) Computed tomographic (CT) pulmonary angiography demonstrates a large pulmonary embolus (white asterisk) within the right main pulmonary artery. Note the large right pleural effusion. (b) CT venography demonstrates a deep vein thrombus producing a filling defect within the left common femoral vein (white arrow) in comparison with the patent right common femoral vein (white arrowhead).*

increased diameter of the affected vein proximally (Fig. 7.5b). By scanning both the chest and lower extremities, the combine CTPA-CTV protocols have been shown to increase thromboembolic disease detection by 15–36 percent when compared with results for CTPA alone.[47,52–54]

Nosocomial and aspiration pneumonia

Nosocomial pneumonias represent 27 percent of all nosocomial infections, accounting for over US$4.5 billion in annual healthcare costs in the United States alone.[55] Mechanical ventilation in the ICU increases the risk of pneumonia by up to 21-fold, with risk increasing in a linear fashion proportional to the duration of mechanical ventilation.[56] The majority of ventilator-associated pneumonia is secondary to aspiration of oropharyngeal or gastric secretions into the distal airways where both chemical pneumonitis and pulmonary infection can occur.

Portable chest radiography has a sensitivity of 87–100 percent in detecting nosocomial pneumonias in the presence of alveolar infiltrates.[57] When alveolar infiltrates from aspiration pneumonia are present, they are typically located along the posterior segments of the lungs in the supine patient. However, because alveolar infiltrates are common in critically ill patients who have no pneumonia, portable chest radiography has a specificity of only 27–35 percent for pneumonia.[56,58–60] Thus, it is generally accepted that portable chest radiography alone is not accurate for the diagnosis of nosocomial pneumonias. The clinical diagnosis of nosocomial pneumonia is traditionally made using a combination of findings including fever, leukocytosis, purulent tracheal secretions, radiographic alveolar infiltrate, and secretion microbiology.[61] Other nonspecific radiologic findings seen with nosocomial pneumonias include air bronchogram signs, progressive alveolar opacification, and abscess or cavity formation within an opacification (Fig. 7.6).[56]

Atelectasis

Atelectasis is frequently seen in ICU patients, and can be classified as obstructive, nonobstructive, or platelike. Obstructive atelectasis in the ICU commonly occurs following endotracheal tube malposition or bronchial obstruction by a mucus plug.[62] Initially, the pulmonic circulation perfuses the airless lung, which results in ventilation/perfusion mismatch and hypoxemia. Subsequently, the pulmonic circulation absorbs the alveolar gas, leading to retraction of the involved lung within hours. As the atelectatic lung collapses, the heart and mediastinum shift toward the atelectatic area, the ipsilateral diaphragm becomes elevated, and the affected lung becomes opacified on the chest radiograph. If the obstruction is removed promptly, the lung reinflates to its normal state. On occasion, blood flow to the area may not return to normal, and can mimic pulmonary embolism.[63] If the obstruction persists, complications including infection, fibrosis, and bronchiectasis may occur. Thus it is crucial to alert clinicians when acute lung opacification or endotracheal tube malposition is encountered on the chest radiograph.

Nonobstructive atelectasis results from loss of contact between the visceral and parietal pleura, which commonly occurs as a result of pleural effusions, pneumothorax, scarring, or adjacent mass effect. On chest radiographs, this type of atelectasis is found adjacent to the underlying process such as a pleural effusion or pneumothorax. On CT scans, pleural effusion is seen in the dependent lobes more commonly than pneumothorax, which affects the nondependent lobes. In the postsurgical setting, general anesthesia and surgical manipulation lead to diaphragmatic dysfunction and diminished surfactant activity, leading to segmental basilar atelectasis.[64,65]

Platelike or subsegmental atelectasis results from buckling of subpleural lung, which commonly occurs during hypoventilation and other persistent low-volume states. As its name suggests, this type of atelectasis appears platelike on

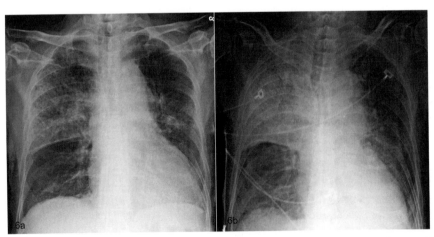

Figure 7.6 *(a) Chest radiograph of a febrile patient demonstrating opacification of the right upper lobe, consistent with pneumonia. (b) Chest radiograph of the same patient obtained 2 days later demonstrating the progressive opacification of the right upper lobe that is characteristic of lobar pneumonias.*

chest radiographs. These small areas of atelectasis occur because of inadequate regional ventilation and abnormalities in surfactant formation from hypoxia, ischemia, oxygen toxicity, and other toxic exposures.[66,67]

Prolonged atelectasis may worsen hypoxemia through shunting of the pulmonic circulation, and may predispose the patient to nosocomial pneumonia.[68,69] The mainstay of treatment for atelectasis in ICU patients has been tracheobronchial suctioning and, on some occasions, chest physiotherapy and bronchoscopy.[70,71] Recognition of atelectasis and its potential cause on chest radiography is particularly important for the critically ill patient who already has a reduced cardiopulmonary reserve.

Pleural effusions and empyema

Pleural effusions can be found in up to 60 percent of ICU patients.[72] In the ICU, pleural effusions can be seen in both supine and semi-erect chest radiographs, both of which are less sensitive than lateral erect radiographs. Evaluation of pleural effusions is important because many cases are noninfectious and rapidly improve with treatment of the underlying disease. Noninfectious causes of pleural effusions include heart failure, fluid overload, malignancy, hypoalbuminemia, postoperative, and atelectasis.[73,74]

Several large prospective studies of medical ICU patients have found that 18–62 percent of pleural effusions were infectious in etiology, and would benefit from diagnostic thoracentesis.[73,74] Pleural infection occurs in three stages:

1. An exudative simple parapneumonic effusion that is typically treated with antibiotics.
2. A complex parapneumonic effusion or empyema that is typically drained percutaneously.
3. Finally, pleural fibrosis that is typically treated with thoracotomy and decortication.[75]

During pleural infection, radiographs typically show a loculated pleural effusion with air–fluid levels (Fig. 7.7). Occasionally, an empyema may appear as a rounded pleural mass, similar in appearance to lung cancer or mesothelioma. If pleural infection is suspected, lateral decubitus radiographs have been recommended to detect small amounts of pleural fluid, especially in critically ill patients who are unable to provide standard upright views.[76,77] If loculations are suspected, based either on the appearance of the chest radiograph or on the inability to completely drain the fluid, then a chest CT can be performed to define the pleural anatomy and to guide thoracentesis.

In a prospective study of 1640 medical ICU patients, Tu *et al.* found that portable ultrasound-guided thoracentesis in febrile patients is a safe and useful method for diagnosing thoracic empyema. Tu *et al.* also described three sonographic patterns associated with infected pleural effusions: homogeneously echogenic; complex nonseptated and relatively hyperechoic; and complex septated.[74]

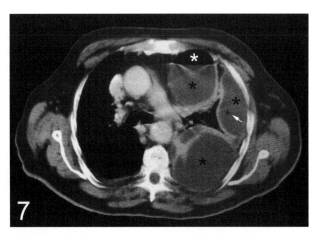

Figure 7.7 *Computed tomography scan of a patient with an empyema demonstrates multiple loculated collections of gas (white asterisk) and fluid (black asterisks) within the left hemithorax. Also note the presence of small gas bubbles (white arrow) within the collections.*

SUPPORT DEVICES

Several complications may arise from malpositioned ICU support devices such as endotracheal tubes, tracheostomy tubes, enteric tubes, pulmonary artery catheters, intraaortic balloon pump, and central venous catheter. Clinical examination alone is often insufficient to appropriately position or locate these support devices. Portable radiographs of the chest or abdomen are often required to localize these devices and identify any complications that may arise from their placement.

Endotracheal tubes and tracheostomy tubes

The endotracheal tube (ETT) is the most commonly placed support device in the ICU patient and portable chest radiography is the standard imaging modality to evaluate ETT position. The ideal position of the ETT is 3–4 cm above the carina. Flexion and extension of the patient's neck results in migration of the tip of the ETT up to 2 cm in the inferior and superior directions.[78] When the ETT is malpositioned within a mainstem bronchus, complete atelectasis of the contralateral lung often occurs, accompanied by difficulties with mechanical ventilation (Fig. 7.8). When the ETT is malpositioned within the superior trachea, there is a risk of accidental extubation and vocal cord injury (Fig. 7.9).

Malposition of the ETT occurs in approximately 15 percent of patients and, in one of the more recent reviews of 101 patient intubations, Lotano *et al.* recommended the use of routine post-intubation chest radiography for detection of ETT malposition, for which clinical diagnosis is unreliable.[79] Lotano *et al.* also concluded that, in the absence of specific pulmonary complications, an immediate or 'stat' post-intubation chest radiograph is not indicated.[79] This is

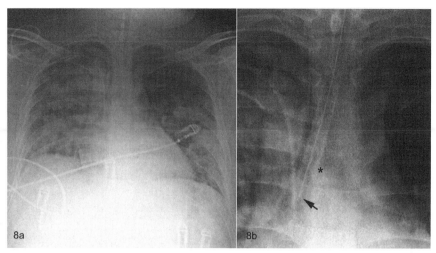

Figure 7.8 *(a) Chest radiograph demonstrating an inadvertent intubation of the right mainstem bronchus in this patient with pulmonary edema. (b) Magnified view of the mediastinum from the same radiograph demonstrating the relationship between the malpositioned endotracheal tube tip (arrow) and the carina (asterisk).*

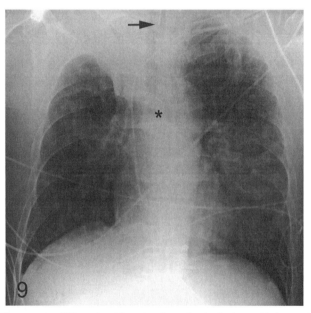

Figure 7.9 *This malpositioned endotracheal tube (arrow) is located above the thoracic inlet, over 9 cm superior to the carina (asterisk).*

somewhat counterintuitive, as it is often difficult to identify specific pulmonary complications on the basis of clinical examination alone. Furthermore, ICU patients often have large bilateral pleural effusions that can mask or mimic asymmetric breath sounds. Thus, the ACR Appropriateness Criteria recommends an immediate chest radiograph for all patients after intubation.[4]

Tracheostomy tubes are typically inserted percutaneously and are rarely malpositioned in the modern ICU. Several studies have found that the few abnormalities identified on posttracheostomy radiographs do not affect patient management, thus not warranting the cost of routine posttracheostomy radiography.[80–82]

Enteric tubes

The most commonly placed enteric tubes in the ICU setting are the Dobhoff feeding tube and the nasogastric tube (NGT). The feeding tube is a small-bore catheter that is primarily used for feeding or drug administration, whereas the NGT is a larger-bore catheter that has additional functions including gastric decompression and drainage. The ideal position for the tip of the feeding tube is distal to the pylorus.[83] When the feeding tube tip is positioned proximal to the pylorus, there is an increased likelihood of gastroesophageal reflux. The ideal tip position of the NGT is the mid to distal stomach. Many serious complications can occur as a result of enteric tube malposition. Respiratory failure and death can occur as a result of airway placement and intrapulmonary feeding.[84,85] Pneumothorax and mediastinitis can occur after pleural space or mediastinal placement.[86] Esophageal and gastric perforation have also been reported (Fig. 7.10).[87,88] It is generally accepted that the accurate localization of the enteric tube tip is crucial prior to initiating tube feeds. Thus, an abdominal radiograph is required immediately after each enteric tube placement or repositioning. If the enteric tube tip is not visible on the abdominal radiograph, a stat chest radiograph should be obtained to identify any pulmonary complications arising from the malpositioned enteric tube (Fig. 7.11). The ACR Appropriateness Criteria recommends obtaining a chest radiograph after enteric tube placement, especially in the critically ill patient.[4]

Chest tube and pleural catheter

Chest tubes have been in use for over 60 years. In today's ICU, chest tubes and pleural catheters are used to treat pneumothoraces and hydrothoraces following iatrogenic or

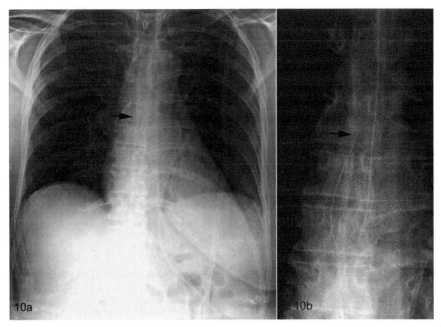

Figure 7.10 *(a) Chest radiograph demonstrating a stiff nasogastric tube that is coiled within the mid-esophagus (arrow), placing the patient at risk for esophageal perforation. (b) Magnified view of the same radiograph, delineating the malpositioned nasogastric tube tip that is pointing superiorly (arrow).*

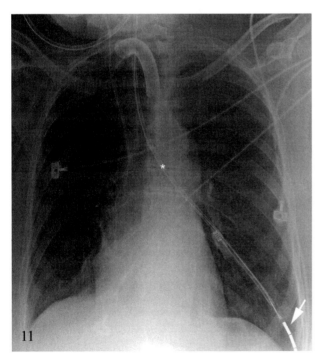

Figure 7.11 *Chest radiograph demonstrating a feeding tube tip (arrow) that was inadvertently placed into the left lower lobe through the left mainstem bronchus (asterisk).*

infarction, diaphragmatic injury, and visceral perforation.[89] On plain radiographs, the chest tube tip and its side holes should be within the pleural space. The side hole of the chest tube is designed to improve the drainage efficiency of the tube. Malpositioning of the chest tube or its side hole outside of the pleural space results in an air leak. This air leak is seen radiographically as a persistent or worsening pneumothorax or pleural effusion. Increased pulmonary density along the chest tube or kinking of the chest tube should alert the radiologist to the possibility of lung injury or entrapment.[90] Malpositioning of the chest tube too far medially within the thoracic cavity has also been reported to cause a contralateral pneumothorax as well as esophageal and cardiac perforations.[91–93] The ACR Appropriateness Criteria recommends a chest radiograph after initial chest tube placement.[4] Chest tubes that are not definitively within the pleural space on chest radiographs may be malpositioned inferior to the diaphragm and can result in abdominal organ injury.[94] Chest tubes may also be malpositioned within the subcutaneous tissues of the chest wall. Computed tomography may be necessary to locate the chest tube tip when the chest radiograph is equivocal (Fig. 7.12).

Central venous catheter

Central venous catheters (CVCs) have been in use for almost 50 years, and are increasingly common with the ICU patients requiring multiple intravenous medications. Their complications are classified as either mechanical or infectious.

traumatic causes. They are also commonly used for drainage of pus, bile, or chylous effusions. Due to the more rigid nature of chest tubes, their complications during insertion include hemorrhage, pulmonary contusion, pulmonary

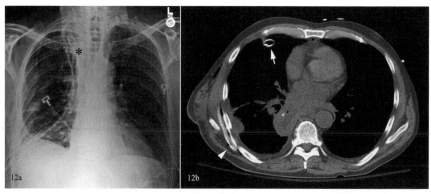

Figure 7.12 *(a) The two chest tubes (asterisks) appear to be in proper position within the right hemithorax on chest radiograph. (b) Computed tomography scan of the same patient performed on the same day demonstrates one chest tube appropriately within the right pleural space (arrow) while the other chest tube is malpositioned within the subcutaneous tissues of the right posterolateral chest wall (arrowhead).*

Mechanical complications include pneumothorax, cardiac arrhythmia, air embolism, hemothorax, and retained guidewires.[95] Among these complications, pneumothorax is encountered most commonly, at a rate of about 0.2–2 percent, depending on operator expertise and site of catheter insertion.[96,97] Due to its low complication rates, several studies have found that there is essentially no benefit in performing routine radiographs after a technically successful right internal jugular CVC placement.[98–100] Nevertheless, the ACR Appropriateness Criteria states that there is good evidence to support obtaining a chest radiograph after initial CVC placement, and that follow-up radiographs are recommended only if complications are suspected clinically.[4]

Infectious complications consist primarily of catheter-related bacteremia, which occurs in about 20 percent of central venous catheters.[101] The underlying mechanism for bacterial colonization of CVCs is thrombus formation. Predisposing factors to catheter infection include underlying disease, catheter composition, indwelling time, insertion site, insertion technique, and catheter care. Many of the currently produced CVCs are impregnated with antibiotics or antiseptics that reduce the risk of infection by up to 70 percent compared with traditional catheters.[102] A recent randomized controlled study of 346 CVCs has also suggested that antibiotic impregnation of long-term-use CVCs may obviate the need for subcutaneous tunneling.[103]

Pulmonary artery catheter

Pulmonary artery catheters have been in use for over 30 years as a hemodynamic monitoring device in the ICU. In a recent randomized trial consisting of 1041 ICU patients, it was found that 10 percent of catheter placements led to complications.[104] Older studies have found complications rates of up to 19 percent when the catheter is introduced via a jugular approach.[105] Death has been a rarely reported complication.[106] The ideal location of the pulmonary artery catheter tip is in the main pulmonary artery, within 2 cm proximal to its bifurcation. The catheter tip should not extend

distal to the proximal interlobar arteries when the balloon is deflated (Fig. 7.13). Catheter malposition has been associated with vascular trauma and thromboembolic events.[107] The most common complications of pulmonary artery catheter placement identifiable on portable radiographs include pneumothorax, hemothorax, and retained guidewires within the femoral vein and inferior vena cava.[104] Thus, the ACR Appropriateness Criteria suggests that chest radiography be performed after placement or manipulation of the pulmonary artery catheter.[4]

Intraaortic balloon pump

The intraaortic balloon pump (IABP) has been in use for almost 40 years, providing temporary circulatory support during cardiac ischemia, shock, and multisystem failure. In

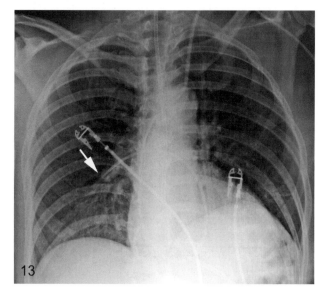

Figure 7.13 *Chest radiograph demonstrating a pulmonary artery catheter that is positioned just proximal to the region of the interlobar arteries (arrow). A more distal placement would increase the risk for vascular trauma and thromboembolic events.*

recent years, the most common complications of IABP placement are vascular complications such as retroperitoneal hematomas and limb ischemia in about 3 percent.[108,109] This frequency has decreased in comparison to prior estimates of about 18 percent, possibly due to improved patient selection prior to IABP placement and careful radiographic assessment.[110,111] The tip of the IABP should be positioned within the aortic arch distal to the origin of the left subclavian artery. The inferior end of the IABP should be positioned proximal to the origin of the renal arteries. Malposition or migration of the IABP can compromise blood flow to the left subclavian artery or renal arteries, which are rare complications. Thus, a chest radiograph should always follow IABP placement or manipulation.

CONCLUSION

Imaging of respiratory emergencies in the intensive care unit (ICU) is a constant challenge due to the increasing complexity of medical and surgical ICU patients. Technological advancements in PACS, cross-sectional imaging, and image-guided interventional procedures have increased the clinical demand for radiologic imaging in both the emergency department and in the ICU. In the near future, improvements in radiation dose-reduction technologies, image-processing algorithms, and our understanding of pulmonary complications will further enhance the efficacy and safety of radiologic imaging of the critically ill patient.

Key learning points

- Respiratory emergencies represent a spectrum of life-threatening cardiopulmonary conditions that are commonly encountered in the emergency room and ICU.

- With the deployment of PACS, multidetector-row CT scanners, and image-guided interventions, radiology has evolved technologically to meet the challenges of today's emergency room and ICU.

- Imaging in the ICU is traditionally performed using both routine and nonroutine radiography, allowing physicians to monitor both clinical progress and unexpected complications.

- Combined with a familiarity with common respiratory emergencies, vigilant radiologic monitoring frequently detects life-threatening pathology that is clinically occult.

- Rapid advancements in radiation dose-reduction technologies and image processing algorithms are underway to further improve imaging safety and efficacy.

REFERENCES

1. Henschke CI, Pasternack GS, Schroeder S, *et al.* Bedside chest radiography: diagnostic efficacy. *Radiology* 1983; **149**: 23–6.

2. Strain DS, Kinasewitz GT, Vereen LE, George RB. Value of routine daily chest x-rays in the medical intensive care unit. *Crit Care Med* 1985; **13**: 534–6.

3. Graat ME, Stoker J, Vroom MB, Schultz MJ. Can we abandon daily routine chest radiography in intensive care patients? *J Intensive Care Med* 2005; **20**: 238–46.

4. Tocino I, Westcott J, Davis SD, *et al.* Routine daily portable x-ray. American College of Radiology. ACR Appropriateness Criteria. *Radiology* 2000; **215**(Suppl): 621–6.

5. McCunn M, Mirvis S, Reynolds N, Cottingham C. Physician utilization of a portable computed tomography scanner in the intensive care unit. *Crit Care Med* 2000; **28**: 3808–13.

6. Mayo-Smith WW, Rhea JT, Smith WJ, *et al.* Transportable versus fixed platform CT scanners: comparison of costs. *Radiology* 2003; **226**: 63–8.

7. Matson MB, Jarosz JM, Gallacher D, *et al.* Evaluation of head examinations produced with a mobile CT unit. *Br J Radiol* 1999; **72**: 631–6.

8. Chahine-Malus N, Stewart T, Lapinsky SE, *et al.* Utility of routine chest radiographs in a medical-surgical intensive care unit: a quality assurance survey. *Crit Care* 2001; **5**: 271–5.

9. Kim PK, Gracias VH, Maidment AD, *et al.* Cumulative radiation dose caused by radiologic studies in critically ill trauma patients. *J Trauma* 2004; **57**: 510–14.

10. Kalra MK, Maher MM, Toth TL, *et al.* Strategies for CT radiation dose optimization. *Radiology* 2004; **230**: 619–28.

11. Aberle DR, Wiener-Kronish JP, Webb WR, Matthay MA. Hydrostatic versus increased permeability pulmonary edema: diagnosis based on radiographic criteria in critically ill patients. *Radiology* 1988; **168**: 73–9.

12. Gropper MA, Wiener-Kronish JP, Hashimoto S. Acute cardiogenic pulmonary edema. *Clin Chest Med* 1994; **15**: 501–15.

13. Gluecker T, Capasso P, Schnyder P, *et al.* Clinical and radiologic features of pulmonary edema. *Radiographics* 1999; **19**: 1507–31.

14. Goss CH, Brower RG, Hudson LD, Rubenfeld GD; ARDS Network. Incidence of acute lung injury in the United States. *Crit Care Med* 2003; **31**: 1607–11.

15. Goodman LR, Fumagalli R, Tagliabue P, *et al.* Adult respiratory distress syndrome due to pulmonary and extrapulmonary causes: CT, clinical, and functional correlations. *Radiology* 1999; **213**: 545–52.

✱ 16. Bernard GR, Artigas A, Brigham KL, *et al.* The American-European Consensus Conference on ARDS. Definitions, mechanisms, relevant outcomes, and clinical trial coordination. *Am J Respir Crit Care Med* 1994; **149**: 818–24.

◆ 17. Bernard GR. Acute respiratory distress syndrome: a historical perspective. *Am J Respir Crit Care Med* 2005; **172**: 798–806.

18. Sporer KA, Dorn E. Heroin-related noncardiogenic pulmonary edema: a case series. *Chest* 2001; **120**: 1628–32.

19. Mann H, Ward JH, Samlowski WE. Vascular leak syndrome associated with interleukin-2: chest radiographic manifestations. *Radiology* 1990; **176**: 191–4.

20. Gabry AL, Ledoux X, Mozziconacci M, Martin C. High-altitude pulmonary edema at moderate altitude (<2,400 m; 7,870 feet): a series of 52 patients. *Chest* 2003; **123**: 49–53.

21. Smith WS, Matthay MA. Evidence for a hydrostatic mechanism in human neurogenic pulmonary edema. *Chest* 1997; **111**: 1326–33.

22. Gammon RB, Shin MS, Buchalter SE. Pulmonary barotrauma in mechanical ventilation. Patterns and risk factors. *Chest* 1992; **102**: 568–72.

◆ 23. Ricard JD. Barotrauma during mechanical ventilation: why aren't we seeing any more? *Intensive Care Med* 2004; **30**: 533–5.

24. Boussarsar M, Thierry G, Jaber S, *et al.* Relationship between ventilatory settings and barotrauma in the acute respiratory distress syndrome. *Intensive Care Med* 2002; **28**: 406–13.

25. de Latorre FJ, Tomasa A, Klamburg J, *et al.* Incidence of pneumothorax and pneumomediastinum in patients with aspiration pneumonia requiring ventilatory support. *Chest* 1977; **72**: 141–4.

26. Kollef MH. Risk factors for the misdiagnosis of pneumothorax in the intensive care unit. *Crit Care Med* 1991; **19**: 906–10.

27. Plewa MC, Ledrick D, Sferra JJ. Delayed tension pneumothorax complicating central venous catheterization and positive pressure ventilation. *Am J Emerg Med* 1995; **13**: 532–5.

28. Gordon R. The deep sulcus sign. *Radiology* 1980; **136**: 25–7.

29. Levin B. The continuous diaphragm sign: a newly recognized sign of pneumomediastinum. *Clin Radiol* 1973; **24**: 337–8.

30. Zylak CM, Standen JR, Barnes GR, Zylak CJ. Pneumomediastinum revisited. *Radiographics* 2000; **20**: 1043–57. [Erratum in: *Radiographics* 2001; **21**: 1616.]

31. Bridges KG, Welch G, Silver M, *et al.* CT detection of occult pneumothorax in multiple trauma patients. *J Emerg Med* 1993; **11**: 179–86.

32. Amato MB, Barbas CS, Medeiros DM, *et al.* Effect of a protective-ventilation strategy on mortality in the acute respiratory distress syndrome. *N Engl J Med* 1998; **338**: 347–54.

33. Anzueto A, Frutos-Vivar F, Esteban A, *et al.* Incidence, risk factors and outcome of barotrauma in mechanically ventilated patients. *Intensive Care Med* 2004; **30**: 612–19.

34. Moser KM, LeMoine JR, Nachtwey FJ, Spragg RG. Deep venous thrombosis and pulmonary embolism. Frequency in a respiratory intensive care unit. *JAMA* 1981; **246**: 1422–4.

35. Cullen DJ, Nemeskal AR. The autopsy incidence of acute pulmonary embolism in critically ill surgical patients. *Intensive Care Med* 1986; **12**: 399–403.

36. Major KM, Wilson M, Nishi GK, *et al.* The incidence of thromboembolism in the surgical intensive care unit. *Am Surg* 2003; **69**: 857–61.

✱ 37. British Thoracic Society Standards of Care Committee Pulmonary Embolism Guideline Development Group. *Thorax* 2003; **58**: 470–83.

◆ 38. Remy-Jardin M, Mastora I, Remy J. Pulmonary embolus imaging with multislice CT. *Radiol Clin North Am* 2003; **41**: 507–19.

39. Powell T, Muller NL. Imaging of acute pulmonary thromboembolism: should spiral computed tomography replace the ventilation-perfusion scan? *Clin Chest Med* 2003; **24**: 29–38.

◆ 40. Johnson MS. Current strategies for the diagnosis of pulmonary embolus. *J Vasc Interv Radiol* 2002; **13**: 13–23.

◆ 41. Kanne JP, Lalani TA. Role of computed tomography and magnetic resonance imaging for deep venous thrombosis and pulmonary embolism. *Circulation* 2004; **109**(Suppl): 15–21.

42. Donato AA, Scheirer JJ, Atwell MS, *et al.* Clinical outcomes in patients with suspected acute

pulmonary embolism and negative helical computed tomographic results in whom anticoagulation was withheld. *Arch Intern Med* 2003; **163**: 2033–8.

43. Moores LK, Jackson WL Jr, Shorr AF, Jackson JL. Meta-analysis: outcomes in patients with suspected pulmonary embolism managed with computed tomographic pulmonary angiography. *Ann Intern Med* 2004; **141**: 866–74.

44. Krestan CR, Klein N, Fleischmann D, *et al.* Value of negative spiral CT angiography in patients with suspected acute PE: analysis of PE occurrence and outcome. *Eur Radiol* 2004; **14**: 93–8.

45. van Rossum AB, van Houwelingen HC, Kieft GJ, Pattynama PM. Prevalence of deep vein thrombosis in suspected and proven pulmonary embolism: a meta-analysis. *Br J Radiol* 1998; **71**: 1260–5.

◆ 46. Katz DS, Loud PA, Hurewitz AN, *et al.* CT venography in suspected pulmonary thromboembolism. *Semin Ultrasound CT MR* 2004; **25**: 67–80.

47. Cham MD, Yankelevitz DF, Henschke CI. Thromboembolic disease detection at indirect CT venography versus CT pulmonary angiography. *Radiology* 2005; **234**: 591–4.

48. Garg K, Kemp JL, Wojcik D, *et al.* Thromboembolic disease: comparison of combined CT pulmonary angiography and venography with bilateral leg sonography in 70 patients. *AJR Am J Roentgenol* 2000; **175**: 997–1001.

49. Lim KE, Hsu WC, Hsu YY, *et al.* Deep venous thrombosis: comparison of indirect multidetector CT venography and sonography of lower extremities in 26 patients. *Clin Imaging* 2004; **28**: 439–44.

50. Taffoni MJ, Ravenel JG, Ackerman SJ. Prospective comparison of indirect CT venography versus venous sonography in ICU patients. *AJR Am J Roentgenol* 2005; **185**: 457–62.

51. Begemann PG, Bonacker M, Kemper J, *et al.* Evaluation of the deep venous system in patients with suspected pulmonary embolism with multi-detector CT: a prospective study in comparison to Doppler sonography. *J Comput Assist Tomogr* 2003; **27**: 399–409.

52. Cham MD, Yankelevitz DF, Shaham D, *et al.* Deep venous thrombosis: detection by using indirect CT venography. *Radiology* 2000; **216**: 744–51.

53. Loud PA, Katz DS, Bruce DA, *et al.* Deep venous thrombosis with suspected pulmonary embolism: detection with combined CT venography and pulmonary angiography. *Radiology* 2001; **219**: 498–502.

54. Richman PB, Wood J, Kasper DM, *et al.* Contribution of indirect computed tomography venography to computed tomography angiography of the chest for the diagnosis of thromboembolic disease in two United States emergency departments. *J Thromb Haemost* 2003; **1**: 652–7.

◆ 55. Napolitano LM. Hospital-acquired and ventilator-associated pneumonia: what's new in diagnosis and treatment? *Am J Surg* 2003; **186**: 4S–14S; discussion 31S–34S.

56. Garrard CS, A'Court CD. The diagnosis of pneumonia in the critically ill. *Chest* 1995; **108**(Suppl): 17S–25S.

57. Wunderink RG. Radiologic diagnosis of ventilator-associated pneumonia. *Chest* 2000; **117**(Suppl 2): 188S–190S.

58. Wunderink RG, Woldenberg LS, Zeiss J, *et al.* The radiologic diagnosis of autopsy-proven ventilator-associated pneumonia. *Chest* 1992; **101**: 458–63.

59. Winer-Muram HT, Rubin SA, Ellis JV, *et al.* Pneumonia and ARDS in patients receiving mechanical ventilation: diagnostic accuracy of chest radiography. *Radiology* 1993; **188**: 479–85.

60. Lefcoe MS, Fox GA, Leasa DJ, *et al.* Accuracy of portable chest radiography in the critical care setting. Diagnosis of pneumonia based on quantitative cultures obtained from protected brush catheter. *Chest* 1994; **105**: 885–7.

◆ 61. Baughman RP. Diagnosis of ventilator-associated pneumonia. *Curr Opin Crit Care* 2003; **9**: 397–402.

62. Nair SR, Pearson SB. Images in clinical medicine. Mucous plug in the bronchus causing lung collapse. *N Engl J Med* 2002; **347**: 1079.

63. Bray ST, Johnstone WH, Dee PM, *et al.* The 'mucous plug syndrome'. A pulmonary embolism mimic. *Clin Nucl Med* 1984; **9**: 513–18.

64. Uzieblo M, Welsh R, Pursel SE, Chmielewski GW. Incidence and significance of lobar atelectasis in thoracic surgical patients. *Am Surg* 2000; **66**: 476–80.

◆ 65. Magnusson L, Spahn DR. New concepts of atelectasis during general anaesthesia. *Br J Anaesth* 2003; **91**: 61–72.

66. Joffe N, Simon M. Pulmonary oxygen toxicity in the adult. *Radiology* 1969; **92**: 460–5.

67. Westcott JL, Cole S. Plate atelectasis. *Radiology* 1985; **155**: 1–9.

68. Brooks-Brunn JA. Postoperative atelectasis and pneumonia: risk factors. *Am J Crit Care* 1995; **4**: 340–9.

69. van Kaam AH, Lachmann RA, Herting E, *et al.* Reducing atelectasis attenuates bacterial growth and translocation in experimental pneumonia. *Am J Respir Crit Care Med* 2004; **169**: 1046–53.

70. Kreider ME, Lipson DA. Bronchoscopy for atelectasis in the ICU: a case report and review of the literature. *Chest* 2003; **124**: 344–50.

71. Schindler MB. Treatment of atelectasis: where is the evidence? *Crit Care* 2005; **9**: 341–2.

72. Mattison LE, Coppage L, Alderman DF, *et al.* Pleural effusions in the medical ICU: prevalence, causes, and clinical implications. *Chest* 1997; **111**: 1018–23.

73. Fartoukh M, Azoulay E, Galliot R, *et al.* Clinically documented pleural effusions in medical ICU patients: how useful is routine thoracentesis? *Chest* 2002; **121**: 178–84.

74. Tu CY, Hsu WH, Hsia TC, *et al.* Pleural effusions in febrile medical ICU patients: chest ultrasound study. *Chest* 2004; **126**: 1274–80.

◆ 75. Chapman SJ, Davies RJ. Recent advances in parapneumonic effusion and empyema. *Curr Opin Pulm Med* 2004; **10**: 299–304.

◆ 76. Colice GL, Curtis A, Deslauriers J, *et al.* Medical and surgical treatment of parapneumonic effusions: an evidence-based guideline. *Chest* 2000; **118**: 1158–71. [Erratum in: *Chest* 2001; **119**: 319.]

77. Metersky ML. Is the lateral decubitus radiograph necessary for the management of a parapneumonic pleural effusion? *Chest* 2003; **124**: 1129–32.

78. Conrardy PA, Goodman LR, Lainge F, Singer MM. Alteration of endotracheal tube position. Flexion and extension of the neck. *Crit Care Med* 1976; **4**: 7–12.

79. Lotano R, Gerber D, Aseron C, *et al.* Utility of postintubation chest radiographs in the intensive care unit. *Crit Care* 2000; **4**: 50–3.

80. Hoehne F, Ozaeta M, Chung R. Routine chest X-ray after percutaneous tracheostomy is unnecessary. *Am Surg* 2005; **71**: 51–3.

81. Tyroch AH, Kaups K, Lorenzo M, *et al.* Routine chest radiograph is not indicated after open tracheostomy: a multicenter perspective. *Am Surg* 2002; **68**: 80–2.

82. Tarnoff M, Moncure M, Jones F, *et al.* The value of routine posttracheostomy chest radiography. *Chest* 1998; **113**: 1647–9.

83. Rees RG, Payne-James JJ, King C, Silk DB. Spontaneous transpyloric passage and performance of 'fine bore' polyurethane feeding tubes: a controlled clinical trial. *JPEN J Parenter Enteral Nutr* 1988; **12**: 469–72.

84. Harvey PB, Bull PT, Harris DL. Accidental intrapulmonary Clinifeed. *Anaesthesia* 1981; **36**: 518–22.

85. Odocha O, Lowery RC Jr, Mezghebe HM, *et al.* Tracheopleuropulmonary injuries following enteral tube insertion. *J Natl Med Assoc* 1989; **81**: 275–81.

86. Hand RW, Kempster M, Levy JH, *et al.* Inadvertent transbronchial insertion of narrow-bore feeding tubes into the pleural space. *JAMA* 1984; **251**: 2396–7.

87. McWey RE, Curry NS, Schabel SI, Reines HD. Complications of nasoenteric feeding tubes. *Am J Surg* 1988; **155**: 253–7.

● 88. Siegle RL, Rabinowitz JG, Sarasohn C. Intestinal perforations secondary to nasojejunal feeding tubes. *AJR Am J Roentgenol* 1976; **126**: 1229–32.

◆ 89. Gilbert TB, McGrath BJ, Soberman M. Chest tubes: indications, placement, management, and complications. *J Intensive Care Med* 1993; **8**: 73–86.

● 90. Peterson WP, Whiteneck GG, Gerhart KA. Chest tubes, lung entrapment, and failure to wean from the ventilator. Report of three patients with quadriplegia. *Chest* 1994; **105**: 1292–4.

● 91. Gerard PS, Kaldawi E, Litani V, *et al.* Right-sided pneumothorax as a result of a left-sided chest tube. *Chest* 1993; **103**: 1602–3.

● 92. Johnson JF, Wright DR. Chest tube perforation of esophagus following repair of esophageal atresia. *J Pediatr Surg* 1990; **25**: 1227–30.

● 93. Meisel S, Ram Z, Priel I, *et al.* Another complication of thoracostomy – perforation of the right atrium. *Chest* 1990; **98**: 772–3.

◆ 94. Gayer G, Rozenman J, Hoffmann C, *et al.* CT diagnosis of malpositioned chest tubes. *Br J Radiol* 2000; **73**: 786–90.

◆ 95. Polderman KH, Girbes AJ. Central venous catheter use. Part 1: mechanical complications. *Intensive Care Med* 2002; **28**: 1–17.

● 96. Hagley MT, Martin B, Gast P, Traeger SM. Infectious and mechanical complications of central venous catheters placed by percutaneous venipuncture and over guidewires. *Crit Care Med* 1992; **20**: 1426–30.

● 97. Kincaid EH, Davis PW, Chang MC, *et al.* 'Blind' placement of long-term central venous access devices: report of 589 consecutive procedures. *Am Surg* 1999; **65**: 520–3; discussion 523–4.

● 98. Lucey B, Varghese JC, Haslam P, Lee MJ. Routine chest radiographs after central line insertion: mandatory postprocedural evaluation or unnecessary waste of resources? *Cardiovasc Intervent Radiol* 1999; **22**: 381–4.

99. Sanabria A, Henao C, Bonilla R, *et al.* Routine chest roentgenogram after central venous catheter insertion is not always necessary. *Am J Surg* 2003; **186**: 35–9.

100. Lessnau KD. Is chest radiography necessary after uncomplicated insertion of a triple-lumen catheter in the right internal jugular vein, using the anterior approach? *Chest* 2005; **127**: 220–3.

101. Polderman KH, Girbes AR. Central venous catheter use. Part 2: infectious complications. *Intensive Care Med* 2002; **28**: 18–28.

102. Darouiche RO, Raad II, Heard SO, *et al.* A comparison of two antimicrobial-impregnated central venous catheters. Catheter Study Group. *N Engl J Med* 1999; **340**: 1–8.

103. Darouiche RO, Berger DH, Khardori N, *et al.* Comparison of antimicrobial impregnation with tunneling of long-term central venous catheters: a randomized controlled trial. *Ann Surg* 2005; **242**: 193–200.

104. Harvey S, Harrison DA, Singer M, *et al.* PAC-Man study collaboration. Assessment of the clinical effectiveness of pulmonary artery catheters in management of patients in intensive care (PAC-Man): a randomised controlled trial. *Lancet* 2005; **366**: 472–7.

105. Kaiser CW, Koornick AR, Smith N, Soroff HS. Choice of route for central venous cannulation: subclavian or internal jugular vein? A prospective randomized study. *J Surg Oncol* 1981; **17**: 345–54.

106. Robin ED. Death by pulmonary artery flow-directed catheter: time for a moratorium? *Chest* 1987; **92**: 727–31.

107. Coulter TD, Wiedemann HP. Complications of hemodynamic monitoring. *Clin Chest Med* 1999; **20**: 249–67.

108. Kang N, Edwards M, Larbalestier R. Preoperative intraaortic balloon pumps in high-risk patients undergoing open heart surgery. *Ann Thorac Surg* 2001; **72**: 54–7.

109. Davidson J, Baumgariner F, Omari B, Milliken J. Intra-aortic balloon pump: indications and complications. *J Natl Med Assoc* 1998; **90**: 137–40.

110. Kantrowitz A, Wasfie T, Freed PS, *et al.* Intraaortic balloon pumping 1967 through 1982: analysis of complications in 733 patients. *Am J Cardiol* 1986; **57**: 976–83.

111. Funk M, Ford CF, Foell DW, *et al.* Frequency of long-term lower limb ischemia associated with intraaortic balloon pump use. *Am J Cardiol* 1992; **70**: 1195–9.

8

Bronchoscopy

ANUP BANERJEE, PRAVEEN N MATHUR

INTRODUCTION

Bronchoscopy has been in use since over a century ago when Gustav Killian of Freiburg, Germany used a rigid endoscope to extract a pork bone from the trachea of a German farmer.[1] The flexible fiberoptic bronchoscope was first developed by Shigeto Ikeda of the National Cancer Institute, Tokyo, in 1964 and became commercially available in 1967.[2] Bronchoscopy is currently the most commonly used invasive procedure in the practice of pulmonary medicine and has helped in the development of newer concepts in diagnosis and management of pulmonary diseases.

This chapter discusses the various indications, contraindications, use of premedication, sedation and anesthesia, complications and care of bronchoscope, with special emphasis on use of bronchoscopy in respiratory emergencies.

EQUIPMENT

Both rigid and flexible bronchoscopes have undergone several modifications. Fiberoptic bronchoscopes have essentially replaced rigid bronchoscopes. A survey by the American College of Chest Physicians (ACCP) in 1991 indicated that less than 10 percent of doctors used rigid bronchoscopes in their practice.[3] In fact there are few bronchoscopic procedures that cannot be accomplished with the flexible bronchoscope. Fiberoptic bronchoscopes come

in different sizes depending on their distal end: pediatric scope (3.5–3.6 mm, 1.2 mm working channel); small adult (4.9 mm, 2.2 mm working channel); and standard adult (5.9–6.0 mm, 2.2–2.8 mm working channel). A flexible bronchoscope with a larger working channel allows the use of larger biopsy forceps, laser fibers, balloon catheters, and other instruments.

Rigid bronchoscopy is relatively more invasive and is usually performed under general anesthestic with adequate sedation and muscle relaxants. The procedure may be performed in an endoscopy suite with available anesthesia, but is more appropriately performed in an operating suite.

INDICATIONS (Boxes 8.1–8.3)

Although the American Thoracic Society,[4] ACCP,[5] and the British Thoracic Society[6] have guidelines for bronchoscopy, the ultimate value of the procedure depends on the experience and expert judgment of the clinician.

CONTRAINDICATIONS

Absolute contraindications for bronchoscopy are limited and consist primarily of refractory hypoxemia or unstable cardiac arrhythmia. Relative contraindications depends on risk of procedure (Box 8.4).

Box 8.1 Indications of bronchoscopy

Diagnostic indications (this includes evaluation of symptoms, suspected conditions, or radiological findings):

- Unexplained cough, localized wheeze, or stridor
- Hemoptysis
- Hoarseness of voice or vocal cord paralysis
- Diaphragmatic paralysis
- Chest trauma
- Inhalation injury
  - Thermal
  - Chemical
- Tracheoesophageal or bronchopleural fistula
- Graft rejection in transplant patients
- Postoperative assessment of tracheal, tracheobronchial, bronchial anastomosis, and stump
- Abnormal chest radiograph
  - Paratracheal/hilar/mediastinal nodes
  - Pleural effusion
  - Parenchymal mass/nodule
  - Etiology of pneumonia
  - Persistent pneumothorax

Therapeutic indications:

- Foreign body
- Atelectasis secondary to mucus plug after failure to remove by noninvasive technique
- Removal of endobronchial lesion
  - Laser therapy: neodymium:yttrium aluminum garnet (Nd:YAG), potassium-titanyl-phosphate (KTP)
  - Cryotherapy
  - Electrosurgery
  - Argon photocoagulation
- Delivery of brachytherapy, photodynamic therapy
- Stent placement
- Aspiration of cysts
  - Bronchogenic
  - Mediastinal cysts
- Assist in intubation, confirm tube placement
- Assist in percutaneous tracheostomy

Box 8.2 Indications for bronchoscopy in an intensive care unit

- Difficult intubation: placement or change of endotracheal tube
- Evaluation of upper airway at extubation
- Evaluation of ventilator-associated pneumonia
- Pulmonary toilet
  - Excessive secretions
  - Lobar collapse

Box 8.3 Indications for rigid bronchoscopy

- Massive hemoptysis
- Foreign body retrieval
- Dilation of tracheal or bronchial strictures
- Placement of airway stents
- Tumor ablation

Box 8.4 Relative contraindications to bronchoscopy

- Lack of patient cooperation
- Unstable bronchial asthma
- Recent myocardial infarction (within 6 weeks) or unstable angina
- Respiratory insufficiency associated with hypoxemia or hypercarbia
- Partial tracheal obstruction
- Debility and advanced age
- Untreated tuberculosis
- Conditions with increased bleeding risk particularly with biopsy
  - Pulmonary hypertension
  - Coagulopathy
  - Uremia (increased risk of bleeding with biopsy)
  - Obstruction of the superior vena cava

PREPARATION FOR BRONCHOSCOPY

Although many practitioners perform routine pre-bronchoscopy testing, its effectiveness has not been established. The ACCP survey of bronchoscopists in North America found that chest imaging study, complete blood cell count, platelet count and prothrombin time were some of the routine pre-bronchoscopy screening tests that were commonly obtained.[3] Patients with chronic obstructive pulmonary disease, particularly with severe disease, should be evaluated carefully before bronchoscopy with arterial blood gases. A good history and physical exam still play a key role in the safety and success of the procedure. Verbal and written patient information has been shown to improve tolerance of the procedure and should be provided to the patient.[7]

Premedication and sedation

Although it is possible in many cases to perform flexible bronchoscopy without using sedatives, it is a common practice to routinely sedate patients before this procedure. A combination of a short-acting benzodiazepine, such as midazolam, and narcotics is highly preferred. Midazolam not only provides sedation but also creates amnesia.[8] Opioids enhance the effects of benzodiazepines and also act as a cough suppressant. Use of atropine to reduce secretions and minimize cough has been widely debated. In a recent study, 217 patients were randomized to receive atropine, glycopyrrolate, or saline placebo.[9] There were no significant differences in secretion control, cough suppression or overall patient comfort between each group. Use of music to create a soothing environment has been studied with conflicting results. Asthmatic patients should be premedicated with bronchodilators before bronchoscopy. Prophylactic antibiotics should be given before rigid bronchoscopy and should be considered in all high-risk patients, particularly those who have prosthetic heart valve, previous history of endocarditis, or are asplenic.[10]

Anesthesia

Rigid bronchoscopy is usually performed in the operating suite under the guidance of an anesthetist, as general anesthesia is required. Flexible bronchoscopy can be performed under local anesthesia. Topical lidocaine is the most commonly used agent because of its safety compared with other agents. There have been case reports of myocardial ischemia with topical cocaine, and it should be avoided.[11]

Topical lidocaine is used in the form of nasal gel when the nose is used as the route of bronchoscopy. Liquid lidocaine, used as spray or via an atomizer, helps in anesthetizing the upper airway and reducing laryngospasm and cough during the procedure. Lidocaine is absorbed into the systemic circulation and can lead to complications when used in higher doses.[12] Approximately 50 percent is absorbed when applied as nasal gel with 35 percent oral bioavailability. Seizure activity, agitation, and hypotension have been reported with topical lidocaine use. Toxicity is more common in elderly patients particularly in those with impaired hepatic function, as lidocaine is predominantly metabolized in the liver.[13] The 2001 British Thoracic Society guidelines suggest limiting the dose to approximately to 8.2 mg/kg in adults (approximately 29 mL of 2 percent solution for a 70 kg patient).[6] On rare occasions the use of topical lidocaine or benzocaine can cause methemoglobinemia.[14] This complication should be considered if there is a rapid drop in oxygen saturation as measured by pulse oximetry and should be confirmed by arterial blood gas cooximetry.

TREATMENT/MANAGEMENT

Hemoptysis

Bronchoscopy plays an important role in evaluation and management of hemoptysis. Massive hemoptysis is defined as more than 200 mL of bleeding in 24 hours or bleeding causing respiratory compromise and needing intubation, and it may have a fatal outcome if not managed adequately.[15] Bronchoscopy and computed tomography are complementary to localizing lung lesions and possible sources of bleeding.[16,17] The common causes of massive hemoptysis include tuberculosis, bronchiectasis, lung abscess, invasive fungal infections, aspergilloma, foreign body, broncholiths, and malignancies.[18] It can also manifest in several rheumatologic diseases with vasculitis.[19]

The initial priorities in treating such patients include maintenance of airway, optimizing oxygenation, and stabilizing hemodynamic status. The immediate cause of death is usually asphyxiation from pooling of blood in the airways. If the bleeding site is known, the patient should be placed with the bleeding lung in the dependent position. Patients should be electively intubated if there is any danger of airway compromise. Urgent bronchoscopy should be performed in unstable patients as it plays a key role in identifying the site of lesion and directs therapy. In various studies early bronchoscopy identified the site of bleeding in more than 90 percent patients.[20]

In patients with localized active bleeding, control of the airway may be obtained during the procedure with topical therapy, endobronchial tamponade, or selective intubation of normal lung. Double lumen intubation may be helpful if a skilled physician is available. If visualization is difficult because of bleeding, rigid bronchoscopy or emergent arteriography is indicated. Rigid bronchoscopy enables easier removal of blood and clot, localization of the site of bleed, and attempting tamponade. Fogarty balloon-tipped catheters have been successfully used to tamponade bleeding and remove big clots compromising the airway.[21]

Bronchial artery embolization has emerged as an excellent alternative in cases where bronchoscopy fails to control the bleed. It is highly effective and the risks encountered during surgery can be avoided. Surgery is always an option if everything else fails. However, surgery is primarily recommended in patients with massive hemoptysis caused by trauma, arteriovenous malformation, or leaking thoracic aneurysm with bronchial communication.

Inhalation injuries

Estimates show that fire and burns account for approximately 5500 deaths per year, although there has been significant decline in trend from 1971 to 1991.[22] This may be attributed to better understanding of management of burn victims including aggressive fluid resuscitation, early excision of burn wounds, and advances in nutrition, antibiotics, and critical care.

Various studies have attributed age and body surface area as major risk factors for mortality.[23–25] However, recent studies have emphasized the presence of inhalation injury as one of the major factors contributing to mortality from burns. Bronchoscopy helps in confirming the diagnosis of inhalation injury, aids in management, and can also be helpful in securing a difficult airway.

In a large study conducted in Canada, 1705 burn patients, admitted between 1977 and 1987, were analyzed for inhalation injury.[23] Inhalation injury was noted in 124 patients (7.3 percent) by bronchoscopy. Overall survival rate was 95.9 percent. Inhalation injury accounted for 34 percent of deaths, independent of age and total body surface area. The maximum detrimental effects of inhalation injury occurred when it coexisted with moderate (15–29 percent) to large surface area burns (>30 percent). Inhalation burns were also associated with prolonged hospital stay compared with cutaneous burns.

In another large study, the impact of inhalation injury, burn size, and age on overall outcome following burn injuries was examined in 1447 consecutive burn patients over a period of 5.5 years.[24] The presence of inhalation injury, increasing burn size, and advanced age were all associated with increased mortality. Inhalation injury was noted in 19.6 percent of patients. The overall mortality for all patients was 9.5 percent and inhalation injury accounted for 31 percent of mortality. These findings were confirmed by a retrospective review of patients with acute burn injuries, which included 1665 patients admitted between 1990 and 1994 to Massachusetts General Hospital and the Shriners Burns Institute in Boston, Massachusetts.[25] The three most important risk factors identified for death included age greater than 60 years, more than 40 percent of body surface area burns, and presence of inhalation injury.

Inhalation injury should be suspected based on clinical history of closed-space exposure, facial burns, singed nasal hairs, and carbonaceous debris in the mouth, pharynx, or sputum. A third of patients with inhalation injury, however, may not present with facial burns.[26] Smoke inhalation can cause injury by various mechanisms including thermal injury, direct toxic effect on airways, carbon monoxide poisoning, and hypoxia. Thermal injury is usually limited to the supraglottic region, but may cause significant erythema, ulceration, and edema. Upper airway edema typically presents within the first 24 hours and may cause asphyxiation. Patients should be monitored for respiratory compromise including stridor, respiratory distress, or hypoxia. A careful exam for erythema or blisters of the oropharynx should be done. In presence of any these signs early intubation is warranted. A large lumen endotracheal tube is preferred as it helps in management of secretions. Upper airway edema usually resolves by 3–5 days.

Carbon monoxide poisoning is thought to be the most common cause of death in inhalation injury. Carbon monoxide is formed by the incomplete combustion of carbon containing compounds. The symptoms include headache, nausea, altered cognition, seizures, cardiac dysrhythmias, angina, and heart failure. If clinically suspected, the patient should be treated with 100 percent oxygen. The diagnosis can be confirmed by measuring carbon monoxide levels by cooximetry of the arterial blood gas sample.

Common substances in house fire smoke include chlorine, formalin, acrolein, phosgene, nitrogen oxides, and sulfur dioxide, and they have toxic effects on the bronchial mucosa. Particles less than 4 μm in diameter can reach the distal airways and are more dangerous. The acute inflammatory response to local injury may present as cough, wheezing with severe bronchospasm, dyspnea, and bronchorrhea. This may be noted 12–36 hours after the exposure to inhalation injury. There may be mucosal necrosis and airway occlusion from soot and debris. There is also loss of ciliary function, and intrapulmonary shunting develops as a result of interstitial and alveolar edema.

The chest radiograph is a poor predictor of inhalation injury and may show normal findings in a patient with inhalation injury.[27] However, the presence of pulmonary infiltrates upon initial evaluation may indicate a poorer prognosis. Pulmonary hygiene is of utmost importance and bronchoscopy aids in suctioning soot and thick secretions. Infection of the denuded material can lead to tracheobronchitis or pneumonia needing prolonged mechanical ventilation and a complicated course.

Foreign body

Foreign body aspiration can be life-threatening, requiring early intervention. It is more commonly seen in children but can also occur in adults. Retrospective studies showed that the peak incidence in children occurred during the second year of life, and in adults it was noted to be in the sixth decade.[28,29] Nearly all series showed male predominance.

Peanuts are usually the most common aspirated foreign body in children.[30] Others are various nuts, sunflower seeds, popcorn husk, kernel corn and other food particles, and parts of toys. In adults the nature of the foreign body has been found to be variable and includes pins, vegetable matter, and bone fragments. Loss of consciousness, alcohol, sedative use, dental procedures, and neurologic disorders may predispose to aspiration.[31] Patients usually present with sudden onset of choking sensation, intractable cough, and vomiting. There may be associated fever, wheezing, and breathlessness. The foreign body is usually located in the proximal airways in children. In contrast it is usually found in the distal airways in adults, more commonly the right bronchial tree.

Presentation in children is usually early, whereas in adults it is usually delayed. Patients are usually more symptomatic if the foreign body is lodged in the trachea. A chest radiograph may show normal findings on initial investigation, and a high index of suspicion should always warrant adequate intervention. Atelectasis secondary to obstruction is the most common abnormality noted in adults in the chest radiograph. Patients sometimes present after 1 year with findings of lung abscess or bronchiectasis.

Although rigid bronchoscopy has been the gold standard for extraction of aspirated foreign bodies in children, successful removal of foreign bodies with flexible bronchoscopy was reported in 24 of 39 children (62 percent) in a review.[30] Another prospective study reviewed 83 consecutive children with suspected airway foreign bodies.[32] History of acute asphyxia, findings of radioopaque foreign body, and unilateral decreased breath sounds along with obstructive emphysema were found to have high positive predictive value. The authors recommended the use of rigid bronchoscopy in such patients. A rigid bronchoscope helps in maintaining airway as it works in a similar fashion to the an endotracheal tube and also provides larger conduit to remove the foreign body. However, lack of availability of equipment and trained personnel have limited its use.

The standard flexible bronchoscope has been used more frequently in treating adults with foreign body aspiration.[29,32,34] The flexible bronchoscope has the advantage of allowing retrieval of foreign bodies that have migrated to deeper subsegmental bronchi. Once the foreign body is located various types of instruments including forceps, baskets, snares, grasping claws, and balloon-tipped catheters can be used for retrieval. If the foreign body is round, smooth forceps are preferred compared with an irregular foreign body for which alligator forceps are usually preferred. Alternatively, a cryotherapy probe can be used to retract a foreign body.

Complications reported during removal of foreign body include bleeding from manipulation of granulation tissue and dislodgment of the foreign body more distally. Few patients develop stridor and cough after rigid bronchoscopy, which is thought to be from post-bronchoscopy laryngeal edema.

In summary, retrieval of a foreign body can be attempted with a flexible bronchoscope in both children and adults. General anesthesia and endotracheal intubation is recommended to secure the airway. A rigid bronchoscope should be available along with skilled operator, so that in the case of failure with the flexible scope, the procedure can be accomplished in the same setting, and complications if any, can be handled adequately.

Atelectasis in the intensive care unit

Atelectasis is one of the common complications seen in the intensive care unit (ICU). It may cause worsening of hypoxemia and predispose to infection. Bronchoscopy is frequently used in ICUs along with other modes of therapy such as suctioning, mucolytic agents, kinetic beds, mechanical vibration devices. In a recent review of literature of bronchoscopy for atelectasis in ICU patients, Kreider and Lipson looked at efficacy, safety, and advantage of bronchoscopy over other modes of therapy.[35] The effectiveness of bronchoscopy varied from 19 percent to 89 percent.

In Lindholm et al.'s[36] case series of 52 patients who had undergone 71 fiberoptic bronchoscopy procedures in the ICU, 81 percent (43/53) demonstrated improvement on follow-up chest radiograph if secretions were noted during the procedure, versus 22 percent (4/18) if secretions were absent. Weinstein et al. reviewed 43 bronchoscopies with lavages, performed in six patients for atelectasis as seen in chest radiograph.[37] Although no obvious mucus plug was noted, 81 percent (35/43) had improvement in PaO_2/PAO_2 ratio and 63 percent (27/43) had improvement in static lung compliance. The authors suggested that lavages have additional yield if there is no obvious central mucus plugging. In a larger case series, Stevens et al. studied 297 bronchoscopies that had been performed in 223 ICU patients.[38] In 118 patients bronchoscopy was performed for atelectasis seen in the chest radiograph; 79 percent (93/118) were noted to have improvement, based on follow-up radiograph or reduction in the alveolar–arterial oxygen gradient. However, among patients who had bronchoscopy for retained secretions, only 44 percent (31/70) showed improvement. In another case series, Snow and Lucas reviewed 76 bronchocopies performed on 51 patients in surgical ICU;[39] 35 patients had lobar atelectasis and 8 patients had subsegmental atelectasis. Radiographic improvement was seen in 89 percent (31/35) of patients with lobar atelectasis versus 56 percent (5/9) of patients with subsegmental atelectasis. Olopade and Prakash retrospectively reviewed 90 patients in the Mayo Clinic ICU, who had had bronchoscopy for atelectasis.[40] Interestingly, only 19 percent (17/90) had an improvement seen in chest radiographs or oxygenation by 72 hours.

The above studies suggest that a subgroup of patients with lobar atelectasis might respond better than those with retained secretions or subsegmental atelectasis. This is presumably because these patients have large central plugs that can be removed easily with bronchoscopy. In addition, these studies suggest that bronchioalveolar lavage may be of additional benefit for clearing more distal mucus plugs. Some authors have advocated the use of insufflation in addition to standard bronchoscopy.[41] As insufflation was performed in only a few studies after initial bronchoscopy failed, benefit of insufflation over bronchoscopy alone remains unclear.

Not many studies have compared the rate of success between bronchoscopy and other modalities for treatment of atelectasis. In one trial, Marini et al. randomized 31 consecutive patients with lobar atelectasis to emergent bronchoscopy or chest physiotherapy.[42] Fourteen patients were randomized to emergent bronchoscopy and then chest therapy every 4 hours for 48 hours. Seventeen patients received chest therapy every 4 hours. Patients who failed chest therapy in the first 24 hours underwent bronchoscopy. The authors found no significant difference in the rate of resolution of atelectasis with bronchoscopy versus chest therapy at either 24 or 48 hours.

Although bronchoscopy is a relatively safe procedure, in critically ill patients it can cause worsening hypoxemia, hypercapnia, increase in end-inspiratory and end-expiratory pressures, and hemodynamic changes.[36,43] Studies have also demonstrated marked elevation of intracranial pressure[44] and worsening of cardiac ischemia by electrocardiographic monitoring during bronchoscopy in such patients, although the clinical significance is not clear. Hence, indication for bronchoscopy in such patients largely depends on overall assessment of the patient.

Difficult airway

Flexible bronchoscopy has become an important tool in evaluation of difficult airway and managing difficult intubations. It is of great importance in care of critically ill trauma patients with suspected airway damage or cervical injury. Bronchoscopic inspection also helps in proper positioning of the endotracheal tube. It is also advisable to do bronchoscopy-guided intubation in patients with failed extubation when upper airway edema is suspected.

Stent migration

With recent advances in interventional bronchoscopy, there has been a rise in the use of endoprosthetic stents for management of central airway obstruction. Various types are available: metallic (self-expandable metallic airway stents [SEMS]), silicone (Dumon stents), and hybrid stents. The choice of stent depends on the operator's preference and the underlying lesion. Rigid bronchoscopy is essential for placement of silicone airway stents, where as SEMS can be placed with a flexible bronchoscope.

One of the main potential complications associated with stent placement is stent migration. In one retrospective analysis of 46 patients, Dumon silicone stent was compared with screw thread stent.[45] There was a trend toward higher rate of migration with the Dumon stent compared with the screw thread stent, in particular in benign tracheal stenosis. In another retrospective analysis of 82 patients with SEMS, the overall migration rate was found to be 4.7 percent.[46]

Complications associated with stent removal include hemoptysis, laryngeal edema, respiratory failure needing intubation, and bronchial perforation. Stent removal needs operator expertise and is usually done in operation suite, under general anesthesia.

COMPLICATIONS

Complications associated with bronchoscopy are quite uncommon and usually minor in nature. This has been shown in multiple surveys involving large number of procedures. However, there may be underreporting of the incidence of complications as many questionnaires were answered based on recall rather than actual recorded data. The two major complications include bleeding and pneumothorax and are usually related to transbronchial

biopsies. A summary of the various studies that have looked into the incidence of major and minor complications and mortality from bronchoscopy follows.

Credle et al. in 1974 were the first to review the complications of fiberoptic bronchoscopy.[47] They surveyed 250 physicians, and 78 percent responded with a total of over 24 000 procedures. Mortality was 0.01 percent and the incidence of major complications was 0.08 percent. This was followed by another larger survey by Suratt et al., which included 1041 physicians.[48] Thirty-one percent responded, with a total of 48 000 procedures. Mortality was 0.03 percent and the incidence of major complications was 0.3 percent.

Pereira et al. conducted the first prospective study, involving 908 patients. Mortality was 0.44 percent, and the rate of major complications was 1.65 percent and minor complications was 6.5 percent.[49] A survey of 40 000 bronchoscopies in UK revealed a mortality of 0.04 percent and a major complication rate of 0.12 percent.[50] In 1991, an ACCP survey of North America, which included 53 639 bronchoscopies done in 1989, showed a minor complication rate of 10 percent or less for 80 percent of respondents. Only 3.5 percent of physicians reported a major complication rate of more than 5 percent.[4] In another review of 3096 bronchoscopies over 9 years at the Cleveland Clinic, which included biopsy or brushing, the incidence of significant bleeding was found to be 1.9 percent.[51] In a retrospective review by Pue et al. of 4273 bronchoscopies in a university hospital, which included 2493 lavages and 173 transbronchial biopsies, no mortality was noted and the overall rate of major and minor complications was 0.5 percent and 0.8 percent, respectively.[52] Four percent of patients with transbronchial biopsy developed pneumothorax and 2.8 percent developed significant bleeding (greater than 50 mL).

Another potential complication of bronchoscopy is infection. Although fever has been frequently reported following bronchoscopy, there are few studies or case reports of bacteremia.[53,54] In a recent prospective study involving 518 bronchoscopies in immunocompetent adult patients, fever was reported in 5 percent with no bacteremia.[55] The fever was transient in nature and subsided within 1 day. The severity of bleeding was identified as an independent risk factor. Bronchioalveolar lavage, the amount of saline solution or drug administered, and the dose of lidocaine instilled, were also identified as risk factors. In another prospective study involving bronchoscopy in 91 immunocompetent children, 48 percent developed fever within 24 hours of the procedure, however bacteremia was absent.[56] The systemic inflammatory response has been postulated to be a cause of fever, as increase in total leukocyte count and proinflammatory cytokines such as tumor necrosis factor α have been reported during bronchoscopy.[57]

Infections can result from cross-contamination between patients. Contamination of bronchoscopes and sterilizing equipment has been associated with transmission of infection or pseudoinfection with various mycobacteria including

Mycobacterium chelonae, M. xenopi, and *M. abscessus*.[58–60] In 2001, multiple outbreaks of *Pseudomonas aeruginosa* were linked to defects in the biopsy port of the bronchoscope, which prevented adequate sterilization.[61] Premedication may cause hypotension, tachycardia, nausea, vomiting, allergic reaction, and respiratory depression. Lidocaine used as local anesthetic can cause laryngospasm, bronchospasm, seizures, arrhythmias, and rarely methemoglobinemia.

Hypoxemia is commonly noted during bronchoscopy. It usually develops after administration of sedation and is easily reversed with use of supplemental oxygen. Oxygen supplementation and sedation should be used with caution with patients who are carbon dioxide retainers, as it may further worsen carbon dioxide retention and cause hypercapnic respiratory failure. Patients with hypoxemia should also be monitored for cardiac arrhythmias.

POST-PROCEDURE CARE

Most complications occur early, so patients should be closely monitored for 2–4 hours after the procedure. Feeding should be avoided until the effects of sedation has resolved. Most centers obtain a chest radiograph following transbronchial biopsy, however, occasionally pneumothorax may develop much later.

CARE OF EQUIPMENT

Adequate precautions during the use of the instrument and familiarity with the care of the bronchoscope can prevent most of the damage. A biteguard should always be used when a transoral approach is implemented. Disinfection of bronchoscopes should be done by trained staff and preferably in a dedicated room. Commonly used disinfectant solutions include activated dialdehydex (Cide), 2 percent alkaline glutaraldehyde (Cidex 7), and alkaline glutaraldehyde plus alkaline phenate buffer (Sporicidin). *M. tuberculosis, P. aeruginosa*, and many viruses are destroyed within 10 minutes with 2 percent glutaraldehyde. Disinfection with inadequate solutions has been associated with contamination and should be avoided.

Key learning points

- Bronchoscopy should be avoided if possible in patients with severe hypoxia and recent myocardial infarction (6 weeks).

- Transbronchial biopsy should be avoided in patients with increased risk of bleeding (coagulopathy, pulmonary hypertension, uremia).

- Asthmatic patients should be premedicated with bronchodilators before bronchoscopy.

- Oxygen supplementation and sedation should be used with caution in patients who are carbon dioxide retainers, as it may further worsen carbon dioxide retention and cause hypercapnic respiratory failure.

- Antibiotic prophylaxis should be considered in all high-risk patients, particularly those who have history of endocarditis or asplenia, or have prosthetic heart valves.

- Higher doses of lidocaine are associated with seizures and cardiac arrhythmias and additional caution should be used in elderly patients and those with hepatic and cardiac problems.

- Early bronchoscopy along with computed tomography is helpful in identifying site of bleed in patients with hemoptysis.

- Inhalation injury is one of the major factors affecting morbidity and mortality from burns. Bronchoscopy helps in confirming the diagnosis of inhalation injury and aids in the management.

- Carbon monoxide poisoning is thought to be the most common cause of death in inhalation injury.

- Upper airway edema secondary to burns typically presents within the first 24 hours and may cause asphyxiation.

- The chest radiograph is a poor diagnostic modality for inhalation injury and may show normal findings in a patient with inhalation injury.

- Foreign body aspiration in adults may go undiagnosed and may present later with bronchiectasis or lung abscess.

- Although rigid bronchoscopy has been considered the gold standard for retrieval of foreign bodies, recent studies suggests that it can be successfully attempted with flexible bronchoscopy.

- Patients with lobar atelectasis might respond better with bronchoscopy as compared with patients with subsegmental atelectasis.

- Bronchoscopy in critically ill patients can cause worsening of hypoxemia, hypercapnia, hemodynamic changes, rise in intracranial pressure, and worsening of cardiac ischemia. Indication of bronchoscopy depends on overall assessment of the patient.

- Bronchoscopy is useful in the evaluation and management of difficult airway including difficult intubation and patients with suspected airway and cervical injury.

- Contamination of bronchoscopes and sterilization equipment has been associated with transmission of infection or pseudoinfection with various mycobacteria including *M. chelonae, M. xenopi*, and *M. abscessus*.

REFERENCES

1. Killian G. Meeting of the Society of Physicians of Freiburg. Dec 17, 1897. *Munchen Med Wschr* 1989; **45**: 378.

2. Sackner MA. Bronchofiberoscopy. *Am Rev Respir Dis* 1975; **111**: 62–88.

3. Prakash UB, Offord KP, Stubbs SE. Bronchoscopy in North America: The ACCP survey. *Chest* 1991; **100**: 1668–75.

4. Guidelines for fiberoptic bronchoscopy in adults. American Thoracic Society. Medical Section of the American Lung Association. *Am Rev Respir Dis* 1987; **136**: 1066.

5. Ernst A, Silverstri GA, Johnstone D. Interventional pulmonary procedures: Guidelines from the American College of Chest Physicians. *Chest* 2003; **123**: 1693–717.

6. British Thoracic Society guidelines on diagnostic flexible bronchoscopy. *Thorax* 2001; 56 Suppl 1:i1–i21.

7. Poi PJH, Chuah SY, Srinivas P, Liam CK. Common fears of patients undergoing bronchoscopy. *Eur Respir J* 1998; **11**: 1147–9.

8. Williams TJ, Nicoulet I, Coleman E, *et al.* Safety and patient acceptability of intravenous midazolam for fiberoptic bronchoscopy. *Respir Med* 1994; **88**: 305–7.

9. Cowl CT, Prakash UB, Kruger BR. The role of anticholinergics in bronchoscopy: A randomized clinical trial. *Chest* 2000; **118**: 188–92.

10. Dajani AS, Taubert KA, Wilson *et al.* Prevention of bacterial endocardities: Recommendations by the American Heart Association. *JAMA* 1997; **277**: 1794–801.

11. Osula S, Stockton P, Abdelaziz MM, Walshaw MJ. Intratracheal cocaine induced myocardial infarction: an unusual complication of fiberoptic bronchoscopy. *Thorax* 2003; **58**: 733–4.

12. Loukides S, Katsoulis K, Tsarpalis K, *et al.* Serum concentrations of lignocaine before, during and after fiberoptic bronchoscopy. *Respiration* 2000; **67**: 13–17.

13. Wu FL, Razzaghi A, Souney PF. Seizure after lidocaine for bronchoscopy: Case report and review of the use of lidocaine in airway anesthesia. *Pharmacotherapy* 1993; **13**: 72–8.

14. Karim A, Ahmed S, Siddiqui R, *et al.* Methemoglobinemia complicating topical lidocaine used during endoscopic procedures. *Am J Med* 2001; **111**: 150–3.

15. Crocco JA, Rooney JJ, Fankushen DS. Massive hemoptysis. *Arch Intern Med* 1968; **121**: 495–8.

16. Naidich DP, Funt S, Ettenger NA, *et al.* Hemoptysis: CT bronchoscopic correlations in 58 cases. *Radiology* 1990; **177**: 357–62.

17. Hirshberg B, Biran I, Glazer M, *et al.* Hemoptysis: Etiology, evaluation and outcome in tertiary referral hospital. *Chest* 1997; **112**: 440–4.

18. Ramakantan R, Bandekar VG, Gandhi MS, *et al.* Massive hemoptysis due to pulmonary tuberculosis: Control with bronchial artery embolization. *Radiology* 1996; **200**: 691–4.

19. Odeh M, Best LA, Kerner H, *et al.* Localized Wegener's granulomatosis relapsing as diffuse massive intra-alveolar hemorrhage. *Chest* 1993; **104**: 955–6.

20. Smiddy JF, Elliot RC. The evaluation of hemoptysis with fiberoptic bronchoscopy. *Chest* 1973; **64**: 158–62.

21. Saw EC, Gottlieb LS, Yokoyama T, *et al.* Flexible fiberoptic bronchoscopy and endobronchial tamponade in the management of massive hemoptysis. *Chest* 1976; **70**: 589–91.

22. Brigham PA, McLoughlin E. Burn incidence and medical care use in the United States: estimates, trends, and data sources. *J Burn Care Rehabil* 1996; **17**: 95–107.

23. Tredget EE, Shankowsky HA, Taerum TV, *et al.* The role of inhalation injury in burn trauma. A Canadian experience. *Ann Surg* 1990; **212**: 720–7.

24. Smith DL, Cairns BA, *et al.* Effects of inhalation injury, burn size, and age on mortality: a study of 1447 consecutive burn patients. *J Trauma* 1994; **37**: 655–9.

25. Saffle JR, Davis B, Williams P. Recent outcomes in the treatment of burn injury in the United States: a report from the American Burn Association Patient Registry. *J Burn Care Rehabil* 1995; **16**: 219–32.

26. Ryan, CM, Schoenfeld, DA, Thorpe, *et al.* Objective estimates of the probability of death from burn injuries. *N Engl J Med* 1998; **338**: 363.

27. Herndon DN, Langer F, Thompson P, *et al.* Pulmonary injury in burned patients. *Surg Clin North Am* 1987; **67**: 31–46.

28. Pruitt B, Cioffi W, Shimazu T *et al.* Evaluation and management of patients with inhalation injury. *J Trauma* 1990; **30**: S63.

29. WAS 34Chen CH, Lai CL, Tsai TT, *et al.* Foreign body aspiration into the lower airway in Chinese adults. *Chest* 1997; **112**: 129–33.

30. Baharloo F, Veyckemans F, Francis C, *et al.* Tracheobronchial foreign bodies: Presentation and management in children and adults. *Chest* 1999; **115:** 1357–62.

31. Swanson K L, Prakash UBS, Midthun DE, *et al.* Flexible bronchoscopic management of airway foreign bodies in children. *Chest* 2002; **121:** 1695–700.

32. Limper AH, Prakash UB. Tracheobronchial foreign bodies in adults. *Ann Intern Med* 1990; **112:** 604–9.

33. Martinot A, Closset M, Marquette CH, *et al.* Indications for flexible versus rigid bronchoscopy in children with suspected foreign-body aspiration. *Am J Respir Crit Care Med* 1997; **155:** 1676–9.

34. Debeljak A, Sorli J, Music E, *et al.* Bronchoscopic removal of foreign bodies in adults: experience with patients from 1974–1998. *Eur Respir J* 1999; **14:** 792–5.

35. Kreider ME, Lipson DA. Bronchoscopy for atelectasis in the ICU. *Chest* 2003; **124:** 344–50.

36. Lindholm CE, Ollman B, Snyder J, *et al.* Flexible bronchoscopy in critical care medicine: diagnosis, therapy, and complications. *Crit Care Med* 1974; **2:** 250–61.

37. Weinstein HJ, Bone RC, Ruth WE. Pulmonary lavage in patients treated with mechanical ventilation. *Chest* 1977; **72:** 583–7.

38. Stevens RP, Lillington GA, Parsons G. Fiberoptic bronchoscopy in the intensive care unit. *Heart Lung* 1981; **10:** 1037–45.

39. Snow N, Lucas A. Bronchoscopy in the critically ill surgical patient. *Am Surg* 1984; **50:** 441–5.

40. Olopade CO, Prakash UB. Bronchoscopy in the critical care unit. *Mayo Clinic Proc* 1989; **64:** 1255–63.

41. Tsao TC-Y, Tsai Y-H, Lan R-S, *et al.* Treatment for collapsed lung in critically ill patients: selective intrabronchial air insufflation using the fiberoptic bronchoscope. *Chest* 1990; **97:** 435–8.

42. Marini JJ, Pierson DJ, Hudson LD. Acute lobar atelectasis: a prospective comparison of fiberoptic bronchoscopy and respiratory therapy. *Am Rev Respir Dis* 1979; **119:** 971–8.

43. Matsushima Y, Jones RL, King EG, *et al.* Alterations in pulmonary mechanics and gas exchange during routine fiberoptic bronchoscopy. *Chest* 1984; **86:** 184–8.

44. Kerwin A, Croce M, Timmons S, *et al.* Effects of fiberoptic bronchoscopy on intracranial pressure I patients with brain injury, a prospective clinical study. *J Trauma* 2000; **48:** 878–82.

45. Noppen M, Meysman M, Claes I, *et al.* Screw-thread vs Dumon Endoprosthesis in the management of tracheal stenosis. *Chest* 1999; **115:** 532–5.

46. Saad P C, Murthy S, Krizmanich G, Mehta AC. Self-expandable metallic airway stents and flexible bronchoscopy. *Chest* 2003; **124:** 1993–9.

47. Credle WF, Smiddy JF, Elliot RC. Complications of fiberoptic bronchoscopy. *Am Rev Respir Dis* 1974; **109:** 67–72.

48. Suratt PM, Smiddy JF, Gruber B. Deaths and complications associated with fiberoptic bronchoscopy. *Chest* 1976; **69:** 747–51.

49. Pereira W Jr, Kovnat DM, Snider GL. A prospective cooperative study of complications following flexible fiberoptic bronchoscopy. *Chest* 1978; **73:** 813–16.

50. Simpson FG, Arnold AG, Purvis A, *et al.* Postal survey of bronchoscopic practice by physicians in the United Kingdom. *Thorax* 1986; **41:** 311–17.

51. Cordasco EM Jr, Mehta AC, Ahmad M. Bronchoscopically induced bleeding: A summary of nine years' Cleveland Clinic experience and review of the literature. *Chest* 1991; **100:** 1141–7.

52. Pue CA, Pacht ER. Complications of fiberoptic bronchoscopy at a university hospital. *Chest* 1995; **107:** 430–2.

53. Yigla M, Oren I, Bentur L, *et al.* Incidence of bacteremia following fiberoptic bronchoscopy. *Eur Respir J* 1999; **14:** 789–91.

54. Gillis S, Dann EJ, Berkman N, *et al.* Fatal *Haemophilus influenzae* septicemia following bronchoscopy in a splenectomized patient. *Chest* 1993; **104:** 1607–9.

55. Um SW, Choi CM, Lee CT, *et al.* Prospective analysis of clinical characteristics and risk factors of postbronchoscopy fever. *Chest* 2004; **125:** 945–52.

56. Picard E, Schwartz S, Goldberg S, *et al.* A prospective study of fever and bacteremia after flexible bronchoscopy in children. *Chest* 2000; **117:** 573–7.

57. Standiford TJ, Kunkel SL, Strieter RM. Elevated serum levels of tumor necrosis factor-alpha after bronchoscopy and bronchoalveolar lavage. *Chest* 1991; **99:** 1529–30.

58. Campagnaro RL, Teichtahl H, Dwyer B. A pseudoepidemic of *Mycobacterium chelonae*: contamination of a bronchoscope and autocleaner. *Aust N Z J Med* 1994; **24:** 693.

59. Bennett SN, Peterson DE, Johnson DR, *et al.*

Bronchoscopy associated *Mycobacterium xenopi* pseudoinfections. *Am J Respir Crit Care Med* 1994; **150**: 245–50.

60. Maloney, S, Welbel S, Daves B, *et al. Mycobacterium abscessus* pseudoinfection traced to an automated endoscope washer: utility of epidemiologic and laboratory investigation. *J Infect Dis* 1994; **169**: 1166–9.

61. Srinivasan A, Wolfenden LL, Song X, *et al.* An outbreak of *Pseudomonas aeruginosa* infections associated with flexible bronchoscopes. *N Engl J Med* 2003; **348**: 221–7.

9

Chest tubes and thoracoscopy

ROBERT LODDENKEMPER, WOLFGANG FRANK

INTRODUCTION

Respiratory emergencies requiring management with chest tubes or thoracoscopy usually involve conditions that interfere with lung expansion by causing either lung collapse or lung compression. Pneumothorax and effusion (pleural or pericardial), or more generally, intrathoracic displacing processes, are the common denominator of these conditions, which may occur in combination (seropneumothorax), have an acute or prolonged onset, and may also interfere with cardiac performance.

Drainage for empyema was known to Hippocrates' disciples in the ancient times. However, chest tube thoracostomy, based on the concept of artificial pneumothorax, is essentially a development of the nineteenth century (Carson 1821, Hewett 1876, Forlanini 1882, Buelau 1891).[1] Ever since the 1920s it has undergone continual improvement in close connection with the development of thoracic surgery and thoracoscopy (Jacobaeus 1910, Graham 1918, Lilienthal 1922, Roe 1958, Munnel 1975).[1-3]

In Western populations currently the overall combined incidence of pneumothorax and significant pleural effusion that may need an invasive diagnostic or therapeutic intervention is around 200/100 000.[4] About every tenth of these may eventually require chest tube emergency management.[5,6] Surgical and traumatic indications contribute an equally large proportion. Mechanical factors – or their elimination – obviously represent crucial management issues in these conditions, but other issues, such as control of pneumonia or sepsis (as in empyema) and bronchial obstruction (as in cancer) or hemorrhage (as in trauma), may significantly contribute or even prevail. Pleural interventions in these types of respiratory emergency have three aims: (i) instant palliation and symptom relief, (ii) long-term or permanent disease control, and (iii) establishment of diagnosis of the underlying condition. Thoracoscopy (pleuroscopy), whenever feasible, adds a unique dimension to chest tube management by allowing visualization of the pleural cavity. Therefore, it is an excellent tool for optimizing pleural interventions in terms of superior diagnostic and therapeutic results.

COMMON INDICATIONS AND CLINICAL PRESENTATION

An overview of the indications and their approximate incidence is presented in Table 9.1. The most common indication is pneumothorax followed by tension, bilateral, and hemopneumothorax, and air dissection in the soft tissues. Salient indications related to intrathoracic displacement include: profuse effusion due to a number of causes, and most important, infectious pleurisy (empyema/parapneumonic effusion) and hemothorax.

Chest tube management is a basic component of the procedure in elective and emergency thoracic surgery. There are a few absolute contraindications to tube thoracostomy, most importantly untreated coagulopathy and end-stage, high-risk disease states such as in advanced cancer, where the invasive nature of the intervention would appear inappropriate. Relative contraindications include situations where small-bore catheters or palliative thoracentesis may suffice to control the condition, such as in a small spontaneous pneumothorax or in medically nonresponsive transudative effusion.

Table 9.1   *Indications for chest tube management and their relative incidence*

Indication	Disease/condition	Frequency (%)
Pneumothorax	Spontaneous, traumatic	30
Pleural effusion Inflammatory	Empyema, parapneumonic effusion, tuberculosis and others	23
Malignant	Bronchial carcinoma, metastatic, mesothelioma, others	
Hemothorax	Trauma, malignancy, others	
Chylothorax	Trauma, malignant, others	
Transudates	Hepatic, cardiac, renal disease	
Elective thoracic surgery related	Diagnostic and resective formal thoracotomy, video-assisted thoracoscopic surgery	25
Other than pleural	Trauma, malignancy, air dissection, infection	2
Pericardium Lung Mediastinum Soft tissue		

The main symptoms in all of these conditions consist of varying degrees and combinations of dyspnea, cough, and pain. The correlation between the amount of displacement of the chest volume and the symptoms, however, may be remarkably loose. In primary pneumothorax even a complete unilateral lung collapse may cause few symptoms as opposed to severe life-threatening respiratory distress (PO_2 <50 mm Hg) that may be provoked by just a small pneumothorax in individuals with significant pre-existent pulmonary morbidity such as chronic obstructive pulmonary disease or interstitial lung disease. Similarly, fluid amounts even up to 2 L may go unnoticed in long-standing effusion, whereas short-term profuse effusion as in acute hemothorax clearly presents a life-threatening complication. Compressive processes, including tension pneumothorax with mediastinal shift, will invariably produce respiratory and circulatory distress. A similar mechanism occurs in severe mediastinal emphysema. Signs and symptoms of coexistent or underlying systemic or organ disease may modify the clinical presentation, most importantly infection (pneumonia, empyema, sepsis) and malignancy (pulmonary and others).

PHYSIOLOGIC CONSIDERATIONS: THE RATIONALE OF CHEST TUBE MANAGEMENT

Chest tubes are basically designed to drain the pleural space and to restore lung expansion, whenever a substantial amount of air or liquid has penetrated there. Only in exceptional circumstances may chest tubes be inserted in locations other than the pleural space, such as an intrapulmonary cavity, the pericardium, soft tissue, or the mediastinum. Apart from their basic draining function, chest tubes may have additional interventional aims such as delivering pharmacologic agents or clearing the pleura of secretions by lysis and/or irrigation protocols. Indeed, the indications and aims of chest tube management often merge into each other (Table 9.2). To meet these aims chest tube management must include a suction device to overcome the pulmonary recoil force and to mobilize secretions. A reasonable level of suction to maintain lung expansion against its physiologic recoil force can be achieved with the gravity and posture-modified negative pressure normally present in the pleura. This varies between −4 cm H_2O and −8 cm H_2O throughout the respiratory cycle. It may, however, reach −21 cm H_2O in deep inspiration at the 90 percent total lung capacity (TLC) level and ≥40 cm H_2O with forced expiratory maneuvers.[7] Thus routinely, a suction force of approximately −20 cm H_2O appears to be reasonable and safe to counterbalance the physiologically occurring negative pressures. In clinical practice, however, suction devices must provide a significantly higher negative pressure reserve to also accommodate decreased lung compliance as occurs in lung consolidation or trapped lung due to membranes. Higher negative pressures may also be required to overcome increased resistance to suction as in the presence of tenacious or clotted secretions.

Table 9.2   *Aims and functions of chest drains*

Aims	Function
Air evacuation, lung expansion active fluid mobilization	Suction
Fluid (exudate, secretion, blood) clearance	Drainage
Pharmacologic effects (pleurodesis, fibrinolysis)	Instillation
Resolution, clearance of thick secretions	Irrigation

No adverse pulmonary effects have been noted with short-term increase in suction forces to as high as −80 cm H_2O as long as the lung does not remain completely detached from the chest wall and the negative pressure is thus transmitted to the mediastinum to produce mediastinal shift.[8] If a chest drain is to be operated without suction, the pleural cavity must be sealed against the ambient pressure with an external valve device. One of these, which is often used in pneumothorax treatment, is a Heimlich maneuver flutter valve; the most simple, effective and reliable device, however, is a classic water seal. The device preserves the negative pleural pressure and prevents access of air/fluid to the pleural space. However, it will allow the air/fluid to exit whenever there is a positive intrathoracic pressure (cm H_2O) that exceeds the depth of immersion (cm H_2O) of the tube in a water bottle.

TECHNICAL AND PROCEDURAL APPROACHES

Chest tube specification: small-bore catheters versus large-bore drains, optimum tube design and material

On the basis of the physiologic requirements discussed in the previous section specific criteria can be laid down to warrant successful, state-of-the-art chest tube therapy. First, the components of a chest tube suction set need to be defined. These include an appropriate arrangement of: a chest tube; a connection piece; a fluid collection device; and an optional suction-generating system. Figure 9.1 illustrates the chest drainage components, including a properly placed chest tube and combined suction/fluid collection system.

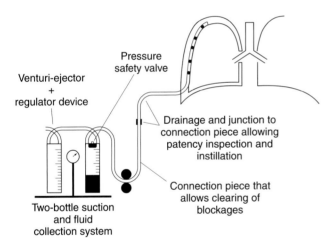

Figure 9.1 *Schematic representation of standard components of a chest drainage system including optimally positioned drainage, connection piece and Venturi-ejector-operated two-bottle suction/fluid collection system.*

Second, the most critical issue with regard to the entire system concerns the length and diameter of the intrathoracic tube portion. Box 9.1 provides a detailed explanation of how to calculate the required tube size based on flow-dynamic criteria and clinical demands.[9] On the assumption of -10 cm H_2O as the lowest acceptable suction force and the empiric requirement of an airflow up to 15 L/min (regardless of laminar or turbulent flow conditions) to be accommodated by the system in the case of major pulmonary air leaks (bronchopleural fistula), the minimal required internal

diameter of the tube system is 5.87 mm. This corresponds to a standardized external tube size of 24 Fr.

The length of the tube should not exceed 70 cm. Due to the exponential inverse relation between resistance and the tube radius, tube sizes smaller than 20 Fr would require disproportionately higher suction forces to handle high flow rates. Because large tubes are also advantageous in the management of thick viscous or clotty secretions, the recommendations for a standard tube call for a tube size of 24–28 Fr and a length of no more than 70 cm. The 24 cm intrathoracic portion should be open at the distal end and fenestrated up to a distance of about 18 cm to allow effective suction across a large surface of the pleural space. In general an ideal chest tube needs to be: anti-adhesive and transparent to prevent plugging and allow visual control of patency; supple and smooth enough to cause only minor patient discomfort; and stiff enough to prevent kinking and occlusion. These physicochemical properties are best provided by polyvinylchloride (PVC) products, and to a lesser extent also by silicone.

Box 9.1 What about chest tube size?

Flow dynamics:

- Poiseuille's law: $\dfrac{P}{Q}$ (R) $= \dfrac{8l\eta}{\pi r^4}$ (laminar)

- Fanning equation: $\dfrac{P}{Q}$ (R) $= \dfrac{fl}{\pi^2 r^5}$ (turbulent)

Actually occurring flow (Q) demands: <1–16 L/min

Required tube size (Fr), internal diameter (mm) and length at a standard suction level of -10 cm H_2O
- To deliver 10 L/min: 20 Fr (4.72 cm) <70 cm
- To deliver 15 L/min: 24 Fr (5.87 cm) <70 cm

where $P =$ pressure; $Q =$ flow; $R =$ resistance; $l =$ length; $\eta =$ viscosity coefficient; $r =$ radius; f = friction coefficient.

Third, different criteria apply to the extrathoracic large-bore connecting piece to the secretion collection system. This is appropriately made of rubber to allow manipulation by a roller-clamp or manually for mobilization of fibrin deposits or clots ('milking').

A summary of the essential criteria for the entire suction and air/fluid-conducting system is given in Box 9.2. Although the criteria recommended above are for 'all-round' standardized chest tube and equipment, small-bore Teflon catheters (8–14 Fr) continue to be widely used for reasons of obviously easier handling and purportedly better patient compliance.

Variously sized small-bore catheter systems are commercially available as full scale insertion kits, including either an outer introductory trocar-cannula or a needle

Box 9.2 Specifications of 'all-round' chest tubes

Intrathoracic section (chest tube)

- PVC or silicone
- Caliber >24 Fr, length <70 cm
- Sterile
- Transparent
- Soft and tissue-compatible
- Nonadhesive
- Resistant to kinking and occlusion
- Fenestrated for at least 18 cm and distance-marked intrathoracic section
- Radioopaque or contrast line-equipped

Extrathoracic section (connection piece)

- Rubber
- Disposable
- Large-bore, length <2 m
- Collapse-resistant up to 80 cm H_2O suction pressure
- Full elastic to allow 'milking' manually or by roller clamp
- Only few and large size adapters

guidewire set. The airflow in the system will usually vary between 2 L/min and 5 L/min flow depending on caliber, length, and fenestration design.[9] There is good evidence that they are sufficient to control a large proportion of uncomplicated pneumothoraces and low viscosity serous effusions such as transudates; however, they will often have limitations in unforeseen complications and interventional demands. In addition, in case of adhesions and loculations it may be difficult to control the catheter tip at insertion and to achieve an optimum position, which is true even when a Seldinger guidewire technique is used. Thus the pros and cons of small-bore catheters versus large-bore drains should be critically weighed according to the criteria in Table 9.3.

The individual choice will certainly vary with the indication, but often also depends on logistics and the interventionalist's skills and opinion, thus raising the question: Is chest drainage a surgeon's or a pulmonologist's job?

Procedures in chest tube management: who inserts and how and where to insert a chest tube?

Procedures can vary and opinion is divided about how and where to introduce a chest tube and who can do it optimally. In particular, differences in opinion may be about the preferred approach (medical or surgical), tube caliber issues, and related technical questions. Who is in charge of tube drainage management should not, within reason, be a specialty- or profession-linked consideration but rather should be based on qualification criteria. Large-bore trocar intervention may give the distinct impression of being a surgical intervention, but qualified and skilled pulmonologists with training and experience in pleuroscopy may be equally able to do it. According to a large American survey published in 1995 this was so for at least 60 percent of pulmonologists,[10] a figure that has likely substantially increased subsequently. It has been shown that well-trained physicians perform tube thoracostomy with only a 3 percent early and 8 percent late complication rate.[11] Most hospitals have custom-designed sterile kits for chest tube insertion that are deployed on emergency intervention trays. These kits can be reasonably standardized to contain the components listed in Box 9.3 but may also be expanded to include full-scale pleuroscopy equipment.

A chest drain is conventionally inserted with the patient in the lateral decubitus position, particularly in the high-dependency patient or the patient being ventilated. In the low-dependency conscious patient it may be inserted in the sitting upright and supported position. Premedication with atropine may prevent vagovasal syncope; an anxiolytic such as diazepam/midazolam may or may not be given depending on the patient. Informed consent in keeping with respective

Table 9.3　*What is the optimum tube equipment? Small-bore catheters vs. large-bore drains*

Tube size	Pros	Cons
Catheters – 8–14 Fv ± Heimlich flutter valve	Easy to insert No conditioning required Good patient tolerance Mobile patient Allows safe emergency intervention in less experienced hands	Prone to obturation and kinking Difficult to maneuver endothoracically even when guidewire Poor patency control and patency-conditioning Poorly compatible with thick secretions, blood, major air leaks and irrigation/instillation protocols
Large-bore drains ≥ 24 Fv ± continuous suction	Excellent patency control and patency conditioning Good compatibility with thick secretions, blood, major air leaks and any intervention Combination with pleuroscopy results in optimum efficacy	Higher technical demands Lower patient tolerance Limited patient mobility More prone to local complications such as infection and surgical emphysema

Box 9.3 Suggested components of a large-bore chest tube insertion kit

Basic equipment

- Povidone iodine solution
- Gauze swabs and sterile gloves
- Sterile towels and drapes
- Lidocaine hydrochloride solution 1% or 2%
- Syringes (5–20 mL)
- Needles (21–25 gauge)
- Scalpel
- Kelly clamps
- Trocar/sleeve system with sharp and blunt obturator or tube/stylet system
- Single- and double-lumen chest tubes (24–28 Fr)
- Surgical needle holder
- Silk suture with needle
- Scissors and surgical pince
- Sterile dressing
- Transparent tape or film
- Connection piece to wall suction and adaptor

Additional pleuroscopy equipment

- Portable high-power cold light source (200 W)
- Rigid 0° and angled vision scopes (4 mm and 9 mm)
- Forceps
- Sterile gown
- Anticondense vision scope conditioning (chemical or thermal)
- Biopsy-processing facilities (normal saline/formalin) flasks, smear carriers
- Optional: video equipment
- Optional: high performance engine-powered suction system

national/regional guidelines should be taken from the conscious patient prior to administration of sedative drugs.

The entry point is carefully cleansed with povidone iodine solution and covered with a fenestrated adhesive drape. Local anesthesia, 1–2 percent lidocaine, should be generously applied, infiltrating the skin, the relevant costal interspace and the rib edges in particular, but avoiding damage to the subcostal vasculature/nerve bundle. The infiltrating needle may be used as a probe to warn of a too-shallow subcostal space. Aspiration of air or free fluid will confirm safe insertion of the needle and the correct entry point. The undisputed preference for large-bore tubes clearly favors external trocar-sleeve or internal stylet-based techniques that allow penetration of the chest wall to an appropriate depth, e.g. with a 9 mm thoracoscopy-compatible external diameter sleeve. Both penetration techniques involve a sharp-tipped instrument, emphasizing the need of perfect imaging control of the air/fluid space underneath to prevent laceration of the lung and neighboring organs. The trocar/sleeve technique

requires a skin incision of no more than 1 cm. In a more traditional surgical approach a superficial skin incision of about 3 cm is followed by blunt dissection along with careful digital exploration and dissection of the muscle planes down to the pleura.[12] The chest drain should smoothly fit into the prepared port. It should never be forcefully inserted. A radiograph or fluoroscopy is a basic requirement for guiding drain insertion, but ultrasonography in particular is extremely helpful. It can identify loculations or adhesions even within fluid collections and thus help avoid trauma to the underlying lung.

Too little attention is often given to an appropriate fixation of the drain and the external dressing. Although purse-string sutures are no longer used, the tube should be fixed and sutured with a double knot placed close to the surrounding skin (to prevent bypassing air/fluid leakage) and should penetrate the chest wall at an acute angle, to avoid any kinking at the lower rib edge. The transparent dressing allows efficient routine inspection of the penetration site.

The entry point of drain insertion should be selected based on standardized criteria provided the lung is completely retracted and one is dealing with a large monolocular fluid- or airspace. Favorable and safe points of access are divided into upper and lower sites as shown in Figure 9.2. The most convenient and widely accepted lower entry point is defined with some variability in the fifth–sixth intercostal space in the mid or anterior axillary line, keeping a 3–4 cm safe distance from the diaphragm. This takes into account a usually higher diaphragmatic position after pleural evacuation or when the patient is pressing down. A functionally optimal and well-tolerated intrathoracic position of the tube is achieved by advancing the tip of the drain toward the apico-posterior angle of the pleural cavity.

The alternative apico-posterior access point is in the second paravertebral dorsal intercostal space, and this can be reproducibly and safely identified on the chest as halfway on the line connecting the upper median angle of the scapula and the seventh vertebro-spinal protrusion.[13] This classic surgical approach is best performed with the patient in a stable sitting and forward leaning position. It certainly requires increased effort and skill due to the marked thickness of the chest wall locally, but offers excellent functional results and tolerance of the indwelling drain. A third point, recommended in many emergency manuals, is the apical anterior entry point for small-bore catheters in the second–third intercostal space in the medioclavicular line (Fig. 9.2). In our opinion, the use of this point should be discouraged, especially for large-bore tubes. At this site tubes usually take an unfavorable, too short, and transverse intrathoracic course, and are easily subject to kinking. They may also leave an unsightly scar and with an access point that is too medial to the internal mammary artery may be at risk of laceration.

Insertion sites other than those recommended may be chosen in the presence of loculated pleural spaces depending on the actual situation. At times the insertion of a drain in a

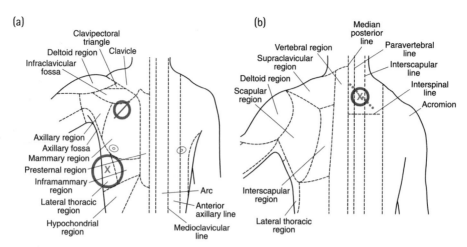

Figure 9.2 *Suggested standard access sites for large-bore chest drainage. (a) anterior basal access (X). Fifth to sixth intercostal space (ICS) in the mid to anterior axillary line. Ø is not routinely recommended: apical anterior access (second to third ICS medioclavicular). (b) Posterior apical access (X). Second intercostal paravertebral space halfway on the connection line between the seventh vertebral protrusion and superior scapular angle.*

strictly subpulmonary, i.e. supradiaphragmatic, cavity may be a technically challenging intervention. Drains should always be placed adjoining to the parietal pleura and interlobar positions avoided. A paramediastinal drain is generally poorly tolerated and should likewise be avoided unless specifically indicated. Once a chest drain has been placed, fixed appropriately, and connected with the conducting tube and suction system, the lung may be immediately reexpanded with increase in the suction force in increments of 5 cm H_2O until 20 cm H_2O is reached, with constant monitoring of the patient's tolerance. This strategy is not undisputed, and some authors advocate spontaneous reexpansion under a no-suction water seal.[9] However, there is no apparent advantage of leaving a lung unexpanded or incompletely expanded (or pleural fluid partially retained) for an uncertain period of time and to give up the instant opportunity to examine lung expandability. Exceptional situations that call for 'permissive', prolonged lung expansion and the actual failure to respond to reexpansion are described in the section on trouble shooting and critical issues later in this chapter.

A major complication during the insertion of a pleural drain is wrong placement, e.g. incorrect entry point resulting in trauma to the lung, spleen, liver, and heart. (Although this complication should practically not occur with expert imaging-controlled technique.) More realistic complications involve infections (empyema), which, in the thoracoscopic and surgical literature, amount to only 1 percent, major bleeding (e.g. by trauma to an intercostal artery) <3 percent, and intercostal nerve damage.[14–17] Soft-tissue surgical emphysema due to provoked cough and pain reactions is not infrequent (about 7 percent) but rarely progresses to become a major problem.[18] Reflexogenic hypotensive circulatory events related to pleural contact with the drainage equipment ('pleura shock') are occasionally seen but are by

definition transitory. There are only sparse combined data on complications covering the entire spectrum of indications including small-bore catheters. In one major review featuring 599 tube thoracotomies in 379 trauma patients the overall rate of complications of large-bore drainage (>24 Fr) was 21 percent.[19]

Options for suction generators and fluid collection devices

A number of devices are available for generation of short- or long-term therapeutic suction gradients. Basically these may be divided into high-performance electro-powered pumps for short-term use only; Venturi-operated, central pressurized air-supply-driven systems (wall suction) for continuous use; and simple gravity-dependent devices, which, however, offer only limited suction reserve. All these systems may be combined with a variety of fluid collection systems, the most simple and classic of which is a two-bottle system as depicted in Figure 9.1, which must also include a positive pressure safety valve. Many technical improvements have occurred over the years with a trend to disposable single-use sets that are increasingly replacing traditional two-bottle hardware. The core element of all of these fully integrated fluid collection/suction systems is a water seal unit, supplemented by a multichamber overflow collection system and positive pressure safety valve devices. The water seal is a highly sensitive indicator of appropriate function of the air/fluid conducting system. Persistent air bubbles after expansion of the lung suggest a visceral pleural leak (unless a technical leak is responsible). With the use of no-suction or low-suction gradients (≤20 cm H_2O) the visible respiratory swing of fluid in the chest tube signals patency of the system and confirms the correct position of the tube in the pleural cavity. A variety of so-called four-component-systems, as schematically depicted and described in Figure 9.3, including (i) a suction generator/control system, (ii) a water seal, (iii) an overflow fluid collection device, and (iv) a manometer monitoring the effective pleural pressure, are currently available. They are generally designed as fully integrated transparent, single use disposable devices, which may optionally be run with or without active suction.[20]

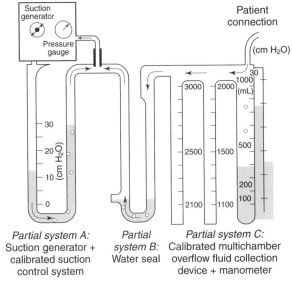

Figure 9.3 *Schematic representation of an integrated suction and fluid collection system. The arrows and bubbles indicate airflow direction, both from the ambient air (suction control system) and from the pleural cavity. If no suction is applied, the system operates as a two-bottle gravity-dependent combined water seal and fluid collection system. The integrated manometer in the fluid collection system (C) allows monitoring of the actual suction applied on the patient (= suction level of system A minus height of the water seal column [system B]). It also acts as a positive pressure safety valve.*

How to measure efficacy, trouble shooting, and when to remove a chest tube

Complete and sustained lung expansion clearly is the foremost important aim of chest tube therapy. However, many factors modify the timing and results of pleural drainage, such as inflammation, pleural fluid production, and lung pathology. One technically important point is if, and eventually for how long, the drainage system should be run with active suction. Whereas in terms of recurrent pneumothorax a general no-suction water-seal regimen appears to be tantamount to the suction strategy, there is good evidence that the total chest tube time and the interval between air leak cessation and tube removal may be significantly shortened with an active regimen.[21,22] In most uncomplicated situations and with free-flowing, serous effusion the pleura will spontaneously drain air and fluid collections. Drainage may also be enhanced by expiratory

efforts of the patient, such as pressing or coughing. However, optimal drainage is certainly not indicated in the presence of loculations, rapid fluid production, and viscous secretions. For the reasons discussed above we favor a permanent low-level standard suction pressure of $-20\,cm\,H_2O$, which virtually does not interfere with patient comfort, increases safety, and requires shorter tube dwell times. Failure of expansion to such suction or early recurrence of lung detachment and fluid retention requires critical analysis of the underlying problem. It may indicate:

- reduced lung compliance (stiff or trapped lung)
- loculated pneumothorax with adhesions
- loculated fluid compartments not communicating with the drainage system
- pulmonary air leak (bronchopleural fistula)
- technical problems such as kinked or plugged tube, water in the filter or excessively long connecting tubes reducing or preventing the creation of a negative pressure within the pleural cavity throughout the respiratory cycle.

If technical reasons are ruled out, specific modifications of the drainage system may be indicated depending on the problem (see list above), including no-suction and water seal management, as set out in the section on 'critical issues'.

Chest tubes should be removed as soon as:

- the lung is completely adherent to the chest wall
- no external suction is required to maintain adherence
- air leaks have closed
- pleural fluid/secretion collections have been cleared
- pleural fluid production or bleeding has ceased
- instillation of agents is not or no more indicated.

These success criteria can be examined any time by imaging, clinical observation, and monitoring of the drainage itself (function control, air/fluid output). In pneumothorax typical duration for successful drainage varies from <3 to 7 days.[21,23] Much longer times may be required in inflammation and malignancy, in particular when fibrinolysis or pleurodesis protocols are involved. In this setting drainage times of up to 12 days are a generally accepted time window for successful therapy.[23–25]

The risk of prolonged tube drainage is contamination and infection. In addition patient discomfort and immobilization caused by unnecessarily prolonged chest drainage must be considered. However, very long-term chest drainage (>2 weeks) may be unavoidable in chronic effusion, such as transudates nonresponsive to medical therapy, failure to pleurodesis or persistent air leaks in spite of adequate therapeutic efforts.

The critical issue in terminating drainage therapy is to safely exclude unrecognized persistent air leakage. To avoid premature removal of a chest tube, we, and others, employ a probationary clamping period, starting with 4 hours and extending to 12 or even up to 24 hours (after complicated pneumothorax). At each step, radiography is used to demonstrate a stable and fully expanded lung adhering to the chest wall. Alternatively, it is common – actually about 50 percent of the members of the American College of Chest Physicians (ACCP) and the British Thoracic Society (BTS) consensus-conference favor this strategy – to use a no-suction water-seal management approach prior to removal.[21,23] However, there is no evidence that this strategy is more advantageous for the prevention of lung detachment than probationary clamping.[21] Importantly, whenever probationary clamping is done without interposition of a positive pressure safety valve, the patient must be closely observed throughout the clamping period; this is particularly important in the patient being ventilated. If a patient with a clamped drain becomes breathless or develops subcutaneous emphysema, the tube must be immediately unclamped and drainage continued.

When clamping has been considered successful and the chest tube is to be removed, special care must be taken not to provoke accidental reentry of air into the pleural space. The best strategy is to withdraw the tube in apnea after cutting the fixing sutures and after unclamping the tube (i.e. under active suction) with brisk manual extraction. Increased resistance to extraction that would necessitate anesthesia or sedation practically never occurs. The skin lesion is then digitally compressed, adapted with a surgical clamp, and protected with a sterile dressing. Except with a large skin lesion, sutures are not usually needed. Although it is not established whether removal should occur in deep inspiratory or expiratory apnea,[23,26] we consider expiration safer, because the positive pleural pressure minimizes the odds for air reentry. Control radiographs 2 hours after removal and the day after help to confirm stable expansion of the lung.

Role of thoracoscopy

Medical thoracoscopy is a traditional investigative pleural procedure in Europe, which was introduced into respiratory medicine as early as in 1910 by Jacobaeus in Sweden.[27] Modern medical thoracoscopy, which should probably, and appropriately, be called pleuroscopy is practiced as a video-supported procedure in almost every major pulmonary center using a single-port technique, almost exclusively under local anesthesia and conscious sedation.[28] It is thus clearly different from much more elaborate surgical thoracoscopic procedures that come under the popular acronym VATS (video-assisted thoracic surgery) and involve double-lumen intubation and general anesthesia.

Pleuroscopy shares essential logistic features with state-of-the-art chest drainage, such as trocar-bound single-port entry and large-bore tubes. Thus visual exploration of the thoracic cavity without additional risk would appear to be an intriguing option in chest drainage management. This is true in elective indications as well as in many situations of high dependency. There are only minor additional logistic requirements to perform pleuroscopy in this clinical setting.

They can be basically reduced to a cold light source, one or two (optionally angled) rigid telescopes and a forceps; a more detailed list is provided in Box 9.3. For induction of conscious sedation (if required at all, depending on the scope of the intervention) a combination of midazolam (2–3 mg intramuscularly) and hydrocodone (7.5–15 mg intramuscularly) may be sufficient, but other protocols including analgesic opioids and neuroleptics are equally good. After the creation of an entry port as described for large-bore drainage, visual exam may reveal a number of findings and allow interventions that may considerably modify and optimize case management. Details of the technique and procedural approach may be obtained from the literature and major reviews.[1,29–35] The salient features and benefits relevant to tube drainage management may be summarized as follows:

- *Option to establish diagnosis by biopsy or microbiologic studies.* Pleuroscopy is the gold standard for the diagnosis of pleural disease with an overall accuracy of 96 percent and a sensitivity ranging from 94 percent to 99 percent with 100 percent specificity, similar to malignant and specific inflammatory disease. [29,30,33,34,36]
- *Staging in primary and secondary spontaneous pneumothorax.* Pleuroscopy allows recognition and quantification of bullous and adhesive changes so that patients with extensive changes may be selected for more efficient surgical therapy. A relevant staging system was developed in the 1980s by Swierenga and Vanderschueren and has successfully been used over subsequent years as a guideline to different management strategies. From a current point of view, the original concept of progressive causative lesions or stages in pneumothorax is no more tenable. In particular there is good evidence that even in the thoracoscopically normal appearing lung, microscopic emphysema-like-changes (ELCs) are usually present. Thus the so-called stage I, i.e. 'normal lung', as often seen in primary pneumothorax, virtually does not exist. However, when the system is modified in terms of describing different types or patterns rather than progressive stages, as shown in Box 9.4, it still provides a valuable basis for therapeutic algorithms.[37] See also the endoscopic examples in Figures 9.4 and 9.5.
- *Assessment of lung expandability.* The practical importance is that in the presence of factors that impede lung expansion, such as air leaks, trapped lung, or consolidation, it is suggested to use modified chest drainage strategies. Direct visualization of air leaks may be difficult in low-stage pneumothorax and when the visceral pleura is inflamed, but it can be facilitated with the use of inhaled dyes such as lipofuscin.[30] Easily spotted trapped lung and consolidation may be extensive and impressive as shown in Figures 9.6 and 9.7.
- *Breaking and blunt dissection of loculations and adhesions.* These procedures may substantially contribute to the

efficacy of drainage by creating an easier-to-treat monolocular cavity. However particular care should be taken to limit dissection procedures to fibrinous adhesions and to spare fibrous-organized or even vascularized changes. An example of extensive loculations in empyema that need to be mechanically broken down is shown in Figure 9.8.

- *Visual control of optimum drainage position.* This helps to prevent otherwise unnoticed ineffective or incorrectly placed chest tubes. Incorrect placement is indeed among the leading causes of dysfunction and complications in tube drainage management.
- *Pleurodesis.* Pleuroscopy can be directly transformed to an intervention by intrathoracoscopic talc poudrage or postthoracoscopic slurry instillation as described later in the respective section. Figure 9.9 shows a pleural cavity after evacuation of effusion followed by talcum poudrage.
- *Fibrinolysis.* Presence of chambers, thick inflammatory membranes, and pus indicate fibrinolysis for debridement of trapped lung.
- *Cautery.* For closure of visible air leaks.

Contraindications (although these would equally apply to elective tube thoracostomy) include severely impaired cardiac performance (left ventricular ejection fraction <35 percent), recent myocardial infarction (<6 weeks), and bleeding disorders (partial prothrombin time >40 s; quick test <60 percent, platelets <40 000/μL).[30]

Box 9.4 The role of pleuroscopy in the evaluation of spontaneous pneumothorax (modified from reference 37)

- Pattern (Type) I (40 percent) – Idiopathic pneumothorax, normal appearing lung
- Pattern (Type) II (12 percent) – Pleural adhesions (may be assicated with hemothorax)
- Pattern (Type) III (31 percent) – Blebs and bullae <2 cm in size
- Pattern (Type) IV (17 percent) – Bullae >2 cm in size

CLINICAL PRACTICE

Critical issues in chest tube management

IMPEDED LUNG EXPANSION

Apart from technical problems and inadequate tube and suction hardware, impeded lung expansion is the major cause of failure and critical problems in chest drainage therapy. The five clinical entities usually responsible for impaired expansion are: trapped lung; consolidation and displacement due to inflamed membranes, loculations, hemorrhage, pneumonic infiltration, or malignant disease; air leaks; and central bronchial obturation (Fig. 9.10, p.134).

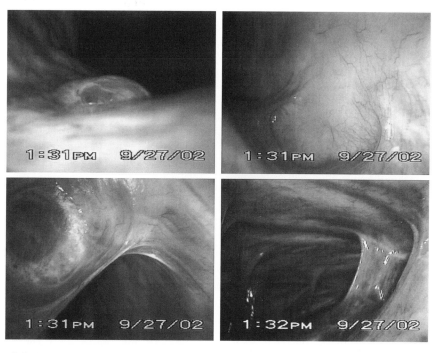

Figure 9.4   *The benefit of pleuroscopy in tube drainage management: otherwise unrecognized Vanderschueren pattern (type) II changes in spontaneous pneumothorax with extensive adhesions.*

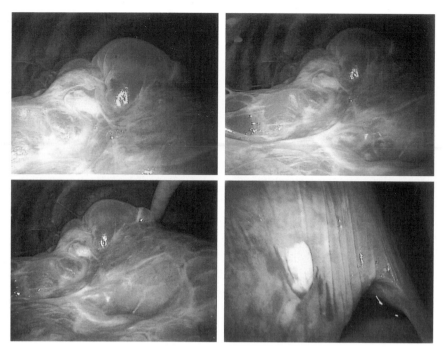

Figure 9.5   *The benefit of pleuroscopy in tube drainage management: extensive Vanderschueren pattern (type) IV changes in spontaneous pneumothorax with numerous bullae >2 cm and a few adhesions.*

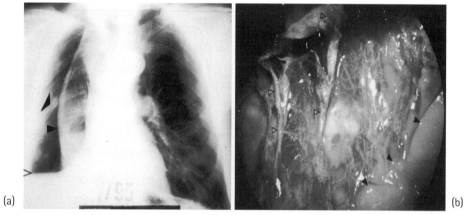

(a)   (b)

Figure 9.6   *The benefit of pleuroscopy in tube drainage management: recognition of trapped lung in empyema. (a) The visceral peel with indwelling chest tube (arrows) being unable to expand the trapped lung post-pleuroscopically is clearly seen; (b) corresponding pleuroscopic aspect of the visceral membrane after breaking of inflammatory chambers (arrows).*

They often occur in combination and aggravate the management problem. Importantly however, impaired expansion may be absolute (irreversible) or relative (reversible) if the underlying condition is amenable to therapy. Each of these conditions requires specific strategies and modifications of chest tube management.

Trapped, displaced, and consolidated lung

Trapped, displaced, and consolidated lung may often be identified prior to chest tube intervention by imaging, but is not infrequently unexpectedly revealed at pleuroscopy. An active strategy for impaired expansion of this type may consist of elevated suction pressures, provided the cause is considered transitory. Caution must be taken not to produce

mediastinal shift, and the patient must be carefully observed under a stepwise increase in suction. In empyema and pneumonia it is generally wiser to adopt a permissive approach: response to pleural fibrinolysis and systemic antibiotic therapy may be excellent, allowing delayed complete expansion of a trapped or consolidated lung after resolution of the inflammatory lesions and membranes.

Air leaks

Air leaks (bronchopleural fistula) may be a challenging and recalcitrant problem in chest tube management. The cause is overwhelmingly pneumothorax and empyema related. The air leak will be apparent by the continuous or discontinuous, often audible, flow passing through the drainage. The

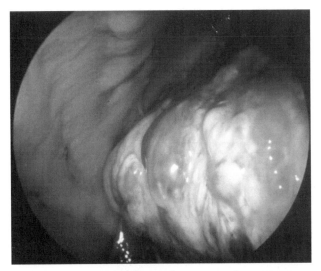

Figure 9.7 *The benefit of pleuroscopy in chest tube management: recognition of impaired pulmonary expansion in malignant consolidation. Evacuation of pleural fluid reveals previously concealed right lower lobe consolidation.*

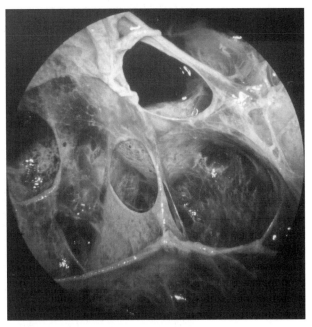

Figure 9.8 *The benefit of pleuroscopy in tube drainage management: recognition and elimination of multiloculation in empyema (same case as Fig. 9.6 prior to breaking and removal of chambers).*

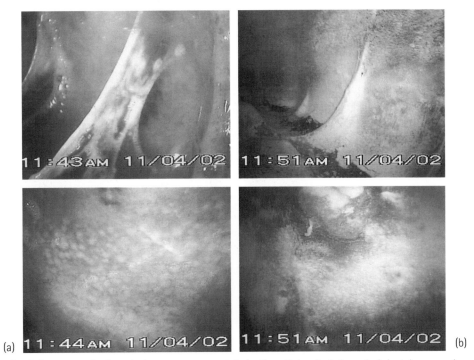

(a)   (b)

Figure 9.9 *The benefit of pleuroscopy in chest drainage management: induction of chemical pleurodesis by talcum poudrage. Pleural situs (a) before and (b) after poudrage.*

volume of air leakage may vary widely from <1 L/min to 16 L/min, e.g. after thoracotomy or in acute respiratory distress syndrome (ARDS). It can be measured by flowmetry incorporated in the drainage system but is also clinically evident from air bubbles passing through the water seal. In the patient being ventilated quantitative assessment is easily done by subtracting expiratory minute volume from inspiratory volume. Standard chest tubes (>24 Fr) will accommodate up to 15 L/min airflow. Attempts to reexpand the lung may merely increase the leak – this is particularly

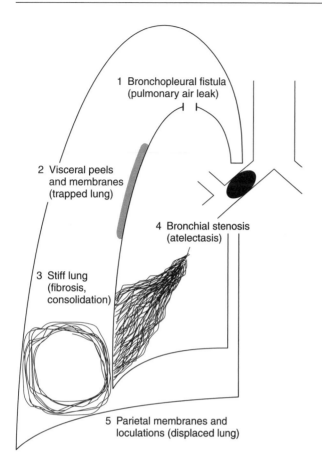

1 Bronchopleural fistula
(pulmonary air leak)

2 Visceral peels
and membranes
(trapped lung)

4 Bronchial stenosis
(atelectasis)

3 Stiff lung
(fibrosis,
consolidation)

5 Parietal membranes and
loculations (displaced lung)

Figure 9.10 *Schematic representation of causes that may impede lung expansion. The causes may occur singly or in combination and may be absolute (irreversible) or relative (transitory). Relative impaired expansion may respond to tolerably increased pleural suction levels or/and interventional approaches such as pleuroscopy, pleural fibrinolysis, and bronchoscopy.*

true in the case of superimposed stiff or trapped lung. In these instances it may be difficult to achieve adequate oxygenation, although the respiratory 'steal' will eliminate carbon dioxide. If the lesion is not too large and the lung can be reexpanded, the air leak will usually cease on reinstitution of pleural contact. In large pleural leaks it may be better to avoid suction and to use the drainage system merely as a safety valve to prevent tension pneumothorax. Delayed lung expansion may be attempted after closure of the defect.

In persistent failure to expand the lung, selective surgical closure, eventually combined with pleurodesis using VATS or formal thoracotomy, may be eventually indicated. Management of bronchopleural fistula in the intensive care setting and in the patient on mechanical ventilation, may require complex strategies with a major focus on measures to reduce ventilator pressure (permissive hypoventilation) to enhance spontaneous closure of the leak.[38] Active 'repair' attempts either bronchoscopically using fibrin sealant (the success rate of which in our experience, however, is only

around 50 percent) or via thoracoscopy, employing cautery or talc pleurodesis, are other approaches. Respirator- and ventilation-pattern modifications such as unilateral or differential bilateral ventilation can be tried but are technically difficult and rarely successful. High frequency jet ventilation and high frequency oscillation therapy are often effective in the temporary stabilization of the difficult patient but surgical closure may still be required when/if the patient survives the acute period.

Bronchial obturation

Bronchial obturation, the last mechanism of impaired expansion, may sometimes not be apparent in the highly dependent patient with profuse effusion, but at times it may be the prevailing emergency. The most adequate and straightforward management strategy for impaired expansion after pleural evacuation would be bronchoscopic interventional control of the obturating lesion.

MASSIVE AND MALIGNANT PLEURAL EFFUSION

Massive effusion may present as a respiratory emergency similar to tension pneumothorax. It primarily requires decompression of the pleural space. Therapeutic thoracentesis meets these urgent demands for relief of respiratory distress and sometimes cardiac congestion. Palliative thoracentesis often follows a diagnostic puncture, but for an explicit therapeutic intention the use of a kit is advised. These devices consist of a modified 16 gauge needle, often housing a spring-loaded blunt internal cannula, a three-way stopcock, a 50–100 mL syringe, a safety valve, and a 2 L collection bag, thus avoiding trauma to the lung, infectious contamination, and air access to the pleura.

There are conflicting views on the amount and the time-setting of fluid removal.[22] Immediate relief will usually result from relatively small quantities (500 mL), but amounts up to 1.5 L are also well tolerated. Unless pleuroscopy is an option, it is better to repeat palliative thoracentesis, rather than to remove too large amounts. There is often concern about the creation of excess negative pleural pressures (-20 cm H_2O or less), but this will occur only with trapped or consolidated lung. Also the risk of reexpansion lung edema is only increased in longstanding (>7 days) compressive collections, when the lung has developed complete atelectasis with surfactant depletion. Fluid removal should then be slowed down to about 500 mL/h and should not exceed 1 L/h.

Massive effusion is frequently associated with malignancy and should therefore, whenever possible, be explored by pleuroscopy with appropriate standard large-bore chest tube drainage thereafter. With the rapid drainage of large fluid amounts (>3000 mL) as required for effective pleuroscopy, it is a wise precaution to counterbalance redistribution of intravasal volume by isotonic volume replacement to prevent hypovolemic circulatory syncope. Large-volume fluid drainage associated with pleuroscopy is not subject to critical negative pleural pressures, because the investigation occurs under ambient air equilibration. Subsequent to visualization and biopsy, again (as with fluid removal from the closed chest) the lung is expanded slowly (within hours) to prevent edema. Distressing, reexpansion-induced cough is common, and may cause complicating surgical emphysema. Premedication with an antitussive opioid such as hydrocodone (as practiced for thoracoscopy) may be useful if there are no contraindications.

In visually evident malignant effusion the induction of pleurodesis by talc poudrage or postthoracoscopic slurry instillation should always be considered. Sometimes, as when the patient is too debilitated to tolerate a more invasive approach such as in end-stage cancer, the treatment of massive effusion must remain restricted to (repeat) therapeutic thoracentesis or to small-catheter drainage.

EMPYEMA AND PARAPNEUMONIC EFFUSION

Empyema and parapneumonic effusion are interrelated, overlapping manifestations of bacterial pleurisy. Their combined incidence accounts for a high proportion (20 percent) of all effusions. Bacterial pleurisy complicates pneumonia from a variety of causes in 20–57 percent cases.[39] Empyema should be suspected in a patient with pulmonary infection in the presence of the following:

- persisting or unexplained fever after adequately treated pneumonia
- persisting elevation of inflammatory markers (C-reactive protein, white blood cell [WBC] count, erythrocyte sedimentation rate)
- history of procedures such as thoracic or esophageal surgery and aspiration
- predisposing morbidity such as alcoholism
- feculent sputum production, suggesting bronchopleural fistula
- imaging findings suggesting pleural membranes and multiloculation.

Frank, clinical empyema is a classic high-dependency indication for thoracostomy. The intervention threshold in parapneumonic effusion used to be less well defined but consensus has been reached about indications over time on the basis of extensive clinical data both from individual studies and metaanalyses by various scientific societies.[23,24,40,41] Thus, in the overall treatment algorithm for the management of bacterial pleurisy, based on clinical criteria and pleural-fluid-derived criteria, thoracostomy with tube drainage is vitally important in the following conditions (Table 9.4):

- frank empyema at thoracentesis
- severe clinical course (sepsis)
- profuse (>2 L), in particular, displacing effusion
- air in the pleural space indicating bronchopleural fistula.

The Light criteria help to establish the diagnosis and classify bacterial pleurisy in the categories of uncomplicated parapneumonic effusion, complicated parapneumonic effusion, and frank empyema.[40–42] Empyema and complicated parapneumonic effusions requiring tube thoracostomy are characterized by low pH (<7.0) and glucose (<2.2 mmol/L [40 mg/dL]), raised lactate dehydrogenase (>10.000 IU/L) and WBC count (>15 × 10^9 /L)), and the bacterial culture will usually be positive.

The current ACCP guidelines basically follow these suggestions although they define four risk and outcome categories:[23]

- Category I – minimal free-flowing effusion with culture and pH being unknown
- Category II – small to moderate free-flowing effusion with negative culture and pH >7.2
- Category III – large free-flowing effusion, loculations and membranes, pH <7.2
- Category IV – category III and evidence of frank pus.

Although category I apparently describes a subdivision of uncomplicated parapneumonic effusion the grading does

Table 9.4 *Indications of tube drainage in bacterial pleurisy*[21,22,39,40]

Empyema/complicated parapneumonic effusion (ACCP categories III and IV)	Intermediate effusion quality (ACCP category II)	Uncomplicated parapneumonic effusion (ACCP categories I and II)
Frank empyema Bacterial culture positive Any effusion amount Mono/multilocular Light criteria: 　Glucose <2.2 mmol/L 　LDH > 10 000 IU/L 　pH <7.00 　Leuckocyte count >15 x 10^9/L 　Air leaks	Serial pleurocentesis + clinical follow-up	Clear serous effusion Bacterial culture negative Effusion < ca.1000 mL Monolocular Light criteria: 　glucose >3.3 mmol/L 　LDH < 10 000 IU/L 　pH >7.20 　leukocyte count <10 x 10^9/L
?		?
Tube drainage required ◄—	—►	Chest tube not required

not abolish the category of indeterminate effusion that needs close clinical follow-up to decide on the appropriate time for thoracostomy intervention as shown in Table 9.4.

A critical issue in chest tube management is the *distinction between empyema and lung abscess*. An abscess will not usually require thoracostomy but presents with a similar pattern both clinically and on imaging. Contrast-enhanced computed tomography (CT) is helpful for making this distinction, using the criteria shown in Box 9.5.

Box 9.5 Differentiating between empyema and lung abscess on a CT scan

Signs favoring empyema

- Signs of lung compression
- Smooth margins of membranes
- Dissection of the thickened visceral and parietal pleura ('split pleura' sign)
- Blunt angle with the chest wall

Signs favoring lung abscess

- Spherical shape with irregular and thicker wall structures
- Absence of lung compression
- Sharp angle with the chest wall
- Visible airway connection
- Demonstration of vasculature around abscess (definite proof)

The management of empyema involves both antibiotics and drainage and may ultimately require surgery. The decision to operate on an empyema, however, remains largely subjective and there are no established objective criteria to define the point at which a patient should proceed to surgery.[23,24] Parenteral antimicrobial therapy should take into consideration clinical features such as feculent empyema (anaerobic) or antibiotic pre-treatment. For local therapy the use of double-lumen catheters with a diameter of at least 20 Fr, is strongly recommended, as this allows closed circuit large-volume irrigation with normal saline ($\pm$ aseptic additives) and instillation of fibrinolytics.

Streptokinase or urokinase is indicated when the following are prominent features of the presenting empyema: difficult to mobilize thick pus with retention of secretions; membranes or loculations; and trapped lung. Fibrinolysis may thus obviate the need for two or more drains in multiloculated empyema. As expected, fibrinolytic therapy will transiently increase pleural production due to resolution of pus and membranes. Therefore in irrigation/fibrinolysis protocols the mostly turbid fluid output may largely exceed the irrigation input and must be continued until clear sterile fluid is obtained and the net fluid production falls below 50–100 mL/day. The value of fibrinolysis has been shown in several controlled prospective studies (albeit with small

patient numbers) in terms of improving drainage results. However, it remains controversial with respect to clinical endpoints such as mortality and rate of surgery.[43–49] A suggested dose is 200 000–250 000 IU of streptokinase to be instilled once or twice daily with the tube being clamped for 2–4 hours; 50 000–100 000 IU have been suggested as an equipotent dose for urokinase. Our protocol using a streptokinase–streptodornase combination is shown in Box 9.6. The value of the streptodornase(DNAse) component is not yet clinically established. However, experimental data point towards a beneficial effect by decreasing the DNA-dependent viscosity of secretions.[46] The fibrinolytic needs to be instilled usually for 5–6 days but may be useful until 2 weeks. Failure, defined as persisting clinical features or ultrasound demonstrated loculations after 2 weeks, occurs in about 15 percent.[47–49] Contraindications to thrombolytics include bronchopleural fistula, significant coagulation disorders or allergy (streptokinase). Prior use of streptokinase (e.g. in acute myocardial infarction) will not invalidate its use but favors urokinase as a safeguard. Adverse effects may occur with both streptokinase and urokinase, including fever ($\geq$38.5 °C) (4 percent) and significant pain (4 percent), but it may be difficult to attribute the symptoms to therapy or to the primary illness.[50] More importantly, previously absent pulmonary air leakage has been seen to develop during fibrinolysis in 9 percent of cases.[50] There are sporadic reports of local intrapleural bleeding, but there is no evidence that intrapleural streptokinase produces systemic fibrinolysis up to a cumulative dose of 1.5 million IU.[51]

Fibrinolytic treatment of empyema may benefit from the initial use of medical thoracoscopy by breaking trapped lung parenchyma and loculations as shown in Figure 9.8. Instillation of antibiotics as an alternative to fibrinolytic therapy has been suggested with the rationale that low

---

Box 9.6 Combined irrigation/instillation protocol for fibrinolytic chest tube management of empyema (our protocol)[50]

(A) Interventional approach

- Ultrasound-guided thoracentesis
- Double lumen irrigation/suction drainage (20–24 Fr, 40 cm)
  - Ultrasound guided
  - Pleuroscopy guided
  - Empyema evacuation (standard suction: 20 cm H_2O)
- Imaging control (radiographic/fluoroscopy/sonography)
- Irrigation using isotonic saline solution with aseptic additives (povidone iodine 2 percent) until recovery of clear irrigation fluid (before and after fibrinolysis)
- Fibrinolytic agent instillation: Varidase® (1 ampule = 100 000 IU streptokinase + 25 000 IU streptodornase) with a 2–4 h clamping period

(B) Empiric and subsequent targeted antibiotic therapy

penetration of systemic antibiotic therapy might provide suboptimal therapy.[52] However, with inflamed pleural membranes, concentrations well above the minimal inhibitory concentrations (MIC) have been demonstrated in empyema fluid (except aminoglycosides) in many studies.[53]

Surgical therapy, increasingly using VATS rather than formal thoracotomy, is indicated when medical treatment fails, although surgical intervention as early as 4–7 days after initiation of medical therapy has been successfully performed and may be considered in severely ill, nonresponsive patients.[54] The limits of medical therapy and criteria of failure are otherwise poorly defined. A 12–14-day period appears to be a generally accepted working compromise in the critical issue of parapneumonic empyema,[24,25] as opposed to the following situations, which unequivocally have been the domain of surgical therapy for a long time:

- encapsulated chronic empyema (empyema necessitans) which may be resected extrapleurally within the encapsulated empyema sack (empyemectomy)
- traumatic or postoperative empyema
- a chronically infected (e.g. pneumonectomy) cavity which may necessitate long-term open management (rib resection).

Even with adequate antibiotic therapy and judicious medical or surgical management, empyema remains a serious condition with mortality varying from 6 percent up to 21 percent depending on the case mix.[55]

HEMOTHORAX

Hemothorax may present as a dramatic condition. Because of distinct management options, the diagnosis needs instant confirmation in doubtful cases. Since sanguinous effusion with hematocrit values as low as 0.05 (5 percent) may appear as blood, the diagnosis of hemothorax requires a pleural fluid hematocrit level of at least 0.5 (50 percent) of the flowing blood. Blunt or penetrating chest trauma is clearly the leading cause, but medical problems such as malignancy, pulmonary infarction, iatrogenic or noniatrogenic bleeding disorders, and spontaneous pneumothorax may be causative in a large proportion of patients. Iatrogenic causes may be suggested by preceding angiography, bioptical chest interventions, incorrect placement of central venous catheters, or induction of anticoagulation.

Treatment basically consists of insertion of a large-bore (≥28 Fr) chest tube with the following options:[56–58]

- removal of blood and subsequent lung expansion to achieve a tamponade effect
- quantitative control of hemorrhage
- to measure the severity of injury to:
- decrease the risk of empyema
- prevent subsequent fibrothorax
- induction of fibrinolytic instillation therapy if needed.

The drainage should be operated with low suction forces as long as lung expansion is incomplete in order to contain intrathoracic bleeding. The value of fibrinolytic therapy in complicated hemothorax is not convincingly established and is discouraged in guidelines of surgical societies.[57] Also, there have been no controlled studies as yet to validate such efforts. It is critically important to recognize the limits beyond which surgical intervention is indicated. The generally accepted limits are:[59,60]

- complete opacification of one hemithorax and signs of compression
- evacuation of >1000 mL immediately after chest drain insertion
- continuous blood flow >200 mL/h delivered for 3 consecutive hours via the drainage
- evidence of hypovolemic shock despite blood volume replacement
- massive intrathoracic clots preventing lung expansion and that require mechanical debulking.

Surgical intervention in the highly dependent hypovolemic or respiratory compromised patient will usually be formal thoracotomy based, but there is now evidence that an early thoracoscopic (VATS) approach (within 72 hours of chest tube placement) in retained traumatic hemothorax is a safe intervention and is superior to multiple chest tube management in regard to the endpoints, length and cost of hospital stay, and the sequelae of trauma.[60]

Administration of antibiotics is advisable for prevention of empyema, specially if there is retention of large amounts of clots. Fortunately the overall incidence of complicating empyema is as low as 1–4 percent when antibiotics are given prophylactically. The preventive effect of cephalosporins and clindamycin has been quantified in one study as reducing the absolute risk of empyema by 5.5–7.1 percent and that of infectious complications in general by 12.1–13.4 percent.[61]

PNEUMOTHORAX

It is common to classify pneumothorax as traumatic and nontraumatic, i.e. spontaneous pneumothorax. Traumatic pneumothorax shows a wide overlap with hemothorax and by and large shares the management options. Spontaneous pneumothorax needs to be first subdivided into primary and secondary spontaneous pneumothorax. In addition the size of lung collapse must be evaluated, since these are the main determinants of treatment algorithm. According to a recent BTS consensus statement spontaneous pneumothorax should be quantified in the categories:

- small – rim of air around the lung ≤1 cm, approximating 27 percent of the hemithorax volume
- moderate – rim of air around lung ≤2 cm approximating 50 percent of the hemithorax volume
- complete – airless lung, separate from the diaphragm.[62]

More pragmatically the division into a 'small' (<2 cm) and a 'large' pneumothorax (≥2 cm) combined with symptom evaluation will suffice to make intervention-relevant treatment decisions. Current majority opinion[21,23,63,64] suggests that:

- Observation alone is appropriate in a small primary spontaneous pneumothorax with few or no symptoms.
- Hospitalization and intervention with aspiration or chest drain is indicated in a small secondary pneumothorax with moderate symptoms (except in small isolated apical pneumothorax).
- Hospitalization and intervention is indicated in any patient with marked symptoms in primary or secondary pneumothorax.

According to recent evidence the interventional strategy in terms of drainage size and technique should depend largely on the clinical background, i.e. primary or secondary pneumothorax and age. In primary spontaneous pneumothorax simple aspiration has been shown to be as effective as tube drainage with success rate of 59–73 percent, when recurrence within 12 months is taken as an endpoint.[65–67] In secondary spontaneous pneumothorax success rates of simple aspiration of 33–67 percent clearly fall short of those in primary pneumothorax. In addition there is a striking age dependency, with the success rate of 70–81 percent in the age group <50 years falling dramatically to 19–31 percent in elderly patients >50 years.[66–68]

Small-bore catheters (<14 Fr) or even simple aspiration via a Teflon cannula is therefore recommended as the first-line treatment for all primary spontaneous pneumothoraces requiring intervention. However, patients with large secondary pneumothoraces, in particular those over 50 years of age, in whom aspiration strategies or small-bore catheters have a high risk of failure, should be appropriately managed with tube thoracostomy as initial treatment, even more so, when fluid production is involved (seropneumothorax). Most physicians feel that large-bore thoracostomy is also adequate in primary pneumothorax, when aspiration or small catheters have failed, and when tension pneumothorax is present. The same applies to respirator-associated pneumothorax which combines features of secondary spontaneous pneumothorax and traumatic pneumothorax (barotrauma). Bilateral pneumothorax is a challenging and distressing but rare complication, and there is a significant association with specific risk situations such as acquired immune deficiency syndrome (AIDS), ARDS, and polytrauma. Persistent air leaks and bronchopleural fistula usually signal the presence of bullous emphysema, adhesions, inflammation (empyema), and interstitial lung disease. They therefore occur rarely in primary spontaneous pneumothorax. Mediastinal emphysema may result from trauma to the mediastinal pleura and major bronchi as well as from air dissection of the pulmonary interstitium subsequent to alveolar rupture. Thus it need not necessarily be preceded by pneumothorax. Limited extension of mediastinal emphysema will remain asymptomatic with only cosmetic importance, but progression, as frequently occurs in the patient being ventilated, will eventually be associated with massive cervical and facial surgical emphysema that may present as a cardiorespiratory emergency. Decompressive measures are then indicated with the introduction of a number of thin needles in the cervical soft tissue. In severe cardiorespiratory distress only mediastinal drainage via surgical cervical mediastinotomy may control the mediastinal air penetration.[69]

Subcutaneous (surgical) emphysema is a fairly frequent complication occurring primarily in pneumothorax and also secondary to tube drainage management. Air penetration at the site of the chest wall injury is largely enhanced by forced breathing maneuvers, in particular coughing. Air dissection and distribution may be massive and disfiguring but rarely amounts to a threatening situation unless it is associated with concomitant massive mediastinal emphysema. Hemothorax related to rupture of vascularized adhesions has been reported to complicate (preferentially secondary) spontaneous pneumothorax in up to 12 percent but will rarely give rise to an emergency surgical intervention.[70] Similar to empyema, multiple drains may be required in all these complications, in particular in multiloculated pneumothorax to control tension pneumothorax, short-term recurrences, and soft tissue air dissection. Ultimately only a surgical intervention via VATS or formal thoracotomy may eliminate intractable bullae and air leaks. Accepted indications for early surgical intervention in pneumothorax (if the patient's performance allows such approach) may thus be summarized as follows:

- second ipsilateral pneumothorax
- first contralateral pneumothorax
- bilateral spontaneous pneumothorax
- persistent air leak (>5–7 days tube drainage) or persistent failure to reexpand
- spontaneous significant hemothorax.

As discussed earlier in the chapter, as in pleural effusion, medical thoracoscopy can contribute significantly to the diagnosis and management. The staging or classification system shown in Box 9.4 provides precise description of endoscopic findings and a rational basis for therapeutic decisions.[37,70]

PLEURODESIS

The term pleurodesis describes an artificially induced fibrotic transformation of the pleural cleft designed to lead to a permanent syndesmosis subsequent to an acute iatrogenic neutrophilic inflammation (sclerotherapy). Except in interventional attempts to close otherwise intractable pulmonary leaks, pleurodesis is strictly not a component of immediate respiratory emergency management. However, it is an important sequential procedure and – regarding indications and technical aspects – in many ways related to chest drainage management. Effective pleurodesis is best achieved by the gold standard procedure of vision-guided (thoracoscopic) installation of talc powder (poudrage), using a hand-bulb-operated device (intrathoracoscopic pleurodesis).[25, 71–74] Doses up to 4–6 g have been evaluated as safe, but talc has been always subject to controversy and anecdotally reported to cause serious side effects (ARDS) or adverse circulatory effects (syncope) believed to be related to some local and systemic absorption of the agent.[75,76] In a comprehensive American survey of 2723 procedures conducted by Sahn, 37 (1.4 percent) acute episodes of respiratory failure could be registered, but only 17 (0.7 percent) of these were with some likelihood actually talc related.[76] The main concern about talc application refers to reports suggesting that systemic absorption and dissipation actually occurs in animal models.[77] A repeat study using French Luzenac talc could not reproduce these findings.[78] Different particle size may be one explanation for the discrepant results, since the particle size of European Luzenac talc is known to be about threefold that of the American preparations.[77] We therefore believe that Luzenac talc within recommended dose schemes is safe enough to justify a broad clinical use. Based on preliminary data an advanced but yet unpublished European multicenter clinical 'talc safety study' is currently underway and from preliminary data very likely to confirm this clinical impression (ref: personal communication). An endoscopic view of thoracoscopic 'talcage' is shown in Figure 9.9.

Talc poudrage has been evaluated in controlled prospective trials and shown to provide ≥90 percent (88–100 percent) long-term control in malignant pleurisy and even ≥95 percent control in pneumothorax.[71–74,80–82] Alternatively, agents such as tetracycline hydrochloride (0.5–1 g) or doxycycline (250–500 mg), can be instilled via the chest tube with reported success rates between 54 percent and 96 percent,[71] with a realistic mean of around 70 percent.[25,71,83] The instillation of talc as a slurry in equivalent doses to poudrage may be both more effective and better tolerated than tetracycline. Bleomycin is another alternative with success rates similar to tetracycline and doxycycline. As it is much more expensive and cytotoxic systemic side effects may occur, its use is not encouraged.

Apart from the potency of the agent, the successful practice of pleurodesis requires the following basic rules and prerequisites to be observed:

- complete removal of pleural fluid
- full lung expansion, i.e. reinstitution of pleural contact
- equal pleural distribution and continuous drainage after instillation of the agent until fluid production ceases.

Whenever and with whatever agent pleurodesis is performed, the use of large-bore drains provides crucial advantages. In talc pleurodesis large drains are mandatory to prevent irreversible plugging of the system by the sometimes clumpy talc and fibrin deposits. Topical analgesia (200–250 mg lidocaine intrapleurally) is a useful option in addition to mandatory systemic opioid analgesia for pleurodesis, since most agents will sometimes cause severe pain. The reported overall complication rate including minor adverse reactions such as fever and discomfort is around 5 percent.[84] The clinical course in pleural effusion is characterized by an exponential fall in the delivered exudation rate over 3–5 days. Talc is deposited only once, whereas tetracycline instillation is repeated daily until the exudation rate falls below 100 mL/day. The chest tube can then be removed. In pneumothorax the indication of 'talcage' must be carefully weighed against highly efficient (minimal invasive) surgical procedures for pleurodesis with the additional option of breaking adhesions and resection of lung parenchyma containing bullae and fistulas.[85–88] Based on the clinical background and endoscopic (or imaging findings) the following recommendations can be reasonably made:

- Favors initial conservative management:
  - advanced age, high morbidity
  - increased anesthetic risk
  - secondary spontaneous pneumothorax
  - limited (Vanderschueren types I and III) lesions at thoracoscopy.
- Favors initial surgical approach:
  - young individuals (<40 years), low morbidity
  - normal anesthetic risk
  - primary spontaneous pneumothorax
  - extensive (Vanderschueren types II and IV) lesions at thoracoscopy.

Chest tubes in locations other than the pleura

Drainage in locations other than the pleura may be rarely required, and usually indicates extraordinary complications and high-dependency situations. Pericardial effusion or hemopericardium is one of these, and malignancy and trauma are by far the leading emergency-relevant causes. Drainage of the pericardium is vitally indicated, when diastolic cardiac dysfunction or complete cardiac tamponade is evident. Fluid amounts ranging from 300 mL to 1000 mL based on ultrasound findings, and depending on the time course of the collection, may precipitate such complication.[89] Pericardial drainage is the intervention of choice, unless in exceptional cases, emergency surgery (in trauma) or pericardial fenestration (in malignancy) is preferred. Pericardial drainage is based on small-bore pigtail catheters ≤14 Fr, which are introduced via a Seldinger introducer set from a substernal entry point (xiphoid angle). The intervention must be carefully guided by ultrasonography and/or fluoroscopy to prevent hemorrhage and perforation of the right ventricle or atrium with subsequent pericardial tamponade as a serious complication.[89]

In malignancy pericardesis, analogous to pleurodesis, is a logical and useful sequential therapy after evacuation of the pericardium, using tetracycline (500 mg) or doxycycline (250–500 mg) as a single daily instillation over the indwelling catheter until fluid production ceases.[90] Intracavitary pulmonary drains are only exceptionally indicated, when a large infected pulmonary cavity (abscess or bulla), nonresponsive to systemic antibiotic therapy and inaccessible to bronchial drainage, needs to be evacuated in the severely ill and toxic patient. The dissemination of infectious secretions to the pleural space may clearly complicate this intervention, precipitating occasionally a combined pleural/intrapulmonary drainage regimen. Such drainage must be specifically run without suction to prevent a ventilatory 'steal'-airflow through bronchial communications. Irrigation maneuvers must be strictly performed with the diseased side dependent for prevention of bronchial overflow and contamination.

Soft tissue and mediastinal drainage are rare interventions, limited to severe surgical conditions such as mechanical or barotrauma (surgical emphysema, mediastinal emphysema) and may then be part of a complicated pneumothorax management. Life-threatening infection in the context of mediastinitis is another such indication where drainage is a component of a general surgical approach depending on the actual cause of infection.[91]

Key learning points

- Conditions that interfere with lung expansion by causing either lung collapse or lung compression require management with chest tubes or thoracoscopy.

- The most common indication is pneumothorax followed by tension, bilateral, hemopneumothorax, and air dissection in the soft tissues.

- Chest tubes are basically designed to drain the pleural space and to restore lung expansion, whenever a substantial amount of air or liquid has penetrated there. Only in exceptional circumstances may chest tubes be inserted in locations other than the pleural space, such as an intrapulmonary cavity, the pericardium, soft tissue, or the mediastinum.

- An ideal chest tube needs to be: anti-adhesive and transparent to prevent plugging and allow visual control of patency; supple and smooth enough to cause only minor patient discomfort; and stiff enough to prevent kinking and occlusion.

- The entry point of drain insertion should be selected based on standardized criteria provided the lung is completely retracted and one is dealing with a large monolocular fluid- or airspace.

- A number of devices are available for generation of short- or long-term therapeutic suction gradients.

- A permanent low-level standard suction pressure does not interfere with patient comfort, increases safety, and requires only short tube dwell times.

- The risk of prolonged tube drainage is increased patient discomfort, contamination and infection.

- The critical issue in terminating drainage therapy is to safely exclude unrecognized persistent air leakage.

- Impeded lung expansion due to a number of extra- and intrapulmonary factors is the major cause of failure and critical problems in chest drainage therapy.

- A critical issue in chest tube management is the *distinction between empyema and lung abscess*. An abscess will not usually require thoracostomy but presents with a similar pattern both clinically and on imaging.

- Small-bore catheters (<14 Fr) or even simple aspiration via a Teflon cannula is recommended as the first-line treatment for all primary spontaneous pneumothoraces requiring intervention.

- Effective pleurodesis is best achieved by the gold standard procedure of vision-guided (thoracoscopic) instillation of talc powder (poudrage), using a hand-bulb-operated device (intrathoracoscopic pleurodesis).

REFERENCES

◆ 1. Brandt HJ, Loddenkemper R, Mai J. History and development of thoracoscopy. In: Brandt HJ, Loddenkemper R, Mai J, eds. *Atlas of Diagnostic Thoracoscopy*. Stuttgart: Thieme, 1985: 2–6.

◆ 2. Roe BB. Physiologic principles of drainage of the pleural space. *Am J Surg* 1958; **96**: 246–53.

◆ 3. Munnel ER, Thomas EK. Current concepts in thoracic drainage systems. *Ann Thorac Surg* 1975; **19**: 261–8.

● 4. Marel M. Epidemiology of pleural effusion. In: Loddenkemper R, Antony VB, eds. *Pleural Diseases. European Respiratory Monographs* 2002; 7: 146–58.

● 5. Melton LJ, Hepper NG, Offord KP. Incidence of spontaneous pneumothorax in Olmstedt Country, Minnesota. *Am Rev Respir Dis* 1979; **120**: 1379–82.

◆ 6. Light RW. Diagnostic approach in a patient with pleural effusion. In: Loddenkemper R, Antony VB, eds. *Pleural Diseases. European Respiratory Monographs* 2002; 7: 131–45.

◆ 7. Comroe JH. Mechanical factors in breathing. In: Comroe JH, ed. *Physiology of Respiration*. Chicago: Year Book, 1975:94–141.

◆ 8. Munnel ER. Thoracic drainage, collective review. *Ann Thorac Surg* 1997; **63**: 1497–502.

● 9. Baumann MH, Strange CH. Treatment of spontaneous pneumothorax. A more aggressive approach? *Chest* 1997; **112**: 789–804.

● 10. Tape TG, Blank LL, Wigton RS. Procedural skills of practicing pulmonologists: a national survey of 1000 members of the American College of Physicians. *Am J Respir Crit Care Med* 1995; **151**: 282–7.

● 11. Collop NA, Kim S, Sahn SA. Analysis of tube thoracostomies performed by pulmonologists at a teaching hospital. *Chest* 1997; **112**: 709–13.

◆ 12. Miller KS, Sahn SA. Chest tubes, indications, technique, management and complications. *Chest* 1987; **91**: 258–64.

◆ 13. Galvin IF, Gibbons JRP, Magout M, *et al.* Placement of an apical chest tube by a posterior approach. *Br J Hosp Med* 1990; **44**: 330–1.

◆ 14. Symbas PN. Chest drainage tubes. *Surg Clin North Am* 1989; **69**: 41–6.

● 15. Loddenkemper R. Thoracoscopy under local anaesthesia. Is it safe? *J Bronchol* 2000; **7**: 207–9.

● 16. Viskum K, Enk B. Complications of thoracoscopy. *Poumon Coeur* 1981; **37**: 25–8.

● 17. Millikan JS, Moore EE, Steiner E, *et al.* Complications of tube thoracostomy for acute trauma. *Am J Surg* 1980; **140**: 738–41.

● 18. Chan L, Reilly KM, Henderson C, *et al.* Complication rates of thoracostomy. *Am J Emerg Med* 1997; **15**: 368–70.

● 19. Etoch SW, Bar-natan MR, Miller FB, Richardsen JD. Tube thoracostomy: factors related to complications. *Arch Surg* 1995; **130**: 521–5.

● 20. Patel PB, Petrini M, Baumann MH. Flow rates and suction levels in commercial pleural drainage units. *Am J Respir Crit Care Med* 2000; **161**: A 400.

✷ 21. Baumann MH, Strange C, Heffner JE, *et al.* Management of spontaneous pneumothorax. An American College of Chest Physicians Delphi Consensus Statement. *Chest* 2001; **119**: 590–602.

● 22. Davis JW, Mackersie RC, Hoyt DB, Garcia J. Randomised study of algorithms for discontinuing tube thoracostomy drainage. *Am J Coll Surg* 1994; **179**: 553–7.

✷ 23. Davies RJO, Gleeson FV, Ali N *et al.* BTS guidelines for the management of pleural disease. *Thorax* 2003; **58**: 18–28.

✷ 24. Colice GL, Curtis A, Deslaurier B, *et al.* Medical and surgical treatment of parapneumonic effusions. An evidence based guideline. *Chest* 2000; **118**: 1158–71.

✷ 25. Antony VB, Loddenkemper R, Astoul P, *et al.* ATS/ERS statement: Management of malignant pleural effusions. *Am J Respir Crit Care Med* 2000; **162**: 1987–901.

● 26. Bell RL, Ovadia P, Abdullah F, *et al.* Chest tube removal: end-inspiration or end-exspiration? *J Trauma* 2001; **50**: 674–7.

● 27. Jacobäus HC. Über die Möglichkeit, die Zystoskopie bei Untersuchung seröser Höhlen anzuwenden Münch. *Med Wschr* 1910; **40**: 2090–2.

● 28. Loddenkemper R. Zur Geschichte und Zukunft der Thorakoskopie. *Pneumologie* 2004; **58**: 42–9.

◆ 29. Menzies R, Charbonneau M. Thoracoscopy for the diagnosis of pleural disease. *Ann Intern Med* 1991; **114**: 271–8.

✷ 30. Boutin C, Viallat JR, Aelony Y. *Practical Thoracoscopy*. Berlin: Springer, 1991.

◆ 31. Loddenkemper R. Thoracoscopy: state of the art. *Eur Respir J* 1998; **11**: 213–21.

◆ 32. Loddenkemper R, Frank W. Invasive pulmonary diagnostic procedures: pleural diagnostic procedures. In: Crapo D, Glassroth J, Kalinski J, *et al.*, eds. *Textbook of Pulmonary Diseases*, 7th ed. Boston: Lippincott Williams & Wilkins, 2004.

◆ 33. Colt HG. Thoracoscopy: window to the pleural space. *Chest* 1999; **116**: 1409–15.

◆ 34. Seijo LM, Sherman DH. Interventional pulmonology. *N Engl J Med* 2001; **344**: 740–9.

◆ 35. Mathur PN. Medical thoracoscopy: the pulmonologists perspective. *Semin Respir Crit Care* 1997; **18**: 803–16.

● 36. Diacon AH, Van de Wal BW, Wyser C, *et al.* Diagnostic tools in tuberculous pleurisy: a direct comparative study. *Eur Respir J* 2003; **22**: 589–91.

● 37. Vanderschueren RG. The role of thoracoscopy in the evaluation and management of pneumothorax. *Lung* (Suppl) 1990: 1122–5.

● 38. The Acute Respiratory Distress Syndrome Network. Ventilation with lower tidal volumes as compared with traditional tidal volumes for acute lung injury and the acute respiratory distress syndrome. *N Engl J Med* 2000; **342**: 1301–8.

◆ 39. Hamm H, Light RW. Paraneumonic effusion and empyema. *Eur Respir J* 1997; **10**: 1150–8.

◆ 40. Poe RH, Marin MG, Israel RH, *et al.* Utility of pleural fluid analysis in predicting tube thoracostomy/decortication in parapneumonic effusions. *Chest* 1991; **100**: 963–7.

41. Heffner JE, Brown LK, Barbieri C, DeLeo JM. Pleural fluid chemical analysis in parapneumonic effusions: a meta-analysis. *Am J Respir Crit Care Med* 1995; **151**: 1700–8.

42. Light RW. A new classification of parapneumonic effusions and empyema. *Chest* 1995; **108**: 299–301.

43. Bouros D, Schiza S, Patsurakis G, *et al.* Intrapleural streptokinase versus urokinase in the treatment of complicated parapneumonic effusions .A prospective, double-blind study. *Am J Respir Crit Care Med* 1997; **155**: 291–5.

44. Chin NK, Lim TK. Controlled trial of intrapleural streptokinase in the treatment of pleural empyema and complicated parapneumonic effusions. *Chest* 1997; **111**: 275–9.

45. Davies RJO, Trail ZC, Gleeson FV. Randomised controlled trial of intra-pleural streptokinase in community acquired pleural infection. *Thorax* 1997; **52**: 416–12.

45a. Tokuda Y, Matsushima D, Stein GD, Miyagi S. Intrapleural fibrinolytic agents for empyema and complicated parapneumonic effusions: a meta-analysis. *Chest* 2006; **129**: 783–90.

46. Simpson G, Roomes D, Heron M. Effects of streptokinase and desoxyribonuclease on the viscosity of human surgical and empyema pus. *Chest* 2000; **117**: 1728–32.

47. Jerez-Sanchez C, Ramirez-Rivera A, Elizalde JJ, *et al.* Intrapleural fibrinolysis with streptokinase as an adjunctive treatment in hemothorax and empyema: a multicenter trial. *Chest* 1996; **109**: 1514–19.

48. Karrny-Jones R, Sorenson V, Horst M, *et al.* Rigid thoracoscopic debridement and continuous pleural irrigation in the management of empyema. *Chest* 1997; **111**: 272–4.

49. Landreneau RJ, Keenan RJ, Hazelrigg SR, *et al.* Thoracoscopy for empyema and hemothorax. *Chest* 1995; **109**: 18–24.

50. Herziger D, Gogolin J, Frank W. Results of medical therapy in empyema. *Pneumologie* 2003; **57**: S23.

51. Davies CWH, Lok S, Davies RJ. The systemic fibrinolytic activity of intrapleural streptokinase. *Am J Respir Crit Care Med* 1998; **157**: 328–30.

52. Storm HKR, Krasnik M, Bang K, Frimodt- Miler N. Treatment of pleural empyema secondary to pneumonia: thoracocentesis regimen versus tube drainage. *Thorax* 1992; **47**: 621–4.

53. Hughes CE, Van Scoy RE. Antibiotic therapy of pleural empyema. *Semin Respir Infect* 1991; **6**: 94–102.

54. Pothula V, Krellenstein DJ. Early aggressive surgical management of parapneumonic empyemas. *Chest* 1994; **105**: 832–6.

55. Alfagame I, Munoz F, Pena N, Umbria S. Empyema of the thorax in adults: etiology, microbiologic findings and management. *Chest* 1993; **103**: 839–43.

56. Shorr RM, Crittenden M, Judeck M, *et al.* Blunt thoracic trauma analysis of 515 patients. *Ann Surg* 1987; **206**: 200–5.

57. Brunner RG, Vinsant GO, Alexander RH, *et al.* The role of antibiotic therapy in the prevention of empyema in patients with isolated chest injury: a prospective study. *J Trauma* 1990; **30**: 1148–53.

58. Wilson JM, Boren CH, Petersen SR, Thomas AN. Traumatic hemothorax: is decortication necessary? *J Thorac Cardiovasc Surg* 1979; **77**: 489–95.

59. Parry GW, Morgan WE, Salama FD. Management of hemothorax. *Ann R Coll Surg Engl* 1996; **78**: 325–6.

60. Meyer DM, Jessen ME, Wait MW. Early evacuation of traumatic retained hemothoraces using thoracoscopy: a prospective randomised trial *Ann Thorac Surg* 1997; **64**: 1396–402.

61. Fallon WF, Wears RL. Prophylactic antibiotics for the prevention of infectious complications including empyema following tube thoracostomy for trauma: results of a metaanalysis. *J Trauma* 1992; **33**: 110–17.

62. Miller AC, Harvey JE (BTS Care Committee). Guidelines for the management of spontaneous pneumothorax. *BMJ* 1993; **307**: 114–16.

63. Seremetis MG. The management of spontaneous pneumothorax. *Chest* 1970; **8**: 57–65.

64. Flint K, Al-Hillawi AH, Johnson NM. Conservative management of spontaneous pneumothorax. *Lancet* 1984; **1**: 687–8.

65. Harvey J, Prescott RJ. Simple aspiration versus intracostal tube drainage for spontaneous pneumothorax in patients with normal lungs. *BMJ* 1994; **309**: 1338–9.

66. Andrivet P, Djedaim K, Teboul JL, *et al.* Spontaneous pneumothorax, comparison of thoracic drainage vs. immediate or delayed needle aspiration. *Chest* 1995; **108**: 335–40.

67. Noppen M, Alexander P, Driesen P, *et al.* Manual aspiration versus chest tube drainage in first episodes of primary spontaneous pneumothorax. A multicenter, prospective, randomized pilot study. *Am J Respir Crit Care Med* 2002; **165**: 1240–4.

● 68. Dines DE, Claget OTI, Payne WS. Spontaneous pneumothorax in emphysema. *Mayo Clin Proc* 1970; **45**: 481–7.

◆ 69. Maunder RJ, Pierson DJ, Hudson LD. Subcutaneous and mediastinal emphysema *Arch Intern Med* 1984; **144**: 1447–53.

● 70. Boutin C, Astoul P, Rey F, Mathur PN. Thoracoscopy in the diagnosis of spontaneous pneumothorax. *Clin Chest Med* 1995; **16**: 497–503.

◆ 71. Walker-Renard PB, Vaughan LM, Sahn SA. Chemical pleurodesis for malignant pleural effusion. *Ann Intern Med* 1994; **120**: 56–64.

● 72. Boutin C, Rey F, Viallat JR. Etude randomisee de l'efficacite du talcage thoracoscopique et de tetracycline dans le traitement des pleuresies cancereuses recedivantes. *Rev Mal Respir* 1985; **2**: 374.

◆ 73. Hartman DL, Gaither JM, Kesler KA, *et al.* Comparison of insufflated talc under thoracoscopic guidance with standard tetracycline and bleomycin pleurodesis for control of malignant pleural effusion. *J Thorac Cardiovasc Surg* 1993; **105**: 743–8.

◆ 74. Rodriguez-Panadero F, Antony VB. Pleurodesis: state of the art. *Eur Respir J* 1997; **10**: 1648–54.

◆ 75. Light R. W Pro/Con editorials. Talc should not be used for pleurodesis. *Am J Respir Crit Care Med* 2000; **162**: 2024–6.

◆ 76. Sahn SA. Pro/Con editorials. Talc should be used for pleurodesis. *Am J Respir Crit Care Med* 2000; **162**: 2023–4.

● 77. Werebe EC, Pazetti R, Milanez de Campos JR, *et al.* Systemic distribution of talc after intrapleural administration in rats. *Chest* 1999; **115**: 190–3.

● 78. Fraticelli A, Robaglia-Schlupp A, Riera H, *et al.* Distribution of calibrated talc after intrapleural administration: an experimental study in rats. *Chest* 2002; **122**: 1737–41.

● 79. Janssen JP, Collier GH, Tschopp JM, *et al.* The European Multicentre Study on the safety of talc in malignant pleural effusion (SOTIM). *Proc Am Thorac Soc* 2006; **3**: A539.

● 80. el Khawand C, Marchandise FX, Mayne A, *et al.* Spontaneous pneumothorax. Results of pleural talc therapy using thoracoscopy. *Rev Mal Respir* 1995; **12**: 275–81.

● 81. Tschopp JM, Boutin C, Astoul P, *et al.*, and the ESMEVAT team. Talcage by medical thoracoscopy for primary spontaneous pneumothorax is more cost-effective than drainage: a randomised study. *Eur Respir J* 2002; **20**: 1003–9.

● 82. Milanez JRC, Vargas FS, Filomeno LTB, *et al.* Intrapleural talc for the prevention of recurrent pneumothorax. *Chest* 1994; **106**: 1162–5.

● 83. Ruckdeschel JC, Moores D, Lee JY, *et al.* Intrapleural therapy for malignant pleural effusions. A randomized comparison of bleomycin and tetracycline. *Chest* 1991; **100**: 1528–35.

● 84. Frank W, Fritzsche A, Raffenberg M, Loddenkemper R. Results of talc pleurodesis in malignant effusion. World Congress of Bronchology, Munich 1993.

● 85. Bresticker MA, Oba J, Locicero J, *et al.* Optimum pleurodesis: a comparison study. *Ann Thorac Surg* 1993; **55**: 364–47.

● 86. Freixinet J, Canalis E, Rivas JJ, *et al.* Surgical treatment of primary spontaneous pneumothorax with video-assisted thoracic surgery. *Eur Respir J* 1997; **10**: 409–11.

● 87. Schramel FMNH, Sutedja TG, Braber JCE, *et al.* Cost-effectiveness of video-assisted thoracoscopic surgery versus conservative treatment for first time or recurrent spontaneous pneumothorax. *Eur Respir J* 1996; **9**: 1821–5.

◆ 88. Shah SS, Cohen AS, Magee PP. Surgery remains a late and underutilised option in the management of spontaneous pneumothorax: should the British Thoracic Society Guidelines be revisited? *Thorax* 1998; **53**(Suppl 4): A52.

● 89. Kopecki SI, Callahan JA, Tajek AJ, *et al.* Percutaneous pericardial catheter drainage: report of 42 consecutive cases. *Am J Cardiol* 1986; **58**: 633–6.

◆ 90. Shephard FA, Ginsberg JS, Evans WR, *et al.* Tetracycline sclerosis in the management of malignant pericardial effusion. *J Clin Oncol* 1983; **3**: 1678–80.

◆ 91. Krizek TJ, Lease JG. Surgical management of suppurative mediastinitis In: Sabiston DC, Jr, ed. *Textbook of Surgery*, 14th ed. Philadelphia: WB Saunders 1991:1796–800.

Diseases and Syndromes

Upper airway infections

MARCIA EPSTEIN, ANGELA KIM, HEMWATTIE SHANTIE JAIMANGAL

INTRODUCTION

The upper respiratory tract is a critical area. It is essential that the clinician recognizes the signs and symptoms of disease presenting in this location as it may herald more serious systemic illness and infection. Indeed this area may serve as the portal of entry for certain infections. Furthermore, the anatomy of this area must be understood. Infections of the upper respiratory tract can rapidly spread to the mediastinum and other critical areas such as the carotid sheath and retropharyngeal space, causing life-threatening complications. This chapter will focus mainly on upper respiratory tract infections where a delay in diagnosis might affect prognosis. These infections include Lemierre syndrome, Ludwig angina, Vincent angina, noma, diphtheria, peritonsillar abscesses, croup, epiglottitis, rabies, and sinusitis with an emphasis on the agents of mucormycosis (Table 10A.1).

OROFACIAL INFECTIONS

Poor orodental hygiene leads to dental caries, periapical abscess, and periodontitis. Although treatable, these diseases predispose to more serious and potentially life-threatening complications if extension into orofacial spaces or deep fascial spaces of the head and neck occurs. Left untreated, dental caries and periodontitis may progress to periapical abscess. In severe cases, Vincent angina, an acute necrotizing ulcerative gingivitis, can result. Most perimandibular dental infections begin as endodontal or periapical infections of which a small proportion progresses to involve the sublingual and/or the submandibular spaces.

Common initiating causes of orofacial infections include pharyngitis, tonsillitis, sinusitis, otitis, and parotitis. Other noninfectious causes include radiation- or chemotherapy-induced mucositis and/or stomatitis.[1] Intravenous drug users who inject into neck vessels may also have infections in deep neck spaces.

Definition and anatomy

Infections spread along paths of least resistance including along fascial planes of connective tissue. In orofacial anatomy, infections of dental or periodontal origin (supporting teeth structures) spread to molar apices (Fig. 10A.1). From here infection extends more medially or laterally above or below anatomic boundaries such as the buccinator muscle resulting in intraoral (formed by the buccinator attachment to maxilla or mandible) or extraoral (outside the buccinator attachment) swelling. In the case of mandibular molar infections, sublingual or submandibular extension occurs depending on spread to above or below the mylohyoid muscle, respectively. Generally, these infections remain localized.

Maxillary molar infections can readily extend to the paranasal sinuses.[3] Periorbital and orbital infections may also result from extension of odontogenic infections usually by way of maxillary premolars and molars.[4] Unlike typical

Table 10A.1   *Upper airway infections – respiratory emergencies*

Entity	Clinical features	Treatment
Ludwig angina	Rapidly spreading cellulitis of the submandibular and sublingual space. Begins in the floor of the mouth	High-dose parental antibiotics, close monitoring of airway, intubation or tracheostomy if necessary, occasionally surgical drainage
Vincent angina	Presents with ulceration, pain, necrosis of gingiva	Antibiotic treatment, local debridement and lavage with oxidizing agent
Noma	Most common in sub-Saharan Africa. Is an acute fulminating, gangrenous infection of oral and facial soft tissue	Treatment of underlying dehydration and malnutrition. High doses of parental antibiotics, usually penicillin
Diphtheria	Forms necrotic membrane and can cause severe edema of the neck. Can have myocardial and neurologic involvement	Diphtheria antitoxin and antibiotics such as penicillin or erythromycin
Lemierre disease	Usually caused by *Fusobacterium necrophorum*. Septic thrombosis of the internal jugular vein with metastatic emboli	Antibiotic treatment with antibiotics active against β-lactamase-resistant anaerobic organisms. Anticoagulation occasionally helpful
Oropharyngeal manifestations of agents of bioterroism	Can mimic more common infections. Agents include *Bacillus anthracis, Francisella tularemia, Yersinia pestis*	In the case of biologic attack antibiotic-resistant patterns are unpredictable. For naturally occurring strains of anthrax the effective antibiotics include penicillin and possibly doxycycline and the fluoroquinolones. The preferred agents for plague are the aminoglycosides or possibly doxycycline. For tularemia aminoglycosides are first line therapy
Croup	Usually of viral etiology. Inspiratory stridor, hoarseness and a brassy cough	Cool mist, racemic epinephrine and steroids
Epiglotittis	Rapidly progressive cellulitis of the epiglottis, usually bacterial. Abrupt onset of fever and sore throat. Leukocytosis usually present	Maintain adequate airway. Prompt administration of antibiotics
Rabies (furious form)	Inability to swallow because of pharyngeal spasm	Supportive care. Usually incurable once symptoms have begun
Mucormycosis (zygomycosis)	Sinusitis, painless necrotic palatal or nasal septal ulcer or eschar	Surgical debridement, amphotercin product and or posaconazole, ± hyperbarbaric oxygen

Modified from Chow AW. Infections of the oral cavity, neck, and head. In: Mandell GE, Bennett JE, Dolin R, eds. *Principles and Practice of Infectious Disease*, 5th ed, vol 1. New York: Churchill Livingstone, 2000: 689–702 with permission from Elsevier.

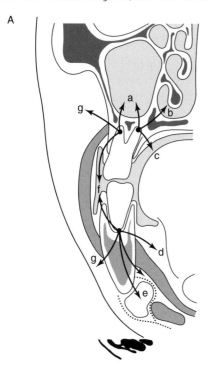

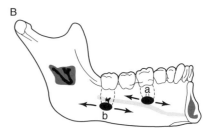

Figure 10A.1   *Routes of spread of odontogenic orofacial infections along planes of least resistance. A: coronal section in the region of the first molar teeth: a, maxillary antrum; b, nasal cavity; c, palatal plate; d, sublingual space (above the mylohyoid muscle); e, submandibular space (below the mylohyoid muscle); f, intraoral presentation with infection spreading through the buccal plates inside the attachment of the buccinator muscle; g, extraoral presentation to buccal space with infection spreading through the buccal plates outside the attachment of the buccinator muscle. B: lingual aspect of the mandible: a, apices of the involved tooth above the mylohyoid muscle, with spread of infection to the sublingual space; b, apices of involved tooth below the mylohyoid muscle, with spread of infection into the submandibular space. (From Chow AW et al.[2].)*

bacterial pathogens, *Actinomyces* species have been associated with cervicofacial infections. This occurs more commonly at the angle of the mandible and extends across tissue planes. Unfortunately this diagnosis is often missed.

Background and epidemiology

Most cases of orofacial infections occur following complications of dental infection or recent dental extraction particularly of the second or third maxillary or mandibular molars. Mandibular fracture or trauma secondary to intubation and bronchoscopy has also been implicated as causative factors.[5]

A few orofacial infections can be classified as potential emergencies. The first is Ludwig angina. Ludwig angina is inflammation of the tissues of the floor of the mouth extending under the tongue. It often occurs following an infection of the roots of the teeth or after dental injury. Swelling of the tissues occurs rapidly and may block the airway or prevent swallowing of saliva. This condition is rarely seen in children but has been documented in young otherwise healthy individuals, and resulted in asphyxiation and death during the pre-antibiotic era.[6] If the diagnosis is made early, Ludwig angina can be cured with proper protection of the breathing passages and adequate antibiotic therapy. Noma, a second potential orofacial emergency infection, is an acute fulminating gangrenous infection of oral and facial soft tissues. Noma is seen in areas of famine and poor hygiene but rarely in industrialized regions. It is not usually of dental origin and it is estimated that 100 000 to 140 000 cases occurs per year with a mortality of 70–90 percent.[7] The third type of infection is termed Vincent angina or trench mouth. This is an acute necrotizing gingivitis extending from the interdental papillae along the gingival margins. It has a predilection for young adults aged 18–25 years, with a predominance among male soldiers. In severe cases, Vincent angina can result in periapical abscess.

Etiology

Typically infections of odontogenic origin are polymicrobial and include normal oral flora such as *Bacteroides*, *Prevotella*, *Fusobacterium*, *Porphyromonas*, *Peptostreptococcus*, microaerophilic streptococci, *Veillonella*, *Actinomyces*, and aerobic streptococci.[1,2] Specifically, the following microbial organisms have been isolated – *Porphyromonas gingivalis*, *Prevotella intermedius*, *Campylobacter pectus*, *Bacteroides forsythus*, *Actinobacillus actinomycetemcomitans*, *Veillonella parvula*, *Fusobacterium nucleatum*, *Fusobacterium alocis*, *Peptostreptococcus micros*, *Peptostreptococcus anaerobius*, *Eubacterium timidum*, *Eubacterium alactolyticum*, *Eubacterium brachy*, β-hemolytic streptococcus, *Capnocytophaga* species, *Staphylococcus* species, Gram-negative enteric pathogens, *Pseudomonas* species, and *Actinomycetes* species.[8,9]

Clinical presentation

In general, a tooth abscess presents with pain, especially during chewing or with extreme changes in temperature. Periodontal infections cause gum swelling and are also painful.[1]

LUDWIG ANGINA

Progression of these infections predisposes to Ludwig angina, a rapidly spreading cellulitis of the submandibular space associated with pain in the floor of the mouth with elevation of the tongue, neck rigidity, trismus, dysphagia, shortness of breath, drooling, and fever. Clinically, it is defined by bilateral involvement of both the sublingual and submandibular spaces. The disease usually follows a mandibular molar infection and often occurs without frank abscess formation. Examination reveals high fever, systemic toxicity, swelling at the floor of the mouth, and, if extensive enough, the tongue is displaced both superiorly and posteriorly.

VINCENT ANGINA

In trench mouth or Vincent angina, an acute ulcerative gingivostomatitis, involvement of the pharyngeal area results in sudden onset of pain, ulceration and necrosis in the gums associated with halitosis, altered taste sensation, fever, malaise, adenopathy, and superficial gray pseudomembrane.

NOMA OR CANCRUM ORIS

More common in areas of sub-Saharan Africa or war-torn regions, is noma or cancrum oris, which begins with ulceration of the mucous membrane and progresses to facial edema and rapid destruction of soft tissue structures and bone. Debilitation and malnourishment are risk factors. Outbreaks of measles infection have been associated with the onset of noma. Acute necrotizing gingivitis may precede development of this disease.[7,10]

In general, mild odontogenic infections are easily treatable and not life-threatening unless extensive involvement of the fascial planes with edema which compromises the airway.

Investigation

Pantomography is useful to determine the presence of abscesses. If possible, extraoral procurement of specimen is preferred, as intraoral specimen collection is often contaminated by normal flora. Gram, acid fast, and fungal stains are important for microbiologic diagnosis and selection of antibiotic therapy.

Treatment

LUDWIG ANGINA

Antibiotics with high doses of ampicillin-sulbactam or penicillin G (12–20 million units daily) plus metronidazole are the mainstay of treatment of Ludwig angina.[1] First generation cephalosporins are alternatives for patients allergic to penicillin, unless complicated by anaphylaxis.[11] However, equally important is frequent and close monitoring for signs and symptoms of airway compromise including access to a bedside tracheostomy tray in case of need for emergent tracheostomy. If during observation, cellulitis progresses, intubation is recommended before airway compromise occurs.[12] Occasionally, surgical decompression and drainage is required.

Parental antibiotics in conjunction with surgical intervention have significantly decreased the mortality from over 50 percent (pre-antibiotic) to 0–4 percent (presently).[13]

VINCENT ANGINA

In addition to appropriate antibiotics, Vincent angina responds to surgical debridement of necrotic and infected tissue. Premature incision and drainage of a not well-demarcated abscess is therapeutically futile.

Antibiotic choices include penicillin, amoxicillin, doxycycline, and clindamycin in patients allergic to penicillin. For slow or nonresponders, broader Gram-negative and anaerobic coverage should be considered (i.e. quinolones, metronidazole).

NOMA OR CANCRUM ORIS

Seen infrequently in the United States and Europe, noma is managed initially with antibiotics such as penicillin and clindamycin along with nutritional support and rehydration. This may be followed by surgical reconstruction as survivors may have facial mutilation, speech and/or chewing deficits, and nasal regurgitation of food.[10]

Complications

Most of the complications are related to airway compromise and the potential for asphyxiation as well as extension of infection intracranially, into the retropharyngeal or pleuropulmonary spaces, periorbitally, into adjacent spaces (sinusitis) or by fascial planes (mediastinitis being the most dreaded complication).[12,14]

PHARYNGITIS

Sore throat, a common complaint among both children and adults, results in numerous visits to primary care and emergency medical physicians. It is defined by inflammation of the pharynx usually by either viral or bacterial microbes. Most cases are either self-limiting or easily treated once the pathogen is identified. Occasionally, severe or inadequately treated cases may progress to potentially life-threatening complications. Diphtheria, Lemierre syndrome and other

unusual pathogens involving the pharyngeal space will be reviewed in this section.

Background and epidemiology

Seasonal variation can dictate the pathogens that are responsible for causing pharyngitis. Streptococcal pharyngitis has a bimodal trend, occurring mostly during winter and spring months whereas coronaviral infections peak during the winter months. Other etiologies are less seasonal and some are sexually transmitted such as *Gonococcus* and human immunodeficiency virus (HIV) infection. Person-to-person transmission of pharyngitis is common, especially among household contacts and those living in close quarters.

Pathogenesis and etiology

Viruses frequently cause pharyngitis. Common viruses include rhinovirus, coronavirus, adenovirus, herpes simplex virus (both types 1 and 2), parainfluenza virus, influenza virus (types A and B), Epstein–Barr virus, cytomegalovirus and HIV. Bacterial causes of pharyngitis include most commonly group A β-hemolytic streptococci, group C and G β-hemolytic streptococci, *Neisseria gonorrhea*, *Corynebacterium diphtheriae*, *Fusobacterium necrophorum*, *Arcanobacterium haemolyticum*, and *Mycoplasma pneumoniae*.[15] Rare, but important, causes include *Bacillus anthracis*, *Yersinia pestis*, and *Francisella tularensis*. Some organisms cause disease by stimulating production of mediators that result in an inflammatory response. Some viruses have direct cytopathic effect and others cause disease indirectly by elaborating toxins.

Diphtheria

BACKGROUND, INCIDENCE, AND EPIDEMIOLOGY

Over the past half century, the number of cases of diphtheria has decreased dramatically, partly due to vaccination.[16] In certain parts of the world, however, the disease still remains endemic. This is seen most notably in the former Soviet Union, the Indian subcontinent, Indonesia, the Philippines, countries of sub-Saharan Africa, the Dominican Republic, Haiti, Ecuador, and Brazil.[17] During the mid 1990s, the diphtheria outbreak in the former Soviet Union was considered an international public health emergency. By 1994, the epidemic had affected all 15 newly independent states with over 157 000 cases and more than 5000 deaths reported.[18]

Humans are the only reservoirs for *C. diphtheriae*, the pathogen responsible for diphtheria. The disease spreads by airborne respiratory droplets or by direct contact with open lesions. Transmission with contaminated fomite contact can also occur. Rare epidemics caused by contaminated milk have been described. Asymptomatic carriers remain the major reservoir for infections to nonimmune subjects.

PATHOGENESIS AND ETIOLOGY

The major virulence of *C. diphtheriae* is attributed to the potent exotoxin it elaborates. The organism itself is not very invasive. It usually sits on the superficial mucosal layers causing only a mild inflammatory reaction. Although local complications such as respiratory obstruction may occur, the majority of the complications are due to the effects of the diphtheria toxin on cardiac, neural, or renal tissues (myocarditis, demyelination, and tubular necrosis, respectively).[19,20] The exotoxin exerts its effect by inhibiting protein synthesis selectively in mammalian cells and not in bacterial cells.

Diphtheria toxin production occurs in strains of *C. diphtheriae* that are lysogenized with bacteriophages containing the structural gene for toxin molecule (Tox(+) strains). Tox(−) strains rarely produce disseminated disease. The toxin consists of two segments A and B. Fragment B attaches to cellular receptors and grants fragment A entrance into the cell where it inhibits protein synthesis. Diphtheria toxin is very potent. A single molecule can stop protein synthesis in a cell within hours. The exotoxin is absorbed into the bloodstream and distributed, resulting in systemic complications.[21]

CLINICAL PRESENTATION

The severity of clinical disease is inversely related to patient's immunization history. After a 2–4 day incubation period, diphtheria usually presents itself as a pharyngitis or tonsillitis. The onset is usually abrupt and a low-grade fever is often present. A membrane develops, typically on one or both tonsils and can extend to involve other parts of the oronasopharynx such as the epiglottis, larynx, and trachea or to the tracheobronchial tree. It is a necrotic coagulum of fibrin, leukocytes, erythrocytes, dead epithelial cells and organisms. The membrane is initially white and glossy but transforms into a dirty gray color with patches of green or black necrosis. The extent of membrane involvement usually correlates with severity of disease. Severe edema and swelling of the neck, trachea, and larynx can lead to respiratory compromise, necessitating intubation. This distortion of the normal contours of the cervical and submental area is often referred to as a 'bull neck' appearance.[22]

Two-thirds of the patients have myocardial involvement; however, only 10–25 percent have clinical signs or symptoms of such involvement. Manifestations include atrioventricular blocks, arrhythmias, heart failure, or circulatory collapse.[23] Approximately three-fourths of patients with severe disease develop neurologic complications. Within a few days of pharyngeal symptoms patients can develop local paralysis of the soft palate and posterior pharyngeal wall. Subsequently cranial neuropathies develop. Peripheral neuritis follows from 10 days to 3 months after the onset of pharyngeal disease. Neurologic dysfunction ranges from mild weakness

with diminished tendon reflexes to complete paralysis.[16,20] Most deaths occur within the first 3 or 4 days from asphyxia or myocarditis.

INVESTIGATION

Rapid diagnosis of diphtheria is difficult and the decision to treat depends on a strong clinical suspicion based on a constellation of findings and history. These include painful tonsillitis, pharyngitis associated with a pseudomembrane, low-grade fever, hoarseness, stridor, palatal paralysis, serosanguineous nasal discharge, cervical adenopathy, cervical swelling, and systemic toxicity.

Cultures should be obtained from the pseudomembrane or beneath its edge. *C. diphtheriae* grows on Loeffler or tellurite selective media (such as Tindale agar). Toxin A subunit production can be demonstrated *in vitro* and *in vivo*. Blood work may reveal moderate leukocytosis and possible thrombocytopenia. Chest radiograph shows subglottic narrowing. Electrocardiography may show ST-T wave changes, heart block and other arrhythmias.

TREATMENT

Diphtheria antitoxin, produced in horses, provides neutralization of circulating toxin. Although it does not neutralize toxin that is already fixed to tissues, it does prevent progression of disease. It is critical that the diphtheria antitoxin is administered once a presumptive diagnosis is made. Up to 7 percent of patients will show some hypersensitivity to the horse protein resulting in serum sickness.[24] In addition, antibiotics such as erythromycin and penicillin are effective by killing the organism and thus preventing further toxin production. This also improves local infection and prevents spread to contacts. The disease is less contagious after 48 hours of treatment.

Prophylaxis for close contacts, especially household contacts, with diphtheria booster vaccine is recommended along with benzathine penicillin. Erythromycin is an alternative for patients allergic to penicillin. In view of the short incubation period of diphtheria (1–6 days) and the delay in bacteriologic diagnosis, all close contacts should be monitored for at least 7 days. Although not all patients will become clinically ill, some will become asymptomatic carriers. Diphtheria toxoid protects against clinical complications but it does not prevent the carrier state. Furthermore, asymptomatic carriers may transmit the organism to susceptible hosts. It is therefore recommended that all contacts should have nasal and pharyngeal swabs regardless of vaccination status.[16,22,24]

The most important measure for preventing diphtheria is an ongoing program of active immunization of all children and booster immunizations of adults. The recommendation is that all children receive a routine series of five doses of diphtheria toxoid (Td)-containing vaccine at ages 2, 4, 6, 12–20 months and between 4 and 6 years. Booster of Td should be given at 11–12 years and at 10-year intervals.[17]

Lemierre syndrome

BACKGROUND AND EPIDEMIOLOGY

Lemierre syndrome, also known as necrobacillosis or postanginal sepsis, is characterized by septic thrombosis of the internal jugular vein with metastatic emboli following an acute oropharyngeal infection.[25] This syndrome is most commonly associated with *Fusobacterium necrophorum*, a Gram-negative anaerobic rod that has the potential to induce thrombosis by releasing lipopolysaccharide endotoxins.[26] Intravenous drug abuse, central intravenous catheterization, hypercoagulability, oropharyngeal infections, and atherosclerosis are also risk factors for developing this syndrome.[27]

Lemierre syndrome can be fatal. Approximately 90 percent of patients with this disease will rapidly progress within 7–15 days of its onset.[28] In the post-antibiotic era, documented cases of Lemierre syndrome have decreased significantly, correlating with a mortality of 4–12 percent.[29] This decrease in mortality rate is attributed to prompt initiation of antibiotic therapy.[30]

PATHOGENESIS AND ETIOLOGY

Pathogens known to cause Lemierre syndrome include *Streptococcus* species, *Bacteroides* species, and *Lactobacillus* species. However, by far the single most common organism isolated in blood cultures is *F. necrophorum*. *Fusobacterium* species are part of the normal oral cavity flora and are concentrated in the gingival crevices, subgingival plaques, large bowel, and the female genital tract.

Loss of mucosal integrity from trauma or hypoxia potentiates the overgrowth of *F. necrophorum* leading to invasion into the blood stream. Elaborated proteolytic enzymes, lipopolysaccharide, endotoxin, leukocidin, and hemagglutinin enable the bacteria to invade regional vessels and cause aggregation of platelets. This leads to internal jugular vein thrombosis, the hallmark of Lemierre syndrome.[31] The internal jugular vein is more commonly involved due to compression or extension of thrombophlebitis of the peritonsillar veins into the jugular vein.[28,32]

CLINICAL PRESENTATION

Lemierre syndrome mostly affects adolescents or young adults, yet, several cases have been reported in children.[25,28,30] Symptoms begin with fever, pharyngitis (most commonly), tonsillitis, or gingivitis. Other predisposing factors include mastoiditis, otitis, dental infections, and parapharyngeal abscesses. The onset of suppurative jugular thrombophlebitis is heralded by a sudden presentation of high fever, rigors, neck pain, and swelling. Similar to other forms of endovascular infection, signs and symptoms of metastatic infection are seen, in particular, pulmonary emboli mimicking pneumonia. These patients present with dyspnea, pleuritis, and occasionally hemoptysis.[25,28] In severe cases, adult respiratory distress syndrome, empyema, and lung abscess have resulted in respiratory compromise requiring mechanical ventilation.[33,34]

In addition to the internal jugular vein, other primary sites of septic thrombophlebitis include the external jugular vein, sigmoid sinuses, and superior vena cava.[29] Metastatic foci or direct extension of infection can lead to septic arthritis of large joints such as the knee, hip, shoulder, ankle, and sternoclavicular joint. Intraabdominal abscesses have also been reported in the liver, spleen and kidney.[30]

INVESTIGATION

History, physical examination, and laboratory studies all support the diagnosis. Blood cultures, especially isolation of *Fusobacterium* species, give clues to the diagnosis. Chest radiography might reveal bilateral nodular infiltrates, pleural effusions, and cavitary lesions.[33] The neck and internal jugular veins can be evaluated by venous duplex ultrasound, computed tomography with contrast, magnetic resonance imaging, magnetic resonance venography, nuclear scintigraphy, or gallium-67 scanning (Figs 10A.2 and 10A.3).

Although contrast venography is the gold standard, this procedure is invasive with associated risks and is therefore not frequently used. Either computed tomography or magnetic resonance imaging is the diagnostic modality of choice.

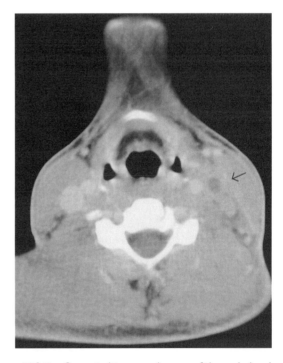

Figure 10A.2 *Computed tomography scan of the neck showing left internal jugular thrombosis (arrow). (Courtesy of Rakesh Shah, MD. North Shore University Hospital, Manhasset, NY.)*

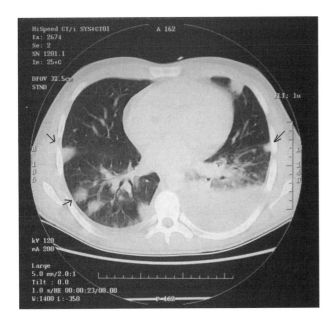

Figure 10A.3 *Computed tomography scan of chest demonstrating multiple metastatic pulmonary emboli (arrows). (Courtesy of Rakesh Shah, MD. North Shore University Hospital, Manhasset, NY.)*

TREATMENT

Prompt initiation of anaerobic coverage with β-lactamase resistant antibiotics and possible surgical drainage is crucial. The most commonly used antibiotics include metronidazole, penicillin, clindamycin, ticarcillin-clavulanate, ampicillin-sulbactam, chloramphenicol, and the carbapenems.[25] Duration of treatment with antibiotics depends on the severity of the infection; however, Lemierre should be treated like most endovascular infections.

Antibiotics initially are administered intravenously for 7–14 days, followed by oral antibiotics for 2–4 weeks.[32] The average duration of antibiotic therapy is 42 days.[25] β-Lactamase production is seen in 23 percent of *F. necrophorum* isolates hence the need for careful selection of appropriate antibiotic.[35,36] Adjunctive anticoagulation therapy has been shown to facilitate the resolution of septic pelvic thrombophlebitis and decrease the progression of the clot, but this remains controversial.[37] If used, the recommended duration is 3 months.[37]

In patients with advanced disease, persistent fevers, recurrent emboli or uncontrolled sepsis, ligation, or embolectomy is indicated. Over the past decade thrombectomy was performed in 9 percent of reported cases.[25]

COMPLICATIONS

Left untreated, Lemierre syndrome can persist as overwhelming sepsis with multiorgan metastatic emboli leading to respiratory distress and possibly death.[38]

OROPHARYNGEAL MANIFESTATIONS OF AGENTS OF BIOTERRORISM AND OTHER UNCOMMON PHARYNGEAL PATHOGENS

In the current climate, the physician must be aware of atypical presentations of agents of bioterrorism. In this section, some of the possible pathogens (*B. anthracis*, *Y. pestis*, and *F. tularensis*) will be discussed. At present the information is limited because of the rarity of these pathogens presenting with oral manifestations of infection.

Anthrax

BACKGROUND

Historically anthrax has been a disease found in animals with occasional serious illness in humans following contact with either an anthrax-infected animal or anthrax-contaminated animal products, or wool sorters. In humans, three types of anthrax infection are described: inhalation, cutaneous, and gastrointestinal.[39] Cutaneous anthrax is the most commonly described. It is postulated that the gastrointestinal form is probably underreported because the diagnosis is often unrecognized. Inhalation anthrax is a rapidly progressive, often fatal infection.

PATHOPHYSIOLOGY AND EPIDEMIOLOGY

A number of factors contribute to the pathogenesis of anthrax. First, *B. anthracis* has a capsule that prevents phagocytosis. Other important features that makes this pathogen virulent is the elaboration of virulent toxins through the production of three proteins – protective antigen, lethal factor, and edema factor – that combine to form two toxins: lethal toxin and edema toxin. The role of protective antigen is to enable the binding of lethal and edema factors to cell membranes and facilitate their transport across the membrane. Edema toxin impairs neutrophil functions and affects water homeostasis causing edema. Lethal factor is believed to cause the release of tumor necrosis factor (TNF)-α and interleukin-1β.[40]

CLINICAL PRESENTATION

Gastrointestinal anthrax occurs following ingestion of insufficiently cooked, contaminated meats or other food products. This can lead to two distinct syndromes, oral pharyngeal, or abdominal anthrax (Fig. 10A.4a–c). The oropharyngeal form of the disease occurs after the germination of anthrax spores in the upper gastrointestinal tract. First ulcers form followed by the development of lymphadenopathy, edema, and sepsis.[40] Patients may complain of a severe sore throat, fever, dysphagia, and sometimes present in respiratory distress secondary to the massive edema and marked lymphadenopathy. Oral ulcers may form a pseudomembrane that may be confused with

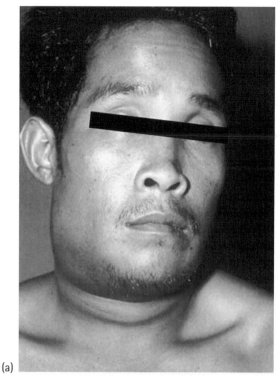

(a)

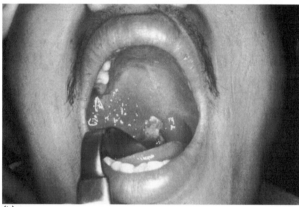

(b)

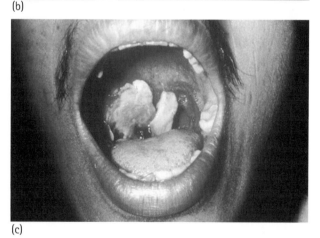

(c)

Figure 10A.4 *(a) A 29-year-old man, 1 day after the symptoms of oropharyngeal anthrax. Marked and painful swelling of right side of neck. (b) Tonsillar swelling and marked edema 5 days after onset of symptoms. (c) Same patient with pseudomembrane 9 days after onset of symptoms. (From Sirisanthana and Brown.[41])*

diphtheria. The pathologic examination of the anthrax lesion in the gastrointestinal tract shows that the mucosa is always involved as well as regional lymph nodes, which enlarge and become hemorrhagic.

Some authors believe that the transit time of the gastrointestinal tract is too rapid to allow spores to cause oropharyngeal anthrax and believe that these cases result from ingestion of large numbers of vegetative bacilli from poorly cooked infected meat, rather than from spores.[40] In 1982, there was an outbreak of 24 cases of oropharyngeal anthrax in northern Thailand from water buffalo meat.[41] The mean incubation period was 42 hours (range 2–144 hours). All the patients (except for one) required hospitalization and were febrile. Painful neck swelling was the presenting complaint. The other common complaints were sore throat, dysphasia, and hoarseness.

INVESTIGATION

Diagnosis of this form of anthrax can be made from culture of the exudates from the mouth sores or biopsy of skin lesions. Gram stain will reveal Gram-positive bacilli. Serological testing may be useful retrospectively. In pulmonary anthrax, a widened mediastinum is seen on chest radiograph.

TREATMENT

Antibiotic resistance patterns in the setting of a biologic attack are unknown. Most naturally occurring strains of anthrax are sensitive to penicillin, doxycycline and the fluoroquinolones, and are all likely to be efficacious. Weapon-grade strains, however, may be selected to be penicillin resistant.[42]

Plague

BACKGROUND AND ETIOLOGY

Plague is an enzootic infection of rats, prairie dogs, ground squirrels, and other rodents worldwide (except Australia).[43] *Y. pestis*, a Gram-negative bacillus belonging to the family Enterobacteriaceae is the cause of plague. It is a nonlactose-fermenter, grows aerobically, and possesses several virulence factors including the production of a lipopolysaccharide endotoxin, the presence of temperature-dependent enzymes coagulase and fibrinolysin and others.[44]

PATHOGENESIS AND CLINICAL PRESENTATION

Human plague usually occurs when plague-infected fleas bite humans who then develop bubonic plague or rarely just sepsis. Either of these can cause secondary pneumonic plague that can then spread the disease via respiratory droplets. A rare form of plague is a pharyngitis that resembles acute tonsillitis. There is anterior cervical adenopathy and the organism can be isolated from the throat or by aspiration of the cervical bubo. This form of plague is felt to result either from the ingestion or inhalation of the plague bacilli.

TREATMENT

Historically streptomycin was the preferred treatment for plague but tetracyclines and the quinolones are probably efficacious as well.[45] Chloramphenicol and the sulfonamides might also be active.

Tularemia

BACKGROUND, ETIOLOGY, EPIDEMIOLOGY, AND PATHOGENESIS

F. tularensis, the etiologic agent of tularemia is one of the most infectious pathogenic bacteria known to mankind. As few as 10 organisms can cause disease. Virulence seems to be attributed to the capsule and citrulline ureides activity.[46] Humans usually acquire tularemia through handling infectious animals or tissues, bites of infected arthropods, inhalation of infective aerosols, or ingestion of infected water, food or soil. Once the bacteria are inoculated into skin or mucous membranes, they multiply and spread to regional lymph nodes and travel to various organs.

CLINICAL PRESENTATION

The different clinical manifestations include ulceroglandular, glandular, oculoglandular, oropharyngeal, pneumonic, typhoidal, and septic forms. The oropharyngeal form of tularemia is usually an exudative pharyngitis or tonsillitis sometimes with ulceration. There can be pronounced cervical or retropharyngeal adenopathy. This form of the disease is usually acquired by consuming contaminated water, food, and less commonly by inhaling contaminated droplets or aerosols.[47]

INVESTIGATION AND TREATMENT

To make the diagnosis of tularemia, the physician must first alert the lab to use special safety procedures. *F. tularensis* grows best in cysteine-enriched broth, thioglycollate broth, cysteine heart blood agar, buffered charcoal yeast agar, and chocolate agar. Cultures should be placed at 37 °C. Serologic confirmation of disease takes at least 10 days.

Aminoglycosides (streptomycin or gentamicin) are the primary first line treatment. Alternative agents include the tetracyclines and quinolones.[47]

PARAPHARYNGEAL, LATERAL NECK, AND LARYNGEAL INFECTIONS

Infections involving parapharyngeal and lateral pharyngeal space arise from oropharyngeal infections (pharyngitis,

tonsillitis, parotitis, otitis media, and mastoiditis) or odontogenic infection.[1,48] Again, the most crucial aspect in diagnosis and management of the neck space infections involves airway assessment.

Anatomy and definition

The cervical fascia divides into superficial and deep cervical fascia, which further subdivides into superficial, visceral (middle or pretracheal), and prevertebral layers. The prevertebral layer again subdivides into alar and prevertebral fascia. Deep spaces in the neck can be categorized into the suprahyoid region composed of the submandibular, sublingual, and lateral pharyngeal spaces; and the infrahyoid region comprised of the retropharyngeal, pretracheal, 'danger', and prevertebral spaces (Fig. 10A.5).

The submandibular and sublingual spaces have been described above. The lateral pharyngeal space bounded by the superficial component of the deep cervical fascia is partitioned into an anterior component (containing fat, lymph nodes, and muscle) and posterior component containing neurovascular structures such as cranial nerves IX through XII, carotid artery, jugular vein, and cervical sympathetic nerve chain.[12,48]

The middle deep fascial layer encloses the visceral components (esophagus, trachea, thyroid).[2] The retropharyngeal space is bounded by the pharynx anteriorly and the alar fascia posteriorly.[49] The deep layer connects the base of the skull and travels anterior to the vertebrae down to the diaphragm. Laterally, it encases the paraspinal muscles. It defines the prevertebral space and posterior wall of the 'danger space' which leads directly to the posterior mediastinum and may result in mediastinitis, a devastating complication associated with increased mortality.

Background and epidemiology

There has been a decrease in incidence of complicated deep neck space infections since the advent of antibiotics and advancement in oral/dental hygiene. Lateral pharyngeal space infections may originate from tonsillitis, pharyngitis, peritonsillar abscess, otitis media, sinusitis, parotitis, and odontogenic infections (mandibular molar infections).[49] Retropharyngeal space infections may result from extension of lateral pharyngeal space infection or from lymphatic spread from deep cervical lymph node infections more commonly seen in children.

Etiology

Peptostreptococcus, other microaerophilic streptococci, *Actinomycetes*, *Bacteroides*, *Fusobacterium*, *Veillonella*, and *Corynebacteria* have all been isolated from clinical specimens of lateral and retropharyngeal space infections. Interestingly,

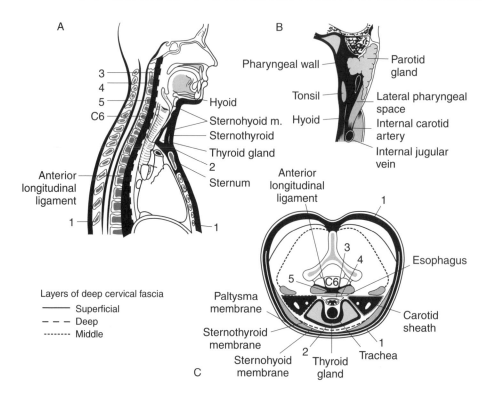

Figure 10A.5 *Relations of lateral pharyngeal, retropharyngeal, and prevertebral spaces to the posterior and anterior layers of the deep cervical fascia. 1: Superficial space; 2: pretracheal space; 3: retropharyngeal space; 4: 'danger' space; 5: prevertebral space. (a) Midsagittal section of the head and neck. (b) Coronal section in the suprahyoid region of the neck. (c) Cross-section of the neck at the level of the thyroid isthmus. (Redrawn from Chow AW. Infections of the oral cavity, neck, and head. In: Mandell GE, Bennett JE, Dolin R, eds.* Principles and Practice of Infectious Disease, *5th ed, vol 1. New York: Churchill Livingstone, 2000:689–702 with permission from Elsevier.)*

Staphylococcus aureus, *M. tuberculosis*, and *Coccidioides immitis* have been isolated in prevertebral space infections as a result of direct extension from vertebral or epidural infections.

Clinical presentation

Patients with *peritonsillar abscess* often present with erythema, edema of the pharynx that may or may not be asymmetric, purulent discharge, and cervical adenitis. Trismus, a feature of anterior but not usually posterior lateral pharyngeal space infections, is accompanied by fever, chills, pain, swelling, dysphasia, and medial displacement of lateral pharyngeal wall.[12,49]

In posterior lateral pharyngeal space infections, swelling may be absent but clinically there may be signs of septicemia, respiratory obstruction, suppurative jugular thrombophlebitis, and involvement of carotid sheath leading to thrombosis of internal jugular vein with cranial nerve findings (Horner syndrome, hoarseness, unilateral tongue paresis). Retropharyngeal space infections are more common in children following suppurative adenitis of the lymph nodes draining nose, nasopharynx, pharynx, middle ear, eustachian tubes, and paranasal sinuses. These lymph nodes regress in adults, therefore, infection often follows traumatic introduction from esophageal instrumentation, foreign bodies, repeated or difficult intubation, or esophageal rupture.[12] Patients present with fever, chills, severe sore throat, dysphasia, dyspnea, drooling, stridor, neck pain, esophageal regurgitation, and bulging posterior pharynx.

'Danger' space involvement presents with septicemia and an otherwise nonfocal examination. Prevertebral space infections often arise from cervical spinal infections (osteomyelitis, blunt trauma, hematogenous seeding) and therefore may involve organisms of nonoral flora.

Investigation

Lateral neck radiographs will reveal compression or deviation of the tracheal air column or gas within the soft tissue. Normally, the retropharyngeal space in both children and adults is <7 mm at the level of C2 and <22 mm at the level of C6.[50] Loss of normal cervical lordosis secondary to muscle spasm may also be seen. If time is available, a computed tomography scan (CT scan) or magnetic resonance imaging (MRI) aid in localization and extent of infection. One retrospective review noted 80 percent sensitivity and 100 percent specificity of lateral neck radiographs and 100 percent sensitivity with only 45 percent specificity of CT scan.[14] This same study also noted a 100 percent positive and 94 percent negative predictive value of lateral neck radiographs and 40 percent and 100 percent, respectively, for CT images. Generally, extraorally obtained specimens are preferable in order to decrease the risk of contamination with resident flora. Gram stain for bacteria as well as acid fast and fungal stains should be performed. Histopathology is also help to determine presence of acute and/or chronic inflammation. If suppurative jugular venous thrombosis is suspected, ultrasonography with Doppler flow imaging should be pursued.[12]

Treatment

Antibiotic treatment with penicillin is the mainstay of therapy. Clindamycin may be substituted in allergic patients. Chloramphenicol is also a possibility.[12] Peritonsillar abscess in patients at risk for recurrence (younger age, history of recurrent symptoms) should undergo tonsillectomy. Older adults do fine with incision and drainage.[51] For lateral and retropharyngeal space infections extraoral and/or intraoral surgical drainage are also critical especially if no improvement is noted despite antibiotics. If an odontogenic focus is identified, dental extraction may also be required. Close monitoring of impending airway compromise is necessary.

Complications

In a review of 196 cases with deep neck space infections, Wang *et al.* found airway compromise in 15 patients of which 8 required emergency tracheotomy, with descending mediastinitis in 5 patients and suppurative jugular venous thrombosis in 2 patients.[48] Other potential complications include pneumonia, epiglottitis, and erosion to the carotid artery with aneurysm formation and rupture.[12] Retropharyngeal space infections with direct extension to superior mediastinum, or by way of the 'danger' space to the posterior mediastinum, can have a mortality rate of as high as 40–50 percent mortality with sepsis.[52]

CROUP

Croup, or laryngotracheobronchitis, consists of a triad of inspiratory stridor, hoarseness, and a brassy cough. These symptoms are caused by the edema and secretions within the larynx and associated obstruction of the subglottic portion of the upper airway.[53] The disease is most often caused by a viral infection and is described predominantly in children,

with rare reports in adults.[54] The viruses implicated are usually seasonal. In the fall parainfluenza viruses are responsible for a large part of the cases; whereas in the winter influenza A and in the spring both influenza B and respiratory syncytial virus predominate. The newly recognized human metapneumovirus has also been implicated as a cause of laryngotracheobronchitis.[55,56] Adenoviruses, and rarely rhinoviruses, enteroviruses, measles, and *M. pneumoniae* can cause croup.

Pathophysiology

Infection and inflammation begin in the nasopharynx and then spread distally to involve all levels of the respiratory tract. Subglottic tracheal edema results in the least distensible portion of the airway, which is the area surrounded by fixed cricoid cartilages. In small children this lumen is normally quite narrow so any further decrease in size greatly increases airway resistance and the work of breathing. In older children with congenital or acquired subglottic stenosis this becomes problematic. There may also be an immunologic component to the problem. Some children experience a hypersensitivity reaction to the insulting virus that influences the clinical manifestations.[57]

Clinical presentation

Most children with croup have a history of an upper respiratory infection for 1–2 days consisting of rhinorrhea, fever, mild sore throat, and slight cough. The onset of croup is heralded by hoarseness and brassy cough. Inspiratory stridor ensues. Typically a child develops a 'barking cough', tachypnea, tachycardia, and use of accessory respiratory muscles.

In most children the course of croup is 3–4 days, although cough may persist for longer. Severe complications are less common since the use of newer modes of therapy such as nebulized racemic epinephrine and steroids. The need for intubation is rare. Other potential complications include pneumothorax, pulmonary edema, and aspiration pneumonia.[58]

Investigation

It is important to distinguish croup from epiglottitis in children. Also important is differentiating croup from other noninfectious causes of stridor such as foreign body aspiration, allergic reactions, and other processes. In general, epiglottitis is presents as a rapid onset, with the child appearing toxic. There is drooling and the absence of a characteristic 'barking cough'. In addition to the presenting clinical differences, radiographs of the neck may be helpful in making a diagnosis. In croup the classic finding is the 'steeple sign' or 'hourglass' sign.[59] Although not consistently visible on radiograph, this sign appears secondary to the wall edema in the subglottic larynx. A pseudo-steeple sign may be present in children without symptoms of croup.

Identification of the specific viral pathogen causing croup can be achieved with viral culture or the newer techniques of rapid viral diagnosis, depending on the virus.

Treatment

Treatment modalities include cool mist, racemic epinephrine, and steroids (oral and/or intramuscular dexamethasone). Previously controversial, the use of steroids is now the standard of care for moderate to severe croup. Steroids reduce hospitalizations, length of illness, and subsequent treatments when compared with placebo. The current treatment recommendation for patients with moderate to severe croup is with oral dexamethasone at a dose of 0.6 mg/kg (maximum 10–12 mg). Intramuscular dexamethasone is reserved for patients with severe respiratory distress or those who are vomiting and are unable to tolerate oral treatment.[60] A recent randomized trial suggested that a single dose of dexamethasone may provide some benefit to children with mild croup treated in an ambulatory setting with more rapid resolution of symptoms and decreased need for further care.[61] A recent study comparing the effect of adding a helium–oxygen mixture versus racemic epinephrine to children with moderate or severe croup already receiving cool, humidified oxygen and 0.6 mg/kg of intramuscular dexamethasone found no difference in improvement.[62]

EPIGLOTTITIS

Epiglottitis, also known as supraglottitis, is a rapidly progressive cellulitis of the epiglottis. The edema of the epiglottis and surrounding structures can potentially cause airway obstruction and asphyxiation.

Background and epidemiology

Historically, epiglottitis was deemed an adult emergency, however in 1950–1980, it became known as a pediatric emergency infection. The most common bacterial pathogen associated with epiglottitis is *Haemophilus influenzae* type b. Prior to the vaccine era, population-based studies showed invasive infection to occur in 40–100 cases/100 000 children under 5 years of age.[63] Since the introduction of *H. influenzae* type b (HiB) conjugated vaccine in the late 1980s, the number of cases declined to 0.7 cases /100 000 of immunized patients.[64,65]

Pathophysiology and etiology

The epiglottis is formed by cartilaginous tissue with a squamous epithelium. Invasion of this epithelium leads to an influx of inflammatory cells and resulting edema. The amount of edema during this acute inflammatory phase in conjunction with the close proximity of the epiglottis to the larynx allows for narrowing and potential obstruction of airflow. The final result is hypoxemia, hypercapnia, acidosis, and cardiorespiratory arrest.

H. influenzae type b was the organism most commonly associated with epiglottitis. Since the HiB vaccine era, *H. influenzae* type b only accounts for 25 percent of the cases.[66] Other pathogens associated with epiglottitis include *Haemophilus parainfluenzae, Strept. pneumoniae, Staph. aureus,* and β-hemolytic streptococci groups A, B, and C. *P. aeruginosa* and *Candida* species are associated with immunocompromised patients with epiglottitis.[5,67,68] In addition, reported cases of varicella zoster viral infections are complicated by Group A streptococcal epiglottitis.[69]

Nonbacterial causes of epiglottitis include viral pathogens such as herpes simplex virus type 1, parainfluenzae virus type 3, and influenza B viruses.[70,71] Acute epiglottitis has also been associated with thermal injury, ingestion of corrosive agents, and graft-versus-host disease.[72,73]

Clinical presentation

In children, supraglottitis usually involves the epiglottis and surrounding tissues, while in adults it may involve the paravertebral soft tissues, the valleculae, the base of the tongue, and the soft palate.[74]

Epiglottitis presents abruptly with sudden onset of fever and sore throat. Dysphagia and drooling are not uncommon. Unlike most forms of pharyngitis, progression of disease occurs rapidly. Children usually appear toxic and ashen gray in color. Signs and symptoms of respiratory distress such as irritability, anxiety, forward lean, and a hyperextended neck with a lifted chin may be present. Speech may sound muffled or hoarse. The presence of inspiratory stridor is an ominous sign. Unlike croup, a barking, spontaneous cough is absent.

Direct inspection of the epiglottis by laryngoscopy confirms the diagnosis; however, this should not be attempted unless the airway can be secured immediately. Although the disease is less severe in adults, the death rate is 3.2 percent higher in adults than in children.[75]

Investigation

In addition to a careful history and physical exam, lateral neck radiographs suggest the diagnosis. The classic findings on radiograph include an enlarged and protruding epiglottitis (the 'thumb' sign) and dilation of the hypopharynx.[75]

Leukocytosis greater than 20 000 cells/mm^3 with a neutrophilic predominance and the presence of bands are common laboratory findings. Most children present with concomitant bacteremia.[75] In adults, approximately 70 percent of blood cultures are negative.[76] Positive blood cultures predict a more fulminant course.

In children, laryngoscopic exam is marked by a large, swollen, cherry-red epiglottitis with surrounding erythema and edema. In adults, the epiglottitis may appear pale or mildly erythematous with edema.[76,77]

Treatment

The two main components of treatment are maintenance of an adequate airway and prompt administration of appropriate antibiotics. If necessary, intubation with a nasotracheal tube is preferred over endotracheal intubation to reduce post-intubation sequelae. If nasotracheal intubation is not possible, then tracheostomy is an alternative. The inhalation anesthetic of choice for intubation was halothane.[78] However, sevoflurane is now being considered because of its efficacy in decreasing laryngospasm.[78] After establishment of a secure airway, blood cultures and cultures of the epiglottitis should be obtained.

Due to the increased incidence of ampicillin-resistant *H. influenzae* among children, cefotaxime, ceftriaxone, or ampicillin-sulbactam should be initiated intravenously. Second and third generation cephalosporins are the class of antibiotics used for adults. Intravenous antibiotics are usually continued for 48–72 hours, followed by a 10-day course of oral antibiotics (trimethoprim-sulfamethoxazole or cefaclor).[77,79,80] Extubation depends on the resolution of edema and the patient's mental status and usually occurs within 1–2 days. Studies of the use of racemic epinephrine and steroids in the treatment of *H. influenzae* infection have not shown a decrease in severity or duration of disease.[79,80]

Children with epiglottitis treated with ceftriaxone or cefotaxime do not need further prophylactic antibiotics with rifampin for eradication of the nasopharyngeal carrier states.[79] Household contacts under 4 years of age who are not immunized or incompletely immunized, nonimmunized children under 12 months of age, or immunocompromised children should receive prophylaxis. Prophylaxis should be given to all household contacts exposed to *H. influenzae* epiglottitis.[81] All nursery and childcare centers where two or more cases are documented within 60 days of occurrence warrant prophylaxis. For children younger than 4 years of age exposed to *H. influenzae* infection, rifampin prophylaxis of 20 mg/kg/day for 4 days should be initiated. Limited data exist for infants younger than 1 month; however, rifampin 10 mg/kg has been used. Adults should receive rifampin 600 mg daily.[81]

Complications

Possible complications include pneumonia, meningitis, cervical adenitis, pericarditis, septic shock, epiglottitis abscess, pneumothorax, pneumomediastinum, and death by asphyxiation.

RABIES

Background and epidemiology

Rabies is a viral infection of the central nervous system that is nearly always fatal without appropriate postexposure prophylaxis. It is found worldwide except for Antarctica and a few island nations.[82] The early manifestations of rabies can be nonspecific and difficult to recognize. The disease can then progress to two distinct forms, furious (encephalitic) and paralytic (dumb) forms. The more common furious form is characterized by upper respiratory findings that some call 'hydrophobia' and 'aerophobia'. It is important to consider rabies in the differential diagnosis when a patient complains of difficulty swallowing liquids. Dysphagia is seen due to pharyngeal spasms.

Pathogenesis

The rabies virus is a bullet-shaped single stranded RNA virus of the Rhabdoviridae family and is highly neurotropic. The virus is usually introduced from rabies-contaminated saliva through the epidermis from the bite of an infected animal. A scratch from a rabid animal, transplantation of an infected cornea or other organ transplant,[83] or inhalation of heavily contaminated material, such as bat droppings, can also cause infection. The rabies virus travels from the site of inoculation via the peripheral nervous system by intraaxonal retrograde transport to the central nervous system (CNS), where it replicates in the gray matter. The virus can then spread centrifugally along afferent sensory nerves to reach other tissues such as the salivary glands, lacrimal glands, adrenal medulla, kidneys, lungs, and other densely innervated tissue. The animal can then spread the disease through the infected saliva. The average incubation period ranges from 10 to 90 days although it may be up to 7 years.[84]

Clinical presentation

Rabies is acute and fulminant encephalitis. There may be a history of animal bite or exposure. The patient may first complain of numbness at the area of the bite or inoculation. Next, the patient may have a nonspecific illness characterized by fever, headache, malaise, nausea, and vomiting. Within a few days the full-blown illness occurs in either the encephalitic or the paralytic form with periods of lucidity alternating with periods of confusion. Patients may present to medical care with complaints of pharyngeal spasms. They may complain of inability to eat or drink because of these painful pharyngeal spasms that can progress to retching, especially when attempting to drink water. Similarly, blowing or fanning air on the chest may induce laryngeal spasm, pharyngeal spasm, or other muscle spasms.[84]

Investigation

It is important to remember rabies in the differential diagnosis of pharyngeal and laryngeal spasms. The diagnosis of rabies is made by demonstration of specific viral antigens, nucleic acid, or infectious virus. Possible specimens include a skin biopsy (especially from the densely innervated nape of the neck), and saliva, cerebral spinal fluid and corneal impressions can be examined for virus.

Treatment

Human rabies is considered incurable and efforts must focus on prevention. After exposure to rabies the combination of local wound treatment (20 percent soap solution, irrigation with a virucidal agent such as povidone-iodine), passive immunization (rabies immune globulin), and vaccination is quite effective. Once symptoms of rabies have begun, despite excellent intensive care support, almost all patients succumb to the disease. In the 1970s, however, there were three isolated case reports of patients who survived the disease.[85–88] More recently, there was a 15-year-old girl who survived rabies infection. This is the first documented recovery from clinical rabies by a patient who had not received either pre- or postexposure prophylaxis. The patient was treated with intravenous ribavirin in an investigational protocol.[89]

ACUTE SINUSITIS

Sinus infections, although not typically considered respiratory tract emergencies, may lead to complications such as cavernous sinus (ethmoid or sphenoid sinuses), superior sagittal sinus (frontal or ethmoid sinuses), and/or sigmoid sinus (mastoid air cells) thrombosis. Other possible complications of sinusitis include meningitis or brain abscesses. In particular, invasive fungal sinusitis caused by zygomycoses is associated with high mortality and prompt diagnosis is crucial. Mucormycosis is a group of diseases caused by fungi that the examining physician must consider in the differential diagnosis in the patient with sinus complaints.

Anatomy and definition

The paranasal sinuses are sterile potential spaces divided into frontal, ethmoid, sphenoid, and maxillary sinuses.[90] Inflammation and edema of the epithelium of one to all of these spaces defines sinusitis. The maxillary sinuses are most easily involved in sinusitis due to the anatomic position of the draining ostium located superiorly. The maxillary, ethmoid, and frontal sinuses all drain into the nasal cavity via the infundibulum. This canal allows clearance of normal amounts of mucus produced by uninflamed epithelium.

Background and epidemiology

The incidence of viral sinusitis follows the seasonal pattern of the causative virus. Viral sinusitis can be complicated by superinfection with bacterial pathogens. Other predisposing factors of acute bacterial sinusitis include allergies, nasal polyps that cause obstruction, swimming and more rarely agammaglobulinemia, human immunodeficiency virus, chronic granulomatous disease, and cystic fibrosis.[91]

Pathophysiology and etiology

Infection of the sinus cavity results from increased mucus production, decreased clearance of mucus, decreased function of the mucociliary epithelium, and engorgement of the vasculature. This combination leads to obstruction of the infundibulum. Common viral causes include rhinovirus, coronaviruses, respiratory syncytial virus, and influenza virus. Typical bacterial pathogens include *Strep. pneumoniae*, *H. influenzae*, *Moraxella catarrhalis*, α-streptococci and *Staph. aureus*. *Aspergillus* species, *Cryptococcus* species, and zygomycoses all cause fungal sinusitis.

Clinical presentation

Signs and symptoms of acute sinusitis are not necessarily specific and include sneezing, rhinorrhea, nasal congestion, fever, headache, and facial pain or pressure. Purulent nasal discharge is also suggestive. Sphenoid sinusitis often presents with retroorbital pain, whereas severe frontal sinusitis can present with forehead swelling secondary to accumulation of pressure. Fungal sinusitis can present with proptosis and bony erosions on computed tomography.

Investigation

Most patients are treated empirically but if failure to respond to antibiotic treatment or fungal sinusitis is suspected then sinus puncture is recommended in order to determine the pathogen; unfortunately, the invasiveness of the procedure precludes its routine use.[91] Computed tomography of the sinuses provides radiologic confirmation with findings of air–fluid levels and mucosal thickening of the epithelium. Magnetic resonance imaging is not economically practical.

Treatment

Therapy should be targeted toward the most commonly isolated pathogens such as *Strep. pneumoniae*, *H. influenza*, *M. catarrhalis*, α-streptococci and *Staph. aureus*. In addition to antibiotics, decongestants, nasal saline, steam inhalation, and mild analgesics all prove helpful.

Treatment options include respiratory fluoroquinolones, high-dose amoxicillin-clavulanate, and azithromycin.[92] The macrolides are still useful but there is documented resistance to this class of drug in *Strep. pneumoniae* and *H. influenzae*.[93] In addition, there is reduced susceptibility of pneumococcus to the penicillins and other antibiotics have to be considered when making an antibiotic selection.[94]

MUCORMYCOSIS (ZYGOMYCOSIS)

Background and epidemiology

Rhinocerebral mucormycosis is a syndrome characterized by sinusitis and a painless, necrotic black palatal or nasal septal ulcer or eschar.[95] The taxonomy of the agents of mucormycosis is now preferably referred to as zygomycosis. Fungi of the order Mucorales are most commonly associated with human infections in North America; however, other fungi of the order Entomophthorales also cause disease compatible with zygomycosis, usually seen outside North America.[96]

Pathophysiology and etiology

Rhizopus species is the most common isolated species of zygomycosis, followed by the *Rhizomucor* species. The pathogens are ubiquitous in the environment and soil, especially in decaying material. These fungi exist as hyphal forms in the environment and in tissue. In the household setting, they can be found on moldy bread. Other species include *Absidia* species, *Apophysomyces* species, *Conidiobolus* species, and *Cunninghamella* species.

Zygomycetes grow rapidly and release numerous spores that once airborne colonize the nasal pathway and possibly the alveoli. In the right host, colonization is followed by germination and subsequent invasion. These fungi possess tropism to the blood vessels and ultimately cause necrosis and infarction of host tissues. In the cutaneous form of disease, the spores invade compromised skin resulting in wound infections, necrotic soft tissue, and possible necrotizing fasciitis.[97]

Box 10A.1 Conditions associated with zygomycosis

- Acquired immune deficiency syndrome (AIDS)
- Diabetes mellitus
- Hematologic malignancies
- Intravenous drug users
- Metabolic acidosis
- Treatment with corticosteroids
- Treatment with deferoxamine
- Trauma and burns
- Solid organ transplant

Most patients with invasive disease have associated underlying diseases (Box 10A.1). Diabetic patients with ketoacidosis, bone marrow and solid organ transplant recipients, and those on corticosteroids or deferoxamine therapy are the groups of patients at most risk.[98,99] Also, gastrointestinal zygomycosis occurs in malnourished patients.[100]

Clinical presentation

There are six clinical presentations of mucormycosis: rhinocerebral, pulmonary, cutaneous/soft tissue, gastrointestinal, central nervous system, and miscellaneous. Rhinocerebral is the most common manifestation of mucormycosis.

RHINOCEREBRAL MUCORMYCOSIS

Rhinocerebral disease present in two forms, rhino-orbitocerebral and rhinomaxillary. This form of mucormycosis is a true upper respiratory tract emergency as early recognition and treatment are critical. Fifty percent of diabetic patients with rhinocerebral mucormycosis will present with ketoacidosis. Neutropenic leukemic patients or neutropenic bone marrow transplant recipients tend to present with rhinomaxillary or pulmonary mucormycosis.[96,97] Rare reports of invasive zygomycosis exist in otherwise immunocompetent individuals.[100]

Presenting symptoms of facial pain, headaches, and fevers are common. Invasion into the orbits causes orbital cellulitis, proptosis, and changes in vision. With disease progression, cranial nerve palsies occur. In the rhinomaxillary form, invasion of sinus blood supply causes thrombosis of the turbinates and subsequent ischemia to the hard palate.[97] Findings of purulent nasal discharge (sometimes black) with black eschar on the turbinates and hard palate may appear afterward. The differentiation of necrotic nasal discharge from dried blood is critical. Cerebral abscess and cavernous sinus and/or internal carotid artery thrombosis are complications seen with rhinocerebral mucormycosis.

Investigation

Swift diagnosis and confirmation by tissue biopsy is crucial. The presence of a black eschar should prompt the clinician toward a diagnosis of zygomycosis. Unfortunately, isolating the pathogen on nasal swab preparations is inadequate diagnostically and tissue biopsy demonstrating presence of invasion by hyphae is required. Typical histopathology stains include potassium hydroxide, hematoxylin-eosin, Grocott methenamine-silver, or periodic acid Schiff (PAS) stains.

In addition to biopsy, in the right clinical setting, sinus radiographs demonstrating mucosal thickening of the orbits and sinuses with or without air–fluid levels are suggestive. Erosion of bone in the orbits or sinuses usually means disease progression. Computed tomography is superior in demonstrating bone destruction and soft tissue involvement. Magnetic resonance imaging can also be helpful.

Treatment

Survival depends on early surgical debridement in addition to amphotericin B (1 mg/kg per day intravenously). This combination of treatment increases the rate of survival to 80 percent.[101] Lipid-formulated antifungals can be substituted in patients who are unable to tolerate standard amphotericin B.[102,103] Unfortunately, azole antifungals and flucytosine are ineffective and should play no role in the treatment of zygomycosis; however, there are data to suggest utility of posaconazole.[98] Results of studies of hyperbaric oxygen are controversial.[104–107]

The key to prevention of mucormycosis depends on control of the underlying predisposing conditions, such as diabetes, metabolic acidosis, and neutropenia.

Complications

The angioinvasive nature of these fungi and the usually immunosuppressed host allow for brain abscess, cavernous sinus thrombosis, internal carotid artery thrombosis, and pulmonary hemorrhage leading to respiratory distress and death. If not managed aggressively and promptly, mortality is high.

Key learning points

- Many oropharyngeal infections arise from dental origin. A complete dental evaluation must be done as part of the initial investigation.

- Consider diphtheria in the returning traveler with a pharyngitis and tonsillar membrane who may not be vaccinated or has not received booster vaccine.

- Oral anthrax may resemble the membrane of diphtheria. However, diphtheria may have associated neurologic and cardiac manifestations.

- In cases of pharyngitis followed by neck pain, pleuritis think of Lemierre syndrome. Check for jugular vein thrombosis.

- Epiglottitis has a rapid onset. In croup, there is usually an antecedent upper respiratory tract infection of 1–2 days' duration. Always consider other causes of stridor such as foreign body obstruction or allergic reaction.

- Patients with rabies may have pharyngeal spasm and inability to drink liquids.

- Consider rhinocerebral mucormycosis in a patient with sinusitis and a painless, necrotic black palatal or nasal septal ulcer or eschar, especially in diabetic and immunocompromised patients.

REFERENCES

1. Chow AW. Infections of the oral cavity, neck, and head. In: Mandell GE, Bennett JE, Dolin R, eds. *Principles and Practice of Infectious Disease*, 6th ed, vol 1. Philadelphia: Churchill Livingstone, 2005: 787–802.

2. Chow AW, Roser SM, Brady FA. Orofacial odontogenic infections. *Ann Intern Med* 1978; **88**: 392.

3. Thadepalli H, Mandal AK. Anatomic basis of head and neck infections. *Infect Dis Clin North Am* 1988; **2**: 21.

4. Bullock JD, Fleishmn JA. The spread of odontogenic infections to the orbit: diagnosis and management. *J Oral Maxillofac Surg* 1985; **43**: 749–55.

5. Lacroix J, Gauhtier M, Lapointe N, *et al. Pseudomonas aeruginosa* supraglottitis in a six-month old child with severe combined immunodeficiency syndrome. *Pediatr Infect Dis J* 1988; **7**: 739–41.

6. Moreland LW, Corey J, McKenzie R. Ludwig's angina: report of a case and review of the literature. *Arch Intern Med* 1988; **148**: 461–6.

7. Berthold P. Noma: a forgotten disease. *Dent Clin North Am* 2003; **47**: 559–74.

8. Tanner A, Stillman N. Oral and dental infections with anaerobic bacteria: clinical features, predominant pathogens, and treatment. *Clin Infect Dis* 1993; **16** (Suppl 4): S304–9.

9. Rams TE, Flynn MF, Slots J. Subgingival microbiologic associations in severe human periodontitis. *Clin Infect Dis* 1997; **25** (Suppl 2): S224–6.

10. Enwonwu CO. Noma: neglected scourge of children in sub-Saharan Africa. *Bull World Health Organ* 1995; **73**: 541.

11. Flynn TR. The swollen face. Severe odontogenic infections. *Emerg Med Clin North Am* 2000; **18**: 481–519.

12. Blomquist IK, Bayer AS. Life-threatening deep fascial space infections of the head and neck. *Infect Dis Clin North Am* 1988; **2**: 237.

13. Busch RF. Ludwig's angina: early aggressive therapy. *Arch Otolaryngol Head Neck Surg* 1999; **125**: 1283–4.

14. Dierks EJ, Meyerhoff WL, Schultz B, Finn R. Fulminant infections of odontogenic origin. *Laryngoscope* 1987; **97**(3 Pt 1): 271–4.

15. Bisno AL. Pharyngitis. In: Mandell GE, Bennett JE, Dolin R, eds. *Principles and Practice of Infectious*

Disease, 6th ed, vol 1. Philadelphia: Churchill Livingstone, 2005: 752–8.

◆ 16. Farizo KM, Strebel PM, Chen RT, *et al.* Fatal respiratory disease due to *Corynebacterium diphtheria*: case report and review of guidelines for management, investigation and control. *Clin Infect Dis* 1993; **16**: 59–68.

17. Centers for Disease Control and Prevention. Fatal respiratory diphtheria in a U.S. traveler to Haiti – Pennsylvania 2003. *MMWR Morb Mortal Wkly Rep* 2004; **52**: 1285–6.

18. Centers for Disease Control and Prevention. Update: Diphtheria epidemic – newly independent state of the Soviet Union. January 1995–March 1996. *MMWR Morb Mortal Wkly Rep* 1996; **45**: 693–7.

◆ 19. Tiley SM, Kociuba KR, Heron LG, Munro R. Infective endocarditis due to nontoxigenic *Corynebacterium diphtheriae*: report of seven cases and review. *Clin Infect Dis* 1999; **16**: 271–5.

20. Doble RA, Tobey DN. Clinical features of diphtheria in the respiratory tract. *JAMA* 1979; **242**: 2197–201.

21. Singh MK, Saba PZ. Diphtheria. www.emedicine.com/EMERG/topic138.htm.

22. MacGregor RR. *Corynebacterium diphtheriae*. In: *Principles and Practice of Infectious Disease*, 6th ed, vol 1. Philadelphia: Churchill Livingstone, 2005: 2457–65.

23. Boyer NH, Weinstein L. Diphtheritic myocarditis. *N Engl J Med* 1948; **239**: 913–19.

24. Centers for Disease Control and Prevention. Diphtheria, tetanus, and pertussis: recommendations for vaccine use and other preventive measures recommendations of the Immunization Practices Advisory Committee (ACIP) *MMWR Morb Mortal Wkly Rep* 1991; **40** (No RR-10): 1–28.

◆ 25. Armstrong AW, Spooner K, Sanders JW. Lemierre's syndrome. *Curr Infect Dis Rep* 2000; **2**: 168–73.

● 26. Strokroos RJ, Manni JJ, de Kruijk JR, *et al.* Lemierre's syndrome and acute mastoiditis. *Arch Otolaryngol Head Neck Surg* 1999; **125**: 589–91.

27. Anand VK, Morrison WV. Thrombophlebitis of the jugular vein. *Ear Nose Throat J* 1987; **66**: 64–9.

28. Sinave CP, Hardy GJ, Fardy PW. The Lemierre syndrome: suppurative thrombophlebitis of the internal jugular vein secondary to oropharyngeal infection. *Medicine* 1989; **68**: 85–94.

◆ 29. Moore BA, Dekle C, Werkhaven J. Bilateral Lemierre's syndrome: a case report and literature review. *Ear Nose Throat J* 2002; **81**: 234–40.

30. Leugers C, Clover R. Lemierre syndrome: postanginal sepsis. *J Am Board Fam Pract* 1995; **8**: 384–91.

31. Stahlman GC, DeBoer DK, Green, NE. *Fusobacterium* osteomyelitis and pyarthrosis: A classic case of Lemierre's syndrome. *J Pediatr Orthop* 1996; **16**: 529–32.

32. Lustig LR, Cusick BC, Cheung SW, *et al.* Lemierre's syndrome: two cases of postanginal sepsis. *Otolaryngol Head Neck Surg* 1995; **112**: 767–72.

33. Palmer AL, Strain JD, Henry DB, *et al.* Postanginal sepsis after oropharyngeal trauma. *Pediatr Infect Dis J* 1995; **14**: 249–51.

34. Barker J, Winer-Muram T, Grey SW. Lemierre syndrome. *South Med J* 1996; **89**: 1021–3.

35. Applebaum PC, Spangler SK, Jacobs MR. Beta lactamase production and susceptibilities to amoxicillin-clavulanate, ticarcillin, ticarcillin-clavulanate, cefoxitin, imipenem, and metronidazole of 320 non-*Bacteroides fragilis bacteroides* isolates and 129 Fusobacteria from 28 US centers. *Antimicrob Agents Chemother* 1990; **34**: 1646–50.

36. Brook I. Infections caused by beta-lactamase-producing *Fusobacterium* sp. in children. *Pediatr Infect Dis J* 1993; **12**: 532–3.

✳ 37. Josey WE, Staggers SR. Heparin therapy in septic pelvic thrombophlebitis: a study of 45 cases. *Am J Obstet Gynecol* 1974; **120**: 228–33.

38. Hughes CE, Spear RK, Shinabarger CE, *et al.* Septic pulmonary emboli complicating mastoiditis: Lemierre's syndrome revisited. *Clin Infect Dis* 1994; **8**: 633–5.

◆ 39. Swartz MN. Recognition and management of anthrax – an update. *N Engl J Med* 2001; **345**: 1621–6.

40. Inglesby TV, O'Toole T, Henderson DA. Anthrax as a biological weapon, 2002: updated recommendations for management. *JAMA* 2002; **287**: 2236–52.

41. Sirisanthana T, Brown A. Anthrax of the gastrointestinal tract. *Emerg Infect Dis* 2002; **8**: 649–51.

42. Inglesby TV, Henderson DA, Bartlett JG, *et al.* Anthrax as a biological weapon – medical and public health management. *JAMA* 1999; **281**: 1735–45.

43. Perry RD, Fetherston JD. *Yersinia pestis* – etiologic agent of plague. *Clin Microbiol Rev* 1997; **1**: 35–6.

44. Butler T, Dennis DT. Yersinia species, including plague. In: Mandell GL, Bennett JE, Dolin R, eds. *Principles and Practice of Infectious Diseases*, 6th ed. Philadelphia: Churchill Livingstone, 2005: 2691–701.

◆ 45. Inglesby TV, Dennis DT, Henderson DA, *et al.* Plague as a biological weapon – medical and public health management. *JAMA* 2000; **283**: 2281–90.

46. Penn RL. *Francisella tularensis.* In: Mandell GL, Bennett JE, Dolin R, eds. *Principles and Practice of Infectious Disease*s, 6th ed. Philadelphia: Churchill Livingstone, 2005: 2674–85.

◆ 47. Dennis DT, Inglesby TV, Henderson DA. Tularemia as a biological weapon – medical and public health management. *JAMA* 2001; **285**: 2763–73.

◆ 48. Wang L-F, Kuo W-R, Tsai S-M, Huang K-J. Characterization of life-threatening deep cervical space infections: a review of one hundred and ninety-six cases. *Am J Otolaryngol* 2003; **24**: 111–17.

49. Pynn BR, Sands T, Pharoah MF. Odontogenic infections: part one. Anatomy and radiology. *Oral Health* 1995; **85**: 7–10, 13–14, 17–18.

50. Barratt BE, Koopmann CF, Jr, Coulthard SW. Retropharyngeal abscess – a ten-year experience. *Laryngoscope* 1984; **April**: 455–63.

51. Parker GS, Tami TA. Management of peritonsillar abscess in the 90s: an update. *Am J Otolaryngol* 1992; **13**: 284–8.

52. Marra S, Hotaling AJ. Deep neck infections. *Am J Otolaryngol* 1996; **17**: 287–98.

53. Mufson M. Viral pharyngitis, laryngitis, croup, and bronchitis. In: Goldman L, Ausiello D, eds. *Cecil Textbook of Medicine*, 22nd ed. Philadelphia: WB Saunders 2004: 1969–71.

54. Woo PC, Young K, Tsang KW, *et al.* Adult croup: a rare but more severe condition. *Respiration* 2000; **67**: 684–8.

55. Williams JV, Harris PA, Tollefson SJ, *et al.* Human meta pneumovirus and lower respiratory tract disease in otherwise healthy infants. *N Engl J Med* 2004; **350**: 443–50.

56. Ho HK. Human metapneumovirus and lower respiratory tract disease in children. *N Engl J Med* 2004; **350**: 1788–90.

57. Urquart GED, Kennedy DH, Ariyawansa JP. Croup associated with parainfluenza type 1 virus: two subpopulations. *BMJ* 1979; **1**: 1604.

58. Hall CB, McBride JT. Acute laryngotracheobronchitis (croup). In: Mandell GL, Bennett JE, Dolin R, eds. *Principles and Practice of Infectious Diseases*, 6th ed. Philadelphia: Churchill Livingstone 2005: 760–6.

59. Salour M. The Steeple sign. *Radiology* 2000; **216**: 428–9.

60. Rittichier KK. The role of corticosteroids in the treatment of croup. *Treat Respir Med* 2004; **3**: 139–45.

61. Bjornson CL, Klassen TP, Williamson J, *et al.* A randomized trial of a single dose of oral dexamethasone for mild croup. *N Engl J Med* 2004; **351**: 1306–13.

62. Weber JE, Chudnofsky, Younger JG, *et al.* A randomized comparison of helium-oxygen mixture (Heliox) and racemic epinephrine for the treatment of moderate to severe croup. *Pediatrics* 2001; **107**: E96.

63. Wenger JD. Epidemiology of *Haemophilus influenzae* type b disease and impact of *Haemophilus influenzae* conjugate vaccines in the United States and Canada. *Ped Infect Dis J* 1998; **17**: S132–6.

64. Shah RK, Roberson DW, Jones DT. Epiglottitis in the *Haemophilus influenzae* type b vaccine era: changing trends. *Laryngoscope* 2004; **114**: 557–60.

65. Cherry, JD. Epiglottitis (supraglottitis). In: Feigin RD, Cherry JD, eds. *Textbook of Pediatric Infectious Diseases*, 4th ed. Philadelphia: WB Saunders, 1998: 218.

66. Westerman EL, Hutton JP. Acute uvulitis associated with epiglottitis. *Arch Otolaryngol Head Neck Surg* 198; **112**: 448–9.

67. Walsh TJ, Gray WC. *Candida* epiglottitis in immunocompromised patients. *Chest* 1987; **91**: 482–5.

68. Myer CM. *Candida* epiglottitis: clinical implications. *Am J Otolaryngol* 1997; **18**: 428–30.

69. Slack CL, Allen GC, Morrison JE, *et al.* Post-varicella epiglottitis and necrotizing fasciitis. *Pediatrics* 2000; **105**: e13.

70. Bogger-Goren S. Acute epiglottitis caused by herpes simplex virus. *Pediatr Infect Dis J* 1987; **6**: 1133–4.

71. Grattan-Smith T, Forer M, Kilham H, Gillis J. Viral supraglottitis. *J Pediatr* 1987; **110**: 434–5.

72. Lai, SH, Wong, KS, Laio SL, Chou YH. Non-infectious epiglottitis in children: two case report. *Int J Pediatr Otorhinolaryngol* 2000; **55**: 57–60.

73. De Diego JI, Prim MP, Hardisson D, *et al.* Graft vs. host disease as a cause if enlargement of the epiglottitis in an immunocompromised child. *Arch Otolaryngol Head Neck Surg* 2001; **127**: 439–41.

74. Rothrock SG, Pignatiello GA, Howard RM. Radiologic diagnosis of epiglottis: Objective criteria for all ages. *Ann Emerg Med* 1990; **19**: 978–82.

75. Burns JE, Hendley JO. Epiglottitis. In: Mandell GL, Bennett J, Dolin R, eds. *Principles and Practice of Infectious Diseases*, 6th ed. Philadelphia: Churchill Livingstone, 2005: 784–6.

76. Mayo-Smith MF, Hirsch PJ, Wordzinskii SF, *et al.* Acute epiglottitis in adults. *N Engl J Med* 1986; **314**: 1133–9.

77. Mace SE. Acute epiglottitis in adults. *Am J Emerg Med* 1985; **3**: 543.

78. Spalding MS, Ala-Kokko TI. The use of inhaled sevoflurane for endotracheal intubation in epiglottitis. *Anesthesiology* 1988; **89**: 1025–6.

79. Stair TO, Hirsch BE. Adult supraglottitis. *Am J Emerg Med* 1985; **3**: 512–18.

80. Guss D, Jackson JE. Recurring epiglottis in an adult. *Ann Emerg Med* 1987; **16**: 441–4.

81. American Academy of Pediatrics. *Haemophilus influenzae* infections. In: *2003 Red Book: Report of the Committee on Infectious Diseases*, 26th ed. Elk Grove Village, IL: American Academy of Pediatrics, 2003: 296.

82. Bleck TP, Rupprecht CE. Rhabdoviruses. In: Mandell GL, Bennett JE, Dolin R, eds. *Principles and Practice of Infectious Disease*, 6th ed. Philadelphia: Churchill Livingstone, 2005: 2047–56.

83. Centers for Disease Control and Prevention. Investigation of rabies infections in organ donor and transplant recipients – Alabama, Arkansas, Oklahoma, and Texas 2004. *MMWR Morb Mortal Wkly Rep* 2004; **53**: 586–9.

84. Basgoz N, Frosch M. A 32 year-old woman with pharyngeal spasms and paresthesia after a dog bite. *N Engl J Med* 1998; **339**: 105–12.

85. Hatwick MA, Weis TT, Stetschulte CJ, *et al.* Recovery from rabies. A case report. *Ann Intern Med* 1972; **76**: 931–42.

86. Porras C, Barboza JJ, Fuenzalida E, *et al.* Recovery from rabies in a man. *Ann Intern Med* 1976; **85**: 44–8.

87. Centers for Disease Control and Prevention. Rabies in a laboratory worker – New York. *MMWR Morb Mortal Wkly Rep* 1977; **26**: 183.

◆ 88. Fishbein DB, Robinson LE. Rabies. *N Engl J Med* 1993; **329**: 1632–8.

● 89. Centers for Disease Control and Prevention. Recovery of a patient from clinical rabies – Wisconsin. *MMWR Morb Mortal Wkly Rep* 2004; **53**: 1171–3.

90. Gwaltney JM. Sinusitis. In: Mandell GE, Bennett JE, Dolin R, eds. *Principles and Practice of Infectious Disease*, 6th ed, vol 1. Philadelphia: Churchill Livingstone, 2005: 772–83.

91. Piccirillo JF. Acute bacterial sinusitis. *N Engl J Med* 2004; **351**: 902–10.

92. Henry DC, Riffer EM, Sokol WN, *et al.* Randomized double-blind study comparing 3- and 6-day regimens of azithromycin with a 10-day amoxicillin-clavulanate regimen for treatment of acute bacterial sinusitis. *Antimicrob Agents Chemother* 2003; **47**: 2770–4.

93. Musher D, Musher RG. Sinusitis. *N Engl J Med* 2005; **352**: 203.

94. Anon JB, Poole MD, Jacobs MR. Sinusitis. *N Engl J Med.* 2005; **352**: 204.

95. DeShazo RD, Chapin K, Swain RE. Fungal sinusitis. *N Engl J Med* 1997; **337**: 254–9.

96. Munoz P, Burillo A, Bouza E. Mold infections after solid organ transplantation. In: Bowden RA, Ljungman P, Paya CV, eds. *Transplant Infections*, 2nd ed. New York: Lippincott Williams & Wilkins, 2003: 483–508.

97. Sugar AM. In: Mandell GE, Bennett JE, Dolin R, eds. *Principles and Practice of Infectious Disease*, 6th ed, vol 1. Philadelphia: Churchill Livingstone, 2005: 2973–84.

98. McNulty JS. Rhinocerebral mucormycosis: Predisposing factors. *Laryngoscope* 1982; **92**: 1140–3.

99. Singh N, Gayowski T, Singh J, *et al.* Invasive gastrointestinal zygomycosis in a liver transplant recipient: case report and review of zygomycosis in solid-organ transplant recipients. *Clin Infect Dis* 1995; **20**: 617–20.

100. Radner AB, Witt MD, Edwards JE. Acute invasive rhinocerebral zygomycosis in an otherwise healthy patient: case report and review. *Clin Infect Dis* 1995; **20**: 163–6.

101. Cagatay AA, Oncu SS, Calangu SS, *et al.* Rhinocerebral mucormycosis treated with 32 gram liposomal amphotericin B and incomplete surgery: a case report. *BMC Infect Dis* 2001; **I**: 22.

102. Strasser MD, Kennedy, RJ. Adam RD. Rhinocerebral mucormycosis. Therapy with amphoterin B lipid complex. *Arch Intern Med* 1996; **156**: 2262.

103. Herbrecht R, Letscher-Bru V, Bowden RA, *et al.* Treatment of 21 cases of invasive mucormycosis with amphotercin B colloidal dispersion. *Eur J Clin Microbiol Infect Dis* 2001; **20**: 460–6.

104. Yohai RA, Bullock JD, Aziz AA, *et al.* Survival factors in rhino-orbital-cerebral mucormycosis. *Surv Ophthalmol* 1994; **39**: 3–22.

105. Ferguson BJ, Mitchell TG, Moon R, *et al.* Adjunctive hyperbaric oxygen for treatment of rhinocerebral mucormycosis. *Rev Infect Dis* 1988; **10**: 551–9.

106. Garcia-Covarrubias L, Barratt DM, Bartlett R, *et al.* Treatment of mucormycosis with adjunctive hyperbaric oxygen – five cases treated at the same institution and review of the literature. *Rev Invest Clin* 2004; **56**: 51–5.

107. Gonzalez CE, Rinaldi MG, Sugar AM. Zygomycosis. *Infect Dis Clin North Am* 2002; **16**: 895–914.

Emergency treatment of community-acquired pneumonia

MAURICIO VALENCIA, ANTONI TORRES

INTRODUCTION

Community-acquired pneumonia (CAP) is a frequent cause of emergency room visits, and although its diagnosis is usually straightforward, certain aspects such as the evaluation of severity and choice of antibiotic treatment influence the prognosis of the patient. Other factors of importance in CAP treatment are respiratory insufficiency and the treatment of the associated sepsis, and the recognition of progressive pneumonia and nonresolving pneumonia (Fig. 10B.1).

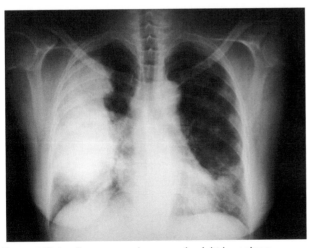

Figure 10B.1 *Pneumococcal pneumonia: right lower lung.*

EVALUATION OF THE PATIENT

Once the patient has been diagnosed with CAP, the next step is to evaluate its severity, which influences the decisions with regard to where the patient must receive treatment, the diagnostic tests to be performed, and the initial, empiric treatment.

The choice of the place where the patient is going to be treated (ambulatory or in hospital) is the first and most important decision in the initial evaluation of a patient with pneumonia. The consequences of this decision are significant and determine the thoroughness of the subsequent exam and investigations, the antibiotic treatment, the costs of the treatment, and the monitoring and wellbeing of the patient. The decision is based on the diverse risk factors (clinical, laboratory tests, and radiologic) that are associated with a poor prognosis or mortality following pneumonia and that necessitate treatment in a hospital setting. Box 10B.1 shows risk factors for a complicated course according to the American Thoracic Society (ATS). The ATS recommends admission of patients with multiple risk factors. Since the clinical evaluation of the severity of the patient's condition depends on the experience of the doctor (the seriousness of the pneumonia is typically overestimated), diverse predictive models have been developed that, although not designed specifically to define the need for hospitalization, can help the clinician to identify patients with a poor prognosis early. The purpose of these rules is to support the decision of the clinician and should not be used as a substitute.

Box 10B.1 Factors of poor prognosis in CAP

Epidemiological and comorbid factors

- Age >65 years
- Chronic obstructive pulmonary disease (COPD) or other pulmonary disease
- Cardiac insufficiency
- Chronic renal failure
- Hepatic disease
- Diabetes mellitus
- Alcoholism
- Malnutrition
- Immunosuppression (including systemic corticosteroids)
- Suspicion of aspiration
- Hospital admission in the last year
- Previous splenectomy

Findings from the physical exam

- Temperature >38.3 °C
- Respiration rate >30/min
- Systolic pressure <90 mm Hg or diastolic <60 mm Hg
- Mental status altered
- Extrapulmonary compromise (septic arthritis, meningitis, etc.)
- Radiologic findings
- Multiple or bilateral lobes affected
- Cavitation
- Pleural effusion

Laboratory findings

- Leukocytosis (>30 × 10^9/L) or leukopenia (<4 × 10^9/L)
- Hematocrit <30% or hemoglobin <9 g/dL
- Pa_{O_2} <60 mm Hg or Sa_{O_2} <90% breathing air at atmospheric pressure
- Creatinine >1.2 mg/dL or blood urea nitrogen >20 mg/dL

The PORT Study: Pneumonia Outcomes Research Team

In this study, Fine et al.[1] developed the Pneumonia Severity Index (PSI), whose principal objective is the identification of patients with CAP who are at low risk for mortality within 30 days and who can be treated on a outpatient basis or with a short period of observation in the emergency room (Box 10B.2). Additionally, it separates patients into five groups according to risk of death. Initially, patients with the lowest risk of death are identified (group 1), based solely on the information provided by their clinical history and physical exam:

- patients under 50 years of age
- without comorbidity (neoplasia, cardiac insufficiency, renal insufficiency, hepatic insufficiency, or cerebrovascular disease)

- no clinical indications of severity (alterations in the consciousness, pulse rate ≥125/min, respiratory rate ≥30/min, systolic blood pressure <90 mm Hg, and temperature <35 °C or ≥40 °C).

Group I patients have a risk of death of between 0.1 and 0.4 percent, and treatment as an outpatient is recommended. In the second step, the patient is classified in categories II–V depending on whether the patient is older than 50, has comorbidities, or has abnormal findings in the physical exam or laboratory tests. Inhospital treatment is recommended for groups IV and V (risk of mortality 9 percent and 27 percent, respectively), whereas patients in category III are candidates for a brief admission to an observation unit given that the risk of deterioration is greater in the first few hours of the initiation of the disease. Patients in group II can be treated on an outpatient basis.

Box 10B.2 PORT risk scale

Assigned point characteristics

- Age:
  - Men: years (= points)
  - Women: years −10
- Nursing home residence +10
- Neoplastic disease +30
- Hepatic disease +20
- Congestive cardiac insufficiency +10
- Cerebrovascular disease +10
- Renal disease +10
- Reduction in level of consciousness +20
- Respiratory rate >30/min +20
- Systolic pressure <90 mmHg +20
- Temperature <35 °C or >40 °C +15
- Pulse >125/min +10
- Arterial pH <7.35 +30
- Blood urea nitrogen >10.7 mmol/L (30 mg/dL) +20
- Na <130 mmol/L +20
- Glucose >13.9 mmol/L (250 mg/dL) +10
- Hematocrit <30% +10
- Pa_{O_2} <60 mm Hg +10
- Pleural effusion +10

The final score of each patient is the total sum obtained according to the scale

- Group II: Score <70 – clinical treatment
- Group III: Score 71-90 – brief admission for observation
- Group IV: Score 91-130 – hospital admission
- Group V: Score >130 – hospital admission

Among the limitations of the index is the great weight placed on the patient's age in the final scoring, which could hide important risks in younger patients and vice versa. The clinician should also value the importance of the psychosocial condition of the patient, which can limit outpatient treatment despite a low risk score. All patients with hypoxemia (defined as an arterial oxygen saturation less than 90 percent or a arterial oxygen partial pressure of less than 60 mm Hg in a room air breathing patient) or severe hemodynamic instability should be admitted no matter which PSI group they belong to. Other indications for admission are metastatic or suppurative complications of the infection such as empyema or bacterial endocarditis.

The British Thoracic Society algorithm

Although the PSI has been validated by multiple studies, its application is so complex that it is impractical at most levels of care. More over, it prioritizes the identification of low-risk patients. The British Thoracic Society (BTS) has derived and validated various rules[2] for the prediction of the severity and identification of patients with severe pneumonia. Based on the original rules (BTS I and II) is the modified BTS (mBTS). Also known as CURB, it is based on the following variables:

- *Confusion*
- *Urea* concentration (>7 mmol/L)
- *Respiratory* rate (≥30/min)
- *Blood* pressure: systolic pressure ≤90 mm Hg

The risk of mortality is based on the number of variables present in the patient, being 1.4 percent for patients with none of the above variables (score 0) and 5.4 percent, 14.2 percent, 32.9 percent, and 14.3 percent for patients with one, two, three, or all variables, respectively.

Besides CURB, another predictive rule named CURB-65 has been validated which simply adds age to the previous variables (≥65 years).[3] The mortality risk of these patients varies from 0.7 percent (score 0) to 40 percent (score 4). It allows the categorizing of patients with pneumonia in three groups:

- Group 1, score 0 or 1, low mortality (1.5 percent)
- Group 2, score 2, intermediate mortality (9.2 percent)
- Group 3, score ≥3, high mortality (22 percent).

Using this score, patients in group 1 can receive outpatient treatment, whereas those in group 2 should be treated under supervised hospital conditions that may include brief admission. For group 3, inhospital treatment is necessary and possibly admission to the intensive care unit (ICU) for patients with a score of 4 or 5 (Fig. 10B.2).

Points in common between the two sets of rules

The two prognostic rules explained above do not take some important factors into consideration, such as the psychosocial environment of the patient (determinant of the treatment conditions), less frequent comorbidities, such as neuromuscular diseases, or preferences of the patient with regard to where they wish to be treated. In fact, most low-risk patients with CAP who are admitted to the hospital prefer outpatient treatment.[4]

In summary, the PORT prognostic rule is useful to identify patients at low risk who could be treated in a clinic setting, whereas the BTS scheme identifies more severely ill patients who must receive hospital care.

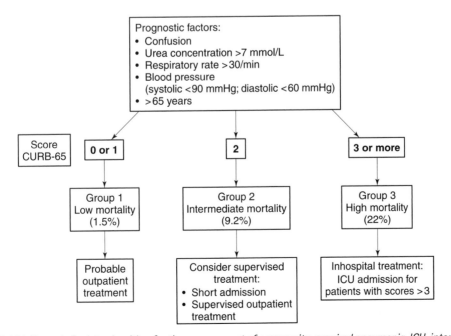

Figure 10B.2   *The British Thoracic Society algorithm for the management of community-acquired pneumonia. ICU, intensive care unit.*

SEVERE COMMUNITY–ACQUIRED PNEUMONIA

Certain aspects of the incidence, etiology, progression, and prognosis of severe CAP are sufficiently different from mild CAP to warrant a specific management plan. Approximately 10 percent of all patients hospitalized for CAP require admission to the ICU, increasing the mortality risk to 50 percent. Although *Streptococcus pneumoniae* is the responsible pathogen in most cases of severe CAP, other microorganisms such as *Legionella* species, *Haemophilus influenzae*, enteric Gram-negative bacilli, *Pseudomonas aeruginosa*, and *Staphylococcus aureus* have special relevance in that this influences the initial, empiric antibiotic treatment.[5,6]

The early identification of patients with severe CAP is of great importance since it facilitates prompt treatment oriented at likely pathogens as well as the establishment of monitoring and support measures. Various guidelines recommend admission to ICU for patients with CAP in the case of a series of indications of a poor prognosis. The ATS guidelines list 10 criteria for severe CAP, grouped into three categories:[7]

- respiratory parameters: respiratory rate (>30/min), PaO_2/FiO_2 <250, and need for mechanical ventilation)
- radiographic parameters: bilateral involvement, multiple affected lobes, and radiological progression >50 percent in 48 hours
- hemodynamic data: systolic blood pressure <90 mm Hg or diastolic <60 mm Hg, need for vasopressive drugs for a period of more than 4 hours, and diuresis <80 mL in 4 hours or renal insufficiency requiring dialysis.

The presence of even one of these 10 factors establishes severe pneumonia, resulting in a recommendation for admission of the patient into the ICU. Subsequent trials have demonstrated the low sensitivity and reduced positive prognostic value of these parameters in individual form.[8,9] Therefore, Ewig *et al.*[8] proposed a modification of the ATS criteria to improve the definition of severe CAP. According to this, three minor criteria are established at the time of admission:

- systolic blood pressure <90 mm Hg
- multiple lobes affected
- PaO_2/FiO_2 <250.

And two major criteria may be present throughout the evolution:

- need for mechanical ventilation
- septic shock.

The presence of two minor criteria or a single major criterion classifies the pneumonia as severe, with a sensitivity and specificity of 78 percent and 94 percent, respectively. A study that aimed to validate the modified ATS rule and the two BTS rules for the prediction of ICU admission and mortality of CAP was published recently.[10] The modified ATS rule achieved a sensitivity of 69 percent (95 percent CI 50.7 to 77.2), specificity of 97 percent (95 percent CI 96.4 to 98.9), positive predictive value of 87 percent (95 percent CI 78.3 to 93.1), and negative predictive value of 94 percent (95 percent CI 91.8 to 95.8) in predicting admission to the ICU. The corresponding predictive indices for mortality were 94 percent (95 percent CI 82.5 to 98.7), 93 percent (95 percent CI 90.6 to 94.7), 49 percent (95 percent CI 38.2 to 59.7), and 99.5 percent (95 percent CI 98.5 to 99.9), respectively. This study confirms the power of the modified ATS rule to predict severe pneumonia in individual patients. If a patient meets the criteria for severe CAP, admission to the ICU is recommended.

Antibiotic treatment

Although ideally the choice of antibiotic treatment should be based on the microbiologic findings, in current clinical practice the choice is empiric. This is because despite existing diagnostic tools (including invasive techniques), the clinician can only establish an etiologic diagnosis in 50 percent of cases; and even less in the emergency room.

An important aspect of the antibiotic treatment of CAP is its early initiation. Available data show a reduction of mortality within 30 days if the patient receives the first dose of antibiotics in the first 8 hours of arriving at the hospital.[10,11] Although this action can negatively influence the microbiologic tests, there is no justification for delaying the antibiotic treatment, which should be effective against pneumococcus, the most frequent causative agent of CAP.

When making the choice of initial, empiric antibiotic treatment, local epidemiologic factors must be kept in mind as well as the particularities of each patient, such as the severity of clinical symptoms, comorbidities, and risk factors for specific pathogens (Box 10B.3).

The ATS[7] guidelines classify patients affected by CAP into four categories as shown in Table 10B.1. In group II patients (more complex outpatients with cardiopulmonary comorbidities or risk factors for specific pathogens) the oral β-lactam must be efficacious and used in an adequate doses in case other risk factors exist that indicate a strain of pneumococcus resistant to penicillin. In hospitalized patients the macrolide can be administered orally or intravenously, depending on the severity of the disease. If anaerobic or pulmonary abscesses are evident, clindamycin or metronidazole should be added. In patients without comorbidity or other risk factors, the efficacy of intravenous azithromycin has been demonstrated in monotherapy, although the relatively low plasma levels of azithromycin are of concern with regard to the treatment of bacteremia. In patients with severe pneumonia the treatment should be stratified according to the presence or absence of risk factors of *P. aeruginosa* (see Box 10B.3).

Box 10B.3 Predisposing factors for infection by specific pathogens

Resistant pneumococcus

- Age >65 years
- Treatment with β-lactams in the last 3 months
- Alcoholism
- Immunosuppressive disease (including treatment with systemic steroids)
- Multiple medical comorbidities
- Contact with school children in daycare centers

Enteric Gram-negative bacteria

- Nursing home residence
- Underlying cardiopulmonary disease
- Multiple concomitant medical conditions
- Recent antibiotic treatment

Pseudomonas aeruginosa

- Bronchiectasis
- Treatment with systemic corticoids (>10 mg prednisone/day)
- Broad-spectrum antibiotics for more than 7 days in the last month
- Malnutrition

In the absence of risk factors, the treatment consists of a β-lactam plus a new generation macrolide (erythromycin is not recommended for this group of patients due to problems of administration and tolerance) or a quinolone (levofloxacin and moxifloxacin). The role of monotherapy (antipneumococcal fluoroquinolone) in severe CAP is doubtful (there are studies that favor it, but these included few patients). If there are risk factors for *Pseudomonas*, the treatment must include two antipseudomonal agents and provide coverage against pneumococcus and *Legionella*. This can be achieved with certain β-lactams such as cefepime, imipenem, meropenem, and piperacillin-tazobactam, and should be accompanied by an antipseudomonal quinolone such as ciprofloxacin or an aminoglycoside. If the patient is allergic to β-lactams, aztreonam can be used in combination with a regimen that includes an aminoglycoside and an antipneumococcal fluoroquinolone.

These recommendations do not take into account the newer antibiotics that have recently appeared (such as telithromycin, linezolid) and the new quinolones (such as gatifloxacin or moxifloxacin) which, although having demonstrated their effectiveness in the treatment of CAP in phase III studies, have not been incorporated into the guidelines of scientific societies.

Telithromycin is the first representative of the ketolide family and was designed to provide an optimal oral therapy for clinical treatment of respiratory infections. It has a wide

Table 10B.1 *Empiric antibiotic treatment in community-acquired pneumonia*

Microorganisms	Treatment
Group I: Outpatients patients with no concomitant diseases or risk factors	
S. pneumoniae	New generation macrolide
M. pneumoniae	
C. pneumoniae	
H. influenzae	
Respiratory virus	
Group II: Outpatients with concomitant diseases or risk factors	
S. pneumoniae	β-Lactam plus macrolide *or*
M. pneumoniae	antipneumococcal
C. pneumoniae	fluoroquinolones only
Mixed infection	
H. influenzae	
Enteric Gram-negative microorganisms	
Respiratory virus	
Group III: Hospitalized patients	
S. pneumoniae	Intravenous β-lactam plus
H. influenzae	macrolide, oral *or* intravenous
M. pneumoniae	*or* antipneumococcal
Mixed infection	fluoroquinolone
Genus *Legionella*	intravenous only
Aspiration (anaerobics)	
Group IVa: Patients admitted to the ICU without risk factors for Pseudomonas aeruginosa	
S. pneumoniae	Intravenous β-lactam plus
Genus *Legionella*	intravenous macrolide *or* an
H. influenzae	intravenous fluoroquinolone
Enteric bacilli	
Gram-negative	
S. aureus	
M. pneumoniae	
Respiratory virus	
Group IVb: Patients admitted to the ICU with risk factors for Pseudomonas aeruginosa	
All previous pathogens	Antipseudomonal β-lactams
P. aeruginosa	plus a fluoroquinolone Intravenous antipseudomonal

antibacterial spectrum with bactericidal activity against the most frequent respiratory pathogens (including atypical and intracellular types). Its activity against resistant pneumococcus is of special interest. Other advantages of telithromycin are its ease of administration (a single daily dose) and its high tolerance. Thus, telithromycin is a good option for monotherapy in clinical treatment of mild to moderate CAP. Linezolid is an oxazolidinone whose antibacterial spectrum primarily consists of Gram-positive bacteria. Its activity against pneumococcus and *S. aureus* is of great interest as is its safety, which makes it an attractive alternative to vancomycin in the hospital setting. The new quinolones feature pharmacodynamic and pharmacokinetic improvements, such as a lower maximum inhibitory concentration for pneumococcus.

Table 10B.2 summarizes the dosages and means of administration of the most frequently used antibiotics in CAP treatment.

Table 10B.2. *Dosage and method of administration of most commonly used antibiotics in the treatment of community-acquired pneumonia*

Antibiotic	Dosage	Administration
Ceftriaxone	1–2 g/24 h	IV
Cefotaxime	1–2 g/8 h	IV
Cefepime	2 g/12 h	IV
Cefuroxime	1.5 g/8 h	IV
Cefuroxime axetil	500 mg/12 h	Oral
Meropenem	1 g/8 h	IV
Imipenem	500 mg/6 h	IV
Piperacillin–tazobactam	4–0.5 g/8 h	IV
Aztreonam	1 g/8 h	IV
Amoxicillin–clavulanate	2–0.2 g/8 h	IV
	75–125 mg/8 h	Oral
Clarithromycin	500 mg/12 h	IV or oral
Azithromycin	500 mg/24 h	IV or oral
Erythromycin	1 g/6 h	IV or oral
Telithromycin	800 mg/24 h	Oral
Levofloxacin	500 mg/24 h	IV or oral
Moxifloxacin	400 mg/24 h	Oral
Ciprofloxacin	400 mg/8–12 h	IV
	500–750 mg/12 h	Oral

IV, intravenous.

RESPIRATORY FAILURE IN PATIENTS WITH PNEUMONIA

Patients with CAP, especially those with some chronic lung diseases, usually manifest arterial hypoxemia to (one extent or another) as a consequence of a secondary shunt effect produced by infiltration of the alveoli by inflammatory exudates. The management of respiratory failure in these patients ranges from conventional oxygen therapy to mechanical ventilation (noninvasive or conventional) depending on the severity of the symptoms.

In the case of hypoxemic nonhypercapnic patients, oxygen therapy must be initiated with Venturi system at high oxygen concentration. If the patient does not improve, a low-flow mask with reservoir is indicated. For hypercapnic patients, the Venturi system is recommended at low concentrations to avoid worsening carbon dioxide retention.[12]

Approximately 60–85 percent of patients with severe pneumonia develop respiratory failure requiring mechanical ventilation. Hypoxemia can be difficult to correct in these patients because of the need for additional positive pressure at the end of the exhalation (positive end-expiratory pressure [PEEP]), especially in those with primarily unilateral pneumonia. This is because the nonaffected lung can become overstretched with no recruitment of alveolar units in the affected lung.[13] A useful strategy is putting the patient in the lateral position with the side with the healthy lung down. This technique improves the ventilation/perfusion ratio by better perfusion of the healthy lung (gravity effect). The improved ventilation of the affected lung can ease the relaxation performance, but this technique is not always effective and carries the risk of inoculating the healthy lung with purulent secretions.[14] For this reason, a conventional ventilation approach with high FiO_2, PEEP test for best oxygenation, and hemodynamic and gasometric monitoring to prevent overstretching of the healthy lung is recommended. Lateral position should be considered only early on for extreme hypoxemia or in stable patients with satisfactory evolution.

About 5 percent of patients with severe CAP develop acute respiratory distress syndrome (ARDS), with a mortality of 70 percent. The ventilatory approach consists of protective ventilation (reduced tidal volume to 6 mL/kg) and high PEEP with the aim to maintain a plateau pressure less than 30 cm H_2O.[15]

Inhalation pharmacologic treatments, such as nitric oxide and prostacyclin, can be considered – especially for severe cases with refractory hypoxemia. Although they improve the gas exchange by reducing the intrapulmonary shunt, they do not improve the survival of these patients.[16] Another strategy for the treatment of severe respiratory failure is the prone position. This strategy improves the ventilation/perfusion ratio and respiratory mechanics with a transitory improvement in gas exchange but without affecting mortality.[17] In the past few years, noninvasive ventilation (NIV) has been increasingly used as an alternative therapy. The first studies of NIV in severe pneumonia were conflicting, but recent studies have demonstrated that NIV reduces the requirement for tracheal intubations and the length of ICU stay, particularly for COPD patients.[18] In a recent study in patients with severe hypoxemic respiratory failure due pneumonia, Ferrer *et al.*[19] demonstrated that NIV, when compared with conventional oxygenation therapy, decreased the rate of intubations, the incidence of septic shock and death in ICU, and improved survival at 90 days. Multivariate analysis demonstrated that the use of NIV was an independently associated factor in decreasing the risk of intubations and death at 90 days.

These positive effects of NIV in hypoxemic respiratory insufficiency are associated with the lower load on respiratory muscles and lower ventilatory efforts. Noninvasive ventilation improves the breathing pattern, reduces the respiratory rate, and increases the tidal volume. Other documented effects are an improvement of the ventilation/perfusion ratio and intrapulmonary shunt with recovery of the gas exchange.

SEPSIS

The pulmonary parenchyma is the largest epithelial surface in the body in contact with the external environment. A specific defense system exists whose objective is to keep it sterile. The first line of pulmonary defense is formed by alveolar macrophages and polymorphonuclear leukocytes, which are regulated by a long list of cytokines whose purpose is to maintain the homeostasis of the immune system. Among the principal cytokines involved are the tumor necrosis factor (TNF) and interleukins (IL)-1, -8, and -12: proinflammatory; and IL-6 and -10: anti-inflammatory. In the case of CAP, initially there is an interaction between components of the microorganism (such as liposaccharide A in the case of Gram-negative bacteria) and the alveolar macrophage, which initiates the immune response, whose objective is to control and eradicate the infection.

This response remains confined to the affected pulmonary parenchyma as a compartmentalized process. Sometimes (either due to the infection itself or the immune system) the infection can overcome the lung and unleash an excessive or uncontrolled systemic inflammatory response that implies the generation and activation of numerous secondary inflammation mediators (prostaglandins, leukotrienes, proteases, and other cytokines) as well as an activation of the coagulation system, creating a procoagulant state.

The clinical manifestation of all this inflammatory and procoagulant activity is known as sepsis (defined as the presence of two or more of the following characteristics: fever or hypothermia, leukocytosis or leukopenia, tachycardia and tachypnea), which can further develop into septic shock and multiple organ failure.[20] Apart from the antibiotic therapy and hemodynamic management, new treatments have been developed for sepsis with the aims of improving the patient's immune system, inhibiting the mediators of inflammation, and preventing the development a procoagulant state. Among those which stand out are systemic steroids, granulocyte colony stimulating factor (G-CSF), and recombinant C protein.

Systemic steroids

Endogenous corticoids play an important role in the regulation of the host response to infection by inhibiting the migration of leukocytes, the adhesion of neutrophils to endothelial cells, and the production of cytokines. They also inhibit macrophage and endothelial cells function. In addition, steroids exert several actions over the cardiovascular system (increase in cardiac expenditure and in arterial tension) and over the metabolism (increase in gluconeogenesis). Their role in supplementary treatment in sepsis was evaluated 30 years ago. However, two older, randomized studies did not demonstrate the benefit of using systemic steroids in terms of survival. Some benefit could be demonstrated only in patients affected by bacterial meningitis and typhoid fever.[21] Notably, in these studies high doses of steroids were given for short periods of time.[22]

Recent trials have been done in septic patients with evaluation of adrenal function. The trials found a relative suprarenal insufficiency in this group of patients. Annane and coworkers showed in a placebo-controlled study that treatment with hydrocortisone at low dosage and fludrocortisone for 7 days significantly reduced the risk of ICU and inhospital mortality in patients with septic shock and relative adrenal insufficiency.[23]

Granulocyte colony stimulating factor

The first cells that respond to the inflammatory mediators produced by the immune system are the polymorphonuclear leukocytes (PMN) or granulocytes, representing the pivotal point in the host response against an infection. Granulocyte colony stimulating factor (G-CSF) is a cytokine produced by activated alveolar macrophages. It recruits and activates granulocytes in the infected lung, as well as stimulating the formation and maturation of new PMNs systemically. Hence, it reinforces the organism's defenses against infection. The concentration of G-CSF increases significantly during bacterial infections, which suggests that this cytokine has a relevant role in the regulation of the inflammatory response. Human recombinant G-CSF maintains the properties of the original cytokine regarding the proliferation and differentiation of neutrophils, and it has been demonstrated that it is effective in reducing bacterial load and improving survival rates in animal models of pneumonia.

Based on preclinical trials results, recent studies have been undertaken of G-CSF as a supplement to antibiotics in the treatment of non-neutropenic patients with pneumonia complicated by sepsis or septic shock. The administration of G-CSF increased the blood concentration of PMN; hastened the radiologic resolution of the pneumonia; reduced the incidence of serious complications such as severe respiratory distress syndrome and disseminated intravascular coagulation (DIC); and it was safe and well tolerated. In a small (18 patients) randomized, placebo-controlled trial of patients with CAP and either septic shock or severe sepsis, there were no differences in types and occurrences of adverse events, including ARDS, or in outcome between the two groups. This trial concluded that more indepth studies are required to determine the benefit of treatment in terms of survival.[24] A multicenter, double-blind, randomized trial showed that the addition of filgrastim to the antibiotic and supportive care treatment of patients with pneumonia complicated by severe sepsis is safe, but not effective in reducing mortality or complications of this infection.[25]

Human recombinant activated protein C

The secondary systemic inflammatory response to infection in sepsis generates a procoagulant state as a consequence of the activation of coagulation and inhibition of fibrinolysis. This state gives rise to diffuse endothelial lesions, multiple organ dysfunction, and death. Activated protein C is an endogenous protein that modulates coagulation (it promotes fibrinolysis and inhibits thrombosis) and the inflammatory response (it inhibits IL-6). The formation of activated protein C in sepsis can be compromised by the effect of inflammatory cytokines, and the reduction of their plasma levels is associated with a higher risk of mortality in patients with sepsis. In a randomized, placebo-controlled study by Bernard *at el.*[26] of nearly 1700 patients, the administration of recombinant human protein C increased the survival rate at 28 days of patients with serious sepsis. However, it was associated with a nonsignificant bleeding risk. The guidelines for management of severe sepsis and septic shock have recommended the use of recombinant human activated protein C in patients at high risk of death (Acute Physiology and Chronic Health Evaluation II ≥25; sepsis-induced multiple organ failure; septic shock or sepsis-induced ARDS; and no absolute contraindication related to bleeding risk or relative contraindication that outweighs the potential benefits).[27] This is a Grade B recommendation based in the previously cited trial.

PROGRESSIVE PNEUMONIA AND NONRESOLVING PNEUMONIA

Clinical improvement in hospitalized CAP patients usually happens within 24–48 hours from the start of antibiotic treatment. Fever usually disappears 2–4 days after starting treatment for pneumococcus infection. Leukocytosis often resolves on the fourth day of treatment, although the pulmonary physical exam findings, such as crackling sounds, can persist in up to 40 percent of patients until after the seventh day. Advanced age, multiple concomitant diseases, severity of the pneumonia, multiple affected lobes, alcoholism, and bacteremia are well-known factors associated with a delay in clinical resolution.[28,29] Radiologic resolution of pneumonia can be slower. Radiographic findings can be seen in almost 40 percent of patients with pneumococcal pneumonia below age 50 and without comorbidities at 4 weeks. The resolution can even be slower in older patients or those with chronic diseases, and the chest

radiograph is normal after 4 weeks in 25 percent of cases only.[30,31]

Progressive pneumonia means clinical deterioration in the first 24 hours of treatment with an increase of 50 percent in pulmonary infiltrates. It is considered a medical emergency with vital implications for the patient requiring a prompt change in the diagnostic and therapeutic strategy (Fig. 10B.3). When clinical improvement of a patient with CAP (without factors that could delay their clinical course) is not adequate by the third day, it is considered to be nonresolving pneumonia. When some of the above mentioned factors that delay the improvement of the pneumonia are present, it is not considered nonresolving until after the fifth day.

The incidence of progressive pneumonia and of nonresolving pneumonia is not well established, but approximately 10 percent of inpatients are considered not to respond adequately to the initial empiric antibiotic treatment, whereas another 60 percent have progressive pneumonia. However, mortality of both groups of patients can be up to three times higher that the general mortality rate of patients admitted for pneumonia.

In the two previously described situations, it is necessary to perform a meticulous reevaluation to identify the possible causes of the poor response. These reasons can be grouped into four categories:

- *Inappropriate choice of antibiotic treatment.* The causative microorganism could be resistant to the initial antibiotic treatment or could have developed resistance over the course of treatment. In this case it is recommended to test the sensitivities of the microorganism in initial cultures and follow-up. Another possibility is that the infection is caused by an agent that is not sensitive to any antimicrobial (such as a virus).
- *Unusual pathogens.* An infection by an unusual pathogen should be suspected when clinical or radiographic signs are persistent. In the differential diagnosis, tuberculosis, fungi (especially in those patients in chronic treatment with steroids),[32] and *Pneumocystis carinii* should be included.
- *Complications of pneumonia.* Up to 10 percent[33] of patients with bacterial pneumonia can develop

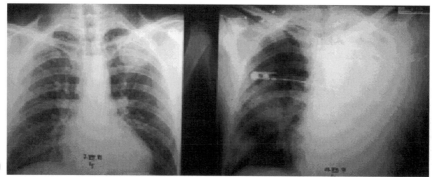

(a)   (b)

Figure 10B.3   *(a,b) Progressive pneumonia: (b) was taken 48 hours after admission.*

metastatic infections such as meningitis, arthritis, endocarditis, pericarditis, peritonitis, cavitation (Figs 10B.4 and 10B.5), and empyema. (Empyema will be dealt with in this chapter also due to its clinical importance.)

- *Noninfectious diseases*. Entities such as pulmonary thromboembolism, congestive cardiac failure, diffuse alveolar hemorrhage, and bronchogenic carcinoma, or inflammatory diseases such as bronchiolitis obliterans with organizing pneumonia, sarcoidosis, eosinophilic pneumonia, and Wegener granulomatosis can clinically mimic pneumonia.

To identify this range of possibilities, it is essential to take an exhaustive clinical history, collect epidemiological data of interest (trips, contact with animals, etc.) and a microbiologic reevaluation, preferably using invasive methods (e.g. bronchoscopy), especially in older patients, smokers, and seriously ill patients.[34,35] Computed axial tomography is also useful in the diagnosis of local complications or when neoplasia and pulmonary infarction are suspected. If the diagnostic evaluation has not been successful and the patient's condition is still severe, consider an open lung biopsy in the affected area of the lung.

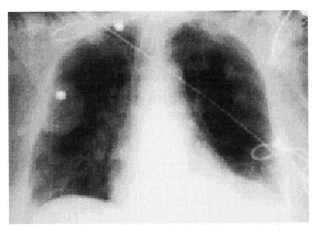

Figure 10B.4 *Pneumonia with cavitation (right upper lung)*

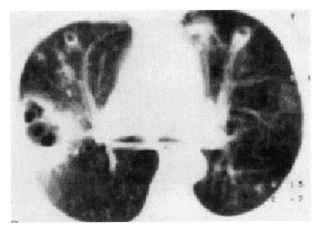

Figure 10B.5 *Pneumonia with cavitation: tomographic image.*

The most frequent cause of progressive pneumonia and of pneumonia that does not respond to treatment is infection. Therefore, after a microbiological reevaluation it is mandatory to consider a change in the initial empiric antibiotic treatment that takes into account the coverage of anaerobes, *P. aeruginosa*, and *S. aureus* and has efficacy against the usual pathogens such as *S. pneumoniae* and *Legionella*. For this reason, treatment with an antipseudomonal β-lactam is recommended (piperacillin-tazobactam, meropenem, imipenem, cefepime) along with an intravenous, antipneumococcal quinolone such as levofloxacin or an intravenous macrolide. If there is suspicion of infection with *P. aeruginosa*, a combination of at least two antipseudomonal antibiotics must be used (an antipseudomonal β-lactam plus ciprofloxacin or an aminoglycoside plus an intravenous macrolide).

PARAPNEUMONIC EFFUSION AND EMPYEMA

More than 57 percent of patients admitted for CAP develop parapneumonic pleural effusion. This complication increases the morbidity and mortality of the pneumonia. It constitutes a medical emergency because it requires diagnostic thoracentesis, which will determine the type of treatment. In some cases it will resolve with the antibiotics alone, whereas in other instances drainage will be necessary.

The therapeutic approach and techniques for treating parapneumonic effusion and empyema have changed in recent years. The recommendations of the American College of Chest Physicians (ACCP)[36] divide patients with pneumonia and pleural effusion into four categories, according to the associated risk of death and need for secondary interventions (Table 10B.3).

In groups 1 and 2 (pleural effusion affecting less than a half hemithorax, with sterile liquid and a pH ≥7.20), pleural drainage is not recommended. If the clinical evolution is not favorable, a second thoracentesis and drainage of the effusion should be considered. In group 3 (pleural effusion that affects more than half of the hemithorax or with Gram's stain and/or cultures positive, or a pH <7.20) and group 4 (presence of gross puss in the pleura), pleural drainage with a thoracotomy tube (28–32 Fr) is recommended. In these patients, drainage is often insufficient for the treatment of the effusion or empyema, especially when there are multiple loculations into the pleural cavity.

In this situations fibrinolytic treatment or surgical excision of infected tissue via thoracotomy or video-thoracoscopy should be strongly considered. This last technique has a comparable effectiveness to thoracotomy and has additional advantages in the postsurgical period.

Table 10B.3 *Treatment of parapneumonic effusion*[35]

Anatomy of the pleural space	Bacteriology	Biochemistry*	Category	Risk of deterioration	Drainage
Minimal free effusion (<10 mm)[§]	Gram stain and culture unknown	pH unknown	Group 1	Very low	No
Moderate free effusion (>10 mm and <1/2 hemithorax)	Gram stain and culture negative	pH ≥7.20	Group 2	Low	No
Massive effusion (>1/2 hemithorax or loculated effusion)	Gram stain or cultures positive	pH <7.20	Group 3	Moderate	Yes
	Frank pus		Group 4	High	Yes

*The pH of pleural liquid should be determined by analysis of arterial gases. If this is not available, the glucose from the pleural fluid can be used with a cut-off point of 60 mg/dL.

[§]Clinical experience indicates that pleural effusion <10 mm does not require thoracentesis.

Key learning points

- The severity of the disease and choice of antibiotic treatment influence the prognosis of CAP.

- Other factors of importance in CAP are the treatment of respiratory insufficiency and the associated sepsis, and the recognition of progressive pneumonia and nonresolving pneumonia.

- Predictive models of severity have been developed (PSI, CURB) that can help the clinician to identify patients with a poor prognosis early.

- Certain aspects of the incidence, etiology, progression, and prognosis of severe CAP are sufficiently different from mild CAP to warrant a specific management plan.

- An important aspect of the antibiotic treatment of CAP is its early initiation. Available data show a reduction of mortality within 30 days if the patient receives the first dose of antibiotics in the first 8 hours of arriving at the hospital.

- When making the choice of initial, empiric antibiotic treatment, local epidemiologic factors must be kept in mind as well as the particularities of each patient, such as the severity of clinical symptoms, comorbidities, and risk factors for specific pathogens.

- In respiratory failure in patients with pneumonia, noninvasive ventilation improves the breathing pattern, reduces the respiratory rate, and increases the tidal volume.

- In patients with sepsis, apart from the antibiotic therapy and hemodynamic management, new treatments have been developed with the aims of improving the patient's immune system, inhibiting the mediators of inflammation, and preventing the development a procoagulant state. Among those which stand out are systemic steroids, granulocyte colony stimulating factor (G-CSF), and recombinant C protein.

- The most frequent cause of progressive pneumonia and of pneumonia that does not respond to treatment is infection.

- Parapneumonic effusion constitutes a medical emergency because it requires diagnostic thoracentesis, which will determine the type of treatment.

REFERENCES

- 1. Fine MJ, Auble TE, Yealy DM, *et al.* A prediction rule to identify low risk patients with community-acquired pneumonia. *N Engl J Med* 1997; **336**: 243–50.

✱ 2. BTS guidelines for the management of community-acquired pneumonia in adults. *Thorax* 2001; **56**(Suppl 4): IV1–64.

- 3. Lim WS, Van der Eerden MM, Laing R, *et al.* Defining community acquired pneumonia severity on presentation to hospital: an international derivation and validation study. *Thorax* 2003; **58**: 377–82.

4. Coley CM, Yi-Hwei L, Medsger AR, *et al.* Preference for home vs. hospital care among low-risk patients with community acquired pneumonia. *Arch Intern Med* 1996; **156**:1565–71.

- 5. Torres A, Serra-Batlles J, Ferrer A, *et al.* Severe community-acquired pneumonia. Epidemiology and prognostic factors. *Am Rev Respir Dis* 1991; **144**: 312–18.

6. Pachón J, Prados MD, Capote F, *et al.* Severe community-acquired pneumonia: aetiology, prognosis and treatment. *Am Rev Respir Dis* 1990; **142**: 366–73.

✱ 7. Ewig S, Ruiz M, Mensa J, *et al.* Severe community-acquired pneumonia: assessment of severity criteria. *Am J Respir Crit Care Med* 1998; **158**: 1102–8.

- 8. Gordon GS, Throop D, Berberian L, *et al.* Validation of the therapeutic recommendations of the American

Thoracic Society (ATS) guidelines for community acquired pneumonia in hospitalised patients. *Chest* 1996; **110**: 55S.

9. Ewig S, De Roux A, Bauer T, *et al.* Validation of predictive rules and indices of severity for community acquired pneumonia. *Thorax* 2004; **59**: 421–7.

● 10. Meehan TP, Fine MJ, Krumholz HM, *et al.* Quality of care process and outcome in elderly patients with pneumonia. *JAMA* 1997; **278**: 2080–4.

11. Niederman MS, Mandell LA. Guidelines for the management of adults with community-acquired pneumonia. Diagnosis, assessment of severity, antimicrobial therapy, and prevention. *Am J Respir Crit Care Med* 2001; **163**: 1730–54.

12. Tang CM, Macfarlane JT. Early management of younger adults dying of community acquired pneumonia. *Respir Med* 1993; **87**: 289–94.

13. Kanarek DJ, Shannon DC. Adverse effect of positive end-expiratory pressure on pulmonary perfusion and arterial oxygenation. *Am Rev Respir Dis* 1975; **112**: 457–9.

14. Ibáñez J, Raurich JM, Abizanda R, *et al.* The effect of lateral position on gas exchange in patients with unilateral lung disease during mechanical ventilation. *Intensive Care Med* 1981; **7**: 231–4.

● 15. The Acute Respiratory Distress Syndrome Network. Ventilation with lower tidal volumes as compared with traditional tidal volumes for acute lung injury and the acute respiratory distress syndrome. *N Engl J Med* 2000; **342**: 1301–8.

16. Michael JR, Barton RG, Saffle JR, *et al.* Inhaled nitric oxide versus conventional therapy. Effect on oxygenation in ARDS. *Am J Respir Crit Care Med* 1998; **157**: 1372–80.

17. Gattinoni L, Tognini G, Pesenti A, *et al.* Effect of prone positioning on the survival of patients with acute respiratory failure. *N Engl J Med*, 2001; **345**: 568–73.

18. Confalonieri M, Potena A, Carbone G, *et al.* Acute respiratory failure in patients with severe community-acquired pneumonia. A prospective randomized evaluation of non-invasive ventilation. *Am J Resp Crit Care Med* 1999; **160**: 1585–91.

● 19. Ferrer M, Esquinas A, Leon M, *et al.* Noninvasive ventilation in severe hypoxemic respiratory failure. A randomized clinical trial. *Am J Respir Crit Care Med* 2003; **168**: 1438–44.

◆ 20. Wheeler AP, Bernard GR. Treating patients with severe sepsis. *N Engl J Med* 1999; **340**: 207–14.

◆ 21. Cronin L, Cook DJ, Carlet J. Corticosteroid treatment for sepsis: a critical appraisal and meta-analysis of the literature. *Crit Care Med* 1995; **23**: 1430–9.

22. Lefering R, Neugebauer EA. Steroid controversy in sepsis and septic shock: a meta-analysis. *Crit Care Med* 1995; **23**: 1294–303.

● 23. Annane D, Sébille V, Charpentier C, *et al.* Effect of treatment with low doses of hydrocortisone and fludrocortisone on mortality in patients with septic shock. *JAMA* 2002; **288**: 862–71.

24. Wunderink R, Leeper KV, Schein R, *et al.* Filgrastim in patients with pneumonia and severe sepsis or septic shock. *Chest* 2001; **119**: 523–9.

25. Root RK, Lodato RF, Patrick W, *et al.* Multicenter, double-blind, placebo-controlled study of the use of filgrastim in patients hospitalized with pneumonia and severe sepsis. *Crit Care Med* 2003; **31**: 367–73.

26. Bernard GR, Vincent JL, Laterre PF, *et al.* Efficacy and safety of recombinant human activated protein C for severe sepsis. *N Engl J Med* 2001; **344**: 699–709.

✱ 27. Dellinger RP, Carlet JM, Masur H, *et al.* Surviving sepsis campaign guidelines for management of severe sepsis and septic shock. *Crit Care Med* 2004; **32**: 858–73.

28. Finkelstein MS, Petkun WM, Freedman ML, Antopol SC. Pneumococcal bacteraemia in adults: age-dependent differences in presentation and in outcome. *J Am Geriatr Soc* 1983; **31**: 19–27.

29. Halm EA, Fine MJ, Marrie TJ, *et al.* Time to clinical stability in patients hospitalized with community-acquired pneumonia: implications for practice guidelines. *JAMA* 1998; **179**: 1452–7.

30. Jay SJ, Johanson WG, Jr, Pierce A. The radiologic resolution of *Streptococcus pneumoniae*. *N Engl J Med* 1975; **293**: 798–801.

31. Mittl RL, Schwab RJ, Duchin JS, *et al.* Radiographic resolution of community acquired pneumonia. *Am J Respir Crit Care Med* 1994; **149**: 630–5.

32. Rodrigues J, Niederman MS, Fein AM, Pai PB. Nonresolving pneumonia in steroid-treated patients with obstructive lung disease. *Am J Med* 1992; **98**: 1322–6.

33. Marrie TJ. Bacteriemic pneumococcal pneumonia: a continuously evolving disease. *J Infect* 1992; **24**: 247–55.

34. Ortqvist A, Kalin M, Lejdeborn L, Lundberg B. Diagnostic fiberoptic bronchoscopy and protected brush culture in patients with community-acquired pneumonia. *Chest* 1990; **97**: 576–82.

35. Feinsilver SH, Fein AM, Niederman MS, Schultz DE, Faegenburg DH. Utility of fiberoptic bronchoscopy in nonresolving pneumonia. *Chest* 1990; **98**: 1322–6.

✱ 36. Colice GL, Curtis A, Deslauriers J, *et al.* Medical and surgical treatment of parapneumonic effusions: an evidence-based guidelines. *Chest* 2000; **18**: 1158–71.

Acute respiratory distress syndrome

NUALA J MEYER, GREGORY A SCHMIDT

INTRODUCTION

Acute respiratory distress syndrome (ARDS) is among the most challenging disease processes faced in pulmonary medicine. It is a condition which can occur without warning, afflicting healthy young individuals as well as the comorbid elderly. Over the past two decades, our understanding of both the pathophysiology as well as the management of ARDS has progressed significantly; nonetheless, its mortality remains high. In this chapter, we review the definitions, clinical features, and epidemiology of ARDS, and discuss the recent advancements in its pathobiology and treatment.

DEFINITION

The term 'respiratory distress syndrome' was first coined in 1967 when a case report of 12 patients with varied initial insults – trauma, infection, and pancreatitis – all developed respiratory distress characterized by tachypnea, hypoxemia, and decreased lung compliance.[1] In the ensuing years, the syndrome remained a clinical diagnosis, recognized as the constellation of symptoms of abject respiratory distress, hypoxemia refractory to supplemental oxygen, and diffuse airspace opacities on chest radiograph. In 1971, the syndrome was referred to as the 'adult respiratory distress syndrome' in part to distinguish it from the hyaline membrane disease observed in neonates, the authors describing the syndrome as a 'nonspecific response to a variety of pulmonary injuries.'[2] The article asserted that the pathologic basis of the disease appeared to be damage to the alveolar capillary membrane, causing leakage of alveolar and interstitial fluid into the alveolar space. Subsequent physicians referred to this phenomenon as 'noncardiogenic pulmonary edema'[3] and many considered a pulmonary artery catheterization vital in order to exclude hydrostatic pulmonary edema before diagnosing a patient with ARDS.

In 1992, clinicians and scientists from the United States and Europe met to discuss the definition of the ARDS for the dual purposes of patient care and study design. The result was an American–European Consensus Conference (AECC) statement published in 1994 which has been widely applied, and which distinguishes severe lung injury from lung injury with less devastating clinical consequences.[4] According to the AECC, acute lung injury (ALI) is defined as the acute onset of impaired gas exchange in which the ratio of arterial oxygen pressure to the fraction of inspired oxygen (PaO_2/FiO_2) is less than 300 mm Hg. Patients with ARDS – and here the authors strongly opined a preference for *acute*, rather than *adult*, respiratory distress syndrome as the syndrome does occur in children – represent those with ALI at the most severe end of the spectrum, in whom the PaO_2/FiO_2 ratio is less than 200 mm Hg. Criteria common to both syndromes are: an acute onset; bilateral lung abnormalities on a frontal chest radiograph; and absence of evidence of left atrial hypertension (see Table 10C.1). By AECC criteria, positive end-expiratory pressure (PEEP) does not affect the calculation of the PaO_2/FiO_2 ratio nor the definition of ALI versus ARDS.

Table 10C.1   *AECC definition of ALI and ARDS[4]*

ALI	Acute onset	$PaO_2/FiO_2 \leqslant 300$	Bilateral infiltrates on chest radiograph	No clinical evidence of left atrial hypertension; or $P_{pw} <18$ mm Hg
ARDS	Acute onset	$PaO_2/FiO_2 \leqslant 200$	Bilateral infiltrates on chest radiograph	No clinical evidence of left atrial hypertension; or $P_{pw} <18$ mm Hg

ALI, acute lung injury; ARDS, acute respiratory distress syndrome; AECC, American–European Consensus Conference.

It has been our experience that many physicians fail to recognize ALI and ARDS until patients have progressed to the most severe form of the disease, and thus miss the opportunity to intervene early in the course of disease. One undeniable advantage of the AECC definition is its absolute simplicity, which frees clinicians from any cumbersome 'burden of proof' such as a proved inciting event or a low pulmonary capillary wedge pressure. Two points deserve mention, however. First, the most commonly cited precipitants of ARDS include sepsis, pneumonia, aspiration, hypertransfusion of blood products, and trauma; with these risks, ARDS warrants the highest consideration.[5–8] Conversely, when encountering respiratory embarrassment in a patient without known precipitants of ARDS, an alternative diagnosis should be actively considered and excluded. Second, we emphasize that the diagnosis of ARDS no longer requires a pulmonary artery (PA) catheterization or pulmonary capillary wedge pressure (P_{pw}). Echocardiography has largely supplanted the PA catheter in diagnosing LV dysfunction and even diastolic dysfunction, and it is now well recognized that low pressure edema can coexist with left ventricular dysfunction.

EPIDEMIOLOGY

Researchers have struggled for several decades to accurately estimate the incidence of ALI and ARDS. Prior to the AECC statement in 1994, multiple definitions for the syndrome were employed, and as ARDS is not a common disease, studies were typically multicenter, expensive, and methodologically difficult. An early estimate was provided by the United States National Heart and Lung Institute Task Force in 1972, when the incidence was estimated at 75 per 100 000 people, or approximately 150 000 cases per year in the United States.[9] The estimate was generated upon convening an expert panel, and was not based upon an epidemiological study. More recently, multiple studies have examined the incidence of ALI/ARDS in several different populations. Studies of specific communities in the United Kingdom, Spain, and the United States reported ARDS incidences of between 1.5 and 8.3 per 100 000 persons.[10–12] These reports are an order of magnitude smaller than the initial estimate provided by the Heart and Lung Task Force, yet they are difficult to compare with one another as they apply inconsistent definitions for ARDS.

The first study to apply the AECC definition to its study population was performed in Scandinavia, where the incidence was significantly higher, at 17.9 per 100 000 for ALI and 13.5 per 100 000 for ARDS.[13] A study of the population of an Ohio health maintenance organization yielded a similar result, with an incidence of 15.3 per 100 000 persons per year.[14] A subsequent study in the United States employed a different epidemiologic strategy: studying the incidence of ARDS cases in 40 referral centers and then adjusting these data for the total number of intensive care unit (ICU) beds in the United States.[15] By this method, the authors reported an annual incidence of 22.4 cases per 100 000 person-years, with a range from between 19 and 96 per 100 000 depending on the method used to calculate available ICU beds. Echoing the higher incidence was a study in Australia, which found an ALI incidence of 34 cases per 100 000 per year, and an ARDS incidence of 28 per 100 000 per year.[16] Occasionally studies are unable to assess an incidence – due to an undefined total population – but are able to measure the prevalence of ARDS among all ICU admissions. One European study found that 6.9 percent of patients entering the ICU met criteria for ARDS, and accounted for 16 percent of patients being mechanically ventilated and 32 percent of hypoxemic patients being mechanically ventilated.[17] Although it is dissatisfying to be unable to reach a more precise assessment, it nevertheless appears that the incidence of ALI is greater than earlier appreciated, is frequently encountered in the ICU, and inflicts a substantial morbid and financial cost.

CLINICAL PRESENTATION

Much attention has been granted to the issue of defining ARDS, but the syndrome itself is protean and often progressive within individual patients. As the disease progresses, distinct stages can be identified based on specific clinical, pathologic, and radiographic criteria.[18] The initial stage, known as the acute or exudative phase, is characterized by the rapid development of respiratory failure, often with cyanosis, arterial hypoxemia refractory to supplemental oxygen, and marked tachypnea. One physiologic correlate of this stage is an increased dead space fraction (V_D/V_T, calculated as the difference between the arterial partial pressure of carbon dioxide ($PaCO_2$) and the mean expired partial pressure of carbon dioxide (P_ECO_2) relative to the $PaCO_2$. Represented mathematically, $V_D/V_T = (PaCO_2 -$

$P_ECO_2)/PaCO_2$.[19] Because the fraction of alveoli participating in gas exchange is reduced in ARDS, the minute ventilation ($\dot{V}_E$) rises, and the clinician will observe patients with extraordinary $\dot{V}_E$ yet with normal or near-normal $PaCO_2$. Lung compliance is also markedly reduced, which will be manifest by unusually high airway pressures with normal or even low tidal volumes. This reduction is not due to stiffness of the lung itself, but rather to the effective loss of functional alveoli owing to extensive consolidation and collapse, leaving a 'baby lung'. Chest radiographs done at this phase show pulmonary edema, and are often indistinguishable from radiographs of patients in cardiogenic, or hydrostatic, pulmonary edema.[20]

Pathologically, one sees diffuse alveolar damage – characterized by alveolar septal thickening, hyaline membranes layered across the alveolar surface, and interstitial edema widening the alveolar spaces – from as early as several days following the onset of respiratory distress.[21] This diffuse injury is thought to compromise the integrity of the alveolar–capillary barrier and causes subsequent leakage of fluid and protein into the alveolar space.[21] For some patients, the severe defect in lung permeability will resolve rapidly, within a week of onset. In many, however, the syndrome progresses into a subacute phase, with similar clinical, physiologic, and radiographic findings evident for 7 days and more.[22] Pathologically, this phase may be distinguished by the development of fibrosing alveolitis, with detectable fibroblasts and collagen within the alveolar septae.[21] Alveolar epithelial type I cells become lost, and are replaced by proliferating alveolar type II cells, which transform the epithelium into a layer of cuboidal cells more resistant to injury.[21] Such changes can be appreciated as early as 5–7 days after the initial respiratory embarrassment.[21]

In a proportion of patients with ARDS, full resolution will occur following the exudative phase, even when prolonged to 10 days or more. In those unfortunate others, however, the syndrome may progress to a proliferative phase, characterized pathologically by extensive fibrosis. Clinically, one observes persistent oxygenation defects, low lung compliance, and high alveolar dead space fraction. Pathologic examination of the lungs is nearly indistinguishable from any form of chronic pulmonary fibrosis, with loss of any normal, recognizable lung architecture.[22] The risks for developing proliferative ARDS are still not well elucidated, and are an area for ongoing investigation.

DIAGNOSTIC STUDIES

Radiographic imaging

Radiographic studies have long been a mainstay of the diagnosis of ALI and ARDS. In the initial description of the syndrome, the radiographic films of all 12 patients were described as 'consistent with pulmonary edema', with bilateral infiltrates.[1] Certain studies have attempted to grade the severity of lung injury in part by the extent of involvement on the frontal chest radiograph.[23] However, the severity score does not predict outcome, and we thus cannot prognosticate based upon a chest radiograph alone. By the AECC definition of ALI, a patient must have bilateral infiltrates on chest radiograph.[4] Patients with unilateral consolidation may still have extreme hypoxemia and a very low PaO_2/FiO_2 ratio, but at least one study would suggest that this population behaves differently from patients with bilateral disease who meet criteria for ALI. A French study found a dramatically lower mortality (41 percent vs. 60 percent) for patients with unilateral radiographic findings and PaO_2/FiO_2 ratio less than 200 compared with those with the similar PaO_2/FIO_2 ratio but bilateral disease.[17]

Although chest radiography is inherent to the diagnosis of ARDS, its ability to discriminate between pulmonary edema on the grounds of increased hydrostatic pressure and that of increased capillary leak edema is an issue of some debate. Milne et al. in 1985 described the cardinal features of cardiogenic pulmonary edema and noncardiogenic edema on the frontal chest radiograph.[24] Hydrostatic, or cardiogenic, edema was marked by an increased cardiac size, enlarged vascular pedicle width (>72 mm), central or homogeneous distribution of edema, pleural effusions, and interstitial changes such as peribronchial cuffs and septal lines.[24] In contrast, increased permeability edema was distinguished by normal cardiac size and vascular pedicle, patchy or peripheral distribution of edema, absent interstitial changes, diminished pulmonary blood volume, and prominent air bronchograms.[24] Milne's criteria are acceptably predictive of cardiogenic edema, yet for permeability edema, their discriminatory value is mediocre at best. A landmark study which scored films by three independent readers who were blinded to the patients' clinical information found that experienced chest radiologists and intensivists correctly identified increased permeability edema in only 60 percent of patients based on the Milne criteria.[20]

Although the chest radiograph can suggest but not prove a diagnosis of ALI, it may be extremely helpful in managing such patients. Recent studies of chest radiographs in patients with ALI found that the portable chest radiograph was useful in predicting intravascular volume.[25,26] In one study, 100 patients with PA catheters underwent portable, supine, digital chest radiography to determine whether the vascular pedicle width (measured by dropping a perpendicular line from the point at which the superior vena cava crosses the right mainstem bronchus across to the point at which the left subclavian artery exits the aortic arch) and cardiothoracic ratio (cardiac silhouette diameter divided by the transverse diameter of the thorax) could predict those patients with P_{pw} ≤18 mm Hg.[25] The authors found that a vascular pedicle width >70 mm and cardiothoracic ratio >0.55 predicted a P_{pw} >18 mm Hg with an accuracy of 70 percent, and a likelihood ratio of 3.1.[25] Interestingly, in 8 of 22 (36 percent) patients with myocardial infarction in this study, the P_{pw} was below 18 mm Hg, whereas in 5 of 10 patients (50 percent) with ARDS, the P_{pw} was greater than 18 mm Hg.[25] Thus, while chest radiography, even portable and supine, is helpful in determining the intravascular volume of patients, it has not proved sensitive in distinguishing cardiogenic from increased permeability edema.

Computed tomography (CT) of the chest has also lent insights to the nature of ALI. Goodman reviewed the utility of CT in examining patients with pulmonary edema in 1996, and observed great inhomogeneity of lung involvement among patients with capillary leak pulmonary edema, even in those whose initial insult was to be caused by systemic processes.[27] Gattoni *et al.* studied CT in humans and animals with capillary leak edema, and demonstrated that the injured lung behaves as though it has three pathologic compartments: one which is relatively normal lung; one with mildly consolidated or atelectatic lung tissue; and the third with dense consolidation.[28] Typically this compartmentalization appears somewhat gravity dependent, with relative sparing of the anterior lobes and more dense consolidation of the posterior fields. Figures 10C.1 and 10C.2 show the radiograph and CT of a 40-year-old man with pneumonia caused by *Klebsiella pneumoniae* who subsequently developed ARDS. Note that despite a relatively uniform appearance to the airspace consolidation on frontal chest radiograph, CT reveals some areas of lung to be quite spared, whereas others are completely consolidated. Figure 10C.3 shows his chest radiograph 3 months after hospital discharge, by which time his hypoxemia had resolved and his baseline performance status had been fully restored.

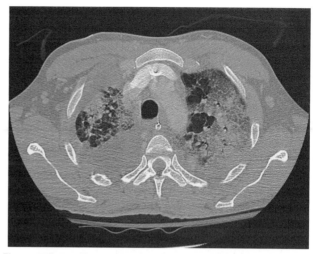

Figure 10C.2   *Chest computed tomography scan of the same patient, revealing inhomogeneous areas of lung consolidation.*

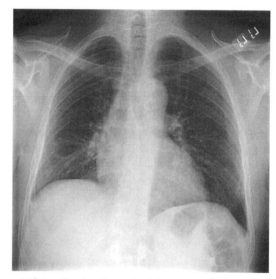

Figure 10C.3   *Chest radiograph of the same patient 3 months later, after full resolution of his acute respiratory distress syndrome.*

Computed tomography is also quite helpful in elucidating the progression of ARDS. After 7–10 days, subpleural cysts, bullae, and emphysematous cysts are more commonly seen.[28] Whether such complications represent a predictable evolution of the disease process or a complication of therapy, particularly mechanical ventilation, is as yet still unknown. When PEEP is applied to lungs which appear consolidated, repeat CT has demonstrated airspace recruitment, visualized as better aeration and less radiographic consolidation, in as little as 15 minutes.[29,30] Lower diaphragms, smaller pulmonary vessels, and the resolution of atelectasis have been reported following the application of PEEP.[30]

Pulmonary artery catheter

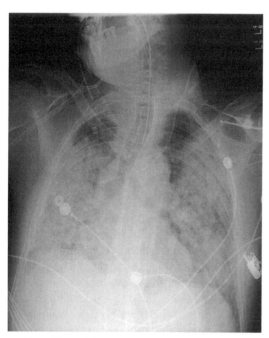

Figure 10C.1   *Frontal chest radiograph of a 40-year-old man with pneumonia and acute respiratory distress syndrome.*

With the introduction in 1970 of flow-directed balloon-tipped pulmonary artery catheters (PACs) capable of measuring P_{pw}, physicians rapidly applied the knowledge of P_{pw} to the diagnosis and management of ARDS. The AECC definition of ALI/ARDS reports that the P_{pw}, if measured, must be below 18 mm Hg.[4] What was once taken for granted as a defining criterion for ARDS has been subject to repeated inquiry, however, as physicians weigh the risks and benefits in their sickest patients. Several observational studies set out to determine whether use of PAC changed management. One study in 1983 found that physicians – whether attending level, critical care fellows, or house staff – were inaccurate in predicting patients' P_{pw} or coronary index, being correct only 42 percent of the time.[31] Insertion of a PAC was associated with an alteration in the administration of fluid, medications, or both in nearly half of all cases in which it was inserted.[31] Countering this assertion of the vital role for PAC were studies which reported that physicians and nurses alike often misinterpreted PAC data; thus, use of PAC raised the potential for misguided management.[32,33] Most alarming, a multicenter trial evaluating the use and safety of PAC reported an excess mortality among patients who received PAC compared with case-matched controls.[34] The study was not ideal in that it used historical case-matched controls rather than a randomized, controlled design, and many physicians pointed out the possibility that the sickest cohort of patients might be the very group whose physicians felt a PAC was necessary. Nonetheless, the study ushered in an era of widespread investigation into the safety and efficacy of PAC, prompting calls from such institutions as the United States Food and Drug Administration and National Heart, Lung, and Blood Institute to establish collaborative groups to study PAC use in varied intensive care settings.[35]

Data on the safety and usefulness of PAC continue to trickle in. In 2003, a collaborative effort from Canada published a trial which randomized high-risk surgical patients either to PAC or 'standard care' – in which most, but not all, patients received a central venous catheter and had free access to echocardiogram (to guide perioperative management) and found no difference in mortality or hospital stay between the two groups.[36] Furthermore, the PAC group had an excess rate of pulmonary embolism which was statistically significant.[36] Later that year, another randomized controlled trial was published from France studying PAC in patients with septic shock and ARDS.[37] This trial differed in that treatment after randomization was not protocol driven, as were most of the prior studies of PAC. Nonetheless, the French study similarly concluded there was no difference in mortality, organ dysfunction, or time in the ICU based upon the use or avoidance of PAC.[37] Once again, most patients in the no-PAC group had central venous catheters and free access to echocardiogram.[37] Importantly, both the Canadian and the French studies found no excess mortality in the PAC group, although the Canadian trial did find excess morbidity, in the form of pulmonary embolism, associated with PAC. As PAC seems to add risk without any proved benefit, we would advocate the use of a central venous catheter with echocardiography as needed to investigate a patient's hemodynamics in ALI. A collaborative effort in the United States is currently studying this approach versus PAC, and may further clarify the issue.

Edema fluid analysis

Very early in the study of ARDS, as investigators appreciated the differences between cardiogenic and increased permeability edema, attention focused upon the edema fluid as a potential diagnostic aid. In an analysis of pulmonary edema fluid from patients with low- and high-pressure pulmonary edema as stratified by history and P_{pw}, one group reported that the ratio of protein in edema fluid to plasma was consistently greater than 0.6 in patients with increased permeability edema, and consistently below 0.6 in those with cardiogenic edema.[38] Edema fluid was obtained by suctioning either through a bronchoscope or directly through the endotracheal tube.[38] Subsequent studies confirmed a low protein ratio in patients with hydrostatic pulmonary edema, and even found that the rate of edema resolution correlated with an increase in edema fluid protein concentration, presumably reflecting increased fluid resorption across the respiratory epithelium.[39] Although not widely used, protein fluid analysis can be extremely helpful in cases where ALI or ARDS coexists with left ventricular dysfunction, and routine measures to exclude congestive heart failure as the etiology of hypoxemia prove problematic. In such a setting, an initial edema-to-serum protein ratio greater than 0.6 should prompt consideration of ALI.

Bronchoscopy and lung biopsy: role in differential diagnosis

Though ARDS is a clinical syndrome which can proceed from numerous primary insults, there exist several distinct disease processes which can mimic the radiographic and clinical symptomatology of ARDS. These are important to recognize, as many are readily treatable. In patients with respiratory distress, yet without risk factors for ALI, bronchoscopy with bronchoalveolar lavage (BAL) or lung biopsy may help to exclude treatable disease. Table 10C.2 later in the section describes several of the more commonly encountered imitators of ARDS, characterized by their profound gas exchange abnormalities and their diffuse radiographic findings.[40]

Among infections, nearly any pneumonia – bacterial, viral, or fungal – can precipitate ARDS; pneumonia is a well-recognized risk factor for the disease.[7–8] This distinction notwithstanding, the pneumonia caused by the fungus *Pneumocystis jiroveci*, the microorganism responsible for pneumocystis pneumonia, uniquely imitates ARDS. As pneumocystis pneumonia is a common acquired immune deficiency syndrome (AIDS)-defining illness, much of what we understand of the organism comes from data on patients with human immunodeficiency virus (HIV), though it is now a well-described infection that occurs as a complication in patients who receive chronic corticosteroid immunosuppression.[41] Early in the AIDS epidemic, infection with *P. carinii* – now renamed *P. jiroveci* to reflect the isolate specific to the human species – carried an extremely poor prognosis, with reports suggesting an inhospital mortality approaching 90 percent for intubated patients with pneumocystis pneumonia.[42,43] With the advent of adjunctive corticosteroid therapy, the mortality from pneumocystis pneumonia in the HIV-positive population has fallen to 10–20 percent; mortality in patients without HIV infection varies between 30 percent and 60 percent.[41] It is now the minority of patients with HIV-related pneumocystis who require intubation and mechanical ventilation; however, this subgroup continues to face a poor prognosis, with recent mortality rates of 38 percent.[42] As the organism does not grow in culture, it is most often detected by staining sputum or bronchoalveolar fluid to detect trophic forms.[41] Induced sputum is the preferred method of diagnosis in patients with HIV, although the practical difficulties of obtaining adequate sample make bronchoscopy with BAL an acceptable first-line alternative. Treatment of pneumocystis pneumonia is typically with trimethoprim-sulfamethoxazole, with the addition of corticosteroids in patients who are hypoxemic (PaO_2 <70 mm Hg).[41]

A number of noninfectious processes also mimic ARDS. Several which deserve mention are acute eosinophilic pneumonia, acute cryptogenic organizing pneumonia, acute hypersensitivity pneumonitis, and diffuse alveolar hemorrhage.[40] Acute eosinophilic pneumonia remains a rare disease, but the largest series to date of 22 patients describes the typical patient as young (mean age 29), previously healthy, and with either an acute or a subacute progression to respiratory failure.[44] All patients had symptoms for less than 1 month, and the majority presented within 1 week complaining of dyspnea, fever, cough, chest pain, and myalgias.[44] In most patients acute eosinophilic pneumonia appears to be idiopathic, but in a minority it may follow recent exposure to cigarettes, medications, or environmental exposure.[40] Bilateral pulmonary infiltrates on chest radiograph were present without exception, and the average PaO_2/FiO_2 ratio was 145, compatible with ARDS. Distinguishing these patients from those with ARDS, however, was their BAL fluid, which showed greater than 50 percent eosinophils; in those with pleural effusions, four of five had elevated eosinophils on body fluid cell count.[44] Interestingly, peripheral blood eosinophilia is typically absent. In addition, the prognosis of patients with acute eosinophilic pneumonia is drastically better than those with ARDS; 100 percent survival was reported in the 2002 review, even for patients who did not receive corticosteroid therapy.[44] Cryptogenic organizing pneumonia (COP) is another pathologic process which can simulate ARDS. Though typically COP follows a subacute course over months, in some patients it can result in an acute progression to respiratory failure in just 3 days.[45] Like the more indolent

form of COP, these patients complain primarily of dyspnea, often with concomitant cough or weight loss, and variable but typically bilateral chest radiograph opacities.[45] For the few patients definitively diagnosed with acute COP, who number approximately 20 in the literature, all required lung biopsy to establish the diagnosis.[45] Transbronchial biopsy is not reliably sensitive to exclude the disease. Patients are treated with corticosteroids much like those with subacute COP, and retrospective data suggest that prognosis is better when corticosteroids are begun early in the course of respiratory failure.[45]

Like organizing pneumonia, hypersensitivity pneumonitis is typically subacute or relapsing, but occasionally presents with acute respiratory failure. Clinically, patients have fever, cough, dyspnea, and leukocytosis – almost indistinguishable from patients with pneumonia – but typically present within 4–6 hours of an organic exposure.[40] Although most patients will improve simply by removal of the offending agent, in certain patients the disease is severe enough to necessitate mechanical ventilation.[40] Respiratory failure can occur either from the primary encounter with antigen or on reexposure.[46] The clinical history can be helpful and suggestive of hypersensitivity pneumonitis, especially for patients with known acute exposure to birds or hay, but numerous inciting antigens have been reported, and in some the cause is never identified.[40] Bronchoscopy yielding a lymphocytic BAL with negative microbiological cultures may suggest the diagnosis, but lung biopsy is often necessary to confirm it.[40] The prognosis for acute hypersensitivity pneumonitis tends to be excellent, either with removal of the offending agent or with corticosteroid therapy.[47] Patients with more chronic hypersensitivity pneumonitis, especially those in whom pulmonary fibrosis is found on biopsy, may have less response to corticosteroids. Finally, diffuse alveolar hemorrhage (DAH) can mimic ARDS. Although hemoptysis is the anticipated symptom, it is absent in up to a third of patients with DAH.[48] It results from inflammatory destruction of arterioles, venules, or alveolar capillaries, thus disrupting the alveolar–capillary barrier and allowing blood to fill the alveolar space.[48] Establishing the cause of DAH is of utmost importance, since many cases are reversible and, left untreated, massive alveolar hemorrhage is life-threatening.[48] Bronchoscopy should be performed early, both to localize the hemorrhage and to exclude airway trauma. In patients without known precipitant of DAH – such as the antiphospholipid syndrome, known connective tissue disease, or coagulopathy – biopsy can be extremely helpful to evaluate for antibasement membrane disease, pulmonary capillaritis, or Wegener granulomatosis.[40] Biopsy can often be accomplished by video-assisted thoracoscopic approach, though open lung biopsy may be preferable in patients who are coagulopathic or in severe distress.[40] Table 10C.2 summarizes common considerations in the differential diagnosis of ARDS.

Table 10C.2   *Differential diagnosis for ALI/ARDS* [40,49,50]

Disease	Diagnostic features
Infectious	
Pneumocystis pneumonia	Sputum or BAL stains for *Pneumocystis jirovecii*
Non–infectious	
Acute eosinophilic pneumonia	BAL = $\geqslant$20% eosinophils
	Fever, myalgias common
Acute cryptogenic organizing pneumonia	Biopsy = proliferating fibroblasts within alveolar ducts and alveoli $\pm$ bronchiolar involvement
Acute hypersensitivity pneumonitis	Biopsy = cellular interstitial pneumonia with bronchiolitis, poorly formed granulomas, intralumenal organizing fibrosis
Diffuse alveolar hemorrhage	BAL = many RBCs and hemosiderin-laden macrophages
	Biopsy recommended to exclude Wegener's granulomatosis, antibasement membrane disease, pulmonary capillaritis

BAL, bronchoalveolar lavage; RBC, red blood cell.

ETIOLOGY

CLINICAL FACTORS

From its very first description, ARDS was recognized as a final common pathway stemming from various initial insults. In the 12 patients initially described, trauma – accompanied by massive transfusion of blood products – sepsis, viral pneumonia, aspiration, and pancreatitis were the offending catalysts.[1] In both prospective and retrospective studies of hospitalized patients, the following risk factors repeatedly emerge as precipitants of ARDS: sepsis, pneumonia, aspiration, trauma (fracture of the pelvis or of multiple long bones), and hypertransfusion of blood products.[5–8]

In 1982, a group attempted to identify risk factors for the development of ARDS by prospectively studying all intubated patients whom they felt were predisposed to the syndrome. Sepsis, aspiration of gastric contents, pulmonary contusion, multiple emergency transfusions, multiple major fractures, near-drowning, pancreatitis, and prolonged hypotension were the 'at risk' conditions identified.[5] Of the 136 patients observed, ARDS developed in 34 percent.[5] Among patients with sepsis, nearly 40 percent developed ARDS, whereas for aspiration and multiple transfusions the rate of ARDS was 30 percent and 24 percent, respectively.[5] In addition, patients with more than one predisposing factor were more likely to meet criteria for ARDS; this was especially true for trauma patients, among whom up to 86 percent of patients with three risk factors developed ARDS.[5] The effect of multiple risk factors has been further verified, with progression to ARDS in trauma patients with sepsis approaching 56 percent in one study.[6] In another, both severity of illness and mortality were positively correlated with the number of risk factors present.[7] The aim of many of these observational studies was to identify the 'at risk' population for ARDS, in order to design therapeutic interventions which could be tested in those patients with the most to gain. Hudson *et al.* reported a sensitivity of 79 percent for diagnosing ARDS based on the following risk factors: sepsis, multiple transfusions, pulmonary contusion, aspiration, near-drowning, multiple fractures, and drug overdose.[6] At the study institution, 21 percent of patients who developed ARDS did not have any of the above risk factors, but did have such conditions as pneumonia, head injury, and subarachnoid hemorrhage.[6] Additional studies have confirmed the importance of pneumonia, pancreatitis, and central nervous system insult in developing ARDS.[7,8] Host factors may also impact the predilection for acute lung injury. Chronic alcohol use,[6,51] chronic lung disease,[6] and underlying hepatic disease[52] have all been reported to increase the incidence of ARDS.

Box 10C.1 lists many of the more common risk factors for the development of ALI and ARDS. Some authors find it helpful to think of the etiologies of ALI as either direct or pulmonary – such as pulmonary contusion, pneumonia, or aspiration – or as indirect/extrapulmonary.[53] Examples of the latter include such risks as sepsis, hypotension, severe trauma, or pancreatitis. Direct or indirect injury to the lung may impart different lung mechanics and could impact the lung's response to therapy, although to date no large trial has prospectively studied therapy in the two groups.

PATHOGENESIS

Acute lung injury and its most severe form, ARDS, result from an inflammatory process in the lung which induces damage to the alveoli, and thus the extrusion of proteinaceous fluid into the alveolar space.[54] In the normal lung, the alveolar–capillary barrier is the juxtaposition of the respiratory epithelial layer against the vascular endothelium. In cardiogenic edema, the greatly increased hydrostatic pressure within the microvasculature is the driving force to extrude fluid across the endothelium into the alveolar space.[38] In noncardiogenic edema, injury to both the vascular endothelium and the respiratory epithelium are

Box 10C.1 Clinical risk factors for ALI

Direct/pulmonary Injury

- Pneumonia: bacterial, viral, or fungal*
- Aspiration of gastric contents*
- Pulmonary contusion
- Fat emboli
- Inhalational injury
- Near-drowning

Indirect/extrapulmonary Injury

- Sepsis*
- Shock*
- Severe trauma*
- Hypertransfusion of blood products
- Acute pancreatitis
- Disseminated intravascular coagulopathy
- Antiphospholipid syndrome
- Drug overdose

*Most common; severe trauma defined as fracture of pelvis or more than one long bone; hypertransfusion defined as greater than 10 units packed red blood cells (PRBC) in 12 hours.

responsible.[18] The vascular endothelium is more permeable than the epithelium even under normal conditions, and in experimental models of ARDS, it becomes yet more leaky in response to endotoxin.[55] Damage to the epithelial barrier is equally important, however. The respiratory epithelial type II cells, which normally comprise only 10 percent of the alveolar surface area, proliferate in response to damage. The normal function of type II cells include fluid and ion transport across the alveolar surface, production of surfactant, and differentiation into the flat type I cells.[18,39] When injury occurs, despite proliferation of type II cells, their normal function is impaired, such that edema is slow to resolve and surfactant production is decreased.[18,56,57]

ARDS has been postulated to result from activation of the complement cascade with elaboration of superoxide radicals by neutrophils; or from a disorder of intravascular coagulation and fibrinolysis; or as the end result of toxic oxygen therapy and shear stresses caused by the ventilator.[18,58] The potential biologic factors driving this epithelial and endothelial injury are legion, and include proinflammatory cytokines such as interleukin (IL)-1, -6, -8, -10 and tumor necrosis factor (TNF)-α; lipid mediators; oxidants; growth factors; coagulation factors; components of the complement system; endothelial products; and vasoactive substances such as nitric oxide.[18,58,59] Parallel to the studies investigating clinical risk factors for ARDS have been multiple investigations to define a molecular marker of early lung injury which might predict which patients will develop ALI.[58] None has yet been successful in finding an easily measured substance with well-defined clinical relevance. Although science has yet to elucidate the precise sequence of events in the generation of diffuse alveolar damage, it seems credible that at its heart, ALI results from an imbalance between mediators of inflammation and repair at the alveolar–capillary barrier. It may be that the patients who survive ARDS are those in whom this balance is restored more effectively, whereas those who succumb have persistent elaboration of inflammatory mediators.

MANAGEMENT

In treating ALI, despite over 30 years of intensive research, no pharmacologic therapy has yet proved efficacious either in limiting the extent of injury or in promoting resolution. The focus of therapy therefore centers on therapy which has proved beneficial: a lung-protective ventilation strategy with appropriate attempts to diagnose and treat the inciting event.

Mechanical ventilation

The vast majority of patients with ARDS, and most with ALI, present with respiratory failure necessitating intubation and mechanical ventilation. Mechanical ventilation serves a multitude of purposes in ARDS, but chief among these is the ability to decrease the body's oxygen consumption by taking over the work of breathing, and to provide PEEP. Early pathologic studies raised the possibility that ventilator support not only healed, but also potentially induced lung injury,[21] thus begging the question of whether oxygen therapy or the ventilator itself damaged the alveolar–capillary membrane. Numerous animal studies reveal that oxygen therapy provokes lung damage ranging from destruction of the alveolar–capillary barrier to severe pneumonitis, and that the injury appears to be mediated by reactive oxygen intermediates.[60]

In studying the nonsurvivors of the extracorporeal membrane oxygenation project in 1979, Pratt et al. found that the degree of pathologic lung findings correlated with the patients' duration of exposure to oxygen therapy.[21] Patients in this group had progressed to fibrosing alveolitis even with as little as 50 percent FiO_2. Physiologic studies in normal subjects found that those given 60 percent oxygen or higher for 3 or more days developed a marked reduction in diffusion capacity.[61] Nonetheless, the toxic threshold of oxygen is controversial, and it may be that injured lungs behave differently on exposure to high-level oxygen than do normal lungs. A retrospective study examining patients receiving high FiO_2 for greater than 48 hours found no significant difference between survivors and nonsurvivors for exposure time to FiO_2 of 0.9 or more.[62] Moreover, the total duration of ventilation with FiO_2 over 0.5 was higher in survivors than nonsurvivors.[62] Nevertheless, a multivariate analysis revealed that exposure of oxygen therapy of 0.9 or more for 4 days was significantly associated with death.[62] Further studies on the relation of lung injury to oxygen and hyperoxia in both normal and impaired lungs are lacking. However, we advocate using the least possible FiO_2 to allow arterial oxygen saturation (SaO_2) of at least 88 percent, or a PaO_2 equal to or greater than 50 mm Hg. These values, although below normal physiologic values, have been tested in large trials of ALI with mortality between 25 percent and 40 percent.[63,64] No absolute threshold for toxic FiO_2 has been established, yet we aim to lower the FiO_2 below 60 percent while meeting the above oxygenation goals, and use PEEP to accomplish this.

While acknowledging the potential toxicity of oxygen therapy, it is equally critical to provide appropriate oxygen delivery to all vital tissues. These conflicting goals of therapy in ARDS have largely been resolved through the use of PEEP, which was perhaps the first recognized therapy for ARDS.[1,2] PEEP has been demonstrated to increase functional residual capacity and appears to recruit collapsed alveoli, thus reducing the fraction of nonaerated lung and improving oxygenation.[2,65] It may be that PEEP decreases ventilator-induced lung injury by decreasing mechanical shear forces caused by repetitive opening and closing of alveoli in atelectatic regions of the lung, or by reducing stretch between aerated and nonaerated regions.[64,66] The effects of PEEP may extend beyond lung mechanics, however; the concept of mechanotransduction – by which physical forces on the cell membrane or receptors are converted to cell-signaling pathways – would suggest that by altering shear forces, PEEP manipulates the lung's inflammatory response.[66] Mechanical ventilation may also injure the lung through overdistension. Because injured alveoli in ALI are subject to increased edema and surfactant dysfunction, the inspiratory pressure necessary to open collapsed alveoli may be significantly increased.[18,66,67] This led many early clinicians to assume that high-volume ventilation – tidal volumes of between 12 mL and 15 mL per kilogram of ideal body weight (IBW) – would improve oxygen transport.[2] However, high volumes and the pressures they transmit may overdistend and damage previously uninjured alveoli, or may trigger production of inflammatory mediators which propagate lung injury or even multisystem organ failure.[66] It was these hypotheses which drove the investigation of ventilatory strategies aimed at minimizing further lung injury.

In 1979, a study used extracorporeal membrane oxygenation to allow reduction of tidal volume to 8–9 mL/kg in the study group, yet showed no change in mortality.[68] Likewise, a randomized clinical trial of extracorporeal carbon dioxide removal paired with low-frequency positive pressure ventilation failed to find any survival benefit.[69] Neither extracorporeal oxygenation nor carbon dioxide removal are considered useful for treatment of ARDS at this time. Normalization of arterial blood gases, and particularly of the $PaCO_2$, was a widely held goal of ventilation as physicians began to treat patients with ARDS. It was only with the publication of a successful approach of permissive

hypercapnia – reducing tidal volume to as low as 5 mL/kg IBW to keep the peak inspiratory pressure below 40 cm H_2O, and allowing the $PaCO_2$ to rise to as much as 70 mm Hg – that strategies to limit tidal volume and permit elevated $PaCO_2$ began to gain acceptance.[70,71] In one important trial, no significant difference in $PaCO_2$ was noted between survivors and nonsurvivors, and despite maximum $PaCO_2$ of as much as 140 mm Hg, no sodium bicarbonate or other alkali therapy was given.[70] The lowest pH recorded was 7.02, and the average pH was 7.23 at the time of maximum $PaCO_2$.[70] Certain patient populations might experience greater harm from respiratory acidosis, such as patients with elevated intracranial pressure and those with active myocardial ischemia. Such patients should be managed differently than the general population with ALI, and their target $PaCO_2$ should be below 45 mm Hg.

A Brazilian group applied these principles in 1998 with a randomized trial of 'open lung ventilation,' which compared traditional ventilation (12 mL/kg IBW tidal volumes and the lowest PEEP for acceptable oxygenation) with a strategy of limiting tidal volume to 6 mL/kg IBW and limiting driving pressure.[67] Driving pressure was maintained by using pressure-preset modes of ventilation, keeping the inspiratory pressure less than 40 cm H_2O and the difference between the inspiratory pressure and PEEP less than 20 cm H_2O.[67] The result was dramatic, despite the small number of patients enrolled; 38 percent of the patients in the protective ventilation/open lung group had died by 28 days compared with 71 percent of patients in the control group.[67] Criticisms of the study were that only 53 patients were enrolled and all at one center; that the control-group mortality was higher than would be predicted; that the mortality difference was only realized at 28 days; and that measurement of the lower inflection point of the pressure-volume curve – which this study used to determine a patient's optimal PEEP – is technically difficult and requires a heavily sedated or paralyzed patient.[18]

Following the publication of the open lung study, the ARDS network (ARDSNet) in the United States completed a large multicenter randomized trial investigating low versus traditional tidal volumes in ALI and ARDS. Patients in the experimental arm received ventilation with 6 mL/kg of predicted IBW or less to maintain their plateau pressure (P_{plat}) below 30 cm H_2O; patients in the traditional arm received 12 mL/kg or less, keeping their P_{plat} below 50 cm H_2O.[63] 861 patients were studied, and the trial was stopped early due to the reduced mortality observed in the low tidal volume group. Whereas 40 percent of patients receiving traditional tidal volumes died, only 31 percent of those receiving low tidal volumes died, and the latter group had an increase in the number of ventilator-free days.[63] It is worth emphasizing that each patient in this trial had his or her tidal volume (V_T) determined by predicted ideal body weight based on sex and height. The formula used to derive IBW for males equaled 50 + 0.91(height in centimeters − 152.4); for females, IBW = 45.5 + 0.91(height in centimeters − 152.4).

Thus for an average man of 177.8 cm (5 feet, 10 inches), IBW = 73 kg, and a protective, 6 mL/kg tidal volume is 438 mL. Likewise, for an average woman of 162.6 cm (5 feet, 4 inches), IBW = 55 kg, and a protective tidal volume is 330 mL. Table 10C.3 demonstrates the IBW for men and women of different height, along with the initial protective tidal volume for patients with ALI. By calculating the tidal volume of 6 mL/kg IBW, one obtains the initial V_T for that patient. However, as in the ARDSNet study, if the P_{plat} is above 30 cm H_2O despite the calculated V_T, tidal volume must be further reduced to as low as 4 mLkg IBW to pursue a lung protective strategy.[63] An interesting secondary endpoint of the study was a failure to demonstrate a difference in the rate of barotrauma between the low- and conventional-V_T groups.[63]

Table 10C.3 *Calculation of ideal body weight (IBW) and lung-protective tidal volume (V_T)*

Height in cm (inches)	IBW (kg)	Initial V_T (6 mL/kg)
Men*		
162.6 (64)	59.2	354 mL
165.1 (65)	61.5	369 mL
167.6 (66)	63.8	383 mL
170.2 (67)	66.1	397 mL
172.2 (68)	68.4	410 mL
175.3 (69)	70.7	424 mL
177.8 (70)	73	438 mL
180.3 (71)	75.3	452 mL
182.9 (72)	77.6	466 mL
185.4 (73)	79.9	479 mL
188.0 (74)	82.2	493 mL
195.6 (75)	84.5	507 mL
Women†		
149.9 (59)	45.5	273 mL
152.4 (60)	45.5	273 mL
154.9 (61)	47.8	287 mL
157.5 (62)	50.1	301 mL
160.0 (63)	52.4	314 mL
162.6 (64)	54.7	328 mL
165.1 (65)	57.0	342 mL
167.6 (66)	59.3	356 mL
170.2 (67)	61.6	370 mL
172.2 (68)	63.9	384 mL
175.3 (69)	66.2	397 mL
177.8 (70)	68.5	411 mL
180.3 (71)	70.8	425 mL

*IBW = 50 + 0.91 (height in cm − 152.4) or 50 + 2.3 (height in inches − 60).

†IBW = 45.5 + 0.91 (height in cm − 152.4) or 50 + 2.3 (height in inches − 60).

The dramatic benefit of reduced tidal volume naturally raises the question as to whether additional benefit can be achieved by further reducing tidal volume. Analysis of unpublished data from patients ventilated with an intermediate tidal volume of 9 mL/kg IBW shows

intermediate survival, supporting the notion of a dose–response relation. These findings have rekindled interest in high-frequency ventilation, not as a rescue mode, but rather as a way to reduce tidal volume to its absolute minimum.

The optimal level of PEEP in the treatment of ALI has also been a topic of considerable investigation. The 1998 AECC reported that PEEP levels which raised airway pressure above the lower inflection point of the lung/chest wall pressure–volume curve – typically 10–15 cm H_2O per the AECC – approached nearly complete recruitment of alveoli.[22] In contrast, in their open lung strategy, Amato *et al.* calculated bedside inspiratory and static pressure-volume curves in each patient, and set each patient's PEEP at 2 cm H_2O above the lower inflection point.[67] By this strategy, PEEP values in the protective ventilation group averaged 16 cm H_2O, compared to 7 cm H_2O for the conventional group, and the protective ventilation group had lower 28-day mortality.[67] To attempt to determine whether tidal volume or PEEP was of greater importance on mortality, ARDSNet recently completed a multicenter randomized trial comparing lower- versus higher-PEEP algorithms for the management of patients with ALI and ARDS.[64] The lower-PEEP group used the same strategy of adjusting PEEP and FiO_2 as did the low tidal volume ARDSNet study; PEEP and FiO_2 were adjusted in discrete steps to maintain SaO_2 between 88 percent and 95 percent, or PaO_2 between 55 mm Hg and 80 mm Hg.[63,64] By this pathway, for an FiO_2 of 1.0, PEEP was between 18 cm H_2O and 24 cm H_2O; for FiO_2 of 0.7 PEEP was 10–14 cm H_2O; and below 0.6 FiO_2, PEEP was below 10 cm H_2O.[64] In contrast, for the higher-PEEP group, PEEP was set at 22–24 cm H_2O for a FiO_2 of 1.0; 20 cm H_2O PEEP for FiO_2 of between 0.5 and 0.8; and PEEP of 12–14 cm H_2O for FiO_2 between 0.3 and 0.5.[64] Both groups were ventilated with a lung protective volume-controlled strategy, using tidal volumes of 6 mL/kg IBW or less and maintaining P_{plat} below 30 cm H_2O. There was no difference in clinical outcome whether a lower- or higher-PEEP pathway was used.[64] Mortality was unchanged between groups, as were the number of days breathing unassisted.[64] Perhaps as importantly, higher levels of PEEP did not impart harm to the 251 patients treated in the experimental arm. Pneumothorax and air leaks occurred with the same frequency in each group, as did circulatory, coagulation, hepatic, or renal failure.[64] Mortality for both groups was approximately 25 percent, significantly lower than previous studies.[63,64,67]

Reduction of PEEP, even for extremely short periods of time, is often met with rapid alveolar derecruitment and a precipitous fall in arterial hemoglobin saturation. Even brief disconnection from the ventilator for airway suctioning or for transport – when patients are often bag-ventilated – can have dramatic consequences to the patient's saturation, and impaired oxygenation may take hours to rectify. In light of this observation, we advocate that suctioning of the endotracheal tube be kept to a minimum after diagnostic samples have been obtained, and that patients be bag-ventilated with PEEP valves during transport. When titrating PEEP as patients' oxygenation status improves, we advocate gradual reduction of PEEP, often in increments of just 1 cm H_2O 30 or 60 minutes following a tolerated reduction in FiO_2 of 0.1.

Noninvasive positive pressure ventilation

With the knowledge that a successful treatment strategy for ALI involves PEEP to abolish cyclic opening and collapsing of the alveoli, and careful attention to tidal volume and P_{plat} to minimize lung overdistension, noninvasive positive pressure ventilation (NIPPV) beckons as a potentially ideal therapy. Using a well-fitting soft mask over either the mouth and nose or the nose alone, both PEEP and pressure support can be applied without the need for an endotracheal tube. Necessary criteria for the institution of NIPPV include a cooperative patient agreeable to application of the mask, preserved ability to protect one's airway, and a facial structure which is amenable to the mask. NIPPV has been well validated as an effective and intubation-sparing intervention for patients with acute exacerbations of chronic obstructive pulmonary disease (COPD) and with cardiogenic pulmonary edema.[71,72] However, early studies of patients with acute respiratory failure randomized either to NIPPV or to conventional oxygen therapy by Venturi mask found no significant reduction in intubation rates, mortality, or ICU length of stay for patients receiving NIPPV.[73,74] In 1998, a study randomized patients with acute hypoxemic respiratory failure – a quarter of whom had ARDS – to either NIPPV or intubation with mechanical ventilation, and found NIPPV to be as effective in improving gas exchange.[75] Moreover, the study found a significant decrease in the number of septic complications for patients who avoided intubation, as well as a shorter ICU length of stay.[75] A retrospective case-matched study found that the rate of nosocomial pneumonia and crude mortality were significantly reduced in patients receiving NIPPV compared with intubated patients.[76]

As perhaps the greatest advantage of NIPPV is its reduction in ventilator-associated pneumonia, the patient population who stand poised to reap its maximum benefit are those at highest risk for infection: immunocompromised patients. When compared with treatment with oxygen alone, NIPPV applied early in the course of respiratory distress has been shown to reduce the need for intubation and the ICU mortality of patients undergoing solid organ transplantation.[77] Hospital mortality did not differ between groups, and reduction in the rate of sepsis for patients receiving NIPPV narrowly missed achieving statistical significance ($P = 0.05$).[77] Subsequently, patients with immunosuppression stemming from medication, hematologic malignancy, or HIV infection, were randomized to early NIPPV or oxygen therapy and were found to have a decreased rate of intubation (odds ratio 0.6), ICU mortality,

and hospital mortality when NIPPV was used.[78] The superiority of NIPPV over conventional oxygen therapy for immunosuppressed patients with acute hypoxemic respiratory failure is thus readily apparent. Less clear, however, is the role of NIPPV in patients with shock, or with ALI. One multicenter prospective cohort study found that failure of NIPPV and progression to intubation was more far more common when patients had ARDS or community-acquired pneumonia causing their respiratory failure (odds ratio 4.77), when sepsis was present on study entry (odds ratio 3.13), or when the PaO_2/FiO_2 ratio was below 150 after 1 hour of NIPPV (odds ratio 3.06).[79] Rates of intubation were similar for patients with pulmonary or extrapulmonary causes of ARDS.[79] A recent randomized trial comparing NIPPV to conventional oxygen therapy in patients with acute hypoxemic respiratory failure disclosed a decreased rate of intubation, decreased ICU mortality, and increased 90-day survival for patients treated with NIPPV, but again found that ARDS was a major risk factor for intubation, with an adjusted odds ratio of 28.5.[80] Not only did the control group in this study undergo intubation more frequently, but control patients were significantly more likely to develop septic shock.[80] Owing to a lack of convincing benefit for NIPPV over conventional intubation and mechanical ventilation in patients with ARDS, we cannot advocate its routine use except for patients with underlying immunosuppression, early in their course of dyspnea.

In summary, our recommended ventilatory approach to a patient with ALI or ARDS is as follows:

- Maintain adequate oxygen delivery, titrating therapy to a pulse oximeter SaO_2 of 88–95 percent or PaO_2 of 55–80 mm Hg. There is no evidence that SaO_2 of 95 percent is superior to 88 percent.
- Minimize oxygen toxicity by using adequate PEEP to allow FiO_2 of below 0.6 as quickly as feasible.
- Titrate PEEP to an adequate oxygen saturation while maintaining inspiratory P_{plat} ≤30 cm H_2O. In general, increase PEEP quickly and withdraw PEEP quite gently.
- Using a volume-controlled mode of ventilation, initial tidal volume should be 6 mLkg IBW *or less*, maintaining P_{plat} ≤30 cm H_2O. Table 10C.3 shows how to calculate IBW. If hypercapnia results, as it does in approximately 10 percent of patients, it is tolerable to $PaCO_2$ levels of up to 80 mm Hg.
- An initial respiratory rate of between 20 and 30 breaths/min is typically sufficient for patients with ALI. Respiratory rate may be titrated to help offset the fall in $\dot{V}_E$ with low V_T, although it is rarely helpful to raise the respiratory rate above 36 breaths/minute. We do not advocate use of sodium bicarbonate to mitigate respiratory acidosis caused by low-V_T strategies.
- Sedation and analgesia to allow patients to tolerate volume-controlled ventilation is necessary and appropriate, but should be lifted daily to assess a patient's neurologic function and need for ventilation.[81] Paralysis

is infrequently necessary and carries substantial risk, so should be avoided when possible.

- Liberation from the ventilator for patients with ARDS is no different than for patients with other forms of respiratory failure, and spontaneous breathing trials should occur at regular intervals once a patient is awake, protecting their airway, and with $FiO_2 \leq 0.4$ and PEEP $\leq 8\,cm\,H_2O$.

Experimental and salvage therapies

In certain patients with severe ARDS, even our validated low-V_T/low P_{plat} approach is unsuccessful. Among the various strategies employed in this situation, several have been proved to be safe and a few may be as effective as our conventional therapy. High-frequency oscillatory ventilation (HFOV) oscillates the lung at a set airway pressure, often a pressure higher than that used in conventional pressure- or volume-controlled ventilation. While oscillating pressures can be measured at the endotracheal tube, in experimental models, the pressure fluctuations at the alveolar level are significantly attenuated.[82] Theoretically, HFOV avoids both lung overdistension and the cyclic collapse/reexpansion of alveoli, the two mechanisms purported to cause ventilator-induced lung injury, by maintaining a constant level of alveolar recruitment.[82] The mechanism of gas exchange in this model of ventilation is not fully understood, but may be due to enhanced axial diffusion of gases.[82] A recent randomized controlled trial found HFOV to have comparable mortality to conventional therapy in patients with ARDS.[82] The 'conventional therapy' group in this trial did not uniformly receive low tidal volume ventilation nor were plateau pressures kept routinely below $30\,cm\,H_2O$, but with these reservations it seems that HFOV is safe for patients with ARDS, and further clinical trials would be fruitful.

Partial liquid ventilation (PLV) employs perfluorocarbon to fill the lungs to a volume approaching functional residual capacity (FRC) and then gas ventilate the lungs with a mechanical ventilator.[83] Because perfluorocarbon is immiscible with aqueous solutions and has a high oxygen and carbon dioxide carrying capacity, it theoretically could improve gas exchange, decrease shunt, and increase lung compliance.[83] A phase I nonrandomized pilot study using PLV in adults with ALI on extracorporeal life support found that although oxygenation did improve, PLV did not cause any significant change in lung function.[84] Subsequently, a prospective randomized pilot study of PLV versus conventional ventilation in 90 patients was completed.[85] In the context of this trial, conventional therapy did not consist of a V_T-limited strategy, but rather aimed for an arterial oxygen saturation greater than 90 percent, a $PaCO_2$ <50 mm Hg, and P_{plat} <45 mm Hg. The trial found no difference between groups for mortality, PaO_2/FiO_2 ratio, or the number of ventilator-free days.[85] It did find a statistically significant

reduction in the rate of progression from ALI to ARDS in the patients with less severe gas exchange derangement at enrollment.[85] At this time, PLV can be considered an experimental therapy, and to date it has not been definitively tested against a lung-protective ventilation strategy.

Inverse ratio ventilation (IRV) is pressure-cycled or volume-cycled ventilation employing a prolonged inspiratory time (I:E ratio ≥ 1) in the hopes of decreasing physiologic dead space and better mixing of alveolar and bronchial gases.[86] In a subset of patients, observational studies suggest that IRV can provide better oxygenation when conventional ventilation is met with refractory hypoxemia. In randomized controlled trials, however, the promise of IRV has not borne out. One study compared ventilation with an I:E ratio of 2:1 to a conventional arm in which I:E equaled 1:2.[87] Tidal volume and PEEP were constant between arms, with each patient acting as their own crossover. After 6 hours, IRV resulted in a lower cardiac index and lower oxygen delivery (DO_2) without altering P_{plat} or PaO_2.[87] $PaCO_2$ was diminished, supporting the notion that IRV enhances elimination of carbon dioxide.[87] The fall in cardiac output may have been as a result of increased intrinsic PEEP – also called auto-PEEP – at the expense of extrinsic or applied PEEP, resulting in a higher mean airway pressure and thus a higher mean alveolar pressure, which impairs venous return.[86] More recently, a study randomized patients to an inverse ratio of I:E of 2:1 or 4:1 versus traditional I:E of 1:2 while keeping mean airway pressure constant, and observed no fall in cardiac output or DO_2 but an actual reduction in both arterial and venous oxygenation.[86] Auto-PEEP was increased by almost $3\,cm\,H_2O$ in the 2:1 arm and over $6\,cm\,H_2O$ in the 4:1 arm.[86] Although it is possible that applying IRV over an extended period of time may recruit a previously collapsed subset of lung tissue, the increase in auto-PEEP without documented improvement in oxygenation leads us to question the utility of IRV.

Extracorporeal gas exchange for either oxygenation or carbon dioxide removal from the bloodstream offers theoretical advantages to patients with ARDS, but several clinical trials have shown it to be ineffective. In 1979, a prospective trial of extracorporeal membrane oxygenation (ECMO) for patients with ARDS detected no survival benefit.[68] Patients enrolled in the trial were severely ill, and the overall mortality was 92 percent across both arms of the study.[68] Extracorporeal carbon dioxide removal ($ECCO_2R$), tested in a randomized controlled trial of 40 patients likewise did not increase survival.[88] In fact, the treatment arm receiving $ECCO_2R$ had a trend toward reduced 30-day survival and had excess bleeding, as extracorporeal support requires anticoagulation.[88] As such, both ECMO and $ECCO_2R$ are best regarded as salvage or heroic therapy for patients in whom all other measures have failed.

One technological advancement generating interest for improved therapy in ARDS is the intravenous oxygenator (IVOX). This is a hollow-fiber membrane oxygenator mounted on a central catheter and inserted into the patient's superior vena cava.[89] In theory, this device is an intracorporeal extrapulmonary gas exchanger.[89] Although no prospective clinical trial using IVOX has yet been published, a phase II trial to establish its safety in patients with ARDS disclosed 50 percent short-term and 60 percent overall mortality.[89] Over the 48 hours studied, patients' average PaO_2/FiO_2 ratio did improve – from 79 at baseline to approximately 120 – although PaO_2/FiO_2 ratio correlates poorly with survival.[89] Complications reported included bleeding with device insertion and deep venous thrombosis in 4 of 20 patients.[89] It will be interesting to observe this technology as it advances, but at present there is no role for IVOX in the treatment for ARDS.

Finally, because ALI causes inhomogeneous distribution of pulmonary consolidation, often with marked gravity dependence, changes in position can considerably impact oxygenation in approximately 75 percent of patients.[27–29,90,91] Repositioning to the decubitus or prone position redistributes lung perfusion and can reduce the plateau airway pressure, despite reducing lung/chest wall compliance.[91] A multicenter randomized trial evaluating prone positioning for 6 hours per day over 10 days found no survival benefit for patients with ALI.[92] However, a significant increase in PaO_2/FiO_2 ratio was observed, and a mortality benefit at 10 days was observed in the sickest patients, though this mortality benefit did not persist beyond discharge from the ICU.[92] Complications from prone position include an increase in pressure sores at the new weight-bearing sites, such as cheekbone, thorax, breast, iliac crest, and knee,[92] as well as the potential for retinal ischemia from pressure on the eye. Surprisingly, prone positioning did not increase the rate of loss of venous or endotracheal access, but did demand a high nursing cost (on average, four people were required to turn each patient) and increased levels of sedation.[92] As such, prone positioning appears safe and may be beneficial in patients with severe, refractory hypoxemia.

Pharmacologic interventions

CIRCULATORY MANAGEMENT

Acute lung injury represents a severe defect of fluid handling at the alveolar–capillary barrier. As such, a strategy of minimizing edema fluid by maintaining the minimum necessary circulating volume has considerable appeal. In animal models of ARDS, lowering the left atrial pressure effectively reduced edema formation.[93,94] In a retrospective review of patients with ARDS and a PAC, patients who underwent a 25 percent reduction in the P_{pw} over the initial 48 hours had a significantly improved survival compared with patients whose P_{pw} did not fall by 25 percent (75 percent vs. 29 percent), even when correcting for severity of illness.[95] A second clinical study, although small, found that reducing the positive fluid balance for critically ill patients was associated with a reduction in the number of days on the ventilator and in the ICU.[96] A large, randomized trial is currently underway to assess a fluid-liberal versus a fluid-conservative approach, guided by PAC versus central venous catheters.[97] Awaiting these data, it seems prudent to attempt to maintain adequate perfusion at the lowest possible intravascular volume.[18] Vasoactive medications are occasionally necessary to attain adequate perfusion.

CORTICOSTEROIDS

As the pathophysiology of ALI came to be recognized as a seemingly unregulated inflammatory response of the lung, many physicians hoped that corticosteroid therapy would prove fruitful in the prevention or treatment of ARDS. One early trial of methylprednisolone in patients with septic shock suggested that although mortality was unchanged for patients receiving steroids, respiratory insufficiency might be less.[98] Two further studies of glucocorticoids in sepsis did not support this finding.[99,100] A randomized trial of methylprednisolone (30 mg/kg every 6 hours) versus placebo for patients with ARDS found no difference in mortality or oxygenation over 45 days.[101] The subgroup of patients with sepsis as the precipitant of ARDS likewise experienced no effect on survival from steroids.[101] A second study comparing methylprednisolone with placebo in patients with sepsis failed to show a reduction in mortality or the development of ARDS.[102] Thus the AECC did not find a role for corticosteroids in treating the acute phase of ALI/ARDS.[22]

In contrast, for the subset of patients with ARDS and prolonged respiratory failure who develop fibroproliferative lung changes, corticosteroid treatment has remained of interest.[103] Meduri and colleagues performed a randomized controlled trial of high-dose, prolonged methylprednisolone therapy in unresolving ARDS and reported reduced mortality and increased successful extubation for patients receiving corticosteroids.[104] Because this was a small study (24 patients) with a high rate of crossover from placebo to treatment arm, there are difficulties in extrapolating this study to all patients with late ARDS. Toward that end, a large clinical trial sponsored by the National Institutes of Health was performed[105] and has been reported at an international meeting, but has not yet been subjected to peer review. This study showed no clear benefit to corticosteroid therapy and no difference in mortality or ICU length of stay. There was, however, a modest reduction in time on the ventilator for those receiving corticosteroids. The results of this trial will surely dampen enthusiasm for steroid treatment of late-stage ARDS, but it remains possible that some adjustment of dose could convert the reduced time on the ventilator to a more meaningful outcome.

INHALED NITRIC OXIDE

Inhaled nitric oxide (iNO) is a local vasodilator typically released from the vascular endothelium. Because iNO binds rapidly and with high affinity to hemoglobin, it is rapidly inactivated in the circulation and causes no systemic vasodilation.[106,107] Theoretically, iNO might have the ideal effect on gas exchange in ARDS, by dilating the pulmonary capillaries of ventilated alveoli yet having no effect on nonventilated, flooded alveoli or on systemic blood pressure.[106] An observational trial of 10 patients with severe ARDS receiving iNO was promising, as iNO significantly increased patients' PaO_2/FiO_2 ratio while lowering the pulmonary artery pressure.[106] Several randomized, controlled trials of iNO versus placebo in patients with ALI/ARDS have found improvement in oxygenation but no change on mortality or duration of mechanical ventilation with the delivery of iNO.[107–109] The PaO_2/FiO_2 ratio of patients receiving iNO tends to improve more rapidly over the first 12–24 hours compared with patients receiving placebo; however beyond 24 hours, PaO_2/FiO_2 ratios of the two groups equalize.[109] Most recently, a randomized trial of low dose iNO – 5 parts per million (ppm) as opposed to the more traditional 10–40 ppm dose – had no effect on mortality or on duration of ventilatory support.[110] Although it may have an experimental role for treating severe refractory hypoxemia, iNO thus cannot be advocated for the treatment of ALI/ARDS. Less selective vasodilators, such as prostaglandin E, have likewise not been found beneficial.[18,111]

SURFACTANT

ARDS has inevitably drawn comparisons to neonatal respiratory distress syndrome, and derangements in surfactant production and function in patients with ARDS clearly contribute to the syndrome's pathogenesis.[56,57] Nonetheless, although synthetic surfactant therapy in premature infants is credited for the largest drop in infant mortality in the United States in 20 years,[112] the benefit of surfactant administration to adults with ALI/ARDS is far less certain. A randomized study of aerosolized surfactant in patients with ARDS caused by sepsis found no significant difference in 30-day mortality or duration of ventilation between surfactant and placebo.[113] Mortality was 60 percent in both groups, and surfactant did not improve oxygenation or peak airway pressure.[113] Addressing concerns that aerosol delivered an insufficient dose of surfactant in the above trial, a pilot study of a novel recombinant surfactant instilled into the lungs of patients with ARDS likewise failed to show a statistically significant effect on mortality or duration of ventilatory support.[114] A larger randomized trial comparing endotracheal-instilled surfactant to placebo found an initial improvement in oxygenation over the first 24 hours with surfactant, but again failed to show any mortality benefit.[115] Synthetic surfactant is therefore not indicated for ARDS.

KETOCONAZOLE

Two randomized, placebo-controlled studies in critically ill surgical patients found ketoconazole, a thromboxane A_2 synthetase inhibitor, significantly decreased the incidence of ARDS.[116,117] One of the studies, performed on 54 surgical patients with sepsis, found that not only was the frequency of ARDS decreased from 64 percent in the placebo group to 15 percent in the ketoconazole group, but that mortality was also reduced.[117] However, a large randomized trial by ARDSNet failed to detect a difference in mortality, ventilator-free days, or organ failure-free days when ketoconazole was given early in the treatment of ALI/ARDS.[118] Thus, there is no role for ketoconazole in treating ALI/ARDS.

OUTCOMES

Mortality

Collecting accurate data on mortality from ARDS has been fraught with many of the same problems which plague incidence studies; difficulties surrounding the definition of the syndrome itself and its reference population can create varied results. In the initial published report of the syndrome in 1967, 7 of 12 patients died.[1] A larger series – 88 patients in three hospitals in Denver, Colorado – recorded a 65 percent mortality in 1983.[3] Villar and Slutsky, studying the population of the Canary Islands in Spain, noted a mortality of 70 percent among those patients with severe hypoxemia (PaO_2/FIO_2 ratio of 110 or less) due to ARDS versus 50 percent for those with PaO_2/FIO_2 ratio of 150 or less.[11] With apparent mortality rates of 50–70 percent, the prognosis for anyone diagnosed with ARDS appeared grim. In 1995 came a glimmer of hope; publishing their hospital's mortality trend over the past decade, a group reported that overall ARDS case fatality had decreased substantially – to under 50 percent.[119] Supporting this assertion, the ARDSNet study of low tidal volumes in ARDS found a mortality of 40 percent for patients receiving traditional ventilation versus 31 percent for those receiving low tidal volume ventilation,[63] and a recent study on PEEP in ARDS reported a mortality of approximately 27 percent.[64]

Even in the recent era of a widely accepted AECC definition of ARDS, however, mortality findings vary between 25 percent and 60 percent. The discrepancy results in part from studying populations with ALI (PaO_2/FIO_2 ratio <300) compared with ARDS (PaO_2/FIO_2 ratio <200). Studying both syndromes, Luhr et al. found that mortality was equivalent; 42 percent for ALI and 41 percent for ARDS.[13] In subsequent studies, results for ALI compared with ARDS have been inconsistent. A 2-month study of Australian ICUs found 32 percent mortality for ALI on the day of diagnosis, 34 percent for ARDS, and 15 percent for patients with ALI who did not progress to ARDS, which represented a minority of ALI cases.[16] Two-thirds of patients with ALI on day 1 progressed to ARDS during their hospital stay.[13] Another prospective observational study performed at multiple ICUs across Europe found 60 percent mortality for patients with ARDS, compared to 31 percent for patients who did not meet criteria for ARDS; this latter group included patients with ALI, patients with unilateral pulmonary infiltrates, and patients with heart failure.[17] A recent study of 460 patients with ALI and ARDS found a striking difference in mortality between the two groups: 18 percent versus 58 percent, respectively.[120] Authors have remarked that the mortality rate reported in randomized controlled trials – such as 27 percent recently reported by the ARDSNet[64] – is often significantly lower than that reported in observational studies,[14,121] which may reflect either tighter adherence to proved lung-protective strategies or exclusion of patients with risky comorbidities.

Causes of mortality in ARDS have likewise evolved over time. Whereas respiratory failure was considered the cause of death in up to 75 percent of patients in early observational studies,[122] subsequent publications recognize the increasing importance of multisystem organ failure, or sepsis. In 1985, Montgomery et al. reported that only 16 percent of all ARDS deaths were directly attributable to respiratory failure.[123] Rather, 73 percent of patients who died 3 or more days after the onset of ARDS succumbed to sepsis, and sepsis was six times more likely in ARDS patients than in critically ill trauma patients without the syndrome.[123] Suchyta et al. prospectively studied 215 patients with ARDS, and found that 40 percent died from respiratory failure and 32 percent from sepsis.[8] It appears that multisystem organ failure (MSOF) and sepsis are thus equally likely as progressive respiratory failure to kill patients with ARDS. Efforts to further impact survival in ARDS may hinge on reducing MSOF in these at-risk patients.

Long-term outcomes

As we document improved acute survival for patients with ALI and ARDS, the necessary corollary is that a larger number of patients are living with the potential for long-term effects of ALI. Early studies focused on the long-term pulmonary function of survivors of ARDS. Despite the severe lung dysfunction in ARDS, most survivors will have normal or nearly normal pulmonary function within 6–12 months.[124] A recent prospective study of over 100 survivors of ARDS found that although FVC and forced expiratory volume in 1 second (FEV_1) improved from below 75 percent of predicted to normal within 6–12 months, the diffusing capacity of carbon monoxide (D_LCO) remained low.[125] Impairment of D_LCO did improve over time, from 63 percent at 3 months to 72 percent of predicted at 12 months, but the abnormality did persist at 12 months.[125] From a functional assessment, patients had a lower than predicted 6-minute walk distance even at 12 months, which the patients attributed to musculoskeletal problems as well as dyspnea.[125] By multivariate analysis, it appeared that the strongest predictor of distance walked in 6 minutes was the absence of corticosteroid therapy, raising the possibility that corticosteroids significantly contribute to the functional impairment of patients with ARDS.[125]

A more difficult outcome to measure is quality of life following ALI. Survivors of ALI/ARDS have reported persistent symptoms such as cough, chest tightness, and wheezing, and score similarly to patients with serious chronic illness on validated health surveys.[126] Although the level of such pulmonary symptomatology is mild in comparison with that of patients with severe COPD, patients recovering from ARDS are persistently more symptomatic than normal controls.[127] Compared with population norms, patients who have survived ARDS report significant reductions in health-related quality of life (HRQoL) measures. One study found that patients' HRQoL scores improved from hospital discharge to 6 months post-discharge, but these scores remained below normal compared with the population at large.[124] Another study found that ARDS patients scored significantly lower on HRQoL measures even when compared with severity-matched critically ill controls, defined as patients in the ICU with sepsis or trauma but without ARDS.[128] Statistically and clinically significant reductions were found in such domains as physical functioning, social functioning, and mental health.[128] When screened for depression, 73 percent of survivors of ARDS in the short term and 25 percent of patients a year after recovery for ARDS scored likely to be depressed.[126] Posttraumatic stress disorder was reported in one study at a frequency of 22 percent in patients who had survived ARDS, notably higher than in age-matched patients undergoing maxillofacial surgery (12 percent) or German soldiers who had served with the United Nations in Cambodia (2 percent).[129] Emphasizing the variability of outcomes in ARDS is the fact that many survivors – up to 70 percent – return to work within 6–12 months, and many return to their original position.[127,129]

DIRECTIONS FOR THE FUTURE

Although substantial progress has been made elucidating the pathophysiology and ventilator management of ALI and ARDS, mortality remains high. Active research abounds in many facets of ALI, both at the basic science and the clinical level, and multicenter efforts in both the United States and Europe are greatly improving and standardizing our patient care. As we further elucidate the complex process of inflammation and repair in the acutely injured lung, we may yet add effective pharmacologic therapies to our arsenal in caring for these acutely ill patients.

Key learning points

- Acute lung injury is an inflammatory process of damage to the alveolar–capillary membrane, which may be incited by a variety of initial insults.

- Acute respiratory distress syndrome describes patients at the most severe end of the spectrum of ALI.

- Both ALI and ARDS are commonly encountered in the ICU, and frequently go unrecognized.

- Clinicians should actively seek an alternative diagnosis when certain 'at-risk' conditions for ARDS – sepsis, pneumonia, aspiration – are absent, since specific, treatable conditions that mimic ARDS may be present.

- Mechanical ventilation is the mainstay of therapy for ALI and ARDS; tidal volumes should be 6 mL/kg of IBW or less, and P_{PLAT} should be kept below 30 cm H_2O.

- Positive end-expiratory pressure should be employed to keep the fraction of inspired oxygen (Fio_2) in the nontoxic range while achieving an arterial oxygen saturation above 87 percent.

- To date, no pharmacologic intervention has been proved to change the outcome of ARDS.

- Mortality in ARDS remains high at nearly 30 percent; long-term sequelae include dyspnea, neuromuscular weakness, and psychologic stress.

REFERENCES

1. Ashbaugh DG, Bigelow DB, Petty TL, Levine BE. Acute respiratory distress in adults. *Lancet* 1967, **2**: 319–23.

2. Petty TL, Ashbaugh DG. The adult respiratory-distress syndrome: clinical features, factors influencing prognosis, and principals of management. *Chest* 1971; **60**: 233–9.

3. Fowler AA, Hamman RF, Good JT, *et al.* Adult respiratory distress syndrome: risk with common predispositions. *Ann Intern Med* 1983: **98**; 593–7.

4. Bernard GB, Artigas A, Brigham KL, *et al.* The American-European Consensus Conference on ARDS: definitions, mechanisms, relevant outcomes, and clinical trial coordination. *Am J Respir Crit Care Med* 1994; **149**: 818–24.

5. Pepe PE, Potkin RT, Hudson LD, *et al.* Clinical predictors of the adult respiratory distress syndrome. *Am J Surg* 1982; **144**: 124–30.

6. Hudson LD, Milberg JA, Anardi D, Maunder RJ. Clinical risks for the development of the acute respiratory distress syndrome. *Am J Respir Crit Care Med* 1995; **151**: 293–301.

7. Sloane PJ, Gee MH, Gottlieb JE, Albertine KH, *et al.*

A multicenter registry of patients with acute respiratory distress syndrome. *Am Rev Respir Dis* 1992; **146**: 419–26.

8. Suchyta MR, Clemmer TP, Elliott CG, *et al.* The adult respiratory distress syndrome: a report of survival and modifying factors. *Chest* 1992; **101**: 1074–9.

9. Conference report: mechanisms of acute respiratory failure. *Am Rev Respir Dis* 1977; **115**: 1071–8.

10. Webster NR, Cohen AT, Nunn JF. Adult respiratory distress syndrome – how many cases in the UK? *Anaesthesia* 1988; **43**: 923–6.

11. Villar J, Slutsky AS. The incidence of the adult respiratory distress syndrome. *Am Rev Respir Dis* 1989; **140**: 814–16.

12. Thomsen GE, Morris AH. Incidence of the adult respiratory distress syndrome in the state of Utah. *Am J Respir Crit Care Med* 1995; **152**: 965–71.

13. Luhr OR, Antonsen A, Karlsson M, *et al.* Incidence and mortality after acute respiratory failure and acute respiratory distress syndrome in Sweden, Denmark, and Iceland. *Am J Respir Crit Care Med* 1999; **159**: 1849–61.

14. Arroliga AC, Ghamra ZW, Perez Tripichio A, *et al.* Incidence of ARDS in an adult population of northeast Ohio. *Chest* 2002; **121**: 1972–6.

15. Goss CH, Brower RG, Hudson LE, Rubenfeld GD. Incidence of acute lung injury in the United States. *Crit Care Med* 2003; **31**: 1607–11.

16. Bernsten AD, Edibam C, Hunt T, Moran J. Incidence and mortality of acute lung injury and the acute respiratory distress syndrome in three Australian states. *Am J Respir Crit Care Med* 2002; **165**: 443–8.

17. Roupie E, Lepage E, Wysocki M, *et al.* Prevalence, etiologies, and outcome of the acute respiratory distress syndrome among hypoxemic ventilated patients. *Intensive Care Med* 1999; **25**: 920–9.

18. Ware LB, Matthay MA. The acute respiratory distress syndrome. *N Engl J Med* 2000; **342**: 1334–49.

19. Lamy M, Fallat RJ, Koeniger E, Dietrich HP, *et al.* Pathologic features and mechanisms of hypoxemia in adult respiratory distress syndrome. *Am Rev Respir Dis* 1976; **114**: 267–84.

20. Aberle DR, Wiener-Kronish JP, Webb WR, Matthay MA. Hydrostatic versus increased permeability pulmonary edema: diagnosis based on radiographic criteria in critically ill patients. *Radiology* 1988; **168**: 73–9.

21. Pratt PC, Vollmer RT, Shelburne JD, Crapo JD. Pulmonary morphology in a multihospital

collaborative extracorporeal membrane oxygenation project. *Am J Pathol* 1979; **95**: 191–214.

✱ 22. Artigas A, Bernard GB, Carlet J, *et al.* The American-European consensus conference on ARDS, Part 2: ventilatory, pharmacologic, supportive therapy, study design strategies, and issues related to recovery and remodeling. *Am J Respir Crit Care Med* 1998; **157**: 1332–47.

23. Murray JF, Matthay MA, Luce JM, Flick MR. An expanded definition of the adult respiratory distress syndrome. *Am Rev Respir Dis* 1988; **138**: 720–3. [Erratum in: *Am Rev Respir Dis* 1989; **139**: 1065.]

24. Milne EN, Pistolesi M, Miniati M, *et al.* The radiologic distinction of cardiogenic and noncardiogenic edema. *Am J Roentgenol* 1985; **144**: 879–94.

25. Ely EW, Smith AC, Chiles C, Aquino SL, *et al.* Radiologic determination of intravascular volume status using portable, digital chest radiography: a prospective investigation in 100 patients. *Crit Care Med* 2001; **29**: 1502–12.

26. Martin GS, Ely ES, Carrol FE, Bernard GR. Findings on the portable chest radiograph correlate with fluid balance in critically ill patients. *Chest* 2002; **122**: 2087–95.

27. Goodman LR. Congestive heart failure and adult respiratory distress syndrome: new insights using computed tomography. *Radiol Clin North Am* 1996; **34**: 33–46.

28. Gattoni L, Bombino M, Pelosi P, *et al.* Lung structure and function in different stages of severe adult respiratory distress syndrome. *JAMA* 1994; **271**: 1772–9.

29. Gattoni L, Pesenti A, Bombino M, *et al.* Relationships between lung computed tomographic density, gas exchange, and PEEP in acute respiratory failure. *Anesthesiology* 1988; **69**: 824–32.

30. Zimmerman JE, Goodman LR, Shahvari MB. Effect of mechanical ventilation and positive end-expiratory pressure (PEEP) on chest radiograph. *AJR* 1979; **133**: 811–15.

31. Connors AF Jr, McCaffree DR, Gray BA. Evaluation of right-heart catheterization in the critically ill patient without acute myocardial infarction. *N Engl J Med* 1983; **308**: 263–7.

32. Iberti TJ, Fischer EP, Leibowitz AB, *et al.* A multicenter study of physicians' knowledge of the pulmonary artery catheter. *JAMA* 1990; **264**: 2928–32.

33. Iberti TJ, Fischer EP, Leibowitz AB, *et al.* Assessment of critical care nurses' knowledge of the pulmonary artery catheter. *Crit Care Med* 1994; **22**: 1674–8.

34. Connors AF Jr, Speroff T, Dawson NV, *et al.* The effectiveness of right heart catheterization in the care of critically ill patients. *JAMA* 1996; **276**: 889–97.

35. Bernard GR, Sopko G, Cerra F, *et al.* Pulmonary artery catheterization and clinical outcomes. *JAMA* 2000; **283**: 2568–72.

36. Sandham JD, Hull RD, Brant RF, *et al.* A randomized, controlled trial of the use of pulmonary-artery catheters in high-risk surgical patients. *N Engl J Med* 2003; **348**: 5–14.

37. Richard C, Warszawski J, Anguel N, *et al.* Early use of the pulmonary artery catheter and outcomes in patients with shock and acute respiratory distress syndrome: a randomized controlled trial. *JAMA* 2003; **290**: 2713–20.

38. Fein A, Grossman RF, Murray JF, *et al.* The value of edema fluid protein measurement in patients with pulmonary edema. *Am J Med* 1979; **67**: 32–8.

39. Matthay MA, Wiener-Kronish JP. Intact epithelial barrier function is critical for the resolution of alveolar edema in humans. *Am Rev Respir Dis* 1990; **142**: 1250–7.

40. Schwartz MI, Albert RK. 'Imitators' of the ARDS: implications for diagnosis and treatment. *Chest* 2004; **125**: 1530–5.

41. Thomas CF, Limper AH. Pneumocystis pneumonia. *N Engl J Med* 2004; **350**: 2487–98.

42. Curtis JR, Yarnold PF, Schwartz DN, *et al.* Improvements in outcomes of acute respiratory failure for patients with human immunodeficiency virus-related *Pneumocystis carinii* pneumonia. *Am J Respir Crit Care Med* 2000; **162**: 393–8.

43. Wachter RM, Luce JM, Turner J, *et al.* Intensive care of patients with the acquired immunodeficiency syndrome: outcomes and changing patterns of utilization. *Am Rev Respir Dis* 1986; **134**: 891–6.

44. Philit F, Etienne-Mastroianni B, Parrot A, *et al.* Idiopathic acute eosinophilic pneumonia: a study of 22 patients. *Am J Respir Crit Care Med* 2002; **166**: 1235–9.

45. Nizami IY, Kissner DG, Visscher DW, Dubaybo BA. Idiopathic bronchiolitis obliterans with organizing pneumonia: an acute and life-threatening syndrome. *Chest* 1995; **108**: 271–7.

46. DaBroi U, Orefice U, Cahalin C, *et al.* ARDS after double extrinsic exposure hypersensitivity pneumonitis. *Intensive Care Med* 1999; **25**: 755–7.

47. Zacharisen MC, Schlueter DP, Kurup VP, Fink JN. The long-term outcome in acute, subacute, and chronic forms of pigeon breeder's disease hypersensitivity pneumonitis. *Ann Allergy Asthma Immunol* 2002; **88**: 175–82.

48. Schwartz MI, Brown KK. Small vessel vasculitis of the lung. *Thorax* 2000; **55**: 502–10.

49. American Thoracic Society/European Respiratory Society. American Thoracic Society/European Respiratory Society International Multidisciplinary Consensus Classification of the Idiopathic Interstitial Pneumonias. *Am J Respir Crit Care Med* 2002; **165**: 277–304.

50. Ryu JH, Myers JL, Swensen SJ. Bronchiolar disorders. *Am J Respir Crit Care Med* 2003; **168**: 1277–92.

51. Moss M, Bucher B, Moore FA *et al.* The role of chronic alcohol abuse in the development of acute respiratory distress syndrome in adults. *JAMA* 1996; **275**: 50–4.

52. Matuschak GM, Rinaldo JE. Organ interactions in the Adult Respiratory Distress Syndrome during sepsis: role of the liver in host defense. *Chest* 1988; **94**: 400–6.

● 53. Gattoni L, Pelosi P, Suter PM, *et al.* Acute respiratory distress syndrome caused by pulmonary and extrapulmonary disease: different syndromes? *Am J Respir Crit Care Med* 1998; **158**: 3–11.

54. Pugin J, Verghese G, Widmer M-C, Matthay MA. The alveolar space is the site of intense inflammatory and profibrotic reactions in the early phase of acute respiratory distress syndrome. *Crit Care Med* 1999; **27**: 304–12.

55. Wiener-Kronish JP, Albertine KH, Matthay MA. Differential responses of the endothelial and epithelial barriers of the lung in sheep to *Escherichia coli* endotoxin. *J Clin Invest* 1991; **88**: 864–75.

56. Greene KE, Wright JR, Steinberg KP, *et al.* Serial changes in surfactant-associated proteins in lung and serum before and after onset of ARDS. *Am J Respir Crit Care Med* 1999; **160**: 1843–50.

57. Lewis JF, Jobe AH. Surfactant and the adult respiratory distress syndrome. *Am Rev Respir Dis* 1993; **147**: 218–33. [Erratum in: *Am Rev Respir Dis* 1993; **147**: 1068.]

58. Connelly KG, Repine JE. Markers for predicting the development of acute respiratory distress syndrome. *Annu Rev Med* 1997; **48**: 429–45.

59. Rinaldo JE, Rogers RM. Adult respiratory-distress syndrome: changing concepts of lung injury and repair. *N Engl J Med* 1982; **306**: 900–9.

60. Mantell LL, Horowitz S, Davis JM, Kazzaz JA. Hyperoxia-induced cell death in the lung – the correlation of apoptosis, necrosis, and inflammation. *Ann N Y Acad Sci* 1999; **887**: 171–80.

61. Kapanci Y, Tosco R, Eggermann J, Gould V. Oxygen pneumonitis in man: light and electron-microscopy morphometric studies. *Chest* **62**: 162–9.

62. Capellier G, Beuret P, Clement G, *et al.* Oxygen tolerance in patients with acute respiratory failure. *Intensive Care Med* 1998; **24**: 422–8.

● 63. The Acute Respiratory Distress Syndrome Network. Ventilation with lower tidal volumes as compared with traditional tidal volumes for acute lung injury and the acute respiratory distress syndrome. *N Engl J Med* 2000; **248**: 1301–8.

● 64. The National Heart, Lung, and Blood Institute ARDS Clinical Trials Network. Higher versus lower positive end-expiratory pressures inpatients with the acute respiratory distress syndrome. *N Engl J Med* 2004; **351**: 327–36.

65. Gattinoni L, Pelosi P, Crotti S, Velenza F. Effects of positive end-expiratory pressure on regional distribution of tidal volume and recruitment in adult respiratory distress syndrome. *Am J Respir Crit Care* 1995; **151**: 1807–14.

66. Slutsky AS, Tremblay LN. Multiple system organ failure: is mechanical ventilation a contributing factor? *Am J Respir Crit Care Med* 1998; **157**: 1721–5.

● 67. Amato MB, Barbas CS, Medeiros DM, *et al.* Effect of a protective-ventilation strategy on mortality in the acute respiratory distress syndrome. *N Engl J Med* 1998; **338**: 347–54.

68. Zapol WM, Snider MT, Hill JD *et al.* Extracorporeal membrane oxygenation in severe acute respiratory failure: a randomized prospective study. *JAMA* 1979; **242**: 2193–6.

69. Morris AH, Wallace CJ, Menlove RL, *et al.* Randomized clinical trial of pressure-controlled inverse ratio ventilation and extracorporeal CO_2 removal for adult respiratory distress syndrome. *Am J Respir Crit Care Med* 1994; **149**: 295–305.

● 70. Hickling KG, Henderson SJ, Jackson R. Low mortality associated with low volume pressure limited ventilation with permissive hypercapnia in severe adult respiratory distress syndrome. *Intensive Care Med* 1990; **16**: 372–7.

71. Brouchard L, Mancebo J, Wysocki M, *et al.* Noninvasive ventilation for acute exacerbations of chronic obstructive pulmonary disease. *N Engl J Med* 1995; **333**: 817–22.

72. Lin M, Yang YF, Chiang HT, *et al.* Reappraisal of continuous positive airway pressure therapy in acute cardiogenic pulmonary edema: short-term results and long-term follow-up. *Chest* 1995; **107**: 1379–86.

73. Wysocki M, Tric L, Wolff MA, *et al.* Noninvasive pressure support ventilation in patients with acute respiratory failure: a randomized comparison with conventional therapy. *Chest* 1995; **107**: 761–8.

74. Delclaux C, L'Her E, Alberti C, *et al.* Treatment of acute hypoxemic nonhypercapnic respiratory insufficiency with continuous positive airway pressure delivered by face mask. *JAMA* 2000; **284**: 2352–60.

75. Antonelli M, Conti G, Rocco M, *et al.* A comparison of noninvasive positive-pressure ventilation and conventional mechanical ventilation in patients with acute respiratory failure. *N Engl J Med* 1998; **339**: 429–35.

76. Girou E, Schortgen F, Delclaux C, *et al.* Association of noninvasive ventilation with nosocomial infections and survival in critically ill patients. *JAMA* 2000; **284**: 2361–7.

77. Antonelli M, Conti G, Bufi M, *et al.* Noninvasive ventilation for treatment of acute respiratory failure in patients undergoing solid organ transplantation. *JAMA* 2000; **283**: 235–41.

78. Hilbert G, Gruson D, Vargas F, *et al.* Noninvasive ventilation in immunosuppressed patients with pulmonary infiltrates, fever, and acute respiratory failure. *N Engl J Med* 2001; **344**: 481–7.

79. Antonelli M, Conti G, Moro ML, *et al.* Predictors of failure of noninvasive positive pressure ventilation in patients with acute hypoxemia respiratory failure: a multi-center study. *Intensive Care Med* 2001; **27**: 1718–28.

80. Ferrer M, Esquinas A, Leon M, *et al.* Noninvasive ventilation in severe hypoxemic respiratory failure. *Am J Respir Crit Care Med* 2003; **168**: 1438–44.

81. Kress JP, Pohlman AS, O'Connor MF, Hall JB. Daily interruption of sedative infusions in critically ill patients undergoing mechanical ventilation. *N Engl J Med* 2000; **342**: 1471–7.

82. Derdak S, Mehta S, Stewart TE, *et al.* High-frequency oscillatory ventilation for acute respiratory distress syndrome in adults. *Am J Respir Crit Care Med* 2002; **166**: 801–8.

83. Hirschl RB, Conrad S, Kaiser R, *et al.* Partial liquid ventilation in adult patients with ARDS: a multicenter phase I – II trial. *Ann Surg* 1998; **228**: 692–700.

84. Hirschl RB, Pranikoff P, Wise C, *et al.* Initial experience with partial liquid ventilation in adult patients with the acute respiratory distress syndrome. *JAMA* 1996; **275**: 383–9.

85. Hirschl RB, Croce M, Gore D, *et al.* Prospective, randomized, controlled pilot study of partial liquid ventilation in adult acute respiratory distress syndrome. *Am J Respir Crit Care Med* 2002; **165**: 781–7.

86. Huang C-C, Shih M-J, Tsai Y-H, *et al.* Effects of inverse ratio ventilation versus positive end-expiratory pressure on gas exchange and gastric intramucosal PCO_2 and pH under constant mean airway pressure in acute respiratory distress syndrome. *Anesthesiology* 2001; **95**: 1182–8.

87. Mercat A, Titiriga M, Anguel N, *et al.* Inverse ratio ventilation (I/E = 2/1) in acute respiratory distress syndrome: a six-hour controlled study. *Am J Respir Crit Care Med* 1997; **155**: 1637–42.

88. Morris AH, Wallace J, Menlove RL, *et al.* Randomized clinical trial of pressure-controlled inverse ratio ventilation and extracorporeal CO_2 removal for adult respiratory distress syndrome. *Am J Respir Crit Care Med* 1994; **149**: 295–305.

89. Conrad SA, Eggerstedt JM, Grier LR, *et al.* Intravenacaval membrane oxygenation and carbon dioxide removal in severe acute respiratory failure. *Chest* 1995; **107**: 1689–97.

◆ 90. Kollef MH, Schuster DP. The acute respiratory distress syndrome. *N Engl J Med* 1995; **332**: 27–37.

91. Pelosi P, Tubiolo D, Mascheroni D, *et al.* Effects of prone position on respiratory mechanics and gas exchange during acute lung injury. *Am J Respir Crit Care Med* 1998; **157**: 387–93.

92. Gattoni L, Tognoni G, Pesenti A, *et al.* Effect of prone positioning on the survival of patients with acute respiratory failure. *N Engl J Med* 2001; **345**: 568–73.

93. Prewitt RM, McCarthy J, Wood LDH. Treatment of acute low-pressure pulmonary edema in dogs: relative effects of hydrostatic and oncotic pressure, nitroprusside, and positive end-expiratory pressure. *J Clin Invest* 1981; **67**: 409–18.

94. Matthay MA, Broaddus VC. Fluid and hemodynamic management in acute lung injury. *Semin Respir Crit Care Med* 1994; **15**: 271–88.

95. Humphrey H, Hall J, Sznajder I, *et al.* Improved survival in ARDS patients associated with a reduction in pulmonary capillary wedge pressure. *Chest* 1990; **97**: 1176–80.

96. Mitchell JP, Schuller D, Calandrino FS, Schuster DP.

Improved outcome based on fluid management in critically ill patients requiring pulmonary artery catheterization. *Am Rev Respir Dis* 1992; **145**: 990–8.

97. Pulmonary Artery Catheter Study (FACCT). ARDS Network website, available at http://www.ardsnet.org/documents/factt.pdf. Accessed July 30, 2004.

98. The Veterans Administration Systemic Sepsis Cooperative Study Group. Effect of high-dose glucocorticoid therapy on mortality in patients with clinical signs of systemic sepsis. *N Engl J Med* 1987; **317**: 659–65.

99. Sprung CL, Caralis PV, Marcial EH, *et al.* The effects of high-dose corticosteroids in patients with septic shock. *N Engl J Med* 1984; **311**: 1137–43.

100. Bone RC, Fisher CJ, Clemmer TP, *et al.* A controlled clinical trial of high-dose methylprednisolone in the treatment of severe sepsis and septic shock. *N Engl J Med* 1987; **317**: 653–8.

101. Bone RC, Fisher Jr CJ, Clemmer TP, *et al.* Early methylprednisolone treatment for septic syndrome and the adult respiratory distress syndrome. *Chest* 1987; **92**: 1032–6.

102. Luce JM, Montgomery AB, Marks JD, *et al.* Ineffectiveness of high-dose methyprednisolone in preventing parenchymal lung injury and improving mortality in patients with septic shock. *Am Rev Respir Dis* 1988; **138**: 62–8.

103. Martin GS, Bernard GR. Acute respiratory distress syndrome: innovative therapies. *Semin Respir Crit Care Med* 2001; **22**: 293–305.

● 104. Meduri GU, Headley AS, Golden E, *et al.* Effect of prolonged methylprednisolone therapy in unresolving acute respiratory distress syndrome. *JAMA* 1998; **280**: 159–65.

105. Late Steroid Rescue Study (LaSRS). ARDS Network website, available at http://www.ardsnet.org/documents/lasrs6200web.pdf (accessed July 30, 2004).

106. Roissant R, Falke K, Lopez F, *et al.* Inhaled nitric oxide for the adult respiratory distress syndrome. *N Engl J Med* 1993; **328**: 399–405.

107. Dellinger RP, Zimmerman JL, Taylor RW, *et al.* Effects of inhaled nitric oxide in patients with acute respiratory distress syndrome: results of a randomized phase II trial. *Crit Care Med* 1998; **26**: 15–23.

● 108. Troncy E, Collet J-P, Shapiro S, *et al.* Inhaled nitric oxide in acute respiratory distress syndrome. *Am J Respir Crit Care Med* 1998; **157**: 1483–8.

109. Micheal JR, Barton RG, Saffle JR, *et al.* Inhaled nitric oxide versus conventional therapy: effect on oxygenation in ARDS. *Am J Respir Crit Care Med* 1998; **157**: 1372–80.

110. Taylor RW, Zimmerman JL, Dellinger RP, *et al.* Low-dose inhaled nitric oxide in patients with acute lung injury. *JAMA* 2004; **291**: 1603–9.

111. Bone RC, Slotman F, Maunder R, *et al.* Randomized double-blind, multicenter study of prostaglandin E_1 in patients with the adult respiratory distress syndrome. *Chest* 1989; **96**: 114–19.

112. Long W, Zucker J, Kraybill E. Symposium on synthetic surfactant II: perspective and commentary. *J Pediatr* 1995; **126**: 1S–4S.

113. Anzueto A, Baughman RP, Guntupalli KK, *et al.* Aerosolized surfactant in adults with sepsis-induced acute respiratory distress syndrome. *N Engl J Med* 1996; **334**: 1417–21.

114. Spragg RG, Lewis JF, Wurst W, *et al.* Treatment of acute respiratory distress syndrome with recombinant surfactant protein C surfactant. *Am J Respir Crit Care Med* 2003; **167**: 1562–6.

115. Spragg RG, Lewis JF, Walmrath H-D, *et al.* Effect of recombinant surfactant protein C-based surfactant on the acute respiratory distress syndrome. *N Engl J Med* 2004; **351**: 884–92.

116. Slotman GJ, Burchard KW, D'Arezzo A, Gann DS. Ketoconazole prevents acute respiratory failure in critically ill surgical patients. *J Trauma* 1988; **28**: 648–54.

117. Yu M, Tomasa G. A double-blind, prospective, randomized trial of ketoconazole, a thromboxane synthetase inhibitor, in the prophylaxis of the adult respiratory distress syndrome. *Crit Care Med* 1993; **21**: 1635–42.

118. The ARDS network authors. Ketoconazole for early treatment of acute lung injury and acute respiratory distress syndrome. *JAMA* 2000; **283**: 1995–2002.

119. Milberg JA, Davis DR, Steinberg KP, Hudson LD. Improved survival of patients with acute respiratory distress syndrome (ARDS). *JAMA* 1995; **273**: 306–9.

120. Brun-Buisson C, Minelli C, Bertolini G, *et al.* Epidemiology and outcome of acute lung injury in European intensive care units: results from the ALIVE study. *Intensive Care Med* 2004; **30**: 51–61.

121. Frutos-Vivar F, Nin N, Esteban A. Epidemiology of acute lung injury and acute respiratory distress syndrome. *Curr Opin Crit Care* 2004; **10**: 1–6.

122. Fowler AA, Hamman RF, Zerbe GO, *et al.* Adult

respiratory distress syndrome: prognosis after onset. *Am Rev Respir Dis* 1985; **132**: 472–8.

123. Montgomery AB, Stager MA, Carrico CJ, Hudson LD. Causes of mortality in patients with the adult respiratory distress syndrome. *Am Rev Respir Dis* 1985; **132**: 485–9.

124. McHugh LG, Milberg JA, Whitcomb ME, *et al.* Recovery of function in survivors of the acute respiratory distress syndrome. *Am J Respir Crit Care Med* 1994; **150**: 90–4.

● 125. Herridge MS, Cheung AM, Tansey CM, *et al.* One-year outcomes in survivors of the acute respiratory distress syndrome. *N Engl J Med* 2003; **348**: 683–93.

126. Weinert CG, Gross CR, Kangas JR, *et al.* Health-related quality of life after acute lung injury. *Am J Respir Crit Care Med* 1997; **156**: 1120–8.

127. Lee CM, Hudson LD. Long-Term outcomes after ARDS. *Semin Respir Crit Care Med* 2001; **22**: 327–36.

128. Davidson TA, Caldwell ES, Curtis JR, *et al.* Reduced quality of life in survivors of acute respiratory distress syndrome compared with critically ill controls. *JAMA* 1999; **281**: 354–60.

129. Schelling G, Stoll C, Haller M, *et al.* Health-related quality of life and posttraumatic stress disorder in survivors of the acute respiratory distress syndrome. *Crit Care Med* 1998; **26**: 651–9.

Tropical pulmonary syndromes

ARUNABH TALWAR, GAUTAM AHLUWALIA

INTRODUCTION

The warm climate and general socioeconomic conditions in tropical countries provide an ideal environment for pathogenic organisms, their vectors, and intermediate hosts to flourish. Tropical pulmonary infections are the leading cause of morbidity and mortality which are attributable to infection. In addition, international travel and changing immigration patterns have made tropical diseases part of the scope of medical practice worldwide. Each year millions of travelers visit tropical countries, and many spend time in the areas where they are at risk for infectious diseases. Thus, today it is essential for any practicing physician to be aware of the common tropical lung diseases.

A physician evaluating pulmonary infection in a returning traveler should have thorough understanding of common causative organisms, epidemiology, and modes of presentation.[1] Although tuberculosis and malaria are the most common infectious diseases in the tropics, this chapter will primarily focus on parasitic diseases (caused by protozoa and helminths such as nematodes, cestodes, trematodes) and specific emerging viral infections encountered in the tropics.

PARASITIC PULMONARY DISORDERS

Parasitic infections must be considered in cases of pulmonary infection in residents of or travelers to endemic areas. The clinical presentation can vary. Whereas paragonimiasis, amebiasis, and echinococcosis usually present with predominantly pleural involvement, the spectrum of pulmonary infiltrates in parasitic infection varies from a mild patch of pneumonitis to acute respiratory distress syndrome (ARDS) resulting in respiratory insufficiency (Table 10D.1).

Helminthic parasites are multicellular metazoan organisms, and infection with a diverse range of these organisms elicits eosinophilia and IgE production, controlled by cytokines secreted by the T-helper (Th)2 lymphocyte.[2] Although peripheral eosinophilia may provide a hematologic clue to the presence of helminthic infection, its sensitivity is not 100 percent. Increased IgE levels seem to correlate with the increasing levels of tissue invasion probably due to the secretion of factors by parasites that stimulate interleukin (IL)-4. Total serum IgE declines after successful treatment. In contrast with infections with helminthic parasites, infections with single-celled protozoan parasites do not characteristically elicit eosinophilia.

Definite evidence of pulmonary involvement in parasitic infections requires demonstration of ova or larvae in the sputum, bronchoalveolar lavage, pleural fluid, or lung tissue, which is not always possible. Thus in all suspected cases, stools should also be evaluated for ova and parasites. Careful examination of cytologic preparations may reveal parasites,[3] ova, or echinococcal hooks.[4] In some cases ova may be found in the sputum but this is more common when parenchymal involvement is present.[5] Serologic tests (e.g. enzyme linked immunosorbent assay [ELISA] and the use of monoclonal antibodies) may be the only diagnostic tool for paragonimiasis, toxocariasis, strongyloidiasis, and amebiasis when parasites or ova cannot be found in samples taken from the respiratory tract or stools.[6] Bronchoscopy is rarely helpful in establishing the diagnosis of parasitic infections[7] but may show evidence of eosinophilia in bronchoalveolar lavage fluid in helminthic infections. Pleural biopsy has a

Table 10D.1 *Parasites causing lung diseases in humans*

Disease	Parasite
Nematodes (roundworms)	
Loeffler syndrome	*Ascaris lumbricoides*
	Ancylostoma braziliense (cutaneous larva migrans)
	Ancylostoma duodenale (hookworm)
	Necator americanus (hookworm)
	Strongyloides stercoralis
	Trichinella spiralis
	Toxocara canis, T. catis (visceral larva migrans)
Chronic cough	*Mammomonogamus* species
	Capillaria species
	Gnathostoma spinigerum
Tropical eosinophilia	*Wuchereria bancrofti* (lymphatic filariasis)
	Brugia malayi
Solitary nodule on radiograph	*Dirofilaria immitis* (dog heartworm)
Cestodes (tape worm)	*Echinococcus granulosus* (hydatid disease)
Lung mass	*Echinococcus multilocularis*
Calcification intercostal muscle	*Cysticercus cellulosae*
Trematodes (flat worm)	
Pleural effusion	*Paragonimus westermani*
Pulmonary infiltrates,	*Schistosoma mansoni*
Pulmonary hypertension	*Schistosoma haematobium*
Loeffler-like syndrome	*Clonorchis sinensis*
	Fasciola hepatica
Arthropod	
Pentastomiasis	*Linguatula serrata*
	Armillifus armilata
Protozoa	
Pleural effusion	*Entamoeba histolytica*
Respiratory failure	*Plasmodium falciparum*
Pulmonary infiltrate	*Toxoplasma gondii*
Kala-azar	*Leishmania donovani*
Bronchiectasis	*Trypanosoma cruzi*

limited role – only rarely is a specific diagnosis of a parasitic infection established.[8]

Protozoa

MALARIA

Malaria is an enormous global public health problem, with nearly 500 million febrile episodes per year and approximately 1 million deaths annually worldwide.[9] Poor primary healthcare, failure of mosquito eradication programs, and emerging drug resistance in endemic areas have all contributed to its morbidity and mortality.

Human malaria is caused by four species of plasmodia: *Plasmodium falciparum, P. vivax, P. ovale,* and *P. malariae*. Human infection by all four plasmodia species occurs by transmission of sporozoites via a bite from an infected anopheles mosquito. Worldwide, most malaria infections are caused by either *P. falciparum* or *P. vivax*, and most malaria-associated deaths are due to *P. falciparum*.[10] Mixed infection with more than one malarial species occurs in 5–7 percent of infections. The severity and manifestations of malarial infestation are usually governed by the infecting species, magnitude of parasitemia, and the cytokines released as a result of the infection.[11]

Pathophysiology

The virulence of *P. falciparum* is attributed to its propensity to produce heavy parasitemia and its ability to adhere to the cells of the vascular endothelium, which leads to sequestration of parasitized red blood cells in the microvasculature of vital organs. The organ-specific sequestration of mature, late-stage *P. falciparum* in deep vascular endothelium has been considered a key process in the pathophysiology of severe malaria, a concept supported by a number of autopsy studies[12] (Fig. 10D.1).

The parasitized red cells develop the property of cytoadherence, which is enhanced by tumor necrosis factor (TNF) and other cytokines.[13] Therefore, noninfected red cells adhere around parasitized red cells forming rosettes and aggravating the mechanical obstruction of small vessels.[14] Similar to sepsis, malaria is associated with release of a variety of toxins that can trigger activation of host immune factors. These include proinflammatory cytokines, oxygen free radicals and nitric oxide, all of which can result in damage to host tissues. Similar to many serious infections raised levels of proinflammatory cytokines correlate with disease severity and outcome.[15,16] The parasites also release various proteins, such as *Plasmodium falciparum* erythrocyte membrane protein 1 (PfEMP-1), on the surface of parasitized red cells. The proteins bind to receptors such as intercellular adhesion molecule (ICAM-1) and CD36 on the endothelium of cerebral venules causing cytoadherence of parasitized cells.[14,17]

Peripheral sequestration of parasitized red blood cells in the capillary bed of end organs along with production of cytokines by the host are responsible for specific complications encountered with *P. falciparum* infection. In African children with cerebral malaria, plasma concentration of TNF-α, IL-1α and other proinflammatory cytokines IL-1β, -6, and -10, have been observed to correlate closely with severity of the disease as reflected by parasitemia, hypoglycemia, case fatality, and neurologic sequelae.[13] They may also be responsible for fever, coagulopathy, and leukocytosis.[13,18,19] Interestingly, the development of cytoadherence is specific to a particular strain. Therefore, cerebral malaria is caused only by *P. falciparum* infection.[20] Similar sequestration of activated neutrophils and parasites in pulmonary microvasculature ultimately results in injury

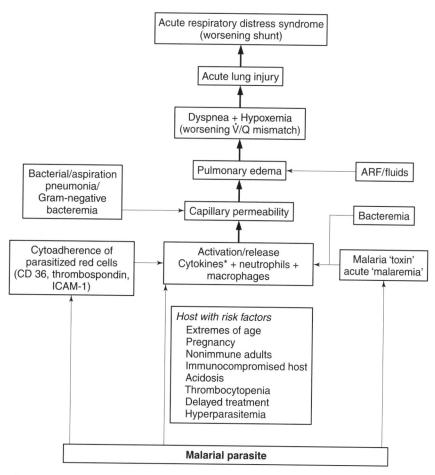

Figure 10D.1   *A schematic summary of the possible pathophysiologic steps in malaria-associated acute lung injury and acute respiratory distress syndrome. *Tumor necrosis factor, interleukin-1, interferon-γ. V̇/Q, ventilation–perfusion; ICAM-1, intercellular adhesion molecule 1, ARF, acute renal failure.*

to the alveolar capillary membrane. This leads to increased pulmonary vascular permeability and explains the development of noncardiogenic pulmonary edema[21] seen in this condition.

The microvascular dysfunction partly explains multiple organ dysfunction syndrome (MODS) associated with severe falciparum malaria. The clinical manifestations of MODS[22] include ARDS (Fig. 10D.2), altered sensorium, and/or acute hepatorenal failure[22] (Box 10D.1). Data from case series of adults admitted with severe falciparum malaria to intensive care units in India,[23] Malaysia,[24] South Africa,[19] and France,[25] all provide evidence of multiorgan failure as major risk factor for death. In severe malaria, mortality is 6.4 percent when one or fewer organs fail but increases to 48.8 percent with dysfunction of two or more organs.[23] The similarity between severe malaria and the pathogenesis of bacterial sepsis is clearly evident. Severe malaria due to *P. falciparum*, like bacterial sepsis, results in a hyperdynamic circulatory state, characterized by tachycardia, high cardiac output, hypotension, and reduced systemic vascular resistance.[13,21,22] In fulminant cases a low cardiac output, high systemic vascular resistance, and

refractory hypotension – similar to a terminal bacterial sepsis – characterize the hemodynamic status. In addition, similar to an episode of severe sepsis there is an activation of the coagulation cascade in the course of severe malaria leading to a depletion of coagulation inhibitors such as protein C.[26,27]

Clinical features

Malaria usually presents as an acute febrile episode. The common complications of severe malaria include disseminated intravascular coagulation, ARDS, hypoglycemia,[28] anemia, acute renal failure,[29] and cerebral malaria[30] (Table 10D.2). In children, metabolic acidosis (often caused by hypovolemia), hypoglycemia, hyperlacticacidemia, severe anemia, seizures, and raised intracranial pressure (ICP) are more common where as in adults, renal failure and acute respiratory failure are more common (Table 10D.3). *P. falciparum* is responsible for the most severe forms of malaria and accounts for approximately 80 percent of deaths due to this disease. Four clinical features that are associated with mortality are: unarousable coma, ARDS, shock, and acidosis.[25]

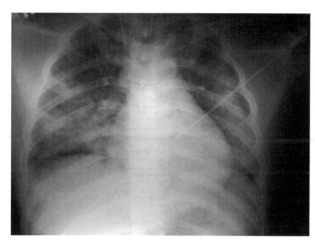

Figure 10D.2 *Acute respiratory distress syndrome in a patient with* Plasmodium falciparum *infection.*

Box 10D.1 Clinical and laboratory features of severe and complicated falciparum malaria in adults

Criteria

- Coma (unarousable coma defines cerebral malaria)
- Impaired consciousness
- Prostration/extreme weakness
- Multiple convulsions
- Hyperbilirubinemia (total bilirubin ≥51.3 µmol/L [3 mg/dL])
- Pulmonary edema
- Acute renal failure
- Severe anemia (in adults, hemoglobin <70 g/L [7 g/dL], hematocrit <0.2 [20 percent]; in children, hemoglobin <70 g/L [7 g/dL], hematocrit <0.15 [15 percent])
- Acute intravascular hemolysis with hemoglobinuria
- Spontaneous bleeding
- Hypoglycemia (whole blood glucose <2.2 mmol/L)
- Shock
- Acidemia/acidosis (pH <7.35/plasma bicarbonate <15 mmol/L)
- Hyperlactemia (plasma lactate >5 mmol/L)
- Parasitemia – ≥4 percent to ≥20 percent (depends on malaria acquired immunity [i.e. ≥4 percent in nonimmune persons])

Data from World Health Organization.[11]

There is a wide range of pulmonary involvement in malaria from asymptomatic respiratory alkalosis with tachypnea to acute respiratory distress syndrome.[32,33] Common presenting symptoms include cough (77 percent), dyspnea (32 percent), expectoration (29 percent) and chest pain (15 percent).[34] The acute lung injury usually occurs a few days into the disease course. It may develop rapidly, even after initial response to antimalarial treatment and clearance of parasitemia. The first indications of this include tachypnea and dyspnea, followed by hypoxemia accompanied by the development of bilateral infiltrates, ultimately resulting in respiratory failure requiring intubation.[35] Patients often have other complications of severe malaria as well.[11]

Table 10D.2 *Clinical features of malaria and possible mechanisms of disease*[150]

Syndrome	Clinical features	Disease mechanisms
Severe anemia	Shock; impaired consciousness; respiratory distress	Reduced RBC production (reduced erythropoietin activity, proinflammatory cytokines); increased RBC destruction (parasite-mediated, erythrophagocytosis, antibody and complement-mediated lysis)
Cerebral complications (cerebral malaria)	Impaired consciousness; convulsions; long-term neurologic deficits	Microvascular obstruction (parasites, platelets, rosettes, microparticles); proinflammatory cytokines; parasite toxins (e.g. GPI)
Metabolic acidosis	Respiratory distress, hypoxia, tachypnea; acidemia; reduced central venous pressure	Reduced tissue perfusion (hypovolemia, reduced cardiac output, anemia); parasite products; parasite products; proinflammatory cytokines; pulmonary pathology (airway obstruction, reduced diffusion)
Other	Hypoglycemia; disseminated intravascular coagulation	Parasite products and/or toxins; proinflammatory cytokines; cytoadherence
Malaria in pregnancy	Placental infection; low birth weight and fetal loss; maternal anemia	Premature delivery and fetal growth restriction; placental mononuclear cell infiltrates and inflammation; proinflammatory cytokines

RBC, red blood cell; GPI, glucosyl phosphatidyl inositol.

Adapted from *Trends in Parasitology*, 20, Mackintosh CL, Beeson JG, Marsh K. Clinical features and pathogenesis of severe malaria. 597–603, © 2004, with permission from Elsevier.[31]

Table 10D.3 *Differences between severe malaria in adults and children*[11]

Symptoms and signs	Adults	Children
Cough	Uncommon	Common in early stage
Convulsion	Indicates cerebral malaria or hypoglycemia	Indicates cerebral malaria, hypoglycemia but may be nonspecific consequence of fever
Duration of symptoms	Several days	Usually 1–2 days
Jaundice	Common	Uncommon
Anemia	Not so common	Common
Pulmonary edema/ARDS	Common	Rare
Acute renal failure	Common	Rare
Hypoglycemia	Common in pregnant women, or with quinine therapy (sometimes may be present without quinine therapy)	Common before treatment
Seizure	Less common	Frequent
Development of unconsciousness	Insidious	Rapid
Coma recovery time	Slow, usually 2–4 days	Rapid (usually 1–2 days)
CSF pressure	Usually normal	Variable, raised
Neurologic sequelae	Uncommon	Occurs in about 10% cases

ARDS, acute respiratory distress syndrome; CSF, cerebrospinal fluid.

Acute respiratory distress syndrome is a devastating constellation of clinical, radiologic, and pathologic signs, characterized by failure of gas exchange and refractory hypoxia. It occurs in 3–30 percent of patients with severe malaria.[35,36] Pulmonary edema due to fluid overload and heart failure secondary to anemia may occur, but this occurs only in a minority of patients. In most patients the physiologic picture is consistent with noncardiogenic pulmonary edema.[32] Both ARDS and ALI usually occur in falciparum malaria but can occasionally occur in vivax or ovale malaria. However, the prognosis of the two clinical situations is vastly different depending on the plasmodial species. In vivax or ovale malaria, patients usually recover whereas in falciparum malaria, mortality is >80 percent.[24,25,37] In all such cases, other common infectious causes of ARDS seen in the tropics should be meticulously ruled out (Box 10D.2).

Diagnosis

Microscopy still remains the investigation of choice for diagnosing malaria. The thick smear is more sensitive in diagnosing malaria, whereas the thin smear allows species differentiation and staging of parasite differentiation. The thin smear also allows quantification of the percentage of parasitized red cells. Mixed plasmodial infection (*P. vivax* and *P. falciparum*) must be excluded by repeated and meticulous examination of blood smears.[39] However, microscopy is operator dependent, requires expertise, and is also time consuming. Therefore rapid assays are being developed to hasten the diagnostic workup, especially in critically ill patients.

Polymerase chain reaction (PCR) techniques, based upon the detection of nucleic acid sequences (DNA or mRNA) specific to *Plasmodium* species have the ability to detect parasitemia levels as low as 5 parasites/µL.[40] The technique has high sensitivity and specificity.[41] The disadvantages of these techniques are that they are expensive, labor intensive, take hours to complete, and require significant technical expertise. However, PCR may ultimately have a role in

---

Box 10D.2 Diseases causing ARDS in tropical areas that require a high index of suspicion (modified from Jindal *et al.*[38])

Bacterial:

- *Mycobacterium tuberculosis*
- *Salmonella*
- *Brucella*
- *Leptospirosis*

Viral:

- Influenza/parainfluenza
- Respiratory syncytial virus
- Dengue
- Measles
- Chicken pox
- Hantavirus
- Epstein–Barr
- Cytomegalovirus

Others:

- Malaria
- *Pneumocystis carinii* infection
- Strongyloidiasis
- Aspiration
- Toxic fumes
- Paraquat poisoning
- Scorpion bites

monitoring the efficacy of antimalarial therapy and diagnosing therapeutic failure at an early stage.[42]

Management

Effective management of severe malaria includes early administration of antimalarial therapy, supportive therapy, and management of complications present at admission or developing during treatment. Hospitalization and parenteral administration of antimalarial agents are necessary for patients with severe malaria.

Antimalarial therapy

All patients with severe malaria are assumed to be resistant to chloroquine irrespective of the clinical presentation. In most developing countries, quinine dihydrochloride is the parenteral agent of choice for treating individuals with severe malaria. The only drug currently approved and available for severe malaria in the United States is quinidine gluconate (Table 10D.4). It is important to appreciate that quinidine is more potent than quinine against malaria, but it is more cardiotoxic.[43] Quinine dihydrochloride may be administered intravenously or intramuscularly. Quinidine gluconate, a class IA antiarrhythmic agent, should be administered intravenously. Both intravenous quinidine and quinine should be delivered by continuous infusion; when they are administered by rapid or bolus injection, they can induce fatal hypotension.[44] Intravenous quinine or quinidine should be administered only during the time the patient is not able to take oral medications.[44] In Asia, a 7-day course of tetracycline or doxycycline is administered to adults and clindamycin to children or pregnant women. In African countries sulfadoxine-pyrimethamine is used but its efficacy

is decreasing. However, it is prudent to administer quinine for at least 5–7 days. Intravenous quinine or quinidine can induce hypoglycemia, which usually occurs 24 hours after treatment is initiated, and most frequently affects pregnant women and children.[44,45]

Artemisinin or qinghaosu (ching-how-soo) is the active principal of the Chinese medicinal herb *Artemisia annua*. Artemisinin derivatives are efficacious and widely used outside of the United States for treating severe malaria. A water-soluble ester called artesunate and two oil-soluble preparations called artemether and arteether are being used. Artemisinin derivatives can also be given via rectal suppository if parenteral therapy is unavailable.[46] The artemisinins have a number of unique properties including their rapid mode of action; their broad range of activity on all asexual and sexual forms of the parasite; their low tendency to induce parasite resistance;[47] relative ease of administration; and potentially fewer side effects, especially hypoglycemia.[48] However, the potential benefit over quinine is blunted by the slow and erratic absorption, especially in patients who are in shock, as artemether and arteether have to be administered intramuscularly.

There is increasing evidence that artemisinin derivatives are better than quinine.[49,50] In the recent individual patient data metaanalysis of 1919 adults and children entered into randomized comparisons of artemether and quinine, mortality was significantly lower in artemether-treated adults.[51] Artesunate is relatively preferred over artemether as it can be administered both by the intravenous as well as intramuscular route. As with quinine, the oral formulation should be instituted as soon as possible.

Table 10D.4   *Recommended regimens for initial parenteral treatment for severe falciparum malaria*

Drug	Loading dose	Maintenance dose	Comments
Quinine dihydrochloride salt (available outside USA) reconstituted in 5% dextrose	20 mg/kg over 4 h followed 8 h later by maintenance dose*	10 mg/kg diluted in 10 ml/kg of 5% dextrose saline IV over 4 h repeated every 8 h*	If hemodialysis is performed, then quinine is administered after dialysis. Monitor blood glucose because of hypoglycemia
Quinidine gluconate (available in USA), reconstituted in normal saline	10 mg/kg IV infused over 1–2 h followed immediately by maintenance dose*	0.02 mg/kg/min continuous infusion*	Electrocardiographic monitoring is mandatory; slow or stop infusion if QRS >25% baseline value or QTc interval >500 ms
Artesunate	2.4 mg/kg IV bolus[†]	1.2 mg/kg IV daily[†]	Artesunic acid 60 mg is dissolved in 0.6 ml 5% NaHCO$_3$, diluted to 3–5 mL 5% glucose, and given immediately by IV bolus injection for at least 3 days followed by oral antimalarial drugs
Artemether	3.2 mg/kg IM[†]	1.6 mg/kg IM daily[†]	
Arteether	2.4 mg/kg IM[†]	2.4 mg/kg IM daily[†]	

*Intravenous medication given for at least 24 hours but oral antimalarial treatment should be substituted as soon as the patient is stable and can take oral therapy to complete the course. In renal failure the dose of the intravenous quinine should not be decreased in the first 48 hours, however if it needs to be given beyond that the dose should be reduced to half or a third of the initial dose.

[†]Parenteral therapy should be given for at least 3 days but oral antimalarial treatment should be substituted as soon as the patient is stable and can take oral therapy to complete the course.

IV, intravenous; IM, intramuscular.

Supportive management

The patients must be managed in a critical care unit for intensive monitoring of cardiorespiratory and neurologic status. Antipyretics and cold sponging adequately control the temperature; hyperpyrexia itself may lead to coma and convulsions. Convulsions, vomiting, and aspiration pneumonia further complicate the clinical condition if adequate care and precautions are not undertaken. Seizures should be controlled by using intravenous diazepam, phenytoin sodium, or phenobarbital. Although phenobarbital is an effective method for controlling convulsions, it increases the risk of respiratory arrest and patients should be closely monitored for this complication.[52]

Hypoglycemia is common in malaria, especially in pregnancy, and if not treated promptly can be fatal.[28] Intravenous 10 percent or 25 percent dextrose followed by continuous dextrose infusion is given until the blood sugar returns to normal. Hypokalemia is a common complication of severe malaria; however, it is often not apparent on admission. On correction of acidosis, plasma potassium decreases precipitously, and thus careful, serial monitoring of serum potassium with adequate supplementation is suggested in patients with severe malaria complicated by acidosis.[53]

Malaria has many features in common with the sepsis syndrome: the high levels of proinflammatory cytokines may be associated with increased vascular permeability, pathologic vasodilatation, and increased loss of intravascular fluids favoring the development of intravascular volume depletion.[54,55] Particularly in children, volume depletion is present at admission in the majority of children with severe malaria complicated by acidosis. Volume expansion corrects the hemodynamic abnormalities and is associated with improved organ function.[56] The widely perceived fear of aggravating increased ICP in cerebral malaria and of precipitating pulmonary edema has resulted in the use of maintenance requirement fluid regimens, with volume expansion only being considered in children who have hypotension or signs of dehydration.[11] Overhydration can be prevented by judicious monitoring of central venous pressure and/or pulmonary artery wedge pressure. To avoid pulmonary edema, the pulmonary capillary wedge pressure should be maintained between 12 mm Hg and 16 mm Hg or the central venous pressure between 10 cm H_2O and 12 cm H_2O. The urine output rate should be kept above 30 mL/h by continuing fluid administration. A reasonable goal is to maintain a mean arterial blood pressure of >60 mm Hg. Deteriorating respiratory status requires mechanical ventilation for adequate management of the airway. Hopefully early positive pressure ventilation with a lung protective strategy by lowering of tidal volumes may help prevent the high mortality associated with ARDS in severe malaria.[49] Vasopressor use is especially important when systemic perfusion pressures are inadequate to maintain organ blood flow.[57] Use of pulmonary toilet, aspiration precautions, patient positioning (including intermittent prone positioning), and recruitment maneuvers are useful therapeutic complements for maintaining functional residual capacity and decreasing shunt. During ventilation, care must be taken to maintain a Pa_{CO_2} below 30 mm Hg since a rise in the carbon dioxide tension may increase ICP and precipitate death.[58]

Associated bacterial sepsis is reported in 10–30 percent of ARDS patients who have malaria.[35,59,60] It has been suggested that the infections early in the course of disease are due to splanchnic ischemia and transmigration of enteric organisms and later may be due to nosocomial infections.[61] Furthermore, a pronounced general immunosuppression has been reported in malaria patients, which may predispose them to opportunistic infections.[62] Bacterial coinfection occurs more commonly in children; it should always be suspected and treated empirically with broad-spectrum antibiotics until the results of cultures are available.

Patients showing early signs of renal failure should be treated conservatively. A meticulous record of fluid requirement is necessary. Patients should undergo early dialysis if the urine output does not increase and there is further deterioration of renal function. In a study performed in Vietnam, mortality in patients with malaria and renal failure was 75 percent without dialysis and 26 percent when dialysis was available.[29] Recent studies have demonstrated a significantly lower mortality with hemofiltration compared with peritoneal dialysis.[44,63] In renal failure the dose of the intravenous quinine should not be decreased in the first 48 hours; however, if it needs to be given beyond that the dose should be reduced to half or a third of the initial dose.[11] Artemisinin drugs do not require any dose modification in the presence of acute renal failure.

Despite appropriate medical treatment, mortality in patients with greater than 10 percent parasitemia ranges from 20 percent to 40 percent when cerebral or renal function is impaired and up to 80 percent in the presence of ARDS.[64] It has been argued that in these cases, the use of exchange transfusion can achieve a prompt reduction in parasitemia, and may improve prognosis. The main advantages of exchange transfusion are rapid correction of the anemia, decrease in the level of parasites, and elimination of several cytokines and parasite toxins. Other advantages are that it ensures an adequate fluid balance and homodynamic status and absence of interference with drug therapy.[64] However, exchange transfusion treatment is still a matter of debate because some authors consider that results similar to those achieved with exchange transfusion can be obtained with chemotherapy alone.[65] The World Health Organization (WHO) guidelines for management of severe falciparum malaria recommend that exchange transfusion be considered in nonimmune individuals only if pathogen-free compatible blood, facilities for safe exchange, and adequate clinical monitoring are available.[11] Outside antimalarial therapy, mechanical ventilation and renal replacement have also played an important role in reducing mortality of this life-threatening condition.[66]

With a mortality of 15–20 percent despite parenteral antimalarial treatment, cerebral malaria is a considerable therapeutic challenge. Raised ICP is frequently detected in African children with cerebral malaria.[67] Treatment of raised ICP remains controversial; mannitol reduces the ICP but no randomized controlled trial has been conducted to show that it reduces sequelae and mortality. Corticosteroids have not been shown to be of any benefit in cerebral malaria and their use is associated with significant side effects.[59]

AMEBIASIS

Amebiasis is an infection caused by the protozoan *Entamoeba histolytica* and it is the third most common cause of death from parasitic diseases after malaria and schistosomiasis.[68] It produces a spectrum of clinical illness ranging from dysentery to abscess of the liver and other organs. Pleuropulmonary involvement is the most frequent complication of amebic liver abscess.

Pathogenesis
Human infection is caused by ingestion of *E. histolytica* cysts in fecally contaminated food and drink. Excystation occurs in the lumen of the small intestine. Trophozoites are formed which adhere to the mucus and epithelial layers. Sometimes active trophozoites burrow deep into the mucosal wall and form flask-shaped ulcers in the mucosa that have a narrow opening toward the gut lumen. Trophozoites may enter the mesenteric veins and reach the liver via the portal circulation; occasionally they enter systemic circulation through the venules of the middle and inferior rectal and vertebral veins, and are deposited in different organs. The lung is the second most common extraintestinal site of amebic involvement after the liver.

Pleuropulmonary involvement, which is reported in 20–30 percent patients, is the most frequent complication of amebic liver abscess.[69] Common clinical presentations include sterile sympathetic effusions, contiguous spread from the liver, and rupture into the pleural space, resulting in amebic empyema.[70] Rarely, a hepatobronchial fistula may cause cough, productive of large amounts of necrotic material. Recently, pulmonary amebiasis presenting as superior vena cava syndrome has been described.[71]

Clinical features
Pleuropulmonary involvement, like amebic liver abscess, occurs predominantly in men. The reported male:female ratio varies from 9:1 to 15:1.[72] Patients with sympathetic pleural effusion frequently experience pleuritic chest pain, referred to the scapula or the shoulder. Most patients have a tender enlarged liver.[73] It is common to auscultate a pleural rub in patients with an amebic liver abscess extending to the pleura. Transdiaphragmatic rupture of hepatic abscess may present with dramatic onset of severe pain, respiratory distress, shock, and sometimes death may occur.[74] The pleural effusion is frequently massive; the rupture into the right pleural space is seen in about 90 percent of patients. Hemoptysis is common; a brisk bout of hemoptysis followed by expectoration of anchovy-saucelike pus indicates that the pus is of hepatic origin. Hemoptysis due to pulmonary infarction may occur as a result of thromboembolism of the lung from the amebic liver abscess.[75]

Diagnosis
The diagnosis should be suspected in all patients from endemic areas with right-sided pleural effusion. Neutrophilic leukocytosis has been observed in 30 percent. Eosinophilia is usually not a feature. Serum alkaline phosphatase level is elevated in more than 75 percent of patients, whereas transaminases are elevated in about 50 percent.[76]

The chest radiograph may show elevation of the right dome of the diaphragm with or without the pleural effusion.[77] Ultrasonography and computed tomography (CT) can also demonstrate a hepatic abscess and the pleural effusion.[78] The pleural effusion is typically described to be like 'chocolate sauce' or 'anchovy paste' in appearance. Diagnosis can be confirmed by demonstration of trophozoites in the pleural effusion, but these are seen in only 10 percent of patients.[76,79] Several tests have been developed for the diagnosis of extraintestinal amebiasis including indirect hemagglutination test, ELISA, and the indirect fluorescent antibody test. The detection of IgM antibodies may be more useful in diagnosing acute cases because antibodies appear early and persist in the serum for a short period of time. The gel diffusion is positive in more than 95 percent of patients with acute invasive disease and reverts to negative after 6–12 months.

Treatment
Metronidazole is currently the drug of choice. Side effects include nausea, anorexia, metallic taste, dizziness, and a disulfiramlike reaction with alcohol. If the pleural effusion is large enough to cause respiratory distress, a therapeutic thoracentesis or tube thoracostomy may be performed. Bacterial superinfection, which is present in up to a third of the patients with amebic empyema, responds to antibiotics therapy. In some of these cases open drainage or decortication may be necessary. After successful treatment of invasive disease, patients should be considered for eradication of the intestinal phase of the disease with a luminal agent such as iodoquinol, diloxanide furoate, or paromomycin (Table 10D.5).

AMERICAN TRYPANOSOMIASIS (CHAGAS DISEASE)

Chagas disease is an endemic disease in Latin America – from Brazil to Argentina – and is caused by the flagellate protozoan parasite, *Trypanosoma cruzi*. It is transmitted to humans by reduviid bugs. Metacyclic forms of the parasite eliminated with insect feces penetrate human skin and

Table 10D.5   *Drugs for treatment of parasitic infections*

Infection	Drug	Adult dosage
Systemic amebiasis, hepatic abscess, lung ascariasis	Metronidazole or Tinidazole*	750 mg tid × 10 days 600 mg bid or 800 mg tid × 5 days
	Mebendazole	100 mg bid × 3 days or 500 mg once
	or	
	Pyrantel pamoate[†]	11 mg/kg once (max 1 g)
	or	
	Albendazole[†]	400 mg once
Filariasis (TPE)	Diethylcarbamazine	6 mg/kg/per day in three doses × 14 days
Paragonimus westermani infection	Praziquantel	75 mg/kg/per day in 3 doses × 2 days
	or	
	Bithionol	30-50 mg/kg on alternate days × 10-15 doses
Hookworm (*Ancylostoma duodenale*) infection	Mebendazole	100 mg bid × 3 days or 500 mg once
	or	
	Pyrantel pamoate[†]	11 mg/kg (max 1 g) × 3 days
	or	
	Albendazole[†]	400 mg once
Schistosoma mansoni infection	Praziquantel	40 mg/kg in two doses × 1 day
Schistosoma hematobium infection	Praziquantel	40 mg/kg/per day in two doses × 1 day
Schistosoma japonicum infection	Praziquantel	60 mg/kg in three doses × 1 day
Strongyloidiasis	Ivermectin	200 μg /kg/per day × 1-2 days
	Thiabendazole	50 mg/kg/per day in two doses × 2 days (max 3 g/d)
Echinococcus granulosus infection	Albendazole	400 mg bid × 28 days, repeat as necessary
Severe malaria	Quinidine gluconate	10 mg/kg loading dose (maximum 600 mg)
		In normal saline slowly over 1–2 hours followed by continuous infusion of 0.02 mg/kg/min until oral therapy can be started
	Quinine dihydrochloride	20 mg/kg loading dose IV in 5% dextrose over 4 h followed by 10 mg/kg over 2–4 h every 8 h (maximum 1800 mg/d) until oral therapy can be started

*Not marketed in the United States.

[†]An approved drug, but considered investigational for this condition by the US Food and Drug Administration.

tid, three times a day; bid, twice a day; IV, intravenous; TPE, Tropical Pulmonary Eosinophilia.

reach the blood from where they disseminate to the other tissues. In the acute form the illness is characterized by fever, inflammation at the portal of entry, acute myocarditis (with or without heart failure), and meningoencephalitis. Chronic disease usually occurs years following the initial infection and results in chronic cardiomyopathy (20–30 percent). Gastrointestinal megasyndromes occur in <10 percent and peripheral nerve involvement in <5 percent. It is believed that the tracheobronchial tree may be affected by the lesions of the autonomic nervous system resulting in dilatation and eventually in bronchiectasis. Esophageal involvement by the parasite results in megaesophagus. Its symptoms are dysphagia, odynophagia, regurgitation, heartburn, and coughing. Aspiration of the liquid content fat commonly results in pneumonia. Congestive cardiomyopathy may result in pulmonary edema, unilateral or bilateral pleural effusions, or pulmonary thromboembolism. Therapy for Chagas disease is unsatisfactory with nifurtimox, the only drug available in the United States.

Nematodes (round worms)

SIMPLE PULMONARY EOSINOPHILIA (LOEFFLER SYNDROME)

Ascaris lumbricoides (roundworms), and *Ancylostoma duodenale* and *Necator americanus* (both hookworms) may cause pulmonary symptoms during their migration through the lung. This acute disorder also known as Loeffler syndrome is most commonly caused by infection with *Ascaris* species.[80] It is characterized by migratory pulmonary infiltrates accompanied by peripheral blood eosinophilia and minimal pulmonary symptoms. *Ascaris* is transmitted via the ingestion of fertilized eggs, whereas hookworm infection occurs via either oral or dermal penetration by infective larvae. The migration of the parasite larvae from the pulmonary capillaries results in low-grade fever, blood streaked sputum, cough, wheezing, dyspnea, and substernal chest discomfort. These symptoms are due to transient allergic pneumonitis that occurs in response to the parasite antigens. Loeffler syndrome generally tends to occur 1–2 weeks after ingestion of the larval eggs.[81] The sputum examination reveals eosinophilia and Charcot-laden crystals. The chest radiograph shows fleeting infiltrates that resolve over a period of days. Ascaris or hookworm ova may be absent from stool at the time of pneumonitis, but larvae can often be seen in sputum or gastric lavage. The appearance of *Ascaris* or hookworm ova in the stool within 3 months of self-limiting eosinophilic pneumonitis suggests this diagnosis.

Occasionally, Loeffler syndrome may be drug induced and approximately a third of cases are idiopathic. Although severity of symptoms correlates with larval burden, this disorder is self-limiting and tends to resolve spontaneously. Symptomatic patients may be treated with bronchodilators. Prevention of infection and treatment of the intestinal phase are the mainstays of management. The drug of choice for intestinal infestation is mebendazole, although pyrantel pamoate or albendazole can also be used. Albendazole is a newer benzimidazole that has similar activity as mebendazole but is given as a single dose. It is not licensed for general use in the United States.

TROPICAL PULMONARY EOSINOPHILIA

Tropical pulmonary eosinophilia results from immunologic hyperresponsiveness to filarial parasites (*Wuchereria bancrofti* and *Brugia malayi*).[82] It is seen mostly in the Indian subcontinent, although it has also been reported from other areas of the world. The disease occurs mostly in males and is characterized by persistent cough and wheezing of insidious onset associated with a striking eosinophilia. The cough is often worse at night with nonproductive sputum. Physical exam reveals minimal pulmonary findings, hepatosplenomegaly, and generalized lymphadenopathy. Radiographs show increased bronchovascular markings and diffuse coarse interstitial infiltrates. However, the radiographic findings may be normal in up to 30 percent of cases. Pulmonary function tests reveal a predominant restrictive pattern together with mild reversible airway obstruction in most patients. The absolute eosinophil count often exceeds 4000/mm³ with elevation in serum IgE levels (above 1000 units/mL) and erythrocyte sedimentation rate. Bronchoalveolar lavage often reveals an intense eosinophilic alveolitis[83] and striking elevation of antifilarial IgE.[83] While filarial antibodies are typically detected, microfilaria cannot be found in the peripheral blood. Tropical pulmonary eosinophilia must be distinguished from other eosinophilic syndromes; this is generally not difficult, given the geographic distribution of the disease and rapid clinical and radiologic response to therapy with diethylcarbamazine.[84] The syndrome has typically been reported to present as 'refractory bronchial asthma', usually in nonimmune individuals (travelers to endemic regions). Despite a 3-week course of diethylcarbamazine, low-grade alveolitis persists in almost half of such patients, and it may be the cause of progressive pulmonary fibrosis seen in many inadequately treated patients.[85] Relapses can occur and are treated with repeat courses of the same drug. Corticosteroids may be helpful in treating the chronic forms of tropical pulmonary eosinophilia.[86]

DIROFILARIA IMMITIS

Human pulmonary dirofilariasis is caused by the dog parasite *Dirofilaria immitis*. Infection occurs when mosquito-borne infective larvae are transmitted to a human. Since humans are not a natural host, the organism does not complete its life cycle and dies before reaching sexual maturity. It is subsequently embolized into the pulmonary arterial circulation causing thrombosis, infarction, and a granulomatous reaction.[87] Most patients are asymptomatic and present with a solitary pulmonary nodule; peripheral eosinophilia is sometimes seen. Surgical resection is both diagnostic and curative.

VISCERAL LARVA MIGRANS

This disease is also called systemic toxocariasis, a zoonotic disease infecting the human viscera by the migrating larvae of the *Toxocara canis* or *T. catis*, the common intestinal ascarids in dogs and cats, respectively. Human beings are accidental hosts who acquire this condition by ingesting eggs in contaminated soil or food. Once ingested the larvae migrate through the intestine via the lymphatics and blood stream to reach other organs, including liver and lungs. The host's immune response to this invasion results in increased levels of eosinophils and IgE, both in the serum and bronchoalveolar lavage. Pulmonary involvement is reported in 20–80 percent of cases[81] and may vary from dry cough and wheezing (mimicking asthma) to respiratory failure.[88] The chest radiograph usually shows unilateral or bilateral migratory infiltrates. The diagnosis of visceral larvae migrans is established by a positive ELISA test for *T. canis* in a patient with history of pica. The condition is usually self-limiting and rarely requires treatment. The role of specific anthelmintic drugs such as mebendazole or albendazole is not established. Preventive measures, such as curbing geophagia and deworming the animal hosts, are important in decreasing the incidence of this condition.

STRONGYLOIDIASIS

Strongyloides stercoralis is a free-living parasite that is endemic throughout the tropics. The larvae of *S. stercoralis* penetrate the skin and enter the blood and lung *en route* to the small intestine to complete their life cycle. Within the small intestine they develop into the adult form and then reenter the blood stream (without going through a soil cycle), causing autoinfection. The most common respiratory manifestation of *S. stercoralis* infection in nonimmunosuppressed hosts is Loeffler syndrome, presenting as transient cough and wheeze, eosinophilia and dyspnea during the migration of the larvae through the lungs. The infection in the gut is usually asymptomatic and can remain undetected for decades. Strongyloidiasis is difficult to diagnose because the parasite load is low and the larvae output is irregular.[89] Several immunodiagnostic assays have been found ineffective in detecting disseminated infections and show cross-reactivity with hookworms, filariae, and schistosomes. Hyperinfection is seen in patients who are immunosuppressed and receiving corticosteroid therapy, resulting in high mortality rates (~90 percent). Almost all deaths due to helminths in the United States result from *S. stercoralis* hyperinfection.[90]

Hyperinfection develops when larvae that have hatched from eggs laid by adult worms in the duodenum develop into the infective stage, repenetrate the bowel and develop into adult forms and spread throughout the body, particularly into the lungs. Patients develop spiking fever, anemia, weight loss, diffuse alveolar infiltrates, and hypoxic respiratory failure resembling ARDS. The larvae are present in sputum, bronchoalveolar lavage, urine, and stool. Gram-negative fecal flora, piggybacking onto the parasites, may cause sepsis.[91] The clinical features alone seldom permit a diagnosis. However, history of travel to an endemic region, even in the remote past, in a patient with multisystem involvement is usual. Thiabendazole (25 mg/kg twice a day × 2 days) has been the drug of choice despite the associated gastrointestinal side effects and high relapse rate.[92] Ivermectin, a potent macrocyclic lactone, which causes paralysis of the nematodes,[93] has been found to be the most effective drug for the treatment of disseminated strongyloidiasis.[94]

PULMONARY TRICHINELLOSIS

Human trichinellosis is an important food-borne zoonosis caused by *Trichinella spiralis*. The parasite undergoes complete development in one host (pig, rat, or man). However, two hosts are required to complete the life cycle and for the preservation of the species from extinction. Humans gets infected after eating raw and partially cooked infected pork which contains larval *Trichinella*. The infective larvae in the pig's muscle are surrounded by a host capsule, which is a modified striated muscle cell known as a 'nurse' cell. In the pig's stomach, the 'nurse' cell is digested and the larvae liberated. The larvae develop into adults (males and females) in the duodenum and jejunum. The newborn larvae produced by female parasites pass through the lymphatics or blood vessels to reach the striated muscles. The larvae undergo encystment in the muscle and a host capsule develops around the larvae. Later on, it may get calcified. The life cycle is completed when infected pig muscle is ingested by a suitable host.

Th-2 cells play an important role in the pathogenesis of the disease. These cells release the cytokines IL-5 and IL-4 which are responsible for eosinophilia and increased IgE production.[95] The common symptoms of trichinellosis are muscle pain, periorbital edema, fever, and diarrhea. Pulmonary symptoms include dyspnea, cough, and pulmonary infiltrates. Dyspnea may be due to the involvement of the diaphragm. Leukocytosis, eosinophilia, and elevated levels of serum muscle enzymes (creatine phosphokinase, lactate dehydrogenase, aldolase, and aminotransferase) are important laboratory findings. ELISA using excretory–secretary antigens for detection of anti-*Trichinella* antibodies may be useful for diagnosis.[96] A definitive diagnosis can be made by muscle biopsy (usually deltoid muscle) that may demonstrate larvae of *T. spiralis*. Symptomatic treatment of trichinellosis includes analgesics and corticosteroids. Specific treatment is with mebendazole or albendazole. Trichinellosis can be prevented by consuming properly cooked pork.

Cestodes (tapeworms)

ECHINOCOCCOSIS (HYDATID DISEASE)

Human echinococcosis is caused by three species of the tapeworm (*Echinococcus granulosus*, *E. multilocularis*, and *E. vogeli*). *E. granulosus* is the most prevalent, producing cystic hydatid disease in about 90 percent of cases. It is most commonly found in sheep- and cattle-raising countries, for the most part in the Middle East, Australia, New Zealand, South America, and central Europe. The disease is particularly common in Lebanon and Greece.[97] The liver (60–70 percent) and the lungs (20–30 percent) are the most frequently involved organs. Pulmonary disease, in particular, appears to be more common in younger individuals.[98]

Pathogenesis

The definitive host for *E. granulosus* is the dog or wolf, and humans are the accidental host. When humans ingest feces containing eggs, larvae emerge in the duodenum, enter the blood, and usually lodge in either the liver or the lung. The parasite grows and may be latent for 10–20 years before producing symptoms. The resulting symptoms depend upon the site, type, and rate of growth of the cystic lesions.[99]

Clinical features

Most patients are asymptomatic, but some may occasionally expectorate the contents of the cyst, or develop symptoms due to compression of the surrounding structures. The cyst may erode the bronchi, mediastinum, or pleural cavity. An air leak between the adventitious and laminated layer of the cyst may give rise to a crescent or 'water-lily' appearance (Fig. 10D.3). The patients may also present with hydatid pulmonary embolism, in which a cyst spontaneously ruptures into the blood stream.[100]

Pleural involvement usually occurs due to rupture of a pulmonary hydatid cyst; often simultaneous rupture into the pleural space and tracheobronchial tree is observed.[101] Since the cyst is not fertile after rupture, pleural hydatidosis is rare.[101] Rarely hepatic cyst rupture into the pleural space may occur. Occasionally sympathetic pleural effusion may

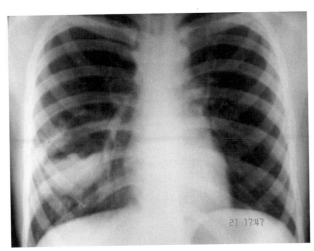

Figure 10D.3   *A chest radiograph showing undulating membrane in a hydatid cyst (water-lily sign).*

accompany a pulmonary or hepatic hydrated cyst.[102] Hepatic cyst rupture into the pleural space is associated with an acute illness characterized by chest pain, cough, respiratory distress, fever, and shock. In half of the patients, simultaneous rupture into the bronchial tree is manifested by expectoration of large quantities of cyst membranes and pus; pulmonary cyst rupture has a similar presentation.[101] In addition, a bronchopleural fistula often produces a hydropneumothorax that may become secondarily infected.

Diagnosis

In endemic areas the diagnosis is established on the basis of the clinical picture, radiologic findings, and serologic tests.[103] Magnetic resonance imaging, CT, and ultrasound reveal a solitary well-defined cyst with thick or thin walls. In up to 30 percent of cases, cysts may be multiple. In cases of rupture of the cyst usual findings include an elevated right hemidiaphragm, moderate right pleural effusion, right lower lobe pneumonitis, and hydropneumothorax.[102,104–106] The definitive diagnosis of pleural echinococcosis is established by the demonstration of echinococcal scolices with hooklets in the pleural fluid stained with toluidine blue. In pleural tissue, a fibrinopurulent exudate with eosinophils is observed.[4] Thoracentesis reveals turbid, yellow fluid with an abundance of polymorphonuclear cells and eosinophils. Casoni skin test and Weinberg complement fixation test are positive in about 70–75 percent of cases.[101] Detection of antibody to specific echinococcal antigens by immunoblotting has the highest degree of specificity.

Treatment

Surgical excision of the cyst is the treatment of choice.[107] An immediate thoracotomy is recommended for patients in whom a hepatic or pulmonary cyst has ruptured into the pleural space. When a hepatic cyst has ruptured, the objectives of surgical treatment are to remove the parasite, to drain the hepatic and pleural cavity, and reexpand the lungs. If the surgical procedure is delayed, decortication may also be required.[108] Patients with hydatid cysts should be treated with antiprotozoal therapy if all cysts cannot be removed or when a cyst has ruptured. The treatment of choice is albendazole 400 mg twice a day for at least 28 days.[109]

Trematodes (flatworms)

PARAGONIMIASIS

Paragonimiasis is a food-borne parasitic disease caused by the trematode *Paragonimus* endemic in certain areas of east and southeast Asia.[110] The pulmonary form is most commonly seen following infection with *Paragonimus westermani* and *P. miyazaki*.

Pathogenesis

Human infection occurs after ingestion of raw or incompletely cooked freshwater crabs or crayfish infected with the metacercaria (larval stage) of the worm.[110] After ingestion, larvae enter the peritoneal cavity through the intestinal wall. They then migrate up and through the peritoneal cavity to the diaphragm, pleural space, and visceral pleura to enter into the lung. Here the larvae mature into adult lung flukes. The eggs produced by mature flukes are expectorated or swallowed and excreted in feces. In the water, eggs develop into ciliated miracidia that infect freshwater snails. Another larval form develops in the snails and is eventually released as cercariae that penetrate crayfish and crabs to complete the cycle.[111]

Clinical features

In the early stages of the infection, patients present with abdominal pain and/or pleuritic chest pain as the larvae penetrate the diaphragm and migrate within the pleural cavity. Cough, malaise, and chest pain may also develop with larval migration within the lung parenchyma. In the lung they mature into adult forms that deposit eggs in the lung parenchyma leading to hemorrhage, necrosis that may present as bronchopneumonia, interstitial pneumonia, bronchitis, bronchiectasis, collapse, fibrosis, pleural thickening, or pleural effusions. Recurrent hemoptysis is a common complaint in late stages of the disease.[112] The sputum typically has a characteristic chocolate color and is composed of a mixture of blood, inflammatory cells, and *Paragonimus* eggs.

Radiologic findings

Radiographic appearances vary with the stage of the infection and the surrounding tissue reaction. The initial finding is patchy airspace consolidation due to hemorrhagic pneumonia caused by migrating larvae. At this stage, pleural effusion or pneumothorax is frequently seen. As larvae mature into adults, cysts form around them. The cysts are filled with hemorrhagic fluid and surrounded by pericystic airspace consolidation, appearing as a localized masslike consolidation on radiographs. Cysts that communicate with adjacent bronchi appear as air cysts within the consolidated lung or as ring shadows. Pleural involvement is represented by pleural effusion (60 percent), hydropneumothorax (30 percent), and pleural thickening (10 percent).[113]

Diagnosis

The diagnosis should be suspected in a patient with history of exposure in an endemic area. It can be established by detection of eggs in the sputum, stool, and bronchoalveolar lavage or biopsy specimen, or a positive anti-*Paragonimus* antibody test. IgE and *P. westermani*-specific-IgE and -IgG levels are elevated and higher in the pleural fluid than in the serum, suggesting that these antibodies are produced in the pleural space.[114] An ELISA is highly sensitive and specific in detecting antibodies; eggs are demonstrable in less than 50 percent of cases.[115] Immunoblot serologic tests may also be helpful.[112] The pleural fluid is frequently eosinophilic and exudative with low glucose (<0.5 mmol/L [10 mg/dL]), low pH (<7.10), and high lactate dehydrogenase (1000 IU/L). The pleural fluid also shows presence of cholesterol crystals, but ova are rare. Peripheral blood and pleural fluid eosinophilia is common.[116,117] Level of IL-5 is increased in the pleural fluid and correlates significantly with the percentage of eosinophils in both pleural effusions and peripheral blood.[117,118]

Treatment

The treatment of choice is praziquantel 25 mg/kg bodyweight three times a day for 3 days. Response to praziquantel can be followed by a downward trend in peripheral eosinophilia, cessation of egg passage in sputum or stool, improvement in chest radiograph appearance, and decreasing antibody titer to *Paragonimus*. For heavy infections a second course may be required. The alternative treatment is bithionol or niclofan. Thoracotomy and decortication may be necessary when pleural surfaces are abnormally thickened and penetration of drugs into the pleural space is insufficient to eradicate infection.[113]

SCHISTOSOMIASIS

Schistosomiasis is a parasite that is carried by freshwater snails in tropical countries around the world. Eggs are passed in human excrement, hatch in water into miracidia and are ingested by the snails. The snails release the cercarial form in water and these rapidly penetrate the skin to localize in various organs. There are two common forms: urinary schistosomiasis (*Schistosomia hematobium*) seen commonly in southeast Asia and intestinal schistosomiasis (*S. mansoni*, *S. japonicum*) seen commonly in the Middle East, central Africa, and South America.

Acute schistosomiasis (Katayama fever) is a febrile response to the parasite in nonimmune persons 6–8 weeks after a heavy first infection. Pulmonary involvement in acute schistosomiasis includes ill-defined nodular pulmonary infiltrates which are believed to be immunologically mediated[119] along with associated eosinophilia. This is usually self-limiting and resolves over 1–2 months. The natural history can be shortened by steroids and praziquantel.

In the chronic stage, granulomatous inflammation of the lung results in pulmonary hypertension. Approximately 25 percent of patients with schistosomal hepatosplenomegaly have clinical evidence of pulmonary disease but less than 5 percent progress to true cor pulmonale.[120] Pulmonary hypertension results from abnormal migration of eggs of either *S. mansoni* from the portal system through portocaval shunts or of *S. hematobium* from vesicle veins to pulmonary vascular beds[121] with granuloma formation around the eggs. Dyspnea on exertion, decreased lung volume, and impaired diffusion are common. Fine nodules along with dilatation of pulmonary arteries is the most common radiographic pattern. Eggs may be detected at times in bronchoalveolar lavage or transbronchial biopsy. Usually ova can be detected in urine (*S. hematobium*) or stool (*S. mansoni* or *S. japonicum*), or bladder or rectal biopsy.

Praziquantel is the drug of choice for the treatment of all forms of schistosomiasis.[122] *S. mansoni* is also sensitive to oxamniquine.[123] Praziquantel (single dose) also appears to be more effective than metrifonate in terms of parasitologic cure of *S. haematobium*, but the reinfection rate is high with both drugs.[124] Initiation of antischistosomal therapy may result in coughing and wheezing accompanied by new infiltrates on chest radiograph, and eosinophilia, because of an immunologic response to antigens from dead worms.[125]

VIRAL PULMONARY INFECTIONS

Hantavirus infections

Hantaviruses are single-stranded, negative-sense RNA viruses that encompass 25 antigenically distinguishable viral species.[126] They are enveloped virus particles, measure 80–115 nm in diameter, and belong to the family Bunyaviridae. Hantavirus pulmonary syndrome (HPS), caused mainly by Sin Nombre virus, is primarily a lung infection; the kidneys and the skin are largely unaffected.[127] Hantaviruses are transmitted by aerosols of rodent excreta, saliva, and urine. The most common mode of transmission is inhalation of dust or dried particles with dried saliva or waste products of an infected rodent.[128]

Hantavirus pulmonary syndrome is characterized by flulike symptoms: fever, myalgias, headache, and cough. Other symptoms can include chills, abdominal pain, diarrhea, and malaise. Subsequent symptoms include coughing and shortness of breath, tachypnea, tachycardia, dizziness, arthralgia, sweating, and back or chest pain.[129] The disease progresses rapidly; further signs can include thrombocytopenia, hypoxemia, and interstitial pulmonary edema. Eventually, the patient experiences hypotension, shock, and respiratory distress. The vast majority of patients with hantavirus pulmonary syndrome have evidence of pleural effusions caused by the rare cardiac dysfunction or alternatively due to the profound vascular leak. The pleural fluid can be a transudate in initial phase (representing cardiopulmonary dysfunction) or an exudate due to capillary leaks.[130]

DIAGNOSIS

Thrombocytopenia, increased immature granulocytes, and large immunoblastoid lymphocytes, accompanied by an elevated white blood cell count, are commonly observed. The partial thromboplastin and prothrombin times are increased. Serum lactate, lactate dehydrogenase, aspartate aminotransferase, and alanine aminotransferase levels are elevated; IgG or IgM to hantavirus strains Seoul, Hantaan, Puumala, Dobrava, and Sin Nombre, may be detected serologically.[131] Chest radiographs show diffuse interstitial pulmonary infiltrates, advancing to alveolar edema with severe bilateral involvement. In severe infection there may be pulmonary secretions with a total protein ratio of edema fluid/serum greater than 80 percent.

TREATMENT

The patients usually need intensive cardiopulmonary support. Treatment with intravenous ribavirin or amantadine may be effective.[132]

Dengue fever

Dengue virus infection is the most common arthropod-borne disease worldwide with an increasing incidence in tropical and subtropical regions.[133] Dengue viruses belong to the family of Flaviviridae and are transmitted by the bite of infected *Aedes* mosquitoes. Dengue virus infection frequently may remain asymptomatic or manifest as nonspecific viral infection. In severe cases of dengue fever, dengue hemorrhagic fever (DHF), and dengue shock syndrome (DSS) are characterized by high and often biphasic fever, malaise, frontal headache, retroorbital pain, arthralgia with backache, myalgia, generalized lymphadenopathy, and a centrifugal macular or maculopapular rash. Laboratory abnormalities include a usually mild elevation of liver enzymes, thrombocytopenia, and abnormal coagulation.[134]

The definition of DHF as established by the World Health Organization includes a denguelike illness with hemoconcentration (hematocrit elevated by >0.2 [20 percent]), marked thrombocytopenia (<100 × 10^9/L), and hemorrhagic manifestations such as petechiae, conjunctival and gingival bleeding, epistaxis, melena, hematuria, and a positive tourniquet test.[135] Up to 30 percent of patients with DHF may progress to DSS as a consequence of increased vascular permeability leading to hypovolemia, hypotension with narrowing of the pulse pressure (<20 mm Hg), and circulatory shock.[136]

DIAGNOSIS

Dengue disease can be verified by virus isolation, detection of viral RNA by reverse transcription PCR, or identification of dengue virus-specific antibodies. A greater than fourfold rise in hemagglutination inhibition, complement fixation, or neutralizing antibody titers provides laboratory confirmation of dengue infection.

CLINICAL FEATURES

Infection with dengue virus frequently may remain asymptomatic or manifest as nonspecific viral infection to increasingly severe conditions that comprise dengue fever, DHF, and DSS. In DSS, an acute increase in capillary permeability results in leakage of plasma into the interstitial space and patients may develop ARDS.[137] There is no specific therapy available for dengue virus infections, and it is important to exclude other treatable diagnoses. Patients at risk for dengue can acquire other diseases with similar clinical features, such as malaria, typhoid fever, and leptospirosis.

TREATMENT

The patients with DSS should receive adequate fluid resuscitation,[138] along with efforts toward correction of coagulopathy and mechanical ventilation. Most patients who present for medical attention before profound shock develops and who receive appropriate fluid therapy will recover quickly.

Severe acute respiratory syndrome

Severe acute respiratory syndrome (SARS) is an emerging infectious disease with a formidable morbidity and mortality. In March 2003 there was a serious outbreak of SARS in Hong Kong.[139] Within a month, the disease also spread to Singapore, Vietnam, Taiwan, Germany, Canada, and the United States. It appears to spread by close person-to-person contact via droplet transmission or fomite. A novel coronavirus (CoV) is now identified as the main pathogen responsible for SARS.[140,141]

CLINICAL FEATURES

The major clinical features on presentation include persistent fever, chills/rigor, myalgia, dry cough, headache, and dizziness. Lymphopenia, thrombocytopenia, prolonged activated partial thromboplastin time, and elevated D-dimer, lactate dehydrogenase, and creatinine kinase levels are common laboratory features of SARS. The radiographic appearance of SARS shares features with other causes of pneumonia. By the onset of fever, almost 80 percent of patients with SARS have abnormal findings on chest radiographs, all of which show airspace consolidation. Old age, presence of comorbid conditions such as diabetes and hepatitis B, and elevated serum lactate dehydrogenase on admission indicate poor prognosis.[142]

DIAGNOSIS

The diagnosis of SARS is based on clinical, epidemiologic, and laboratory criteria that have been laid down by the Centers for Disease Control and Prevention (CDC).[143] The clinical criteria include:

- asymptomatic or mild respiratory illness
- temperature > 38 °C (100.4 °F) and at least one respiratory feature (i.e. cough, dyspnea, difficulty breathing, or hypoxia)
- severe respiratory illness (features of the second criterion and radiographic evidence of pneumonia, the presence of respiratory distress syndrome, autopsy findings consistent with pneumonia, or the presence of respiratory distress syndrome without an identifiable cause).

The epidemiologic criteria include:

- travel (including transit in an airport) within 10 days of the onset of symptoms to an area with current, recently documented, or suspected community transmission of SARS
- close contact within 10 days of the onset of symptoms with a person known or suspected to have SARS infection.

The laboratory criteria include:

- detection of an antibody to SARS-CoV in specimens obtained during acute illness or 21 days after illness onset
- detection SARS-CoV RNA by reverse-transcriptase PCR
- isolation of SARS-CoV.

Since the case definition of SARS is broad, it is important to evaluate patients with suspected SARS for a variety of bacterial and viral pathogens that can cause pneumonia. Specific therapies are available for some of these organisms.

TREATMENT

There is currently no treatment recommended except for meticulous supportive care. Critically ill SARS patients with ARDS experience a potentially fatal, but in some cases self-limiting, clinical course.[144] Several antiviral agents have been tried including ribavirin, oseltamivir, and lopinavir–ritonavir, but the efficacy of these drugs has not been established.[145] Hospitalized patients should be isolated in negative pressure rooms; healthcare workers and visitors should wear masks (preferably N-95 respirator such as used for tuberculosis precautions) to prevent airborne and droplet acquisition and gowns, gloves, and protective eyewear to guard against contact transmission. Since SARS is contagious, prevention measures center on avoidance of exposure and infection control for suspected cases and contacts. The most important element of infection control in the community is for patients with suspected SARS to stay at home and not go out for any reason. The CDC advises that the patient remain at home for a full 10 days after the resolution of fever and other symptoms.

Avian influenza

More than a century ago, avian influenza, also called 'bird flu', was first identified in Italy as a highly lethal viral disease of poultry. Subsequently, it was observed that avian influenza is a global disease. However, the recent epidemic in southeast Asia has brought it in focus due to cross-infection in humans.

PATHOPHYSIOLOGY

All influenza viruses including that of avian influenza belong to the Orthomyxoviridae family. The two surface antigens, hemagglutinin (H) and neuraminidase (N), are used for serologic labeling of influenza viruses. The type description (A, B, or C) depends on the antigenic character of the virus particle. Avian influenza viruses belong to type A. There are 15 hemagglutinin (H) subtypes and 9 neuraminidase (N) subtypes of influenza A viruses. Avian influenza viruses have representatives in all of these subtypes. As of now, all outbreaks of the highly pathogenic form have been caused by influenza A viruses of subtypes H5 and H7. Of the 15 avian influenza virus A subtypes, H5N1 is of particular concern. Types B and C do not affect domestic animals.

Avian influenza virus infection varies from an asymptomatic disease to an acute, fatal illness of the poultry. There is an extensive reservoir of influenza viruses potentially circulating in bird populations. Migratory waterfowl, especially wild duck, is the natural reservoir of avian influenza viruses. However, these birds are also the most resistant to infection. The domestic poultry, including chickens and turkeys, are particularly susceptible to epidemics of rapidly fatal influenza. The immediate source of infection for domestic poultry can seldom be ascertained, but most outbreaks probably start with direct or indirect contact of domestic poultry with water birds. Infected birds excrete virus in high concentration in their stool and also in nasal and ocular discharges. The disease generally spreads rapidly in a flock by direct contact. Live poultry markets amplify the risks. Although avian influenza viruses generally replicate inefficiently in humans, some subtypes of avian influenza can replicate within the human respiratory tract and cause disease.

In 1997, the first documented human infection with an avian influenza virus A H5N1, occurred in Hong Kong resulting in severe respiratory disease in 18 humans with a high mortality of 30 percent.[146] This infection coincided with an epidemic of pathogenic A H5N1 avian influenza virus strain in Hong Kong's poultry population and resulted in high fatality in the poultry stock. Genetic studies determined that the virus had 'jumped' directly from birds to humans due to close contact with live-infected poultry.[147] Data on human to human transmission of avian influenza virus subtype A H5N1 are limited.

CLINICAL FEATURES

The clinical features of A H5N1 avian influenza infection are a spectrum from fever, sore throat, and cough to acute respiratory distress syndrome (ARDS) secondary to viral pneumonia. The incubation period in humans is generally 2–5 days.[148] Risk factors associated with severe disease are older age, delayed admission to hospital, and the presence of pneumonia, leukopenia, and lymphopenia. Complications include multiorgan failure with renal dysfunction and cardiac compromise, pulmonary hemorrhage, pneumo-thorax, and pancytopenia.[148]

DIAGNOSIS

The diagnosis of avian influenza can be made by viral culture, PCR assay for avian influenza A (H5N1) RNA, immunofluorescence test for antigen with the use of monoclonal antibody against H5, or demonstrating a fourfold rise in H5-specific antibody in paired serum samples. The detection of viral RNA by PCR appears to be the most sensitive for diagnosis. Most patients with A H5N1 infection give a history of recent exposure to dead or ill poultry. Thus, a comprehensive travel and epidemiologic history may be of importance in the identification of suspected cases. The differential diagnosis of avian influenza includes atypical pneumonia, typical respiratory virus infections (such as human influenza, respiratory syncytial virus), SARS, and upper respiratory infections associated with conjunctivitis (e.g. adenovirus).

TREATMENT

The treatment of avian influenza is mainly supportive with the simultaneous use of antiviral drugs. These viruses are susceptible to the neuraminidase inhibitors (oseltamivir and zanamivir) but clinical experience with these antivirals to treat A H5N1 is limited. The experience to date is considered inconclusive because the drug was given too late and the numbers were small. Furthermore the optimal dose and duration are unknown and antiviral resistance can occur in N1-containing viruses during therapy.[149,150] The immediate priority to prevent a global epidemic from a highly pathogenic A H5N1 avian influenza virus in birds is to immediately detect and destroy the infected poultry populations, thereby reducing opportunity for human exposure to the virus.

The role of vaccination of people at high risk of exposure to infected poultry using vaccines effective against currently circulating human influenza strains also needs to be emphasized for reducing coinfection of humans with avian influenza and human influenza strains. This decreases the risk of antigenic drift. Obviously, personnel involved in the culling of poultry flocks must be protected with appropriate barrier precautions and receive prophylactic antiviral drugs. At present there are no licensed vaccines against avian influenza, although it is an area of active study.

CONCLUSION

The spectrum of pulmonary disease in tropical region involves a vast gamut of infectious diseases and represents a considerable burden of illness. These pulmonary infections are a significant cause of morbidity and mortality attributable to these infections, and are preventable if appropriate clinical and laboratory tools are in place to facilitate early detection of the pulmonary infections, identification of the pathogen involved, and institution of appropriate therapy. Consequently, there is still great scope for improvement in implementing potentially effective interventions to improve the outcome of pulmonary infections in tropical countries.

Key learning points

- Parasitic infections must be considered in residents of or travelers to endemic areas; knowledge of the geographical distribution of the main parasites involved in the lung diseases and their modes of transmission allows clinicians to suspect possible diagnoses.

- Depending upon the parasite involved, several tools can be used to confirm the diagnosis leading to appropriate treatment.

- Infection with helminthic parasites leads to eosinophilia and IgE production, but infection with single-celled protozoan parasites does not characteristically elicit eosinophilia.

- *P. falciparum* can present with MODS; while in children, metabolic acidosis (often caused by hypovolemia), hypoglycemia, hyperlacticacidemia, severe anemia, seizures, and raised ICP is more common; in adults renal failure and acute respiratory failure are more common.

- Of all the parasitic infections malaria can be prevented by pharmacologic agents, others can be prevented by adequate lifestyle measures adapted to the particular geographic area and by understanding the life cycle of the corresponding parasite.

- A high index of suspicion is required to diagnose emerging viral infections such as SARS and avian influenza.

- Avian influenza (influenza A H5N1) has genetic similarities with the agent of the 1918–19 pandemic. Major differences are a 50 percent mortality and lack of sustained human-human transmission by influenza A H5N1.

- Oseltamivir and zanamivir are active *in vitro* against nearly all strains of A H5N1. Clinical data show no efficacy for treatment, but the data are anecdotal and most patients were treated late in the course.
- Major methods of control of avian influenza today are social distancing (close schools, businesses, and quarantine); treating infected people with antivirals and isolating them; vaccinating contacts, giving them antivirals (ring antivirals), and isolating them.

REFERENCES

1. Laughlin L. Clinical practice in the tropics. In: Strickland G, ed. *Hunter's Tropical Medicine and Emerging Infectious Diseases*. Philadelphia: WB Saunders, 2000: 1–7.

◆ 2. Wilson RA. Immunity and immunoregulation in helminth infections. *Curr Opin Immunol* 1993; **5**: 538–47.

3. Klion AD, Eisenstein EM, Smirniotopoulos TT, *et al.* Pulmonary involvement in loiasis. *Am Rev Respir Dis* 1992; **145**(4 Pt 1): 961–3.

4. Jacobson ES. A case of secondary echinococcosis diagnosed by cytologic examination of pleural fluid and needle biopsy of pleura. *Acta Cytol* 1973; **17**: 76–9.

5. Johnson JR, Falk A, Iber C, Davies S. Paragonimiasis in the United States. A report of nine cases in Hmong immigrants. *Chest* 1982; **82**: 168–71.

◆ 6. Singh B. Molecular methods for diagnosis and epidemiological studies of parasitic infections. *Int J Parasitol* 1997; **27**: 1135–45.

7. Emad A. Exudative eosinophilic pleural effusion due to *Strongyloides stercoralis* in a diabetic man. *South Med J* 1999; **92**: 58–60.

8. Gupta K, Sehgal A, Puri MM, Sidhwa HK. Microfilariae in association with other diseases. A report of six cases. *Acta Cytol* 2002; **46**: 776–8.

9. Filler S, Causer LM, Newman RD, *et al.* Malaria surveillance – United States, 2001. *MMWR Surveill Summ* 2003; **52**: 1–14.

● 10. Severe and complicated malaria. World Health Organization, Division of Control of Tropical Diseases. *Trans R Soc Trop Med Hyg* 1990; **84**(Suppl 2): 1–65.

● 11. Falciparum malaria. World Health Organization, Communicable Diseases Cluster. *Trans R Soc Trop Med Hyg* 2000; **94**(Suppl 1): S1–90.

12. Pongponratn E, Turner GD, Day NP, *et al.* An ultrastructural study of the brain in fatal *Plasmodium falciparum* malaria. *Am J Trop Med Hyg* 2003; **69**: 345–59.

13. Kwiatkowski D, Hill AV, Sambou I, *et al.* TNF concentration in fatal cerebral, non-fatal cerebral, and uncomplicated *Plasmodium falciparum* malaria. *Lancet* 1990; **336**: 1201–4.

14. Baruch DI, Ma XC, Singh HB, *et al.* Identification of a region of PfEMP1 that mediates adherence of *Plasmodium falciparum* infected erythrocytes to CD36: conserved function with variant sequence. *Blood* 1997; **90**: 3766–75.

15. Moormann AM, Sullivan AD, Rochford RA, *et al.* Malaria and pregnancy: placental cytokine expression and its relationship to intrauterine growth retardation. *J Infect Dis* 1999; **180**: 1987–93.

16. Clark IA, Cowden WB. The pathophysiology of falciparum malaria. *Pharmacol Ther* 2003; **99**: 221–60.

17. Reeder JC, Cowman AF, Davern KM, *et al.* The adhesion of *Plasmodium falciparum*-infected erythrocytes to chondroitin sulfate A is mediated by *P. falciparum* erythrocyte membrane protein 1. *Proc Natl Acad Sci U S A* 1999; **96**: 5198–202.

18. Lichtman AR, Mohrcken S, Engelbrecht M, Bigalke M. Pathophysiology of severe forms of falciparum malaria. *Crit Care Med* 1990; **18**: 666–8.

◆ 19. Vogetseder A, Ospelt C, Reindl M, *et al.* Time course of coagulation parameters, cytokines and adhesion molecules in *Plasmodium falciparum* malaria. *Trop Med Int Health* 2004; **9**: 767–73.

20. Pouvelle B, Buffet PA, Lepolard C, *et al.* Cytoadhesion of *Plasmodium falciparum* ring-stage-infected erythrocytes. *Nat Med* 2000; **6**: 1264–8.

21. Charoenpan P, Indraprasit S, Kiatboonsri S, *et al.* Pulmonary edema in severe falciparum malaria. Hemodynamic study and clinicophysiologic correlation. *Chest* 1990; **97**: 1190–7.

● 22. Bruneel F, Gachot B, Timsit JF, *et al.* Shock complicating severe falciparum malaria in European adults. *Intensive Care Med* 1997; **23**: 698–701.

23. Krishnan A, Karnad DR. Severe falciparum malaria: an important cause of multiple organ failure in Indian intensive care unit patients. *Crit Care Med* 2003; **31**: 2278–84.

24. Koh KH, Chew PH, Kiyu A. A retrospective study of malaria infections in an intensive care unit of a general hospital in Malaysia. *Singapore Med J* 2004; **45**: 28–36.

● 25. Bruneel F, Hocqueloux L, Alberti C, *et al.* The clinical spectrum of severe imported falciparum malaria in the intensive care unit: report of 188 cases in adults. *Am J Respir Crit Care Med* 2003; **167**: 684–9.

26. Hemmer CJ, Kern P, Holst FG, *et al.* Activation of the host response in human *Plasmodium falciparum* malaria: relation of parasitemia to tumor necrosis factor/cachectin, thrombin-antithrombin III, and protein C levels. *Am J Med* 1991; **91**: 37–44.

27. Clemens R, Pramoolsinsap C, Lorenz R, *et al.* Activation of the coagulation cascade in severe falciparum malaria through the intrinsic pathway. *Br J Haematol* 1994; **87**: 100–5.

28. Krishna S, Waller FW, ter Kuile F, *et al.* Lactic acidosis and hypoglycaemia in children with severe malaria: pathophysiological and prognostic significance. *Trans R Soc Trop Med Hyg* 1994; **88**: 67–73.

29. Trang TT, Phu NH, Vinh H, *et al.* Acute renal failure in patients with severe falciparum malaria. *Clin Infect Dis* 1992; **15**: 874–80.

30. Mohanty S, Mishra SK, Pati SS, *et al.* Complications and mortality patterns due to *Plasmodium falciparum* malaria in hospitalized adults and children, Rourkela, Orissa, India. *Trans R Soc Trop Med Hyg* 2003; **97**: 69–70.

31. Mackintosh CL, Beeson JG, Marsh K. Clinical features and pathogenesis of severe malaria. *Trends Parasitol* 2004; **20**: 597–603.

32. James MF. Pulmonary damage associated with falciparum malaria: a report of ten cases. *Ann Trop Med Parasitol* 1985; **79**: 123–38.

33. Hovette P, Camara P, Burgel PR, *et al.* [Pulmonary manifestations associated with malaria]. *Rev Pneumol Clin* 1998; **54**: 340–5.

34. Rajput R, Singh H, Singh S, *et al.* Pulmonary manifestations in malaria. *J Indian Med Assoc* 2000; **98**: 612–14.

35. Gachot B, Wolff M, Nissack G, *et al.* Acute lung injury complicating imported *Plasmodium falciparum* malaria. *Chest* 1995; **108**: 746–9.

36. Baud M, Bauchet E, Poilane I, *et al.* Acute respiratory distress syndrome due to falciparum malaria in a pregnant woman. *Intensive Care Med* 1997; **23**: 787–9.

37. Losert H, Schmid K, Wilfing A, *et al.* Experiences with severe *P. falciparum* malaria in the intensive care unit. *Intensive Care Med* 2000; **26**: 195–201.

38. Jindal SK, Aggarwal AN, Gupta D. Adult respiratory distress syndrome in the tropics. *Clin Chest Med* 2002; **23**: 445–55.

39. Perren A, Beretta F, Schubarth P. [ARDS in plasmodium vivax malaria]. *Schweiz Med Wochenschr* 1998; **128**: 1020–3.

40. Postigo M, Mendoza-Leon A, Perez HA. Malaria diagnosis by the polymerase chain reaction: a field study in south-eastern Venezuela. *Trans R Soc Trop Med Hyg* 1998; **92**: 509–11.

41. Hanscheid T. Diagnosis of malaria: a review of alternatives to conventional microscopy. *Clin Lab Haematol* 1999; **21**: 235–45.

42. Ciceron L, Jaureguiberry G, Gay F, Danis M. Development of a *Plasmodium* PCR for monitoring efficacy of antimalarial treatment. *J Clin Microbiol* 1999; **37**: 35–8.

43. Sabchareon A, Chongsuphajaisiddhi T, Sinhasivanon V, *et al.* In vivo and in vitro responses to quinine and quinidine of *Plasmodium falciparum*. *Bull World Health Organ* 1988; **66**: 347–52.

◆ 44. White NJ. The treatment of malaria. *N Engl J Med* 1996; **335**: 800–6.

45. Phillips RE, Looareesuwan S, White NJ, *et al.* Hypoglycaemia and antimalarial drugs: quinidine and release of insulin. *Br Med J (Clin Res Ed)* 1986; **292**: 1319–21.

46. Birku Y, Makonnen E, Bjorkman A. Comparison of rectal artemisinin with intravenous quinine in the treatment of severe malaria in Ethiopia. *East Afr Med J* 1999; **76**: 154–9.

◆ 47. Maitland K, Makanga M, Williams TN. Falciparum malaria: current therapeutic challenges. *Curr Opin Infect Dis* 2004; **17**: 405–12.

48. Tran TH, Day NP, Nguyen HP, *et al.* A controlled trial of artemether or quinine in Vietnamese adults with severe falciparum malaria. *N Engl J Med* 1996; **335**: 76–83.

◆ 49. White NJ. The management of severe falciparum malaria. *Am J Respir Crit Care Med* 2003; **167**: 673–4.

50. Pittler MH, Ernst E. Artemether for severe malaria: a meta-analysis of randomized clinical trials. *Clin Infect Dis* 1999; **28**: 597–601.

51. Artemether-Quinine Meta-analysis Study Group. A meta-analysis using individual patient data of trials comparing artemether with quinine in the treatment of severe falciparum malaria. *Trans R Soc Trop Med Hyg* 2001; **95**: 637–50.

52. Crawley J, Waruiru C, Mithwani S, *et al.* Effect of phenobarbital on seizure frequency and mortality in childhood cerebral malaria: a randomised, controlled intervention study. *Lancet* 2000; **355**: 701–6.

53. Maitland K, Pamba A, Newton CR, *et al.* Hypokalemia in children with severe falciparum malaria. *Pediatr Crit Care Med* 2004; **5**: 81–5.

54. Day NP, Phu NH, Mai NT, *et al.* The pathophysiologic and prognostic significance of acidosis in severe adult malaria. *Crit Care Med* 2000; **28**: 1833–40.

55. Day NP, Hien TT, Schollaardt T, *et al.* The prognostic and pathophysiologic role of pro- and antiinflammatory cytokines in severe malaria. *J Infect Dis* 1999; **180**: 1288–97.

56. Maitland K, Pamba A, Newton CR, Levin M. Response to volume resuscitation in children with severe malaria. *Pediatr Crit Care Med* 2003; **4**: 426–31.

57. Rosenberg AL. Fluid management in patients with acute respiratory distress syndrome. *Respir Care Clin North Am* 2003; **9**: 481–93.

58. Looareesuwan S, Wilairatana P, Krishna S, *et al.* Magnetic resonance imaging of the brain in patients with cerebral malaria. *Clin Infect Dis* 1995; **21**: 300–9.

59. Hoffman SL, Rustama D, Punjabi NH, *et al.* High-dose dexamethasone in quinine-treated patients with cerebral malaria: a double-blind, placebo-controlled trial. *J Infect Dis* 1988; **158**: 325–31.

60. Warrell DA, White NJ, Warrell MJ. Dexamethasone deleterious in cerebral malaria. *Br Med J (Clin Res Ed)* 1982; **285**: 1652.

61. Molyneux ME, Looareesuwan S, Menzies IS, *et al.* Reduced hepatic blood flow and intestinal malabsorption in severe falciparum malaria. *Am J Trop Med Hyg* 1989; **40**: 470–6.

62. Harbarth S, Meyer M, Grau GE, *et al.* Septic shock due to cytomegalovirus infection in acute respiratory distress syndrome after falciparum malaria. *J Travel Med* 1997; **4**: 148–9.

● 63. Phu NH, Hien TT, Mai NT, *et al.* Hemofiltration and peritoneal dialysis in infection-associated acute renal failure in Vietnam. *N Engl J Med* 2002; **347**: 895–902.

● 64. Miller KD, Greenberg AE, Campbell CC. Treatment of severe malaria in the United States with a continuous infusion of quinidine gluconate and exchange transfusion. *N Engl J Med* 1989; **321**: 65–70.

65. Hoontrakoon S, Suputtamongkol Y. Exchange transfusion as an adjunct to the treatment of severe falciparum malaria. *Trop Med Int Health* 1998; **3**: 156–61.

66. Phillips RE, Pasvol G. Anaemia of *Plasmodium falciparum* malaria. *Baillières Clin Haematol* 1992; **5**: 315–30.

67. Newton CR, Crawley J, Sowumni A, *et al.* Intracranial hypertension in Africans with cerebral malaria. *Arch Dis Child* 1997; **76**: 219–26.

68. Walsh JA. Problems in recognition and diagnosis of amebiasis: estimation of the global magnitude of morbidity and mortality. *Rev Infect Dis* 1986; **8**: 228–38.

◆ 69. Mbaye PS, Koffi N, Camara P, *et al.* [Pleuropulmonary manifestations of amebiasis]. *Rev Pneumol Clin* 1998; **54**: 346–52.

70. Herrera-Llerandi R. Thoracic repercussions of amebiasis. *J Thorac Cardiovasc Surg* 1966; **52**: 361–75.

71. Lichtenstein A, Kondo AT, Visvesvara GS, *et al.* Pulmonary amoebiasis presenting as superior vena cava syndrome. *Thorax* 2005; **60**: 350–2.

◆ 72. Charoenratanakul S. Tropical infection and the lung. *Monaldi Arch Chest Dis* 1997; **52**: 376–9.

73. Cameron EW. The treatment of pleuropulmonary amebiasis with metronidazole. *Chest* 1978; **73**: 647–50.

74. Ibarra-Perez C. Thoracic complications of amebic abscess of the liver: report of 501 cases. *Chest* 1981; **79**: 672–7.

75. Thorsen S, Ronne-Rasmussen J, Petersen E, *et al.* Extra-intestinal amebiasis: clinical presentation in a non-endemic setting. *Scand J Infect Dis* 1993; **25**: 747–50.

76. Lyche KD, Jensen WA. Pleuropulmonary amebiasis. *Semin Respir Infect* 1997; **12**: 106–12.

77. Fulton AJ, Picker RH, Cooper RA, Lunzer MR. Pulmonary complication of amoebic liver abscess. *Australas Radiol* 1982; **26**: 60–3.

78. Boultbee JE, Simjee AE, Rooknoodeen F, Engelbrecht HE. Experiences with grey scale ultrasonography in hepatic amoebiasis. *Clin Radiol* 1979; **30**: 683–9.

79. Kubitschek KR, Peters J, Nickeson D, Musher DM. Amebiasis presenting as pleuropulmonary disease. *West J Med* 1985; **142**: 203–7.

◆ 80. Allen JN, Davis WB. Eosinophilic lung diseases. *Am J Respir Crit Care Med* 1994. **150** (5 Pt 1): 1423–38.

81. Chitkara RK, Sarinas PS. Dirofilaria, visceral larva migrans, and tropical pulmonary eosinophilia. *Semin Respir Infect* 1997; **12**: 138–48.

82. Vijayan VK. Tropical pulmonary eosinophilia. *Indian J Chest Dis Allied Sci* 1996; **38**: 169–80.

83. Pinkston P, Vijayan VK, Nutman TB, *et al.* Acute tropical pulmonary eosinophilia. Characterization of the lower respiratory tract inflammation and its response to therapy. *J Clin Invest* 1987; **80**: 216–25.

84. Ong RK, Doyle RL. Tropical pulmonary eosinophilia. *Chest* 1998; **113**: 1673–9.

85. Rom WN, *et al.* Persistent lower respiratory tract inflammation associated with interstitial lung disease in patients with tropical pulmonary eosinophilia following conventional treatment with diethylcarbamazine. *Am Rev Respir Dis* 1990; **142**: 1088–92.

86. Spry CJ, Kumaraswami V. Tropical eosinophilia. *Semin Hematol* 1982; **19**: 107–15.

87. Shah MK. Human pulmonary dirofilariasis: review of the literature. *South Med J* 1999; **92**: 276–9.

88. Bartelink AK, Kortbeek LM, Huidekoper HJ, *et al.* Acute respiratory failure due to *Toxocara* infection. *Lancet* 1993; **342**: 1234.

89. Siddiqui AA, Berk SL. Diagnosis of *Strongyloides stercoralis* infection. *Clin Infect Dis* 2001; **33**: 1040–7.

● 90. Muennig P, Pallin D, Sell RL, Chan MS. The cost effectiveness of strategies for the treatment of intestinal parasites in immigrants. *N Engl J Med* 1999; **340**: 773–9.

91. Gompels MM, Todd J, Peters BS, *et al.* Disseminated strongyloidiasis in AIDS: uncommon but important. *AIDS* 1991; **5**: 329–32.

92. Zaha O, Hirata T, Kinjo F, Saito A. Strongyloidiasis – progress in diagnosis and treatment. *Intern Med* 2000; **39**: 695–700.

93. Ottesen EA, Campbell WC. Ivermectin in human medicine. *J Antimicrob Chemother* 1994; **34**: 195–203.

94. Datry A, Hilmarsdottir I, Mayorga-Sagastume R, *et al.* Treatment of *Strongyloides stercoralis* infection with ivermectin compared with albendazole: results of an open study of 60 cases. *Trans R Soc Trop Med Hyg* 1994; **88**: 344–5.

95. Dessein AJ, Parker WL, James SL, David JR. IgE antibody and resistance to infection. I. Selective suppression of the IgE antibody response in rats diminishes the resistance and the eosinophil response to *Trichinella spiralis* infection. *J Exp Med* 1981; **153**: 423–36.

96. Ljungstrom I, Engvall E, Ruitenberg EJ. Proceedings: ELISA, enzyme linked immunosorbent assay – a new technique for sero-diagnosis of trichinosis. *Parasitology* 1974; **69**: xxiv.

◆ 97. Roberts PP. Parasitic infections of the pleural space. *Semin Respir Infect* 1988; **3**: 362–82.

98. Ozcelik C, Inci I, Toprak M, *et al.* Surgical treatment of pulmonary hydatidosis in children: experience in 92 patients. *J Pediatr Surg* 1994; **29**: 392–5.

99. Jerray M, Benzarti M, Garrouche A, *et al.* Hydatid disease of the lungs. Study of 386 cases. *Am Rev Respir Dis* 1992; **146**: 185–9.

100. Bousnina S, Racil H, Maghraoui O, *et al.* [Hydatid pulmonary embolisms. Seven cases]. *Rev Pneumol Clin* 2005; **61**(1 Pt 1): 31–6.

101. Xanthakis DS, Katsaras E, Efthimiadis M, *et al.* Hydatid cyst of the liver with intrathoracic rupture. *Thorax* 1981; **36**: 497–501.

102. von Sinner W. Pleural complications of hydatid disease (*Echinococcus granulosus*). *Rofo Fortschr Geb Rontgenstr Neuen Bildgeb Verfahr* 1990; **152**: 718–22.

103. Wen H, New RR, Craig PS. Diagnosis and treatment of human hydatidosis. *Br J Clin Pharmacol* 1993; **35**: 565–74.

104. Balikian JP, Mudarris FF. Hydatid disease of the lungs. A roentgenologic study of 50 cases. *Am J Roentgenol Radium Ther Nucl Med* 1974; **122**: 692–707.

105. Balikian JP, Idriss IA, Dagher IK. Hydatid tension pneumothorax. Report of a case. *J Med Liban* 1974; **27**: 551–6.

106. Lewall DB, McCorkell SJ. Rupture of echinococcal cysts: diagnosis, classification, and clinical implications. *AJR Am J Roentgenol* 1986; **146**: 391–4.

107. Cangir AK, Sahin E, Enon S, *et al.* Surgical treatment of pulmonary hydatid cysts in children. *J Pediatr Surg* 2001; **36**: 917–20.

◆ 108. Skerrett SJ. Parasitic infections of the pleural space. *Semin Respir Med* 1992; **13**: 242–58.

109. Drugs for parasitic infections. *Med Lett Drugs Ther* 1998; **40**: 1–12.

110. Yokogawa M. Paragonimus and paragonimiasis. *Adv Parasitol* 1965; **3**: 99–158.

111. Minh VD, Engle P, Greenwood JR, *et al.* Pleural paragonimiasis in a Southeast Asia refugee. *Am Rev Respir Dis* 1981; **124**: 186–8.

112. Blair D, Xu ZB, Agatsuma T. Paragonimiasis and the genus *Paragonimus*. *Adv Parasitol* 1999; **42**: 113–222.

113. Mukae H, Taniguchi H, Matsumoto N, *et al.* Clinicoradiologic features of pleuropulmonary *Paragonimus westermani* on Kyusyu Island, Japan. *Chest* 2001; **120**: 514–20.

114. Sharma OP. The man who loved drunken crabs. A case of pulmonary paragonimiasis. *Chest* 1989; **95**: 670–2.

115. Im JG, Whang HY, Kim WS, *et al.* Pleuropulmonary paragonimiasis: radiologic findings in 71 patients. *AJR Am J Roentgenol* 1992; **159**: 39–43.

116. Yee B, *et al.* Pulmonary paragonimiasis in Southeast Asians living in the central San Joaquin Valley. *West J Med* 1992; **156**: 423–5.

117. Yokogawa M, Kojima S, Araki K, *et al.* Immunoglobulin E: raised levels in sera and pleural exudates of patients with paragonimiasis. *Am J Trop Med Hyg* 1976; **25**: 581–6.

118. Taniguchi H, Mukae H, Matsumoto N, *et al.* Elevated IL-5 levels in pleural fluid of patients with *Paragonimiasis westermani. Clin Exp Immunol* 2001; **123**: 94–8.

119. Doherty JF, Moody AH, Wright SG. Katayama fever: an acute manifestation of schistosomiasis. *BMJ* 1996; **313**: 1071–2.

120. Barrett-Connor E. Parasitic pulmonary disease. *Am Rev Respir Dis* 1982; **126**: 558–63.

121. Morris W, Knauer CM. Cardiopulmonary manifestations of schistosomiasis. *Semin Respir Infect* 1997; **12**: 159–70.

122. Kohler P. The biochemical basis of anthelmintic action and resistance. *Int J Parasitol* 2001; **31**: 336–45.

✱ 123. Saconato H, Attalah A. Interventions for treating *Schistosomiasis mansoni. Cochrane Database Syst Rev* 2000; **2**: CD000528.

✱ 124. Squires N. Interventions for treating *Schistosomiasis hematobium. Cochrane Database Syst Rev* 2000; **2**: CD00053.

125. Greco DB, Pedroso ER, Lambertucci JR, *et al.* Pulmonary involvement in *Schistosomiasis mansoni. Mem Inst Oswaldo Cruz* 1987; **82**(Suppl 4): 221–7.

126. Clement JP. Hantavirus. *Antiviral Res* 2003; **57**(1–2): 121–7.

127. Botten J, Mirowsky K, Kusewitt D, *et al.* Persistent Sin Nombre virus infection in the deer mouse (*Peromyscus maniculatus*) model: sites of replication and strand-specific expression. *J Virol* 2003; **77**: 1540–50.

128. Levy H, Simpson SQ. Hantavirus pulmonary syndrome. *Am J Respir Crit Care Med* 1994; **149**: 1710–13.

129. Boone JD, McGwire KC, Otteson EW, *et al.* Infection dynamics of Sin Nombre virus after a widespread decline in host populations. *Am J Trop Med Hyg* 2002; **67**: 310–18.

130. Bustamante EA, Levy H, Simpson SQ. Pleural fluid characteristics in hantavirus pulmonary syndrome. *Chest* 1997; **112**: 1133–6.

131. Hujakka H, Koistinen V, Kuronen I, *et al.* Diagnostic rapid tests for acute hantavirus infections: specific tests for Hantaan, Dobrava and Puumala viruses versus a hantavirus combination test. *J Virol Methods* 2003; **108**: 117–22.

◆ 132. Lednicky JA. Hantaviruses. a short review. *Arch Pathol Lab Med* 2003; **127**: 30–5.

133. Kautner I, Robinson MJ, Kuhnle U. Dengue virus infection: epidemiology, pathogenesis, clinical presentation, diagnosis, and prevention. *J Pediatr* 1997; **131**: 516–24.

134. Rigau-Perez JG, Clark GG, Gubler DJ, *et al.* Dengue and dengue haemorrhagic fever. *Lancet* 1998; **352**: 971–7.

◆ 135. Ramirez-Ronda CH, Garcia CD. Dengue in the Western Hemisphere. *Infect Dis Clin North Am* 1994; **8**: 107–28.

136. Avirutnan P, Malasit P, Seliger B, *et al.* Dengue virus infection of human endothelial cells leads to chemokine production, complement activation, and apoptosis. *J Immunol* 1998; **161**: 6338–46.

137. Lum LC, Thong MK, Cheah YK, *et al.* Dengue-associated adult respiratory distress syndrome. *Ann Trop Paediatr* 1995; **15**: 335–9.

✱ 138. Wills BA, Nguyen MD, Ha TL, *et al.* Comparison of three fluid solutions for resuscitation in dengue shock syndrome. *N Engl J Med* 2005; **353**: 877–89.

139. Lee N, Hui D, Wu A, *et al.* A major outbreak of severe acute respiratory syndrome in Hong Kong. *N Engl J Med* 2003; **348**: 1986–94.

140. Peiris JS, Lai ST, Poon LL, *et al.* Coronavirus as a possible cause of severe acute respiratory syndrome. *Lancet* 2003; **361**: 1319–25.

● 141. Drosten C, Gunther S, Preiser W, *et al.* Identification of a novel coronavirus in patients with severe acute respiratory syndrome. *N Engl J Med* 2003; **348**: 1967–76.

● 142. Leung GM, Hedley AJ, Ho LM, *et al.* The epidemiology of severe acute respiratory syndrome in the 2003 Hong Kong epidemic: an analysis of all 1755 patients. *Ann Intern Med* 2004; **141**: 662–73.

143. Control, C.f.d. Revised US Surveillance case definition for severe acute respiratory syndrome (SARS) and update on SARS cases – United States and worldwide, December 2003. *MMWR* 2003; **52**: 1202–6.

144. Lew TW, Kwek TK, Tai D, *et al.* Acute respiratory distress syndrome in critically ill patients with severe acute respiratory syndrome. *JAMA* 2003; **290**: 374–80.

◆145. Groneberg DA, Poutanen SM, Low DE, *et al.*
Treatment and vaccines for severe acute respiratory
syndrome. *Lancet Infect Dis* 2005; **5**: 147–55.

●146. Katz JM, Lim W, Bridges CB, *et al.* Antibody
response in individuals infected with avian influenza
A (H5N1) viruses and detection of anti-H5 antibody
among household and social contacts. *J Infect Dis*
1999; **180**: 1763–70.

◆147. Kaye D, Pringle CR. Avian influenza viruses and their
implication for human health. *Clin Infect Dis* 2005;
40: 108–12.

◆148. Beigel JH, Farrar J, Han AM, *et al.* Avian influenza A
(H5N1) infection in humans. *N Engl J Med* 2005;
353: 1374–85.

149. de Jong MD, Tran TT, Truong HK, *et al.* Oseltamivir
resistance during treatment of influenza A (H5N1)
infection. *N Engl J Med* 2005; **353**: 2667–72.

150. Le QM, Kiso M, Someya K, *et al.* Avian flu: isolation
of drug-resistant H5N1 virus. *Nature* 2005; **437**:
1108.

Pleural space infections and empyema

JAY T HEIDECKER, JOHN E HEFFNER, STEVEN A SAHN

INTRODUCTION AND DEFINITIONS

Pleural space infection (parapneumonic effusion and empyema) is common and causes significant morbidity and mortality. Pneumonia is the most common cause of death from infectious disease and with influenza ranks sixth as a cause of mortality in the United States.[1] The incidence of community-acquired pneumonia (CAP) is estimated at 3.5–4 million cases per year with about 20 percent of patients requiring hospitalization.[2] Forty-four percent of hospitalized patients with pneumonia develop parapneumonic effusions,[3] translating into 300 000 to 350 000 parapneumonic effusions per year in the United States. Parapneumonic effusion and empyema can also occur as a consequence of hospital-acquired pneumonia, surgical or iatrogenic complication, trauma, and following tuberculosis infection. Pleural space infection represents consequences ranging from a small pleural effusion due to pneumonia that resolves spontaneously to a multiloculated empyema with thick pus that causes pleural sepsis and trapped lung. Therapeutic options range from observation to thoracotomy with decortication. The choice of therapy depends upon the stage of effusion, the presence or absence of pleural sepsis, the severity of clinical symptoms, and the ability of the patient to tolerate surgery.

The classification of pleural space infection can be confusing. For clarity, an uncomplicated parapneumonic effusion is defined as a pleural effusion occurring in the setting of pneumonia that resolves with antibiotic therapy alone. A complicated parapneumonic effusion is a pleural effusion associated with pneumonia that requires drainage. Empyema is defined as pus in the pleural space.[3] Pleural space drainage can be accomplished by small or large bore chest tubes alone, thoracoscopic surgery, or thoracotomy.

PATHOPHYSIOLOGY OF PLEURAL EFFUSIONS

The pleural space is 10–20 µm in width and encompasses the area between the parietal and visceral pleura. Only the parietal pleura has stomata, which are 2–12 µm openings through which liquid and proteins exit the pleural space.[4,5] The stomata communicate with lymphatic lacunae that drain into collecting lymphatics, which converge into the mediastinal lymph nodes. Pleural fluid, an ultrafiltrate of the interstitium of the parietal pleura, enters the pleural space along a pressure gradient. In normal 30 kg sheep, approximately 7 mL of pleural fluid is produced daily. Pleural lymphatics have the capacity to drain over 20 times the physiologic production of pleural fluid. In humans, pleural lymphatics can remove approximately 500 mL of fluid per day. Clinical pleural effusions develop when pleural fluid production exceeds 500 mL per day, lymphatic drainage becomes impaired, or a combination of these two factors. Increased pleural fluid production occurs as a consequence of increased microvascular hydrostatic forces (congestive heart failure), decreased microvascular oncotic pressure (nephrosis), more negative intrapleural pressure (atelectasis), or altered microvascular permeability (pneumonia). Parapneumonic effusions are prototypical exudative effusions that occur as a result of altered microvascular permeability.[6] Inflammatory mediators cause liquid and protein to leak across capillary barriers into the pleural space at a rate that exceeds the resorptive capacity of pleural lymphatics. The inflammatory process can cause fibrinous debris to deposit along pleural membranes and obstruct lymphatic stomata reducing their resorptive capacity and further contributing to pleural fluid accumulation.

PARAPNEUMONIC EFFUSIONS

The natural history of a parapneumonic effusion evolves over three stages: exudative, fibrinopurulent, and organizing. The exudative stage begins shortly after the onset of the pneumonic process. Neutrophils bind to cell wall components on bacteria in the distal alveoli and secrete interleukin (IL)-1, -6, and -8, tumor necrosis factor (TNF)-α, and platelet activating factor (PAF).[7] Interleukin-8 and PAF recruit neutrophils, which secrete additional cytokines that recruit more neutrophils and increase vascular permeability of both pulmonary and adjacent parietal pleural microvessels. Thus, a neutrophil-predominant, protein-rich fluid with an elevated lactate dehydrogenase is formed in the pleural space.[8] At this stage of a parapneumonic effusion, end-products of the metabolic activity of the pleural fluid can be removed from the pleural space maintaining a pH >7.30 and a glucose >33.3 mmol/L (60 mg/dL).[9] Prompt and appropriate antibiotic therapy controls the inflammatory process and allows normal pleural resorptive mechanisms to resolve the effusion. In the absence of timely and appropriate therapy, the effusion evolves into the fibrinopurulent stage.

The fibrinopurulent stage is characterized by continued exudation of plasma proteins, including coagulation factors, as well as deregulation of fibrinolysis, resulting in altered fibrin turnover, septation, and loculation within the pleural space. The mesothelial cell appears to be an integral component of this process. During the development of a parapneumonic effusion, the mesothelial cell is stimulated by TNF-α, IL-1, lipopolysaccharide, and interferon (INF)-γ.[10] In parapneumonic effusion and empyema, levels of plasminogen activator inhibitor (PAI)-1 and PAI-2 are significantly elevated compare with in patients with pleural fluid from malignancy and congestive heart failure.[11–13] The secretion of PAI-1 and PAI-2 inhibits fibrinolysis and fibrin formation.[14] Because there is a fibrinogen-rich protein exudate already within the pleural space, fibrin strands form, causing loculation. It is likely that during the fibrinopurulent stage, bacteria move from the lung parenchyma into the pleural space, causing heightened inflammation with

increased glycolysis, acid generation, derangement of the fibrinolytic system, and pleural loculation. Extensive loculation can lead to lung entrapment.[15] Radiographically, pleural effusions in this stage will not be completely free flowing. Septations and loculations are often visible by ultrasound and computed tomography (CT).[16]

As the effusion evolves from the exudative to fibrinopurulent stage, glucose metabolism is increased and acid byproducts of glucose metabolism (carbon dioxide and lactic acid) accumulate and result in pleural fluid acidosis. This accumulation of acid results from increased production as well as decreased efflux of acid across the abnormal pleural membranes.[9,17] The postulated mechanism in clinical and experimental empyema is increased glucose utilization by pleural fluid leukocytes and bacteria as opposed to impaired glucose transfer from the blood into the pleural space.[18] The acidification of the pleural space is augmented as septations and loculations isolate dependent regions of the pleural space and limit the ability of acid to efflux across the pleural membranes.

The third stage of a parapneumonic effusion is the organizing stage, which results in a frank empyema. Progression to this stage typically occurs over 2–4 weeks in the absence of adequate treatment of the fibrinopurulent stage. Fibroblasts enter the pleural space and promote collagen deposition on the fibrin skeleton and along the pleural surface. The result is an inelastic pleural peel that limits lung expansion. The empyema fluid (pus) becomes thick with fibrin, cellular debris, and coagulation proteins which often contain viable bacteria.[19] An empyema may resolve with some residual degree of pleural thickening or trapped lung,[20] drain through the chest wall (empyema necessitatis), or drain into the bronchi (bronchopleural fistula).[19]

EPIDEMIOLOGY AND MICROBIOLOGY

Causes of pleural space infection include empyema from a progression of parapneumonic effusions, iatrogenic seeding, chest trauma, tuberculosis, progression of mediastinitis, extension of abdominal infection, spontaneous bacterial pleuritis, septic emboli, and seeding of preexisting pleural effusions during bacteremia. Strange and Sahn[3] reviewed 14 case series published during a 7-year period (1990–1997) and found that 70 percent of empyemas resulted from progression of parapneumonic effusions. Of the 380 causes of empyema in their 24-year experience, Weissberg and Refaely[21] found bacterial empyema occurred as a complication of parapneumonic effusion in 308 patients, and as a complication of tuberculosis in 24 patients and trauma in 15 patients; in 29 the cause was undetermined.

Case studies of empyema in the preantibiotic era demonstrated that the predominant organism was *Streptococcus pneumoniae*.[22] Other case series from the 1950s and 1960s showed a predominance of *Staphylococcus aureus* and Gram-negative rods with rare anaerobic infections.[23] More recently, the microbiology of empyema has shifted toward a predominance of mixed infections with anaerobes.[24–26] The microbiology of empyema, however, depends on the patient population that is studied. In a review of two military hospitals, most cases showed pure cultures of either *Staph. aureus* or *Strep. pneumoniae*.[27] In this study, there were numerous anaerobes recovered; however, they were most often in mixed culture and comprised a minority of cases. The preponderance of pure aerobic isolates was likely due to a relatively young military aged population, so aspiration of oropharyngeal contents is likely less common and development of anaerobic infection rare. In a large series of 584 trauma patients, the number of chest tubes was the greatest predictor for development of posttraumatic empyema, as 92 percent of patients with empyema had multiple chest tubes. *Staph. aureus* was the most common pathogen, being isolated in 74 percent of patients.[28] Methicillin-resistant *Staph. aureus* (MRSA) was the most common organism isolated from patients with postoperative empyema in a large case series.[29] In contrast, in a case series of 72 veterans over a 10-year period, anaerobic infection accounted for 39 percent of empyemas and mixed aerobic, and 8 percent of cases had anaerobic infections.[25] Empyema in this patient population was primarily post pneumonic with a sizable minority of patients being postsurgical. Excluding postoperative settings, anaerobic organisms, streptococcal species, and mixed infections are likely to be the most common pathogens identified. *Legionella*[30]and *Mycoplasma pneumoniae*[31,32] can cause parapneumonic effusions that are usually self-limiting.

Empyema most often represents neglected pleural infection. When patients with parapneumonic effusions are admitted to the hospital and treated appropriately, less than 2 percent progress to an empyema.[33] Unfortunately, patients with established empyema commonly experienced delays in their initial care. Ferguson and coworkers,[34] for instance, noted in a series of 119 patients with established empyema that the average time from symptom onset to presentation to a physician was 5 days. Moreover, admitting physicians considered the diagnosis of empyema in only 29 percent of patients. The average time from initial physician visit to admission for management of empyema was 13 days.[34] Heffner and coworkers[35] observed that practicing physicians often delayed thoracentesis in patients admitted with parapneumonic effusion and that length of hospital stay was prolonged in patients with the longest delays.

CLINICAL MANIFESTATIONS

The signs and symptoms of parapneumonic effusion and empyema are similar to those of pneumonia. The most common symptoms are fever, malaise, cough, dyspnea, and chest pain.[25,29,34,36] Other symptoms that may be associated with parapneumonic effusion and empyema are altered mental status, right upper quadrant pain, and rigors. Physical examination may reveal pyrexia, tachycardia, tachypnea, hypotension, bronchial breath sounds, decreased breath sounds, absent tactile fremitus, and dullness to percussion. Of note, there are patients who may be relatively asymptomatic. In one series, fever and dyspnea occurred in less than 50 percent of patients.[34] Often, patients at risk for empyema are those who cannot mount an effective immune response, and therefore may not manifest fever or have significant symptoms. Predisposing risk factors for development of empyema are listed in Table 10E.1. One reason for the underrecognition of empyema by patients and physicians is the lack of specific symptoms.

Table 10E.1 *Predisposing conditions for empyema (pooled analysis of three large case series**

Systemic causes	Pulmonary causes
Aspiration syndromes[†] = 37	Chronic obstructive pulmonary disease = 33
Alcohol ingestion = 23	Lung cancer = 15
Diabetes mellitus = 16	Previous tuberculosis = 7
Rheumatoid arthritis = 14	Bronchiectasis = 5
Congestive heart failure = 13	Recurrent pneumonia = 2
Dental issues = 12	Pulmonary sequestration = 1
Malignancy NOS = 7	
Immune suppressive drugs = 7	
Malnutrition = 4	
Gastrointestinal hemorrhage = 3	
Systemic lupus erythematosus = 1	

[†]Sedative drugs, neurologic disease, gastroesophageal reflux disease, head and neck cancer, seizure disorder esophageal stricture.

*Smith *et al.*,[29] Civen *et al.*,[26] Ferguson *et al.*,[34] total n = 209 patients.

NOS, not otherwise specified.

CHEST IMAGING

A standard chest radiograph may fail to detect a small parapneumonic effusion. Accumulation of less than 200 mL results in a subpulmonic effusion, which may simulate hemidiaphragm elevation and flattening. In contrast to true diaphragmatic elevation, lung markings are not visible below what appears to be the dome of the diaphragm.[37,38] Accumulation of more than 200 mL of pleural fluid causes blunting of the costophrenic angle. Supine radiographs fail to detect large effusions because of posterior layering. Increased density of a hemithorax without obscuration of vascular markings on a supine radiograph should alert the clinician to the possibility of pleural fluid.[37] Lateral decubitus views assist detection of small effusions. Larger effusions obscure dependent portions of the hemithorax. Pleural effusions that do not shift to the dependent position on a decubitus view are likely loculated and suggest the presence of a complicated parapneumonic effusion or empyema.[37] The presence of loculations requires sampling of the fluid under CT or ultrasound guidance.

Ultrasonography can detect small pleural effusions below radiographic thresholds and guide thoracentesis and chest tube placement.[39] Ultrasound can also differentiate pleural fluid collections from lung tissue and parenchymal masses. Demonstration of dynamic changes of the echo-free space during respiration, visualization of atelectatic or compressed lung that flaps during respiration, and a swirling motion in an echo-free space indicate pleural fluid that can be accessed by thoracentesis.[40] Ultrasonography can also categorize pleural effusions into:

- anechoic – no distinguishing characteristics compatible with a transudate or uncomplicated parapneumonic effusion
- echogenic – debris suggestive of complicated parapneumonic effusion in a patient with pneumonia
- septate – being associated with fibrinous stranding and empyema.[41]

Figures 10E.1 and 10E.2 show the ultrasound appearance of a uniloculated empyema and multiloculated empyema, respectively. In a review of 320 pleural effusions assessed by ultrasonography, transudates were never complex in appearance and a homogeneous complex effusion was indicative of hemorrhagic effusion or empyema. Other classifications and correlations to clinical outcomes were not demonstrable.[42] A poor association exists, however, between the presence of ultrasonographic evidence of septation and the biochemical nature of the effusion or the need for surgical drainage.[16] Ultrasonography is able to reliably exclude the presence of a transudative effusion if it appears complex. However, it cannot reliably differentiate between a simple and complicated exudative effusion. Thus, ultrasonography is not able to definitively characterize the need for tube thoracostomy or surgical intervention in pleural infection.

Computed tomography can enhance the evaluation of parapneumonic effusions and empyema. Figures 10E.3 and 10E.4 show chest CT scans of uniloculated and multiloculated empyema, respectively. Chest CT can detect pleural thickening, lung cavitation, intrapleural gas, fluid loculations, and contrast enhancement of the pleura.[16,43] It can also help differentiate an empyema from a lung abscess.[44] As with ultrasonography, CT can assist the placement of chest tubes in patients with loculated fluid collections. The absence of loculations on chest CT suggests that tube thoracostomy is not needed. Himelman and Callen[43] found in their series of 48 patients that only 10 percent of patients without loculations by CT required tube thoracostomy. In the absence of an air–fluid level in the pleural space that identifies a bronchopleural fistula or a

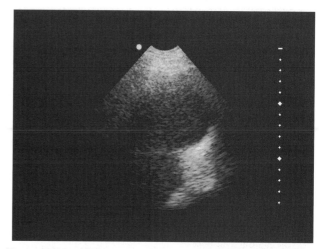

Figure 10E.1 *Ultrasound appearance of a uniloculated empyema under tension caused by* Actinomyces. *Notice the grainy appearance of the effusion. This may indicate that the effusion is either a complicated parapneumonic effusion or an empyema.*

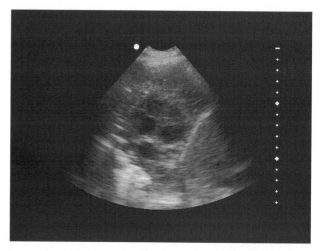

Figure 10E.2 *Ultrasound appearance of a multiloculated empyema. Note the multiple septations seen dividing the pleural effusion. The presence of septations on ultrasound does not necessarily mean the effusion is loculated.*

ruptured esophagus, the presence of loculations on chest CT does not reliably indicate the need for tube thoracostomy.[44] However, CT findings aid clinicians in predicting failure of chest tube drainage. Among patients with empyema or complicated parapneumonic effusions by biochemistry definitions, the presence of loculations had a positive predictive value for failure of drainage of 81 percent (n = 38/47). The positive predictive value for success of drainage in the absence of loculations was 53 percent (n = 28/53).[45] Thus, while there are few specific findings by CT scan that mandate the need for tube thoracostomy, it can be useful in predicting failure of tube thoracostomy.

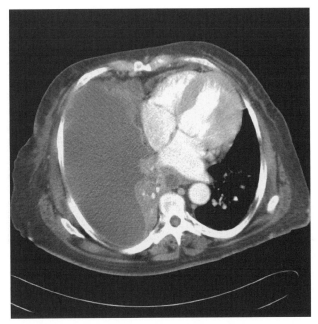

Figure 10E.3 *Computed tomography (CT) scan appearance of the same uniloculated empyema. Note the absence of loculations which correlates with the absence of septations on ultrasound.*

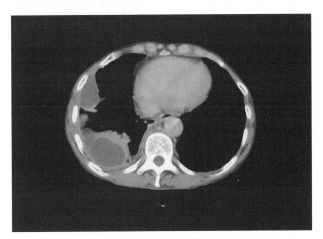

Figure 10E.4 *Computed tomography (CT) scan appearance of a multiloculated empyema. Note the two distinct loculations with pleural thickening and the split pleura sign.*

THORACENTESIS

Pleural fluid analysis provides necessary information to diagnose an empyema (detection of pus), to categorize the stage of a parapneumonic effusion, and to select patients for drainage. The 1962 American Thoracic Society statement defines empyema by the presence of pus in the pleural space. Some clinicians include a positive Gram-stain or growth of an organism in culture in the definition of empyema. Many patients with frank empyema, however, may have negative pleural fluid cultures because of antibiotic therapy or nonviable organisms within grossly purulent pleural exudates. A

diagnostic thoracentesis should be performed for all patients with parapneumonic effusions that layer greater than 1 cm on lateral decubitus film or are loculated. Although treatment with empiric antibiotics should not be delayed, prompt initial thoracentesis is associated with a decreased hospital stay length.[35,46] If available, ultrasonography should be used to guide thoracentesis because of the lower complication rate with this approach.[40] Thoracentesis of loculated pleural effusions should not proceed without ultrasound or CT guidance.

PLEURAL FLUID ANALYSIS

Table 10E.2 lists pleural fluid tests with their diagnostic significance for evaluating a parapneumonic effusion. Parapneumonic effusions may be serous, blood-tinged, bloody, turbid, or frankly purulent in appearance.[47] The presence of purulent fluid at thoracentesis defines an empyema. Malodorous fluid strongly suggests the presence of an anaerobic empyema.[34] Pleural fluid samples should be injected into anaerobic transport bottles for culture studies instead of blood culture bottles.[48] Blood culture bottles overly increase the sensitivity of detecting bacteria and the likelihood of culturing contaminants. The recovery of pus dictates the need for drainage; a positive Gram stain or a positive fluid culture usually require chest tube drainage.[19] An elevated pleural fluid salivary amylase or the finding of food particles confirm an esophageal rupture and a need for thoracostomy.[49]

Pleural fluid pH, glucose, and lactate dehydrogenase (LDH) assist the decision to place a chest tube. Pleural fluid pH and glucose reflect glucose metabolism by bacteria and

Table 10E.2 *Parapneumonic effusion: pleural fluid analysis and significance*

Purulent appearance	Requires drainage
Putrid odor	Anaerobic empyema requiring drainage
Cell count and differential	Neutrophilia indicates acute infection. The degree of leukocytosis is of limited diagnostic import
Glucose	Glucose <22.2–33.3 mmol/L (40–60 mg/dL) suggests need for drainage
pH	<7.30 suggests need for drainage <7.10 most likely requires drainage <6.00 suggests esophageal rupture
Lactate dehydrogenase	>1000 IU/L suggests need for drainage
Positive Gram stain ± culture	Guides antibiotic treatment; suggests need for drainage
Elevated salivary amylase	Diagnostic of esophageal rupture
Food particles or squamous epithelial cells	Diagnostic of esophageal rupture

neutrophils.[18,50] Lactate dehydrogenase is an intracellular enzyme released as intrapleural inflammatory cells undergo autolysis. It is thus a surrogate for the degree of the inflammatory response in a parapneumonic effusion. Several unblinded studies have noted an association between a low pleural fluid pH, low glucose, and high LDH and the clinician's perception that chest tube drainage is needed for patients with parapneumonic effusions. These investigators have reported a high specificity of a pH <7.00 for identifying patients who required drainage of a parapneumonic effusion.[8,9,19,51] The small size of the existing studies and considerable variation between each report, however, have not allowed consensus in selecting an ideal cutoff point for pleural fluid pH for discriminating between complicated and uncomplicated parapneumonic effusions. Consequently, conflicting staging systems using varying pleural fluid pH cut-off values have emerged in the literature (Tables 10E.3 and 10E.4).[52,53]

Heffner and colleagues[17] addressed this issue by performing a metaanalysis of seven studies to evaluate the diagnostic accuracy of pleural fluid pH, glucose, and LDH in predicting the need for drainage and the quality of the primary studies. Patients with empyema, as defined by the authors in their respective studies, were excluded in a separate analysis because the presence of pus requires drainage regardless of pleural fluid test results. Heffner and colleagues found that pleural fluid pH had the highest diagnostic accuracy compared with glucose and LDH and that no single pleural fluid pH clearly discriminates between parapneumonic effusions that require drainage. Thus, a dogmatic acceptance of a pH <7.2 as an absolute indication for tube thoracostomy in parapneumonic effusion is not valid. Rather than using a single cut-off point, they recommended a bayesian approach wherein clinicians considered the pretest probability that a patient required drainage or could not tolerate a delayed drainage if it later

Table 10E.3   *Light staging criteria of parapneumonic effusion and empyema*

Classification	Diagnostic criteria	Suggested therapy
Stage 1 (nonsignificant parapneumonic effusion)	Small <1 cm on lateral decubitus film	Antibiotics – usually not need thoracentesis
Stage 2 (typical parapneumonic effusion)	1 cm pH >7.2, glucose >22.2 mmol/L (40 mg/dL) negative Gram stain, culture	Antibiotics alone
Stage 3 (borderline complicated paraneumonic effusion)	pH 7.0–7.2 ± LDH >1000 IU/L ± glucose >22.2 mmol/L (40 mg/dL) negative Gram stain, culture	Antibiotics with serial thoracentesis, may need tube thoracostomy
Stage 4 (simple complicated parapneumonic effusion)	pH <7 ± glucose <22.2 mmol/L (40 mg/dL) positive Gram stain, culture No pus, not loculated	Antibiotics + tube thoracostomy
Stage 5 (complex complicated parapneumonic effusion)	pH <7 ± glucose <22.2 mmol/L (40 mg/dL) positive Gram stain, culture Multiloculated	Antibiotics + tube thoracostomy + thrombolytics Surgery rarely needed
Stage 6 (simple empyema)	Pus present Single locule or free flowing	Antibiotics + tube thoracostomy ± decortication
Stage 7 (complex empyema)	Pus present Multiple loculi	Antibiotics + tube thoracostomy ± thrombolytics – often needs thoracoscopy and decortication

Adapted from Light.[52]

Table 10E.4   *ACCP staging criteria for parapneumonic effusion and empyema*

Stage	Radiologic appearance		Bacteriology		Pleural fluid analysis	Risk of poor outcome	Drainage
1	A_0 free-flowing <1 cm on decubitus	AND	B_x unknown	AND	C_x pH unknown	Very low	No
2	A_1 free flowing >1cm <½ hemothorax	AND	B_0 negative culture and Gram stain	AND	C_0 pH ≥7.20	Low	No
3	A_2 free-flowing and large (>½ hemithorax), loculated, or thickened parietal pleura	OR	B_1 positive culture and Gram stain	AND	C1 pH <7.20	Moderate	Yes
4			Pus		Pus	High	Yes

Adapted from Colice *et al.*[53]

proved necessary after a course of antibiotic therapy. For instance, a previously healthy, young patient who could tolerate several days of failed antibiotic therapy might not be selected for pleural fluid drainage until pleural fluid pH decreased below 7.20. Conversely, an elderly patient who appeared at high risk for a need for drainage and who could not tolerate a failed course of antibiotics if loculations later occurred might be selected for pleural fluid drainage with a higher pH threshold of 7.30.

Among patients with a low pretest probability for a complicated parapneumonic effusion, a pH value less than 7.21 had an 81 percent sensitivity and 90 percent specificity for needing drainage.[17] More importantly, the positive predictive value was 47 percent and the negative predictive value was 98 percent. Thus, although a negative result (pH >7.21) is reliable at excluding the need for chest tube thoracostomy, only 47 percent of patients with a positive result actually needed tube thoracostomy. The results are similar in higher-risk patients. Using a pleural fluid pH cut-off point of <7.29 for determining the need for drainage, the negative predictive value was 95 percent. In contrast with the low-risk group, however, a pH <7.29 has a 59 percent positive predictive value. In the high-risk group, therefore, 59 percent of patients with a pH <7.29 needed drainage.[17] These data are summarized in Table 10E.5. It should be noted, however, that the primary studies supporting the use of pleural fluid pH had numerous design flaws that limit the application of pleural fluid pH, LDH, and glucose to clinical practice.[17]

Additional pleural fluid tests have value in diagnosis and staging of parapneumonic effusions. Polymerase chain reaction (PCR) of pleural fluid for *Strept. pneumoniae* DNA shows promise in confirming the etiology of parapneumonic effusions. In a small series of patients with clinical or serological pneumonia, Falguera and colleagues[54] found a sensitivity of *Strept. pneumoniae* DNA of 78 percent (7/9) and a negative predictive value 93 percent (39/42). This test appeared to be more sensitive than blood culture, blood PCR, urine antigen, sputum culture, and pleural fluid culture in this series. No data support the utility of pleural fluid PCR, however, for determining the need for pleural fluid drainage. β-Glucuronidase has been evaluated as a method for staging parapneumonic effusions.[55] However, it has no additional discriminating power over LDH in subclassifying exudative effusions. Higher levels of defensins (>5100 ng/mL) are found in patients with empyemas than in those with transudative effusions, parapneumonic effusions, tuberculous effusions, and neoplastic effusions. At a level of 5100 ng/mL, defensins were 100 percent sensitive and specific for the presence of empyema.[56] Defensin levels also correlate with pleural fluid IL-8 levels, which discriminate between empyema and other exudative effusions. This study was limited, however, by the small number of patients (61 total pleural samples) and the low number of patients with parapneumonic effusions (n = 3). A larger series of 219 patients noted discriminative value of pleural fluid IL-8, neutrophil elastase, and myeloperoxidase for separating empyemas from other exudates.[57] However, unlike the defensin levels, there was significant overlap in each test with parapneumonic, tuberculous, and malignant effusions, making these tests less reliable in distinguishing empyema from other exudates.

At a level ≥80 pg/mL or greater, pleural fluid TNF-α has a 78 percent sensitivity and 89 percent specificity for identifying parapneumonic effusions that require drainage in comparison with pleural fluid pH (cut-off point 7.20), which had a sensitivity and specificity of 41 percent and 94 percent, respectively.[58] Pleural fluid LDH (cut-off point 1000 IU/L) had a sensitivity of 74 percent, which was comparable to TNF-α. However, in the metaanalysis by Heffner and coworkers of the available data, elevated LDH levels in low and high likelihood patients had sensitivities of only 41 percent and 71 percent, respectively.[17] Thus, the apparent improved sensitivity of TNF-α for predicting need for drainage requires further confirmation. New diagnostic tests on pleural fluid and their significance are shown in Table 10E.6. Additional studies are needed to determine their clinical utility.

Table 10E.5 *Sensitivity, specificity, positive and negative predictive values of pH, glucose, and LDH in predicting need for drainage*

Patient category*	pH	Glucose (mg/dL)	LDH (IU/L)
Decision threshold			
Low likelihood	<7.22	<79	>2220
High likelihood	<7.3	<99	>620
Sensitivity			
Low likelihood	0.81	0.52	0.41
High likelihood	0.87	0.76	0.71
Specificity			
Low likelihood	0.90	0.86	0.93
High likelihood	0.80	0.66	0.70
Positive predictive value			
Low likelihood	0.47	0.29	0.39
High likelihood	0.59	0.43	0.44
Negative predictive value			
Low likelihood	0.98	0.94	0.93
High likelihood	0.95	0.89	0.88

*Patients were categorized into low and high pre-test likelihoods of a need for pleural fluid drainage.

LDH, lactate dehydrogenase.

Taken from Heffnel *et al.*[17]

ANTIBIOTIC THERAPY

Antibiotic therapy is the cornerstone for managing patients with parapneumonic effusions. Intravenous antibiotic therapy should be initiated as soon as a parapneumonic effusion or empyema is suspected. With the exception of aminoglycosides, most antibiotics

Table 10E.6   *Diagnostic tests and their clinical significance*

Streptococcus pneumoniae DNA PCR (n = 102)	78% sensitive in detecting *S. pneumoniae* empyema 93% specific
Pleural defensin (n = 61)	≥5100 ng/mL 100% sensitivity and specificity for discriminating empyema from uncomplicated parapneumonic effusion
TNF-α (n = 80)	≥80 pg/mL 78% sensitive and 89% specific for discriminating complicated from uncomplicated parapneumonic effusion
β-gluconuridase (n = 123)	Comparable ability of LDH in predicting need for drainage
IL-8, neutrophil elastase, myeloperoxidase (n = 219)	Unable to reliably distinguish complicated and uncomplicated parapneumonic effusion

TNF, tumor necrosis factor; IL, interleukin; LDH, lactate dehydrogenase.

penetrate well into the pleural space. The initial regimen for patients who present from the community with parapneumonic effusions should follow established community acquired pneumonia (CAP) practice guidelines for the selection of antibiotics.[59,60] An intravenous β-lactam with a macrolide or doxycycline or an antipneumococcal fluoroquinolone alone, as recommended by CAP guidelines, should be sufficient for patients who appear to have an uncomplicated parapneumonic effusion without clinical suspicion for aspiration. Patients with empyema or clinical radiographic features of a complicated parapneumonic effusion should be treated with a regimen active against anaerobic bacteria. We recommend clindamycin, piperacillin-tazobactam, or amoxicillin-clavulanic acid for anaerobic coverage because of the absence of resistance to these antibiotics in a case series of patients with anaerobic lung abscess.[61]

For patients at risk for CAP due to *Pseudomonas aeruginosa* (e.g. cystic fibrosis, bronchiectasis) or for those with parapneumonic effusions from a hospital-acquired pneumonia, antipseudomonal coverage should be initiated. For such patients, piperacillin-tazobactam, imipenem, meropenem, cefepime with a macrolide, fluoroquinolone with or without metronidazole, or clindamycin has been recommended.[19,59] Aminoglycosides are less optimal antibiotic choices because of their poor penetration into the pleural space and their inactivation in low pH environments, as exists in empyema pus.[62]

For patients with empyema complicating thoracic surgery, chest instrumentation (e.g. chest tubes), or chest trauma, an antibiotic regimen should include drugs effective against *Staph. aureus*.[28] Similar coverage is required for patients with empyema complicating bronchiectasis. For those who are allergic to penicillin, a quinolone with clindamycin would be a good initial regimen.[2] Antibiotics should be tailored to positive culture results; however, empyema often represents mixed infection. Not all organisms responsible for infection may grow on culture. Thus, the initial empiric antibiotics selected on the basis of clinical factors and guideline recommendations should not be discontinued if suspected pathogens do not grow on culture of pleural fluid.

UNCOMPLICATED PARAPNEUMONIC EFFUSION MANAGEMENT

By definition, an uncomplicated parapneumonic effusion does not require pleural fluid drainage and responds to antibiotic therapy alone. The clinician must evaluate the patient carefully, therefore, to determine the likelihood that an uncomplicated effusion exists and that the patient will not need pleural drainage. The presence of loculations as seen by chest radiograph or CT scan is associated with increased mortality in some studies and an increased probability of failure with antibiotics alone.[43] Patients with large pleural collections are more likely to eventually need surgery.[59] If a patient does not have clinical improvement in symptoms (continued fevers, tachycardia, hypotension) or if a chest radiograph shows worsening of the effusion after 72 hours, alternative treatments such as serial thoracentesis or tube thoracostomy should be performed.[63]

COMPLICATED PARAPNEUMONIC EFFUSION MANAGEMENT

Most complicated parapneumonic effusions require pleural drainage in addition to antibiotic therapy. Numerous studies have documented similar success rates of image-guided smaller catheters and standard large bore chest tubes for complicated parapneumonic effusions.[64,65] Ultrasonographic-directed small-bore chest tubes can be placed into small loculations that may be difficult to reach with blind insertion. CT-guided chest tubes can be placed into apical loculations, loculations abutting the mediastinum, and loculations with underlying lung consolidation.[66] Loculated complicated parapneumonic effusions should be drained with chest tubes in each loculus if possible, depending on the clinical situation. Small-bore chest tubes should be flushed regularly via a three-way valve.[59] The initial management strategies for parapneumonic effusion are shown in Figure 10E.5.

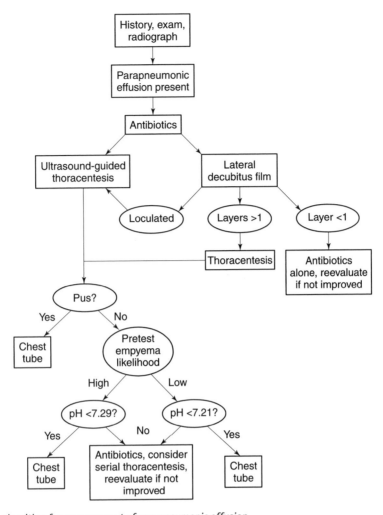

History, exam, radiograph

Parapneumonic effusion present

Antibiotics

Ultrasound-guided thoracentesis

Lateral decubitus film

Loculated   Layers >1   Layer <1

Thoracentesis   Antibiotics alone, reevaluate if not improved

Pus?

Yes   No

Chest tube   Pretest empyema likelihood

High   Low

pH <7.29?   pH <7.21?

Yes   No   Yes

Chest tube   Antibiotics, consider serial thoracentesis, reevaluate if not improved   Chest tube

Figure 10E.5 *Initial decision algorithm for management of parapneumonic effusion.*

EMPYEMA MANAGEMENT

For the patient with empyema, initial therapy should include drainage of the pleural space. The optimal mode of drainage is controversial. Although success with small gauge image guided pig-tail catheters is reported in the literature,[64] a large-bore chest tube is the preferred initial drainage modality of nonloculated empyema.[52] Other options include image-guided placement of a small-bore chest tube and serial thoracentesis. If a large-bore chest tube is placed, there are four techniques: trocar and cannula, trocar chest tube, blunt dissection, and guidewire and dilator. Of these four methods, blunt dissection and guidewire and dilator are the likely safest techniques. Using blunt dissection, one can verify positioning in the pleural space and manually lyse loculations. In general, chest tubes should be inserted in the third to sixth intercostal space and directed posteriorly.[63,67] One disadvantage of blunt dissection is the possibility of creating too large a tunnel with subsequent leakage and secondary infection.[63] Complications associated with chest tube placement are listed in Box 10E.1.

Box 10E.1 Complications of chest tube placement

- Diaphragm perforation
- Spleen, liver, stomach perforation
- Intercostal vein, artery, or nerve laceration
- Internal mammary artery laceration
- Heart perforation
- Aortic perforation
- Vena caval perforation
- Lung perforation
- Phrenic nerve paralysis
- Tension pneumothorax
- Subcutaneous emphysema
- Chest pain
- Secondary pleural infection

Chest tube drainage may be all that is required for uniloculated empyema. However, a significant number of patients with empyema will need surgical drainage. The American College of Chest Physicians (ACCP) pooled data from 21 case series to formulate a consensus statement on management of parapneumonic effusion and empyema. In these patients treated with tube thoracostomy as the primary intervention, a second intervention was required 40 percent of the time.[53] In a small series of patients with empyema, Wait and colleagues[68] found that early treatment of loculated empyema with video-assisted thoracoscopic surgery (VATS) resulted in significantly decreased hospital stay. Thus, many clinicians consider surgical approaches such as VATS and minithoracotomy in the initial management of empyema. However, the data comparing medical and surgical management empyema are limited and of questionable methodological quality. A Cochrane review of all trials comparing medical and surgical therapy of empyema found that most trials were excluded for methodological reasons.[69–71] The only study reviewed was the Wait study and thus definitive conclusions could not be drawn.[72] Certainly, surgical consultation should not be delayed in management of empyema. An algorithm for management of patients with empyema is shown in Figure 10E.6. The primary premise in managing these patients is to initiate an approach that rapidly and effectively drains the pleural space. Delays in completing drainage, regardless of the initial approach selected, contribute to excess morbidity.

EVALUATION OF CHEST TUBE DRAINAGE

When tube thoracostomy is the initial management choice for parapneumonic effusion and empyema, tube output must be monitored carefully. When there is less than 50 mL/day or when a patient's symptoms have not improved, chest radiography or CT scan should be performed to assess adequacy of drainage. If there is residual fluid, the tube should be flushed with sterile saline to ensure patency.[59] If it is kinked, it can be withdrawn slightly to relieve the obstruction. There are commercial dressings available that secure small-bore chest tubes to the chest wall without kinking. Computed tomography is able to demonstrate whether the chest tube is correctly positioned in the fluid collection and whether there are additional loculi that are not in communication with the tube.

In some instances, however, tube thoracostomy alone is inadequate. In a consensus guideline of management of parapneumonic effusions, tube thoracostomy required a second intervention 40 percent of the time.[53] In a patient who does not achieve adequate drainage within a few days, a pulmonologist or thoracic surgeon should be consulted to direct further care if not already involved in placement of the drainage tube.[59] The options available if there is inadequate

drainage include additional chest tubes, intrapleural fibrinolytics, VATS, limited thoracotomy, formal thoracotomy with decortication, and open surgical drainage. The choice of an additional drainage modality depends upon the presence of ongoing pleural sepsis, maturity of the empyema, degree of restriction of lung function from a mature pleural peel, familiarity with the treatment modalities, and debility of the patient.

INTRAPLEURAL FIBRINOLYTICS

Intrapleural fibrinolytics are used when there is occlusion of the chest tube with thick organizing material or when there are multiple pleural loculations that fail to drain.[19] The two fibrinolytics used are urokinase and streptokinase. Streptokinase is dosed by adding 250 000 units to 20–100 mL of normal saline. If urokinase is chosen, 100 000 units are used.[73] The fibrinolytic is then instilled into the pleural space and the chest tube clamped for 2–4 hours.[74,75] The chest tube is then unclamped and returned to suction. Daily or up to three times per day instillations have been used.

The literature regarding the effectiveness of intrapleural fibrinolytics is conflicting. Case series report improvement in the amount of fluid drained,[73–77] radiographic appearance of the pleural space[73,74,77] and clinical outcome.[73,76,77] A randomized, controlled trial of urokinase versus placebo found decrease in duration of hospitalization, duration of pleural drainage and decreased need for VATS compared to normal saline.[73] A Cochrane review of three case series of good methodological quality[73,74,78] found that fibrinolytics appeared to decrease hospital stay, need for surgery, time to defervescence, and improvement in chest radiograph. However, these improvements were not uniform in the studies and the number of patients was small. Therefore, the Cochrane reviewers did not recommend use of intrapleural fibrinolytics for the management of complicated parapneumonic effusion and empyema.[79] A British trial of 500 patients examined the utility of intrapleural fibrinolytic therapy. Preliminary results of 426 patients did not show improvement in mortality rates, need for surgery, or hospital stay.[80] However, this study evaluated all patients with empyema regardless of maturity of the empyema and time from presentation to instillation of fibrinolytics. Thus, there may be a role for fibrinolytics in the setting of empyema in the early fibrinopurulent stage.

Although existing case series do not report bleeding or anaphylaxis with intrapleural fibrinolytic therapy, case reports do exist of localized pleural and systemic bleeding.[81,82] Acute respiratory distress syndrome has also been reported after intrapleural instillation of streptokinase.[83] Streptokinase is a bacterial protein and can, therefore, induce neutralizing antibodies. These antibodies could theoretically interfere with its efficacy and cause anaphylactic reaction if streptokinase is given in subsequent

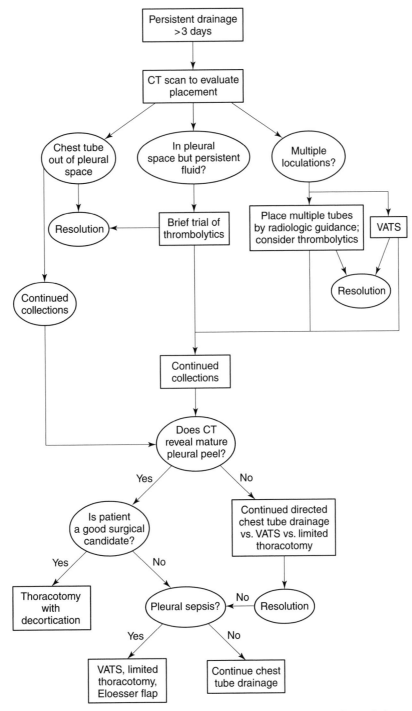

Figure 10E.6 *Decision algorithm for management of parapneumonic effusion or empyema with persistent drainage. CT, computed tomography; VATS, video-assisted thoracoscopic surgery.*

hospitalizations. Patients who have received streptokinase should receive a card indicating their exposure to it and should receive urokinase or tissue plasminogen activator for future thrombolysis. Though not common, intrapleural fibrinolytics can be associated with severe adverse effects.

In the absence of high-grade evidence from adequately performed trials, we limit the use of fibrinolytic therapy to patients with exudative or early fibrinopurulent parapneumonic effusions that do not drain rapidly and completely with chest tube insertion. Parapneumonic effusions in these early stages are more likely to be amenable to fibrinolytic therapy than effusions in the organized stage. We dose streptokinase three times per day, clamping the tube for 2 hours. If we do not achieve radiographic improvement within three doses, we consult thoracic surgery for surgical drainage.

SURGICAL DRAINAGE

Surgical approaches to managing parapneumonic effusions include medical thoracoscopy with directed chest tube placement, VATS with lysis of adhesions, limited thoracotomy, formal thoracotomy with decortication, and rib resection with open drainage. The literature comparing surgical management to more conservative management is limited and often of poor methodological quality. Medical thoracoscopy can be useful in visualizing the pleural space and directing chest tube placement. It is performed under conscious sedation with a local anesthetic and allows visualization of the pleural space and placement of chest tubes under direction visualization. Two trocars are placed into the pleural space and an artificial pneumothorax created. Rigid or flexible thoracoscopes are placed through the trocar and working tools are placed through the other trocar. Extensive pleural adhesions can limit access to the pleural space by medical thoracoscopy, which has its best utility for patients with few loculations or patients with monolocular empyemas and thick pus that could benefit from directed drainage.

Video-assisted thoracoscopy allows lysis of loculations and evacuation of intrapleural debris with limited decortication in selected patients. Patients are selectively intubated and the lung in question is deflated. Multiple intercostal sites are selected for the thoracoscope and multiple endoscopic tools including forceps, scissors, and retractors are employed.[84] In one study, early use of VATS was associated with decreased intensive care unit stay, hospital stay and costs, and increased rate of primary success in patients with loculated parapneumonic effusion or with parapneumonic effusions with a pH <7.2 compared with patients receiving thrombolytic therapy through closed chest tube drainage.[68] Of note in this study, mortality was not improved with early VATS, and all patients in the thrombolytic therapy group could be salvaged with VATS. It is most useful in treatment of multiloculated, parapneumonic effusions in the fibrinopurulent stage. Success of VATS depends on surgical referral occurring before extensive mature intrapleural loculations occur.[85] It is unlikely to return normal lung function to patients who have progressed to the organizing phase and have a thick mature pleural peel limiting the lung's expansion.

A limited, muscle-sparing thoracotomy utilizes a 10 cm incision along the lateral chest wall through which loculations and intrapleural adhesions can be lysed and pus drained with placement of dependent chest tubes under direct visualization. Because only a partial decortication can be performed with a limited thoracotomy, the procedure has limited utility for patients with organized empyemas with significant lung restriction. However, it is a well-tolerated surgery for appropriately selected patients and has a definite role in managing patients with multiloculated complicated parapneumonic effusions and multiloculated empyema who fail more conservative management.

Patients with organized empyemas require a formal thoracotomy with decortication to relieve lung entrapment and restore lung function. A full thoracotomy in this clinical setting, however, has significant mortality risks. In a small series (n = 90) patients requiring formal thoracotomy for empyema had a 10 percent motality.[86] Considering this risk and the ability of directed tube placement, VATS, and limited thoracotomy to control pleural sepsis,[68,86,87] formal thoracotomy should be reserved for patients with acceptable surgical risk who require the release of an extensive pleural peel that limits lung expansion. Patients with persistent pleural sepsis who are not candidates for general anesthesia can be considered for rib resection with open drainage. In this procedure, two ribs are resected under local anesthesia and the pleural space is marsupialized externally allowing long-term pleural drainage.[86]

ADJUNCTIVE TREATMENTS

In addition to effective antibiotic therapy and pleural drainage, there are other therapeutic and diagnostic considerations. If there is a high suspicion for obstructing tumor as the etiology for the empyema, bronchoscopy should be performed. However, in a series of 119 patients with empyema, the incidence of airway obstruction was only 4 percent.[34] Therefore, routine bronchoscopy for empyema is not recommended.[59] If there is lung abscess as the cause of empyema, bronchoscopy may reveal an endobronchial obstruction. In addition, there are reports of successful endobronchial drainage of lung abscess. As such, bronchoscopy can have an adjunctive therapeutic role in empyema secondary to lung abscess. Patients with structural lung disease, such as bronchiectasis, and empyema should use Flutter valves (Axcan Scandipharm, Birmingham, AL) or Acapella valves (DHD Healthcare, Wampsville, NY) to help with sputum clearance. Patients with empyema must have adequate nutrition for normal immune function. These patients are often highly catabolic, so sufficient enteric or parenteral nutrition must be provided.

EMPYEMA IN CHILDREN

Management of empyema in children is similar to adults with some notable exceptions. First, the epidemiology of empyema is different in children than in adults. In general, most children with empyema are healthy and not at risk for anaerobic pathogens as they have less altered mental status, airway protection issues, and aspiration. The most common causative bacterial pathogens are *Staph. aureus*, *Streptococcus* species, *Strep. pneumococcus*, *Haemophilus influenza*, and *P. auruginosa*.[88–90] Anaerobes cause a small percentage of cases of empyema in children. Most patients present with cough, dyspnea, respiratory distress, and fever. Poor feeding is a rare presentation.[89] The second difference between adult and child patients is that mortality from empyema in children in the Western world is now essentially nonexistent. The difference in mortality between adults and children with empyema may be the comorbidities that are often present in adults with parapneumonic effusion and empyema. Most children with empyema are healthy at baseline and recover completely following appropriate therapy. It is unclear whether immediate drainage is necessary in patients who have complicated (by pleural fluid analysis or ultrasound appearance) parapneumonic effusion.

As in adults, children with exudative parapneumonic effusion have been treated successfully with antibiotics alone[89] or with serial thoracentesis as opposed to chest tube placement.[91] Intrapleural fibrinolytics appear to decrease febrile days, need for surgical intervention,[90] and hospital stay,[88] and have a good safety record in children.[92] As mortality is rare from pediatric empyema in the Western world, this endpoint cannot be assessed. Small-bore chest tubes appear effective in draining pediatric empyema and even showed a significant decrease in hospital stay in one study.[88] Surgical options are similar to adults and are indicated for patients with persistent pleural sepsis, multiloculated effusions, and those with a thick, visceral pleural peel and lung entrapment. Limited decortication as well as formal decortication is well tolerated in children and should be pursued when indicated.[93,94]

CONCLUSIONS

Parapneumonic effusion and empyema cause significant morbidity and mortality in the United States despite the advent of effective antibiotic therapy for pneumonia. Patients often present with nonspecific symptoms, such as malaise and fever, which contributes to delayed diagnosis. Underrecognition of pleural infection can cause delays in treatment and allow progression of uncomplicated parapneumonic effusions to more mature and less easily treated stages. Early recognition of empyema with prompt initiation of appropriate antibiotics is critical in minimizing the morbidity associated with a complicated pleural space. The pleural fluid analysis is critical in establishing the presence of a parapneumonic effusion or empyema as well as staging the parapneumonic effusion and should not be delayed. Complicated parapneumonic effusion and empyema can be associated with considerable morbidity which can be avoided with prompt appropriate antibiotics and complete drainage of the pleural space with tube thoracostomy or surgery.

Key learning points

- Signs and symptoms of parapneumonic empyema may be nonspecific and unrecognized by patients and physicians.

- Empyema, the end stage of a parapneumonic effusion, usually results from delayed treatment by the physician or late presentation by the patient.

- When recognized in the exudative stage, parapneumonic effusion can usually be effectively treated with appropriate antibiotics alone.

- Pleural fluid pH and Gram stain are the most useful tests for determining the need for pleural space drainage.

- Clinical likelihood for empyema and a patient's comorbidities should be considered with pleural fluid analysis in staging parapneumonic effusion.

- If fibrinolytics are to be effective, they should be used in the early fibrinopurulent stage.

- Surgical options including medical thoracoscopy, VATS, and thoracotomy should be considered early in patients not responding to conservative therapy and selected according to surgical risk.

REFERENCES

1. US Department of Commerce Bureau of the Census. Monthly vital statistics report. 1997; **45**: 21–4.

2. Bernstein JM. Treatment of community-acquired pneumonia – IDSA guidelines. Infectious Diseases Society of America. *Chest* 1999; **115**: 9S–13S.

◆ 3. Strange C, Sahn SA. The definitions and epidemiology of pleural space infection. *Semin Respir Infect* 1999; **14**: 3–8.

4. Leak LV, Rahil K. Permeability of the diaphragmatic mesothelium: the ultrastructural basis for 'stomata'. *Am J Anat* 1978; **151**: 557–93.

5. Wang NS. The preformed stomas connecting the pleural cavity and the lymphatics in the parietal pleura. *Am Rev Respir Dis* 1975; **111**: 12–20.

◆ 6. Sahn SA. The pathophysiology of pleural effusions. *Annu Rev Med* 1990; **41**: 7–13.

7. Kroegel C, Antony VB. Immunobiology of pleural inflammation: potential implications for pathogenesis, diagnosis and therapy. *Eur Respir J* 1997; **10**: 2411–18.

8. Light RW, Girard WM, Jenkinson SG, *et al.* Parapneumonic effusions. *Am J Med* 1980; **69**: 507–12.

9. Potts DE, Levin DC, Sahn SA. Pleural fluid pH in parapneumonic effusions. *Chest* 1976; **70**: 328–31.

10. Antony VB, Hott JW, Kunkel SL, *et al.* Pleural mesothelial cell expression of C-C (monocyte chemotactic peptide) and C-X-C (interleukin 8) chemokines. *Am J Respir Cell Mol Biol* 1995; **12**: 581–8.

11. Philip-Joet F, Alessi MC, Philip-Joet C, *et al.* Fibrinolytic and inflammatory processes in pleural effusions. *Eur Respir J* 1995; **8**: 1352–6.

● 12. Idell S, Girard W, Koenig KB, *et al.* Abnormalities of pathways of fibrin turnover in the human pleural space. *Am Rev Respir Dis* 1991; **144**: 187–94.

13. Idell S, Zwieb C, Boggaram J, *et al.* Mechanisms of fibrin formation and lysis by human lung fibroblasts: influence of TGF-beta and TNF-alpha. *Am J Physiol* 1992; **263**: L487–94.

14. Idell S, Zwieb C, Kumar A, *et al.* Pathways of fibrin turnover of human pleural mesothelial cells in vitro. *Am J Respir Cell Mol Biol* 1992; **7**: 414–26.

15. Strange C, Tomlinson JR, Wilson C, *et al.* The histology of experimental pleural injury with tetracycline, empyema, and carrageenan. *Exp Mol Pathol* 1989; **51**: 205–19.

16. Kearney SE, Davies CW, Davies RJ, *et al.* Computed tomography and ultrasound in parapneumonic effusions and empyema. *Clin Radiol* 2000; **55**: 542–7.

● 17. Heffner JE, Brown LK, Barbieri C, *et al.* Pleural fluid chemical analysis in parapneumonic effusions. A meta-analysis. *Am J Respir Crit Care Med* 1995; **151**: 1700–8.

● 18. Sahn S. Pathogenesis and clinical features of diseases associated with low pleural fluid glucose. In: Chretein J BJ, Hirsch A, ed. *The Pleura in Health and Disease.* New York: Marcel Dekker, 1985; 267–85.

◆ 19. Sahn SA. Management of complicated parapneumonic effusions. *Am Rev Respir Dis* 1993; **148**: 813–17.

20. Gustafson RA, Murray GF, Warden HE, *et al.* Role of lung decortication in symptomatic empyemas in children. *Ann Thorac Surg* 1990; **49**: 940–6; discussion 946–7.

21. Weissberg D, Refaely Y. Pleural empyema: 24-year experience. *Ann Thorac Surg* 1996; **62**: 1026–9.

22. Finland M, Barnes MW. Changing ecology of acute bacterial empyema: occurrence and mortality at Boston City Hospital during 12 selected years from 1935 to 1972. *J Infect Dis* 1978; **137**: 274–91.

23. Snider GL, Saleh SS. Empyema of the thorax in adults: review of 105 cases. *Dis Chest* 1968; **54**: 410–15.

24. Bartlett JG, Gorbach SL, Thadepalli H, *et al.* Bacteriology of empyema. *Lancet* 1974; **1**: 338–40.

25. Varkey B, Rose HD, Kutty CP, *et al.* Empyema thoracis during a ten-year period. Analysis of 72 cases and comparison to a previous study (1952 to 1967). *Arch Intern Med* 1981; **141**: 1771–6.

26. Civen R, Jousimies-Somer H, Marina M, *et al.* A retrospective review of cases of anaerobic empyema and update of bacteriology. *Clin Infect Dis* 1995; **20**(Suppl 2): S224–9.

27. Brook I, Frazier EH. Aerobic and anaerobic microbiology of empyema. A retrospective review in two military hospitals. *Chest* 1993; **103**: 1502–7.

28. Aguilar MM, Battistella FD, Owings JT, *et al.* Posttraumatic empyema. Risk factor analysis. *Arch Surg* 1997; **132**: 647–50; discussion 650–1.

29. Smith JA, Mullerworth MH, Westlake GW, *et al.* Empyema thoracis: 14-year experience in a teaching center. *Ann Thorac Surg* 1991; **51**: 39–42.

30. Kroboth FJ, Yu VL, Reddy SC, *et al.* Clinicoradiographic correlation with the extent of Legionnaire disease. *AJR Am J Roentgenol* 1983; **141**: 263–8.

31. Fine NL, Smith LR, Sheedy PF. Frequency of pleural effusions in mycoplasma and viral pneumonias. *N Engl J Med* 1970; **283**: 790–3.

32. Mansel JK, Rosenow EC, 3rd, Smith TF, *et al.* *Mycoplasma pneumoniae* pneumonia. *Chest* 1989; **95**: 639–46.

33. Community-acquired pneumonia in adults in British hospitals in 1982–1983: a survey of aetiology, mortality, prognostic factors and outcome. The British Thoracic Society and the Public Health Laboratory Service. *Q J Med* 1987; **62**: 195–220.

● 34. Ferguson AD, Prescott RJ, Selkon JB, *et al.* The clinical course and management of thoracic empyema. *Q J Med* 1996; **89**: 285–9.

35. Heffner JE, McDonald J, Barbieri C, *et al.* Management of parapneumonic effusions. An analysis of physician practice patterns. *Arch Surg* 1995; **130**: 433–8.

36. LeMense GP, Strange C, Sahn SA. Empyema thoracis. Therapeutic management and outcome. *Chest* 1995; **107**: 1532–7.

37. Muller NL. Imaging of the pleura. *Radiology* 1993; **186**: 297–309.

38. Hessen I. The localization of fluid in the free pleura. *Acta Radiol* 1972; **105**: 51–3.

39. O'Moore PV, Mueller PR, Simeone JF, *et al.* Sonographic guidance in diagnostic and therapeutic interventions in the pleural space. *AJR Am J Roentgenol* 1987; **149**: 1–5.

40. Mayo PH, Goltz HR, Tafreshi M, *et al.* Safety of ultrasound-guided thoracentesis in patients receiving mechanical ventilation. *Chest* 2004; **125**: 1059–62.

41. Beckh S, Bolcskei PL, Lessnau KD. Real-time chest ultrasonography: a comprehensive review for the pulmonologist. *Chest* 2002; **122**: 1759–73.

● 42. Yang PC, Luh KT, Chang DB, *et al.* Value of sonography in determining the nature of pleural effusion: analysis of 320 cases. *AJR Am J Roentgenol* 1992; **159**: 29–33.

43. Himelman RB, Callen PW. The prognostic value of loculations in parapneumonic pleural effusions. *Chest* 1986; **90**: 852–6.

44. Stark DD, Federle MP, Goodman PC, *et al.* Differentiating lung abscess and empyema: radiography and computed tomography. *AJR Am J Roentgenol* 1983; **141**: 163–7.

● 45. Huang HC, Chang HY, Chen CW, *et al.* Predicting factors for outcome of tube thoracostomy in complicated parapneumonic effusion for empyema. *Chest* 1999; **115**: 751–6.

46. Ashbaugh DG. Empyema thoracis. Factors influencing morbidity and mortality. *Chest* 1991; **99**: 1162–5.

47. Villena V, Lopez-Encuentra A, Garcia-Lujan R, *et al.* Clinical implications of appearance of pleural fluid at thoracentesis. *Chest* 2004; **125**: 156–9.

48. Morris AJ, Wilson SJ, Marx CE, *et al.* Clinical impact of bacteria and fungi recovered only from broth cultures. *J Clin Microbiol* 1995; **33**: 161–5.

49. Drury M, Anderson W, Heffner JE. Diagnostic value of pleural fluid cytology in occult Boerhaave's syndrome. *Chest* 1992; **102**: 976–8.

● 50. Sahn SA, Reller LB, Taryle DA, *et al.* The contribution of leukocytes and bacteria to the low pH of empyema fluid. *Am Rev Respir Dis* 1983; **128**: 811–15.

51. Poe RH, Marin MG, Israel RH, *et al.* Utility of pleural fluid analysis in predicting tube thoracostomy/decortication in parapneumonic effusions. *Chest* 1991; **100**: 963–7.

52. Light R. Parapneumonic effusions and empyema: Current management strategies. *J Crit Illn* 1995; **10**: 832–9.

✱ 53. Colice GL, Curtis A, Deslauriers J, *et al.* Medical and surgical treatment of parapneumonic effusions: an evidence-based guideline. *Chest* 2000; **118**: 1158–71.

54. Falguera M, Lopez A, Nogues A, *et al.* Evaluation of the polymerase chain reaction method for detection of *Streptococcus pneumoniae* DNA in pleural fluid samples. *Chest* 2002; **122**: 2212–16.

55. Cobben NA, Drent M, Van Dieijen-Visser MP, *et al.* Usefulness of monitoring beta-glucuronidase in pleural effusions. *Clin Biochem* 1999; **32**: 653–8.

56. Ashitani J, Mukae H, Nakazato M, *et al.* Elevated pleural fluid levels of defensins in patients with empyema. *Chest* 1998; **113**: 788–94.

57. Segura RM, Alegre J, Varela E, *et al.* Interleukin-8 and markers of neutrophil degranulation in pleural effusions. *Am J Respir Crit Care Med* 1998; **157**: 1565–72.

58. Porcel JM, Vives M, Esquerda A. Tumor necrosis factor-alpha in pleural fluid: a marker of complicated parapneumonic effusions. *Chest* 2004; **125**: 160–4.

✱ 59. Davies CW, Gleeson FV, Davies RJ. BTS guidelines for the management of pleural infection. *Thorax* 2003; **58** (Suppl 2): 18–28.

✱ 60. Niederman MS. Guidelines for the management of community-acquired pneumonia. Current recommendations and antibiotic selection issues. *Med Clin North Am* 2001; **85**: 1493–509.

61. Hammond JM, Potgieter PD, Hanslo D, *et al.* The etiology and antimicrobial susceptibility patterns of microorganisms in acute community-acquired lung abscess. *Chest* 1995; **108**: 937–41.

62. Shohet I, Yellin A, Meyerovitch J, *et al.* Pharmacokinetics and therapeutic efficacy of gentamicin in an experimental pleural empyema rabbit model. *Antimicrob Agents Chemother* 1987; **31**: 982–5.

63. Munnell ER. Thoracic drainage. *Ann Thorac Surg* 1997; **63**: 1497–502.

64. Silverman SG, Mueller PR, Saini S, *et al.* Thoracic empyema: management with image-guided catheter drainage. *Radiology* 1988; **169**: 5–9.

65. van Sonnenberg E, Nakamoto SK, Mueller PR, *et al.* CT- and ultrasound-guided catheter drainage of empyemas after chest-tube failure. *Radiology* 1984; **151**: 349–53.

66. Klein JS, Schultz S, Heffner JE. Interventional radiology of the chest: image-guided percutaneous drainage of pleural effusions, lung abscess, and pneumothorax. *AJR Am J Roentgenol* 1995; **164**: 581–8.

67. Symbas PN. Chest drainage tubes. *Surg Clin North Am* 1989; **69**: 41–6.

68. Wait MA, Sharma S, Hohn J, *et al.* A randomized trial of empyema therapy. *Chest* 1997; **111**: 1548–51.

69. Lim TK, Chin NK. Empirical treatment with fibrinolysis and early surgery reduces the duration of hospitalization in pleural sepsis. *Eur Respir J* 1999; **13**: 514–18.

70. Sasse S, Nguyen TK, Mulligan M, *et al.* The effects of early chest tube placement on empyema resolution. *Chest* 1997; **111**: 1679–83.

71. Lee SH, Lee SY, Park SM, *et al.* A comparative study of three therapeutic modalities in loculated tuberculous pleural effusions. *Tuberculosis and Respiratory Diseases* 1996; **43**: 683–92.

◆ 72. Coote N. Surgical versus non-surgical management of pleural empyema. *Cochrane Database Syst Rev* 2002:CD001956.

73. Bouros D, Schiza S, Tzanakis N, *et al.* Intrapleural urokinase versus normal saline in the treatment of complicated parapneumonic effusions and empyema. A randomized, double-blind study. *Am J Respir Crit Care Med* 1999; **159**: 37–42.

74. Davies RJ, Traill ZC, Gleeson FV. Randomised controlled trial of intrapleural streptokinase in community acquired pleural infection. *Thorax* 1997; **52**: 416–21.

75. Chin NK, Lim TK. Controlled trial of intrapleural streptokinase in the treatment of pleural empyema and complicated parapneumonic effusions. *Chest* 1997; **111**: 275–9.

76. Diacon AH, Theron J, Schuurmans MM, *et al.* Intrapleural streptokinase for empyema and complicated parapneumonic effusions. *Am J Respir Crit Care Med* 2004; **170**: 49–53.

77. Jerjes-Sanchez C, Ramirez-Rivera A, Elizalde JJ, *et al.* Intrapleural fibrinolysis with streptokinase as an adjunctive treatment in hemothorax and empyema: a multicenter trial. *Chest* 1996; **109**: 1514–19.

78. Tuncozgur B, Ustunsoy H, Sivrikoz MC, *et al.* Intrapleural urokinase in the management of parapneumonic empyema: a randomised controlled trial. *Int J Clin Pract* 2001; **55**: 658–60.

◆ 79. Cameron R, Davies HR. Intra-pleural fibrinolytic therapy versus conservative management in the treatment of parapneumonic effusions and empyema. *Cochrane Database Syst Rev* 2004:CD002312.

● 80. Davies RJ, Maskell NA, Nunn AJ, *et al.* Preliminary result from the UK MRC/BTS randomised trial of streptokinase v placebo in pleural infection (the MRC/BTS MIST trial, ICTN 39138989. *Am J Respir Crit Care Med* 2004; **169**: A861.

81. Porter J, Banning AP. Intrapleural streptokinase. *Thorax* 1998; **53**: 720.

82. Temes RT, Follis F, Kessler RM, *et al.* Intrapleural fibrinolytics in management of empyema thoracis. *Chest* 1996; **110**: 102–6.

83. Frye MD, Jarratt M, Sahn SA. Acute hypoxemic respiratory failure following intrapleural thrombolytic therapy for hemothorax. *Chest* 1994; **105**: 1595–6.

84. Landreneau RJ, Keenan RJ, Hazelrigg SR, *et al.* Thoracoscopy for empyema and hemothorax. *Chest* 1996; **109**: 18–24.

85. Waller DA, McConnell SA, Rajesh PB. Delayed referral reduces the success of video-assisted thoracoscopic surgery for spontaneous pneumothorax. *Respir Med* 1998; **92**: 246–9.

86. Pothula V, Krellenstein DJ. Early aggressive surgical management of parapneumonic empyemas. *Chest* 1994; **105**: 832–6.

87. Moulton JS, Benkert RE, Weisiger KH, *et al.* Treatment of complicated pleural fluid collections with image-guided drainage and intracavitary urokinase. *Chest* 1995; **108**: 1252–9.

88. Thomson AH, Hull J, Kumar MR, *et al.* Randomised trial of intrapleural urokinase in the treatment of childhood empyema. *Thorax* 2002; **57**: 343–7.

89. Chan W, Keyser-Gauvin E, Davis GM, *et al.* Empyema thoracis in children: a 26-year review of the Montreal Children's Hospital experience. *J Pediatr Surg* 1997; **32**: 870–2.

90. Yao CT, Wu JM, Liu CC, *et al.* Treatment of complicated parapneumonic pleural effusion with intrapleural streptokinase in children. *Chest* 2004; **125**: 566–71.

91. Shoseyov D, Bibi H, Shatzberg G, *et al.* Short-term course and outcome of treatments of pleural empyema in pediatric patients: repeated ultrasound-guided needle thoracocentesis vs chest tube drainage. *Chest* 2002; **121**: 836–40.

92. Kilic N, Celebi S, Gurpinar A, *et al.* Management of thoracic empyema in children. *Pediatr Surg Int* 2002; **18**: 21–3.

93. Kosloske AM, Cartwright KC. The controversial role of decortication in the management of pediatric empyema. *J Thorac Cardiovasc Surg* 1988; **96**: 166–70.

94. Hoff SJ, Neblett WW, Edwards KM, *et al.* Parapneumonic empyema in children: decortication hastens recovery in patients with severe pleural infections. *Pediatr Infect Dis J* 1991; **10**: 194–9.

Diving-related injuries and decompressive syndromes

ALEXANDRE R ABREU, BRUCE P KRIEGER

INTRODUCTION

Since antiquity, man has felt a yearning to explore the underwater environment that covers most of our planet. Over 2500 years ago, Herodotus described how Scyllis used a hollow reed as a snorkel to remain submerged and avoid capture by his enemies. The first diving bell was invented in 1530 and by 1650, von Guericke had developed an air pump to simulate high-altitude environments.[1] Twenty years later, Sir Robert Boyle described decompression sickness (DCS) when he observed bubbles floating in the vitreous humor of animals exposed to von Guericke's hypobaric chamber.[1] During the early nineteenth century, William James developed and Augustus Siebe manufactured the first diving suits with a surface air supply. In the mid-1800s, DCS was recognized in men working in the compressed gas environments of caissons and tunnels in France. Paul Bert (1833–86) hypothesized that 'caisson disease' resulted from the development of nitrogen bubbles in body tissues after recompression from a hyperbaric exposure.[2] During World War II, significant advances were accomplished, including:

- Jacques Cousteau and Emile Gagnon's development of the self-contained breathing apparatus (scuba) which is a demand regulator that delivers breaths at the ambient pressure to which the diver is exposed.
- Refinement of hyperbaric chamber treatment techniques.
- Behnke's recognition of a link between the syndromes of aviators, divers, and caisson workers.[3]

Cousteau and Gagnon's scuba gear has enabled a rapidly growing number of recreational divers around the world to experience the thrills and potential dangers of diving. Over the past few decades, the demand to discover minerals and oil under the ocean floor has pushed hyperbaric exposures to increasing depths and potential hazards. In this chapter, the incidence, physiology, clinical presentation, and treatment of hyperbaric-related injuries will be elucidated.

DEFINITIONS AND INCIDENCE

As of the beginning of this millennium, more than 10 million diving certificates had been issued worldwide.[2,3] Despite the growing ranks of recreational divers, the number of diving-related injuries has remained at 0.53–3.4 incidents per 10 000 dives over the past decade.[4] These injuries are secondary to dysbarism, which is the term used to describe the pathologic changes that occur to a human when exposed to an alternobaric (altered environmental pressure) change.[1] There are two major injurious manifestations of dysbarism – barotrauma and DCS. Decompression illness (DCI) and decompression disorders are terms that encompass both conditions.[4] Whereas DCS refers to syndromes that are the consequence of bubble formation and embolization, the barotrauma of diving is due to the expansion of a gas in an enclosed space, such as the inner ear or an obstructed alveolus.

The incidence of DCI has been estimated to be 1–2.28 cases per 10 000 dives.[3,5] The most frequent dysbaric disorder is DCS. It occurs upon an aviator's or diver's return from an alternobaric exposure. The neuromuscular system is most frequently involved. Ocular symptoms occur in approximately 7 percent of all DCS cases.[6] Serious pulmonary manifestations (the chokes) have been reported in 2–8 percent of DCS incidences.[7] Although barotrauma is not as frequent as DCS, certain manifestations, such a tension pneumothorax with or without an arterial gas embolus (AGE), are potentially fatal. Other consequences of diving-related barotrauma, such as middle ear disease, are less serious, but can occur in up to 30 percent of first-time divers.[8,9]

Dysbaric osteonecrosis is a late sequelae of exposure to hyperbaric conditions that was first described at the beginning of the twentieth century in caisson workers. Caissons are chambers that are used to construct bridge foundations and tunnel connections in the bedrock of a body of water or tunnel. Air is pumped into the caisson at 3–6 atmosphere (atm) to displace the water and allow construction to be performed underwater. Caisson disease was later described in divers and rarely in aviators exposed to hypobaric conditions. In divers, the prevalence of caisson disease correlates with the exposure dose. The Medical Research Council Decompression Sickness Registry in the United Kingdom noted an incidence of 4.2 percent in 4980 commercial divers over a 10-year period.[1] The disease has been reported after even a single hyperbaric exposure.

PHYSIOLOGIC EFFECTS OF DIVING

Physiologic basis of dysbarism

Because the major component of the human body is water, it is nearly incompressible. In contrast, the gases located in body cavities (lungs, sinuses, middle ear, intestine, and others) are altered by three factors (pressure, volume, and temperature) according to Boyle's, Dalton's, and Henry's gas laws. Together, these laws describe the behavior of a gas under alternobaric conditions according to the ideal gas law:

$$PV = nRT$$

where P = pressure; V = volume; n = number of moles of gas; R = universal gas constant, T = absolute temperature.[8]

Boyle's law ($P_1V_1 = P_2V_2$) explains the pathophysiology of diving-related barotrauma. The law states that the volume of a given gas varies inversely to its pressure at a constant temperature.[10,11] At sea level, the human body is exposed to a barometric pressure of 760 mm Hg of pressure, which is equivalent to 1 atm (14.7 psi or 100 kPa). When submerged, this pressure increases linearly by 1 atm for every 10 m (33 feet) of sea water. For example, under 10 m of sea water, the absolute pressure is 2 atmosphere absolute units (ATA). As the barometric pressure increases, there will be a proportional reduction in the volume of gas in a given cavity.

Therefore, at a depth of 10 m (2 atm), the volume in a closed space will be 50 percent of the volume at the surface. If a diver has a lung volume of 6 L, then during a breath-hold dive to 10 m (2 atm), the lung volume would be compressed to 3 L.[11] Similarly, air located in any body cavity will be compressed during descent and expand during ascent. In contrast with a breath-hold dive, when divers use a scuba valve, their lung volume is maintained at the ambient pressure to which they are exposed. Therefore, at 10 m underwater with a scuba valve, the same diver's lung volume would be maintained at 6 L but under hyperbaric (2 ATA) conditions (Fig. 11A.1). During ascent, the lung volume of scuba divers could potentially double if they failed to exhale, which would expose them to the risk of barotrauma (for example, a pneumothorax). However, a pneumothorax rarely occurs during a breath-hold dive since the lung capacity cannot expand above the initial volume (for example, 6 L) that was present at the surface before the dive.

Gas pressures are predictably affected during diving. At sea level, the partial pressure of nitrogen (P_N) is 600 mm Hg and the partial pressure of oxygen (P_{O_2}) is 160 mm Hg. At a 20 m depth (3 ATA), the P_N will increase to 1800 mm Hg and the P_{O_2} to 480 mm Hg (Table 11A.1). Henry's law states that at a given temperature, the mass of a gas dissolved in a given volume of solvent is directly proportional to the pressure of the gas with which it is in equilibrium. Thus, as pressure increases during scuba diving, more nitrogen is dissolved in the body. Since nitrogen is five times more soluble in fat than it is in water, its removal from the human body during ascent is prolonged.[12,13] The dissolved nitrogen in tissue increases proportionally to the ambient pressure, exposure time, and to the diver's fat tissue content. During ascent from a dive, the ambient pressure decreases. This pressure gradient favors the release of gas bubbles from their supersaturated state in tissues.

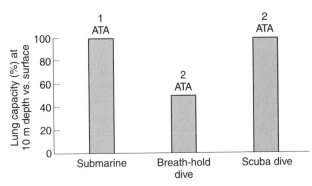

Figure 11A.1 *Boyle's law explains the effect of hyperbaric conditions on lung volumes in a submarine, during a breath-hold dive, and when a scuba valve is used. At a depth of 10 m, the ambient pressure is 2 ATA (atmosphere absolute) except when protected by the shell of a submarine. The lung volume of a breath-hold diver will be halved at 10 m but will be normal in a submarine (100 percent of the lung capacity at the surface) and also 100 percent if a scuba valve is used.*

Table 11A.1 *Gas pressures and bubble volume under hyperbaric conditions*

Distance from sea level (m)	Pressure (ATA)	Po_2 (mm Hg)	P_N (mm Hg)	P total (mm Hg)	Bubble volume (%)
0	1.0	160	600	760	100
−10	2.0	320	1200	1520	50
−20	3.0	480	1800	2280	33
−30	4.0	640	2400	3040	25

ATA, atmosphere absolute; Po_2, oxygen tension; P_N, nitrogen tension; P total, total gas tension.

Henry's law not only provides the physiologic basis for understanding DCS, but also explains why bubbles form when a bottle of champagne is uncorked. Since the spinal cord has a nitrogen elimination half-life of 8–9 minutes[14] versus <1 minute for the cortical gray matter, spinal cord lesions are the most common form of DCS. Dalton's law of partial pressures states that in a mixture of gases, the total pressure (P_T) is the sum of the partial pressures of each of the component gases:

$$P_T = P_1 + P_2 + P_3 + \dots P_n.$$

As ambient pressure increases, the total pressure of the gas mixture increases;[15] conversely, as barometric pressure declines at high altitudes, Po_2 will decline. Dalton's law explains the basis for hyperbaric treatment of dive-related complications.

Cardiopulmonary consequences of diving

The previous section explained how the gas laws predict DCS and barotrauma during diving. This section will explain the cardiopulmonary consequences of the changes that gases undergo during ascent and descent.

The head-out immersion model has been studied extensively to measure changes that occur during submersion. As the subject is immersed up to the neck, venous return is augmented due to the elevated pressures that surround the extremities and abdominal compartment. This stimulates the release of atrial natriuretic factor which promotes diuresis and sodium loss.[16] The increase in intrathoracic pressure results in decreases in the vital capacity and expiratory reserve volume and a 60 percent increase in the work of breathing due to an increase in the nonelastic airways resistance. A form of 'negative-pressure breathing' also occurs since the thorax is hyperbaric relative to the mouth which remains at ambient pressure. During a breath-hold dive, 'negative-pressure breathing' does not occur since the whole body is exposed to the same hyperbaric conditions although lung volumes will still diminish according to Boyle's law.

In contrast, a scuba valve maintains pressure within the respiratory tract at the ambient pressure to which the diver is exposed. As such, the diver is exposed to a hyperoxic breathing mixture that is denser than atmospheric air. This results in diminished expiratory flow rates and increased work of breathing.[7] In addition, the scuba gear (mouthpieces, masks, and helmets) adds to the diver's dead space which further increases the required ventilation for adequate gas exchange.

Studies of elite breath-hold divers and submarine escape training instructors have noted a blunted response to hypercapnia, thus allowing longer times underwater without the need to surface. However, if an untrained individual hyperventilates before a breath-hold dive, they may drown due to hypoxia-induced syncope while submerged, dubbed the 'shallow water blackout syndrome'.[7] This is due to retarding the brainstem's hypercapnic stimulus by depleting the body's carbon dioxide reserves during the pre-dive hyperventilation.

Physiologic effects of gas embolization

Gas embolization to the heart and pulmonary vasculature results in mechanical as well as secondary effects due to release of mediators. Similarly, gas bubbles that form within tissues and their vasculature have mechanical and mediator-induced injurious effects. An air embolus may cause mechanical obstruction ('air-lock' phenomenon) of the right heart or pulmonary arterial system which could result in acute right heart failure and death. If the obstruction is only partial, the vortex flow around the embolus is postulated to cause a blood-froth mixture that can activate platelets and enhance fibrin formation as well as activate complement and the kinin system.[1] Nitrogen bubbles can also activate the clotting cascade[17] and interact with the vascular endothelium to induce an inflammatory response.[18] The damaged capillaries become permeable to edema fluid that compresses the microvasculature and reduces tissue oxygenation. The activated neutrophils, platelets, and complement may lead to pathology that is similar to reperfusion injury.[18–21] These changes may persist even after recompression has eliminated the bubbles. Nitrogen bubbles may also mechanically occlude veins, arteries, and lymphatics.

After air, oxygen, or nitrogen gas emboli occur, airways resistance (R_{aw}) increases. If the bubbles are filled with carbon dioxide or inert gases such as helium, neon, argon, or xenon, the resistance does not significantly change.[2] The changes in R_{aw} and pulmonary vascular resistance result in maldistribution of ventilation ($\dot{V}$) to perfusion (Q) which results in hypoxemia (due to low $\dot{V}$/Q units) as well as increased areas of dead space (elevated $\dot{V}$/Q ratios). In areas of high $\dot{V}$/Q, there is a 'washout' of carbon dioxide from poorly or nonperfused alveoli, which results in a decline in end-tidal carbon dioxide. This decline will be exaggerated if the cardiac output is concomitantly low.

Miscellaneous effects of dysbarism

CARBON MONOXIDE TOXICITY

A diver may be exposed to high levels of carbon monoxide if their air tank was contaminated during the filling process. Hemoglobin has a greater affinity for carbon monoxide than for oxygen. Thus, in the presence of carbon monoxide, oxygen is displaced from hemoglobin resulting in elevated levels of carboxyhemoglobin and lower levels of oxyhemoglobin even though the oxygen tension in the blood may be normal or even elevated (if supplemental oxygen is being utilized by the patient). Since oxygen delivery is directly related to oxyhemoglobin and only weakly related to oxygen tension, the displacement of oxyhemoglobin by carboxyhemoglobin will result in a decrease in oxygen delivery to the tissues.

CARBON DIOXIDE TOXICITY

Carbon dioxide increases with exercise. It can accumulate to a toxic level in a diver who intentionally hypoventilates to conserve air, takes shallow breathes, uses a tight wetsuit or jacket (restriction), or if significant intrapulmonary gas exchange abnormalities exist.[22] The risk is increased when a closed or semi-closed circuit rebreathing apparatus is used by commercial divers.

OXYGEN TOXICITY

Because of the hyperbaric condition beneath the water's surface, all divers are exposed to relatively high oxygen concentrations. However, oxygen toxicity rarely occurs unless the diver is using a hyperoxic gas mixture termed 'nitrox.' In an effort to prolong the safety of prolonged dives relative to nitrogen supersaturation (DCI), nitrox tanks contain lower concentrations of nitrogen and higher oxygen concentrations (usually 32–36 percent). If scuba enthusiasts do not limit their dive to shallow depths, the combination of hyperbaric conditions and hyperoxia may result in acute oxygen toxicity.

NITROGEN NARCOSIS AND HIGH–PRESSURE NERVOUS SYNDROME

Nitrogen has high lipid solubility. Therefore, when divers are under hyperbaric conditions, nitrogen supersaturates their brain tissue and exerts a narcotic effect. The hyperbaric conditions themselves, especially with the deeper depths that nitrox allows, may cause disturbances in neural transmission. These disturbances allow enhancement of synaptic transmission and actually can antagonize the effects of anesthesia and nitrogen narcosis.[23,24]

PULMONARY EDEMA

Pulmonary edema has been reported to occur rarely in swimmers during strenuous military training or even during the course of a safe dive.[25–28] Although the cause has not been fully clarified, it does not appear to be related to barotrauma or DCS. Various unproved theories have been proposed to explain this occurrence including micro-aspiration, increased fluid in the intravascular space,[27,29] dry air delivered from the scuba device, and as a result of falling oxygen tension as a diver surfaces. Its incidence is not dependent on left ventricular systolic or diastolic dysfunction, plasma levels of epinephrine, norepinephrine, cortisol, aldosterone, renin, or atrial natriuretic peptides.[26]

CLINICAL PRESENTATIONS

Barotrauma

Barotrauma is the consequence of compression or expansion of a gas-filled cavity during descent or ascent. Barotrauma can occur in any enclosed area of the body, including spaces around the diving equipment (mask, wet suit) or body cavities (lungs, pleura, intestines, middle ear, sinuses, dental caries or fillings). The most severe cases of pulmonary barotrauma are seen after an uncontrolled ascent and the most feared sequela is when bubbles escape from the pulmonary vasculature and cause arterial gas embolism (AGE).[30]

Pulmonary barotrauma of ascent

Given that there is a relatively high likelihood of death, pulmonary barotrauma during a scuba dive ascent is the most severe form of barotrauma. Boyle's law explains how this form of barotrauma may occur during ascent from a scuba dive. If exhalation is restricted during ascent either because the diver fails to exhale rapidly enough or the gas is trapped due to an airway obstruction, the enclosed, hyperbaric, lung volume will expand beyond its original volume at the surface (Fig. 11A.1). When transpulmonary (intratracheal minus alveolar) pressure exceeds 100 cm H_2O, gas can escape from the alveolar space and cause lung rupture. If the gas tracks along the perivascular sheath, a pneumomediastinum[31–33] or subcutaneous emphysema of the neck and upper chest[22,34] will occur. If the air escapes into the pleural, pericardial, or peritoneal spaces, then a pneumothorax,[32] pneumopericardium, or pneumoperitoneum may result. The disruption of the alveolar–capillary membrane may cause alveolar hemorrhage,[35] or allow gas to escape via the pulmonary veins or through a patent foramen ovale resulting in an arterial gas embolus.[36]

Pneumothorax usually presents as sudden pleuritic chest pain and dyspnea associated with tachypnea, decreased breath sounds, and hyperresonance to percussion over the affected lung.[37] If its size increases and intrathoracic tension develops, hemodynamic compromise may result in shock and death. If a pneumomediastinum accompanies subcutaneous emphysema, then the patient may note dysphagia, odynophagia, cough, dyspnea, and pleuritic chest pain. If air escapes into the pericardial sac (pneumopericardium), a harsh pericardial rub (Hamman crunch) may be auscultated.[1] Even if the expansion of gas does not result in alveolar rupture, overdistension of the lung can result in hemoptysis. Although subcutaneous emphysema may resolve spontaneously,[22] the concern that DCS may also be present requires transfer to a specialized recompression chamber (see section on treatment). The risk of pulmonary barotrauma of ascent has been associated with the presence of airway obstruction,[38] bullous disease,[39] increased transpulmonary and transatrial pressures, lower mid-expiratory flow (MEF) rates at 50 or 25 percent of vital capacity,[31] pleural adhesions,[31,40] reductions in MEF_{25} of more that 20 percent of the predictive values,[31] and the presence of an intracardiac shunt.[41]

MIDDLE EAR BAROTRAUMA

Middle ear barotrauma (MEB) may also occur during ascent due to failure of the expanding gas to vent through the eustachian tube.[9] The diagnosis of MEB is made by a Weber test, in which there will be an increase in bone conduction on the affected side. Otoscopic examination may also reveal an erythematous, retracted, or ruptured tympanic membrane.[11,22]

Pulmonary barotrauma of descent

Although the barotrauma of descent is usually not life-threatening, a breath-hold diver can still experience serious complications during a rapid descent. The acute change in atmospheric pressures during a fast, breath-hold descent may lead to a rapid decrease in lung volume (lung squeeze) which can mechanically disrupt the delicate alveolar–capillary membrane. This results in alveolar exudation and hemorrhage with resulting cough, dyspnea, and hemoptysis.[42,43] Pulmonary edema has also been reported in scuba divers[28] and in swimmers during vigorous exercise.[44]

A mask squeeze occurs during descent when the diver fails to exhale through the nose. This results in a vacuum effect that may lead to engorgement of periorbital and ocular blood vessels resulting in swelling and subconjunctival hemorrhage.[22,45,46]

External ear barotrauma usually occurs during descent due to occlusion of the external auditory canal by cerumen, earplugs, hoods, or masks. The increase in ambient pressure precipitates petechial hemorrhages within the ear canal[22] which causes otalgia and ear fullness.

Barotrauma of the middle ear is the most common disorder experienced by the first-time divers.[8,9] If the eustachian tube does not allow air to enter the middle ear during descent, the middle ear is unable to equalize pressures

with the ambient environment. It usually presents as a sensation of pressure followed by otalgia, tinnitus, nausea, transient conductive hearing loss, vertigo, and reversible facial nerve palsy.[11,12,22] Risk factors for this complication include inappropriate equalization techniques, upper respiratory infections, allergic rhinitis, and anatomic deformities or variations.[9,11,47] The tympanic membrane may rupture which can result in vertigo. Rarely, this can lead to life-threatening disorientation while underwater.[12,48]

Inner ear barotrauma is the result of forceful efforts to equalize middle ear pressure during descent when the eustachian tube is occluded. Inner ear barotrauma may rupture the inner ear membrane and create a labyrinthine window fistula.[22,49,50] The customary symptoms of inner ear barotrauma include sensory-neural deafness, tinnitus, vertigo, nausea, and emesis. Fistula formation is a medical emergency that needs to be differentiated from inner ear decompression sickness, which occurs after surfacing.

Paranasal sinus barotrauma is the second most common malady affecting divers.[9,11] It is twice as common during descent than ascent. Blockage of the sinus ostia[11] may cause chronic dysfunction of the nasal or paranasal sinuses that results in paranasal sinus mucosal hypertrophy.[51] Since the maxillary sinuses are commonly involved, symptoms usually include frontal sinus pain and epistaxis.[45,52]

Decompression sickness

Since the diagnosis of DCS is based on clinical symptoms, it may be confused with barotrauma. However, the complications of barotrauma are evident within minutes of surfacing, whereas the symptoms of DCS are usually evident only after 1–6 hours. Therefore, any neurologic or cardiovascular signs or symptoms that occur within the first 15 minutes after a diver reaches the surface are assumed to be due to barotrauma or AGE.[1]

Symptoms of DCS include limb pain (the bends), fatigue, malaise, and various neurologic syndromes. Bubbles may travel through the pulmonary arterial system and become lodged within the pulmonary microvasculature, leading to a less common pulmonary form of DCI (the chokes). Precursors to DCS include stasis, dehydration, and a rapid ascent.[53] The manifestations can be accentuated by obstructive airway disease.[54]

To prioritize the severity and thus medical urgency of DCS, it is divided into two types (I and II). Type I (the bends) manifests as a deep, aching, and poorly localized musculoskeletal pain,[11,55] which arises over approximately 1 hour after surfacing, with symptoms increasing during the next 36 hours. The affected limb is usually held in a semi-flexed position by the diver because of a dull, aching pain. The pain may be preceded by paresthesias and a less intense sensation referred to as 'the niggles'. Joint pain is due to supersaturation and separation of nitrogen within poorly perfused, periarticular, tight connective tissue during decompression.[11] Rash and lymphedema are secondary to bubble formation in the skin and lymphatics.[56]

When cardiorespiratory or neurologic symptoms occur, it is termed type II DCS. The symptoms may appear within 10–30 minutes or many days after ascent.[11] Neurologic injury is felt to be secondary to the thrombogenic effect of bubbles in the epidural venous plexus surrounding the spinal cord which causes venous stasis and spinal cord ischemia.[56] Around 90 percent of divers in this category are symptomatic.[57] It may cause paresthesias, paraplegia, bladder paralysis, fecal incontinence, priapism, and referred abdominal pain. Spinal cord lesions are the most common type of involvement with limb paresthesias being the most common symptom.[58] Other manifestations include paralysis, vertigo, ataxia, speech disturbance, unconsciousness, skin dysesthesias, and visual or cognitive deficits.[12,45,59] Psychiatric manifestations may also be present.[60]

The cardiopulmonary manifestations of DCI are due to the migration of bubbles. If an anatomic shunt, such as a patent foramen ovale, is present, the bubbles may invade the systemic arterial circulation and lead to cardiovascular and neurologic abnormalities due to AGE.[61,62] The risk of neurologic deficits are increased in divers with a patent foramen ovale, atrial septal defect, or pulmonary arteriovenous fistula.[63,64] If the bubbles lodge within the pulmonary vasculature (pulmonary venous emboli – the 'chokes'), then chest tightness, cough, dyspnea, pulmonary hypertension, pulmonary edema, and systemic hypotension may result. Frequently, gas bubbles are detected in the venous circulation by ultrasonography but do not cause any hemodynamic instability.[65]

Dysbaric osteonecrosis (caisson disease)

Symptoms, if they arise, may not appear for months or even years after exposure to dysbaric conditions. The most common symptom is arthritic pain that may advance to severe osteoarthritis and disability if the juxtaarticular surfaces are involved. However, if the shaft of a long bone is involved, there may be no symptoms. In these cases, the only findings are radiographic and include necrotic areas and evidence of repair (thickened trabeculae). Rarely, mesenchymal malignancies (fibrous histiocytomas or osteosarcomas) have been reported in areas of necrosis.[66]

Arterial gas embolus

The most feared and fatal form of DCI is AGE, the second most common cause of death in divers (drowning is the leading cause).[67] Although the pathophysiology and treatment of AGE and DCS are similar, the source of the gas bubbles differ. Whereas DCS requires a change to a lower ambient pressure and an anatomic right-to-left shunt, AGE can occur isobarically from gas escaping along the pulmonary perivascular sheath due to a tension pneumothorax or pneumomediastinum or through a shunt. Ninety-five percent of divers who develop AGE manifest isolated central nervous system symptoms whereas cardiovascular collapse is more frequent in aviators who develop AGE. The AGE-related hemodynamic collapse is due to a coronary artery embolus or neurogenic-mediated hypertension if the embolus lodges within a cerebral artery. There is a direct relation between serum creatine kinase activity and the severity of AGE.[68] Computed tomographic or nuclear magnetic resonance scans are less sensitive than the clinical evaluation.[68]

Neurologic symptoms and signs of AGE are diverse and almost invariably occur immediately after the diver surfaces. A feeling of apprehension and confusion is rapidly followed by sensory disturbances which may progress to aphasia, hemiplegia, cortical blindness, hemianopsias, confusion, coma, and seizures depending on the affected intracerebral artery.[1] A rare, but classic, sign of AGE is a sharply demarcated area of pallor on the tongue (Lieberman sign). Other classic signs include marbling of the skin of the upper body and gas bubbles in the retinal arteries.[69] Symptoms of AGE improve within minutes in 60 percent of victims due to redistribution of the emboli. Fifteen percent of individuals recover spontaneously within an hour. However, late relapses have been described and are thought to be due to the delayed effects of inflammatory mediators. Five percent of AGE victims die almost immediately upon surfacing.

Miscellaneous syndromes caused by dysbarism

CARBON MONOXIDE TOXICITY

The symptoms of acute carbon monoxide poisoning correlate with the percentage of carboxyhemoglobin. It may present as headache, dizziness, nausea, dyspnea weakness, tachycardia, visual disturbances, confusion, syncope, seizure, coma, cardiopulmonary dysfunction, and death.[70]

OXYGEN TOXICITY

Oxygen toxicity usually presents with nausea, dizziness, central chest pain, paresthesias, auditory hallucinations, visual disturbances, focal seizures, irritability, and disorientation. Fatal generalized seizures may occur.[22,71] After 12 hours of oxygen exposure, lung congestion, pulmonary edema, and atelectasis may develop.[22]

NITROGEN NARCOSIS AND HIGH-PRESSURE NERVOUS SYNDROME

The clinical picture of nitrogen narcosis mimics alcohol intoxication and was termed 'rapture of the depths' by Cousteau. At depths of 20–30 m, it may present as euphoria, lightheadedness, weakness, clumsiness, and impaired memory and judgment. At higher atmospheric pressures, disorientation and loss of consciousness may be seen[22] which is associated with a high risk of drowning. The narcosis usually resolves spontaneously during decompression. There is individual susceptibility to the narcotic effects of high nitrogen concentrations as well as risk factors that may exacerbate the symptoms (cold water, fatigue, strenuous activity, sedative or alcohol consumption).

High-pressure nervous syndrome presents with signs and symptoms of hyperexcitability of the central nervous system. Symptoms include headache, vertigo, euphoria, nausea, and fatigue. Signs that have been reported include myoclonus, hyperreflexia, tremors, and decreased manual dexterity.[24]

PULMONARY EDEMA

The first symptom that develops when pulmonary edema occurs is a cough that worsens as the diver ascends. Weakness, chest discomfort, orthopnea, wheezing, dizziness and hemoptysis may occur. The symptoms may persist for 48 hours after the dive. The chest radiographic appearance is similar to that in the acute respiratory distress syndrome. Although it is more common in older adults and in hypertensive patients, there is no clear association with systolic dysfunction. Cold, prior respiratory infection, or water inhalation may be precipitating factors. Individuals with a history of pulmonary edema should be advised against diving[54] since recurrence is seen in many cases. It usually resolves spontaneously.[10]

MANAGEMENT AND PREVENTION OF THE COMPLICATIONS OF DIVING

Hyperbaric treatment

Type II decompression sickness and the barotrauma of ascent should be considered to be medical emergencies. Urgent recompression in a hyperbaric chamber while breathing 100 percent oxygen followed by a controlled ascent is used to diminish the size of bubbles regardless of their origins. In addition, breathing 100 percent oxygen produces a gradient by which inert gas bubbles may diffuse from saturated tissues. Currently there are over 400 hyperbaric chambers in the United States,[36] but more than half of those are monoplace (one person) chambers. Although monoplace chambers are not ideal to treat the most critically ill divers who require bedside attention in a multiperson chamber, they can recompress to 3 ATA which is enough to treat most cases of DCI and AGE.[55] Treatment should be started promptly using tables established by the US Navy.[55] Details of hyperbaric therapy are beyond the scope of this chapter. Specialized training is required to administer hyperbaric treatment. If a hyperbaric facility is not easily accessible, the diver should be transported immediately to a facility where it can be provided since favorable results can still be expected.[72] Some diving spots have portable monoplace recompression chambers, which were developed to treat high-altitude

pulmonary edema. If air transportation by helicopter is preferred over ground transportation, the altitude should not exceed 300 m unless the aircraft is fully pressurized in order to avoid hypobaric cabin conditions.[73] Treatment with hyperbaric oxygen for DCS can be extremely effective (>95 percent success) if begun early. However, 30–50 percent of DCS victims require repeat recompression for relapses that may occur days after the initial event.[74]

Decompression sickness

Treatment of DCS depends on the severity of the presenting symptoms. In type I DCS, symptoms may disappear once the diver reaches the surface and the partial pressure equilibrates. If needed, recompression may become necessary. Type II DCS and AGE should always be treated in a recompression chamber in order to reduce bubble size and morbidity. In most cases, immediate treatment with hydration and 100 percent FiO_2 should be started.[43] The high concentration of inspired oxygen promotes better diffusion of the inert gas into the tissue and therefore decreases the bubble size.[22,75] It also slightly improves oxygen delivery to the poorly perfused tissues. Some authors advocate the use of the Trendelenburg and left lateral decubitus position to avoid hypotension and to try to 'trap' bubbles in the right atrium of the heart. However, neither the position of the patient nor the use of corticosteroid or anticoagulants have been proved to be of significant benefit in treating DCS.[22] Once a diver experiences an episode of DCS, there are no uniform criteria for when it is safe to return to recreational diving. The diver is expected to avoid diving for at least 4 weeks after all symptoms have disappeared completely.[54] If symptoms remain or if AGE occurred, then diving should be completely avoided.

Barotrauma of ascent

As noted earlier in this chapter, the barotrauma of ascent includes multiple complications including pneumothorax, pneumomediastinum, pneumopericardium, and subcutaneous emphysema. All effected divers should be evaluated for treatment in a recompression chamber. After surfacing, a pneumothorax may continue to expand and develop into a tension pneumothorax that causes hemodynamic instability. If this occurs, emergent needle decompression and chest tube placement may be necessary.[11,37] Pneumomediastinum and subcutaneous emphysema usually resolve spontaneously.[22]

Barotrauma of descent

The treatment of MEB includes the use of topical or systemic vasoconstrictors and antihistamines.[11,22] Myringotomy may be required and in cases of tympanic membrane perforation, prophylactic antibiotics may be used.[9,12] A decreased incidence of MEB has been reported when pseudoephedrine hydrochloride (60 mg) is given 30 minutes before diving.[47]

Inner ear barotrauma is a medical emergency and should be differentiated from inner ear decompression sickness which occurs during ascent or after surfacing. A specialist's evaluation is usually required and primary treatment consists of bed rest, head elevation, and stool softeners.[11,76] Some experts recommend early surgical exploration if the fistula does not heal spontaneously within 5–10 days.[22,50] Treatment of paranasal barotrauma includes the use of topical or systemic decongestants or adrenergic agents and antibiotics in cases of purulent discharge.[11]

Toxicities from carbon monoxide, carbon dioxide, and nitrogen

The treatment of carbon monoxide toxicity is based on the use of supplemental oxygen, ventilatory support, and cardiac monitoring for dysrhythmias. Hyperbaric oxygen therapy has been recommended by the Undersea and Hyperbaric Medical Society when the patient is unconscious, or exhibits neurologic symptoms, cardiovascular dysfunction, or severe acidosis.[70] Nitrogen narcosis and carbon dioxide toxicity usually resolve spontaneously after the diver surfaces.

Prevention of diving complications

Ideally, the complications of diving should be avoided by proper medical screening, strict adherence to dive tables, use of safe equipment, and proper techniques. All diving candidates require a medical evaluation prior to diving. The evaluation should focus on conditions that may limit the candidate's ability to exercise or diseases that may be exacerbated by strenuous activity in a cold, dry, hyperbaric, confined environment. The major contraindications include various pulmonary and cardiovascular diseases.[77] Box 11A.1 lists conditions that may disqualify individuals from diving. Scuba certifying organizations, the Occupational Safety and Health Administration, and the US Navy have published guidelines concerning pre-dive medical evaluations.[58] In addition, any condition that precludes the use of hyperbaric oxygen therapy should disqualify the candidate from diving.

Individuals who are affected by conditions that predisposed them to the development of a pneumothorax should not dive. These include cystic fibrosis, histiocytosis X, Ehlers–Danlos syndrome, the presence of lung bullae, or a previous history of a spontaneous pneumothorax.[78]

Insulin-dependent diabetes mellitus and epilepsy can lead to loss of conscious resulting in drowning. Various articles in the literature maintain that it is safe for diabetic patients to dive.[79–82] Epilepsy is still a contraindication for diving except in those people who have a history of febrile seizures ending prior to the age of 5 years.[83]

> **Box 11A.1 Cardiopulmonary conditions that predispose to diving complications**
>
> Pulmonary diseases
>
> - Obstructive lung diseases
>   - Asthma
>   - Bronchiectasis
>   - Emphysema
>   - Chronic obstructive pulmonary diseases
> - Increased risk of pulmonary barotrauma
>   - Previous pneumothorax
>   - Previous thoracic surgery
>   - Cystic lung diseases
>   - Bullous lung diseases
> - History of pulmonary hemorrhage
>
> Cardiac diseases
>
> - Patent foramen ovale
> - Unrepaired intracardiac defects
> - Exercise-induced tachyarrhythmias
> - Uncontrolled dysrhythmias
>
> Miscellaneous
>
> - Previous arterial gas embolus
> - Sequelae from decompression sickness
> - Recurrent seizures
> - Recurrent episodes of syncope

Asthma

Asthma is present in 5 percent of the American population[84] and, according to various surveys, in a similar percentage of recreational scuba divers.[85] When considering the safety of allowing an individual with asthma to dive, guidelines vary according to specific countries and medical associations. In England, most divers with asthma are allowed to dive if they do not have cold-induced asthma and have not required the use of a bronchodilator within 48 hours of diving. In addition, the diver needs to show physiologic stability as evidenced by a stable peak expiratory flow rate (<20 percent diurnal variability).[54] The position of the French Federation for Submarine Sports and Education is that asthma is an absolute contraindication for scuba diving.[86] The South Pacific Underwater Medicine Society recommends a provocation test with exercise or saline to exclude the presence of asthma because of their concern that asthmatics have a higher relative risk of developing DCS. The American Lung Association of California maintains that dive applicants should be evaluated for the presence of asthma by history and physical examination. Data from the Divers Alert Network have shown that the risk of AGE and DCI is not increased in people with asthma when compared with the nonasthmatic population if there is no current exacerbation of asthma. At the present time, it is recommended that the assessment of asthmatic divers be individualized, with active participation of the diving candidate in the final decision and commitment to dive safely.[87]

Key learning points

- Most of the complications of diving are secondary to the changes that occur when an individual is exposed to environmental pressure changes.

- These environmental pressure changes are predicted according to the ideal gas equation.

- Diving-related injuries are usually due to the formation of bubbles or the expansion of air pockets in the body.

- Treatment of serious, diving-related injuries requires recompression and controlled decompression in a hyperbaric chamber.

- Symptoms or signs that occur within a few minutes of surfacing from a dive are usually due to barotrauma of ascent or AGE and should be treated as medical emergencies.

- Potential divers need to be medically screened for diseases that may predispose them to barotrauma or cardiopulmonary complications during strenuous activity in a cold, hyperbaric, environment.

REFERENCES

1. de la Hoz RE, Krieger B. Dysbarism. In: Rom W, ed. *Environmental and Occupational Medicine*, 3rd ed. Philadelphia: Lippincott-Raven, 1998: 1359–75.

◆ 2. Wilson MM, Curley FJ. Gas embolism: Part I. Venous gas emboli. *J Intensive Care Med* 1996; **11**: 182–204.

● 3. Behnke A. Decompression sickness incident to deep sea diving and high altitude ascent. *Medicine* 1945; **24**: 381–402.

4. Smith DJ, Francis TJ, Pethybridge RJ, *et al.* An evaluation of the classification of decompression disorders. *Undersea Biomed Res* 1993; **20**: 17–18.

5. Bove AA. Risk of decompression sickness with patent foramen ovale. *Undersea Hyperb Med* 1998; **25**: 175–8.

6. Butler FK, Jr. Diving and hyperbaric ophthalmology. *Surv Ophthalmol* 1995; **39**: 347–66.

◆ 7. de la Hoz RE, Krieger B. Dysbarism. *Clin Pulm Med* 1998; **5**: 329–36.

8. Brown M, Jones J, Krohmer J. Pseudoephedrine for the prevention of barotitis media: a controlled clinical trial in underwater divers. *Ann Emerg Med* 1992; **21**: 849–52.

✱ 9. Neblett LM. Otolaryngology and sport scuba diving. Update and guidelines. *Ann Otol Rhinol Laryngol Suppl* 1985; **115**: 1–12.

10. Bove AA. *Diving Medicine*, 3rd ed. Philadelphia: WB Saunders, 1997.

◆ 11. Melamed YS, Shupak A, Bitterman, H. Medical problems associated with underwater diving. *N Engl J Med* 1992: 30–5.

◆ 12. Replogle WH, Sanders SD, Keeton JE, Phillips DM. Scuba diving injuries. *Am Fam Physician* 1988; **37**: 135–42.

13. Doolete DJ, Mitchell SJ. The physiological kinetics of nitrogen and the prevention of decompression sickness. *Clin Pharmacokinet* 2001; **40**: 1–14.

14. Wilmshurst P, Bryson P. Relationship between the clinical features of neurological decompression illness and its causes. *Clin Sci (Lond)* 2000; **99**: 65–75.

15. Brylske A. The gas laws. A guide for the mathematically challenged. *Dive Training* 1997; **September**: 26–34.

16. Liner MH. Cardiovascular and pulmonary responses to breath-hold diving in humans. *Acta Physiol Scand* 1994; **151**(Suppl 620): 1–32.

17. Hills BA. Supersaturation by counterperfusion and diffusion of gases. *J Appl Physiol* 1977; **42**: 758–60.

18. Levin LL, Stewart GJ, Lynch PR, Bove AA. Blood and blood vessel wall changes induced by decompression sickness in dogs. *J Appl Physiol* 1981; **50**: 944–9.

19. Zamboni WA, Roth AC, Russell RC, *et al.* Morphologic analysis of the microcirculation during reperfusion of ischemic skeletal muscle and the effect of hyperbaric oxygen. *Plast Reconstr Surg* 1993; **91**: 1110–23.

20. Ward CA, McCullough D, Fraser WD. Relation between complement activation and susceptibility to decompression sickness. *J Appl Physiol* 1987; **62**: 1160–6.

21. Helps SC, Gorman DF. Air embolism of the brain in rabbits pretreated with mechlorethamine. *Stroke* 1991; **22**: 351–4.

◆ 22. Moon RE. Treatment of diving emergencies. *Crit Care Clin* 1999; **15**: 429–56.

23. Madsen J, Hink J, Hyldegaard O. Diving physiology and pathophysiology. *Clin Physiol* 1994; **14**: 597–626.

24. Jain NN. High-pressure neurological syndrome (HPNS). *Acta Neurol Scand* 1994; **90**: 45–50.

25. Wilmshurst PT, Nuri M, Crowther A, Webb-Peploe MM. Cold-induced pulmonary oedema in scuba divers and swimmers and subsequent development of hypertension. *Lancet* 1989; **1**: 62–5.

26. Pons M, Blickenstorfer D, Oechslin E, *et al.* Pulmonary oedema in healthy persons during scuba-diving and swimming. *Eur Respir J* 1995; **8**: 762–7.

27. Hampson NB, Dunford RG. Pulmonary edema of scuba divers. *Undersea Hyperb Med* 1997; **24**: 29–33.

28. Slade JB, Jr, Hattori T, Ray CS, *et al.* Pulmonary edema associated with scuba diving: case reports and review. *Chest* 2001; **120**: 1686–94.

29. Arborelius M, Jr, Ballidin UI, Lilja B, Lundgren CE. Hemodynamic changes in man during immersion with the head above water. *Aerosp Med* 1972; **43**: 592–8.

30. Dutka AJ. A review of the pathophysiology and potential application of experimental therapies for cerebral ischemia to the treatment of cerebral arterial gas embolism. *Undersea Biomed Res* 1985; **12**: 403–21.

◆ 31. Tetzlaff K, Reuter M, Leplow B, Heller M, Bettinghausen E. Risk factors for pulmonary barotrauma in divers. *Chest* 1997; **112**: 654–9.

32. Friehs I, Friehs GM, Friehs GB. Air embolism with bilateral pneumothorax after a five-meter dive. *Undersea Hyperb Med* 1993; **20**: 155–7.

33. Blood C, Hoiberg A. Analyses of variables underlying US Navy diving accidents. *Undersea Biomed Res* 1985; **12**: 351–60.

34. Boettger ML. Scuba diving emergencies: pulmonary overpressure accidents and decompression sickness. *Ann Emerg Med* 1983; **12**: 563–7.

35. Balk M, Goldman JM. Alveolar hemorrhage as a manifestation of pulmonary barotrauma after scuba diving. *Ann Emerg Med* 1990; **19**: 930–4.

36. Neuman TS, Jacoby I, Bove AA. Fatal pulmonary barotrauma due to obstruction of the central circulation with air. *J Emerg Med* 1998; **16**: 413–17.

● 37. Edmond C, Lowry C, Pannefather J. Barotrauma. In: Edmond C, Lowry C, Pannafather J, eds. *Diving and Subaquatic Medicine*, 2nd ed. Mosman, NSW, Australia: Diving Medical Centre, 1983: 93–127.

38. Weiss LD, Van Meter KW. Cerebral air embolism in asthmatic scuba divers in a swimming pool. *Chest* 1995; **107**: 1653–4.

39. Mellem H, Emhjellen S, Horgen O. Pulmonary barotrauma and arterial gas embolism caused by an emphysematous bulla in a SCUBA diver. *Aviat Space Environ Med* 1990; **61**: 559–62.

40. Calder IM. Autopsy and experimental observations on factors leading to barotrauma in man. *Undersea Biomed Res* 1985; **12**: 165–82.

41. Wilmshurst P. Patent foramen ovale and decompression illness. *SPUMS J* 1997; **27**: 82–3.

42. Strauss MB, Wright PW. Thoracic squeeze diving casualty. *Aerosp Med* 1971; **42**: 673–5.

43. Leitch DR, Green RD. Pulmonary barotrauma in divers and the treatment of cerebral arterial gas embolism. *Aviat Space Environ Med* 1986; **57**(10 Pt 1): 931–8.

44. Weiler-Ravell D, Shupak A, Goldenberg I, *et al.* Pulmonary oedema and hemoptysis induced by strenuous swimming. *BMJ* 1995; **311**: 361–2.

45. Chesire Jr WP, Ott MC. Headache in divers. *Headache* 2001; **41**: 235–47.

46. Elliot DH, Moon RE. *Manifestations of Decompression Disorders*, 4th ed. Philadelphia: WB Saunders, 1993.

47. Uzun C, Adali MK, Tas A, *et al.* Use of the nine-step inflation/defation test as the predictor of middle ear barotraumain sports scuba divers. *Br J Audiol* 2000; **34**: 153–63.

48. Uzun C, Adali MK, Koten M, *et al.* Relationship between mastoid pneumatization and middle ear barotrauma in divers. *Laryngoscope* 2002; **112**: 287–91.

49. Farmer JC, Jr. Diving injuries to the inner ear. *Ann Otol Rhinol Laryngol Suppl* 1977; **86**(1 Pt 3 Suppl 36): 1–20.

50. Farmer JC, Jr. *The Physiology and Medicine of Diving*, 3rd ed. San Pedro: Best Publishing, 1982.

51. Yanagawa Y, Okada Y, Ishida K, *et al.* Magnetic resonance imaging of the paranasal sinuses in divers. *Aviat Space Environ Med* 1998; **69**: 50–2.

52. Weissman B, Green RS, Roberts PT. Frontal sinus barotrauma. *Laryngoscope* 1972; **82**: 2160–8.

53. Bove AA, Hallenbeck JM, Elliott DH. Changes in blood and plasma volumes in dogs during decompression sickness. *Aerosp Med* 1974; **45**: 49–55.

✱ 54. British Thoracic Society guidelines on respiratory aspects of fitness for diving. *Thorax* 2003; **58**: 3–13.

55. Strauss MB, Borer RC, Jr. Diving medicine: contemporary topics and their controversies. *Am J Emerg Med* 2001; **19**: 232–8.

56. Gerriets T, Tetzlaff K, Liceni T, *et al.* Arteriovenous bubbles following cold water sport dives: relation to right-to-left shunting. *Neurology* 2000; **55**: 1741–3.

57. Francis TJ, Pearson RR, Robertson AG, *et al.* Central nervous system decompression sickness: latency of 1070 human cases. *Undersea Biomed Res* 1988; **15**: 403–17.

◆ 58. Strauss RH. Diving medicine. *Am Rev Respir Dis* 1979; **119**: 1001–23.

59. Newton HB. Neurologic complications of scuba diving. *Am Fam Physician* 2001; **63**: 2211–18.

60. Hopkins RO, Weaver LK. Acute psychosis associated with diving. *Undersea Hyperb Med* 2001; **28**: 145–8.

61. Wilmshurst P, Davidson C, O'Connell G, Byrne C. Role of cardiorespiratory abnormalities, smoking and dive characteristics in the manifestations of neurological decompression illness. *Clin Sci (Lond)* 1994; **86**: 297–303.

62. Bove AA, Hallenbeck JM, Elliott DH. Circulatory responses to venous air embolism and decompression sickness in dogs. *Undersea Biomed Res* 1974; **1**: 207–20.

63. Hagen PT, Scholz DG, Edwards WD. Incidence and size of patent foramen ovale during the first 10 decades of life: an autopsy study of 965 normal hearts. *Mayo Clin Proc* 1984; **59**: 17–20.

64. Wilmshurst P, Nightingale S. Relationship between migraine and cardiac and pulmonary right-to-left shunts. *Clin Sci (Lond)* 2001; **100**: 215–20.

65. Brubakk AO, Eftedal O. Comparison of three different ultrasonic methods for quantification of intravascular gas bubbles. *Undersea Hyperb Med* 2001; **28**: 131–6.

66. Torres FX, Kyriakos M. Bone infarct-associated osteosarcoma. *Cancer* 1992; **70**: 2418–30.

67. Bradley ME. *Diving Medicine*. Philadelphia: WB Saunders, 1990.

● 68. Smith RM, Newman TS. Elevation of serum creatine kinase in divers with arterial gas embolization. *N Engl J Med* 1994; **330**: 19–24.

◆ 69. Wilson MM CF. Gas embolism: Part II. Arterial gas embolism and decompression sickness. *J Intensive Care Med* 1996; **11**: 261–83.

70. Varon J, Marik PE, Fromm RE, Gueler A. Carbon monoxide poisoning: a review for clinicians. *J Emerg Med* 1999; **17**: 87–93.

71. Clark JM, Thom SR. Toxicity of oxygen, carbon dioxide, and carbon monoxide. In: Bove AA, ed. *Bove and Davis' Diving Medicine*, 3rd ed. Philadelphia: WB Saunders, 1997: 131–45.

72. Halpern P, Greenstein A, Melamed Y, *et al.* Spinal decompression sickness with delayed onset, delayed treatment, and full recovery. *Br Med J (Clin Res Ed)* 1982; **284**: 1014.

73. Tetzlaff K, Shank ES, Muth CM. Evaluation and management of decompression illness-an intensivist's perspective. *Intensive Care Med* 2003; **29**: 2128–36.

74. Moon RE, Vann RD, Bennett PB. The physiology of decompression illness. *Sci Am* 1995; **273**: 70–7.

75. Annane D, Trouche G, Delisle F, *et al.* Effects of mechanical ventilation with normobaric oxygen therapy on the rate of air removal from cerebral arteries. *Crit Care Med* 1994; **22**: 851–7.

76. Parell GJ, Becker GD. Conservative management of inner ear barotrauma resulting from scuba diving. *Otolaryngol Head Neck Surg* 1985; **93**: 393–7.

77. Caruso JL, Uguccioni DM, Dovenbarger JA. Fatalities related to cardiovascular disease in the recreational diving population. *Undersea Hyperb Med* 1997; **24**: 26.

78. Simpson G. Primary lung bullae and scuba diving. *SPUMS J* 1998; **28**: 10–12.

79. Uguccioni DM, Pollock NW, Dovenbarger JA. Blood glucose response to single and repetitive dives in insulin-requiring diabetics. A preliminary report. *Undersea Hyperb Med* 1998; **25**(Suppl): 52.

80. Bryson P, Edge C, Gimby A. SCUBA diving and diabetes: Collecting definitive data from a covert population of recreational divers. Interim observations from a long term on-going prospective study. *Undersea Hyperb Med* 1998; **25**(Suppl): 61–6.

81. Lerch M, Lutrop C, Thurm U. Diabetes and diving: Can the risk of hypoglycaemia be barred? *SPUMS J* 1996; **26**: 61–6.

82. Williamson JA. Some diabetics are fit to dive, but which ones? The Australian experience and SPUMS policies. *SPUMS J* 1996; **26**: 70–2.

83. Mclver NKI. Neurology and mental fitness. In: Elliot DH, ed. *Medical Assessment of Fitness to Dive*. Surrey, England: Biomedical Seminars, 1995: 213–14.

84. Glen S, White S, Douglas J. Medical supervision of sport diving in Scotland: reassessing the need for routine medical examinations. *Br J Sports Med* 2000; **34**: 375–8.

◆ 85. Koehle M, Lloyd-Smith R, McKenzie D, Taunton J.

Asthma and recreational SCUBA diving: a systematic review. *Sports Med* 2003; **33**: 109–16.

86. Coetmeur D, Briens E, Dassonville J, Vergne M. [Asthma and scuba diving Absolute contraindication? in all asthma patients?] [In French]. *Rev Mal Respir* 2001; **18**(4 Pt 1): 381–6.

87. Krieger B. Diving: what to tell the patient with asthma and why. *Curr Opin Pulm Med* 2001; **7**: 32–8.

High-altitude diseases (HACE/HAPE)

COLIN K GRISSOM

INTRODUCTION

Oxygen delivery to the tissues depends on an adequate supply of oxygen at each step of the oxygen transport chain from the inspired air to the mitochondria. The atmospheric pressure and inspired partial pressure of oxygen (Table 11B.1) predictably decrease with increasing altitude (Table 11B.2). Humans at high altitude must overcome the disadvantage of ambient hypoxia by making a number of adaptations through a process called acclimatization to optimize the availability of oxygen to the tissues. In unacclimatized people ascending to a high altitude, failure of the body to adapt to the stress of hypobaric hypoxia may lead to the cerebral and pulmonary syndromes of high-altitude illness. Acute mountain sickness (AMS) and high-altitude cerebral edema (HACE) refer to the cerebral disorders, and high-altitude pulmonary edema (HAPE) to the pulmonary abnormalities. Although there is a great deal of individual variability and overlap in these disorders, this chapter deals with the cerebral and pulmonary disorders separately.

Table 11B.1 *Physiologic terms*

Symbol	Term
P_B	Barometric pressure (mm Hg)
Po_2	Partial pressure of oxygen
Pio_2	Inspired $Po_2 = [0.21 \times (P_B - 47 \text{ mm Hg}^*)]$
PAo_2	Po_2 in alveolus
$Paco_2$	Partial pressure of carbon dioxide in arterial blood
Pao_2	Po_2 in arterial blood
$Sao_2 \%$	Arterial oxygen saturation % ($Hbo2$/total $Hb \times 100$)
R	Respiratory quotient (CO_2 produced/O_2 consumed)
$PAo2 = Pio_2 - Paco_2/R$	Alveolar gas equation (simplified form)

*Vapor pressure of H_2O at 37°C.

Table 11B.2 *Approximate barometric pressure, inspired partial pressure of oxygen, and partial pressure of arterial oxygen and carbon dioxide at various altitudes for acclimatized people[1-4]*

Altitude		Barometric pressure (mm Hg)	Pio_2 (mm Hg)	Pao_2 (mm Hg)	$Paco_2$ (mm Hg)
Meters	**Feet**				
Sea Level		760	150	90	40
1524	5000	635	124	75	36
2743	9000	550	106	60	33
4572	15 000	430	80	52	25
6000	19 685	355	64	41	20
8000	26 240	280	49	37	13
8848	29 029	253	43	30	11

ACUTE MOUNTAIN SICKNESS AND HIGH-ALTITUDE CEREBRAL EDEMA

Definitions

Acute mountain sickness is a neurologic syndrome that occurs after acute ascent to altitudes greater than 2000 m. Headache as the prominent feature associated with one or more nonspecific symptoms of malaise, gastrointestinal upset, lightheadedness, dizziness, or disturbed sleep. Although symptoms of AMS usually resolve without sequelae, AMS can progress to life-threatening HACE, which is the severe progression of brain pathophysiology that occurs in AMS. HACE occurs at altitudes greater than 3000 m and is characterized by an altered level of consciousness and ataxia, and without treatment progresses to obtundation, coma, and death due to brainstem herniation.[1,2,5]

Incidence/epidemiology

Susceptibility to AMS increases with higher altitude and faster rates of ascent (Table 11B.3). In Summit County, Colorado, 25 percent of travelers who ascend from low altitude to ski resorts at 2000–3000 m develop AMS.[6] On Mt Rainier, Washington, nearly two-thirds of climbers who rapidly ascend from sea level to the summit at 4400 m over 1–3 days develop AMS.[7] A prior history of AMS, residence at altitudes below 900 m, and obesity all increase susceptibility to AMS.[6] Physical fitness is not protective against AMS.[12] Men and women are equally susceptible to AMS,[13] and incidence in children is similar to adults.[14] Older people, however, are less susceptible to AMS.[6,15]

The exact incidence of HACE is not clear because it is much less common than AMS and there are few reports in the literature. Incidence of HACE in trekkers in Nepal at altitudes of 4243–5500 m was reported to be 1 percent overall, but 3.4 percent among those who had AMS.[9] It is much more common in those with HAPE, occurring in 13–20 percent of people presenting with HAPE.[16] Based on studies of HAPE, incidence of HACE is estimated to be less

than 0.1 percent in Mt Rainier climbers[1,7] and less than 1 percent in climbers on Mt McKinley (6195 m), Alaska.[1,11]

Etiology

In high-altitude illness neurohumoral and hemodynamic responses occur in the brain, lungs, and peripheral tissues that result in fluid retention, overperfusion of microvascular beds, and extravasation of fluid into the extravascular space. Symptoms of AMS suggest a primary neurologic syndrome, and current concepts of pathophysiology emphasize a cerebral etiology. Using various neuroimaging techniques brain edema has been observed in severe AMS,[17,18] suggesting that AMS is the precursor to HACE. In milder cases of AMS, however, edema has not been observed on brain computed tomography (CT).[18] Proposed causes for brain swelling in AMS include increased blood flow and brain blood volume, extravasation of fluid from the intravascular to the extravascular space, neuronal cell swelling, or a combination of these. One or more of these etiologies leads to severe cerebral edema in HACE.[16] A study using brain magnetic resonance imaging (MRI) in subjects after 32 hours at a simulated altitude of 4572 m showed brain swelling likely due to increased cerebral blood flow,[19] but brain swelling did not correlate with symptoms of AMS. In another study brain MRI showed no increase in brain swelling in subjects exposed to 4500 m for 10 hours.[20] Brain swelling may not occur acutely, but may be delayed for 12–24 hours after ascent, similar to the time course of increased cerebral blood flow after ascent to high altitude.[21] Cerebral blood flow increases on ascent to high altitude, probably because the vasodilator effect of hypoxemia outweighs the vasoconstrictor effect of hypocapnia resulting from hyperventilation. Increased cerebral blood flow may increase brain volume and contribute to AMS. Symptoms of AMS, however, have not been shown to correlate with increased cerebral blood flow.[22,23] One hypothesis to explain these discrepancies proposes that people who develop AMS have less ability to compensate for swelling of the brain that occurs on ascent to high altitude. Those with a lower ratio of cranial cerebrospinal fluid (CSF) to brain volume are less

Table 11B.3 *Incidence of high altitude illness*

Study group	Sleeping altitude (m)	Maximum altitude reached (m)	Average rate of ascent to sleeping altitude (days)	AMS (%)	HAPE or HACE (%)	Reference
Colorado skiers	2000–3000	3500	1–2	25	0.01	6, 8
Mt Everest trekkers	3000–5200	5500	1–2 (fly)	47	1.6	9, 10
			10–13 (walk)	23	0.05	
Mt Rainier climbers	3000	4392	1–2	67	0.1	7
Mt McKinley climbers	3000–5000	6195	4–7	30	1	11

AMS, acute mountain sickness; HAPE/HACE, high-altitude pulmonary/cerebral edema.

(Modified from *Wilderness Medicine*, 4th ed., Auerbach PS, 2001, with permission from Elsevier.[2])

able to compensate for swelling through the displacement of CSF, and are more likely to have AMS.[17]

Systemic fluid retention and weight gain also occur in AMS.[24] Individuals who are susceptible to AMS have an exaggerated aldosterone and antidiuretic hormone response on ascent different from that of well-acclimatizing individuals who have low antidiuretic hormone and a diuresis.[25] A shift of fluid from the extracellular space to the interstitial and intracellular compartments occurs normally during the initial few days at high altitude, but it may be accentuated and prolonged in people with hypoventilation and AMS.[26] Fluid shifts also may explain pulmonary dysfunction and relative hypoxemia in some people with AMS, which may be a precursor of overt HAPE. Pulmonary pathophysiology in AMS includes hypoventilation,[26,27] gas-exchange abnormalities,[28,29] decreased diffusing capacity,[30] and pulmonary mechanical dysfunction.[7] Individuals with a blunted hypoxic ventilatory response may be more predisposed to fluid retention and AMS.[26,27] One study found that climbers at 4200 m on Mt McKinley, Alaska, who were more hypoxemic than other normally acclimatizing climbers were more likely to get AMS higher on the mountain.[31] This suggests that individuals who do not mount a sufficient ventilatory response are more hypoxemic and are more likely to develop AMS.

Autopsies of HACE victims have shown gross cerebral edema with herniation and small petechial hemorrhages.[24,32] Brain CT in HACE shows small ventricles, disappearance of

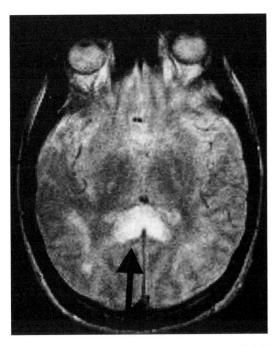

Figure 11B.1 *Magnetic resonance image of patient with high-altitude cerebral edema. Increased T2 signal in splenium of corpus callosum (arrow) indicates edema. (Reprinted from* Wilderness Medicine, *4th ed., Auerbach PS, 2001, with permission from Elsevier.[2])*

sulci, and a diffuse low-density appearance of the entire cerebrum, indicating cerebral edema.[33] More recently MRI studies in 7 of 9 patients with HACE after evacuation from high altitude showed intense T2 signal in white matter areas, especially the splenium of the corpus callosum (Fig. 11B.1), and no gray matter abnormalities.[34] These findings suggest that the predominant pathophysiologic mechanism in HACE is a vasogenic cerebral edema with movement of fluid and protein out of the vascular compartment likely due to increased permeability of the blood–brain barrier. In this study all patients completely recovered, and repeat MRI in four patients available for follow-up showed complete resolution of changes. The possibility must be considered that cytotoxic edema may coexist with vasogenic edema in the pathogenesis of HACE. Definitive imaging studies to distinguish cytotoxic from vasogenic edema during HACE will be necessary to answer this question.[16]

Clinical presentation

The Lake Louise Consensus Group defined AMS as the presence of headache in an unacclimatized person who has recently ascended to high altitude and who has one or more of the following: gastrointestinal symptoms (anorexia, nausea, or vomiting), fatigue or weakness, dizziness or lightheadedness, or difficulty sleeping.[35] The headache usually begins shortly after ascent (6–24 hours), is more severe in the morning, and is treatable with mild analgesics. Some people show signs of fluid retention with facial or peripheral edema,[10,36] or focal crackles on lung auscultation,[10] although these signs may also be present in the absence of AMS after ascent to high altitude. Resting heart rate is elevated in AMS[36] and body temperature is mildly elevated.[37] Tachypnea is not a distinguishing feature of AMS because it occurs in all people after ascent to high altitude. Signs and symptoms of AMS usually resolve over several days with rest and mild analgesics as acclimatization occurs. Although symptoms of AMS usually resolve without sequelae, AMS can progress to HACE and/or HAPE, which can be life-threatening.

Usually HACE occurs at altitudes greater than 3000 m and is less common than HAPE, however, severe HAPE and HACE may occur simultaneously. High-attitude cerebral edema is characterized by progression of global cerebral signs and symptoms in a person with AMS or HAPE. Focal neurologic signs may occur, but prompt consideration of another diagnosis. Because the symptoms of AMS are similar yet milder than those of HACE, it is reasonable to assume that HACE is the severe progression of AMS pathophysiology. HACE is distinguished from AMS by a severe headache, an altered level of consciousness, and ataxia. Progression of symptoms from severe AMS to HACE may include drowsiness, apathy, confusion, and ataxia progressing to being obtunded and nonambulatory. Auditory and visual hallucinations may occur, but are uncommon. Seizures are rare. Papilledema is common suggesting cerebral edema. Retinal hemorrhages are also common, but may be an incidental finding at altitudes over 5000 m because they are also observed in people who are not ill.[16] The condition may rapidly progress from confusion to obtundation and coma followed by death, and therefore lifesaving immediate treatment with descent is mandatory. In addition to descent, treatment with supplemental oxygen and dexamethasone is recommended.

Patients with HACE will likely require hospitalization after evacuation and descent from high altitude. A complete evaluation will help to exclude other diagnoses including meningitis, encephalitis, stroke, and cerebral hemorrhage. Diagnostic studies include serum electrolytes, complete blood count, and a lumbar puncture with appropriate CSF studies to rule out infection after a brain CT or MRI. Because of the association of HACE with HAPE, a chest radiograph and arterial oxygen saturation should be evaluated. In one series of severely ill hospitalized patients with HACE, 11 of 13 also had HAPE.[38]

Imaging studies may be helpful for diagnosis. On CT scans there is attenuation of signal, either diffusely or in the white matter, with compression of sulci and flattening of gyri.[16] However, MRI is more valuable both to identify the characteristic findings to confirm HACE and to exclude other pathology. T2 and especially diffusion-weighted MRI reveal increased signal in the white matter, particularly in the splenium of the corpus callosum.[34] Although this finding is not pathognomonic, in the setting of recent ascent to altitude it can be considered confirmatory.

Treatment/management

PREVENTION OF ACUTE MOUNTAIN SICKNESS

The best strategy for the prevention of AMS is a gradual ascent to allow time for acclimatization. Suggested guidelines are to limit the increase in sleeping altitude to a 600 m elevation gain over a 24-hour period once above 2500 m and to add an extra day for acclimatization, without an increase in sleeping altitude, after every 600–1200 m gained.[39] In one study a gradual ascent over 4 days to 3500 m, as compared with a 1-hour ascent, decreased the incidence and severity of acute mountain sickness by 41 percent.[40] Pharmacologic prophylaxis using acetazolamide or dexamethasone is well proven to prevent AMS, and is recommended for people who experience recurrent AMS on ascent to high altitude or for people who must ascend rapidly – such as in a rescue operation (Table 11B.4).

Acetazolamide, a carbonic anhydrase inhibitor, is the primary drug recommended for aiding acclimatization and preventing AMS. Acetazolamide eradicates periodic breathing and arterial oxygen desaturation during sleep at high altitudes[41,42] at a low dose of 125 mg before bedtime, which is sufficient to stimulate ventilation.[43] The drug also stimulates ventilation at rest and during exercise by inducing a renal excretion of bicarbonate causing a metabolic acidosis with compensatory hyperventilation, which may facilitate acclimatization. Acetazolamide lowers CSF pressure by decreasing CSF formation. Which of these effects is responsible for the drug's efficacy is not known. Side effects of acetazolamide are minimal and include peripheral, self-limited paresthesias, polyuria, and altered taste. A rare side effect is visual disturbance with myopia which is reversible upon discontinuation. Multiple studies have demonstrated the efficacy of acetazolamide for the prevention of AMS,[7,9,44,45] but the appropriate dose is controversial. One review recommends 250 mg three times a day[46] as a minimum effective dose. Recent studies, however, report that doses of 250 mg twice a day[47] or 125 mg twice a day[48] were effective for prevention of AMS. Many experts suggest that a dose of 250 mg twice a day is efficacious and results in fewer side effects than 250 mg three times a day.[21,39] Individuals who are allergic to sulfa drugs should not take acetazolamide.

Many studies have demonstrated the efficacy of dexamethasone in prevention of AMS.[49–52] Dexamethasone 4 mg two to three times a day is recommended; lower doses have not been shown to be effective.[52,53] Dexamethasone taken in combination with acetazolamide may be more effective at preventing AMS than either drug alone,[54,55] and

Table 11B.4   *Prevention of acute mountain sickness (AMS)*

Agent	Dose	Comments
Gradual ascent	Average gain of 600 m altitude per day above 2500 m	Sleeping altitude is more important than daytime altitude for risk of AMS
Acetazolamide	250 mg orally two to three times a day starting the day before ascent	Recommended only for those people with a history of recurrent AMS on ascent to altitude, contraindicated if person has sulfa allergy
Dexamethasone	4 mg orally two to three times a day starting the day before ascent	Alternative to acetazolamide, recommended if rapid ascent to altitude is required, such as in rescue operations
Ginkgo biloba	80–120 mg orally twice daily starting 5 days before ascent	Requires more study. If proved efficacious *Ginkgo biloba* has the advantage of no side effects compared with acetazolamide and dexamethasone. May increase bleeding risk if taken with anticoagulant or antiplatelet drugs

this combination might be considered in situations where rapid ascent to high altitude is required in unacclimatized persons, such as in rescue operations. There are no data to suggest that dexamethasone facilitates acclimatization and discontinuation of the drug while at high altitude may result in a rebound of altitude illness.[53] The mechanism of dexamethasone in preventing AMS is not known, but it may stabilize the endothelium of the microvascular circulation and prevent capillary leak.

A newer, and more controversial, alternative for pharmacologic prophylaxis of AMS is *Ginkgo biloba*. Studies have been conflicting regarding efficacy. In small randomized controlled studies *Ginkgo biloba* was found to be effective in preventing AMS[56,57] and in reducing severity.[58] In a study comparing *Ginkgo biloba* to acetazolamide in prevention of AMS in a Himalayan trekking population, however, *Ginkgo biloba* was not effective but acetazolamide 250 mg twice daily was effective.[47] The possible mechanism for efficacy of *Ginkgo biloba* is unknown but may involve modulation of neurotransmitters and mitochondrial adenosine triphosphate (ATP) production, promotion of neuronal glucose uptake, reduction of edema, or increase in erythrocyte deformability. At this point, the efficacy of *Ginkgo biloba* for prevention of AMS remains uncertain and further studies are required.

TREATMENT OF ACUTE MOUNTAIN SICKNESS

Successful management of AMS involves recognition and appropriate treatment (Table 11B.5). If the awareness of and suspicion for AMS are keen enough, then AMS usually will not progress and can be treated with conservative measures, such as rest, mild analgesics (aspirin, acetaminophen [paracetamol], codeine), and antiemetics (prochlorperazine). Sedatives, narcotics, and alcohol should be avoided because they may suppress ventilation and mask worsening symptoms. If the patient seems more ill with worsening headache or any other clear neurologic signs, especially ataxia, then this situation should be considered serious, and they should descend as quickly as possible. Even a few hundred meters may be helpful. If conditions do not permit descent, then oxygen, if available, is a good temporizing measure.

Both acetazolamide and dexamethasone are effective for treating AMS. A small, randomized, placebo-controlled study showed that acetazolamide 250 mg in two doses 8 hours apart reduced severity of AMS within 24 hours.[29] Several randomized controlled studies have shown dexamethasone effective for treating AMS[18,59,60] and a dose of 4 mg every 6 hours is recommended.

Lightweight (6.8 kg [15 lb]) portable hyperbaric bags operated with a foot pump and capable of pressurizing to about 13.7 kPa (2 psi) are also available for treatment of AMS. These provide a physiologic descent of about 2000 m. Several studies have shown portable hyperbaric bags to improve symptoms of AMS.[60–63] Short-term pressurization, however, provides no long-term benefit, because once pressurization ceases rebound AMS usually occurs. Still, in remote areas the portable hyperbaric bag provides an excellent, reusable alternative to oxygen.

The best treatment for AMS is prevention, including slow, gradual ascent. Maintenance of fluids to ensure a normal urine output and adequate calories in carbohydrates are time-honored tactics. The notion that forced overhydration is beneficial in AMS has no scientific basis and may lead to hyponatremia and worsening AMS or even HACE.

TREATMENT OF HIGH-ALTITUDE CEREBRAL EDEMA

Early recognition is essential because HACE, more than any other altitude illness, can rapidly progress to death. Evacuation of a person ill with HACE is easier and safer if HACE is recognized early while the victim is still ambulatory and can aid in their own descent. If HACE is recognized early symptoms may improve with descent, although neurologic abnormalities, particularly ataxia, may be slow to recover after descent. The clinical course of HACE varies with the duration and severity of illness prior to evacuation and treatment. In a mountaineering or trekking situation immediate descent is the primary treatment. Oxygen and dexamethasone (8 mg to 12 mg) by any route available immediately, then 4 mg every 6 hours until symptoms resolve) should be started as soon as possible and are used as adjunctive therapy with descent. Although no controlled clinical trials exist evaluating dexamethasone for the

Table 11B.5   *Treatment of acute mountain sickness (AMS)*

Agent	Dose	Comments
Descent	Decrease altitude until symptoms resolve	Recommended if AMS symptoms progress to ataxia or an altered level of consciousness
Oxygen	Low flow nasal cannula to keep Sao_2 >90%	Simulates descent, may be used for sleep as an adjunct to treatment of mild to moderate AMS
Acetazolamide	250 mg orally two to three times a day	Contraindicated in people with sulfa allergy
Dexamethasone	4 mg orally three times a day	Alternative to acetazolamide, recommended for more severe symptoms of AMS
Portable hyperbaric bag	30–60 minutes of pressurization or until symptoms resolve	Effective at relieving symptoms of AMS by simulating descent of about 1524 m but rebound AMS usually occurs within hours after treatment

Table 11B.6 *Treatment of high altitude cerebral edema (HACE)*

Agent	Dose	Comments
Descent	Descend in altitude until symptoms resolve	Descent is mandatory and may be lifesaving, early recognition of HACE is essential so that descent may be undertaken while the patient is still ambulatory
Oxygen	Titrate flow to keep Sa_{O_2} >90%	Useful treatment adjunct to descent and simulates descent in situations where descent is delayed
Dexamethasone	8 mg by any route available, then 4 mg every 6 hours	Useful treatment adjunct to descent
Portable hyperbaric bag	Pressurization until descent is possible	May be an effective temporizing treatment if descent is delayed because of weather or terrain conditions

treatment of HACE, studies do demonstrate that dexamethasone is effective in treating severe AMS,[18,53,54] and it seems reasonable to use dexamethasone for treatment of HACE given the proposed similar pathophysiology. Any pharmacologic treatment for HACE should be considered as an adjunct to descent and oxygen (Table 11B.6). Oxygen and dexamethasone have been lifesaving measures for treatment of HACE at 4200 m on Mt McKinley in situations where descent by helicopter evacuation was delayed due to weather. A portable hyperbaric bag may also be helpful but should never delay descent if the patient is ambulatory or transportable. A problematic feature of the portable hyperbaric bag for treatment of HACE in the field is loss of access to a patient with an abnormal mental status.

Once evacuation to a lower altitude has occurred patients with HACE will most likely require hospitalization. In one report of nine patients with HACE the average hospital stay was 6 days.[34] Severely ill comatose patients may require intubation for airway protection and a catheter for bladder drainage. The osmotic diuretic mannitol, or the loop diuretic furosemide, may be useful for treatment of severe cerebral edema, although no clinical studies have evaluated these drugs for treatment of HACE. Patients with HACE typically have spontaneous hyperventilation and a respiratory alkalosis and induced hyperventilation may cause cerebral vasoconstriction and ischemia. Induced hyperventilation causing cerebral vasoconstriction in order to decrease intracranial pressure (ICP) should therefore be reserved for treatment of impending herniation.[64,65] At high altitude treatment with oxygen alone reduces cerebral blood flow and ICP.[16] Adequate intravascular volume and euvolemia should be maintained to ensure adequate cerebral perfusion. Hypovolemia should be avoided particularly if mannitol and furosemide are used for treatment, and intravenous isotonic or hypertonic crystalloid may be required to maintain adequate intravascular volume. In severely ill patients with HACE monitoring central venous pressure may helpful to guide fluid management. Systemic hypertension is an appropriate physiologic response to maintain cerebral perfusion pressure in the setting of increased ICP and should be treated cautiously. A cerebral perfusion pressure (CPP = mean arterial pressure – ICP) of greater than 65 cm H_2O is

optimal, and systemic blood pressure management is guided by monitoring ICP to target an adequate mean arterial pressure to maintain cerebral perfusion pressure, or in the absence of an ICP, monitor targeting a mean arterial pressure >90 mm Hg.[64,65] Most patients with HACE who survive evacuation from high altitude to hospital admission recover completely, although prolonged recovery time and presumed permanent impairment are reported.[16]

HIGH-ALTITUDE PULMONARY EDEMA

Definitions

High-altitude pulmonary edema (HAPE) is a noncardiogenic pulmonary edema that afflicts susceptible people who ascend to altitudes above 2500 m and remain there for 24–48 hours or longer. Onset of symptoms is within a few days after ascent to high altitude, and may be preceded by AMS. As HAPE progresses, incidence of concurrent HACE increases.

Incidence/epidemiology

The incidence of HAPE increases with faster ascent rates and higher altitude, and has been reported as high as 15 percent in Indian troops airlifted from sea level to altitudes between 3500 m and 5500 m.[24] A lower 1–2 percent incidence is estimated in climbers making a more gradual ascent to 6150 m on Mt McKinley in Alaska,[11] or 0.01 percent in visitors to ski resorts in the Rocky Mountains at altitudes of 2500–3000 m.[8] Sleeping altitude is more important than daytime altitude where activities occur in determining the risk of HAPE. In a recent study, however, a series of patients with HAPE who presented to a hospital in the French Alps were skiing at altitudes of 1400–2400 m but sleeping at altitudes of 900–1800 m,[66] raising the possibility that HAPE may be more common at altitudes less than 2500 m than previously thought. Other factors contributing to the development of HAPE include male sex, exertion, cold ambient temperature, preexisting upper respiratory infection, or a prior history of HAPE.[67]

Etiology

High-altitude pulmonary edema may be an extension of the normal process of accumulation of lung interstitial edema that occurs on acute ascent to altitude.[68] Additionally, many asymptomatic people have crackles on chest auscultation that resolve with further acclimatization. These findings suggest any person may develop HAPE if exertion, ascent rate, and altitude are great enough. Immunogenetic factors,[69] exaggerated hypoxic pulmonary vasoconstriction,[70,71] or a blunted hypoxic ventilatory response,[72] however, make some people more susceptible to HAPE.

HAPE was described as a unique clinical syndrome in 1960[73,74] and subsequent studies showed that HAPE is a form of noncardiogenic pulmonary edema associated with pulmonary hypertension.[75] People susceptible to HAPE have a blunted hypoxic ventilatory response[67] and an exaggerated hypoxic pulmonary vasoconstrictor response that leads to elevated pulmonary artery pressures at high altitude.[70,71] People susceptible to HAPE have augmented sympathetic activation,[76] increased release of the pulmonary vasoconstrictor endothelin-1,[77] and decreased synthesis of the pulmonary vasodilator nitric oxide.[78,79] Exaggerated pulmonary vasoconstriction in people susceptible to HAPE also leads to redistribution of blood flow in the lungs from the bases to the apices.[80] The concept that overperfusion of a vasoconstricted pulmonary vascular bed contributes to the pathophysiology of HAPE is supported by the high susceptibility for HAPE in people with congenital absence of the right pulmonary artery.[81] The role of pulmonary hypertension in HAPE is supported by the efficacy of nifedipine in prevention[82] and inhaled nitric oxide in treatment.[83] The importance of sympathetic tone in the pulmonary vascular bed in HAPE is supported by the finding that intravenous phentolamine, a short acting α-adrenergic blocker, decreases pulmonary vascular resistance and improves gas exchange in people ill with HAPE.[84]

Hypoxic pulmonary vasoconstriction, overperfusion, and increased pulmonary hypertension are clearly associated with the pathophysiology of HAPE. A recent study also suggests that in HAPE pulmonary capillary pressure is elevated whereas pulmonary capillary wedge pressure is normal.[85] Increased pulmonary capillary pressure may occur because of pulmonary venular vasoconstriction or uneven hypoxic pulmonary vasoconstriction resulting in recruitment and overdistension of some parts of the pulmonary vascular bed.[86] Increased pulmonary capillary pressure results in stress failure of the pulmonary capillary endothelium due to increased capillary transmural pressure.[87] This mechanical injury to pulmonary capillary endothelial cells occurs in a patchy rather than diffuse pattern very early in the course of HAPE and is sufficient to cause alveolar hemorrhage.[88,89] The increased permeability of the pulmonary capillary endothelium results in an exudative edema with alveolar flooding. Findings in bronchoalveolar lavage (BAL) fluid from cases of HAPE show high concentrations of proteins and red blood cells early in HAPE,[89] and persistently high BAL protein concentrations with increasing inflammatory cells and inflammatory mediators later in the course of HAPE.[90–93]

An inflammatory response follows mechanical injury to pulmonary capillary endothelial cells in HAPE. Inflammatory markers in BAL fluid from climbers with HAPE include increased leukocytes, primarily macrophages, and increased markers of inflammation including thromboxane B$_2$, a mediator of pulmonary hypertension, and leukotriene B$_4$, a potent chemotactic factor for leukocytes,[90,91] and increased concentrations of interleukin (IL)-1β, -6, and -8, and tumor necrosis factor (TNF)-α.[92,93] Increased urinary leukotrienes have also been reported in HAPE.[94] The inflammatory response possibly follows mechanical pulmonary endothelial cell injury in HAPE because urinary leukotrienes and other inflammatory markers in BAL fluid are not increased early in the course of HAPE.[89,95]

Preliminary evidence shows that people susceptible to HAPE may have impairment of sodium and fluid clearance from alveoli,[96] which would lead to a predisposition for development and retention of alveolar edema. Alternatively, a theory describing the very high protein content in BAL fluid in HAPE, higher than that observed in the acute respiratory distress syndrome (ARDS) (Fig. 11B.2), proposes a healthy and intact alveolar epithelium that actively pumps water out of flooded alveoli faster than protein via the Na$^+$K$^+$ ATPase.[97] In both cardiogenic and noncardiogenic pulmonary edema, increased alveolar protein concentration is associated with better outcome presumably because injury to the alveolar epithelium is limited.[98] In HAPE, endothelial cell injury may be limited to isolated areas of overperfused pulmonary capillaries. Therefore, areas of capillary

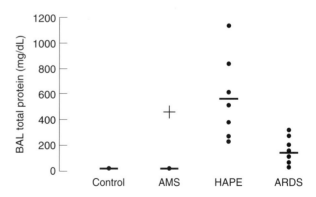

Figure 11B.2 *Protein concentration in bronchoalveolar lavage (BAL) fluid in individual subjects (dark circles) and group means (horizontal bars) in groups (left to right) healthy controls at high altitude (n = 5), acute mountain sickness (AMS) (n = 5), high-altitude pulmonary edema (HAPE) (n = 7), and the acute respiratory distress syndrome (ARDS) at sea level (n = 15). The + indicates a climber with AMS and acute bronchitis who had a higher BAL total protein than the other 5 subjects with AMS. (Data from references 88 and 90.)*

permeability are patchy rather than extensive, and the alveolar epithelium is relatively spared. This is consistent with the easy reversibility of HAPE with appropriate therapy compared with ARDS where inflammation and endothelial permeability undergo a prolonged course of recovery.

Studies of the leukocyte adhesion molecules, E-selectin and P-selectin, in plasma and BAL fluid in HAPE suggest that endothelial cell activation, platelet activation, and neutrophil recruitment in the lung in HAPE are not as extensive as in ARDS. Plasma concentrations of soluble E-selectin are mildly elevated after ascent to high altitude and in HAPE.[99] P-selectin is not elevated in plasma[99] or BAL fluid[92] in HAPE but is markedly elevated in ARDS,[100] suggesting that endothelial cell injury and platelet activation in HAPE are not as extensive as in ARDS. In early HAPE, compared with ARDS, the initial process appears to be patchy rather than diffuse and the initial inflammatory response consists of predominately macrophages rather than neutrophils.

An inflammatory response in the lung may cause increased capillary permeability and allow leakage of fluid into alveoli at lower hydrostatic pressures. Animal studies suggest that inflammation may predispose the lung to increased capillary permeability at high altitude. Rats injected with endotoxin have increased lung edema after exposure to high altitude[101] and rats pretreated with dexamethasone are protected from lung leak on exposure to high altitude.[102] A preexisting respiratory infection during ascent to high altitude is known to increase susceptibility to HAPE in humans.[103] Inflammation, therefore, may 'prime' the pulmonary endothelium to mechanical injury and increase susceptibility to HAPE on ascent to high altitude.

Autopsy studies clearly show inflammation in terminal HAPE. Autopsy specimens from people dying of HAPE show diffuse lung edema, neutrophilic alveolitis, focal alveolar hemorrhages, thrombi in small pulmonary arteries, and alveolar hyaline membranes.[104] Right ventricular and atrial dilation with a normal left ventricle and atrium are also observed. Histologically, these findings are consistent with diffuse alveolar damage, the hallmark of ARDS. Terminal HAPE, therefore, has much in common with ARDS.

Clinical presentation

Typical symptoms of HAPE are dyspnea, decreased exercise tolerance, and a dry cough that progresses to a cough productive of pink frothy sputum in severe cases. Frank hemoptysis is uncommon. Headache and nausea, typical symptoms of AMS, are common. Signs include cyanosis, tachycardia, tachypnea, low-grade fever, and crackles on lung auscultation.[105] The chest radiograph shows patchy bilateral, or unilateral in early HAPE, linear and confluent opacities with a normal cardiac silhouette (Fig. 11B.3).[105,106] The degree of hypoxemia depends on the altitude where HAPE occurs. In one study, in patients with HAPE at 2928 m the mean arterial oxygen saturation was 74 percent (range

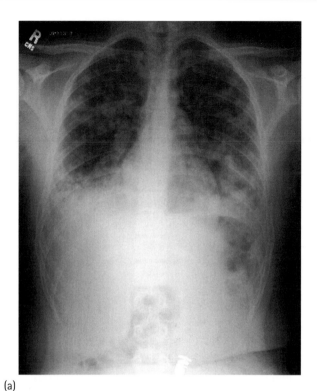

(a)

(b)

Figure 11B.3 *(a) Chest radiograph of a 15-year-old boy after helicopter evacuation from an altitude of 3352 m. for high-altitude pulmonary edema. The chest radiograph shows dense bilateral patchy alveolar infiltrative change and normal cardiac and mediastinal width. (b) Chest radiograph of the same patient after 1 day of treatment with supplemental oxygen delivered by nasal cannula at a flow rate of 4 L/min. The chest radiograph shows improvement in bilateral infiltrates.*

38–93),[105] whereas in two other studies of climbers with HAPE at 4200 m mean arterial oxygen saturation was 64 percent (range 50–75) compared with healthy climbers at that altitude with a mean (standard deviation) arterial oxygen saturation of 86 (3) percent.[90,99] If symptoms are recognized early enough, while the patient is still ambulatory, descent is an effective treatment. Most patients recover fully, and many are able to re-ascend to high altitude within a fortnight. This observation is important, as it implies that the lung architecture is preserved even after severe edema.

REENTRY PULMONARY EDEMA

Long-time residents at high altitudes may be more susceptible to high-altitude pulmonary edema if they descend to a low altitude and reascend. Young people (children and teenagers) may be more susceptible, especially if descent and ascent are rapid. Cases have been reported from South America (6.4 percent incidence)[107] and Leadville, Colorado.[108] The cause of reentry HAPE is not known, but it may be secondary to a hypermuscularization and subsequent hyperreactivity of the pulmonary vasculature to hypoxia on re-ascent.[1]

Treatment/management

The best way to prevent HAPE is to allow sufficient time for acclimatization. Even people susceptible to HAPE can dramatically reduce the incidence of HAPE by ascending gradually over days.[109] It is not always possible, however, for climbers, trekkers, or tourists to ascend at a pace that is slow enough to prevent HAPE. Therefore, HAPE will remain an important clinical problem for physicians to recognize and treat.

Because of the low incidence and unpredictability of HAPE, controlled clinical studies and pharmacologic trials have been difficult to conduct. No studies have been done using acetazolamide or dexamethasone in the prevention or treatment of HAPE. One randomized controlled study has shown nifedipine effective in preventing HAPE.[82] Nifedipine

has also been studied for treatment of HAPE where it improved gas exchange in some, but not all, of the subjects.[110] Another randomized controlled study showed that an inhaled long-acting β-agonist (salmeterol) was effective in preventing HAPE in susceptible people.[96] The authors suggested that β-adrenergic stimulation of alveolar transepithelial sodium transport improved fluid clearance from alveoli. In light of these studies, people susceptible to HAPE, who have to ascend quickly to high altitude should take an extended release preparation of nifedipine and use an inhaled β-agonist (Table 11B.7). Other pharmacological agents that decrease pulmonary artery pressure may be useful for prevention or as an adjunct to treatment of HAPE. A recent study showed that oral sildenafil decreased pulmonary artery pressure and improved exercise capacity in normal persons at high altitude.[111] Whether sildenafil is effective in preventing or treating HAPE requires further study.

The most important step in the treatment of HAPE is its early recognition. In remote settings, individuals should descend while they are still able to walk. A descent of 500–1000 m may be all that is necessary to prevent progression of this potentially fatal disease and actually result in resolution. Oxygen administration, if available, and rest are also helpful but should not delay descent. Careful administration of nifedipine may be a useful adjunctive therapy in addition to descent or oxygen. In remote areas where supplemental oxygen is unavailable or in limited supply, and when rapid descent may be impossible because of terrain or weather conditions, treatment with pressurization in a portable hyperbaric bag may be lifesaving.[112]

In areas where medical help is available, such as recreational ski locations, some patients with HAPE may be treated with supplemental oxygen rather than evacuation to a lower altitude. Treatment of HAPE with supplemental oxygen delivered by nasal cannula or face mask results in immediate improvement in subjective symptoms, arterial oxygen saturation, and objective pulmonary artery hemodynamic parameters of a lower pulmonary artery pressure and pulmonary vascular resistance[75,85,113] (Table 11B.8). Patients

Table 11B.7 *Prevention and treatment of high-altitude pulmonary edema (HAPE)*

Agent	Dose	Comments
Descent	Descend in altitude until symptoms resolve	Treatment of choice in mountaineering or trekking situations
Oxygen	Titrate flow to keep Sao_2 >90%	Simulates descent, may be used as the primary treatment at moderate altitude where medical care is available (ski resorts)
Nifedipine	30–60 mg sustained release preparation once a day starting the day before ascent for prevention, same dose once a day as an adjunct for treatment	Effective in preventing HAPE in people with a prior history of HAPE. For treatment of HAPE, useful only as an adjunct to definitive treatment with descent or oxygen
Salmeterol	125 µg inhaled twice a day starting 1 day prior to ascent	May be useful for prevention of HAPE in susceptible people
Portable hyperbaric bag	Pressurization until descent is possible	May be an effective temporizing treatment if descent is impossible because of weather or terrain conditions

whose clinical presentation is of the mild or moderate degree, whose oxygen saturation can be improved to greater than 90 percent by the administration of oxygen, and who have family or friends to watch them, can stay at high altitude using low-flow oxygen therapy and rest.[105] Daily follow-up is recommended for patients treated with supplemental oxygen at the same altitude where HAPE occurred.

People with a prior history of a single episode of HAPE should ascend more gradually to high altitude and be aware of symptoms so that HAPE may be treated with early descent. Nifedipine and salmeterol are recommended for prophylaxis of HAPE in people with a prior history of HAPE. Those with a history of more than one episode of HAPE, or HAPE occurring at under 2500 m, should have an evaluation for causes of pulmonary hypertension, increased pulmonary vascular resistance, or intrapulmonary or intracardiac right-to-left shunt.

Table 11B.8 *Hemodynamic and gas exchange parameters in 14 patients with high altitude pulmonary edema at 3600 m before and after treatment with supplemental oxygen*

	Room air rest	50% oxygen breathing
Arterial oxygen saturation (%)	67 ± 4	94 ± 1
Pa_{O_2} (mm Hg)	35 ± 3	81 ± 6
Pa_{CO_2} (mm Hg)	26 ± 1	27 ± 1
Respiratory rate (breaths/min)	31 ± 2	29 ± 2
Mean pulmonary artery pressure (mm Hg)	34 ± 2	24 ± 2
Mean pulmonary artery wedge pressure (mm Hg)	4 ± 1	3 ± 1
Mean right atrial pressure (mm Hg)	2 ± 1	2 ± 1
Heart rate (beats/min)	114 ± 3	105 ± 3
Cardiac index (L/min/m^2)	3.7 ± 0.2	3.3 ± 0.2
Mean arterial pressure (mm Hg)	80 ± 3	84 ± 3

Data expressed as mean ± SEM (from reference 113).

Key learning points

- AMS and HACE are cerebral disorders that occur after acute ascent to high altitude and have a common spectrum of pathophysiology with AMS being the milder form and HACE being the severe.

- Characteristic features of AMS include headache and at least one symptom from among fatigue, gastrointestinal upset, dizziness or lightheadedness, or disturbed sleep. It is usually self-limited and resolves with halting ascent and rest.

- High-altitude cerebral edema occurs in the setting of AMS and is characterized by an altered level of consciousness and ataxia, and may progress to obtundation, coma, and death without treatment.

- The best prevention for AMS and HACE is gradual ascent allowing adequate time for acclimatization.

- The recommended pharmacologic prophylaxis for AMS in people with a prior history of AMS on similar ascents to high altitude is acetazolamide at a dose of 250 mg twice a day starting the day before ascent. An alternative is dexamethasone at a dose of 4 mg every 8 hours. Both drugs are continued for several days after reaching high altitude. On an extended trekking or mountaineering expedition the advantage to acetazolamide over dexamethasone is that it can be started and stopped as dictated by the ascent profile. Repeated courses of dexamethasone may interfere with adrenal axis function.

- In addition to halting ascent and resting, pharmacologic treatment for AMS includes acetazolamide 250 mg two to three times a day or dexamethasone 4 mg three to four times a day.

- If AMS progresses despite halting ascent, or HACE develops, then immediate descent is mandatory. The latter should be treated with supplemental oxygen, dexamethasone 8 mg by any route available then 4 mg every 6 hours, and immediate descent. HACE may progress to coma requiring intubation for airway protection and treatment of elevated intracranial pressure if indicated.

- HAPE is a form of noncardiogenic pulmonary edema that occurs after acute ascent to altitudes higher than 2500 m.

- The pathophysiology of HAPE includes uneven hypoxic pulmonary vasoconstriction, pulmonary hypertension, overperfusion of the pulmonary vascular bed, increased capillary pressure, mechanical stress failure of pulmonary endothelial cells, and an exudative pulmonary edema due to leakage of fluid, protein, and red blood cells in patchy areas of the pulmonary circulation.

- The clinical presentation of HAPE includes decreased exercise tolerance, dyspnea, a dry cough that progresses to a cough productive of pink frothy sputum, low-grade fever, tachypnea, tachycardia, hypoxemia, crackles on lung auscultation, and patchy bilateral alveolar infiltrates with a normal cardiac silhouette on chest radiograph.

- The best prevention for HAPE is gradual ascent allowing adequate time for acclimatization. Pharmacologic prophylaxis for susceptible people who have had at least one prior episode of HAPE includes oral nifedipine or inhaled salmeterol.

- The mainstay of treatment for HAPE is immediate descent or supplemental oxygen. Descent of as little as 500–1000 m can result in marked improvement. Treatment with supplemental oxygen alone without descent is possible in areas with medical facilities at moderate altitude, but requires continuous oxygen for days until all indications of pulmonary edema resolve. Nifedipine may be used as an adjunct to primary treatment with descent or oxygen.

REFERENCES

◆ 1. Schoene RB, Hackett PH, Hornbein TF. High altitude. In: Murray JF, Nadel JA, eds. *Textbook of Respiratory Medicine*, 3rd ed. New York: WB Saunders, 2000: 1915–50.

◆ 2. Hackett PH, Roach RC. High altitude medicine. In: Auerbach PS, ed. *Wilderness Medicine* 4th ed. St Louis, MO: Mosby, 2001: 2–43.

● 3. Sutton JR, Reeves JT, Wagner PD, *et al.* Operation Everest II: oxygen transport during exercise at extreme simulated altitude. *J Appl Physiol* 1988; **64**: 1309–21.

4. Morris AH, Kanner RE, Crapo RO, Gardner RM. *Clinical Pulmonary Function Testing: A Manual of Uniform Laboratory Procedures*, 2nd ed. Salt Lake City: Intermountain Thoracic Society, 1984.

5. Grissom CK, Schoene RB. Adaptation and maladaptation to high altitude. In: Crapo JD, Glassroth J, Karlinsky J, King TE, Jr, eds. *Baum's Textbook of Pulmonary Diseases*, 7th ed. Philadelphia: Lippincott Williams & Wilkins, 2004: 1005–23.

● 6. Honigman B, Theis MK, Kosiol-McLain J, *et al.* Acute mountain sickness in a general tourist population at moderate altitudes. *Ann Intern Med* 1993; **118**: 587–92.

● 7. Larson EB, Roach RC, Schoene RB, Hornbein TF. Acute mountain sickness and acetazolamide: Clinical efficacy and effect on ventilation. *JAMA* 1982; **248**: 328–32.

8. Sophocles AM. High-altitude pulmonary edema in Vail, Colorado, 1975–1982. *West J Med* 1986; **144**: 569–73.

● 9. Hackett PH, Rennie D, Levine HD. The incidence, importance, and prophylaxis of acute mountain sickness. *Lancet* 1976; **2**: 1149–55.

10. Hackett PH, Rennie ID. Rales, peripheral edema, retinal hemorrhage and acute mountain sickness *Am J Med* 1979; **67**: 214–18.

11. Hackett PH, Roach RC, Schoene RB, *et al.* The Denali medical research project, 1982–1985. *Am Alpine J* 1986; **28**: 129–37.

12. Honigman B, Read M, Lezotte D, Roach RC. Sea-level physical activity and acute mountain sickness at moderate altitude. *West J Med* 1995; **163**: 117–21.

◆ 13. Bartsch P, Roach R. Acute mountain sickness and high-altitude cerebral edema. In: Hornbein TF, Schoene RB, eds. *High Altitude, An Exploration of Human Adaptation.* From: *Lung Biology in Health and Disease*, Lenfant C, exec ed. New York: Marcel Dekker, 2001: 731–76.

✱ 14. Pollard AJ, Niermeyer S, Barry P, *et al.* Children at high altitude: an international consensus statement by an ad hoc committee of the International Society for Mountain Medicine, March 12, 2001. *High Alt Med Biol* 2001; **2**: 389–403.

15. Roach RC, Houston CS, Honigman B, *et al.* How well do older persons tolerate moderate altitude? *West J Med* 1995; **162**: 32–6.

◆ 16. Hackett PH, Roach RC. High altitude cerebral edema. *High Alt Med Biol* 2004: **5**: 36–46.

17. Hackett PH. High altitude cerebral edema and acute mountain sickness: a pathophysiological update. In: Roach RC, Wagner PD, Hackett PH, eds. *Hypoxia: Into the Next Millennium*, vol. 474 of *Advances in Experimental Medicine and Biology*. New York: Kluwer Academic/Plenum, 1999: 23–45.

● 18. Levine BD, Yoshimura K, Kobayashi T, *et al.* Dexamethasone in the treatment of acute mountain sickness. *N Engl J Med* 1989; **321**: 1707–13.

19. Morocz IA, Zientara GP, Gudbjartsson H, *et al.* Volumetric quantification of brain swelling after hypobaric hypoxia exposure. *Experimental Neurology* 2001; **168**: 96–104.

20. Fischer R, Vollmar C, Thiere M, *et al.* No evidence of cerebral oedema in severe acute mountain sickness. *Cephalagia* 2004; **24**: 66–71.

21. Bartsch P, Bailey DM, Berger MM, *et al.* Acute mountain sickness: controversies and advances. *High Alt Med Biol* 2004; **5**: 110–24.

22. Baumgartner RW, Spyridopoulos I, Bartsch P, *et al.* Acute mountain sickness is not related to cerebral blood flow: a decompression chamber study. *J Appl Physiol* 1999; **86**: 1578–82.

23. Jensen JB, Wright AD, Lassen NA, *et al.* Cerebral blood flow in acute mountain sickness. *J Appl Physiol* 1990; **69**: 430–3.

24. Singh I, Khanna PK, Srivastava MC, *et al.* Acute mountain sickness. *New Engl J Med* 1969; **280**: 175–84.

25. Bartsch P, Maggiorini M, Schobersberger W, *et al.* Enhanced exercise-induced rise of aldosterone and vasopressin preceding mountain sickness. *J Appl Physiol* 1991; **711**: 136–43.

26. Hackett PH, Rennie ID, Hofmeiser SE, *et al.* Fluid retention and relative hypoventilation in acute mountain sickness. *Respiration* 1982; **43**:321–9.

27. Moore LG, Harrison GL, McCullough RE, *et al.* Low acute hypoxic ventilatory response and hypoxic depression in acute altitude sickness. *J Appl Physiol* 1986; **60**: 1407–12.

28. Sutton JR, Bryan AC, Gray GW, *et al.* Pulmonary gas exchange in acute mountain sickness. *Aviat Space Environ Med* 1976; **47**: 1032–7.

● 29. Grissom CK, Roach RC, Sarnquist FH, Hackett PH. Acetazolamide in the treatment of acute mountain sickness: Clinical efficacy and effect on gas exchange. *Ann Intern Med* 1992; **116**: 461.

30. Ge Ri-Li, Matsuzawa Y, Takeoka M, *et al.* Low pulmonary diffusing capacity in subjects with acute mountain sickness. *Chest* 1997; **111**: 58–64.

31. Roach RC, Greene ER, Schoene RB, Hackett PH. Arterial oxygen saturation for prediction of acute mountain sickness. *Aviat Space Environ Med* 1998; **69**: 1182–5.

32. Dickinson J, Heath D, Gosney J, Williams D. Altitude-related deaths in seven trekkers in the Himalayas. *Thorax* 1983; **38**: 646–56.

33. Kobayashi T, Koyama S, Kubo K, *et al.* Clinical features of patients with high altitude pulmonary edema in Japan. *Chest* 1987; **92**: 814–21.

● 34. Hackett PH, Yarnell PR, Hill R, *et al.* High altitude cerebral edema evaluated with magnetic resonance imaging, clinical correlation and pathophysiology. *JAMA* 1998; **280**: 1920–5.

✱ 35. Roach RC, Bartsch P, Hackett PH, *et al.* The Lake Louise acute mountain sickness scoring system. In: Sutton JR, Houston CS, Coates G, eds. *Hypoxia and Molecular Medicine* Burlington, VT: Charles S Houston, 1993: 272–4.

36. Bartsch P, Shaw S, Franciolli M, *et al.* Atrial natriuretic peptide in acute mountain sickness. *J Appl Physiol* 1988; **65**: 1929–37.

37. Maggiorini M, Bartsch P, Oelz O. Association between raised body temperature and acute mountain sickness: cross sectional study. *BMJ* 1997; **315**: 403–4.

38. Yarnell PR, Heit J, Hackett PH. High altitude cerebral edema (HACE): the Denver/front rang experience. *Semin Neurol* 2000; **20**: 209–17.

◆ 39. Hackett PH, Roach RC. High altitude illness. *N Engl J Med* 2001; **345**: 107–14.

40. Purkayastha SS, Ray US, Arora BS, *et al.* Acclimatization at high altitude in gradual and acute induction. *J Appl Physiol* 1995; **79**: 487–92.

● 41. Sutton JR, Houston CS, Mansell AL, *et al.* Effect of acetazolamide on hypoxia during sleep at high altitude. *N Engl J Med* 1979; **301**: 1329–31.

42. Hackett PH, Roach RC, Harrison GL, *et al.* Respiratory stimulants and sleep periodic breathing at high altitude. Almitrine versus acetazolamide. *Am Rev Respir Dis* 1987; **135**: 896–8.

43. Swenson ER, Leatham KL, Roach RC, *et al.* Renal carbonic anhydrase inhibition reduces high altitude periodic breathing. *Respir Physiol* 1991; **86**: 333–43.

44. Gray GW, Bryan AC, Frayser R, *et al.* Control of acute mountain sickness. *Aerosp Med* 1971; **42**: 81–4.

45. Greene MK, Kerr AM, McIntosh IB, Prescott RJ. Acetazolamide in prevention of acute mountain sickness: a double blind controlled cross-over study. *Br Med J (Clin Res Ed)* 1981; **283**: 811–13.

46. Dumont L, Mardirosoff C, Tramer MR. Efficacy and harm of pharmacological prevention of acute mountain sickness: quantitative systematic review. *BMJ* 2000; **321**: 267–72.

47. Gertsch JH, Basnyat B, Johnson EW, *et al.* Randomized, double blind, placebo controlled comparison of ginkgo biloba and acetazolamide for prevention of acute mountain sickness among Himalayan trekkers: the prevention of high altitude illness trial (PHAIT). *BMJ* 2004; **7443**: 797.

48. Basnyat B, Gertsch JH, Johnson EW, *et al.* Efficacy of low-dose acetazolamide (125 mg BID) for the prophylaxis of acute mountain sickness: a prospective, double-blind, randomized placebo-controlled trial. *High Alt Med Biol* 2003; **4**: 45–52.

● 49. Johnson TS, Rock PB, Fulco CS, *et al.* Prevention of acute mountain sickness by dexamethasone. *N Engl J Med* 1984; **310**: 683–6.

50. Ellsworth AJ, Meyer EF, Larson EB. Acetazolamide or dexamethasone use versus placebo to prevent acute mountain sickness on Mt. Rainier. *West J Med* 1991; **154**: 289–93.

51. Ellsworth AJ, Larson EB, Strickland D. A randomized trial of dexamethasone and acetazolamide for acute mountain sickness prophylaxis. *Am J Med* 1987; **83**: 1024.

52. Rock PB, Johnson TS, Larsen RF, *et al.* Dexamethasone as prophylaxis for acute mountain sickness, effect of dose level. *Chest* 1989; **95**: 568–73.

● 53. Hackett PH, Roach RC, Wood RA, *et al.* Dexamethasone for prevention and treatment of acute mountain sickness. *Aviat Space Environ Med* 1988; **59**: 950–4.

54. Bernhard WN, Schalick LM, Delaney PA, *et al.*

Acetazolamide plus low-dose dexamethasone is better than acetazolamide alone to ameliorate symptoms of acute mountain sickness. *Aviat Space Environ Med* 1998; **69**: 883–6.

55. Zell SC, Goodman PH. Acetazolamide and dexamethasone in the prevention of acute mountain sickness. *West J Med* 1988; **148**: 541–5.

56. Roncin JP, Schwartz F, D'Arbigny P. EGb 761 in control of acute mountain sickness and vascular reactivity to cold exposure. *Aviat Space Environ Med* 1996; **67**: 445–52.

57. Maakestad K, Leadbetter G, Olson S, *et al.* Ginkgo biloba reduces incidence and severity of acute mountain sickness (abstract). *Wilderness Environ Med* 2001; **12**: 51.

58. Gertsch JH, Seto TB, Mor J, Onopa J. Ginkgo biloba for the prevention of severe acute mountain sickness (AMS) starting one day before rapid ascent. *High Alt Med Biol* 2002; **3**: 29–36.

59. Ferrazzini G, Maggiorini M, Kriemler S, *et al.* Successful treatment of acute mountain sickness with dexamethasone. *BMJ* 1987; **294**: 1380–2.

60. Keller HR, Maggiorini M, Bartsch P, Oelz O. Simulated descent v dexamethasone in treatment of acute mountain sickness: a randomised trial. *BMJ* 1995; **310**: 1232–5.

61. Bartsch P, Merki B, Hofstetter D, *et al.* Treatment of acute mountain sickness by simulated descent: a randomised controlled trial. *BMJ* 1993; **306**: 1098–101.

62. Kasic JF, Yaron M, Nicholas R, *et al.* Treatment of acute mountain sickness: hyperbaric versus oxygen therapy. *Ann Emerg Med* 1991; **20**: 1109–12.

63. Kayser B, Herry JP, Bartsch P. Pressurization and acute mountain sickness. *Aviat Space Environ Med* 1993; **64**: 928–31.

64. Marik PE, Varon J, Trask T. Management of head trauma. *Chest* 2002; **122**: 699–711.

65. The brain trauma foundation. The American Association of Neurological Surgeons. The joint section on neurotrauma and critical care. Critical pathway for the treatment of established intracranial hypertension. *J Neurotrauma* 2000; **17**: 537–8.

66. Gabry AL, Ledoux X, Mozziconacci M, Martin C. High altitude pulmonary edema at moderate altitude (<2400 m; 7870 feet), a series of 52 patients. *Chest* 2003; **123**: 49–53.

♦ 67. Schoene RB, Swenson ER, Hultgren HN. High altitude pulmonary edema. In: Hornbein TF, Schoene RB, eds. *High Altitude, An Exploration of Human Adaptation.* From: *Lung Biology in Health and Disease*, Lenfant C, exec ed. New York: Marcel Dekker, 2001: 777–814.

68. Cremona G, Asnaghi R, Baderna P, *et al.* Pulmonary extravascular fluid accumulation in recreational climbers: a prospective study. *Lancet* 2002; **359**: 303–9.

69. Hanaoka M, Kubo K, Yamazaki Y, *et al.* Association of high altitude pulmonary edema with the major histocompatibility complex. *Circulation* 1998; **97**: 1124–8.

● 70. Hultgren HN, Grover RF, Hartley LH. Abnormal circulatory responses to high altitude in subjects with a previous history of high altitude pulmonary edema. *Circulation* 1971; **44**: 759–70.

71. Kawashima A, Kubo K, Kobayashi T, Sekiguchi M. Hemodynamic responses to acute hypoxia, hypobaria, and exercise in subjects susceptible to high altitude pulmonary edema. *J Appl Physiol* 1989; **67**: 1982–9.

72. Hackett PH, Roach RC, Schoene RB, *et al.* Abnormal control of ventilation in high altitude pulmonary edema. *J Appl Physiol* 1988; **64**: 1268–72.

● 73. Houston CS. Acute pulmonary edema of high altitude. *N Engl J Med* 1960; **263**: 478–80.

74. Hultgren H, Spickard W. Medical experiences in Peru. *Stanford Med Bull* 1960; **18**: 76–95.

75. Hultgren HN, Lopez CE, Lundberg E, Miller H. Physiologic studies of pulmonary edema at high altitude. *Circulation* 1964; **29**: 393–408.

76. Duplain H, Vollenweider L, Delabays A, *et al.* Augmented sympathetic activation during short term hypoxia and high altitude exposure in subjects susceptible to high altitude pulmonary edema. *Circulation* 1999; **99**: 1713–18.

77. Sartori C, Vollenweider L, Loffler BM, *et al.* Exaggerated endothelin release in high altitude pulmonary edema. *Circulation* 1999; **99**: 2665–8.

78. Duplain H, Sartori C, Lepori M, *et al.* Exhaled nitric oxide in high altitude pulmonary edema, role in the regulation of pulmonary vascular tone and evidence for a role against inflammation. *Am J Respir Crit Care Med* 2000; **162**: 221–4.

79. Busch T, Bartsch P, Pappert D, *et al.* Hypoxia decreases exhaled nitric oxide in mountaineers susceptible to high-altitude pulmonary edema. *Am J Respir Crit Care Med* 2001; **163**: 368–73.

80. Hanaoka M, Tanaka M, Ge RL, *et al.* Hypoxia induced pulmonary blood redistribution in subjects

with a history of high altitude pulmonary edema. *Circulation* 2000; **101**: 1418–22.

81. Hackett PH, Creagh CE, Grover RF, *et al*. High altitude pulmonary edema in persons without the right pulmonary artery. *N Engl J Med* 1980; **302**: 1070–3.

82. Bartsch P, Maggiorini M, Ritter M, *et al*. Prevention of high-altitude pulmonary edema by nifedipine. *N Engl J Med* 1991; **325**: 1284–9.

83. Scherrer U, Vollenweider L, Delabays A, *et al*. Inhaled nitric oxide for high-altitude pulmonary edema. *N Engl J Med* 1996; **334**: 624–9.

84. Hackett PH, Roach RC, Hartig GS, *et al*. The effect of vasodilators on pulmonary hemodynamics in high altitude pulmonary edema, a comparison. *Int J Sports Med* 1992; **13**: S68–71.

85. Maggiorini M, Melot C, Pierre S, *et al*. High altitude pulmonary edema is initially caused by an increase in capillary pressure. *Circulation* 2001; **103**: 2078–83.

86. Hultgren HN. High altitude pulmonary edema. In Staub N, ed. *Lung Water and Solute Exchange.* New York: Marcel Dekker, 1978: 437–69.

87. West JB, Colice GL, Lee YJ, *et al*. Pathogenesis of high-altitude pulmonary oedema: direct evidence of stress failure of pulmonary capillaries. *Eur Respir J* 1995; **8**: 523–9.

88. Grissom CK, Albertine KH, Elstad MR. Alveolar haemorrhage in a case of high altitude pulmonary oedema. *Thorax* 2000; **55**: 167–9.

89. Swenson ER, Maggiorini M, Mongovin S, *et al*. Pathogenesis of high-altitude pulmonary edema, inflammation is not an etiologic factor. *JAMA* 2002; **287**; 2228–35.

90. Schoene RB, Swenson ER, Pizzo CJ, *et al*. The lung at high altitude, bronchoalveolar lavage in acute mountain sickness and pulmonary edema. *J Appl Physiol* 1988; **64**: 2605–13.

91. Schoene RB, Hackett PH, Henderson WR, *et al*. High altitude pulmonary edema, characteristics of lung lavage fluid. *JAMA* 1986; **256**: 63–9.

92. Kubo K, Hanaoka M, Yamaguchi S, *et al*. Cytokines in bronchoalveolar lavage fluid in patients with high altitude pulmonary oedema at moderate altitude in Japan. *Thorax* 1996; **51**: 739–42.

93. Kubo K, Hanaoka M, Hayano T, *et al*. Inflammatory cytokines in BAL fluid and pulmonary hemodynamics in high altitude pulmonary edema. *Respir Physiol* 1998; **111**: 301–10.

94. Kaminsky DA, Jones K, Schoene RB, Voelkel NF.

Urinary leukotriene E4 levels in high-altitude pulmonary edema. *Chest* 1996; **110**: 939–45.

95. Bartsch P, Eichenberger U, Ballmer PE, *et al*. Urinary leukotriene E4 levels are not increased prior to high altitude pulmonary edema. *Chest* 2000; **117**: 1393–8.

96. Sartori C, Allemann Y, Duplain H, *et al*. Salmeterol for the prevention of high-altitude pulmonary edema. *N Engl J Med* 2002; **346**: 1631–6.

97. Grissom CK, Elstad MR. The pathophysiology of high altitude pulmonary edema. *Wilderness Environ Med* 1999; **10**: 88–92.

98. Matthay MA, Wiener-Kronish JP. Intact epithelial barrier function is critical for the resolution of alveolar edema in humans. *Am Rev Resp Dis* 1990; **142**: 1250–7.

99. Grissom CK, Zimmerman GA, Whatley RE. Endothelial selectins in acute mountain sickness and high-altitude pulmonary edema. *Chest* 1997; **112**: 1572–8.

100. Sakamaki F, Ishizaka A, Handa M, *et al*. Soluble form of P-selectin in plasma is elevated in acute lung injury. *Am J Respir Crit Care Med* 1995; **151**: 1821–6.

101. Ono S, Westcott JY, Chang SW, Viekjek NF. Endotoxin priming followed by high altitude causes pulmonary edema in rats. *J Appl Physiol* 1993; **74**: 1534–42.

102. Stelzner TJ, O'Brien RF, Sato K, *et al*. Hypoxia-induced increases in pulmonary transvascular protein escape in rats. *J Clin Invest* 1988; **82**: 1840–7.

103. Durmowicz AG, Noordeweir E, Nicholas R, Reeves, JT. Inflammatory processes may predispose children to high-altitude pulmonary edema. *J Pediatr* 1997; **130**: 838–40.

104. Hultgren HN, Wilson R, Kosek JC. Lung pathology in high-altitude pulmonary edema. *Wilderness Environ Med* 1997; **8**: 218–20.

105. Hultgren HN, Honigman B, Theis K, Nicholas D. High altitude pulmonary edema at a ski resort. *West J Med* 1996; **164**: 222–7.

106. Vock P, Fretz C, Franciolli M, Bartsch P. High altitude pulmonary edema: findings at high altitude chest radiography and physical examination. *Radiology* 1989; **170**: 661–6.

107. Hultgren HN, Marticorena EA. High altitude pulmonary edema: Epidemiologic observations in Peru. *Chest* 1978; **74**: 372–6.

108. Scoggin CH, Hyers TM, Reeves JT, Grover RF. High altitude pulmonary edema in the children and young adults of Leadville, Colorado. *N Engl J Med* 1977; **297**: 1269–73.

109. Bartsch P. High altitude pulmonary edema. *Med Sci Sports Exerc* 1999; **31**: S23–7.

110. Oelz O, Maggiorini M, Ritter M, *et al.* Nifedipine for high altitude pulmonary edema. *Lancet* 1989; **2**: 1241–4.

111. Ghofrani HA, Reichenberger F, Kohstall MG, *et al.* Sildenafil increased exercise capacity during hypoxia at low altitude and at Mount Everest base camp. *Ann Intern Med* 2004; **141**: 169–77.

112. Hackett PH, Roach RC, Goldberg S, *et al.* A portable, fabric hyperbaric chamber for treatment of high altitude pulmonary edema [abstract]. In Sutton JR, Coates G, Remmers JE, eds. *Hypoxia: The Adaptations.* Philadelphia: BC Decker, 1990: 291.

113. Anand IS, Prasad BA, Chugh SS, *et al.* Effects of inhaled nitric oxide and oxygen in high-altitude pulmonary edema. *Circulation* 1998; **98**: 2441–5.

Drug-induced respiratory emergencies

PHILIPPE BONNIAUD, CLIO CAMUS, AHMAD JIBBAOUI, KABEYA KAZAMBU, NICOLAS BAUDOUIN, PASCAL FOUCHER, PHILIPPE CAMUS

INTRODUCTION

Drugs (i.e. therapeutic drugs, investigative drugs labeled with radioactive substances, illicit substances, and herbals) and radiation therapy can acutely injure the respiratory system (i.e. the lung, airways, and pleura) in many ways, causing distinctive clinicopathologic patterns of involvement with, sometimes, acute chest symptoms and respiratory failure.[1] Drugs can cause *direct* respiratory injury from an increase in the therapeutic efficacy of the drug, which goes hand in hand with drug dosing. For instance, overdosing of anticoagulants can produce alveolar hemorrhage, and an overdose of diltiazem may produce pulmonary edema. To some extent, such dose-related adverse effects can be predicted. Other mechanisms of direct injury from drugs include allergy, hypersensitivity, and idiosyncrasy, which occur only in a few predisposed individuals and are more difficult to predict. Drugs can also *indirectly* injure the respiratory system. For instance, immunosuppressive drugs predispose patients to the development of opportunistic pulmonary infections that may cause acute lung injury and consequent respiratory failure. Although not specifically covered in the present chapter,[2] pulmonary infections are high on the list of differential diagnoses in patients who develop diffuse pulmonary infiltrates while being treated with drugs. Indirect respiratory injury also includes drug-induced myocardial injury and acute systemic hypertension, and valvular heart involvement, which also may cause acute pulmonary edema. Imaging techniques, medical or surgical procedures in the chest or in distant organs, barotrauma,

infusion of stem cell, bone marrow transplantation, and solid organ (including lung) transplantation can also produce acute respiratory involvement.

This chapter deals with respiratory emergencies resulting from treatment with therapeutic drugs. Acute symptoms related to adverse respiratory effects of illicit drugs,[3,4] silicone,[5] radiation therapy,[6] herbals,[7] chemicals,[8,9] medical procedures,[10] and drug-induced neuromuscular impairment[11] are beyond the scope of this chapter. Similarly, terminal aggravation of longstanding chronic drug-induced conditions such as pulmonary fibrosis are not specific to the drug etiology and are not particularly covered here.

DEFINITION, DIAGNOSTIC CRITERIA

Drug-induced respiratory emergencies are characterized by the rapid or sudden development of acute symptoms such as dyspnea or chest pain in relation to acute respiratory involvement, leading patients to seek medical attention (emergency departments or intensive care units). Drug-induced respiratory emergencies are diagnosed by exclusion. Ideally, drug-induced respiratory disease:

- occurs during or after (not before) treatment with the causal drug
- other causes for respiratory involvement are adequately ruled out
- withdrawal of drug therapy is followed by improvement.

Drug-induced respiratory emergencies occur as acute upper or lower airway obstruction, diffuse parenchymal involvement (noncardiogenic pulmonary edema, and the group of infiltrative lung diseases [ILD]), vascular obstruction, pleural effusion, pneumothorax, mediastinal compression, chest pain, or coughing. Therefore, a high index of suspicion for this etiology is needed in emergency and intensive care medicine. Restoration of airway patency, proper fluid management, treatment with oxygen or a helium–oxygen mixture, ventilatory support, early and selective withdrawal of drug therapy, epinephrine, and corticosteroid therapy are the mainstays of management, along with emergent discontinuation of the suspected agent. Care must also be taken to avoid inadvertent rechallenge with the drug, as relapse may occur.

Criteria for the diagnosis of drug-induced respiratory disease include:[12,13]

1. Correct identification of the drug
   This requires a meticulous history of exposure to all drugs, including therapeutic drugs, and over-the-counter and self-medications. In the context of emergency care, it often is useful to ask relatives, the pharmacist, and the family physician for further information about the drugs the patient has been taking. In patients in whom uncertainty remains, blood, urine, and tissue samples should be taken early to measure levels of suspected drugs.
2. Temporal eligibility
   The onset of symptoms should follow, not pre-date, initiation of treatment with the specific drug. Some drug-induced reactions are characterized by a short or very short latency period, which immediately suggests the etiology. The latency period may be as short as a few seconds or minutes (as in non-steroidal anti-inflammatory drug [NSAID]-, aspirin-, or β-blocker-induced bronchospasm and in drug-mediated anaphylaxis), a few hours (as in hydrochlorothiazide-induced pulmonary edema), or a few days (as in acute nitrofurantoin and amiodarone pulmonary toxicity). The latency period extends to months or years with methotrexate, gold, or chemotherapeutic drugs. There is no apparent correlation between drug dosage, route of administration (oral, intravenous, intraarterial, inhaled, intrathecal, intrapleural, and topical), length of time into treatment, and the likelihood of developing acute drug-induced respiratory involvement. Generally, despite close monitoring and follow-up of lung function, late drug-induced respiratory emergencies occur unexpectedly and are difficult to predict.
3. Single- or multidrug regimens
   Ideally, drug-induced respiratory disease occurs in patients exposed to a single agent. Often, however, patients are given more than one drug that possibly causes acute lung injury, e.g. treatment for neoplasia. This creates confusion regarding which drug is responsible for the respiratory problem, unless there is a distinct pattern of involvement that enables easier

recognition, e.g. association of NSAIDs and acute bronchospasm, chemotherapeutic agents and noncardiac pulmonary edema, methotrexate and fulminant ILD, minocycline and acute eosinophilic pneumonia. A list of drugs causing lung injury along with the resulting patterns of involvement is available on the internet (www.pneumotox.com).[1]

4. Characteristic pattern of reaction to a specific drug
   The clinical, imaging, and histopathologic pattern of acute reaction should match earlier descriptions of reactions to the specific drug. Several drugs produce a distinct pattern of involvement enabling easy recognition of the drug-induced condition. Often, however, the histopathologic background of the respiratory reaction remains unknown because patients are either too ill to undergo invasive investigations or because withdrawal of drug therapy as the first step in management is followed by remission of all signs and symptoms.
5. Exclusion of other causes
   Causes of respiratory emergencies other than drugs should be ruled out with enough confidence. The differential diagnosis is complex in patients who already have a disease that may involve the lung, and who present with parenchymal lung disease while being treated with multiple suspect drugs and radiation therapy. Meticulous exclusion of an infectious etiology, and of other causes for the ILD is required. Diagnostic workup is easier in patients who develop acute bronchospasm or pulmonary edema, because these patterns of involvement generally occur in close association with exposure to the drug and also because the corresponding list of differentials is narrower.
6. Remission of signs and symptoms with withdrawal of the drug
   This criterion is not always fulfilled because, once initiated, acute respiratory reactions may seem to follow a course independent from drug therapy withdrawal.
7. Identification of drug in body fluids
   When a reaction to therapy – or to illicit drugs – is suspected, measurements of drug levels should be performed as soon as possible after admission. Quantification of drug in blood, urine, or body tissues may help in elucidating the cause of an acute respiratory distress or in establishing the cause of death in forensic medicine.
8. Recurrence with rechallenge
   Recurrence with rechallenge is central to the diagnosis of drug reactions. This seldom is performed intentionally, however, as symptoms of relapse may be more severe and lead to death. Rechallenge with a crucial drug or graded challenge with the deliberate purpose of inducing tolerance (e.g. with NSAIDs, aspirin, or sulfa drugs) may be contemplated in selected cases.

EPIDEMIOLOGY

Adverse reactions to drugs account for about 3 percent of hospital admissions, and it is estimated that about 5 percent of adverse drug reactions involve the respiratory system. Bronchospasm,[14] anaphylaxis,[15] hemorrhage,[16] and acute infiltrative lung disease including pulmonary edema emerge as the most significant life-threatening reactions to drugs. Among 9112 references of drug-induced and iatrogenic respiratory reactions in the Pneumotox® repository,[1] 1264 (13.9 percent) were 'acute', 931 (10.2 percent) were 'severe', and 405 (4.4 percent) led to death. In 151 reports of recurrence of pulmonary symptoms following rechallenge with the drug, there were 11 fatalities (7.3 percent). The clinical manifestation of the respiratory emergency was parenchymal involvement in 53 percent of reports (acute noneosinophilic infiltrative lung disease 25 percent; acute eosinophilic lung disease 15 percent; acute pulmonary edema 8 percent; alveolar hemorrhage 5 percent), airway reactions in 33 percent of cases (acute bronchospasm 28 percent; upper airway obstruction 5 percent), pleural involvement in 11 percent, thromboembolic disease in 2 percent, and miscellaneous conditions in the remainder.

PATTERNS OF DRUG–INDUCED RESPIRATORY EMERGENCIES

Drug-induced respiratory emergencies may result from involvement of the upper or lower airways, lung parenchyma, pulmonary circulation, pleura, mediastinum, pericardium, or heart. Involvement is in the form of inflammation, edema, a cellular infiltrate, thromboembolism, fat embolism, effusion, hematoma or hemorrhage, producing impairment of gas exchange or compression of a major airway, lung, or heart.

The radiographic appearance of drug-induced respiratory emergencies depends on the primary localization of the pathologic process. For instance, acute drug-induced diffuse parenchymal involvement (e.g. infiltrative lung disease, pulmonary edema, alveolar hemorrhage), or acute pleural or pericardial effusion cause visible changes on the chest radiograph, high-resolution computed tomography (HRCT) and/or ultrasound.[1] In contrast, only subtle changes are present on imaging in patients with drug-induced upper airway involvement or bronchospasm, in the form of reduction in central airway caliber, and/or air trapping. Although changes on imaging, if present, are useful in the diagnosis of drug-induced respiratory emergencies, there is little correlation between the nature or extent of visible changes on imaging and the severity of symptoms such as dyspnea or chest pain, or impairment of gas exchange.

Upper airway obstruction

The typical patient with drug-induced upper airway obstruction seeks medical attention in the emergency room for the acute symptoms of stridor and asphyxia.[17] Early symptoms include sore throat, which can be mistaken for upper respiratory tract infection, mild edema of tongue and/or lips, or change in voice. Later, laborious or noisy breathing, hoarseness or stridor develops. The rate of progression of airway narrowing and of the corresponding symptoms is unpredictable. The disease may suddenly and inexplicably accelerate, causing acute airway compromise, asphyxia, and death in a short period of time. Early recognition is warranted, particularly in patients who are being treated with drugs such as angiotensin-converting enzyme inhibitors (ACEIs). If the disease is not recognized, the drug is not withdrawn, and appropriate therapy is not given, airway narrowing may be so severe, that attempts at endotracheal intubation may fail because it is impossible to correctly identify the air passage.[18] In cases with severe angioedema and impending life-threatening respiratory failure, emergent tracheostomy can be required.

ANGIOEDEMA

It has been known for about 20 years that ACEIs produce angioedema, but recent reports suggest an increasing role for these drugs in the causation of acute angioedema with consequent upper airway obstruction. Current estimates suggest that ACEIs account for about half the cases of angioedema.[19] Less common inducers of angioedema include oral and parenteral amiodarone, inhibitors of angiotensin II (sartans), azathioprine, β-lactams, chlorpropamide, corticosteroids, erythromycin, loratadine, levopromazine, NSAIDs, inhibitors of cyclooxygenase 2 (coxibs), methotrexate, metoclopramide, omeprazole, psyllium, radiographic contrast media, and sulfasalazine.[20] There is no known association of ACEI-induced angioedema with ACEI-induced cough.

No clinical profile reliably identifies which patients are at risk for this adverse effect, except being an African American woman, having a history of upper airway trauma or, perhaps a lupus diathesis, being an atopic, or having demonstrated an earlier, even mild reaction with these agents.[21] A few cases have occurred intraoperatively. Angioedema and upper airway obstruction develop within 12 hours following the first administration of the drug in about a third of patients or after a few weeks of treatment, also in a third of patients.[17,22] Angioedema induced by ACEIs may develop without much notice after months or years into treatment, with no identifiable triggering factor (also in about a third of patients). In patients who develop the condition late into treatment, it is not uncommon to elicit a history of prior episodes of spontaneously resolving tongue swelling (known as 'episodic macroglossia') or hoarseness.[23] These should be interpreted as warning symptoms equivalent to angioedema and, when recognized in time, should dictate drug withdrawal; ACEI-induced angioedema may resolve despite the patient continuing treatment with the drug, erroneously prompting an alternative cause.

Initially patients complain of pruritus and/or edema of the lips or mouth floor, and dysphagia. The pathology has a special predilection for the tongue. In mild cases, the condition manifests itself with sore throat, slight facial or intraoral edema, macroglossia, or drooling of saliva. The edema may resolve, wax and wane, or precede to more pronounced adverse angioedematous reactions and breathing difficulties by hours, days, or months. Edema in distant organs and episodes of abdominal pain can occur, and are misleading. Contrary to hereditary forms of angioedema, assays of C1-esterase inhibitor levels and C4 are normal.[24] In severe cases, which represent about 10 percent of all cases of ACEI-induced angioedema, there is rapidly evolving edema of various parts of the upper air passages, alone or in combination. The severity of tongue edema may render orotracheal intubation impossible, requiring emergent insertion of an artificial airway *via* tracheostomy. Less often, the laryngeal or tracheal walls are involved. Rarely, bronchospasm develops or anaphylaxis in association with angioedema.

Angioedema is a life-threatening reaction. About 40 percent of patients with angioedema require admission to the ICU, and mortality is up to 5 percent. A recent study described seven fatal cases of ACEI-induced angioedema in African American men and women aged 50–65 years, who were autopsied.[18] Massive edema of the tongue was present in all cases, with only a fraction of patients displaying associated laryngeal or pharyngeal swelling.

Generally, drug withdrawal and treatment with intravenous corticosteroids, antihistamines and, in severe cases, epinephrine, is followed by improvement. Most patients can be discharged after 24–48 hours but in a few, symptoms progress despite optimized medical therapy, necessitating emergency intubation. A rebound phenomenon following successful medical therapy occasionally has been described, dictating appropriate follow-up before discharge. Rechallenge with the drug would expose patients to recurrence of symptoms after variable periods of time and is, therefore, contraindicated. Once even minor angioedema is attributed to an ACEI, an alternative class of medication should be chosen, as relapse with increasing severity can occur at any time. The angioedema that occurs in association with ACEI is mechanism based rather than drug based, so it may occur in the same patient with a different ACEI. Hence treatment with any other ACEI should be regarded as contraindicated. Contrary to expectations based on bradykinin-associated mechanism of involvement, treatment with an angiotensin II receptor antagonist also may be complicated by severe angioedema,[25] although this is less common. Thus therapy with an angiotensin II receptor antagonist in patients with a history of angioedema should be started with caution, and only if no alternative exists. Individuals with a history of idiopathic angioedema probably should not be given an ACEI.

ANAPHYLAXIS

Anaphylaxis is an explosive reaction, which results from IgE-mediated release of preformed mediators in response to insect stings, antigens, foods (e.g. nuts), and drugs. Anaphylaxis is not rare, and every physician should be prepared to manage the condition properly. A recent study reported 712 cases of drug-induced anaphylactic and anaphylactoid reactions seen in different institutions over a 2-year time period.[15] In another study in the United States, 142 cases were seen in a single institution in 1 year.[26] Early measurements of serum histamine and tryptase, and IgE testing are used to confirm the diagnosis of anaphylaxis, as opposed to anaphylactoid reactions.[15,27] Clinical manifestations include the rapid onset of urticaria, itching of the nose or palate, diaphoresis, abdominal cramping, vomiting, diarrhea, ocular symptoms, wheeze bronchospasm, and hypotension. A full-blown reaction is characterized by laryngeal and/or tracheal edema, bronchospasm, frothy sputum at the mouth, hemoptysis, internal organ edema, circulatory collapse, loss of consciousness, shock and seizures, followed by cardiac arrest. If not managed properly and aggressively, anaphylaxis may lead to death within minutes of exposure to the causative agent. Autopsy studies of fatal anaphylaxis cases indicate edema of the epiglottis, larynx and trachea, pulmonary hyperinflation, pulmonary edema, and alveolar hemorrhage.

Drugs may be the cause in 20–40 percent of anaphylactic episodes. Exposure to analgesics, anesthetic agents, antibiotics (amoxicillin, chlorhexidine, ciprofloxacin, dipyrone, penicillin, sulfamides, sulfamethoxazole-trimethoprim, vancomycin), aprotinin, aspirin, calcium and phosphate replacements, several chemotherapeutic agents, colloid plasma expanders, cortisone, coxibs, curares, fluorescein, immunoglobulins, infliximab, latex, lepirudin, methotrexate, NSAIDs (e.g. diclofenac), opioids, oxaliplatin, patent blue, heterologous proteins, psyllium, radiographic contrast media, blood transfusion, and allergen immunotherapy can lead to anaphylaxis.[1,26–33] Most accidents occur following exposure to analgesics, NSAIDs, radiographic contrast agents, and antibiotics.[27,32] Females and atopic individuals are at greater risk of developing the reaction. A study in the UK indicated that half of the 20 yearly deaths from anaphylaxis were caused by drugs.[28] The time to respiratory or cardiac arrest averaged 5 minutes. Even though about a third of the patients were successfully resuscitated, most suffered hypoxic brain damage and died within 30 hours of the accident. Anaphylaxis was sometimes mistaken for panic attack or hysteria, and both diagnosis and treatment were unnecessarily delayed. Complications of treatment included pulmonary edema related to epinephrine or to fluid overload, or other adverse reactions to epinephrine such as vomiting and aspiration of gastric content, and myocardial infarction.

Management of anaphylaxis requires preparedness, alertness, immediate recognition, and administration of fluids and appropriate drugs. Treatment of the full-blown reaction includes rapid correction of hypovolemia through a central line and parenteral epinephrine to be repeated every 15 minutes, until blood pressure is restored and stabilized, high-dose parenteral corticosteroids, and correction of cardiac arrhythmias.[34] Early and adequate access to the airway is crucial, because when significant laryngeal edema has developed, attempts at orotracheal intubation may fail (as in angioedema).

ANTICOAGULANT-INDUCED HEMATOMA

Treatment with heparin, fibrinolytic agents, oral anticoagulants (e.g. warfarin), and platelet surface receptor inhibitors (e.g. abciximab, ticlopidine) can produce profuse hemoptysis, diffuse alveolar hemorrhage (see below), hemothorax, and hemopericardium. Anticoagulants, at large, also can produce a variety of cervical and mediastinal hematomas, potentially causing life-threatening large airway compression, while causing insignificant blood loss.[35–40] Anticoagulant-induced hematomas have a reputation for producing misleading symptoms and being difficult to diagnose. Life-threatening hematomas can involve the tongue, sublingual area, floor of the mouth (causing a pseudo-Ludwig phenomenon, with elevation of the tongue and floor of mouth, leading to airway compromise), tonsils, valleculae, arytenoids, laryngeal wall, vocal cords, thyroid, retropharyngeal or mediastinal space. Although the onset of hematomas may be triggered by sneezing, violent coughing, a Valsalva maneuver, or insertion of a central venous line, most seem to occur spontaneously.

At an early stage, patients complain of vague symptoms such as sore throat and/or a change in voice. These symptoms can be mistaken as mild angioedema or nonspecific upper respiratory tract infection. Sore throat should always be taken seriously in the patient receiving oral anticoagulation therapy. The pharyngeal area should be examined and fiberoptic bronchoscopy should be performed at the slightest doubt. Early symptoms are followed in a few days by expansion of the hematoma into the sublingual, oral, cervical, retropharyngeal or mediastinal space, causing life-threatening airway compromise.[41] Examination of the oral cavity may reveal a reddish submucosal swelling involving the floor of the mouth and the ventral aspect of the tongue, or the whole tongue. Subcutaneous bruising may be present on the neck, which may progressively spread down to the upper chest. Digital examination may reveal induration of the tongue or floor of the mouth, or anterior displacement of the posterior pharyngeal wall in patients with retropharyngeal hematomas. Appearances on imaging include anterior displacement of the posterior aspect of the pharynx or tracheal wall on a lateral radiograph of the neck or chest. A CT study may show the hematoma and resulting compression of the airway lumen. Other cases are revealed on endoscopy, which may show submucosal hematoma of the laryngeal or tracheal wall bulging toward the lumen. In many patients, coagulation studies indicate values above the accepted therapeutic range,[41,42] with international normalized ratios (INRs) up to 50 or more. Inexplicably, in some patients, coagulation studies have been within the accepted therapeutic range. Management includes control of the airway, reversal of the coagulopathy and surgical evacuation or needle aspiration of the hematoma, if indicated.

UVULITIS

A large swollen uvula (uvulitis) with partial upper airway obstruction was reported to have developed in a young man after smoking cannabis. His symptoms resolved with cessation of exposure and administration of corticosteroids and antihistamines.[43] Inhalation of heated vapors and fumes of crack and amfetamines also may cause oropharyngeal and/or laryngotracheal burn.[44,45]

DRUG-INDUCED VOCAL CORD DYSFUNCTION

Inhalation of amphotericin B or eucalyptus can cause vocal cord dysfunction,[46] a condition characterized by adduction of vocal cords during inspiration, obstructing breathing. The condition is suggested by noisy inspiratory dyspnea. Diagnosis is confirmed on laryngoscopy, which reveals adduction of the vocal cords synchronous with inspiration during tidal breathing or forceful inspiration.

PHARMACOBEZOAR

Pharmacobezoar is an aggregate of a medicinal substance (pills/tablets) which, when present in the esophagus, may cause esophageal damage and tracheal compression.[47,48]

Catastrophic bronchospasm

Catastrophic bronchospasm is a common, sudden, and severe adverse effect of drugs such as aspirin, NSAIDs, and β-blockers.[1,49,50] The condition may rapidly progress to the 'locked lung', causing acute respiratory failure, hypoxic brain damage and death.

ASPIRIN AND NSAIDS

Treatment with aspirin and other NSAIDs which have anti-cyclooxygenase-1 (COX-1) activity account for most cases of drug-induced sudden severe bronchospasm.[51,52] A fraction of patients who are naturally intolerant to these drugs may adversely react to the administration of small amounts of the above drugs, in the form of catastrophic bronchospasm. The gravity of this form of drug-induced bronchoconstriction resides in its unpredictability, explosive nature and rapid progression of the asthmatic attack, its possible association with anaphylaxis, and the consequent respiratory failure. Although most accidents occur after oral intake or parenteral injections, dermal applications and ophthalmic preparations also can elicit acute asthma attacks.

In the typical patient prone to catastrophic drug-induced bronchospasm, the asthma develops in the third or fourth decade of life. The disease is more common in women, in a ratio of about 2:1. Typically, rhinitis precedes the clinical onset of the asthma, with aspirin sensitivity becoming apparent only subsequently. In one study, the asthma was often difficult to control, with about 50 percent of those afflicted requiring regular treatment with oral corticosteroids.[53] Prevalence of NSAID sensitivity is greater in patients with a history of severe asthma attack(s), and is estimated that approximately 10 percent of patients admitted to the ICU for an acute asthma attack requiring mechanical ventilation have previous exposure to asthma-triggering drugs.[54] Although typically nasal symptoms and a history of asthma usually pre-date exposure to aspirin or NSAIDs by years, in a few patients drug-induced bronchospasm occurs *de novo*, producing sudden catastrophic bronchospasm as the response to the first intake of a single tablet or less of aspirin or of other NSAIDs with COX-1 inhibitory properties. The weak COX-1 inhibitors acetaminophen (paracetamol) and salsalate trigger bronchospasms in higher concentrations. The preferential COX-2 inhibitors nimesulide and meloxicam cross-react poorly with aspirin or the classic NSAIDs. The selective COX-2 inhibitors (celecoxib, rofecoxib, etoricoxib) cross-react with aspirin in only 1.5–2 percent of NSAID-sensitive individuals. Occasionally, the response is anaphylactoid, with urticaria, severe nasal symptoms, angioedema, abdominal cramping, diarrhea, a choking sensation, loss of consciousness, shock, upper airway compromise, and severe bronchoconstriction leading to the 'locked lung', hypoxia, and death within minutes of exposure to the drug. Treatment of acute bronchospasm induced by the above drugs may require antihistamines, H_2 blockers, corticosteroids, β_2-receptor agonists, epinephrine, and mechanical ventilation.

Following the bronchospasm episode, the history often is straightforward enough and a controlled challenge test is unnecessary. In patients with less severe reactions, when the association is less clear, or when treatment with an NSAID or aspirin is desirable, a controlled challenge test using minute starting doses is considered. Since an acute reaction can develop at any time, the graded challenge test should be conducted close to an ICU, with the patient having venous access in place, and drugs and equipment for bronchospasm, anaphylaxis, and resuscitation readily available. Desensitization to aspirin/NSAIDs can be practiced in patients who are intolerant but need these drugs for the treatment of their underlying condition.[55] Several protocols are available.[56] Since tolerance to aspirin and cross-tolerance to other NSAIDs depends on the continued presence of the drug, uninterrupted treatment is needed to maintain the desensitized state as, otherwise, sensitivity returns in a few days.[57]

Aspirin/NSAID-exacerbated asthma seldom resolves spontaneously.[58] Thus, patients with a clear history of intolerance should be formally advised to avoid all aspirin-containing products and all other COX-1 inhibitors. They should be given a comprehensive list of prohibited drugs to keep with them at all times. Acetaminophen and COX-2 inhibitors pose a substantially lower risk, although cross-reactions have been described. Leukotriene receptor antagonists inconsistently antagonize aspirin-induced bronchospasm.

Β-BLOCKERS

Acute severe bronchospasm and death still occur in asthma, following exposure to β-blockers, especially the older and less selective ones such as propranolol.[59] Thus, β-blockers should be regarded as contraindicated in asthma, regardless of their route of administration. Ophthalmic preparations of β-blockers also can cause bronchospasm. Short-term treatment with cardioselective β_1-blockers is considered safe in patients with moderate asthma or chronic obstructive pulmonary disease, but many argue against this, pointing out that the likelihood and magnitude of bronchospasm during treatment with β-blockers is difficult to predict in the individual patient. Although patients may not exhibit significant bronchospasm when challenged with β-blockers in the clinic, they may experience a severe episode later during chronic treatment with the drug, due to the unstable nature of the asthma, or after an encounter with an asthma trigger. Long-term treatment with β-blockers may increase the risk of anaphylactoid reactions to radiographic contrast material, or to anesthetic agents.[60] Furthermore, β-blockers may blunt the therapeutic response to β_2-receptor agonists, should these drugs be required for the treatment of an acute asthma attack or anaphylaxis.[60]

OTHER DRUGS

Angiotensin-converting enzyme inhibitors, adenosine, antibiotics, cyclophosphamide, interferon α, interleukin-2, methotrexate, narcotics, penicillamine, pentamidine, propofol, propylthiouracil, ribavirin, and radiographic contrast material can also lead to severe bronchospasm.[50] Inhaled drugs (e.g. amphotericin B, pentamidine, *N*-acetyl-cysteine and, less often, inhaled bronchodilators and corticosteroids) can cause an acute asthmatic attack. There is no pathophysiologic link with aspirin/NSAID-exacerbated bronchospasm. Recent evidence points to the use of inhaled heroin as a major cause of sudden severe asthma requiring emergency visits.[61]

Vinblastine and vinorelbine can induced acute chest tightness with or without evidence for bronchospasm.[62] Rechallenge is followed by relapse of signs and symptoms of the condition. Patients who develop such symptoms during treatment with vinca alkaloids may experience residual respiratory impairment, in the form of chronic restrictive lung function defect and hypoxemia, which responds only partially to corticosteroid therapy.[62]

Hypersensitivity reactions

Life-threatening hypersensitivity and infusion reactions can develop during or shortly after the infusion of chemotherapeutic drugs and novel biologic agents.[63] Causal drugs include L-asparaginase, bortezomib, carboplatin, cetuximab, cisplatinum, cyclophosphamide, docetaxel, etoposide, ifosfamide, infliximab, methotrexate, paclitaxel, procarbazine, teniposide, and rituximab. Signs and symptoms include swelling at the injection site, dizziness, nasal stuffiness, dyspnea, wheezing, chest tightness, laryngospasm, abdominal pain, pruritus, skin rash, fever, chills and, in severe cases, hypotension, loss of consciousness, and shock. Depending on the patient, features of this condition may overlap with those of angioedema, noncardiogenic pulmonary edema, capillary leak syndrome, or acute bronchospasm. Management of full-blown hypersensitivity reactions includes corticosteroids and antihistamines. Epinephrine is used to treat severe reactions. Preventive measures include slowing the injection rate, corticosteroids, and antihistamines. Most instances of hypersensitivity and infusion reactions resolve on discontinuation of the drug and with appropriate medication. Prudent rechallenge may not lead to relapse, especially if corticosteroid therapy is given as prophylaxis,[63] enabling continuation of treatment with an essential chemotherapeutic drug.

Acute infiltrative lung disease

Infiltrative lung disease (ILD) is a group of conditions characterized by interstitial and alveolar inflammation, edema, hemorrhage, or fibrosis. Infiltrative lung disease is suspected when rapidly progressive dyspnea, widespread pulmonary opacities, and respiratory failure develop in a patient receiving an eligible drug, and in whom an infection has been appropriately ruled out by bronchoalveolar lavage (BAL) and other tests. The diagnosis is confirmed by lung biopsy, but this test is not required or feasible in all patients.[64]

Many drugs can cause acute ILD.[1] The disease manifests itself with cough, dyspnea, fever and, sometimes, respiratory failure. Acute drug-induced ILD may develop shortly after administration of the culpable drug (e.g. hydrochlorothiazide-induced pulmonary edema), a few hours or days later (e.g. chemotherapy-induced diffuse alveolar damage, acute nitrofurantoin lung, minocycline-induced eosinophilic pneumonia) or, inexplicably, after months to years into treatment (e.g. methotrexate pneumonitis, gold lung, acute amiodarone pulmonary toxicity).

Imaging is notoriously inaccurate in predicting the histopathologic background of drug-induced ILD and in differentiating drug-induced pneumonitis from an infection.[65] Therefore, it is crucial to rule out all treatable diseases, including an infection; BAL should be done as soon as is possible. Should a lung biopsy be considered, a window of opportunity should be determined before irreversible respiratory failure has occurred. Histopathologic appearances include interstitial or alveolar edema, various kinds of ILD, and alveolar hemorrhage. However, not all patients will undergo a confirmatory lung biopsy because the pattern of reaction may be suggestive of the drug etiology, or because drug withdrawal is quickly followed by improvement, or because the patient is judged too ill to undergo the procedure safely. Acute drug-induced conditions in which the lung biopsy may be superfluous include transient pulmonary infiltrates, noncardiac pulmonary edema, methotrexate lung, amiodarone pulmonary toxicity, and eosinophilic pneumonia. Usually, these conditions can be confidently diagnosed by exclusion, using the combination of BAL findings, drug therapy withdrawal and empiric corticosteroid therapy. In patients with a background of advanced malignancy, who develop pulmonary infiltrates during treatment with eligible drugs, the risk of open lung biopsy is often judged to outweigh the expected benefit. These patients are treated empirically with antibiotics and high-dose corticosteroid therapy.

There are few treatment options besides corticosteroid therapy. Outcome depends on (i) drug, with chemotherapeutic agents being associated with poorer outcome, (ii) pattern of lung response, with diffuse alveolar damage and accelerated pulmonary fibrosis being more severe, and (iii) the background condition, with solid and hematologic malignancies having a more severe outlook. Drug-induced pulmonary complications, particularly those associated with chemotherapy, may negatively impact on the management of neoplastic disease, if a change in therapy is required toward a less efficacious or more toxic regimen.

TRANSIENT PULMONARY INFILTRATES

Transient pulmonary infiltrates are usually associated with mild symptoms. In some patients, transient pulmonary infiltrates coexist with fever, cough, and acute chest pain or dyspnea. Transient pulmonary infiltrates can occur following infusion of various chemotherapeutic drugs and allied agents (antithymocyte globulin, bortezomib, cytarabine, docetaxel, gemcitabine, interleukin 2, mitomycin C, paclitaxel), in bone marrow or stem cell transplant recipients, or during treatment with *trans*-retinoic acid (ATRA), arsenium trioxide, hydrochlorothiazide, minocycline, and nitrofurantoin.[1,66–70] Appearances on imaging include a diffuse haze or ground-glass pattern, vague fluffy opacities and, on CT, lobular septal thickening or ground-glass pattern. Bronchoalveolar lavage should be performed early to rule out any infection. Pathologic documentation is rarely obtained, since the condition often is self-limiting, and symptoms and radiographic abnormalities improve or resolve in a few hours or days after withdrawal of drug therapy.

Depending on severity of symptoms and impact on gas exchange, corticosteroid therapy may be required. Histopathologic evidence in a limited number of cases links transient pulmonary infiltrates with noncardiac pulmonary edema or mild vasculitis, suggesting drug-induced vascular leak. Rechallenge with the drug generally produces relapse of signs and symptoms of the reaction. Rechallenge is not recommended for diagnostic purposes, as the reaction may be more severe, producing acute pulmonary edema, diffuse alveolar damage, or an acute respiratory distress syndrome (ARDS) picture. Development of pulmonary infiltrates may be prevented by treatment with corticosteroid drugs as a prophylaxis, enabling resumption of treatment with an essential drug.

PULMONARY EDEMA

Pulmonary edema is characterized by fluid in the interstitium or alveoli of the lung, causing dyspnea, diffuse interstitial or alveolar pulmonary opacities, and respiratory failure. In severe cases, frothy sputum is present at the mouth or in ventilator tubings. The vast majority of cases of drug-induced pulmonary edema are noncardiac in nature. Classic causal agents include epinephrine, amphotericin B, narcotic analgesics, L-asparaginase, aspirin, high-dose β_2-receptor agonists in pregnant women, calcium channel blockers, chemotherapeutic and biologic agents (the anti-CD25 mAb basiliximab, cyclophosphamide, docetaxel, gemcitabine, interleukin 2, infliximab, muromonab CD3), colchicine, hydrochlorothiazide, intrathecal methotrexate, nifedipine, nitrofurantoin, NSAIDs, opioids, oxytocin/vasopressin, phenylephrine, propofol, quinine, and radiographic contrast material.[1] Pulmonary edema may occur as a complication of drug overdose with tricyclic antidepressants,[71] heroin (the so-called 'heroin lung'),[72] and verapamil.[73] Pulmonary edema also has been described in the context of pulmonary hypertension with the use of nifedipine, prostacyclin, or nitric oxide.[74] Pulmonary edema may complicate hyperacute gold, methotrexate, or nitrofurantoin cellular infiltrative lung disease. A detailed list is available in a recent review.[75] Pulmonary edema may result from exposure to drugs which cause contractile dysfunction or acute myocardial injury (e.g. doxorubicin, β-blockers, verapamil, propofol, vasopressin), or induce acute systemic hypertension (epinephrine). General anesthesia, medical and surgical procedures at a distant site (e.g. intraarterial hepatic chemotherapy or chemoembolization, liposuction) can also provoke acute pulmonary edema.[76–79]

Onset is generally shortly after administration of regular therapeutic doses of the suspected drug. Less often, pulmonary edema develops later during chronic treatment with the therapeutic agent. Patients who develop pulmonary edema during treatment with interleukin-2, gemcitabine, docetaxel and, possibly, other chemotherapeutic agents, may present with the features of generalized capillary leak syndrome, which include weight gain, pleural effusion, and pedal edema. On imaging, early cases of drug-induced pulmonary edema are characterized by linear opacities suggestive of interstitial edema. Later cases show the features of full-blown edema, with widespread alveolar shadowing.[9,80–82] Most cases of drug-induced pulmonary edema are noncardiac, and likely result from drug-induced increase in pulmonary capillary permeability. This is confirmed by the normalcy of heart size, cardiac ultrasound, and pulmonary capillary wedge pressure measurements.

A lung biopsy is rarely performed in this condition. Histopathologic appearances include widespread, bland edema with proteinaceous fluid filling most of the alveolar lumens, along with a normal or moderately edematous interstitium. A cellular interstitial infiltrate is not conspicuous. Hyaline membranes, which are diagnostic of diffuse alveolar damage, and a dysplastic epithelium may be present.[83–87] There may be clinical and histopathological overlap with, and transition from, transient pulmonary infiltrates, frank pulmonary edema, and diffuse alveolar damage, especially in patients treated with chemotherapeutic agents.

Management includes discontinuation of drug, corticosteroid therapy and, in severe cases, ventilatory support. Diuretic therapy is reserved for cases with documented fluid overload. Since drug-induced vascular leak causes fluid loss and dehydration, this may be further aggravated by diuresis, producing hypotension and circulatory collapse. The effect of corticosteroids has not been evaluated. Pretreatment with corticosteroids has been shown to attenuate or abolish the symptoms associated with rechallenge, enabling continuation of treatment in some cases.

Transfusion-related acute lung injury (TRALI) and the ATRA syndrome are two distinct patterns of iatrogenic pulmonary edema.

TRANSFUSION-RELATED ACUTE LUNG INJURY

This is life-threatening pattern of noncardiogenic pulmonary edema, which results from transfusion of whole blood, red blood cells, platelets, or fresh frozen plasma.[88] Less often, immunoglobulins or stem cells produce the syndrome. It is a major cause of transfusion-related death, and generally results from complement-mediated binding of antileukocyte, antineutrophil, or anti-HLA antibodies from the donor with the recipient's leukocytes.[89] Less common mechanisms for TRALI include antileukocyte antibodies of recipient origin agglutinating donor leukocytes, and shelf aging of blood products, leading to accumulation of lipid-derived platelet-activating-factorlike substances. Proper recognition of TRALI is important. The responsible donor, generally a multiparous woman with high titers of antileukocyte antibody, should be identified. Blood and blood products from that particular donor should be quarantined and, generally, the donor should be deferred from further blood donation, and TRALI should be reported to safety agencies.[90] The incidence of TRALI in the United States is between 0.08 percent and 0.16 percent of all blood transfusions. Typically, symptoms of TRALI develop within 2–6 hours of the transfusion, sometimes earlier, in the form of abrupt respiratory failure, with rigors, dyspnea, tachypnea, cyanosis, hypotension, mild peripheral eosinophilia, and diffuse alveolar opacities corresponding to fluid leakage. It may manifest as sudden hypoxemia in a patient on the respirator, concomitant with or shortly after transfusion of blood or infusion of fresh frozen plasma.[91,92] The main competing diagnoses of TRALI are overload pulmonary edema, cardiogenic pulmonary edema, and a blood-borne infection.[93] Investigation in TRALI reveals an antibody in one of the donors in the majority of cases.[94] Management of TRALI includes judicious fluid management and oxygen therapy. Mechanical ventilation is required in about three out of four patients. The role of corticosteroid therapy is unclear. Diuretics should be used with caution, as TRALI often is associated with low blood pressure, and vigorous diuresis may cause deterioration of the hemodynamic status.[95] Most patients with TRALI will recover within 96 hours; mortality is 5–15 percent. Recognition of TRALI should lead to prompt examination for antibodies in donors whose blood or fractions were given within 6 hours prior to the accident.[96] A recent look-back study following a fatal case of TRALI indicated that administration of blood from the implicated donor had produced 15 previous adverse reactions in 14 patients, of which 8 were severe.[96] Only two were reported to the regional blood collection facility, and the donor had not been excluded from blood donation.[96]

The role of screening blood donors for antibody may not be useful, as not all blood products with antibodies will produce TRALI. Moreover, antibody-negative blood may not be entirely safe.

ALL *TRANS*-RETINOIC ACID

Arsenium trioxide (AsO$_3$) and ATRA are used to induce remission in acute promyelocytic leukemia. Both drugs can produce a pattern of pulmonary edema, grouped under the eponym 'ATRA syndrome'.[97] Administration of ATRA is often followed in the first day or days by an increase in the number of maturing myeloid cells and neutrophils. Patients with neutrophil counts above 10 000/mL are at risk, especially if there was a recent and rapid rise in neutrophils.[98] Treatment with ATRA may be temporally associated with the development of fever, weight gain, pleuritic chest pain, pleural or pericardial effusion, lower extremity edema, dyspnea, pulmonary infiltrates, frank pulmonary edema, alveolar hemorrhage, or an ARDS picture.[97] The incidence in one study was 9 cases in 35 patients receiving ATRA, the syndrome was preceded by an increase in circulating neutrophil counts in 6, and the condition was deemed unusual in leukopenic patients.[90] Radiographic studies indicate pleural effusions, ill-defined infiltrates, ground-glass opacities, and lung nodules which may progress to diffuse alveolar shadows.[99] The ATRA syndrome differs from other forms of drug-induced pulmonary edema with regard to the background condition and the presence of blast cells and promyelocytes containing Auer rods in lung tissue or in BAL.[90] Generally, patients improve with high-dose corticosteroids. Incidence of the ATRA syndrome has decreased since the prophylactic use of dexamethasone.

DIFFUSE ALVEOLAR DAMAGE

The typical patient with diffuse alveolar damage presents with dyspnea of recent onset, diffuse pulmonary infiltrates and volume loss on imaging, and acute respiratory failure. Diffuse alveolar damage is defined histopathologically by the presence of hyaline membranes, and accurate diagnosis of this condition requires examination of a lung biopsy specimen. Diffuse alveolar damage is mostly observed as a complication of treatment with chemotherapeutic agents (azathioprine, bleomycin, bortezomib, busulfan, chlorambucil, cyclophosphamide, cytosine-arabinoside, docetaxel, etoposide, fludarabine, gemcitabine, imatinib, irinotecan [CPT-11], melphalan, 6-mercaptopurine, methotrexate, mitomycin C, the nitrosamines: bischlorethyl nitrosourea [BCNU], CCNU and chloroethyl-cyclohexyl nitrosourea, and paclitaxel), targeted therapy (erlotinib, gefitinib, imatinib), biologic modifiers (interleukin-2, tumor necrosis factor (TNF)-α, infliximab), radiation therapy to the chest in the context of bone marrow or stem cell transplantation, and a few noncytotoxic agents (amiodarone, BCG therapy, colony-stimulating factors, gold, γ-interferon, mefloquine, nitrofurantoin, ATRA, sirolimus, and ticlopidine).[85,100–109] Diffuse alveolar damage occurs with greater frequency and severity following treatment with high-dose or multiagent chemotherapy regimens, as opposed to treatment with a single agent. It also can occur as a complication of overdoses with aspirin, carbamazepine, narcotics, and psychotropic agents. Contrary to old beliefs, diffuse alveolar damage may develop after intravenous, intrathecal (e.g. methotrexate), and oral administration of drugs (e.g. gefitinib). Concurrent or earlier radiation or oxygen therapy and, possibly, an increasing number of lines of chemotherapy may augment the risk of developing the condition.

Appearances on HRCT include interlobular or intralobular thickenings, a diffuse haze, ground-glass appearance, and white-out with air bronchograms.[65,87,110,111] Bronchoalveolar lavage should be done early to rule out an infection. The main problem in the patient suspected of having diffuse alveolar damage is to decide whether and when a lung biopsy is required to confirm the diagnosis, and whether this will lead to change in treatment that may improve the outcome. While the lung biopsy may enable exclusion of causes for the ILD other than drugs with greater certainty, this test may not solve the issue, since diffuse alveolar damage may result from causes other than drugs. On histopathological examination, there are hyaline membranes reflecting intraalveolar fibrin and loss of surfactant, desquamation of alveolar cells, pneumocyte dysplasia, and interstitial inflammation.[112]

Once the diagnosis of drug-induced diffuse alveolar damage is suggested or confirmed, and in the absence of a documented infection, corticosteroid therapy is advised. Both the response to corticosteroid therapy and outcome are unpredictable. Patients may improve, or develop a pattern of rapidly progressive pulmonary fibrosis or an ARDS picture.

ACUTE CHEMOTHERAPY LUNG

The typical patient with chemotherapy lung presents with diffuse pulmonary infiltrates and respiratory failure, during or shortly after treatment of hematologic malignancies (leukemias, Hodgkin disease, non-Hodgkin lymphoma), solid tumors (breast carcinoma, lung cancer) with single agent (e.g. bleomycin, busulfan, chlorambucil, cyclophosphamide, gemcitabine, melphalan, mitomycin, nitrosoureas, procarbazine), or multiagent chemotherapy regimens.[113] Chemotherapy lung may share features with and be difficult to distinguish from diffuse alveolar damage. Careful exclusion of infection and other causes is essential. Acute chemotherapy lung generally develops in less than 5 percent of patients, and it is estimated that drug toxicity accounts for about 15 percent of all causes for pulmonary infiltrates in this setting.[114] However, an increase in drug dosing, substitution of one drug with another drug intended to augment therapeutic efficacy, even when the dose of each agent taken separately is considered safe, may increase the rate of incidence of the condition to an unacceptable 50 percent.[115,116] Chest radiation therapy, total body irradiation, oxygen, and treatment with colony-stimulating-factors may synergize the pulmonary toxicity of chemotherapeutic agents. It is particularly difficult to separate the effects of drugs and radiation therapy in the pathogenesis of ILD in bone marrow or stem cell transplant recipients, and the condition in this context is referred to as the idiopathic pulmonary syndrome.

Depending on the patient and time of diagnosis, acute chemotherapy lung may have overlapping features with drug-induced pulmonary edema, diffuse alveolar damage, early pulmonary fibrosis or, less often, cellular interstitial pneumonia or eosinophilic pneumonia. The BAL findings include an increase in the percentage and activity of neutrophils, lymphocytes, or both cell types.[117] Lung biopsy is reserved for patients with an atypical presentation, or those who do not improve on empiric treatment.[118] Histopathologic features include interstitial edema, fibrosis, and the alveolar changes of atelectasis, exudation, alveolar edema, accumulation of macrophages and debris, acute fibrinous organizing pneumonia, hyaline membrane formation (diffuse alveolar damage), a dysplastic epithelium, and less often, a pattern of alveolar proteinosis. Interstitial inflammation generally is not conspicuous.[12] Although it is difficult to establish the contribution of each drug to this syndrome in patients exposed to multiple suspect drugs, this is important, as identification of the responsible agent may allow discontinuation of that specific agent, rather than the entire regimen.

Many patients respond favorably to drug discontinuation and high-dose corticosteroid therapy.[119] For example, in 65 patients with hematologic malignancies who had received a carmustine-based conditioning regimen prior to bone marrow transplantation, 17 (26 percent) developed acute pulmonary infiltrates thought to be due to drugs. Fifteen responded to corticosteroids, and only one died of ILD.[120] In patients who respond favorably, corticosteroids should be tapered slowly to avoid recurrence, which may evolve into fatal respiratory failure.[121] Outcome is worse in patients who have received total body irradiation.[122]

A peculiar form of chemotherapy lung can develop after the first course of chemotherapy in patients with acute leukemia and high blast cell counts. Massive lysis and stasis of leukemic cells within pulmonary capillaries produces widespread opacities, acute respiratory failure, and an ARDS picture. Some patients develop tumor lysis syndrome with hyperuricemia, hypocalcemia, hyperkalemia, hyperphosphatemia, azotemia, and multiple organ dysfunction.[123,124]

ACUTE CELLULAR INTERSTITIAL PNEUMONIA

Methotrexate pneumonitis typifies acute drug-induced cellular interstitial pneumonia. The condition develops after a few weeks or years into treatment in 0.3–11.6 percent of patients exposed to the drug for the treatment of hematologic malignancies or, more often now, rheumatoid arthritis.[125,126] Risk factors include advanced age, diabetes, hypoalbuminemia, a background of rheumatoid lung involvement and, possibly, the use of novel drugs, including etanercept and infliximab. The disease may be preceded by a dry cough, dyspnea, fever, and a normal chest radiograph for a few days or 1–2 weeks. Then the disease accelerates, producing rapidly progressive, dense and diffuse alveolar shadowing and volume loss, which characterize full-blown illness.[127] Blood or tissue eosinophilia may be present but are not conspicuous, and methotrexate pneumonitis is not an eosinophilic pneumonia. Diagnostic criteria[128] include dyspnea of acute onset, fever >38 °C, respiratory rate >28/min, the presence of diffuse radiographic abnormalities, a white blood cell count above 15 000/μL, negative blood, sputum, BAL stains and cultures for microorganisms, a restrictive lung function defect and reduced diffusing capacity, a PaO_2 <50 mm Hg on room air, and evidence for interstitial lung disease on a lung biopsy specimen.[128] The disease is deemed definite, probable or possible if six, five, or four criteria are fulfilled, respectively.

Infection with *Pneumocystis jiroveci*, cytomegalovirus, *Cryptococcus*, *Herpes zoster*, and *Nocardia* has been particularly associated with chronic treatment with methotrexate.[20] Thus, it is essential to rule out an infection, as opportunistic pneumonias are similar to methotrexate lung, with no real clinical or radiological discriminators. The BAL can be performed in most patients suspected of having methotrexate lung, if provision is made to correct the hypoxemia that almost invariably occurs during the procedure. In methotrexate lung, BAL shows elevated CD4+ or CD8+ lymphocyte counts, depending on time into the disease, and prior use of corticosteroids.[129]

Noninvasive management includes drug withdrawal and high-dose intravenous corticosteroid therapy. *Pneumocystis* pneumonia with low microorganism burden can be particularly difficult to distinguish from methotrexate lung, and some advocate the addition of appropriate antibiotic coverage. Open lung biopsy is now rarely done to diagnose methotrexate lung. Histologic findings indicate a combination of interstitial inflammation, fibrosis, ill-defined granulomas, and tissue eosinophilia.[125] In predominantly granulomatous methotrexate lung, the involvement is patchy, with intervening areas of normal tissue or tissue showing moderate cellular interstitial pneumonia.[125] Type 2 cell hyperplasia is present, but this feature is less prominent than with other chemotherapeutic agents or alkylating drugs. Alveolar edema, diffuse alveolar damage, and alveolar hemorrhage characterize those cases with hyperacute methotrexate lung.

Following corticosteroid therapy, the chest radiograph and HRCT findings and pulmonary function improve significantly over a few weeks, and continue to improve toward normal over several months. Pulmonary fibrosis as a complication of acute methotrexate lung is quite unusual. Mortality of 15 percent in a recent study underlines the need for early and careful management of this condition.[130] Even though one paper reported that in a fraction of patients the disease did not relapse following rechallenge, reexposure is contraindicated, as death may ensue.[130]

Several of the clinical and imaging features that characterize acute methotrexate lung, except granulomas on histopathology, are also found in gold lung.[131] The condition also has an acute course, produces diffuse infiltrates with respiratory failure and cellular interstitial pneumonia on histology. There is marked lymphocytosis in the BAL, and gold lung also may simulate an infection, which must be ruled out by BAL and other tests. Gold lung responds to withdrawal of drug therapy and corticosteroid therapy, and rechallenge with the drug produces relapse of the disease. Overall, gold lung has a less severe course than methotrexate lung. Cases of gold lung have decreased sharply, paralleling the loss of popularity of this compound in the management of rheumatoid arthritis in many countries.

Cladribine, nitrofurantoin, interferon α, venlafaxine, and a few other drugs can produce a pattern of acute interstitial pneumonia with respiratory failure clinically similar to methotrexate lung, but the incidence is low.[1] Acute pneumonitis may also occur shortly after onset of antiretroviral therapy in human immunodeficiency virus positive individuals, in the form of diffuse opacities and respiratory failure, prompting alternate diagnoses.[132]

Cavitary BCG-therapy can produce an acute granulomatous pulmonary reaction with, sometimes, alveolar damage, causing acute respiratory failure.[133]

ACUTE EOSINOPHILIC PNEUMONIA

Acute eosinophilic pneumonia (AEP) may be difficult to distinguish clinically and on imaging from acute noneosinophilic cellular interstitial pneumonia.[134] Acute eosinophilic pneumonia should be considered as a possible diagnosis when a previously healthy person presents with acute respiratory failure of unknown origin. Collectively, drugs are a significant cause of AEP and include amitriptyline, carbamazepine, chloroquine, ciprofloxacin, fludarabine, illicit drugs, infliximab, interleukin-2, minocycline, nitrofurantoin,

several NSAIDs, phenytoin, progesterone, sertraline, sulfasalazine, tenidap, tobacco smoke, troleandomycin, tryptophan, and venlafaxine.[1] Most cases of drug-induced AEP are described in young people on chronic treatment with minocycline for acne vulgaris,[135] or in patients on antidepressive medications. On imaging, there is dense bilateral linear or alveolar shadowing, which may predominate in upper subpleural regions of the lung. Bilateral pleural effusion and lymph node enlargement may be present as associated features. Ideally, AEP is diagnosed by eosinophilia in blood, BAL, and lung tissue. However, eosinophilia may be absent from blood, since circulating eosinophils can be quickly suppressed by corticosteroid drugs. This should be taken into consideration when the diagnosis of AEP is being considered. Bronchoalveolar lavage is an essential diagnostic tool in this condition and usually there is a marked increase in eosinophils. Other causes of eosinophilia, including parasitic infestation, should be ruled out carefully. A lung biopsy is rarely needed for the diagnosis of this condition. Histopathologic features include a dense cellular infiltrate, which consists of eosinophils admixed with other inflammatory cells.[12] There may be overlapping of histopathologic features of AEP and organizing pneumonia. Drug-induced AEP generally responds to drug therapy withdrawal and corticosteroid therapy, but tends to relapse if the patient is rechallenged with the drug.[135]

Eosinophilic pneumonia, sometimes severe, is a feature of two systemic conditions which can be caused by drugs: the Churg–Strauss and drug hypersensitivity syndromes:

- Reports describe the occurrence of Churg–Strauss syndrome in patients receiving leukotriene receptor antagonists (montelukast, pranlukast, zafirlukast), zileuton, macrolide antibiotics and desensitization. Patients presented with peripheral eosinophilia, pulmonary infiltrates, cardiomyopathy, muscle pain, mononeuritis multiplex, and, less often, digestive or dermatologic involvement was present.[136] Treatment includes drug therapy withdrawal and corticosteroids.
- Drug hypersensitivity syndrome (DHS) is a life-threatening syndrome with many possible patterns and significant morbidity.[20] The drug hypersensitivity syndrome or drug rash and eosinophilia systemic syndrome (DRESS) is characterized by fever, a cutaneous rash, eosinophilia, and internal organ involvement such as hepatitis, myocarditis, nephritis, or acute pneumonitis.[137–141] Presentations include dermatologic, hematologic (eosinophilia, atypical lymphocytosis, anemia, thrombocytopenia, leukemic reactions), lymphatic, and internal organ involvement which can mimic systemic diseases or an infection. Causal drugs include allopurinol, aromatic anticonvulsants, particularly carbamazepine and phenytoin, minocycline, and sulfonamides. Less often, the condition is caused by abacavir, atenolol, azathioprine, bupropion, captopril, chrysotherapy, diltiazem, leflunomide, nevirapine, oxicams, sulfasalazine, and trimethoprim. Onset is

gradual, with fever as a common early feature of drug hypersensitivity syndrome, followed by a widespread and longlasting papulopustular, erythematous skin eruption, which may progress to exfoliative dermatitis. The severity or extent of the skin-related changes do not correlate well with the severity or extent of internal organ involvement, which may remain nearly asymptomatic or be life threatening. Multiple organ dysfunction can occur as a manifestation of DHS. Treatment consists of immediate withdrawal of all suspect drugs, followed by supportive care and corticosteroid therapy. Drug withdrawal is generally followed by significant improvement in a few days; however, in a few patients, the disease may persist, or accelerate without known reason a few weeks after drug therapy withdrawal. Despite appropriate management with corticosteroid therapy and supportive care, the mortality rate is about 10 percent from internal organ failure or superimposed infection. Relapse may occur as the dose of corticosteroids is tapered, and treatment may need to be continued for months. Patients who develop DHS/DRESS must avoid reexposure to the causative medication and to related aromatic compounds (phenytoin, carbamazepine, phenobarbital), since rechallenge may produce relapse with increased severity.[137] Because genetic factors are suspected in the pathogenesis of drug hypersensitivity, relatives of the affected patient should be instructed to avoid similar medications.

ACUTE AMIODARONE PULMONARY TOXICITY

Amiodarone pulmonary toxicity (APT) may manifest itself as acute ILD, with cardiogenic pulmonary edema, diffuse alveolar hemorrhage and an infection as major competing diagnoses. Judicious use of imaging, diuresis, cardiac ultrasound, and BAL helps distinguish between these entities. In contrast to cardiac pulmonary edema, radiographic appearances of APT change little following diuresis.

Classic APT

Classic APT during long-term treatment with amiodarone may present acutely in up to 40 percent of patients with ATP in the form of cough, fever, dyspnea, and diffuse alveolar opacities.[142,143] Appearances on imaging include multiple bilateral fluffy alveolar opacities, which may exhibit high-attenuation numbers on HRCT, due the high iodine content of both amiodarone and metabolite, which are sequestered in lung tissues. Diagnosis is by exclusion, with BAL typically disclosing a greater increase in lymphocytes, compared with the more common insidious form of APT.[142] Classic changes in the form of dyslipidic inclusions in alveolar macrophages help relate the condition to treatment with amiodarone. A noninvasive approach using drug therapy withdrawal, substitution of another antiarrhythmic agent for amiodarone, and corticosteroid therapy may be preferred to

the invasive approach using the lung biopsy.[144] The response to corticosteroid therapy is good, and often is more rapid and convincing than in classic APT.

Acute APT

Acute APT is a severe illness, which is difficult to diagnose reliably. Acute APT can occur a few days after loading with high-dose intravenous amiodarone, especially in the postoperative setting, where the drug is thought to have an important, although underrecognized, role in inducing ARDS.[145,146] Failure to withdraw the drug early exposes to the risk of rapidly progressive APT.[146] Preoperative pulmonary abnormalities, anesthesia, exposure to high concentrations of oxygen, and mechanical ventilation may synergize APT.[147] Acute APT preferentially develops after thoracic or open heart surgery, or following insertion of an implantatable automatic defibrillator, with an incidence rate up to 25 percent in some studies.[148] Patients who have recently undergone resectional surgery for lung cancer are at greater risk, because of reduced ventilatory reserve postoperatively. One study was stopped before completion, due to excessive pulmonary toxicity in patients treated with amiodarone.[149] Abrupt withdrawal of corticosteroid therapy in the patient on long-term amiodarone may exacerbate latent APT, causing acute disease.[150] Acute APT manifests with dyspnea and diffuse interstitial, alveolar or mixed opacities, volume loss, severe hypoxemia or an ARDS picture.[151] Preexisting pathology, e.g. postoperative pneumonia or atelectasis, may mask its development. Pulmonary edema, pulmonary embolism, and a coincidental infection must be ruled out.

Diuresis and, status permitting, measurement of lung function and of diffusing capacity, imaging (including HRCT and contrast-enhanced CT), cardiac ultrasound, measurement of pulmonary capillary wedge pressure and BAL are used to distinguish APT from the above conditions. Foamy alveolar macrophages may be present in the BAL, even after only a few days on the drug.[146] Open lung biopsy may be required to confirm the diagnosis. Histopathological findings in acute APT include diffuse or resolving alveolar damage and/or organizing pneumonia, alveolar fibrin, interstitial edema and fibrosis superimposed on a background of dyslipidosis, with accumulation of alveolar or interstitial foam cells, suggesting APT.[145,150,152] In patients deemed too ill to undergo the procedure, drug therapy is withdrawn and empiric treatment with high-dose corticosteroid therapy is given. This may translate into marked and sustained improvement.[151] A mortality of 50 percent in acute APT despite drug withdrawal and high-dose corticosteroid therapy underscores the need for early recognition and aggressive management of this condition.

ACUTE ORGANIZING PNEUMONIA

Patients with acute organizing pneumonia present with a pattern of peribronchovascular or diffuse pulmonary opacities, and acute respiratory failure.[153,154] Drugs causing the syndrome include antineoplastic chemotherapy, interferon α and β, methotrexate, minocycline, penicillamine and statins.[1] Acute organizing pneumonia also occurs as a manifestation of graft-versus-host disease in bone marrow transplant recipients.[155,156] The condition is rare and can be life threatening. On histologic examination, there are widespread buds of connective tissue within distal airspaces, along with interstitial inflammation and preservation of the general lung architecture. Complete obliteration of airspaces can occur, causing severe respiratory failure and death. Distinguishing acute organizing pneumonia due to drugs, as opposed to organizing pneumonia occurring as a manifestation of background conditions such as rheumatoid arthritis, polymyalgia rheumatica, and ulcerative colitis often is problematic. Drug therapy withdrawal and corticosteroid therapy are indicated.[20]

Acute fibrinous organizing pneumonia is a newly recognized histopathologic entity,[157] which also can cause acute respiratory distress. It shares features with organizing pneumonia, including a background of connective tissue disease and exposure to amiodarone.[157] On histologic examination, there is the dominant pattern of intraalveolar fibrin and organizing pneumonia, type 2 pneumocyte hyperplasia, interstitial edema, and acute or chronic inflammation.

ACCELERATED PULMONARY FIBROSIS

The accelerated variant of pulmonary fibrosis is also known as acute interstitial pneumonia or the Hamman and Rich syndrome. Circumstantial evidence associates development of accelerated pulmonary fibrosis with exposure to amiodarone, bleomycin, danazol, interferon gamma and penicillamine.[158–162] This condition has been particularly associated with treatment of rheumatoid arthritis with infliximab and methotrexate.[158,161] The role of drugs is difficult to evaluate, because accelerated pulmonary fibrosis can also occur as a manifestation of rheumatoid lung, without being related to drugs.[163] The outcome of accelerated lung fibrosis is poor, despite drug therapy withdrawal and institution of high-dose corticosteroid therapy.

ACUTE ALVEOLAR HEMORRHAGE

Diffuse alveolar hemorrhage (DAH) is an unusual complication of drugs, which may or may not be associated with histologically demonstrable capillaritis.[164] The BAL is a reliable diagnostic tool, hence a lung biopsy rarely is performed in patients with this condition. Drugs causing DAH include oral anticoagulants (warfarin), abciximab, allopurinol, aspirin, azathioprine, clopidogrel, fibrinolytic agents, heparin, methotrexate, penicillamine and in the context of bone marrow or stem cell transplantation.[1,164] Occasionally, alveolar hemorrhage occurs as a complication of hyperacute gold, methotrexate, or nitrofurantoin lung. Hydralazine, penicillamine, propylthiouracil and, less often,

azathioprine, leflunomide, and phenytoin can produce a pneumo-renal syndrome, which mimics Goodpasture or Wegener granulomatosis.[20] Patients with alveolar hemorrhage from these agents may present with a perinuclear antineutrophilic cytoplasmic antibodies (ANCA) staining pattern having a antimyeloperoxidase, lactoferrin, or elastase specificity, in contrast with the cytoplasmic ANCA staining pattern and antiproteinase 3 specificity of naturally occurring Wegener.[20] Antiglomerular basement membrane antibodies are rarely found in drug-induced alveolar hemorrhage, as opposed to naturally occurring Goodpasture disease.

Alveolar hemorrhage can be rapidly progressive, requiring expeditious management to avoid irreversible intraalveolar clotting and organization, which may cause irreversible respiratory failure. Full-blown disease may cause general symptoms, arthralgias, dyspnea, diffuse alveolar infiltrates, which may assume a batwing distribution, and profound blood loss and anemia. Hemoptysis is an inconsistent feature in acute alveolar hemorrhage. An increase in the diffusing capacity has been found in a few patients, but is not a reliable finding. The BAL is hemorrhagic and demonstrates increased staining in sequential aliquots and, microscopically, there in an increase in the numbers of red cells. Hemosiderin-laden macrophages are not found initially in acute alveolar hemorrhage and, if present, indicate a background of subacute bleeding. A full panel of autoantibodies is essential in all cases, to classify drug-induced alveolar hemorrhage (autoimmune versus non-autoimmune), and distinguish drug-induced alveolar hemorrhage from naturally occurring conditions.[20,164]

Drug causality is suggested when DAH occurs during treatment with drugs which intentionally produce coagulation defects, even though coagulation studies are within an acceptable therapeutic range.[165] Otherwise, causality assessment is more difficult, because alveolar hemorrhage can occur in so many systemic conditions. A temporal association of drug exposure, p-ANCA titers, and alveolar hemorrhage is consistent with the drug etiology. A change in ANCA specificity in a patient with Wegener granulomatosis during follow-up may indicate drug-induced disease, rather than relapse of the background condition.[166]

Withdrawal of drug therapy is generally advised and may suffice in patients with anticoagulant-induced bleeding. Patients with other forms of DAH and extensive or persistent bleeding, or evidence for renal failure are considered for treatment with corticosteroids or immunosuppressive agents, in a manner similar to autoimmune disease.[20]

Hemolytic uremic syndrome

The hemolytic uremic syndrome is a complication that is relatively specific for mitomycin and gemcitabine, as opposed to other chemotherapeutic agents.[167–171] The syndrome has also been observed in malignant lymphoma, following treatment with BCNU, etoposide, ara-C, and cyclophosphamide.[172] Hemolytic uremic syndrome usually develops 4–8 weeks after completion of mitomycin-based chemotherapy regimens.[167] Some patients develop the disease after a latent period of up to 9 months after termination of treatment.[167] Incidence ranges between 2 percent and 10 percent. Patients present with rapidly evolving Coombs-negative hemolytic anemia, red cell fragmentation, thrombocytopenia, reticulocytosis, systemic hypertension or hypotension, neurologic involvement, irreversible renal failure, pulmonary hypertension, noncardiogenic pulmonary edema, alveolar hemorrhage, or an ARDS picture. All features of the disease may not be present at the same time. Blood transfusions, even in small amounts, may trigger the onset of, aggravate, or lead to relapse of the syndrome. Histologic examination of lung specimen shows intravascular thrombi, alveolar edema, and hemorrhage. Treatment consists of withdrawal of drug therapy, plasmapheresis, and high-dose corticosteroid therapy. In patients who receive mitomycin or gemcitabine, hemoglobin and creatinine levels and urinalysis should be monitored, as subtle changes may indicate early disease.[171] Regular monitoring of hemoglobin and creatinine levels are recommended in patients who have received mitomycin or more than 10 courses of gemcitabine in the recent past, to detect subclinical hemolytic uremic syndrome.[171]

Acute chest pain

Acute chest pain can occur during infusions of bleomycin, simulating acute cardiac, pericardial, or pulmonary events.[173] Radiographic evidence of a small pleural effusion and electrocardiographic changes suggestive of pericarditis can be evidenced. The syndrome is self-limiting. Symptoms resolve following drug therapy withdrawal and analgesics, and may not recur with further courses of the drug.

Episodes of acute transfixation of or excruciating chest pain or subacute chest tightness have been reported during treatment with ATRA, bumetanide, dextran-70, etoposide, intravenous immunoglobulins, mesalazine, methotrexate, propylthiouracil, quinine sulfate, and statins. Acute chest pain is a possible manifestation of ergoline-induced pleural involvement,[174] and in patients with the drug lupus syndrome.[175,176]

Treatment with etoposide or 5-fluorouracil can induce acute anginal chest pain with electrocardiographic changes suggestive of ischemia. These may be related to coronary spasm.[177,178] However, symptoms are poorly relieved by coronary vasodilators.[179] Triptans used in the treatment of migraine can induce acute angina-like chest pain.[180,181] Excruciating chest pain has been described as a manifestation of pneumonitis to minocycline,[135] in cocaine and marijuana users,[182,183] following liquid acrylate embolization of brain arteriovenous malformations[184] and after endoscopic injection sclerotherapy of esophageal varices with cyanoacrylate.[185]

Pulmonary embolism

An increased incidence of pulmonary thromboembolism has been observed during treatment with aprotinin, ATRA, antipsychotic drugs, chemotherapy for Hodgkin disease and solid tumors, clozapine, oral contraceptives, intravenous immunoglobulins, infliximab, olanzapine, risperidone, and thalidomide.[1,186,187] Pulmonary embolism has occurred in a few patients with drug-induced lupus associated with antiphospholipid antibodies.

Calcium phosphate replacement therapy may cause crystal precipitation in the pulmonary circulation, causing widespread obstruction, acute chest tightness and life-threatening pulmonary hypertension and respiratory failure.[188] Total parenteral nutrition,[189] intravenous lipids,[190] administration of drugs solubilized in lipids (e.g. propofol), injection of iodized oil for intraarterial chemoembolization of hepatocellular carcinoma,[191] and liposuction[192,193] may cause fat embolism, diffuse pulmonary opacities, and life-threatening respiratory failure.

Percutaneous vertebroplasty with methacrylate may be complicated by egress and migration of cement fat and bone marrow to the paravertebral plexuses, inferior vena cava and pulmonary circulation, causing life-threatening embolism of foreign material and catastrophic respiratory failure. The condition is diagnosed by the presence of radioopaque material in paravertebral veins, and pulmonary circulation on imaging, and/or in the right atrium or ventricle on ultrasound.[194–196]

Acute lone cough

An increasing number of drugs can cause chronic cough. The typical patient with drug-induced cough is the one being treated with long-term ACEIs.[197] Patients may attend the emergency room for longstanding, annoying cough, or in relation to complications of chronic cough such as incontinence, rib fracture, or pneumothorax.[198] A meticulous drug history is warranted, as the cough will disappear in a few days or weeks after drug discontinuation, and may recur as a manifestation of a drug class effect after rechallenge with any ACEI. Cough persisting after ACEI withdrawal should raise the suspicion of another cause, particularly lung cancer.

Propofol and isoflurane may induce violent coughing in the operating or recovery room,[199,200] raising difficult diagnostic issues.

Miscellaneous conditions

Several drugs can cause pleural effusion or hemothorax, causing compression, silent blood loss, and acute symptoms. The subject has been reviewed recently.[201–203]

Key learning points

- Therapeutic drugs and radiation therapy can acutely injure the respiratory system in many ways, with distinctive clinicopathologic patterns of involvement and, sometimes, acute chest symptoms and respiratory failure.

- Direct respiratory injury from an increase in the therapeutic efficacy of the drug. Indirect injury can also occur, for instance immunosuppressive drugs predispose patients to the development of opportunistic pulmonary infections that may cause acute lung injury and consequent respiratory failure.

- Drug-induced respiratory emergencies are characterized by the rapid or sudden development of acute symptoms such as dyspnea or chest pain in relation to acute respiratory involvement.

- Drug-induced respiratory emergencies are diagnosed by exclusion.

- They may result from involvement of the upper or lower airways, lung parenchyma, pulmonary circulation, pleura, mediastinum, pericardium, or heart.

- There may be inflammation, edema, a cellular infiltrate, thromboembolism, fat embolism, effusion, hematoma or hemorrhage, producing impairment of gas exchange or compression of a major airway, lung, or heart.

- The radiographic appearance of drug-induced respiratory emergencies will depend on the primary localization of the pathologic process.

REFERENCES

1. Pneumotox® website. Produced by P Foucher – Ph Camus. www.pneumotox.com, last update: March, 2006.

2. White DA. Drug-induced pulmonary infection. *Clin Chest Med* 2004; **25**: 179–88.

3. Wolff AJ, O'Donnell AE. Pulmonary effects of illicit drug use. *Clin Chest Med* 2004; **25**: 203–16.

4. Wilson KC, Saukkonen JJ. Acute respiratory failure from abused substances. *J Intensive Care Med* 2004; **19**: 183–93.

5. Duong T, Schonfeld AJ, Yungbluth M, Slotten R. Acute pneumopathy in a nonsurgical transsexual. Silicone emboli to the lung. *Chest* 1998; **113**: 1127–9.

6. Abid SH, Malhotra V, Perry MC. Radiation-induced and chemotherapy-induced pulmonary injury. *Curr Opin Oncol* 2001; **13**: 242–8.

7. Ernst E. Harmless herbs? A review of the recent literature. *Am J Med* 1998; **104**: 170–8.

8. Talbot AR, Shaiw MH, Huang JS, *et al.* Intentional self-poisoning with glyphosate containing herbicides (Roundup): a review of 93 cases. *Hum Exp Toxicol* 1991; **10**: 1–8.

9. Park CH, Kim KI, Park SK, Lee CH. Carbamate poisoning: High resolution CT and pathologic findings. *J Comput Assist Tomogr* 2000; **24**: 52–4.

10. Plataki M, Bouros D. Iatrogenic and rare pleural effusion. In: Bouros D, ed. *Pleural Disorders.* New York: Marcel Dekker, 2004: 897–913.

11. Similowski T, Straus C. Iatrogenic-induced dysfunction of the neuromuscular respiratory system. *Clin Chest Med* 2004; **25**: 155–66.

12. Flieder DB, Travis WD. Pathologic characteristics of drug-induced lung disease. *Clin Chest Med* 2004; **25**: 37–46.

13. Camus P, Bonniaud P, Fanton A, *et al.* Drug-induced and iatrogenic infiltrative lung disease. *Clin Chest Med* 2004; **25**: 479–519, vi.

14. Ibanez L, Laporte JR, Carne X. Adverse drug reactions leading to hospital admission. *Drug Saf* 1991; **6**: 450–9.

15. Mertes PM, Laxenaire MC. Anaphylactic and anaphylactoid reactions occurring during anaesthesia in France. Seventh epidemiologic survey (January 2001–December 2002). *Ann Fr Anesth Reanim* 2004; **23**: 1133–43.

16. Shapiro S, Slone D, Lewis GP, Jick H. Fatal drug reactions among medical inpatients. *JAMA* 1971; **216**: 467–72.

17. Sondhi D, Lippmann M, Murali G. Airway compromise due to angiotensin-converting enzyme inhibitor-induced angioedema: clinical experience at a large community teaching hospital. *Chest* 2004; **126**: 400–4.

18. Dean DE, Schultz DL, Powers RH. Asphyxia due to angiotensin converting enzyme (ACE) inhibitor mediated angioedema of the tongue during the treatment of hypertensive heart disease. *J Forensic Sci* 2001; **46**: 1239–43.

19. Cohen EG, Soliman AMS. Changing trends in angioedema. *Ann Otol Rhinol Laryngol* 2001; **110**: 701–6.

20. Camus P. Drug-induced respiratory disease in connective tissue diseases. In: Wells AU, Denton CP, eds. *Handbook of Systemic Autoimmune Diseases Part VI: Pulmonary Involvement in Systemic Autoimmune Diseases.* Vol. 2: Elsevier BV, 2004: 247–94.

21. Roberts JR, Wuerz RC. Clinical characteristics of angiotensin-converting enzyme inhibitor-induced angioedema. *Ann Emerg Med* 1991; **20**: 119–22.

22. Schuster C, Reinhart WH, Hartmann K, Kuhn M. Angioödem unter ACE-Hemmern und Angiotensin-II-receptor-Antagonisten: Analyse von 98 Fällen. *Schweiz Med Wochenschr* 1999; **129**: 362–9.

23. Israili ZH, Hall WD. Cough and angioneurotic edema associated with angiotensin-converting enzyme inhibitor therapy. *Ann Intern Med* 1992; **117**: 234–42.

24. Seidman MD, Lewandowski CA, Sarpa JR, *et al.* Angioedema related to angiotensin-converting enzyme inhibitors. *Otolaryngol Head Neck Surg* 1990; **102**: 727–31.

25. Chiu AG, Krowiak EJ, Deeb ZE. Angioedema associated with angiotensin II receptor antagonists: challenging our knowledge of angioedema and its etiology. *Laryngoscope* 2001; **111**: 1729–31.

26. Brown AF, McKinnon D, Chu K. Emergency department anaphylaxis: A review of 142 patients in a single year. *J Allergy Clin Immunol* 2001; **108**: 861–6.

27. Gruchalla RS, Pirmohamed M. Clinical practice. Antibiotic allergy. *N Engl J Med* 2006; **354**: 601–9.

28. Pumphrey RSH. Lessons from management of anaphylaxis from a study of fatal reactions. *Clin Exp Allergy* 2000; **30**: 1144–50.

29. Shanholtz C. Acute life-threatening toxicity of cancer treatment. *Crit Care Clin* 2001; **17**: 483–502.

30. Berkes EA. Anaphylactic and anaphylactoid reactions to aspirin and other NSAIDs. *Clin Rev Allergy Immunol* 2003; **24**: 137–47.

31. Shepherd GM. Hypersensitivity reactions to drugs: evaluation and management. *Mt Sinai J Med* 2003; **70**: 113–25.

32. Sicherer SH. Advances in anaphylaxis and hypersensitivity reactions to foods, drugs, and insect venom. *J Allergy Clin Immunol* 2003; **111**: S829–34.

33. Amin HS, Liss GM, Bernstein DI. Evaluation of near-fatal reactions to allergen immunotherapy injections. *J Allergy Clin Immunol* 2006; **117**: 169–75.

34. Leung DY, Shanahan WR, Jr, Li XM, Sampson HA. New approaches for the treatment of anaphylaxis. *Novartis Found Symp* 2004; **257**: 248–60; discussion 260–74, 276–85.

35. Kaplinsky N, Deutsch V, Har Zahav V, Frankl O. Mediastinal bleeding during anticoagulant simulating dissecting hematoma. *Harefuah* 1978; **94**: 172–3.

36. Turetz F, Steinberg H, Kahn A. Spontaneous anterior mediastinal hematoma: a complication of heparin therapy. *J Am Med Womens Assoc* 1979; **34**: 85–8.

37. al-Fallouji HK, Snow DG, Kuo MJ, Johnson PJ. Spontaneous retropharyngeal haematoma: two cases and a review of the literature. *J Laryngol Otol* 1993; **107**: 649–50.

38. Kaynar AM, Bhavani-Shankar K, Mushlin PS. Lingual hematoma as a potential cause of upper airway obstruction. *Anesth Analg* 1999; **89**: 1573–5.

39. Shojania KG. Coumadin-induced lingual hemorrhage mimicking angioedema. *Am J Med* 2000; **109**: 77–8.

40. Ahmed J, Philpott J, Lew GS, Blunt D. Airway obstruction: a rare complication of thrombolytic therapy. *J Laryngol Otol* 2005; **119**: 819–21.

41. Gupta MK, McClymont LG, El-Hakim H. Case of sublingual hematoma threatening airway obstruction. *Med Sci Monit* 2003; **9**: CS95–7.

42. Götte K, Hormann K. Dyspnea caused by spontaneous hematoma of the oropharynx and larynx during marcumar therapy. *HNO* 2001; **49**: 220–3.

43. Boyce SH, Quigley MA. Uvulitis and partial upper airway obstruction following cannabis inhalation. *Emerg Med (Fremantle)* 2002; **14**: 106–8.

44. O'Donnell AE, Selig J, Aravamuthan M, Richardson MSA. Pulmonary complications associated with illicit drug use. An update. *Chest* 1995; **108**: 460–3.

45. White MC, Reynolds F. Sudden airway obstruction following inhalation drug abuse. *Br J Anaesth* 1999; **82**: 808.

46. Huggins JT, Kaplan A, Martin-Harris B, Sahn SA. Eucalyptus as a specific irritant causing vocal cord dysfunction. *Ann Allergy Asthma Immunol* 2004; **93**: 299–303.

47. Perry PA, Dean BS, Krenzelok EP. Drug-induced esophageal injury. *J Toxicol Clin Toxicol* 1989; **27**: 281–6.

48. Stack PE, Thomas E. Pharmacobezoar: an evolving new entity. *Dig Dis* 1995; **13**: 356–64.

49. Plaza V, Serrano J, Picado C, Sanchis J. Frequency and clinical characteristics of rapid-onset fatal and near-fatal asthma. *Eur Respir J* 2002; **19**: 846–52.

50. Babu KS, Marshall BG. Drug-induced airways diseases. *Clin Chest Med* 2004; **25**: 113–22.

51. Babu KS, Salvi SS. Aspirin and asthma. *Chest* 2000; **118**: 1470–6.

52. Szczeklik A, Nizankowska E, Duplaga M. Natural history of aspirin-induced asthma. *Eur Respir J* 2000; **16**: 432–8.

53. Mascia K, Haselkorn T, Deniz YM, *et al.* Aspirin sensitivity and severity of asthma: Evidence for irreversible airway obstruction in patients with severe or difficult-to-treat asthma. *J Allergy Clin Immunol* 2005; **116**: 970–5.

54. Marquette CH, Saulnier F, Leroy O, *et al.* Long-term prognosis of near-fatal asthma. A 6-year follow-up study of 145 asthmatic patients who underwent mechanical ventilation for a near-fatal attack of asthma. *Am Rev Respir Dis* 1992; **146**: 76–81.

55. Berges-Gimeno MP, Simon RA, Stevenson DD. Long-term treatment with aspirin desensitization in asthmatic patients with aspirin-exacerbated respiratory disease. *J Allergy Clin Immunol* 2003; **111**: 180–6.

56. Ramanuja S, Breall JA, Kalaria VG. Approach to 'aspirin allergy' in cardiovascular patients. *Circulation* 2004; **110**: e1–4.

57. Pleskow WW, Stevenson DD, Mathison DA, *et al.* Aspirin desensitization in aspirin-sensitive asthmatic patients: clinical manifestations and characterization of the refractory period. *J Allergy Clin Immunol* 1982; **69**: 11–19.

58. Rosado A, Vives R, Gonzalez R, Rodriguez J. Can NSAIDs intolerance disappear? A study of three cases. *Allergy* 2003; **58**: 689–90.

59. Fallowfield JM, Marlow HF. Propranolol is contraindicated in asthma. *BMJ* 1996; **313**: 1486.

60. Lang DM, Alpern MB, Visintainer PF, Smith ST. Elevated risk of anaphylactoid reaction from radiographic contrast media is associated with both beta-blocker exposure and cardiovascular disorders. *Arch Intern Med* 1993; **153**: 2033–40.

61. Krantz AJ, Hershow RC, Prachand N, *et al.* Heroin insufflation as a trigger for patients with life-threatening asthma. *Chest* 2003; **123**: 510–17.

62. Rivera MP, Kris MG, Gralla RJ, White DA. Syndrome of acute dyspnea related to combined mitomycin plus vinca alkaloid chemotherapy. *Am J Clin Oncol* 1995; **18**: 245–50.

63. Shepherd GM. Hypersensitivity reactions to chemotherapeutic drugs. *Clin Rev Allergy Immunol* 2003; **24**: 253–62.

64. Camus P. Drug-induced infiltrative lung diseases. In: Schwarz MI, King TEJ, eds. *Infiltrative Lung Diseases*, 4th ed. Hamilton, ON: BC Dekker, Inc; 2003: 485–534.

65. Cleverley JR, Screaton NJ, Hiorns MP, *et al.* Drug-induced lung disease: high-resolution CT and histological findings. *Clin Radiol* 2002; **57**: 292–9.

66. Glauser FL, DeBlois G, Bechard D, *et al.* Cardiopulmonary toxicity of adoptive immunotherapy. *Am J Med Sci* 1988; **296**: 406–12.

67. Ramanathan RK, Belani CP. Transient pulmonary infiltrates: a hypersensitivity reaction to paclitaxel. *Ann Intern Med* 1996; **124**: 278.

68. Maillard N, Foucher P, Caillot D, *et al.* Transient pulmonary infiltrates during treatment with anti-thymocyte globulin. *Respiration* 1999; **66**: 279–82.

69. Krantz MJ, Dart RC, Mehler PS. Transient pulmonary infiltrates possibly induced by quinine sulfate. *Pharmacotherapy* 2002; **22**: 775–8.

70. Karacan O, Eyüboglu FO, Akcay S, Özyilkan Ö. Acute interstitial pneumopathy associated with docetaxel hypersensitivity. *Onkologie* 2004; **27**: 563–5.

71. Varnell RM, Godwin JD, Richardson ML, Vincent JM. Adult respiratory distress syndrome from overdose of tricyclic antidepressants. *Radiology* 1989; **170**: 667–70.

72. Silber R, Clerkin EP. Pulmonary edema in acute heroin poisoning. Report of four cases. *Am J Med* 1959; **27**: 187–92.

73. Brass BJ, Winchester-Penny S, Lipper BL. Massive verapamil overdose complicated by noncardiogenic pulmonary edema. *Am J Emerg Med* 1996; **14**: 459–61.

74. Chaouat A, Kessler R, Weitzenblum E. Pulmonary oedema and pleural effusion in two patients with primary pulmonary hypertension treated with calcium channel blockers. *Heart* 1996; **75**: 383.

75. Lee-Chiong TLJ, Matthay RA. Drug-induced pulmonary edema and acute respiratory distress syndrome. *Clin Chest Med* 2004; **25**: 95–104.

76. Doria C, Mandal AL, Scott VL, *et al.* Noncardiogenic pulmonary edema induced by a molecular adsorbent recirculating system: case report. *J Artificial Organs* 2003; **6**: 282–5.

77. Sickmann K, Seider R, Dahm M, Nold H. Negative pressure pulmonary edema. *Anaesthesist* 2005; **54**: 1197–200.

78. Hong SJ, Lee JY, Choi JH, *et al.* Pulmonary edema following laparoscopic bariatric surgery. *Obes Surg* 2005; **15**: 1202–6.

79. Westreich R, Sampson I, Shaari CM, Lawson W. Negative-pressure pulmonary edema after routine septorhinoplasty – Discussion of pathophysiology,

treatment, and prevention. *Arch Facial Plast Surg* 2006; **8**: 8–15.

80. Bouachour G, Varache N, Szapiro N, *et al.* Noncardiogenic pulmonary edema resulting from intravascular administration of contrast material. *AJR Am J Roentgenol* 1991; **157**: 255–6.

81. Paul RE, George G. Fatal noncardiogenic pulmonary edema after intravenous nonionic radiographic contrast. *Lancet* 2002; **359**: 1037–8.

82. Franquet T, Muller NL, Lee KS, *et al.* High-resolution CT and pathologic findings of noninfectious pulmonary complications after hematopoietic stem cell transplantation. *AJR Am J Roentgenol* 2005; **184**: 629–37.

83. Shearer P, Katz J, Bozeman P, *et al.* Pulmonary insufficiency complicating therapy with high dose cytosine arabinoside in five pediatric patients with relapsed acute myelogenous leukemia. *Cancer* 1994; **74**: 1953–8.

84. Pavlakis N, Bell DR, Millward MJ, Levi JA. Fatal pulmonary toxicity resulting from treatment with gemcitabine. *Cancer* 1997; **80**: 286–91.

85. Gonzolez ER, Cole T, Grimes MM, Fink RA, Fowler AAI. Recurrent ARDS in an 39-year-old woman with migraine headaches. *Chest* 1998; **114**: 919–22.

86. Semba S, Moriya T, Youssef EM, Sasano H. An autopsy case of ovarian hyperstimulation syndrome with massive pulmonary edema and pleural effusion. *Pathol Int* 2000; **50**: 549–52.

87. Erasmus JJ, McAdams HP, Rossi SE. Drug-induced lung injury. *Semin Roentgenol* 2002; **37**: 72–81.

88. Kopko PM, Popovsky MA. Pulmonary injury from transfusion-related acute lung injury. *Clin Chest Med* 2004; **25**: 105–13.

89. Popovsky MA. Transfusion and lung injury. *Transfus Clin Biol* 2001; **8**: 272–7.

90. Camus P, Costabel U. Drug-induced respiratory disease in patients with hematological diseases. *Semin Respir Crit Care Med* 2005; **26**: 458–81.

91. Dubois M, Lotze MT, Diamond WJ, *et al.* Pulmonary shunting during leukoagglutinin-induced noncardiac pulmonary edema. *JAMA* 1980; **244**: 2186–9.

92. Yost CS, Matthay MA, Gropper MA. Etiology of acute pulmonary edema during liver transplantation. *Chest* 2001; **119**: 219–23.

93. Popovsky MA. Transfusion and the lung: circulatory overload and acute lung injury. *Vox Sang* 2004; **87**: 62–5.

94. Gajic O, Moore SB. Transfusion-related acute lung injury. *Mayo Clin Proc* 2005; **80**: 766–70.

95. Levy GJ, Shabot MM, Hart ME, *et al.* Transfusion-associated noncardiogenic pulmonary edema. Report of a case and a warning regarding treatment. *Transfusion* 1986; **26**: 278–81.

96. Kopko PM, Marshall CS, MacKenzie MR, *et al.* Transfusion-related acute lung injury. Report of a clinical look-back investigation. *JAMA* 2002; **287**: 1968–71.

97. Frankel SR, Eardley A, Lauwers G, *et al.* The 'retinoic acid syndrome' in acute promyelocytic leukemia. *Ann Intern Med* 1992; **117**: 292–6.

98. Vosburgh E. Pulmonary leukostasis secondary to all-trans retinoic acid in the treatment of acute promyelocytic leukemia in first relapse. *Leukemia* 1992; **6**: 608–10.

99. Davis BA, Cervi P, Amin Z, *et al.* Retinoic acid syndrome: pulmonary computed tomography (CT) findings. *Leuk Lymphoma* 1996; **23**: 113–17.

100. Krous HF, Hamlin WB. Pulmonary toxicity due to bleomycin. Report of a case. *Arch Pathol* 1973; **95**: 407–10.

101. Litam JP, Dail DH, Spitzer G, *et al.* Early pulmonary toxicity after administration of high-dose BCNU. *Cancer Treat Rep* 1981; **65**: 39–43.

102. Andersson BS, Luna BS, Yee C, *et al.* Fatal pulmonary failure complicating high-dose cytosine arabinoside therapy in acute leukemia. *Cancer* 1990; **65**: 1079–84.

103. Mack U, Schmidt K, Heine M. Fatal diffuse alveolar damage after gold medication. *Pneumologie* 1994; **48**: 405–8.

104. Dai MS, Ho CL, Chen YC, *et al.* Acute respiratory distress syndrome following intrathecal methotrexate administration: a case report and review of literature. *Ann Hematol* 2000; **79**: 696–9.

105. Savici D, Katzenstein ALA. Diffuse alveolar damage and recurrent respiratory failure: Report of 6 cases. *Hum Pathol* 2001; **32**: 1398–402.

106. Kramer N, Chuzhin Y, Kaufman LD, *et al.* Methotrexate pneumonitis after initiation of infliximab therapy for rheumatoid arthritis. *Arthritis Rheum* 2002; **47**: 670–1.

107. Oon PC, Jerng JS, Kao HL, *et al.* Diffuse alveolar damage associated with ticlopidine use: a case report. *J Formos Med Assoc* 2003; **102**: 262–5.

108. Manito N, Kaplinsky EJ, Bernat R, *et al.* Fatal interstitial pneumonitis associated with sirolimus

therapy in a heart transplant recipient. *J Heart Lung Transplant* 2004; **23**: 780–2.

109. Seto T, Seki N, Uematsu K, *et al.* Gefitinib-induced lung injury successfully treated with high-dose corticosteroids. *Respirology* 2006; **11**: 113–16.

110. Johkoh T, Itoh H, Müller NL, *et al.* Crazy-paving appearance at thin-section CT: Spectrum of disease and pathologic findings. *Radiology* 1999; **211**: 155–60.

111. Rossi SE, Erasmus JJ, McAdams P, *et al.* Pulmonary drug toxicity: radiologic and pathologic manifestations. *RadioGraphics* 2000; **5**: 1245–59.

112. Roychowdhury M, Pambuccian SE, Aslan DL, *et al.* Pulmonary complications after bone marrow transplantation. An autopsy study from a large transplantation center. *Arch Pathol Lab Med* 2005; **129**: 366–71.

113. Limper AH. Chemotherapy-induced lung disease. *Clin Chest Med* 2004; **25**: 53–64.

114. Mulabecirovic A, Gaulhofer P, Auner HW, *et al.* Pulmonary infiltrates in patients with haematologic malignancies: transbronchial lung biopsy increases the diagnostic yield with respect to neoplastic infiltrates and toxic pneumonitis. *Ann Hematol* 2004; **83**: 420–2.

115. Brockstein BE, Smiley C, Al-Sadir J, Williams SF. Cardiac and pulmonary toxicity in patients undergoing high-dose chemotherapy for lymphoma and breast cancer: prognostic factors. *Bone Marrow Transplant* 2000; **25**: 885–94.

116. Friedberg JW, Neuberg D, Kim H, *et al.* Gemcitabine added to doxorubicin, bleomycin, and vinblastine for the treatment of de novo Hodgkin disease. Unacceptable acute pulmonary toxicity. *Cancer* 2003; **98**: 978–82.

117. Bhalla KS, Wilczynski SW, Abushamaa AM, *et al.* Pulmonary toxicity of induction chemotherapy prior to standard or high-dose chemotherapy with autologous hematopoietic support. *Am J Respir Crit Care Med* 2000; **161**: 17–25.

118. Dai MS, Lee SC, Ho CL, *et al.* Impact of open lung biopsy for undiagnosed pulmonary infiltrates in patients with hematological malignancies. *Am J Hematol* 2001; **68**: 87–90.

119. Kalaycioglu M, Kavuru M, Tuason L, Bolwell B. Empiric prednisone therapy for pulmonary toxic reaction after high-dose chemotherapy containing carmustine. *Chest* 1995; **107**: 482–7.

120. Alessandrino EP, Bernasconi P, Colombo A, *et al.* Pulmonary toxicity following carmustine-based preparative regimens and autologous peripheral blood progenitor cell transplantation in hematological malignancies. *Bone Marrow Transplant* 2000; **25**: 309–13.

121. Richter JE, Hastedt R, Dalton JF, *et al.* Pulmonary toxicity of bischloronitrosourea. Report of a case with transient response to corticosteroid therapy. *Cancer* 1979; **43**: 1607–12.

122. Carruthers SA, Wallington M. Total body irradiation and pneumonitis risk: a review of outcomes. *Br J Cancer* 2004; **90**: 2080–4.

123. Tryka AF, Godleski JJ, Fanta CH. Leukemic cell lysis pneumopathy. A complication of treated myeloblastic leukemia. *Cancer* 1982; **50**: 2763–70.

124. Lester WA, Hull DR, Fegan CD, Morris TCM. Respiratory failure during induction chemotherapy for acute myelomonocytic leukaemia (FABM4Eo) with Ara-C and all-trans retinoic acid. *Br J Haematol* 2000; **109**: 847–50.

125. Imokawa S, Colby TV, Leslie KO, Helmers RA. Methotrexate pneumonitis: review of the literature and histopathological findings in nine patients. *Eur Respir J* 2000; **15**: 373–81.

126. Zisman DA, McCune WJ, Tino G, Lynch JPI. Drug-induced pneumonitis: the role of methotrexate. *Sarcoidosis Vasc Diffuse Lung Dis* 2001; **18**: 243–52.

127. Cannon GW. Methotrexate pulmonary toxicity. *Rheum Dis Clin North Am* 1997; **23**: 917–37.

128. Clearkin R, Corris PA, Thomas SHL. Methotrexate pneumonitis in a patient with rheumatoid arthritis. *Postgrad Med J* 1997; **73**: 603–4.

129. Fuhrman C, Parrot A, Wislez M, *et al.* Spectrum of CD4 to CD8 T-cell ratios in lymphocytic alveolitis associated with methotrexate-induced pneumonitis. *Am J Respir Crit Care Med* 2001; **164**: 1186–91.

130. Kremer JM, Alarcon GS, Weinblatt ME, *et al.* Clinical, laboratory, radiographic, and histopathologic features of methotrexate-associated lung injury in patients with rheumatoid arthritis. *Arthritis Rheum* 1997; **40**: 1829–37.

131. Tomioka H, King TEJ. Gold-induced pulmonary disease: Clinical features, outcome, and differentiation from rheumatoid lung disease. *Am J Respir Crit Care Med* 1997; **155**: 1011–20.

132. Goldsack NR, Allen S, Lipman MCI. Adult respiratory distress syndrome as a severe immune reconstitution disease following the commencement of highly active antiretroviral therapy. *Sex Transm Infect* 2003; **79**: 337–8.

133. Tan L, Testa G, Yung T. Diffuse alveolar damage in BCGosis: A rare complication of intravesical bacillus Calmette-Guérin therapy for transitional cell carcinoma. *Pathology* 1999; **31**: 55–6.

134. Allen JN. Drug-induced eosinophilic lung disease. *Clin Chest Med* 2004; **25**: 77–88.

135. Sitbon O, Bidel N, Dussopt C, *et al.* Minocycline pneumonitis and eosinophilia: a report on 8 patients. *Arch Intern Med* 1994; **154**: 1633–40.

136. Oberndorfer S, Beate U, Sabine U, *et al.* Churg Strauss syndrome during treatment of bronchial asthma with a leucotriene receptor antagonist presenting with polyneuropathy. *Neurologia* 2004; **19**: 134–8.

137. de Vriese ASP, Philippe J, Van Renterghem DM, *et al.* Carbamazepine hypersensitivity syndrome: report of 4 cases and review of the literature. *Medicine (Baltimore)* 1995; **74**: 144–50.

138. Bocquet H, Bagot M, Roujeau JC. Drug-induced pseudolymphoma and drug hypersensitivity syndrome (Drug Rash with Eosinophilia and Systemic Symptoms: DRESS). *Semin Cutan Med Surg* 1996; **15**: 250–7.

139. Bourezane Y, Salard D, Hoen B, *et al.* DRESS (Drug Rash with Eosinophilia and Systemic Symptoms) syndrome associated with nevirapine therapy. *Clin Infect Dis* 1998; **27**: 1321–2.

140. Grasset L, Guy C, Ollagnier M. Cyclines and acne: pay attention to adverse drug reactions! A recent literature review. *Rev Med Interne (Paris)* 2003; **24**: 305–16.

141. Marrakchi C, Kanoun F, Kilani B, *et al.* Allopurinol induced DRESS syndrome. *Rev Med Interne* 2004; **25**: 252–4.

142. Kennedy JI, Myers JL, Plumb VJ, Fulmer JD. Amiodarone pulmonary toxicity. Clinical, radiologic and pathologic correlations. *Arch Intern Med* 1987; **147**: 50–5.

143. Ansoborlo P, Constans J, Le Métayer P, Conri C. Pneumopathy caused by amiodarone in internal medicine: eight cases. *Rev Med Interne (Paris)* 1993; **14**: 698–704.

144. Malhorta A, Muse VV, Mark EJ. An 82-year-old man with dyspnea and pulmonary abnormalities. Case Records of the Massachusetts General Hospital – Case 12 – 2003. *N Engl J Med* 2003; **348**: 1574–85.

145. Donaldson L, Grant IS, Naysmith MR, Thomas JS. Acute amiodarone-induced lung toxicity. *Intensive Care Med* 1998; **24**: 626–30.

146. Handschin AE, Lardinois D, Schneiter D, *et al.* Acute amiodarone-induced pulmonary toxicity following lung resection. *Respiration* 2003; **70**: 310–12.

147. Saussine M, Colson P, Alauzen M, Mary H. Postoperative acute respiratory distress syndrome. A complication of amiodarone associated with 100 percent oxygen ventilation. *Chest* 1992; **102**: 980–1.

148. Hawthorne HR, Wood MA, Stambler BS, *et al.* Can amiodarone pulmonary toxicity be predicted in patients undergoing implantable cardioverter defibrillator implantation? *Pace* 1993; **16**: 2241–9.

149. van Mieghem W, Coolen L, Malysse I, *et al.* Amiodarone and the development of ARDS after lung surgery. *Chest* 1994; **105**: 1642–5.

150. Charles PE, Doise JM, Quenot JP, *et al.* Amiodarone-related acute respiratory distress syndrome following sudden withdrawal of steroids. *Respiration* 2006; **73**: 248–9.

151. Alonso-Fernandez A, Alvarez-Sala R, Mediano O, *et al.* Late postoperative amiodarone pulmonary toxicity. *An Med Interna* 2003; **20**: 419–20.

152. Kharabsheh S, Abendroth CS, Kozak M. Fatal pulmonary toxicity occurring within two weeks of initiation of amiodarone. *Am J Cardiol* 2002; **89**: 896–8.

153. Cohen AJ, King TE, Jr, Downey GP. Rapidly progressive bronchiolitis obliterans with organizing pneumonia. *Am J Respir Crit Care Med* 1994; **149**: 1670–5.

154. Nizami IY, Kissner DG, Vissher DW, Dubaybo BA. Idiopathic bronchiolitis obliterans with organizing pneumonia. An acute and life-threatening syndrome. *Chest* 1995; **108**: 271–7.

155. Baron FA, Hermanne J-P, Dowlati A, *et al.* Bronchiolitis obliterans organizing pneumonia and ulcerative colitis after allogeneic bone marrow transplantation. *Bone Marrow Transplant* 1998; **21**: 951–4.

156. Afessa B, Peters SG. Chronic lung disease after hematopoietic stem cell transplantation. *Clin Chest Med* 2005; **26**: 571–586, vi.

157. Beasley MB, Franks TJ, Galvin JR, *et al.* Acute fibrinous and organizing pneumonia. A histologic pattern of lung injury and possible variant of diffuse alveolar damage. *Arch Pathol Lab Med* 2002; **126**: 1064–70.

158. Coblyn JS, Weinblatt M. Acute interstitial pneumonitis and hypoxemia associated with rheumatoid arthritis. *Med Times* 1981; **109**: 58–62.

159. Leng PH, Murillo B, Fraire A. Acute interstitial pneumonitis occurring after consolidation chemotherapy with high-dose cytarabine for acute myelogenous leukemia. *Chest* 1999; **116**: 409–10.

160. Attar EC, Ervin T, Janicek M, *et al.* Acute interstitial pneumonitis related to gemcitabine. *J Clin Oncol* 2000; **18**: 697–8.

161. Ostor AJ, Crisp AJ, Somerville MF, Scott DG. Fatal exacerbation of rheumatoid arthritis associated fibrosing alveolitis in patients given infliximab. *BMJ* 2004; **329**: 1266.

162. Pakhale S, Moltyaner Y, Chamberlain D, Lazar N. Rapidly progressive pulmonary fibrosis in a patient treated with danazol for idiopathic thrombocytopenic purpura. *Can Respir J* 2004; **11**: 55–7.

163. Pratt DS, Schwartz MI, May JJ, Dreisin RB. Rapidly fatal pulmonary fibrosis: the accelerated variant of interstitial pneumonitis. *Thorax* 1979; **34**: 587–93.

164. Schwarz MI, Fontenot AP. Drug-induced diffuse alveolar hemorrhage syndromes and vasculitis. *Clin Chest Med* 2004; **25**: 133–40.

165. Rostand RA, Feldman RL, Block ER. Massive hemothorax complicating heparin anticoagulation for pulmonary embolus. *South Med J* 1977; **70**: 1128–30.

166. Choi HK, Merkel PA, Cohen-Tervaert JW, *et al.* Alternating antineutrophil cytoplasmic antibody specificity. Drug-induced vasculitis in a patient with Wegener's granulomatosis. *Arthritis Rheum* 1999; **42**: 384–8.

167. Rabadi SJ, Khandekar JD, Miller HJ. Mitomycin-induced hemolytic uremic syndrome: case presentation and review of the literature. *Cancer Treat Rep* 1982; **66**: 1244–7.

168. van der Lelie H, Baars JW, Rodenhuis S, *et al.* Hemolytic uremic syndrome after high dose chemotherapy with autologous stem cell support. *Cancer* 1995; **76**: 2338–42.

169. Teixeira L, Debourdeau P, Zammit C, *et al.* Gemcitabine-induced thrombotic microangiopathy. *Presse Med* 2002; **31**: 740–2.

170. Walter RB, Joerger M, Pestalozzi BC. Gemcitabine-associated hemolytic-uremic syndrome. *Am J Kidney Dis* 2002; **40**: 1–6.

171. Desramé J, Duvic C, Bredin C, *et al.* Hemolytic uremic syndrome as a complication of gemcitabine treatment: report of six cases and review of the literature. *Rev Med Interne (Paris)* 2005; **26**: 179–88.

172. Carlson K, Smedmyr B, Hagberg H, *et al.* Haemolytic uraemic syndrome and renal dysfunction following BEAC (BCNU, etoposide, ara-C, cyclophosphamide) +/- TBI and autologous BMT for malignant lymphomas. *Bone Marrow Transplant* 1993; **11**: 205–8.

173. White DA, Schwartzberg LS, Kris MG, Bosl GJ. Acute chest pain syndrome during bleomycin infusions. *Cancer* 1987; **59**: 1582–5.

174. Zijlstra EE, Wilson JHP, Ouwendijk RJT. Pleural fibrosis associated with ergotamine therapy. *Eur J Intern Med* 1990; **1**: 245–7.

175. Bateman DE. Carbamazepine induced systemic lupus erythematosus: case report. *Br Med J* 1985; **291**: 632–3.

176. Rubin RL. Drug-induced lupus. *Toxicology* 2005; **209**: 135–47.

177. Yano S, Shimada K. Vasospastic angina after chemotherapy by with carboplatin and etoposide in a patient with lung cancer. *Jpn Circulation J* 1996; **60**: 185–8.

178. Tsibiribi P, Descotes J, Lombard-Bohas C, *et al.* Cardiotoxicity of 5-fluorouracil in 1350 patients with no prior history of heart disease. *Bull Cancer* 2006; **93**: E27–30.

179. Cristofini P, Desnos M, Guenot O, *et al.* Cardiotoxicity of 5-fluorouracil: coronary spasm? Apropos of 2 cases with normal coronarography. *Ann Med Interne (Paris)* 1989; **140**: 9–13.

180. Dodick DW. Triptans and chest symptoms: the role of pulmonary vasoconstriction. *Cephalalgia* 2004; **24**: 298–304.

181. Uyarel H, Erden I, Cam N. Acute migraine attack, angina-like chest pain with documented ST-segment elevation and slow coronary flow. *Acta Cardiologica* 2005; **60**: 221–3.

182. Rich JA, Singer DE. Cocaine-related symptoms in patients presenting to an urban emergency department. *Ann Emerg Med* 1991; **20**: 616–21.

183. Olshaker JS. Cocaine chest pain. *Emerg Med Clin North Am* 1994; **12**: 391–6.

184. Pelz DM, Lownie SP, Fox AJ, Hutton LC. Symptomatic pulmonary complications from liquid acrylate embolization of brain arteriovenous malformations. *Am J Neuroradiol* 1995; **16**: 19–26.

185. Zeller FA, Cannan CR, Prakash UB. Thoracic manifestations after esophageal variceal sclerotherapy. *Mayo Clin Proc* 1991; **66**: 727–32.

186. Lauque D, Mazieres J, Rouzaud P, *et al.* Pulmonary

embolism in patients taking estrogen-progestagen oral contraceptives. *Presse Med* 1998; **27**: 1566–9.

187. Opatrny L, Warner MN. Risk of thrombosis in patients with malignancy and heparin-induced thrombocytopenia. *Am J Hematol* 2004; **76**: 240–4.

188. Shay DK, Fann LM, Jarvis WR. Respiratory distress and sudden death associated with receipt of a peripheral parenteral nutrition admixture. *Infect Control Hosp Epidemiol* 1997; **18**: 814–17.

189. Reedy JS, Kuhlman JE, Voytovich M. Microvascular pulmonary emboli secondary to precipitated crystals in a patient receiving total parenteral nutrition. A case report and description of the high-resolution CT findings. *Chest* 1999; **115**: 892–5.

190. Wesson DE, Rich RH, Zlotkin SH, Pencharz PB. Fat overload syndrome causing respiratory insufficiency. *J Pediatr Surg* 1984; **19**: 777–8.

191. Czauderna P, Zbrzezniak G, Narozanski W, *et al.* Pulmonary embolism: a fatal complication of arterial chemoembolization for advanced hepatocellular carcinoma. *J Pediatr Surg* 2005; **40**: 1647–50.

192. Fourme T, Vieillard-Baron A, Loubières Y, *et al.* Early fat embolism after liposuction. *Anesthesiology* 1998; **89**: 782–4.

193. Rothmann C, Ruschel N, Streiff R, *et al.* Fat pulmonary embolism after liposuction. *Ann Fr Anesth Reanim* 2006; **25**: 189–92.

194. Koessler MJ, Aebli N, Pitto RP. Fat and bone marrow embolism during percutaneous vertebroplasty. *Anesth Analg* 2003; **97**: 293.

195. Yoo KY, Jeong SW, Yoon W, Lee J. Acute respiratory distress syndrome associated with pulmonary cement embolism following percutaneous vertebroplasty with polymethylmethacrylate. *Spine* 2004; **29**: E294–7.

196. Righini M, Sekoranja L, Le GG, *et al.* Pulmonary cement embolism after vertebroplasty. *Thromb Haemost* 2006; **95**: 388–9.

197. Dicpinigaitis PV. Angiotensin-converting enzyme inhibitor-induced cough: ACCP evidence-based clinical practice guidelines. *Chest* 2006; **129**: 169S–173S.

198. Aggarwal P, Wali JP. Enalapril-induced cough in the emergency department. *J Emerg Med* 1992; **10**: 689–91.

199. Yemen TA. Small doses of sufentanil will produce violent coughing in young children. *Anesthesiology* 1998; **89**: 271–2.

200. Mitra S, Sinha PK, Anand LK, Gombar KK. Propofol-induced violent coughing. *Anaesthesia* 2000; **55**: 707–8.

201. Morelock SY, Sahn SA. Drugs and the pleura. *Chest* 1999; **116**: 212–21.

202. Huggins JT, Sahn SA. Drug-induced pleural disease. *Clin Chest Med* 2004; **25**: 141–54.

203. Camus P. Drug-induced pleural disease. In: Bouros D, ed. *Pleural Disorders*. New York: Marcel Dekker, 2004: 317–52.

Pneumothorax

JOHN E HEFFNER, JOHN T HUGGINS, STEVEN A SAHN

INTRODUCTION

Pneumothoraces occur in a variety of clinical settings and affect a heterogeneous population of patients. Each episode of pneumothorax, however, represents a potentially life-threatening respiratory emergency that requires prompt diagnosis and a thoughtful management approach. This strategy depends on a clear understanding of the type of pneumothorax that has occurred, its expected clinical course, and the patient's likelihood to experience a recurrence and ability to tolerate a recurrence were one to occur.

DEFINITIONS

A pneumothorax occurs when air collects within the pleural space. The presence of a pneumothorax indicates that either the visceral or parietal pleural membrane has been disrupted to allow air to flow from the atmosphere or an air-containing visceral structure into the pleural space.

Pneumothoraces are classified as spontaneous, traumatic, or iatrogenic (Box 12.1). Spontaneous pneumothoraces occur in the absence of any apparent traumatic injury to the chest. Traumatic pneumothoraces result from penetrating or blunt chest trauma or barotrauma, as occurs in scuba diving. Iatrogenic pneumothoraces are associated with procedures that injure pleural membranes or damage air-containing intrathoracic structures. Spontaneous pneumothoraces are further subdivided into primary (PSP) and secondary (SSP) pneumothoraces. Primary spontaneous pneumothoraces occur in patients without clinically apparent preexisting lung disease. Secondary spontaneous pneumothoraces occur in patients with a wide variety of underlying focal or diffuse pulmonary diseases that predispose to rupture of the airspaces and dissection of air through tissue planes into the pleural space.

Normal intrapleural pressures range from $-3.4\,cm\,H_2O$ during expiration to $-8\,cm\,H_2O$ during inspiration. Patients with persistent air leaks into the pleural space may develop

---

Box 12.1 Classification of pneumothorax

Spontaneous

- Primary – no clinical evidence of underlying lung disease
- Secondary – clinically apparent lung disease present

Traumatic

- Penetrating chest injury
- Blunt chest trauma
- Raised airway pressures (scuba diving)

Iatrogenic

- Transthoracic needle aspiration of the lung
- Placement of catheters into thoracic vasculature
- Thoracentesis and pleural biopsy
- Barotrauma related to mechanical ventilation
- Perforation of the esophagus

increasingly positive intrapleural pressures that compress intrathoracic structures and cause a tension pneumothorax.

INCIDENCE AND EPIDEMIOLOGY

Primary spontaneous pneumothorax occurs in 7.4–18 men and 1.2–6 women per 100 000 population per year.[1,2] Smoking increases risk 20-fold in men.[3] Peak occurrence is in tall, thin men younger than 30 years of age.

Secondary spontaneous pneumothorax has been reported to occur in 6.3 male and 2.0 female individuals per 100 000 population per year.[1] Patients most commonly present in the seventh decade of life, which parallels the age of peak prevalence of chronic lung disease in the general population. Patients with early-onset lung disease (e.g. cystic fibrosis and human immunodeficiency virus infection with *Pneumocystis carinii* pneumonia) present at an earlier age.[4] Major examples of the underlying lung conditions associated with

---

Box 12.2 Lung diseases associated with secondary spontaneous pneumothorax

Airway disease

- Chronic obstructive pulmonary disease
- Cystic fibrosis
- Status asthmaticus

Infectious lung disease

- *Pneumocystis carinii* pneumonia
- Necrotizing pneumonia

Interstitial lung disease

- Lymphangioleiomyomatosis
- Tuberous sclerosis
- Langerhans cell granulomatosis
- Sarcoidosis
- Idiopathic pulmonary fibrosis

Connective tissue disease

- Rheumatoid arthritis
- Ankylosing spondylitis
- Polymyositis and dermatomyositis
- Scleroderma
- Marfan syndrome
- Ehlers–Danlos syndrome

Cancer

- Sarcoma
- Lung cancer

Thoracic endometriosis (catamenial pneumothorax)

---

pneumothorax are listed in Box 12.2, with each category listed in decreasing order of frequency.

ETIOLOGY

Although the absence of clinically apparent lung disease is a defining feature of PSP, 56 percent to 100 percent of patients when examined by chest computed tomography or during surgery have apical, subpleural blebs.[5–10] The etiology of these blebs is unclear, but they may result from small airways inflammation from smoking that creates a ball-valve effect with hyperinflation and barotrauma to subpleural alveoli.[11] Some experts speculate that PSP occurs by rupture of these blebs with dissection of air along the bronchovascular sheath into the mediastinum with secondary rupture into the pleural space.[11,12] It is unclear that the detection of blebs or bullae by CT can guide decisions for surgery to prevent recurrence in patients after their first episode of PSP.[8] One study, however, found that 27 percent of patients with PSP and CT evidence of blebs in a contralateral lung experienced a contralateral pneumothorax within 5 years.[13] Secondary pneumothoraces result from pulmonary parenchymal defects associated with acute and chronic lung diseases that predispose patients to alveolar rupture. Airway obstruction increases the risk of pneumothorax from alveolar overdistension and localized air trapping.

Traumatic pneumothoraces occur from penetrating chest injuries that perforate the visceral pleura. They also occur with blunt chest trauma, which can cause sudden increases in airway pressure that rupture alveoli or injure the pulmonary parenchyma by shock waves that spread through the lung causing pulmonary lacerations. Barotrauma is another cause of traumatic pneumothorax that can occur with changes in ambient barometric pressures (scuba diving) or during positive pressure mechanical ventilation when ventilator assisted breaths overdistend and rupture alveoli.

CLINICAL PRESENTATION

Air within the pleural space compromises pulmonary function, because the ipsilateral lung operates at a decreased functional residual volume and tidal volume. The degree of respiratory compromise depends on the size of the pneumothorax and the severity of any underlying cardiopulmonary disease. Patients with normal lung function may tolerate a large pneumothorax with only minimal respiratory symptoms. Conversely, patients with severe baseline pulmonary impairment may have extreme dyspnea and life-threatening respiratory failure with small pneumothoraces.[14]

Most patients with PSP present with the sudden onset of pleuritic chest pain and dyspnea, which is usually mild because of the normal underlying lung function.[15] Even with the persistence of the pneumothorax, symptoms spontaneously improve or resolve within 24 hours. Patients may have mild tachycardia and tachypnea with a chest exam that varies with the size of the pneumothorax. A small pneumothorax (<20 percent of the volume of a hemithorax) usually does not cause abnormal chest findings. Large pneumothoraces produce increased chest resonance, decreased fremitus, and diminished breath sounds. Patients with SSP present with varying degrees of chest pain and dyspnea. Dyspnea may be profound even with small pneumothoraces depending on the severity of the underlying lung disease.[14,16,17] Physical findings are similar to those associated with PSP although patients with SSP are more likely to have evidence of cardiopulmonary compromise, such as hypoxemia, hypotension, cyanosis, labored breathing, altered mental status, and hypercapnia.[16–18]

With severe pneumothoraces, shift of mediastinal structures away from the pressurized hemithorax, depression of the ipsilateral diaphragm, decreased respiratory system compliance, and decreased venous return to the heart can depress cardiac output, cause respiratory failure, and rapidly progress to cardiopulmonary arrest. Patients with a tension pneumothorax may appear hemodynamically stable until they decompensate with sudden cardiopulmonary collapse.[19] Patients undergoing mechanical ventilation in the intensive care unit (ICU) are at special risk for a tension pneumothorax. In the presence of a bronchopleural fistula, positive pressure breaths increase the pressure gradient for inspired gases to enter the pleural space and raise intrapleural pressures. Pneumothoraces in patients being ventilated, therefore, are always managed aggressively with placement of an intercostal thoracostomy tube.

Patients without ongoing air leaks may spontaneously resolve a pneumothorax by reabsorption of intrapleural air. Approximately 1.25 percent of intrapleural gas can be reabsorbed across pleural membranes each day due to the gas pressure gradient between the pneumothorax and bloodstream.[20] A 15 percent pneumothorax, therefore, requires 12 days to reabsorb spontaneously.

Patients with spontaneous pneumothoraces have a high rate of spontaneous recurrence. From 16 percent to 52 percent of patients with PSP will have a recurrence[21,22] and 50 percent to 80 percent of patients will have a second recurrence. Approximately 40 percent to 50 percent of patients with an initial secondary spontaneous pneumothorax will have a recurrence.[21–23] Pneumothorax recurrence is especially concerning for patients with underlying lung disease considering that each episode may represent a life-threatening event. Management of pneumothorax, therefore, requires consideration of recurrence prevention in addition to initial management to reexpand the lung. The only intervention that can decrease the probability of a recurrence is one of the several techniques available to produce pleurodesis. Different management approaches to reexpand the lung, such as placement of a chest tube, removal of pleural air by a small

catheter or needle, or observation have no effect on the rate of pneumothorax recurrence. Decisions for pleurodesis rest on the probability of a recurrence and the probable risk to the patient if a repeated pneumothorax occurred.

INVESTIGATIONS

A standard posterioanterior and lateral chest radiograph is the initial diagnostic study for ambulatory patients with symptoms compatible with a pneumothorax. Demonstration of intrapleural air and a thin (<1 mm thick) visceral pleural stripe displaced away from the chest wall confirms the diagnosis. A 100 percent pneumothorax results in a perimediastinal density that consists of the airless lung (Fig. 12.1). Some clinicians recommend an expiratory chest radiograph for evaluation of suspected small pneumothoraces because compressed lung during expiration results in a greater difference in radiographic density between the lung and adjacent air-containing pleural space.[24,25] Other clinicians, however, argue that expiratory chest radiographs add little to the diagnostic accuracy of pneumothorax detection and should not be routinely obtained.[26] A decubitus film with the involved hemithorax in the nondependent position assists diagnosis for small pneumothoraces by allowing air to collect along the lateral chest wall. Cadaver studies indicate that lateral decubitus views have a similar sensitivity for detecting pneumothoraces

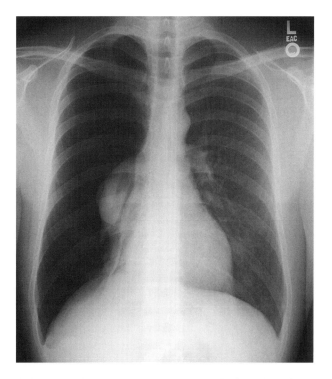

Figure 12.1 *Posteroanterior chest radiograph of a patient with a right-sided primary spontaneous pneumothorax. The lung appears completely collapsed as a right perimediastinal density.*

as chest CT.[27] In a blinded comparative study, however, Beres and Goodman demonstrated that radiologists detected 21 percent more pneumothoraces by examining the upright, expiratory radiographs compared with the decubitus exams.[25]

Detection of pneumothorax is problematic in critically ill patients in an ICU where portable chest films are obtained. Placement of a film or digital cassette against a patient's back for a portable chest radiograph may produce skin folds that simulate the radiographic appearance of a pneumothorax. A pneumothorax can be excluded, however, by noting the absence of the white, visceral pleural line that follows the contour of the chest wall. Supine and semi-recumbent portable chest radiographs in critically ill patients may not show a pleural line because intrapleural air collects in anteromedial and subpulmonic recesses rather than rising to the apex as with upright radiographs.[28] A high index of suspicion for pneumothorax is required by carefully examining the chest radiograph for auxiliary signs of pneumothorax (Figs 12.2 and 12.3; Box 12.3). Unfortunately, these signs are missed by radiologists in 30 percent and critical care physicians in 32 percent of instances, which increases the risk that diagnosis of a pneumothorax will be delayed until a tension pneumothorax occurs.[28–30] Tension pneumothoraces on chest radiographs demonstrate shift of mediastinal and diaphragmatic structures away from the pneumothorax (Fig. 12.4).

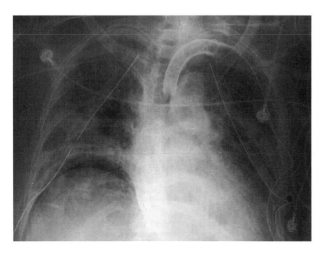

Figure 12.2   *Chest radiograph of a critically ill patient with a right-sided pneumothorax as demonstrated by a basilar collection of pleural air.*

Box 12.3 Chest radiographic signs that indicate or suggest a pneumothorax

- Evidence of air between the lung and chest wall
- Appearance of visceral pleural line shifted medially from the chest wall
- Hyperlucent hemithorax
- Contralateral mediastinal shift and diaphragmatic depression
- Loculated pneumothorax with localized hyperlucency lateral to or overlying the lung
- Deep costophrenic sulcus
- Pneumomediastinum
- Subcutaneous air
- Increased lucency over the upper quadrant of the abdomen
- Unusually sharp definition of the anterior diaphragmatic surface
- Interstitial pulmonary parenchymal air (rarely visualized)

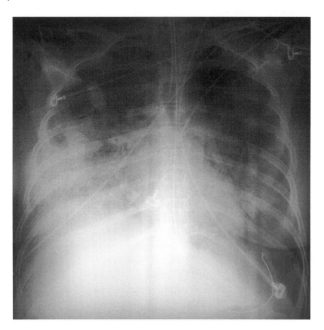

Figure 12.3   *Chest radiograph of a critically ill patient with a left-sided pneumothorax as demonstrated by the deep sulcus sign.*

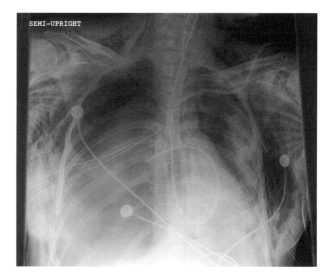

Figure 12.4   *Chest radiograph showing a right-sided tension pneumothorax with contralateral mediastinal shift to the left and diaphragmatic depression. Extensive subcutaneous emphysema is also noted.*

Portable chest radiographs may not detect pneumothoraces in patients with blunt and penetrating chest trauma because of the complexity of associated radiographic findings. The only radiographic manifestations of pneumothorax in these clinical settings may be indirect signs, such as pneumomediastinum or subcutaneous emphysema.

Ambulatory patients with emphysema may have bullae adjacent to the chest wall that can simulate pneumothorax. Most pneumothoraces, however, have a convex margin facing out toward the chest wall, while bullae have a concave surface. Waitches and coworkers described a 'double-wall sign' for detecting pneumothorax in patients with giant bullous emphysema.[31] Patients often require chest CT to discriminate between these two conditions and to avoid placement of an unnecessary intercostal thoracostomy tube.[32]

Findings on the standard chest radiograph can allow an estimation of the size of a pneumothorax. Collins and colleagues showed that a formula based on measurements from a standard inspiratory chest radiograph correlated closely with pneumothorax size as determined on a spiral CT scan (Fig. 12.5).[33] Most clinicians, however, find these systems awkward and use semi-quantitative measures of pneumothorax size that gauge the distance from the lung to the chest wall. One system describes pneumothoraces as small (<2 cm lung-to-chest wall distance) or large (>2 cm lung-to-chest wall distance).[34]

Chest CT is helpful in identifying or excluding small loculated pneumothoraces in patients with underlying lung disease (such as cystic fibrosis) that may obscure a rim of pleural air or simulate a pneumothorax by the presence of parenchymal cystic, cavitary, or bullous disease. Chest CT is also valuable in critically ill patients for detecting pleural air, which commonly collects in intrathoracic recesses that are not clearly imaged with supine radiographs. Chest CT is superior to standard chest radiographs in evaluating patients with blunt and penetrating chest trauma for the presence of pneumothorax.[35,36] Chest CT may suggest the presence of tracheobronchial rupture as a cause of pneumothorax by demonstrating an abnormal course of the mainstem bronchus or a 'fallen lung' sign. The latter sign demonstrates a collapsed lung in a dependent position, hanging on the hilum only by its vascular attachments.[37] Chest CT assists the evaluation of suspected chest tube misplacement that may be more likely to occur in emergency and critical care settings.

Bedside ultrasonography has emerged as an effective imaging modality for the rapid detection of pneumothorax in emergency and critical care settings to expedite patient resuscitation.[38–41] Ultrasonography had a sensitivity of 95 percent and a specificity of 91 percent for pneumothorax detection when used in critically ill patients in a medical ICU.[39] Rowan and coworkers demonstrated in trauma patients that ultrasonography was more sensitive than supine chest radiography and as sensitive as CT in the detection of traumatic pneumothoraces.[42] Dulchavsky and colleagues demonstrated similar utility of ultrasonography for patients with blunt and penetrating chest trauma.[41]

MANAGEMENT

The management of pneumothorax requires a high index of diagnostic suspicion based on a patient's clinical presentation, a rapid diagnosis with an appropriate chest imaging study, selection of a therapeutic approach for reexpanding the lung, and determination if an intervention is needed to prevent a recurrence. The initial management of pneumothorax depends on the existence and severity of underlying lung disease, the degree of cardiopulmonary symptoms on initial presentation, the presence or risk of a tension pneumothorax, and the existence of a persistent air leak. This section will review general considerations of care applicable to all patients with pneumothorax. Following sections will review specific approaches for patients with different types of pneumothorax.

Oxygen

High concentrations of inspired oxygen displace nitrogen from the bloodstream and increase the gradient for nitrogen from the pleural to the vascular space. This increased nitrogen gradient increases the reabsorption rate of intrapleural gas and the rapidity of resolution of a spontaneous pneumothorax by a factor of 4.[20] Supplemental

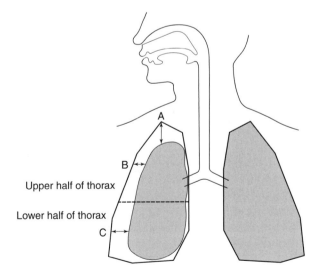

Figure 12.5 *Method for estimating pneumothorax size from a standard inspiratory chest radiograph. The hemithorax is divided into upper and lower halves. Measurements of the distance from the lung to inner chest wall in centimeters are taken at the apex of the chest (A) and midway in the upper (B) and lower (C) halves of the hemithorax. The percentage size of the pneumothorax = 4.2 + [4.7 × (A + B + C)].*

oxygen, therefore, should be administered to all hospitalized patients treated for pneumothorax.

Observation

Some patients who are clinically stable with a first-time, small PSP may be observed for pneumothorax resolution without a pleural drainage procedure. Reliable patients with ready access to emergency care may be discharged from an emergency department if the pneumothorax has not progressed after 6 hours of observation.[43] Close follow-up is required to ensure complete resolution of the pneumothorax. Patients should be thoroughly educated regarding the possibility of a recurrence and lifestyle issues to prevent serious complications if a pneumothorax were to recur (see below).

Most patients with SSP benefit from a pleurodesis procedure during hospitalization for the initial pneumothorax,[43] because a recurrent pneumothorax has lethal potential. Patients with small secondary pneumothoraces who refuse pleurodesis or have a poor prognosis may be carefully observed in an inpatient setting for stability of the pneumothorax. Observation is not appropriate for critically ill or trauma patients who develop a pneumothorax.

Simple catheter aspiration

Simple aspiration is performed by placing a small-caliber catheter into the pleural space with the withdrawal of air by a syringe. Simple aspiration may be successful in avoiding tube thoracostomy for 70–90 percent of patients with PSP.[44–46] Air is withdrawn until resistance is felt in drawing back on the syringe plunger and no more air can be removed. The need to aspirate more than 2.5 L of air predicts failure of this approach.[44] Simple aspiration has no utility for patients managed in the ICU with pneumothorax or patients with pneumothoraces due to trauma. Because of a low success rate (~30 percent) in older patients (>50 years) and patients with underlying lung disease,[47] simple aspiration has little utility in patients with SSP. Simple aspiration can be performed in the emergency department for patients with PSP with discharge of asymptomatic and previously healthy patients after a period of observation with close follow-up.

Tube thoracostomy

Placement of a tube thoracostomy for drainage of air from the pleural space is the primary mode of management for most patients who develop a pneumothorax. Tube thoracostomy is indicated for patients with PSP who fail simple aspiration, most patients with SSP, and all patients with traumatic pneumothoraces.

Various types of tube are used for intercostal drainage. In the absence of large air leaks, patients can be managed with a

10–14 Fr chest catheter placed in the anterior axillary or midclavicular line. Tubes can be placed with or without a Seldinger technique.[48] Appropriate candidates are patients with spontaneous pneumothorax or patients with a traumatic pneumothorax due to needle puncture of the lung (iatrogenic) who do not have intrapleural blood or large volumes of proteinaceous pleural fluid that could obstruct the tubes. Success of small-caliber tubes in these clinical settings is equivalent to larger (>20 Fr) chest tubes with success rates over 85 percent in appropriate patients.[49–53] Larger bore chest tubes (20–24 Fr) can be placed for patients who fail therapy with a small-caliber tube.

Larger-caliber tubes (20–36 Fr) are indicated for initial pleural drainage for patients who have traumatic pneumothorax due to penetrating and nonpenetrating injuries and patients who develop a pneumothorax while undergoing positive pressure ventilation. In all of these settings, large air leaks may exceed the flow capacity of small-caliber tubes and create risk of a tension pneumothorax. Patients with a hemopneumothorax after chest trauma require larger chest tubes (>4 Fr) to drain and monitor intrapleural blood.

Various methods exist for creating a one-way seal to prevent air from entering the chest through a thoracostomy tube. Patients with small air leaks and minimal fluid drainage can be managed with a Heimlich flutter valve attached to the end of the thoracostomy tube.[53–55] Attachment of a fluid collection bag with an exhaust valve for air has been successfully used for patients with pneumothorax who also drain pleural fluid.[56] Tension pneumothorax can occur if the valve becomes clogged with inspissated fluid drainage or if it is attached in error in a reversed orientation.[57] Heimlich valves allow patients with ongoing small air leaks to be discharged with outpatient follow-up. This use has application for patients who develop pneumothorax after needle biopsy of the lung,[58] patients with terminal conditions complicated by persistent pneumothorax,[59–61] and stable patients with a PSP.[54]

The traditional method for hospitalized patients to establish a one-way seal is with the use of an underwater drainage unit. These devices contain three elements:

- an underwater seal that prevents inflow of ambient air back into the chest and allows monitoring for an air leak as demonstrated by air bubbling through the unit
- a fluid collection chamber
- a suction chamber that allows adjustment of any negative pressure applied to the pleural space.

The resistance of these units to the flow of air from the pleural space varies by the manufacturer and unit model.[62] Pneumothoraces may fail to resolve and tension pneumothoraces may develop if the air leak through a bronchopleural fistula is greater than the flow capacity of the drainage unit.[62–64] Flow limitations may be clinically relevant for patients with large ongoing air leaks especially in the setting of positive pressure ventilation. Underwater drainage units are indicated for patients with pneumothorax who have large air leaks or who are draining volumes of pleural fluid that could obstruct the Heimlich flutter valve.

Placement of a thoracostomy tube anywhere within the hemithorax is acceptable for most patients with a pneumothorax in that air drains from an uncomplicated pleural space even when a chest tube is placed within a lobar fissure or in a dependent position.[65] Patients with acute edematous lung disease undergoing mechanical ventilation, however, may experience an ipsilateral recurrence of a pneumothorax when tubes are placed into interlobar fissures possibly because edematous lung occludes chest tube drainage ports.[66]

Suction applied to a newly placed chest tube is not required to promote lung reexpansion.[67] Theoretic concern exists that suction may perpetuate a bronchopleural fistula and air leak, although no comparative studies have examined this concern. Recent, prospective, randomized controlled trials of similar clinical settings to pneumothorax, post-lobectomy and post-thoracoscopy air leaks, support the practice of not routinely using suction by demonstrating that patients managed with water seal after surgery had a shorter period of air leak compared with those who had suction.[68–70] Only patients with large air leaks benefited from suction.[69] Chest tube suction is usually applied for pneumothorax when air leaks fail to resolve within 48 hours even if the lung has fully expanded to the chest wall.[34] Suction should be limited to 10–20 cm H_2O negative pressure by adjusting the fluid level or needle valve in a water seal unit.

Thoracostomy tubes should remain in place until the lung is fully reexpanded and the air leak has resolved. When these goals are achieved, the patient should be observed for 12–24 hours after resolution of the air leak to ensure that the pneumothorax will not recur. The chest tube is pulled when a final chest radiograph after the observation period confirms that the lung has remained expanded.

Some clinicians clamp the chest tube for the 12–24 hours after resolution of the air leak to establish that a small, unobserved air leak does not remain.[43,71] Other physicians promote a cardinal rule that chest tubes should never be clamped because a persistent air leak may result in a tension pneumothorax, and clamping a tube has no utility if the air leak has already resolved.[72] This debate can be resolved by individualizing care. Patients with a brief interval of a small air leak can undergo chest tube removal after resolution of an air leak for 12–24 hours with little risk that the pneumothorax will recur. Patients who have had a difficult clinical course with a prolonged or intermittent air leak may benefit from a final period of observation with the chest tube clamped to ensure resolution of the air leak. One should consider in this circumstance that pulling the chest tube does not differ from clamping the tube in regard to the risk of a tension pneumothorax. If physicians clamp chest tubes before removal, nursing staff must closely monitor the patient and immediately unclamp the tube at the first signs of respiratory distress.

Surgery and pleurodesis

Surgery for patients with pneumothorax has two primary objectives:

- management of persistent air leaks for patients in whom the pneumothorax does not resolve with chest tube drainage alone
- performance of a pleurodesis with or without resection or sealing of sources of air leaks, such as apical blebs, to prevent pneumothorax recurrence.

Several procedures exist to accomplish these goals. Open thoracotomy through a posterolateral incision with resection, stapling, or oversuturing of apical blebs is the historical approach to managing persistent air leaks.[73] Either pleural abrasion or parietal pleurectomy is performed to create a pleural symphysis to prevent pneumothorax recurrence.[74,75] Because of the postoperative morbidity of open thoracotomy related to the size of the incision, in the 1970s surgical techniques were developed that used smaller incisions. A limited, transaxillary thoracotomy employs a 6 cm incision in the axilla that spares major thoracic muscles yet provides adequate access for apical pleurectomy or pleural abrasion with stapling of apical blebs and bullae.[76–79] Both of these thoracotomy procedures provide effective therapy for persistent air leaks with a recurrence rate of less than 0.5 percent.[77,80]

Further efforts to develop minimally invasive techniques for treating pneumothorax resulted in the application of video-assisted thoracic surgery (VATS) to pneumothorax care.[6,81–83] This technique allows endoscopic stapling of apical blebs and bullae or partial pleurectomy. Pleurodesis can be performed by several techniques that include pleural abrasion or the insufflation of talc. Although VATS has become the preferred surgical technique for pneumothorax management in many centers,[43] only two randomized controlled trials have compared the outcomes from VATS with those of transaxillary thoracotomy.[75,84] These studies have not demonstrated any advantages of VATS in terms of resolution or recurrence rates of pneumothorax, operative times, or perioperative morbidity. Surgeons using VATS may have difficulty obtaining adequate access to the apical regions of the lung in patients with extensive blebs and bullae so that air leaks can be missed.[76] It appears that VATS is an acceptable surgical technique with a low rate of pneumothorax recurrence (<2 percent) for patients with PSP who do not have extensive apical blebs or bullae.[85] Limited transaxillary thoracotomy, however, may be the preferred technique for patients with secondary spontaneous pneumothorax who appear to require wide access to the apex of the lungs.[75] The role of VATS in pneumothorax treatment requires further study with larger randomized controlled trials.

Medical thoracoscopy with talc insufflation or pleural abrasion and resection of apical bullae less than 2 cm in size is a more limited procedure performed with local anesthesia through a single insertion site for instruments in the chest.[86–88]

Although no randomized controlled trials exist comparing medical thoracoscopy with VATS or limited thoracotomy, it has been reported to be successful in resolving air leaks and preventing recurrences in patients with PSP.[87,89,90] Patients can be converted to VATS with three insertion ports or a limited transaxillary thoracotomy if blebs larger than 2 cm are noted during medical thoracoscopy.

Chemical pleurodesis entails the instillation of various sclerosing agents, such as doxycycline or talc, through an intercostal thoracostomy tube to resolve or prevent a recurrence of a pneumothorax. Chemical pleurodesis is rarely effective in resolving persistent air leaks. Animal models suggest chemical pleurodesis can be successful in the presence of an air leak if the lung is fully reexpanded against the chest wall,[91] which is not often achieved in humans with ongoing air leaks. The recurrence rate with tetracycline pleurodesis is 25 percent,[21] which is well below the rates associated with surgical pleurodesis. Chemical pleurodesis for the management of pneumothorax is now reserved for patients who cannot or choose not to undergo surgery, such as some patients with end-stage human immunodeficiency virus (HIV) infection.[92]

Specific management issues for PSP

A small PSP (<15 percent) in patients with minimal symptoms can be observed for spontaneous resolution. After 6 hours of observation in an emergency department, young, healthy patients with a small PSP may be discharged with outpatient follow-up if their pneumothorax is not increasing in size. A larger or expanding PSP can be treated with simple aspiration[46] or insertion of a small-bore (7–14 Fr) intercostal catheter.[50,51,93,94] Many physicians prefer simple aspiration for PSP, because it can be performed in the emergency department with discharge, and follow-up if the pneumothorax resolves and does not recur in 6 hours.

Initial treatment with a small-bore catheter or placement of a small-bore catheter after a patient fails simple aspiration allows ambulation and discharge for compliant patients with attachment of a Heimlich flutter valve.[50,95] Catheter drainage is successful in 90 percent of patients with a first-time PSP.[96] Resolution of the air leak occurs within the first several days for 75 percent of patients and after 7–15 days in 80–90 percent of patients.[97,98] A surgical procedure to resolve the pneumothorax, therefore, is not needed in the large majority of patients. For the minority who have a persistent air leak after 7 days of chest tube drainage, a surgical procedure to resolve the pneumothorax and prevent a recurrence is justified.[11]

No empiric data guide the timing of a surgical procedure to prevent a recurrence of a PSP. Traditionally, most physicians have not recommended a pleurodesis procedure after the first pneumothorax because only 30–50 percent of patients have a recurrence. Pleurodesis is recommended, however, after the first recurrence because 50–80 percent will experience a third pneumothorax. This conservative

approach has been challenged by recent decision analyses of pneumothorax management.[99,100] In a prospective study, Tschopp and coworkers found that thoracoscopy with talcage was more cost-effective than tube thoracoscopy followed by follow-up observation for patients with PSP who failed simple aspiration.[99] Morimoto and colleagues did a decision analysis and determined that surgical thoracoscopy was the preferred therapy in terms of quality-adjusted life expectancy after the first episode of PSP in young men who failed simple aspiration.[100] Both of these analyses, however, demonstrate that treatment decisions need to be carefully individualized on the basis of patient wishes, available techniques for pleurodesis within an institution, and the institutional outcomes (success rates, morbidity, and mortality) of these techniques. Patients with occupations or interests that would put them at risk with a first recurrence, such as pilots or wilderness backpackers, are advised to have pleurodesis after the first pneumothorax.

Specific management issues for SSP

Simple aspiration has little utility in patients with SSP because of low success rates (~30 percent) and the high rate of pneumothorax recurrence even with successful initial aspiration.[47] Initial management requires consideration of combined goals of lung reexpansion and recurrence prevention. Because a recurrence in patients with moderate to severe underlying lung disease represents a potentially lethal event, many experts recommend a pleurodesis procedure with the first occurrence of a pneumothorax. If this approach is adopted, stable patients with tolerable respiratory symptoms can be referred for urgent VATS or limited thoracotomy without initial chest tube placement. Unstable or more seriously symptomatic patients can be managed with chest thoracostomy in preparation for pleurodesis.

If pleurodesis will be deferred until the first recurrence, patients are managed with chest thoracostomy. Patients with persistent air leaks are referred for surgical pleurodesis with resection, oversuturing, or stapling of the source of the air leaks. Timing of surgery for these patients requires individualization of care. In those patients with persistent air leaks, only 60–79 percent had resolved by the 15th day of chest tube drainage.[97,98] Many physicians, therefore, begin discussing surgery after 5–7 days of drainage and perform the procedure in good operative candidates at the first opportunity. Terminally ill patients or patients with excessive operative risk are managed with long-term intercostal catheters with Heimlich flutter valves.

Specific management issues for traumatic pneumothorax

Traumatic pneumothoraces occur in patients who sustain trauma and iatrogenic penetrating injuries to the chest wall or airways and in patients who experience marked increases in airway pressures that rupture lung tissue, as occurs with blunt chest trauma and mechanical ventilation. The specific manifestations and approaches to management of these varied conditions are beyond the scope of this chapter. In general, patients are treated with chest tube drainage with surgical interventions to repair bronchopleural fistulas reserved for those who fail initial management.

Pneumothoraces in patients managed in the ICU present special challenges to diagnosis because of concomitant cardiopulmonary conditions that can obscure the clinical and radiographic manifestations of pneumothorax. Kollef and coworkers reported that the following clinical features identify critically ill patients with pneumothorax who are at risk of misdiagnosis:

- mechanical ventilation
- an atypical radiographic location of the pneumothorax
- altered mental status
- development of pneumothorax after peak physician staffing hours.[29]

COMPLICATIONS

In addition to the cardiopulmonary complications of pneumothorax previously discussed, complications can result from pneumothorax management. Chest tube insertion is associated with several important complications. Misplaced intercostal tubes can perforate the lung, other intrathoracic structures including vasculature, and intraabdominal viscera.[101] Impingement of venous and cardiac structures can compromise cardiac output and cause cardiopulmonary arrest.[102] Chest tube misplacement occurs most commonly during emergency chest tube placement. Up to 3 percent of chest tubes placed for emergency indications are inserted into an extrathoracic location, and 6 percent are inserted into the lungs.[103] Interlobar positioning is a common occurrence that can in some circumstances interfere with drainage of intrapleural air.[66,104] Chest CT is the most accurate imaging technique to identify misplaced chest tubes.[105]

Pleural infections occur in 1–6 percent of patients undergoing chest tube placement with the highest risk in patients receiving chest tubes for trauma.[106] Reexpansion pulmonary edema in the ipsilateral lung due to increased pulmonary vascular permeability may occur with rapid drainage of pleural air.[107,108] Most patients with this condition have minor symptoms of dyspnea with primarily a radiographic expression of lung edema.[109] Up to 20 percent of patients may have a lethal outcome, however, with young age, a large pneumothorax, and long duration of collapse being risk factors for reexpansion pulmonary edema.[110] Slow

removal of intrapleural air in patients with large, chronic pneumothoraces and avoidance of chest tube suction in the first 48 hours of chest tube placement may decrease the incidence of reexpansion pulmonary edema.

The introduction of talc into the pleural space for pleurodesis has been reported to cause acute edematous lung injury.[111] This incidence of this complication, however, is low (<1 percent) and may not be due to talc *per se*.

FUTURE DIRECTIONS OF THERAPY

Minimally invasive techniques, such as medical thoracoscopy and VATS, have advanced the treatment of spontaneous pneumothorax. The adoption of smaller-caliber catheters as opposed to standard surgical chest tubes have also improved the early management of pneumothorax. Future advances in care depend on clinical trials and decision analyses that will assist clinicians in individualizing care for the heterogeneous population of patients who present with pneumothorax. The emergence of clinical practice guidelines on pneumothorax care has assisted the standardization of treatment decisions. But further understanding of the impact of different modalities of care on recurrence rates, quality of life, cost, and time to resolution will improve the clinician's ability to adopt ideal therapy for the individual patient.

Key learning points

- Pneumothoraces are classified as spontaneous or traumatic, with spontaneous pneumothoraces being classified as either primary in patients without clinically apparent lung disease or secondary in patients with a variety of parenchymal lung disorders.

- Spontaneous pneumothoraces occur as a result of air-trapping within lung regions that cause alveolar rupture.

- The management of spontaneous pneumothorax depends on its underlying etiology. Spontaneous primary pneumothoraces often respond to observation or conservative therapy and secondary pneumothoraces require definitive therapy to prevent life-threatening recurrences.

- Pneumothoraces commonly recur in patients with spontaneous pneumothorax with the likelihood of recurrence increasing with each subsequent pneumothorax.

- Pleurodesis causes a symphysis of the parietal with visceral pleurae and is indicated for patients with a high probability of recurrence or a risk of life-threatening complications were a pneumothorax to recur.

REFERENCES

1. Melton LJ, 3rd, Hepper NG, Offord KP. Incidence of spontaneous pneumothorax in Olmsted County, Minnesota: 1950 to 1974. *Am Rev Respir Dis* 1979; **120**: 1379–82.

2. Bense L, Eklund G, Wiman LG. Smoking and the increased risk of contracting spontaneous pneumothorax. *Chest* 1987; **92**: 1009–12.

3. Gobbel WGJ, Jr, RWG, Nelson IA, Daniel RAJ. Spontaneous pneumothorax. *J Thorac Cardiovasc Surg* 1963; **46**: 331–45.

4. Primrose WR. Spontaneous pneumothorax: a retrospective review of aetiology, pathogenesis and management. *Scott Med J* 1984; **29**: 15–20.

5. Nkere UU, Griffin SC, Fountain SW. Pleural abrasion: a new method of pleurodesis. *Thorax* 1991; **46**: 596–8.

6. Hazelrigg SR, Landreneau RJ, Mack M, *et al.* Thoracoscopic stapled resection for spontaneous pneumothorax. *J Thorac Cardiovasc Surg* 1993; **105**: 389–92.

7. Inderbitzi RG, Leiser A, Furrer M, Althaus U. Three years' experience in video-assisted thoracic surgery (VATS) for spontaneous pneumothorax. *J Thorac Cardiovasc Surg* 1994; **107**: 1410–15.

8. Smit HJ, Wienk MA, Schreurs AJ, *et al.* Do bullae indicate a predisposition to recurrent pneumothorax? *Br J Radiol* 2000; **73**: 356–9.

9. Mitlehner W, Friedrich M, Dissmann W. Value of computer tomography in the detection of bullae and blebs in patients with primary spontaneous pneumothorax. *Respiration* 1992; **59**: 221–7.

10. Lesur O, Delorme N, Fromaget JM, *et al.* Computed tomography in the etiologic assessment of idiopathic spontaneous pneumothorax. *Chest* 1990; **98**: 341–7.

11. Sahn SA, Heffner JE. Spontaneous pneumothorax. *N Engl J Med* 2000; **342**: 868–74.

12. Ohata M, Suzuki H. Pathogenesis of spontaneous pneumothorax. With special reference to the ultrastructure of emphysematous bullae. *Chest* 1980; **77**: 771–6.

13. Sihoe AD, Yim AP, Lee TW, *et al.* Can CT scanning be used to select patients with unilateral primary spontaneous pneumothorax for bilateral surgery? *Chest* 2000; **118**: 380–3.

14. Tanaka F, Itoh M, Esaki H, *et al.* Secondary spontaneous pneumothorax. *Ann Thorac Surg* 1993; **55**: 372–6.

15. Seremetis MG. The management of spontaneous pneumothorax. *Chest* 1970; **57**: 65–8.

16. Dines DE, Clagett OT, Payne WS. Spontaneous pneumothorax in emphysema. *Mayo Clin Proc* 1970; **45**: 481–7.

17. Shields TW, Oilschlager GA. Spontaneous pneumothorax in patients 40 years of age and older. *Ann Thorac Surg* 1966; **2**: 377–383.

18. George RB, Herbert SJ, Shames JM, *et al.* Pneumothorax complicating pulmonary emphysema. *JAMA* 1975; **234**: 389–93.

19. Holloway VJ, Harris JK. Spontaneous pneumothorax: is it under tension? *J Accid Emerg Med* 2000; **17**: 222–3.

20. Northfield TC. Oxygen therapy for spontaneous pneumothorax. *Br Med J* 1971; **4**: 86–8.

21. Light RW, O'Hara VS, Moritz TE, *et al.* Intrapleural tetracycline for the prevention of recurrent spontaneous pneumothorax. Results of a Department of Veterans Affairs cooperative study. *JAMA* 1990; **264**: 2224–30.

22. Lippert HL, Lund O, Blegvad S, Larsen HV. Independent risk factors for cumulative recurrence rate after first spontaneous pneumothorax. *Eur Respir J* 1991; **4**: 324–31.

23. Videm V, Pillgram-Larsen J, Ellingsen O, *et al.* Spontaneous pneumothorax in chronic obstructive pulmonary disease: complications, treatment and recurrences. *Eur J Respir Dis* 1987; **71**: 365–71.

24. Bradley M, Williams C, Walshaw MJ. The value of routine expiratory chest films in the diagnosis of pneumothorax. *Arch Emerg Med* 1991; **8**: 115–16.

25. Beres RA, Goodman LR. Pneumothorax: detection with upright versus decubitus radiography. *Radiology* 1993; **186**: 19–22.

26. Schramel FM, Golding RP, Haakman CD, *et al.* Expiratory chest radiographs do not improve visibility of small apical pneumothoraces by enhanced contrast. *Eur Respir J* 1996; **9**: 406–9.

27. Carr JJ, Reed JC, Choplin RH, *et al.* Plain and computed radiography for detecting experimentally induced pneumothorax in cadavers: implications for detection in patients. *Radiology* 1992; **183**: 193–9.

28. Tocino IM, Miller MH, Fairfax WR. Distribution of pneumothorax in the supine and semirecumbent critically ill adult. *AJR Am J Roentgenol* 1985; **144**: 901–5.

29. Kollef MH. Risk factors for the misdiagnosis of pneumothorax in the intensive care unit. *Crit Care Med* 1991; **19**: 906–10.

30. Kollef MH. The effect of an increased index of suspicion on the diagnosis of pneumothorax in the critically ill. *Mil Med* 1992; **157**: 591–3.

31. Waitches GM, Stern EJ, Dubinsky TJ. Usefulness of the double-wall sign in detecting pneumothorax in patients with giant bullous emphysema. *AJR Am J Roentgenol* 2000; **174**: 1765–8.

32. Bourgouin P, Cousineau G, Lemire P, Hebert G. Computed tomography used to exclude pneumothorax in bullous lung disease. *J Can Assoc Radiol* 1985; **36**: 341–2.

33. Collins CD, Lopez A, Mathie A, Wood V, Jackson JE, Roddie ME. Quantification of pneumothorax size on chest radiographs using interpleural distances: regression analysis based on volume measurements from helical CT. *AJR Am J Roentgenol* 1995; **165**: 1127–30.

◆ 34. Henry M, Arnold T, Harvey J. BTS guidelines for the management of spontaneous pneumothorax. *Thorax* 2003; **58**(Suppl 2): ii39–ii52.

35. Guerrero-Lopez F, Vazquez-Mata G, Alcazar-Romero PP, *et al.* Evaluation of the utility of computed tomography in the initial assessment of the critical care patient with chest trauma. *Crit Care Med* 2000; **28**: 1370–5.

36. Omert L, Yeaney WW, Protetch J. Efficacy of thoracic computerized tomography in blunt chest trauma. *Am Surg* 2001; **67**: 660–4.

37. Wintermark M, Schnyder P, Wicky S. Blunt traumatic rupture of a mainstem bronchus: spiral CT demonstration of the 'fallen lung' sign. *Eur Radiol* 2001; **11**: 409–11.

38. Sistrom CL, Reiheld CT, Gay SB, Wallace KK. Detection and estimation of the volume of pneumothorax using real-time sonography: efficacy determined by receiver operating characteristic analysis. *AJR Am J Roentgenol* 1996; **166**: 317–21.

39. Lichtenstein DA, Menu Y. A bedside ultrasound sign ruling out pneumothorax in the critically ill. Lung sliding. *Chest* 1995; **108**: 1345–8.

40. Chan SS. Emergency bedside ultrasound to detect pneumothorax. *Acad Emerg Med* 2003; **10**: 91–4.

41. Dulchavsky SA, Schwarz KL, Kirkpatrick AW, *et al.* Prospective evaluation of thoracic ultrasound in the detection of pneumothorax. *J Trauma* 2001; **50**: 201–5.

42. Rowan KR, Kirkpatrick AW, Liu D, *et al.* Traumatic pneumothorax detection with thoracic US: correlation with chest radiography and CT – initial experience. *Radiology* 2002; **225**: 210–14.

◆ 43. Baumann MH, Strange C, Heffner JE, *et al.* Management of spontaneous pneumothorax: an American College of Chest Physicians Delphi consensus statement. *Chest* 2001; **119**: 590–602.

◆ 44. Soulsby T. British Thoracic Society guidelines for the management of spontaneous pneumothorax: do we comply with them and do they work? *J Accid Emerg Med* 1998; **15**: 317–21.

45. Packham S, Jaiswal P. Spontaneous pneumothorax: use of aspiration and outcomes of management by respiratory and general physicians. *Postgrad Med J* 2003; **79**: 345–7.

46. Noppen M, Alexander P, Driesen P, Slabbynck H, Verstraeten A. Manual aspiration versus chest tube drainage in first episodes of primary spontaneous pneumothorax: a multicenter, prospective, randomized pilot study. *Am J Respir Crit Care Med* 2002; **165**: 1240–4.

● 47. Archer GJ, Hamilton AA, Upadhyay R, Finlay M, Grace PM. Results of simple aspiration of pneumothoraces. *Br J Dis Chest* 1985; **79**: 177–82.

48. Argall J, Desmond J. Seldinger technique chest drains and complication rate. *Emerg Med J* 2003; **20**: 169–70.

● 49. Bevelaqua FA, Aranda C. Management of spontaneous pneumothorax with small lumen catheter manual aspiration. *Chest* 1982; **81**: 693–4.

50. Conces DJ, Tarver RD, Gray WC, Pearcy EA. Treatment of pneumothoraces utilizing small caliber chest tubes. *Chest* 1988; **94**: 55–7.

51. Minami H, Saka H, Senda K, *et al.* Small caliber catheter drainage for spontaneous pneumothorax. *Am J Med Sci* 1992; **304**: 345–7.

52. Tattersall DJ, Traill ZC, Gleeson FV. Chest drains: does size matter? *Clin Radiol* 2000; **55**: 415–21.

53. Niemi T, Hannukainen J, Aarnio P. Use of the Heimlich valve for treating pneumothorax [in process citation]. *Ann Chir Gynaecol* 1999; **88**: 36–7.

54. Campisi P, Voitk AJ. Outpatient treatment of spontaneous pneumothorax in a community hospital using a Heimlich flutter valve: a case series. *J Emerg Med* 1997; **15**: 115–19.

● 55. Bernstein A, Waqaruddin M, Shah M. Management of spontaneous pneumothorax using a Heimlich flutter valve. *Thorax* 1973; **28**: 386–9.

56. Lodi R, Stefani A. A new portable chest drainage device. *Ann Thorac Surg* 2000; **69**: 998–1001.

57. Spouge AR, Thomas HA. Tension pneumothorax

after reversal of a Heimlich valve. *AJR Am J Roentgenol* 1992; **158**: 763–4.

58. Dennie CJ, Matzinger FR, Marriner JR, Maziak DE. Transthoracic needle biopsy of the lung: results of early discharge in 506 outpatients. *Radiology* 2001; **219**: 247–51.

59. Trachiotis GD, Vricella LA, Alyono D, *et al.* Management of AIDS-related pneumothorax. *Ann Thorac Surg* 1996; **62**: 1608–13.

60. Vricella LA, Trachiotis GD. Heimlich valve in the management of pneumothorax in patients with advanced AIDS. *Chest* 2001; **120**: 15–18.

61. Van Hengel P, Van de Bergh JH. Heimlich valve treatment and outpatient management of bilateral metastatic pneumothorax. *Chest* 1994; **105**: 1586–7.

62. Baumann MH, Patel PB, Roney CW, Petrini MF. Comparison of function of commercially available pleural drainage units and catheters. *Chest* 2003; **123**: 1878–86.

63. Capps JS, Tyler ML, Rusch VW, Pierson DJ. Potential of chest drainage units to evacuate broncho-pleural air leaks. *Chest* 1985; **88**: 57S.

64. Baumann MH. What size chest tube? What drainage system is ideal? And other chest tube management questions. *Curr Opin Pulm Med* 2003; **9**: 276–81.

65. Curtin JJ, Goodman LR, Quebbeman EJ, Haasler GB. Thoracostomy tubes after acute chest injury: relationship between location in a pleural fissure and function. *AJR Am J Roentgenol* 1994; **163**: 1339–42.

66. Heffner JE, McDonald J, Barbieri C. Recurrent pneumothoraces in ventilated patients despite ipsilateral chest tubes. *Chest* 1995; **108**: 1053–8.

67. So SY, Yu DY. Catheter drainage of spontaneous pneumothorax: suction or no suction, early or late removal? *Thorax* 1982; **37**: 46–8.

68. Marshall MB, Deeb ME, Bleier JI, *et al.* Suction vs water seal after pulmonary resection: a randomized prospective study. *Chest* 2002; **121**: 831–5.

69. Cerfolio RJ, Bass C, Katholi CR. Prospective randomized trial compares suction versus water seal for air leaks. *Ann Thorac Surg* 2001; **71**: 1613–17.

70. Ayed AK. Suction versus water seal after thoracoscopy for primary spontaneous pneumothorax: prospective randomized study. *Ann Thorac Surg* 2003; **75**: 1593–6.

71. Gupta N. Pneumothorax: is chest tube clamp necessary before removal? *Chest* 2001; **119**: 1292–3.

72. Weissberg D, Refaely Y. Pneumothorax: experience with 1,199 patients. *Chest* 2000; **117**: 1279–85.

73. Saha SP, Arrants JE, Kosa A, Lee WH, Jr. Management of spontaneous pneumothorax. *Ann Thorac Surg* 1975; **19**: 561–4.

74. Thevenet F, Gamondes JP, Bodzongo D, Balawi A. Spontaneous and recurrent pneumothorax. Surgical treatment. Apropos of 278 cases. *Ann Chir* 1992; **46**: 165–9.

75. Waller DA, Forty J, Morritt GN. Video-assisted thoracoscopic surgery versus thoracotomy for spontaneous pneumothorax. *Ann Thorac Surg* 1994; **58**: 372–6.

76. Horio H, Nomori H, Fuyuno G, Kobayashi R, Suemasu K. Limited axillary thoracotomy vs video-assisted thoracoscopic surgery for spontaneous pneumothorax. *Surg Endosc* 1998; **12**: 1155–8.

77. Murray KD, Matheny RG, Howanitz EP, Myerowitz PD. A limited axillary thoracotomy as primary treatment for recurrent spontaneous pneumothorax. *Chest* 1993; **103**: 137–42.

78. Becker RM, Munro DD. Transaxillary minithoracotomy: the optimal approach for certain pulmonary and mediastinal lesions. *Ann Thorac Surg* 1976; **22**: 254–9.

79. Deslauriers J, Beaulieu M, Despres JP, *et al.* Transaxillary pleurectomy for treatment of spontaneous pneumothorax. *Ann Thorac Surg* 1980; **30**: 569–74.

80. Weeden D, Smith G. Surgical experience in the management of spontaneous pneumothorax. *Thorax* 1983; **38**: 737–43.

81. Cannon WB, Vierra MA, Cannon A. Thoracoscopy for spontaneous pneumothorax. *Ann Thorac Surg* 1993; **56**: 686–7.

82. Inderbitzi R, Furrer M. The surgical treatment of spontaneous pneumothorax by video-thoracoscopy. *Thorac Cardiovasc Surg* 1992; **40**: 330–3.

83. Nathanson LK, Shimi SM, Wood RA, Cuschieri A. Videothoracoscopic ligation of bulla and pleurectomy for spontaneous pneumothorax. *Ann Thorac Surg* 1991; **52**: 316–19.

84. Kim KH, Kim HK, Han JY, *et al.* Transaxillary minithoracotomy versus video-assisted thoracic surgery for spontaneous pneumothorax. *Ann Thorac Surg* 1996; **61**: 1510–12.

85. Yim AP, Liu HP. Video assisted thoracoscopic management of primary spontaneous pneumothorax. *Surg Laparosc Endosc* 1997; **7**: 236–40.

86. Boutin C, Loddenkemper R, Astoul P. Diagnostic and therapeutic thoracoscopy: techniques and indications in pulmonary medicine. *Tubercle Lung Dis* 1993; **74**: 225–39.

◆ 87. Boutin C, Astoul P, Rey F, Mathur PN. Thoracoscopy in the diagnosis and treatment of spontaneous pneumothorax. *Clin Chest Med* 1995; **16**: 497–503.

◆ 88. Mathur PN, Astoul P, Boutin C. Medical thoracoscopy. Technical details. *Clin Chest Med* 1995; **16**: 479–86.

89. Tschopp JM, Brutsche M, Frey JG. Treatment of complicated spontaneous pneumothorax by simple talc pleurodesis under thoracoscopy and local anaesthesia. *Thorax* 1997; **52**: 329–32.

90. Milanez JR, Vargas FS, Filomeno LT, *et al.* Intrapleural talc for the prevention of recurrent pneumothorax. *Chest* 1994; **106**: 1162–5.

91. Macoviak JA, Stephenson LW, Ochs R, Edmunds LH, Jr. Tetracycline pleurodesis during active pulmonary-pleural air leak for prevention of recurrent pneumothorax. *Chest* 1982; **81**: 78–81.

92. Read CA, Reddy VD, O'Mara TE, Richardson MS. Doxycycline pleurodesis for pneumothorax in patients with AIDS. *Chest* 1994; **105**: 823–5.

93. Martin T, Fontana G, Olak J, Ferguson M. Use of pleural catheter for the management of simple pneumothorax. *Chest* 1996; **110**: 1169–72.

94. Casola G, vanSonnenberg E, Keightley A, *et al.* Pneumothorax: radiologic treatment with small catheters. *Radiology* 1988; **166**(1 Pt 1): 89–91.

95. Ponn RB, Silverman HJ, Federico JA. Outpatient chest tube management. *Ann Thorac Surg* 1997; **64**: 1437–40.

96. Jain SK, Al-Kattan KM, Hamdy MG. Spontaneous pneumothorax: determinants of surgical intervention. *J Cardiovasc Surg (Torino)* 1998; **39**: 107–11.

97. Chee CB, Abisheganaden J, Yeo JK, *et al.* Persistent air-leak in spontaneous pneumothorax – clinical course and outcome. *Respir Med* 1998; **92**: 757–61.

98. Schoenenberger RA, Haefeli WE, Weiss P, Ritz RF. Timing of invasive procedures in therapy for primary and secondary spontaneous pneumothorax. *Arch Surg* 1991; **126**: 764–6.

99. Tschopp JM, Boutin C, Astoul P, *et al.* Talcage by medical thoracoscopy for primary spontaneous pneumothorax is more cost-effective than drainage: a randomised study. *Eur Respir J* 2002; **20**: 1003–9.

● 100. Morimoto T, Fukui T, Koyama H, *et al.* Optimal strategy for the first episode of primary spontaneous pneumothorax in young men. A decision analysis. *J Gen Intern Med* 2002; **17**: 193–202.

◆ 101. Miller KS, Sahn SA. Chest tubes. Indications, technique, management and complications. *Chest* 1987; **91**: 258–64.

102. Hesselink DA, Van Der Klooster JM, Bac EH, *et al.* Cardiac tamponade secondary to chest tube placement. *Eur J Emerg Med* 2001; **8**: 237–9.

103. Baldt MM, Bankier AA, Germann PS, *et al.* Complications after emergency tube thoracostomy: assessment with CT. *Radiology* 1995; **195**: 539–43.

104. Maurer JR, Friedman PJ, Wing VW. Thoracostomy tube in an interlobar fissure: radiologic recognition of a potential problem. *AJR Am J Roentgenol* 1982; **139**: 1155–61.

105. Gayer G, Rozenman J, Hoffmann C, *et al.* CT diagnosis of malpositioned chest tubes. *Br J Radiol* 2000; **73**: 786–90.

106. Chan L, Reilly KM, Henderson C, *et al.* Complication rates of tube thoracostomy. *Am J Emerg Med* 1997; **15**: 368–70.

107. Shanahan MX, Monk I, Richards HJ. Unilateral pulmonary oedema following re-expansion of pneumothorax. *Anaesth Intensive Care* 1975; **3**: 19–30.

● 108. Steckel RJ. Unilateral pulmonary edema after pneumothorax. *N Engl J Med* 1973; **289**: 621–2.

109. Matsuura Y, Nomimura T, Murakami H, *et al.* Clinical analysis of reexpansion pulmonary edema. *Chest* 1991; **100**: 1562–6.

◆ 110. Sherman SC. Reexpansion pulmonary edema: a case report and review of the current literature. *J Emerg Med* 2003; **24**: 23–7.

111. Scalzetti EM. Unilateral pulmonary edema after talc pleurodesis. *J Thorac Imaging* 2001; **16**: 99–102.

Pulmonary embolism

VICTOR F TAPSON, STEVEN DEITELZWEIG

INTRODUCTION

Syndromes characterized by embolization of material into the pulmonary venous circulation causing cardiopulmonary dysfunction are of special interest to the critical care practitioner. This chapter focuses on venous thromboembolic disease with a particular emphasis on pulmonary embolism (PE). Emboli of nonthrombotic material (e.g. fat, amniotic fluid, air, septic material, and tumor) are also discussed. Although prevention is a crucial issue and will be discussed, diagnosis and treatment will be major considerations based upon the respiratory emergency focus.

Most frequently, PE results from proximal lower extremity deep venous thrombosis (DVT), but upper extremity thrombi (particularly common in patients with central venous catheters) may also embolize. Despite recent advances in the prevention, diagnosis, and treatment of venous thromboembolism (VTE), PE is frequently missed and often fatal. Suspected PE is a common consideration in the emergency department as well as in hospitalized patients or those already in the intensive care unit. Patients may present with a wide range of symptoms including dyspnea, chest pain, cough, hemoptysis, and syncope. In the intensive care unit, a critically ill patient may present with a sudden change in oxygenation or hemodynamics. Identifying the presence of risk factors for VTE is key in suspecting the diagnosis and identifying prophylactic needs. Accurate diagnosis followed by effective therapy unequivocally reduces the morbidity and mortality of PE. Instituting appropriate prophylaxis is crucial.

EPIDEMIOLOGY

Venous thromboembolism is a major cause of morbidity and mortality worldwide. Pulmonary embolism afflicts over 500 000 Americans annually, causing 10 percent of all inhospital deaths, and remains the single most important cause of maternal deaths associated with live births in the United States. Given that only a third of proximal DVT cases are clinically recognized, the actual rate may be as high as 2 million per year. It is also estimated that 600 000 patients develop PE in the United States each year and that 60 000–200 000 die from PE.[1–4] Unfortunately, autopsy studies continue to show that most cases of fatal PE are not recognized and diagnosed.[5,6]

While acute fatal PE is our primary concern, there are long-term, morbid sequelae of DVT including postthrombotic syndrome characterized by chronic pain, edema, or ulceration of the lower extremities. This may develop in 30 percent of patients within 8 years of an initial venous thrombotic event and results in substantial cost for its management.[7] Chronic thromboembolic pulmonary hypertension represents another severe result of acute VTE. A recent Italian study suggests that the incidence of chronic thromboembolic pulmonary hypertension after known acute PE was 1 percent at 6 months, 3.1 percent at 1 year, and 3.8 percent at 2 years,[8] which appears higher than previously expected.

PATHOGENESIS

Venous thrombi commonly form along the valve cusps within the soleal sinuses of the calf. These thrombi may quickly overwhelm the endogenous fibrinolytic system. The propensity of a thrombus to propagate and/or embolize is greatest during the first 7 days. Once the thrombus is fully organized, there is less opportunity for propagation. Later, during recanalization, peripheral sinuses appear between the thrombus and the vein wall. The dilation and coalescence of these sinuses in addition to the onset of thrombus fibrosis further augments irregular and often irreversible injury to the intima. The concomitant valve damage can potentiate chronic venous insufficiency, postthrombotic syndrome, and/or recurrent venous thrombosis.

The risk of developing VTE is directly related to the three pathologic factors first identified by Rudolph Virchow in the nineteenth century. These include venous endothelial damage, localized or systemic hypercoagulability, and stasis of venous blood.[9] Risk factors for VTE are derived from these and a list is offered in Box 13A.1.

Ventilation/perfusion ($\dot{V}Q$) mismatch is the principal physiologic effect of PE, and leads to hypoxemia in 85 percent of patients. The hemodynamic response to PE is variable depending on the degree of occlusion of the pulmonary arterial bed, and on underlying cardiovascular disease. The resultant decrease in the cross-sectional area of the pulmonary arterial bed causes an increase in the pulmonary vascular resistance. This impedes right ventricular outflow and reduces left ventricular preload, decreasing cardiac output. In patients without underlying cardiopulmonary disease, greater than 50 percent obstruction of the pulmonary circulation is generally required for a significant increase in the mean pulmonary arterial pressure. Patients with underlying cardiopulmonary disease have less physiologic reserve. When the extent of obstruction of the pulmonary circulation approaches 75 percent, the right ventricle must generate a systolic pressure in excess of 50 mm Hg and a mean pulmonary artery pressure of greater than 40 mm Hg to preserve pulmonary perfusion. A normal right ventricle cannot achieve this and fails.[11]

DIAGNOSING VENOUS THROMBOEMBOLISM: PRELIMINARY TESTING

The key to the diagnosis of DVT and PE begins with clinical suspicion. The diagnostic technology for acute DVT has

---

Box 13A.1 Risk factors for venous thromboembolism

- Increasing age (>40 years)
- Prolonged immobility
- Stroke
- Paralysis
- Previous venous thromboembolism
- Cancer and its treatment
- Major surgery (especially involving the abdomen, pelvis, lower extremities)
- Trauma (particularly fractures of the pelvis, hip, leg)
- Congenital or acquired thrombophilic disorders (e.g. activated protein C resistance, antiphospholipid antibodies, protein C and S deficiency, antithrombin deficiency, dysfibrinogenemia)
- Severe infection
- Obesity
- Varicose veins
- Congestive heart failure
- Indwelling central venous catheters
- Inflammatory bowel disease
- Nephrotic syndrome
- Pregnancy
- Estrogen use
- Recent myocardial infarction
- Chronic respiratory disease

Used with permission from Deitelzweig SB, Vanscoy GJ, Niccolai CS, Rihn TL. Venous thrombolemboism prevention with LMWHs in medical and orthopedic surgery patients. *Ann Pharmacother* 2003:37;402–11.[10]

---

evolved considerably with the advent of compression ultrasound. For PE, $\dot{V}Q$ scanning, often followed by pulmonary arteriography, had been the gold standard approach for decades. Spiral (helical) computed tomography (CT) is now the procedure of choice for suspected PE at most US medical centers. The presence of risk factors as part of the history and physical examination generally guides further diagnostic testing in the setting of suspected VTE. A diagnostic algorithm for suspected acute PE is presented in Figure 13A.1.

History and physical exam

The history and physical exam are notoriously insensitive and nonspecific for the clinical diagnosis of both DVT and PE. Clinical studies have established that DVT cannot be reliably diagnosed based upon the history and physical exam even in high-risk patients.[12,13] Patients may or may not experience erythema, warmth, pain, swelling, or tenderness.

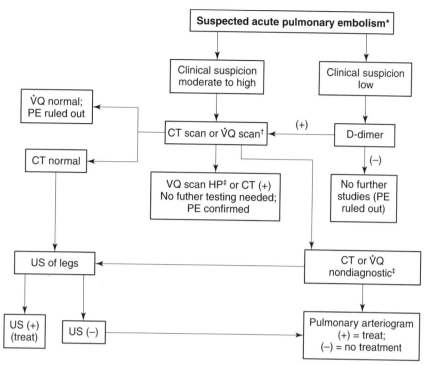

Figure 13A.1   *Algorithm for the diagnostic approach to suspected acute pulmonary embolism. PE, pulmonary embolism; V̇Q = ventilation–perfusion; CT, computed tomography; US, compression ultrasound; HP, high probability.*
*Level of clinical suspicion may affect algorithm.
†The optimal scenario for V̇Q scan is patient with clear chest radiograph and no underlying cardiopulmonary disease. Patients with significant renal insufficiency should undergo a V̇Q scan instead of CT. Chest CT can be performed together with CT venography which may enhance sensitivity.
‡ In setting of prior PE, a HP V̇Q scan may reflect the previous PE. In this case, prior V̇Q scans should be reviewed whenever possible.

Homans sign (pain elicited by dorsiflexion of the foot) is neither sensitive nor specific for DVT. When present, however, any of these findings merit further evaluation despite their lack of specificity. Based upon controlled clinical trials, it should be emphasized that clinical suspicion may imply the need for further evaluation but cannot, by itself, be relied upon to confirm or exclude the diagnosis of DVT.

Pulmonary embolism should always be considered whenever unexplained dyspnea is present. Dyspnea, pleuritic chest pain, and hemoptysis are common in PE, but are nonspecific.[14] Anxiety, lightheadedness, sudden hypotension, and syncope are all symptoms which may be caused by PE but may also result from a number of other disorders. Tachypnea and tachycardia are the most common signs of PE but are also nonspecific. The cardiac and pulmonary physical exams are nonspecific. Clinical suspicion has been shown to be a more useful parameter when considered in conjunction with V̇Q scanning.[15] Diagnostic efforts for suspected PE may be appropriate even in the setting of alternative explanations if risk factors and the clinical setting are suggestive. Dyspnea and tachypnea with clear lung fields and hypoxemia could be

attributed to a flare of chronic obstructive lung disease or asthma when underlying PE may be present.

A subset of patients from the Prospective Investigation of Pulmonary Embolism Diagnosis (PIOPED)[14] without preexisting cardiac or pulmonary disease were evaluated to determine the frequency of clinical characteristics in patients due solely to PE. Dyspnea, tachypnea, or pleuritic pain was present in 97 percent of patients found to have PE. Symptoms and signs of acute PE, and their frequency based upon the PIOPED study are presented in Tables 13A.1 and 13A.2. The frequency of specific symptoms and signs were similar whether underlying cardiopulmonary disease was present or not.

ACUTE PULMONARY EMBOLISM: DIAGNOSTIC TESTING

Chest radiography

Most patients with acute PE have an abnormal but nondiagnostic chest radiograph. Classic findings of

Table 13A.1   *Symptoms of acute pulmonary embolism**

	All patients (%) (n = 383)	No previous cardiopulmonary disease (%) (n = 117)
Dyspnea	78	73
Pleuritic chest pain	59	66
Cough	43	37
Leg pain	27	26
Hemoptysis	16	13
Palpitations	13	10
Wheezing	14	9
Anginalike pain	6	4

*The symptoms listed above are based on data from the Prospective Investigation of Pulmonary Embolism (PIOPED) study and modified from tables presented in Stein PD, ed. *Pulmonary Embolism.* Baltimore: Williams and Wilkins, 1996.[15]

Table 13A.2   *Signs of acute pulmonary embolism**

	All patients (%) (n = 383)	No previous cardiopulmonary disease (%) (n = 117)
Tachypnea (20/min)	73	70
Crackles	55	51
Tachycardia (>100/min)	30	30
Leg swelling	31	28
Loud P2[†]	23	23
DVT[‡]	15	11
Wheezes	11	5
Diaphoresis	10	11
Temperature (≥38.5)	7	7
Pleural rub	4	3
Fourth heart sound	–	24
Third heart sound	5	3
Cyanosis	3	1
Homans sign	3	4
Right ventricular lift	–	4

*The clinical signs listed above are based upon data from the Prospective Investigation of Pulmonary Embolism (PIOPED) study and modified from tables presented in Stein PD, (ed). *Pulmonary Embolism.* Williams and Wilkins, Baltimore 1996.[16]

[†]P2 = pulmonic component of second heart sound.

[‡]DVT, deep vein thrombosis.

pulmonary infarction such as a juxtapleural wedge-shaped opacity at the costophrenic angle indicating pulmonary infarction (Hampton hump) or decreased vascularity (Westermark sign) suggest the diagnosis but are infrequent. Common but nonspecific radiographic findings include atelectasis, pleural effusion, pulmonary infiltrates, and elevation of a hemidiaphragm. A normal chest radiograph in the setting of severe dyspnea and hypoxemia without

evidence of bronchospasm or anatomic shunt strongly suggests PE. However, the chest radiograph should not be used to conclusively diagnose or exclude PE. Pneumonia, congestive heart failure, pneumothorax, or rib fracture may cause symptoms similar to acute PE, and should be considered. The presence of musculoskeletal or cardiopulmonary disease does not necessarily *exclude* the possibility of acute PE. In PIOPED,[14–16] the chest radiograph was abnormal in 98 of 117 (84 percent) patients with no preexisting cardiopulmonary disease, with the most common abnormalities being atelectasis and/or parenchymal abnormalities occurring in 79 of 117 (68 percent) individuals. Either dyspnea, tachypnea, pleuritic pain, atelectasis, or a parenchymal abnormality on the chest radiograph was present in 115 of 117 (98 percent) patients with proved PE.

Electrocardiography

The electrocardiogram (EKG) cannot be used to diagnose acute PE. The findings are generally nonspecific and include T wave changes, ST-segment abnormalities, and left or right axis deviation. In the Urokinase Pulmonary Embolism Trial (UPET) electrocardiographic abnormalities were demonstrated in 87 percent of patients with proved PE without underlying cardiac or pulmonary disease.[17] These findings were not specific for PE, however. Even with massive or submassive PE, manifestations such as the S1Q3T3 pattern, right bundle branch block, P wave pulmonale or right axis deviation occurred only in 26 percent of patients. The low frequency of specific EKG changes associated with PE was confirmed in the PIOPED study.[14] Nonspecific ST-segment or T wave changes were the most common EKG abnormalities and were noted in 44 of 89 (49 percent) patients. T wave inversion in the precordial leads may correlate with more severe right ventricular dysfunction.

Arterial blood gas analysis

Hypoxemia is common in acute PE. Certain individuals, particularly young patients without underlying lung disease may have a normal Pa_{O_2}. In the PIOPED subset of patients suspected of PE without preexisting cardiopulmonary disease, patients with and without PE could not be distinguished based upon the arterial blood gas value or the alveolar–arterial (A–a) difference.[14] Of note, the A–a difference was increased by more than 20 mm Hg in 76 of 88 (86 percent) patients with PE, but it can be normal. In a retrospective study of hospitalized patients with acute PE, the Pa_{O_2} was greater than 80 mm Hg in 29 percent of patients less than 40 years of age compared with 3 percent in the older group.[18] The A–a difference was elevated in all patients, with the P_{CO_2} usually low. It is important to realize that an *elevated* P_{CO_2} (caused for example, by preexisting lung disease, or a metabolic alkalosis), does *not* rule out the possibility of acute PE. In a critically ill, intubated, ventilated, sedated patient, a change in oxygenation may serve as the only clue to the diagnosis of acute PE.

D–dimer testing

D-dimer testing has been extensively evaluated in the setting of suspected acute DVT and PE. The D-dimer represents a specific derivative of cross-linked fibrin, and a normal enzyme-linked immunosorbent assay (ELISA) is extremely sensitive in excluding PE when the clinical probability is low. When a positive D-dimer level is defined as 500 μg/L or greater, the sensitivity and specificity for PE have been shown to be 98 percent and 39 percent, respectively.[19] However, many clinical conditions in addition to acute thromboembolism are associated with an elevated D-dimer level. Although the sensitivity of the D-dimer appears high, the specificity is not high enough to be diagnostic. D-dimer testing in conjunction with other parameters or used with predictive scores may increase the diagnostic utility.

A negative D-dimer assay together with a respiratory rate <20 breaths/min, and a Po_2 >80 mm Hg, has proved to be sensitive in ruling out acute PE.[20] A recent comprehensive review of the various D-dimer assays and clinical trial results reinforces the above findings.[21] Unfortunately, particularly in patients with underlying disease, D-dimer testing is substantially limited by poor specificity.

Clinical probability scores based upon certain simple clinical parameters have been used together with a negative SimpliRed D-dimer test (a rapid red blood cell agglutination D-dimer assay), to help to exclude PE. In a recent prospective clinical trial, the SimpliRED assay was used together with a simplified scoring system utilizing parameters that were readily available in the emergency department.[22] The Geneva score, which includes chest radiograph and arterial blood gas information, has also proved useful.[23] These scoring systems are not, however, commonly used in clinical practice.

Cardiac troponin

Acute PE may be associated with elevated cardiac troponin levels and both troponin T and troponin I levels have been found to be elevated in acute PE.[24–28] The likelihood of a positive test is higher in more massive PE in which myocyte injury due to right ventricular strain might be expected. A recent investigation suggested that an elevated level might be of prognostic value.[27] In this study of 38 patients with acute PE, 18 (47 percent) had elevated cardiac troponin I levels. Of the 18 patients, 12 (67 percent) had right ventricular dilation/hypokinesis compared with only 3 (15 percent) without elevation of troponin I ($P = 0.004$). Lack of sensitivity and specificity for PE limit the utility of the test but in a clinically compatible setting, an elevated value might serve as a clue to the diagnosis of PE and lead to further investigation.

Brain natriuretic peptide

Plasma brain natriuretic peptide levels may be a supplementary tool for evaluating right ventricular function in patients with acute PE. Its exact utility is yet unclear and currently under evaluation. This test may be abnormal in the setting of either right and left ventricular enlargement of any cause so that chronic left or right heart failure would limit specificity.

Imaging techniques and algorithms in suspected acute pulmonary embolism

Spiral CT and V̇Q scanning are the most common diagnostic tests used specifically for suspected PE. Low or intermediate probability (nondiagnostic) V̇Q scans are common in patients subsequently proved to have PE. On the basis of well-designed, prospective clinical trials, when the V̇Q scan is nondiagnostic, it should be interpreted together with the index of clinical suspicion.[15] In the PIOPED study, the utility of V̇Q scanning combined with clinical assessment of patients with suspected PE was prospectively evaluated.[15] Patients with confirmed PE had scans which were high, intermediate, or low probability, as did most patients without PE. Although the specificity of high-probability scans was 97 percent, the sensitivity was only 41 percent. Of interest, 33 percent of patients with intermediate-probability scans and 12 percent of patients with low-probability scans were definitively diagnosed with PE by pulmonary arteriography. When the clinical suspicion of PE was considered very high, PE was found to be present in 96 percent of patients with high probability scans, 66 percent of patients with intermediate scans, and 40 percent of patients with low probability scans. Thus, if the clinical scenario suggests PE, the diagnosis of PE should be rigorously pursued even when the lung scan is low or intermediate probability (i.e. nondiagnostic). Patients with previous PE or certain parenchymal lung diseases may have high-probability scans. When the V̇Q scan is normal, PE is effectively excluded.

Several potential diagnostic pathways may be appropriate after a nondiagnostic V̇Q scan. Pulmonary arteriography (the gold standard) should be considered. Another option is to do lower extremity studies. If in the setting of a nondiagnostic V̇Q scan a leg ultrasound is performed and is positive for DVT, treatment can be instituted and no additional studies are needed, unless there is a history of previous DVT in the same region. When the ultrasound is negative, PE cannot, however, be definitively ruled out since the ultrasound is not adequately sensitive when there are no symptoms or signs of DVT on examination. In the setting of low clinical probability, a negative ELISA D-dimer strongly suggests the absence of VTE. Additional imaging should be performed, however, when the clinical setting suggests that PE is likely.

Another diagnostic option is to start with a contrast-enhanced spiral CT scan. The use of CT scanning for suspected PE has increased significantly over the past decade. It is sometimes positive in the face of a nondiagnostic V̇Q scan. Spiral CT may reveal emboli in the main, lobar, or segmental pulmonary arteries with >80 percent sensitivity and specificity. Examples of bilateral, central PE imaged by spiral CT are shown in Figure 13A.2. Studies evaluating spiral CT to determine sensitivity and specificity for acute PE have revealed a range of 53 percent to 100 percent and 81 percent to 97 percent, respectively, for these parameters.[29–36] Different study designs, patient exclusion criteria, levels of experience, and reading protocols have accounted for some of the differences. Thus, although the results of clinical trials with CT have been generally encouraging, it is important to realize that CT does not have perfect sensitivity nor specificity and the clinical implications of an erroneous diagnosis are important.

One recent large, prospective spiral CT study from Switzerland suggested a lower sensitivity for acute PE than many previous studies.[37] Patients were excluded if they had a negative D-dimer result. The sensitivity of CT for acute PE was 70 percent and in 4 percent the study was inconclusive. Results such as this suggest that a negative CT does not exclude all PE, but it would still appear unlikely that large emboli would be missed. The sensitivity for PE in smaller (subsegmental) vessels remains suboptimal, and the importance of such small emboli also is controversial. A potential concern would be a patient with small, potentially harmless undiscovered subsegmental emboli in whom potentially fatal residual DVT might be present. Not treating could also result in recurrent PE, or possibly contribute to the development of postphlebitic syndrome. Thus, as with V̇Q scanning, considering leg studies in a patient with high clinical suspicion for acute PE and a negative or

nondiagnostic CT would appear prudent. In one prospective study, patients with suspected PE, a negative chest CT and negative ultrasound of the legs had very good outcomes without a significant number of recurrences.[38]

With the advent of multidetector CT scanners (now 64-row detector scanners are available) CT can be performed more quickly and with a shorter breath-hold although this technologic advance may not actually enhance sensitivity or specificity, significantly. The outcome of patients with a negative CT scan has been evaluated and appears to be good,[39] but few studies have actually evaluated outcome in the setting of a negative CT without additional studies. Perrier and associates[40] studied the potential clinical use of a diagnostic strategy for ruling out PE on the basis of D-dimer testing and multidetector-row CT without lower-limb ultrasonography. The proportion of patients with proximal DVT despite negative findings on multidetector CT was low (0.9 percent; 95 percent confidence interval 0.3 to 2.7). Therefore, the improvement of the overall detection rate of PE by ultrasonography was marginal, and the 3-month thromboembolic risk in patients left untreated if PE had been ruled out on the sole basis of a negative multidetector CT scan would have been 1.5 percent (95 percent confidence interval 0.9 to 2.7), similar to that of pulmonary angiography. The authors suggested that a larger outcome study is needed before this approach can be adopted.[40] A key advantage of spiral CT over V̇Q scanning in suspected PE is the ability to define alternative nonvascular pathology including musculoskeletal abnormalities, airway pathology, lymphadenopathy, malignancy, and other parenchymal abnormalities as well as pleural and pericardial disease.[36] The most common relative contraindications to performing contrast-enhanced spiral CT scanning are renal insufficiency and contrast allergy. Additional prospective, randomized clinical trials comparing CT with the standard diagnostic approach to PE are currently underway. In PIOPED II, sponsored by the National Institutes of Health, more than 1000 patients with suspected PE have undergone extensive testing for suspected PE to determine the sensitivity of CT, particularly when CT scanning of the legs (CT venography) is included. These data are pending publication. Previous studies have suggested the potential for diagnosing either DVT, PE, or both with one contrast injection.[41] The advantages and limitations of spiral CT scanning for suspected acute PE are listed in Box 13A.2.

Magnetic resonance imaging (MRI) has been used to evaluate clinically suspected PE[32,42,43] but is still not widely used. This technique has several potential advantages, including excellent sensitivity and specificity for the diagnosis of DVT,[44] allowing the simultaneous and accurate detection of both PE and DVT. However, the test takes much longer than CT and is more confining; it is often not well tolerated in critically ill patients with respiratory distress. In view of relatively frequent contraindications to CT scanning such as renal insufficiency, further study of MRI for PE appears warranted.

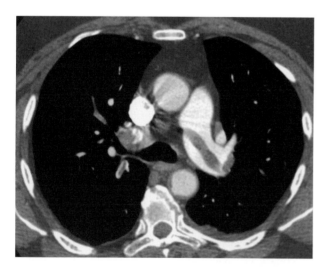

Figure 13A.2 *Massive pulmonary embolism demonstrated by contrast-enhanced spiral computed tomography. The square resides in the center of the large filling defect in the left pulmonary artery.*

Box 13A.2 Advantages and limitations of spiral CT for the diagnosis of acute PE

Advantages

- Availability
- Sensitivity for central emboli*
- Specificity*
- Relative rapidity of procedure
- Diagnosis of other disease entities
- Multiplanar reformation (three-dimensional)
- Safety
- Advancing technology
- Nondiagnostic readings less common†
- Potential for CT venography

Limitations

- Intravenous contrast required
- Not portable
- Reader expertise required
- Imperfect sensitivity and specificity
- More expensive than V̇Q scanning
- Morbid obesity may prevent scanning

Relative contraindications

- Renal insufficiency‡
- Contrast allergy

*In clinical trials to date, high sensitivity and specificity have been limited to emboli in the main, lobar, and segmental vessels. Compared with low or indeterminate probability V̇Q scans, the specificity is superior. Sensitivity is inadequate for subsegmental vessels.

†CT scans are nondiagnostic in 10 percent or less cases (much lower than for V̇Q scans).

‡Mild renal insufficiency is not a contraindication.

Echocardiography

Echocardiography can often be obtained more rapidly than other imaging studies and may reveal findings which strongly support hemodynamically significant PE.[45] Patients with PE often have underlying cardiopulmonary disease such as chronic obstructive lung disease so that the use of right ventricular dilation and hypokinesis to implicate PE is limited. Valuable clues can often be elicited, however. Direct visualization of massive PE may occasionally be possible, particularly if transesophageal echocardiography is performed. Echocardiography is sometimes used to gauge the extent of right ventricular dysfunction in the setting of proved acute PE (see treatment section). Intravascular ultrasound has been used to directly visualize proximal emboli at the bedside.[46]

ACUTE DEEP VENOUS THROMBOSIS: DIAGNOSTIC TESTING

As with suspected acute PE, suspected DVT requires clinical evaluation coupled with objective testing. Compression ultrasound is by far the most common technique utilized in the setting of suspected DVT. As with PE, DVT cannot be reliably diagnosed by history and physical exam, and requires further evaluation.

Compression ultrasound

Over a decade ago, the sensitivity and specificity of compression ultrasound for symptomatic proximal DVT proved to be well above 90 percent and numerous subsequent prospective trials have verified this.[47–49] Limitations were also recognized, including the insensitivity for asymptomatic DVT, operator dependence, difficulty in accurately distinguishing acute from chronic DVT in symptomatic patients, and the insensitivity for thrombosis below the knee.[50,51] Certain patient factors such as plaster casts or morbid obesity affect the ability to visualize the deep veins. It is clear that sensitivity is reduced in the setting of screening asymptomatic legs, often because thrombi are less extensive.[51] Ultrasound is relatively inexpensive and is the preferred diagnostic modality for a straightforward case of symptomatic suspected proximal DVT. An approach that has been successfully tested is that of serial ultrasonography when the initial study is negative in a symptomatic patient.[52] However, concerns about compliance and inconvenience have limited this practice. Thus, high-quality evidence from multiple, prospective, randomized clinical trials indicates that compression ultrasound is highly sensitive and specific for symptomatic, proximal acute DVT, but insensitive for asymptomatic acute DVT and calf DVT.

Upper extremity thrombosis is common in patients who are critically ill or in patients with cancer and is most frequently related to a central venous catheter. Other risks include compression or invasion by local or metastatic neoplasm, transvenous pacemaker, or effort-induced thrombosis. Each can generally be diagnosed by compression ultrasound and can also result in acute PE.[53,54] Effort-induced (primary subclavian vein) upper extremity thrombosis (Paget–Schroetter syndrome) often affects young, healthy active people and may recur.[55,56] An extensive review of clinical trials examining the sensitivity and specificity of ultrasound techniques for suspected acute DVT is provided in the American Thoracic Society consensus statement on the diagnostic approach to acute venous thromboembolism.[57]

Contrast venography

Contrast venography remains the gold standard technique for the diagnosis of DVT, but it is no longer used as the initial diagnostic test. Although ultrasound has excellent sensitivity for proximal DVT in patients with symptomatic suspected DVT, it is clearly less sensitive than contrast venography for calf DVT. Venography is an option when noninvasive testing is nondiagnostic or impossible to perform. It is generally safe and accurate but is an invasive procedure which may result in superficial phlebitis or hypersensitivity reactions.[57]

Magnetic resonance imaging and computed tomography

Magnetic resonance imaging is being used increasingly to diagnose DVT and appears to be an accurate noninvasive alternative to venography. A major advantage of this technique is excellent resolution of the inferior vena cava and pelvic veins. High-quality evidence from several prospective, well-designed clinical trials indicates that it is sensitive and specific for acute proximal DVT.[58,59] It appears to be at least as accurate as contrast venography or ultrasound imaging for proximal DVT and perhaps more sensitive for pelvic vein thrombosis. It offers the opportunity for simultaneous bilateral lower extremity imaging and it may accurately distinguish acute from chronic DVT.[58,59] This technique is not yet widely used for diagnosing DVT and, as is the case with PE, MRI radiologists with experience are instrumental in maximizing accuracy.

Although there are limited data evaluating the sensitivity of MRI for calf DVT, a sensitivity of only 87 percent was demonstrated in one prospective study suggesting that venography may be superior for this location.[59] Spiral CT has also been studied for suspected acute DVT. The contrast dye from the bolus injected for lung imaging is followed into the deep veins of the legs for viewing. Initial data are promising,[41] and the utility of 'CT venography' has been further studied in PIOPED II with results pending publication. These techniques may fit into diagnostic algorithms for DVT and PE but at present these algorithms are generally institution specific depending upon resources and expertise with certain techniques. When a patient with suspected PE has a nondiagnostic lung study and lower extremity imaging is pursued, ultrasound remains the most common diagnostic modality. Although lower extremity MRI might be more sensitive, it has not been prospectively compared in the setting of suspected PE.

TREATMENT OF ACUTE VENOUS THROMBOEMBOLISM

Several pharmacologic and nonpharmacologic options have been studied for the treatment of VTE with different efficacy and safety results. Treatment options include unfractionated heparin (UFH), low-molecular-weight heparin (LMWH), direct anti-Xa and thrombin inhibitors, warfarin, thrombolytic therapy, inferior vena cava filter placement, and

surgical embolectomy. An early question that was addressed by Barritt and Jordan in the first prospective randomized anticoagulation trial in patients with acute venous thromboembolism in 1960 involved the need for anticoagulation in patients with acute PE.[60] This trial was stopped prematurely after only 35 patients were enrolled; the mortality rate from PE in the untreated group was >25 percent compared with no deaths from PE in the anticoagulation group. Treatment of acute VTE is imperative; anticoagulation has been proved to reduce mortality in acute PE.

The goals of VTE treatment are not just limited to prevention of thrombus propagation, embolization, and recurrence. Today's management must consider the potential to prevent postthrombotic (chronic venous insufficiency) syndrome as well as the potential to prevent chronic thromboembolic pulmonary hypertension. There are two phases in the treatment of patients with symptomatic VTE: acute or initial treatment and chronic treatment (secondary prophylaxis). Acute phase treatment options include continuous intravenous UFH infusion, subcutaneous LMWH, the penta saccharide fondaparinux, direct thrombin inhibitors, the use of an inferior vena caval filter (IVCF), and thrombolytic therapy. Acute therapy will be our focus here.

Unfractionated heparin

All heparins are heterogeneous mixtures of glycosaminoglycans derived from animal products that catalyze the blood enzyme antithrombin. Unfractionated heparin has a narrow therapeutic window and has been cited as a common cause of drug-related deaths in hospitalized patients. When VTE is diagnosed or strongly suspected, anticoagulation should be promptly instituted unless contraindications exist. Confirmatory testing should always be planned if anticoagulation is to be continued. Heparins exert a prompt antithrombotic effect preventing thrombus growth. Although neither heparin nor LMWH directly prevent the development of acute PE or dissolve thrombus, they allow the fibrinolytic system to act unopposed and more readily reduces the size of the thromboembolic burden.[61] While thrombus growth can be prevented, early recurrence can develop even in the setting of therapeutic anticoagulation.

With the institution of continuous intravenous heparin, the activated partial thromboplastin time (aPTT) should be aggressively followed at 6-hour intervals until it is consistently in the therapeutic range of 1.5–2.0 times control values.[62] This range corresponds to a heparin level of 0.2–0.4 U/mL as measured by protamine sulfate titration. In general, heparin should be administered as an intravenous bolus of 5000 units followed by a maintenance dose of at least 30 000 to 40 000 U/24 h by continuous infusion. The lower dose is administered if the patient is considered at high risk for bleeding. This aggressive approach decreases the risk of subtherapeutic anticoagulation, and although supratherapeutic levels are sometimes achieved initially, bleeding complications do not appear to be increased.[63] In patients requiring large daily doses of UFH without achieving a therapeutic aPTT (heparin-resistant patients), the dose of heparin should be adjusted by measuring the anti-Xa level because of a dissociation between the aPTT and heparin concentration.[64]

More recent data continue to support aggressive heparin dosing. An alternative regimen consisting of a bolus of 80 U/kg followed by 18 U/kg per hour has been recommended.[65] This weight-adjusted approach is recommended in the recent American College of Chest Physicians (ACCP) Consensus Conference on Antithrombotic Therapy.[66] Warfarin therapy may be initiated as soon as the APTT is therapeutic and heparin should be maintained until a therapeutic international normalized ratio of 2.0–3.0 has been overlapped with a therapeutic APTT for two consecutive days. While proximal lower extremity thrombus is more likely to result in PE, calf thrombi should either be followed for proximal extension over 10–14 days with noninvasive testing or anticoagulation should be instituted.[67] Documented proximal DVT or PE should be treated for at least 3 months.[67] Longer treatment is appropriate when significant risk factors persist. Both short and long-term anticoagulation guidelines are outlined in the ACCP Consensus Conference guidelines.[68]

Bleeding with UFH can be managed by discontinuation and observation as the half-life is only 90 minutes on reversal with 1 mg per 100 U of UFH of protamine sulfate. Side effects of protamine sulfate administration are anaphylaxis, hypotension, and possibly bleeding. Equimolar concentrations of protamine sulfate neutralize anti-IIa activity but only partially neutralize the anti-Xa activity of LMWHs, probably because protamine sulfate does not bind to very low-molecular-weight components. However, it appears very reasonable to use this drug in the setting of bleeding on LMWH.

Low-molecular-weight heparin

The LMWH preparations have emerged as very advantageous options for the acute management of VTE. These are chemically or enzymatically depolymerizations of UFH and they possess a number of significant differences and advantages over UFH including favorable pharmacokinetics with 90 percent bioavailability at both low (prophylaxis) and high (treatment) doses (Table 13A.3 and Box 13A.3). A prolonged half-life independent of dose allows for subcutaneous injection once or twice daily with a predictable dose response, most often without monitoring (anti-Xa level). In fact, these drugs are so bioavailable and have such predictable responses, that, with the exception of certain high-risk situations, no dose monitoring is necessary. LMWHs have fewer pentasaccharide units (the high-affinity binding sites for antithrombin), and the anti-factor Xa to IIa ratio is 2:1 to 4:1 for LMWHs as opposed to 1:1 for UFH.[68]

The efficacy and safety of LMWH for treatment of established acute proximal DVT using recurrent symptomatic VTE as the primary outcome measure is established.[68–76] The incidence of DVT and recurrent bleeding in these trials indicates that LMWH preparations are at least as effective and as safe as UFH. These agents can be administered once or twice per day subcutaneously even at therapeutic doses and do not require monitoring of the aPTT. Factor Xa levels appear reasonable to monitor in certain settings such as in obese patients, very small patients (<40 kg) and in those with renal insufficiency. There is no proved benefit in monitoring other patients.

In two large randomized (Canadian and European) trials performed more than a decade ago, patients were randomized to therapy with LMWH initiated at home (or

Table 13A.3 *A comparison of low molecular weight heparin (LMWH) with unfractionated heparin (UFH)*

Characteristic	UFH	LMWH
Mean molecular weight	12 000–15 000	4000–6000
Protein binding	Substantial	Minimal
Anti-Xa activity	Substantial	Substantial
Anti-IIa activity	Substantial	Minimal
Platelet inhibition	Substantial	Minimal
Vascular permeability	Moderate	None
Microvascular permeability	Substantial	Minimal

Box 13A.3 Potential advantages of LMWH over UFH

Prophylactic and therapeutic advantages

- Comparable or superior efficacy
- Comparable or superior safety
- Superior bioavailability
- Once or twice daily dosing
- Lower incidence of heparin-induced thrombocytopenia

Other therapeutic advantages

- No laboratory monitoring*
- Less phlebotomy
- Subcutaneous administration
- Earlier ambulation
- Home therapy in certain patient subsets

*Measurement of anti-factor Xa levels is recommended in significantly obese patients, very small patients (e.g. <40 kg), and patients with renal insufficiency.

If renal insufficiency is stable, and creatinine clearance is >30 mL/min, no adjustments in dose need to be made. If it is stable and <30 mL/min, the therapeutic dose of enoxaparin is decreased from 1 mg/kg every 12 hours to 1 mg/kg every 24 hours.

continued at home after a brief hospitalization) versus UFH administered in the hospital[68,69] with comparable rates of recurrent VTE. A number of outpatient studies have followed these two pivotal trials. Metaanalytic studies have examined the use of LMWH compared with UFH in the initial treatment of acute proximal DVT.[71–74] Although there was overlap between these analyses, they have helped to confirm the efficacy and safety of LMWH for the treatment of established DVT. In the United States, at the present time, two LMWH preparations are approved by the US Food and Drug Administration (FDA) for use in patients presenting with DVT with or without acute PE. Enoxaparin is approved for both inpatient and outpatient use at a dose of 1 mg/kg subcutaneously every 12 hours, or at 1.5 mg/kg once daily for inpatient use. The latter regimens were both proved effective in a large study of inpatients in which both doses were as effective and as safe as UFH.[75] The second preparation, tinzaparin, is administered as 175 U once daily, with the FDA approval being based upon therapy of inpatients. Although neither drug is approved by the FDA for use in acute PE, tinzaparin has proved effective in a large, randomized European trial of patients with PE.[76] Although dalteparin is approved for several prophylactic indications, it is not approved for the treatment of established VTE in the United States. The pentasaccharide, fondaparinux, is approved for patients presenting with either acute DVT or PE.[77] It should be noted that the prophylactic doses of LMWH preparations agents differ from the doses used for treating active disease. Outpatient therapy of acute DVT reduces the substantial cost of hospitalization.

A serious potential adverse effect with all forms of heparin (particularly UFH) is heparin-induced thrombocytopenia (HIT). This disorder occurs at an incidence of 3.5 percent with UFH and 0.6 percent with LMWH.[78] Typically after at least 5 days of heparin administration, a 50 percent reduction in the platelet count when compared with pretreatment platelet counts, or an absolute reduction to $100\,000/mm^3$ suggests the development of HIT. This is an antigen–antibody reaction between heparin and platelet factor 4. The problem with HIT relates to thrombin activation and thrombosis; bleeding is not generally the clinical concern. If HIT develops, there should be a very low threshold for administration of a direct thrombin inhibitor even in the absence of confirmed thrombosis. The incidence of HIT appears to be significantly lower with LMWH compared with UFH but it should be understood that this complication can occur due to either preparation. The direct thrombin inhibitors (argatroban and lepirudin) are approved for use for heparin-induced thrombocytopenia (HIT) in the United States.

The LMWHs appear to be less often associated with major hemorrhage than UFH, probably due to the complexities of UFH administration which involves pump infusion, varying techniques and laboratory reagents, dosing manipulation, and intrinsic pharmacologic properties and the more predictable bioavailability of LMWH.[79] Absolute contraindications to anticoagulant therapy include intracranial hemorrhage, active internal bleeding, malignant hypertension, intracranial neoplasm, and recent and significant trauma or surgery. Contraindications may be relative and require clinical judgment.

MASSIVE PULMONARY EMBOLISM

The definition of massive PE has not been standardized and universally accepted. Most clinicians would agree that massive PE could be defined as PE resulting in:

- hemodynamic compromise
- significant right ventricular dysfunction
- the need for a high inspired oxygen concentration
- significant anatomic obstruction of the pulmonary arterial bed.

Concomitant cardiopulmonary disease may blur the extent to which the PE itself is causing the above findings, but the most crucial issue may be the severity of the decompensation/level of reserve and not the precise contribution by PE. An issue which is rarely considered in clinical trials is the extent of remaining thrombotic burden that has not embolized or yet reached the lung. This might very well have a substantial impact on patient outcome. Because patients with massive PE may be too unstable for transport portable perfusion scanning may be useful in such individuals since the chances for a high probability diagnostic scan are much higher with massive PE. Echocardiography would be even more likely to reveal dramatic right ventricular dilation and dysfunction, which in the absence of other potential causes would suggest (but not prove) the diagnosis of acute PE. Potential therapeutic implications of such findings will be discussed subsequently.

Once massive PE with hypotension and/or severe hypoxemia is suspected, aggressive supportive treatment should be initiated immediately. Cautious infusion of intravenous saline may augment preload and improve impaired right ventricular function. Dopamine or norepinephrine are the favored vasopressors if hypotension persists.[80] Dobutamine may boost right ventricular output, but as an 'inodilator', may worsen hypotension. Supplemental oxygen, intubation, and mechanical ventilation are instituted as needed to support respiratory failure.

Thrombolytic therapy

Early trials established that thrombolytic agents accelerate clot lysis and reduce clot burden.[81–86] These agents activate plasminogen to form plasmin, which then results in fibrinolysis as well as fibrinogenolysis. Defining those patients in whom the benefit of a rapid reduction in clot burden outweighs the increased hemorrhagic risk of thrombolytic therapy may be difficult. There are three FDA-approved thrombolytic agent regimens for acute PE utilizing weight-based monograms (Box 13A.4). Potential indications are listed in Box 13A.5.

The case for thrombolytic use is strongest in patients with massive PE complicated by shock, which occurs in about 10 percent of PE patients and where the mortality rate may be 25 percent. Thrombolysis in these patients results in a more rapid resolution of abnormal right ventricular function.[85,87] A recent prospective, randomized, clinical trial demonstrated that patients with acute PE without hypotension but with right ventricular dysfunction on echocardiogram had less need for escalation of therapy (i.e. repeat thrombolytic administration) when given thrombolytic therapy plus heparin versus heparin alone.[88] No clear data have shown one thrombolytic agent as superior to the others, though shorter infusion regimens and even bolus dosing may be favored in the case of massive PE. There is no clear consensus on whether or not heparin should be continued during thrombolytic infusion. At least one randomized trial has reported low bleeding rates with tissue-plasminogen activator and concomitant heparin.[88]

Thrombolytic therapy is contraindicated in patients at high risk for hemorrhage as both the lysis of hemostatic fibrin plugs and fibrinogenolysis can lead to severe bleeding (Box 13A.6). Intracranial hemorrhage is the most devastating complication of thrombolytic therapy and is generally stated to occur in about 2 percent of patients. Invasive procedures should be minimized as bleeding commonly occurs at sites of pulmonary arteriography or arterial line placement. Retroperitoneal hemorrhage may result from a vascular puncture above the inguinal ligament and is often clinically silent but may be life-threatening. The decision for thrombolysis should be made on a case-by-case basis. There should be a lower threshold to administer thrombolytic therapy in the setting of a relative contraindication if a patient is extremely unstable from life-threatening PE. Pulmonary embolectomy may be appropriate in patients with massive embolism in whom thrombolytic therapy is contraindicated.

Catheter-directed and systemic thrombolytic therapy have been investigated. For DVT, a catheter-directed dissolution of the thrombus can be performed by an interventional physician; however, this route of administration and dosing strategy has not yet been approved by the FDA. Thrombolysis can be considered in acute DVT (less than 28 days old). Bjarnason et al.[89] reported a 66–100 percent lysis rate compared with only 33 percent if the thrombus was present for more than 4 weeks. Theoretically, this will result in preservation of venous valvular function and a reduced incidence of postthrombotic syndrome. Therefore, thrombolytic therapy may be considered for those patients with iliofemoral DVT, phlegmasia cerulea dolens, young patients with increased risk for postthrombotic syndrome, and patients with upper extremity venous thrombosis.[90] Mechanical thrombectomy

---

Box 13A.4 Thrombolytic therapy for acute venous thromboembolism: approved regimens

- Streptokinase: 250 000 U IV (loading dose over 30 min); then 100 000 U/h for 24 hours*
- Urokinase: 4400 U/kg (2000 U/lb) IV (loading dose over 10 min); then 4400 U/kg per hour (2000 U/lb per hour) for 12–24 hours
- Tissue-type plasminogen activator: 100 mg IV over 2 hours

*Streptokinase administered over 24–72 hours at this loading dose and rate has also been approved for use in patients with extensive DVT.

Box 13A.5 Thrombolytic therapy for acute venous thromboembolism: potential indications*

- Hypotension related to PE†
- Severe hypoxemia
- Massive anatomic (saddle) embolism
- Right ventricular dysfunction associated with PE
- Extensive deep vein thrombosis

*These potential indications may be isolated or occur together.

†This indication is widely accepted. All indications require careful review of contraindications to thrombolytic therapy.

Box 13A.6 Thrombolytic therapy for acute venous thromboembolism: contraindications*

Absolute

- Intracranial tumor or hemorrhagic stroke
- Recent head trauma or cranial surgery
- Active or recent internal bleeding

Relative

- Thrombocytopenia or coagulopathy
- Uncontrolled severe hypertension
- Cardiopulmonary resuscitation
- Surgery or biopsy within the previous 10 days

*Assessment of contraindications often requires considerable clinical judgment. Whether enough time has passed after surgery depends on the specific surgical procedure, assessment of the surgical site, and the severity of the pulmonary embolism (PE). Massive PE with severe hypotension requiring vasoactive medications might suggest that risk/benefit favors thrombolytics in many circumstances.

devices have recently been evaluated for therapy of large occlusive acute venous thrombi either in the lower extremities or pulmonary vasculature.

Vena cava interruption

Inferior vena caval filters placement can be performed to minimize the risk of PE from lower extremity thrombi. The experience from one center over several decades has been reviewed.[91] The primary indications for IVCF placement include contraindications to anticoagulation, recurrent emboli while on adequate therapy, and significant bleeding during anticoagulation. Filters can also be placed in the setting of massive PE when it is believed that any further emboli might be lethal. A number of filter designs exist and can be inserted via the jugular or femoral veins. Rare complications include insertion-related complications, filter migration, direct thrombus extension through the filter, and IVC thrombosis. Recently, temporary filters have been used in patients in whom the risk of bleeding appears to be short term. These can be left indwelling as permanent devices, or it may be retrieved when the clinical need for mechanical IVC interruption no longer exists. Retrieval can take place up to 2 weeks in most cases but longer placement (several months) with successful retrieval has been documented. However, larger multicenter clinical studies are needed to determine the safety of more extended removal.

Surgical embolectomy

While surgical embolectomy is most commonly performed for chronic thromboembolic pulmonary hypertension, rare circumstances warrant its consideration in acute PE. A candidate for acute embolectomy should have a documented massive PE with refractory shock, failure of/or contraindication to thrombolytic therapy, and the availability of an experienced surgical team.

UPPER EXTREMITY THROMBOSIS

Upper extremity thrombosis is common in critically ill patients and is most frequently related to a central venous catheter.[92,93] The clinical manifestations are edema, dilated collateral circulation, and pain. The thrombosis can be located in the subclavian, axillary, or brachial vein. It may lead to complications, such as chronic obstructive edema and PE. Complications from upper-extremity DVT are less frequent than from lower-extremity DVT, but they should not be overlooked. They should generally be treated similarly to uncomplicated DVT but with an added emphasis on prompt catheter removal once the diagnosis is established.[92,93] The risk of clot embolization with catheter

removal is outweighed by the risk for chronic thrombotic complications and potential infection.

AMBULATION AND ACUTE VENOUS THROMBOEMBOLISM

Historically, strict bedrest for several days has been recommended in addition to anticoagulation in patients with VTE to help prevent thrombi from embolizing. With the advent of LMWH and its use in ambulatory patients, the benefit of immobilization has been challenged. In two small randomized studies with limited sample sizes, bedrest as an additional measure to anticoagulation was not shown to reduce the incidence of silent PE as detected by lung scanning.[94,95] In another randomized study of limited size the rate of resolution of pain and swelling was significantly faster when patients were managed with early ambulation and leg compression compared with bedrest.[96] The efficacy of using a compression bandage combined with ambulation was evaluated in 1289 patients with acute DVT most of whom were treated with LMWH.[97] A low incidence of recurrent and fatal PE was observed in the study, suggesting that mobile patients with DVT do not require bedrest. Patients with substantial pain and swelling may benefit from bedrest for a limited period while inflammation subsides.

PROPHYLAXIS FOR VENOUS THROMBOEMBOLISM

Timely and appropriate prophylaxis is essential to minimize VTE events. Multiple risk factors for VTE have been identified and are used to stratify both surgical and medical patients according to their overall risk (see Box 13A.1). Similar to major surgery, acute hospitalization for a medical indication poses a substantial risk of thromboembolic complications.

Measures to prevent VTE appear to be grossly underutilized.[3,98] A substantial reduction in the incidence of DVT can be achieved when patients at risk receive appropriate prophylaxis. In one of the highest risk settings, total hip or knee replacement, the risk is 50 percent or greater without prophylaxis. While a detailed review of prophylaxis indications can be found in the ACCP most recent set of recommendations,[99] it is important to recognize that certain clinical settings are particularly high risk for acute VTE including trauma, spinal cord injury, and orthopedic surgery (particularly total joint replacement and hip fracture surgery). The superiority of LMWH over UFH has been demonstrated in these settings, and extending the duration of prophylaxis to approximately a month after surgery further reduces the DVT rate in total hip replacement.[100] Unfractionated heparin is not recommended in total joint replacement.

Hospitalized general medical patients are also clearly at risk for VTE. Anticoagulant prophylaxis should always be strongly considered as the rate of DVT, based upon a venographic endpoint is as high as 15 percent in medical patients receiving placebo.[101] Much of the information defining the role of UFH for VTE prophylaxis in medical patients has been extrapolated from data and experience from the surgical population. Older clinical trials support the use of anticoagulant prophylaxis in the general medical patient population, but these trials were performed in patient populations likely to differ from currently hospitalized patient populations.

The rate of DVT, including proximal DVT is statistically significantly lower when LMWH is administered compared with placebo.[101,102] At present, two LMWH preparations (enoxaparin and dalteparin) have been approved by the FDA in the United States for prevention of VTE in medical patients. Four key clinical trials have compared the efficacy and safety of low-dose UFH to a LMWH for VTE prophylaxis in medical patients at risk.[103–106] Each trial studied the same treatment regimens, enoxaparin 40 mg subcutaneously daily and UFH 5000 units subcutaneously three times daily. The PRINCE (PRevention IN Cardiopulmonary Disease with Enoxaparin) trial involved 64 centers and evaluated 665 patients with severe respiratory diseases and New York Heart Association (NYHA) classification III/IV heart failure.[103] The patients were randomized to either daily enoxaparin or low-dose UFH every 8 hours for approximately 10 days. Enoxaparin proved at least as effective as UFH, and in the subgroup analysis of patients with heart failure, enoxaparin demonstrated a statistically significant reduction in VTE compared with low-dose UFH. Thus, the LMWH preparation compared favorably with UFH even when the heparin dose was optimal at 5000 units every 8 hours. The incidence of major hemorrhage, was low and comparable between the groups. However, injection site hematomas were more common in patients receiving low-dose UFH than enoxaparin.

Although 5000 units of heparin every 12 hours has been commonly used, there are fewer data to support this preventive regimen in medical patients. In fact, two studies evaluating mortality among medical patients who received either UFH 5000 U subcutaneously twice daily or no prophylaxis yielded conflicting results.[107,108] Bergmann et al.[109] found that a lower daily dose of enoxaparin, 20 mg, was comparable with UFH 5000 U subcutaneously every 12 hours in a nonselect group of hospitalized elderly medical patients with limited mobility. Considering that the efficacy of enoxaparin 20 mg subcutaneously daily in moderately ill medical patients was found to be comparable with placebo in the MEDENOX (prophylaxis in MEDical patients with ENOXaparin) trial[101] the results of this study raise questions regarding the common practice of prescribing UFH every 12 hours in at-risk medical patients except perhaps in very small individuals. However, without a direct comparison of enoxaparin with every 12 hours UFH, no firm conclusions can be drawn.

Intermittent pneumatic compression devices should be utilized when pharmacologic prophylaxis is contraindicated. Both methods combined would be reasonable in patients deemed to be at exceptionally high risk, but an additional reduction in risk in such patients has not been well substantiated. Each hospitalized patient should be assessed for the need for such prophylactic measures and all hospitals should strongly consider formulating their own written guidelines for each particular clinical setting, based upon the available medical literature.[99]

RISK STRATIFICATION

An individual's underlying VTE risk factors appear to be as important as the acute clinical condition precipitating the hospitalization and need to be assessed through a VTE risk/benefit analysis. Critically ill patients always qualify for prophylaxis based upon markedly reduced mobility and multiple risk factors. Independent risk factors including stroke, myocardial infarction, cancer, conditions requiring critical care, total knee or hip replacement and spinal cord injury define the highest thromboembolic risk populations.[99] The moderate risk groups, characterized by DVT rates of 17.1 percent, includes patients with severe cardiopulmonary diseases including NYHA classification III/IV heart failure, pulmonary infection or respiratory failure. Respiratory failure may result from community or nosocomial pneumonia, chronic obstructive lung disease, acute respiratory distress syndrome, pulmonary hypertension, or interstitial lung disease.

Prolonged immobility or reduced mobility are two additional independent VTE risk factors that require consideration when assessing the patient's overall VTE risk.[99] Immobility as a parameter for risk assessment is not meant to imply complete or total bed rest but functional impairment. This reinforces that in a contemporary hospital medicine practice, the majority of patients have multiple risk factors for VTE. These risk factors are additive and need to be acknowledged at the time of admission so that appropriate prophylaxis is initiated in a timely manner. Risk assessment protocols to systematically identify and evaluate patients who require prophylaxis are useful in guiding physicians and electronic alert systems have proved to increase the rates of prophylaxis used.[110] The challenge is to ensure that these recommendations become an integral component of day-to-day practice for the at-risk medical patients.

In summary, practice guidelines are necessary to assist healthcare providers to address the clinical conundrums posed by the medically ill patient with immobility admitted to our healthcare institutions. Sound clinical evidence supports the benefit of prophylaxis for medical patients at risk for VTE. Although fewer clinical trials have been conducted in the critically ill patient population, the medical patient data are compelling and certainly suggest that at least the level of aggressiveness proved in these patients should be extrapolated to the critically ill medical patient population. The surgical and trauma population have been studied in far more detail.

NONTHROMBOTIC PULMONARY EMBOLI

Via venous blood return to the lungs, the pulmonary vascular bed is exposed to a variety of potentially obstructing substances. These substances may be exogenous or endogenous in origin, and may result in various clinical consequences including dyspnea, chest pain, hypoxemia, and sometimes death. Nonthrombotic sources of emboli include fat embolism, amniotic fluid embolism, air embolism, schistosomiasis, septic embolism, and tumor embolism.[111–115]

Fat embolism

Fat embolism most commonly occurs in the setting of the traumatic fracture of long bones.[111] A more impressive clinical syndrome usually results when multiple fractures of larger bones are involved. However, orthopedic procedures and trauma to other fat replete tissues such as the liver or subcutaneous tissue may result in similar consequences. After the inciting event, there is generally a delay of 24–48 hours, before symptoms develop. As neutral fat enters the vascular system, the triad of dyspnea, petechiae, and mental confusion may develop. It is unknown why the syndrome develops in some patients and not in others, even with comparable extents of injury.

The obstruction of vessels by neutral fat particles as well as the deleterious effects of fatty acids released from neutral fat by lipases account for the pathophysiologic consequences of fat embolism.[105] These free fatty acids cause a diffuse vasculitis with capillary leakage from cerebral, pulmonary, and other vascular beds. The diagnosis is made from the clinical and radiographic findings in the setting of risk factors such as surgery or trauma. Fat droplets by oil red O stain in bronchoalveolar lavage fluid may be suggestive of fat embolism but clinical studies to date suggest that this finding is neither sensitive nor specific. Treatment is generally supportive, including oxygen and mechanical ventilation and the prognosis is generally good. Therapy with corticosteroids remains controversial. Steroid prophylaxis has been suggested in high-risk patients.

Amniotic fluid embolism

Although amniotic fluid embolism is uncommon, it represents one of the leading causes of maternal death in the United States.[112] During or after a generally uncomplicated spontaneous or cesarean delivery, amniotic fluid may access to uterine venous channels and then to the maternal pulmonary and general circulations. There are no identifiable risk factors in either the patients or the fetus. The syndrome is heralded by the sudden onset of severe respiratory distress, and hypotension and death frequently result. The thromboplastic activity of amniotic fluid causes injury to the pulmonary vasculature followed by extensive fibrin deposition. A consumptive coagulopathy ensues with marked hypofibrinogenemia. Left ventricular dysfunction may result from the potential myocardial depressant effect of amniotic fluid. The resulting pulmonary edema may be both hydrostatic and noncardiogenic.

The differential diagnosis includes PE, septic and hemorrhagic shock, venous air embolism, aspiration pneumonia, congestive heart failure (from acute myocardial infarction or other causes), placentae abruptio, and ruptured uterus. The diagnosis should be suspected based upon the clinical picture. Examination of the pulmonary arterial blood may or may not reveal the amorphous fragments of vernix caseosa, squamous cells or mucin. The administration of heparin, antifibrinolytic agents such as α-aminocaproic acid, and cryoprecipitate have been suggested for treatment. However, the primary treatment is supportive with oxygen and mechanical ventilation. Even with aggressive support, maternal mortality may be as high as 80 percent.

Air embolism

Air embolism most commonly results from a variety of invasive surgical and medical procedures now available, from indwelling venous and arterial catheters, and from thoracic and other forms of trauma.[113,114] With venous embolism in the setting of a patent foramen ovale, embolization to the coronary or cerebral circulation is a great concern. In the absence of a patent foramen ovale, the lungs can filter modest amounts of air, but large single or continuous episodes of air embolism can still gain access to the systemic arterial circulation. The presentation may include dyspnea, wheezing, chest pain, cough, agitation, confusion, tachycardia, and/or hypotension. A 'mill wheel murmur' (air in the right ventricle) may sometimes be auscultated. Hypoxemia and hypercapnia are present in more severe cases and the chest radiograph may reveal pulmonary edema or air–fluid levels. Upon recognition of the syndrome, the patient should be placed in the Trendelenburg/left lateral decubitus position and administered 100 percent oxygen. If a central venous catheter is in place near the right atrium, air aspiration should be attempted. Occasionally, hyperbaric oxygen is indicated. Anticonvulsants are administered in the presence of seizures. Prevention of air embolism as well as a high index of suspicion when it occurs, are crucial.

Schistosomiasis

This parasitic disorder causes severe pulmonary vascular obstruction and pulmonary hypertension via both anatomic obstruction by the organism itself and an inflammatory vasculitic response to the organism.[115] In endemic areas such as Egypt, schistosomal disease is a common cause of pulmonary hypertension and cor pulmonale. The liver is generally involved quite extensively before pulmonary involvement occurs. The disease is refractory to treatment unless it is detected prior to the development of extensive hepatic and pulmonary inflammation.

Septic embolism

Illicit intravenous drug abuse is by far the most common cause of septic embolism. Prior to the drug era, this entity was nearly always a complication of septic pelvic thrombophlebitis due to both septic abortion and postpartum uterine infection. Infections secondary to indwelling intravenous catheters are increasingly common as well. Subcutaneous injections can cause local infections that subsequently invade peripheral veins.

Other emboli

Pulmonary embolic phenomena may develop from a variety of other substances.[114] Malignant cells may enter and adhere to pulmonary vessels, mimicking PE. Brain tissue may travel to the lungs after head trauma, or liver cells, after abdominal trauma. Bone marrow has been reported in lung tissue after cardiopulmonary resuscitation. Noninfectious vasculitic-thrombotic complications also occur in intravenous drug users. Materials such as talc used to 'cut' heroin or cocaine may occasionally themselves provoke vascular inflammation and secondary thrombosis. Perfusion scans can demonstrate segmental or smaller defects. Distinguishing these from emboli due to DVT can be difficult. Repetitive insults can lead to chronic pulmonary hypertension.

CONCLUSION

Venous thromboembolism continues to be one of the most vexing respiratory emergencies. But the field continues to evolve. The diagnosis of DVT and PE must be established as rapidly and reliably as possible. There are times when therapy should even be considered prior to establishing a firm diagnosis, if there is a high clinical suspicion and low perceived risk of bleeding. It is feasible that early treatment may not only reduce the risk of recurrent PE but also reduce the likelihood of the development of significant sequelae such as chronic thromboembolic pulmonary hypertension or postthrombotic syndrome.

The advent of LMWH has revolutionized the approach to prevention and treatment of VTE and has greatly facilitated outpatient therapy. Thrombolytic therapy should be strongly considered in appropriate settings with due caution. Therapy

with appropriate anticoagulants, thrombolysis, or other catheter-based or surgical interventional maneuvers must be applied with an evidence-based approach, when possible. Novel therapies will likely emerge to again revolutionize our management of this disease with the availability of effective and safe oral agents. Perhaps most crucial, is that we place a clear emphasis on the prevention of this prevalent disorder, and improving the current rates of VTE prophylaxis. This option promotes patient satisfaction and potentially reduces cost to the healthcare system.

Key learning points

- Patients with VTE often have readily identifiable risk factors which may lower the clinical suspicion.

- The symptoms and signs of acute DVT and PE are nonspecific, making clinical suspicion important.

- Establishing an accurate diagnosis of VTE with objective testing is essential.

- Neither chest radiographic, the EKG, nor arterial blood gas findings testing are specific for acute PE, and if clinical suspicion for acute PE is high in the setting of a negative chest CT, additional testing should be done.

- Clear advantages of LMWH over standard UFH for treatment of acute VTE include greater bioavailability, subcutaneous administration, less need for monitoring, and a lower rate of HIT.

- Thrombolytic therapy should be strongly considered for acute PE in the setting of hypotension. It should also be considered when there is severe hypoxemia or right ventricular dysfunction but contraindications must always be carefully reviewed.

- Every patient admitted to the hospital should be considered for VTE prophylaxis. It will be appropriate for most.

REFERENCES

- 1. Dalen JE, Alpert JS. Natural history of pulmonary embolism. *Prog Cardiovasc Dis* 1975; **17**: 257–70.

- 2. Lindblad B, Eriksson A, Bergquist D. Autopsy-verified pulmonary embolism in a surgical department: Analysis of the period from 1951 to 1988. *Br J Surg* 1991; **78**: 849–52.

   3. Anderson FA, Wheeler HB. Venous thromboembolism: Risk factors and prophylaxis. *Clin Chest Med* 1995; **16**: 235–51.

- 4. Alpert JS, Smith R, Carlson J. Mortality in patients

treated for pulmonary embolism. *JAMA* 1976; **236**: 1477–80.

5. Rubinstein I, Murray D, Hoffstein V. Fatal pulmonary emboli in hospitalized patients. An autopsy study. *Arch Intern Med* 1988; **148**: 1425–6.

6. Stein PD, Henry JW. Prevalence of acute pulmonary embolism among patients in a general hospital and at autopsy. *Chest* 1995; **108**: 978–81.

7. Prandoni P, Lensing AWA, Prins M, *et al.* What is the outcome of the post thrombotic syndrome? *Thrombos Haemost* 1999; **82**: 1196–7.

● 8. Pengo V, Lensing AWA, Prins MH, *et al.* Incidence of chronic thromboembolic pulmonary hypertension after pulmonary embolism. *N Engl J Med* 2004; **350**: 2257–64.

● 9. von Virchow R. Weitere Untersuchungen ueber die Verstopfung der Lungenarterien und ihre Folge. *Traube's Beitraege exp path u Physiol* 1846; **2**: 21–31.

10. Deitelzweig SB, Vanscoy GJ, Niccolai CS, Rihn TL. Venous thromboembolism prevention with LMWHs in medical and orthopedic surgery patients. *Ann Pharmacother* 2003; **37**: 402–11.

11. Benotti JR, Dalen JE. The natural history of pulmonary embolism. *Clin Chest Med* 1984; **5**: 403.

12. Wheeler HB. Diagnosis of deep venous thrombosis: review of clinical evaluation and impedance plethysmography. *Am J Surg* 1985; **150**(Suppl): 7–13.

13. Leclerc JR, Illescas F, Jarzem P. Diagnosis of deep vein thrombosis. In: Leclerc JR, ed. *Venous Thromboembolic Disorders*. Philadelphia: Lea and Febiger, 1991: 176–228.

14. Stein PD, Terrin ML, Hales CA, *et al.* Clinical, laboratory, roentgenographic and electrocardiographic findings in patients with acute pulmonary embolism and no pre-existing cardiac or pulmonary disease. *Chest* 1991; **100**: 598–603.

● 15. The PIOPED investigators. Value of the ventilation/perfusion scan in acute pulmonary embolism. Results of the prospective investigation of pulmonary embolism diagnosis. *JAMA* 1990; **263**: 2753–9.

16. Stein PD, ed. *Pulmonary Embolism*. Baltimore: Williams and Wilkins, 1996.

● 17. The Urokinase Pulmonary Embolism Trial; A national cooperative study. *Circulation* 1973; **47**(Suppl II): 1–108.

18. Green RM, Meyer TJ, Dunn M, Glassroth J. Pulmonary embolism in younger adults. *Chest* 1992; **101**: 1507–11.

19. Bounameaux H, Cirafici P, DeMoerloose P, *et al.* Measurement of D-dimer in plasma as diagnostic aid in suspected pulmonary embolism. *Lancet* 1991; **337**: 196.

20. Egermayer P, Town GI, Turner JG, *et al.* Usefulness of D-dimer, blood gas, and respiratory rate measurements for excluding pulmonary embolism. *Thorax* 1998; **53**: 830–4.

◆ 21. Ahearn GS, Bounameaux H. The role of the D-dimer in the diagnosis of venous thromboembolism. *Semin Respir Crit Care Med* 2000; **21**: 521–36.

● 22. Wells PS, Anderson DR, Rodger M, *et al.* Excluding pulmonary embolism at the bedside without diagnostic imaging: management of patients with suspected pulmonary embolism presenting to the emergency department by using a simple clinical model and D-dimer. *Ann Intern Med* 2001; **135**: 98–107.

● 23. Wicki J, Perneger T, Junod A, *et al.* Assessing clinical probability of pulmonary embolism in the emergency ward: a simple score. *Arch Intern Med* 2001; **161**: 92–7.

24. Pacouret G, Schellenberg F, Hamel E, *et al.* Troponine I dans l'embolie pulmonaire aigue massive: resultants d'une serie prospective. *Presse Med* 1998; **27**: 1627.

25. Giannitsis E, Müller-Bardoff M, Kurowski V, *et al.* Independent prognostic value of cardiac troponin T in patients with confirmed pulmonary embolism. *Circulation* 2000; **102**: 211–17.

26. Meyer T, Binder L, Hruska N, *et al.* Cardiac troponin I elevation in acute pulmonary embolism is associated with right ventricular dysfunction. *J Am Coll Cardiol* 2000; **36**: 1632–6.

27. Mehta NJ, Jani K, Khan IA. Clinical usefulness and prognostic value of elevated cardiac troponin I levels in acute pulmonary embolism. *Am Heart J* 2003; **145**: 821–5.

28. Douketis JD, Crowther MA, Stanton EB, Ginsberg JS. Elevated cardiac troponin levels in patients with submassive pulmonary embolism. *Arch Intern Med* 2002; **162**: 79–81.

29. Remy-Jardin M, Remy J, Wattinne L, Giraud F. Central pulmonary thromboembolism: Diagnosis with spiral volumetric CT with the single-breath-hold technique. Comparison with pulmonary angiography. *Radiology* 1992; **185**: 381–7.

30. Remy-Jardin MJ, Remy J, Deschildre F, *et al.* Diagnosis of acute pulmonary embolism with spiral CT: comparison with pulmonary angiography and scintigraphy. *Radiology* 1996; **200**: 699–706.

31. Goodman LR, Curtin JJ, Mewissen MW, *et al.* Detection of pulmonary embolism in patients with unresolved clinical and scintigraphic diagnosis: helical CT versus angiography. *AJR Am J Roentgenol* 1995; **164**: 1369–74.

32. Sostman HD, Layish DT, Tapson VF, *et al.* Prospective comparison of helical CT and MR imaging in patients with clinically suspected pulmonary embolism. *J Magn Reson Imaging* 1996; **6**: 275–81.

33. Mayo JR, Remy-Jardin M, Muller NL, *et al.* Pulmonary embolism: prospective comparison of spiral CT with ventilation-perfusion scintigraphy. *Radiology* 1997; **205**: 447–52.

34. Drucker EA, Rivitz SM, Shepard JO, *et al.* Acute pulmonary embolism: assessment of helical CT for diagnosis. *Radiology* 1998; **209**: 235–41.

35. Garg K, Sieler H, Welsh CH, *et al.* Clinical validity of helical CT being interpreted as negative for pulmonary embolism: implications for patient treatment. *AJR Am J Roentgenol* 1999; **172**: 1627–31.

36. Holbert JM, Costello P, Federle MP. Role of spiral computed tomography in the diagnosis of pulmonary embolism in the emergency department. *Ann Emerg Med* 1999; **33**: 520–8.

37. Perrier A, Howarth N, Didier D, *et al.* Performance of helical computed tomography in unselected outpatients with suspected pulmonary embolism. *Ann Intern Med* 2001; **135**: 88–97.

38. Ferretti GR, Bosson J-L, Buffaz P-D, *et al.* Acute pulmonary embolism: role of helical CT in 164 patients with intermediate probability at ventilation-perfusion scintigraphy and normal results at duplex US of the legs. *Radiology* 1997; **205**: 453–8.

39. Swensen SJ, Sheedy PF, Ryu JH, *et al.* Outcomes after withholding anticoagulation from patients with suspected acute pulmonary embolism and negative computed tomographic findings: A cohort study. *Mayo Clin Proc* 2002; **77**: 130–8.

40. Perrier A, Roy P-M, Sanchez O, *et al.* Multidetector-row computed tomography in suspected pulmonary embolism. *N Engl J Med* 2005; **352**: 1760–8.

41. Loud PA, Katz DS, Klippenstein DL, *et al.* Combined CT venography and pulmonary angiography in suspected thromboembolic disease: Diagnostic accuracy for deep venous evaluation. *AJR Am J Roentgenol* 2000; **174**: 61–5.

42. Meaney JFM, Weg JG, Chenevert TL, *et al.* Diagnosis of pulmonary embolism with magnetic resonance angiography. *N Engl J Med* 1997; **336**: 1422–7.

43. Tapson VF. Pulmonary embolism–new diagnostic approaches. *N Engl J Med* 1997; **336**: 1449–51.

44. Evans AJ, Tapson VF, Sostman HD, *et al.* The diagnosis of deep venous thrombosis: A prospective comparison of venography and magnetic resonance imaging. *Chest* 1992; **102**: 120S.

45. Come PC. Echocardiographic evaluation of pulmonary embolism and its response to therapeutic interventions. *Chest* 1992; **101**: 151S-162S.

46. Tapson VF, Davidson CJ, Kisslo KB, Stack RS. Rapid visualization of massive pulmonary emboli utilizing intravascular ultrasound. *Chest* 1994; **105**: 888–90.

47. Lensing AW, Levi MM, Buller HR, *et al.* Diagnosis of deep-vein thrombosis using an objective Doppler method. *Ann Intern Med* 1990; **113**: 9–13.

48. Killewich LA, Bedford GR, Beach KW, Strandness DE. Diagnosis of deep venous thrombosis: A prospective study comparing duplex scanning to contrast venography. *Circulation* 1989; **79**: 810–14.

49. Burke B, Sostman HD, Carroll BA, Witty LA. The diagnostic approach to deep venous thrombosis: which technique? *Clin Chest Med* 1995; **16**: 253–68.

50. Baxter GM, Duffy P, Partridge E. Colour flow imaging of calf vein thrombosis. *Clin Radiol* 1992; **46**: 198–201.

● 51. Davidson BL, Elliott CG, Lensing AWA. Low accuracy of color Doppler ultrasound in the detection of proximal leg vein thrombosis in asymptomatic high-risk patients. *Ann Intern Med* 1992; **117**: 735–8.

52. Heijboer H, Buller HR, Lensing AWA, *et al.* A comparison of real-time compression ultrasonography with impedance plethysmography for the diagnosis of deep-vein thrombosis in symptomatic outpatients. *N Engl J Med* 1993; **329**: 1365–9.

53. Haire WD, Lynch TG, Lieberman RP, *et al.* Utility of duplex ultrasound in the diagnosis of asymptomatic catheter-induced subclavian vein thrombosis. *J Ultrasound Med* 1991; **10**: 493–6.

54. Prandoni P, Polistena P, Bernardi E, *et al.* Upper-extremity deep vein thrombosis. Risk factors, diagnosis, and complications. *Arch Intern Med* 1997; **157**: 57–62.

55. Kreienberg PB, Chang BB, Darling RC III, *et al.* Long-term results in patients treated with thrombolysis, thoracic inlet decompression, and subclavian vein stenting for Paget-Schroetter syndrome. *J Vasc Surg* 2001; S100–5.

● 56. Paget J. Clinical lectures and essays. In: Anonymous. London: Longman's and Green,1875.

57. Tapson VF, Carroll BA, Davidson BL, *et al.* The diagnostic approach to acute venous thromboembolism. Clinical Practice Guideline. American Thoracic Society. *Am J Respir Crit Care Med* 1999; **160**: 1043–66.

58. Evans AJ, Sostman HD, Witty LA, *et al.* Detection of deep venous thrombosis: prospective comparison of MR imaging and sonography. *J Magn Reson Imaging* 1996; **6**: 44–51.

59. Evans AJ, Sostman HD, Knelson MH, *et al.* Detection of deep venous thrombosis: prospective comparison of magnetic resonance imaging to contrast venography *AJR Am J Roentgenol* 1993; **161**: 131–9.

60. Barritt DW, Jordan SC. Anticoagulant drugs in the treatment of pulmonary embolism. A controlled trial. *Lancet* 1960; **1**: 1309–12.

61. Hull R, Raskob G, Rosenbloom D, *et al.* Optimal therapeutic level of heparin therapy in patients with venous thrombosis. *Arch Intern Med* 1992; **152**: 1589–95.

62. Hirsh J, Dalen JE, Deykin D, Poller L. Heparin and low-molecular-weight heparin: mechanisms of action, pharmacokinetics, dosing, monitoring, efficacy and safety. *Chest* (Suppl) 2001; **119**: 64S–94S.

63. Hull RD, Raskob GE, Hirsh J, *et al.* Continuous intravenous heparin compared with intermittent subcutaneous heparin in the initial treatment of proximal vein thrombosis. *N Engl J Med* 1986; **315**: 1109–14.

64. Levine MN, Hirsh J, Gent M, *et al.* A randomized trial comparing activated thromboplastin time with heparin assay in patients with acute venous thromboembolism requiring large daily doses of heparin. *Arch Intern Med* 1994; **154**: 49–56.

65. Raschke RA, Reilly BM, Guidry JR, *et al.* The weight-based heparin dosing nomogram compared with a "standard care" nomogram. *Ann Intern Med* 1993; **119**: 874.

66. Buller HR, Agnelli G, Hull RD, *et al.* Antithrombotic therapy for venous thromboembolic disease. The Seventh ACCP Conference on Antithrombotic Therapy. *Chest* 2004; **126**: 401–28S.

67. Lagerstedt CI, Olsson C-G, Fagher BO, Oqvist BW. Need for long-term anticoagulant treatment in symptomatic calf-vein thrombosis. *Lancet* 1985; **2**: 515–18.

68. Hirsh J, Raschke R. Heparin and low molecular weight heparin. The Seventh ACCP Conference on Antithrombotic Therapy. *Chest* 2004; **126**: 188–203S.

69. Levine M, Gent M, Hirsh J, *et al.* A comparison of low molecular-weight-heparin administered primarily at home with unfractionated heparin administered in the hospital for proximal deep vein thrombosis. *N Engl J Med* 1996; **334**: 677–81.

70. Koopman MM, Prandoni P, Piovella F, *et al.* Low molecular-weight-heparin versus heparin for proximal deep vein thrombosis. *N Engl J Med* 1996; **334**: 682–7.

71. Dolovich LR, Ginsberg JS, Douketis JD, *et al.* A meta-analysis comparing low molecular weight heparins with unfractionated heparin in the treatment of venous thromboembolism. *Arch Intern Med* 2000; **160**: 181–8.

72. Siragusa S, Cosmi B, Piovella F, *et al.* Low-molecular-weight heparins and unfractionated heparin in the treatment of patients with acute venous thromboembolism: results of a meta-analysis. *Am J Med* 1996; **100**: 269–77.

73. Lensing AWA Lensing AWA, Prins MH, Davidson BL, Hirsh J. Treatment of deep venous thrombosis with low-molecular-weight heparins: a meta-analysis. *Arch Intern Med* 1995; **155**: 601–7.

74. Leizorovicz A, Simonneau G, Decousus H, Boissel JP. Comparison of efficacy and safety of low molecular weight heparins and unfractionated heparin in initial treatment of deep venous thrombosis. *BMJ* 1994; **309**: 299–304.

75. Merli G, Spiro T, Olsson C G, Abildgaard U, *et al.* Subcutaneous enoxaparin once or twice daily compared with intravenous unfractionated heparin for treatment of venous thromboembolic disease. *Ann Intern Med* 2001; **134**: 191–202.

76. Simmoneau G, Sors H, Charbonnier B, *et al.* A comparison of low-molecular-weight heparin with unfractionated heparin for acute pulmonary embolism. The THESEE Study Group. *N Engl J Med* 1997; **337**: 663–9.

77. The Matisse Investigators. Subcutaneous fondaparinux versus intravenous unfractionated heparin in the initial treatment of pulmonary embolism. *N Engl J Med* 2003; **349**: 1695–702.

78. Warkentin TE, Greinacher A. Heparin-induced thrombocytopenia: recognition, treatment, and prevention. The Seventh ACCP Conference on Antithrombotic and Thrombolytic Therapy. *Chest* 2004; **126**: 311S–337S.

79. Gould MK, Dembitzer AD, Doyle RL, *et al.* Low-molecular-weight heparins compared with unfractionated heparin for treatment of acute deep

venous thrombosis. A meta-analysis of randomized, controlled trials. *Ann Intern Med* 1999; **130**: 800–9.

80. Layish DT, Tapson VF. Pharmacologic hemodynamic support in massive pulmonary embolism. *Chest* 1997; **111**: 218–24.

81. Urokinase pulmonary embolism trial: phase 1 results; a cooperative study. *JAMA* 1970; **214**: 2163–72.

82. Urokinase-streptokinase embolism trial: phase 2 results; a cooperative study. *JAMA* 1974; **229**: 1606–13.

83. Marder, VJ. The use of thrombolytic agents: choice of patient, drug administration, laboratory monitoring. *Ann Intern Med* 1979; **90**: 802–8.

● 84. Goldhaber SZ, Kessler CM, Heit J, *et al.* Randomised controlled trial of recombinant tissue plasminogen activator versus urokinase in the treatment of acute pulmonary embolism. *Lancet* 1988; **2**: 293–8.

85. Goldhaber, SZ, Haire, WD, Feldstein, ML, *et al.* Alteplase versus heparin in acute pulmonary embolism: randomised trial assessing right-ventricular function and pulmonary perfusion. *Lancet* 1993; **341**: 507–11.

86. Goldhaber, SZ, Agnelli, G, Levine, MN. Reduced dose bolus alteplase vs conventional alteplase infusion for pulmonary embolism thrombolysis: an international multicenter randomized trial: The Bolus Alteplase Pulmonary Embolism Group. *Chest* 1994; **106**: 718–24.

87. Meneveau, N, Schiele, F, Vuillemenot, A, *et al.* Streptokinase vs alteplase in massive pulmonary embolism: a randomized trial assessing right heart haemodynamics and pulmonary vascular obstruction. *Eur Heart J* 1997; **18**: 1141–8.

● 88. Konstantinides S, Geibel A, Heusel G, Heinrich F, Kasper W. Heparin plus alteplase compared with heparin alone in patients with submassive pulmonary embolism. *N Engl J Med* 2002; **347**: 1143–50.

89. Bjarnason H, Kruse JR, Asinger DA, *et al.* Iliofemoral deep venous thrombosis: Safety and efficacy outcome during 5 years of catheter-directed thrombolytic therapy. *J Vasc Interv Radiol* 1997; **8**: 405–18.

90. Semba CP, Dake MD. Iliofemoral deep venous thrombosis: Aggressive therapy with catheter-directed thrombolysis. *Radiology* 1994; **191**: 487–94.

91. Athanasoulis CA, Kaufman JA, Halpern EF, *et al.* Inferior vena caval filters: review of a 26-year single-center clinical experience. *Radiology* 2000; **216**: 54–66.

92. Lindblad B, Tengborn L, Bergqvist D. Deep vein thrombosis of the axillary-subclavian veins: epidemiologic data, effects of different types of treatment and late sequelae. *Eur J Vasc Surg* 1988; **2**: 161–5.

93. Marinella, MA, Kathula SK, Markert RJ. Spectrum of upper-extremity deep venous thrombosis in a community teaching hospital. *Heart Lung* 2000; **29**: 113–17.

94. Schellong SM, Schwarz T, Kropp J, *et al.* Bed rest in deep vein thrombosis and the incidence of scintigraphic pulmonary embolism. *Thromb Haemost* 1999; **82**(Suppl): 127–9.

95. Aschwanden M, Labs KH, Engel H, *et al.* Acute deep vein thrombosis: early mobilization does not increase the frequency of pulmonary embolism. *Thromb Haemost* 2001; **85**: 42–6.

96. Partsch H, Blattler W. Compression and walking versus bed rest in the treatment of proximal deep venous thrombosis with low molecular weight heparin. *J Vasc Surg* 2000; **32**: 861–9.

97. Partsch, H. Therapy of deep vein thrombosis with low molecular weight heparin, leg compression and immediate ambulation. *Vasa* 2001; **30**: 195–204.

98. Goldhaber SZ, Tapson VF. A prospective registry of 5,451 patients with ultrasound confirmed deep vein thrombosis. *Am J Cardiol* 2004; **93**: 259–62.

✱ 99. Geerts WH, Pineo GF, Heit JA, *et al.* Prevention of Venous Thromboembolism: The Seventh ACCP Conference on Antithrombotic Therapy. *Chest* 2004; **126**: 338–400S.

100. Comp PC, Spiro T, Friedman, RJ, *et al.* Prolonged enoxaparin therapy to prevent venous thromboembolism after primary hip or knee replacement. *J Bone Joint Surg* 2001; **83A**: 336–45.

● 101. Samama MM, Cohen AT, Darmon J-Y, *et al.* A comparison of enoxaparin with placebo for the prevention of venous thromboembolism in acutely ill medical patients. *N Engl J Med* 1999; **341**: 793–800.

102. Leizorovicz A, Cohen AT, Turpie AGG, *et al.* A randomized placebo controlled trial of dalteparin for the prevention of venous thromboembolism in 3706 acutely ill medical patients: the PREVENT medical thromboprophylaxis study. *J Thromb Haemost* 2003; **1**(Suppl): OC396.

103. Kleber F, Witt C, Vogel G, *et al.* Randomized comparison of enoxaparin with unfractionated heparin for the prevention of venous thromboembolism in medical patients with heart

failure or severe respiratory disease. *Am Heart J* 2003; **145**: 614–21.

104. Lechler E, Schramm W, Flosbach CW, *et al.* The venous thrombotic risk in non-surgical patients: Epidemiological data and efficacy/ safety profile of a low molecular weight heparin (enoxaparin). The PRIME study. *Haemostasis* 1996; **26**(Suppl 2): 49–56.

105. Harenberg J, Shomacker U, Flosbach CW, Spiro T. Enoxaparin is superior to unfractionated heparin in the prevention of thromboembolic events in medical patients at increased risk of thromboembolism (abstract). *Blood* 1999; **94**(Suppl 1): 399a.

106. Hillbom J, Enla T, Flosbach CW, *et al.* Enoxaparin, a low molecular weight heparin, is superior to heparin in patients with acute atherothrombotic stroke (abstract). *Stroke* 1998; **29**: 304.

107. Garlund B. Randomised, controlled trial of low-dose heparin for prevention of pulmonary embolism in patients with infectious diseases. The heparin prophylaxis study group. *Lancet* 1996; **347**: 1357–61.

108. Halkin H, Goldberg J, Modan M, Modan B. Reduction of mortality in general medical in-patients by low-dose heparin prophylaxis. *Ann Intern Med* 1982; **96**: 561–5.

109. Bergmann JF, Neuhart E. A multicenter randomized double-blind study of enoxaparin compared with unfractionated heparin in the prevention of venous thromboembolic disease in elderly in-patients bedridden for an acute medical illness. The Enoxaparin in Medicine Study Group. *Thromb Haemost* 1996; **76**: 529–34.

● 110. Kucher N, Koo S, Quiroz R, *et al.* Electronic alerts to prevent venous thromboembolism among hospitalized patients. *N Engl J Med* 2005; **352**: 969–77.

111. Johnson MJ, Lucas GL. Fat embolism syndrome. *Orthopedics* 1996; **19**: 41–8.

112. Martin RW. Amniotic fluid embolism. *Clin Obstet Gynecol* 1996; **39**: 101–6.

113. Vesely TM. Air embolism during insertion of central venous catheters. *J Vasc Intervent Radiol* 2001; **12**: 1291–5.

114. King MB, Harmon KR. Unusual forms of pulmonary embolism. *Clin Chest Med* 1994; **15**: 561–80.

115. Morris W, Knauer CM. Cardiopulmonary manifestations of schistosomiasis. *Semin Respir Infect* 1997; **12**: 159–70.

Management of massive hemoptysis

SEAN T DEVINE, MICHAEL LIPPMANN

INTRODUCTION

The purpose of this chapter is to review the entity of massive hemoptysis. We review the history and physical exam, the differential diagnosis, the diagnostic evaluation, and potential therapies of massive hemoptysis.

DEFINITION AND ANATOMY

The definition of hemoptysis is not precise, and authors' opinions vary. However, the one common variable is the time span of 24 hours. Hemoptysis may be grouped into three categories:

- mild hemoptysis – <100 mL of blood in 24 hours
- moderate hemoptysis – <600 mL of blood in 24 hours
- massive hemoptysis – >600 mL of blood in 24 hours.

The amount and rate of bleeding and overall medical condition are important factors in the management of hemoptysis. For example, the patient who bleeds more than 600 mL in 6 hours has a mortality approaching 70 percent, and the patient with severe emphysema who bleeds only 100 mL will be significantly compromised. Fortunately, massive hemoptysis accounts for only 1.5 percent of hemoptysis cases.[1]

To understand the nature of hemoptysis, a brief review of the circulation of the lung is necessary.[2] The bronchial circulation is the source of hemoptysis in 90 percent of cases. The bronchial vessels typically originate from the aorta or the intercostal arteries; however, there is a great deal of variation. Typically, one bronchial artery supplies the right lung and two supply the left lung. It is not uncommon for the bronchial artery supply to have anastomotic connections with the pulmonary circulation. The bronchial arteries receive approximately 1 percent of cardiac output. This circulation becomes hypertrophied in conditions that increase its circulation (congenital heart disease) or in inflammatory states such as bronchiectasis or infections. When this occurs, the bronchial arterial supply can comprise 7 percent of the cardiac output. The blood that supplies the trachea and first several bronchial segments typically drains into the right heart via the azygos and hemiazygos veins. The blood that supplies the remaining bronchi drains into the left heart and contributes to venous admixture.

The pulmonary circulation is an infrequent contributor to hemoptysis. Instances in which it is the source of bleeding include common entities such as pulmonary infarcts and arteriovenous (AV) malformations to rare causes such as pulmonary artery agenesis and Rasmussen aneurysms.

HISTORY AND PHYSICAL EXAM

The history and physical exam are often normal, but the presence of certain signs and symptoms can offer insight into potential causes. The presence of a fever tends to indicate a infectious or vasculitic process; a wheeze or rhonchus in a fixed location suggests an obstructing carcinoma; a friction rub may indicate pulmonary thromboembolic disease; an ear, nose, and throat exam may reveal a bleeding source of the upper airway; cutaneous lesions may indicate a bleeding diathesis, trauma, or AV malformations, and a diastolic murmur could point to mitral stenosis.

Occasionally, a patient may experience pain or a warm feeling on the side of the hemoptysis, thus allowing self-localization of the bleeding. This, however, must always be confirmed by objective testing. It is occasionally difficult to differentiate between hemoptysis, epistaxis, and hematemesis. Epistaxis is frequently bright red because of its arterial origin and is associated with the spitting up rather than coughing of blood. Hematemesis is usually darker, resembling coffee grounds and occasionally mixed with food. Vigorous vomiting is often present. If measured the pH may be somewhat acidic in fresh hematemesis but will become buffered with time. With epistaxis, it assumes normal arterial values.

LABORATORY TESTS

A sputum Gram and acid-fast stain, complete blood count, coagulation profile, electrolytes, blood urea nitrogen/creatinine, and a urinalysis should be obtained to evaluate for an underlying infection, bleeding diathesis, a pulmonary–renal syndrome, or a paraneoplastic syndrome. When a collagen vascular disease, vasculitis or Goodpasture syndrome is suspected, further confirmatory testing may need to be done including an antinuclear antibody, c- and p-antineutrophilic cytoplasmic antibodies, antiglomerular basement membrane (GBM) antibodies. If human immunodeficiency virus (HIV) infection is suspected, testing is recommended.

DIAGNOSTIC EVALUATION

In the patient with massive hemoptysis, localization of the bleeding site is of the utmost importance. The diagnostic evaluation includes one or more of the following: chest radiograph, high-resolution computed tomography (CT) scan, fiberoptic bronchoscopy, rigid bronchoscopy, and angiography.

The chest radiograph is the most readily available diagnostic tool, but it has limitations. The usefulness of the radiograph is probably greatest when a pneumonia, cavitating lesion, lung abscess, or large cancer is present. Depending on the series reviewed, the chest radiograph localizes the site of bleeding between 46 percent and 82 percent of the time.[3–6] The inability of the chest radiograph to properly localize the site of the bleeding may be the result of aspiration of blood throughout the respiratory tree.

There is some controversy whether fiberoptic bronchoscopy or CT scanning of the chest should be the next step. Bronchoscopy should probably be the next step in the management of massive hemoptysis. It provides several initial advantages over CT:

- It is usually more readily available.
- It can be performed at the bedside.
- It has the ability to be a therapeutic maneuver (selective intubation and control of bleeding).
- If the chest radiograph is abnormal, it has a high likelihood of identifying the site of bleeding.

Bronchoscopy should be viewed as complementing CT. When both modalities are used, the positive yield is over 90 percent.[3] Several authors have advocated obtaining a high-resolution CT scan prior to or in place of bronchoscopy.[6,7] Most of these studies included minor and moderate amounts of hemoptysis. In addition, the studies based these recommendations on the fact that CT scans identified the cause and location more often than bronchoscopy. Although these parameters are important, CT does not offer a therapeutic intervention and is potentially hazardous for an unstable patient. It should be undertaken once the patient is stabilized to further define a treatment plan such as surgical resection.

DIFFERENTIAL DIAGNOSIS

The differential diagnosis of hemoptysis is extensive; however, it can be compartmentalized into the following etiologies: infectious, neoplastic, immunologic, vascular, and miscellaneous, including iatrogenic (Box 13B.1).

The most common causes of nonmassive hemoptysis are bronchitis, bronchiectasis, and lung cancer.[8] The most common cause of massive hemoptysis worldwide is active pulmonary tuberculosis.[9] In a recent retrospective study from Turkey, Fidan et al. reported that the most common causes of hemoptysis were lung cancer (34.2 percent), bronchiectasis (25 percent), and tuberculosis (17.6 percent).[10] Massive hemoptysis was most commonly associated with the latter two. Hirshberg et al.[3] reported that bronchiectasis (20 percent), lung cancer (19 percent), bronchitis (18 percent), and pneumonia (16 percent) were the most frequently identified causes of hemoptysis. Massive hemoptysis was most likely due to pneumonia (24 percent) and bronchiectasis (20 percent). The most recent series from the United States is by Johnston and Reisz.[11] In their retrospective review of 148 patients with hemoptysis, the most common causes were bronchitis (37 percent), bronchogenic carcinoma (19 percent), tuberculosis (7 percent), and pneumonia (5 percent). In this series, bronchiectasis was a far less common cause of massive hemoptysis (4 percent of the cases). Tuberculosis was still an important cause of massive hemoptysis in 18 percent of cases.

Box 13B.1 Differential diagnosis of hemoptysis

Infection

- Bronchitis
- Bronchiectasis
- Pneumonia
- Lung abscess
- Tuberculosis
- Fungi
- Parasites
- Tracheitis
- *Stachybotrys atra* infections

Neoplastic

- Primary lung cancer
- Bronchial adenoma
- Metastatic disease

Immunologic

- Goodpasture syndrome
- Idiopathic pulmonary renal syndrome
- IgA nephropathy
- Wegener's granulomatosis
- Polyarteritis nodosa
- Pemphigoid
- Henoch–Schönlein purpura
- Medication-induced thrombocytopenia
- Pulmonary hemosiderosis
- Systemic lupus erythematosus (SLE)
- Alveolar proteinosis
- Pulmonary Langerhans cell histiocytosis
- Scleroderma
- Behçet disease
- Microscopic polyangiitis
- Mixed cryoglobulinemia

Vascular

- AV malformations
- Primary pulmonary hypertension
- Pulmonary emboli
- Congenital heart disease
- Eisenmenger complex
- Aortic aneurysms
- Mitral stenosis
- Sequestration
- Pulmonary artery agenesis

Miscellaneous/iatrogenic

- Factitious
- Septic pulmonary emboli
- Bleeding diathesis
  - Anticoagulation, antiplatelet agents

- Trauma
  - Tracheobronchial tears
- Procedure induced
  - Bronchoscopy
  - Pulmonary artery catheters
  - Tracheal-innominate artery fistula
- Amyloidosis
- Idiopathic pulmonary hemorrhage
- Toxic alveolar hemorrhage

The most common infectious agents responsible for massive hemoptysis include tuberculosis, fungi, and bacterial pneumonia that may be associated with a lung abscess.[12–16] The presence of hemoptysis in tuberculosis typically indicates extensive involvement. It is also more common with chronic tuberculosis than acute tuberculosis. Chronic tuberculosis can lead to hemoptysis in several ways: it can lead to bronchiectasis, a pulmonary artery aneurysm near a cavity (Rasmussen aneurysm) or a broncholith that has eroded the wall of a bronchus. Furthermore, it can cavitate, thus predisposing to the development of an aspergilloma. Approximately 50–80 percent of patients with an aspergilloma will develop hemoptysis. On CT scan, a halo sign may be visualized (Fig. 13B.1). The hemoptysis is a result of the *Aspergillus* eroding the walls of blood vessels or release of a potent hemolysin. Although it is usually minimal in quantity, it can be massive and life-threatening.[12,17]

Bronchiectasis may be caused by any chronic inflammatory process. The array of implicated infectious agents include: tuberculosis, adenovirus, influenza, mycobacterium avium complex, HIV, measles, and pertussis.[13] Heroin use has also been implicated in the development of bronchiectasis. The pathophysiology of this is probably related to aspiration, infection, and pulmonary edema. Several case reports have described hemoptysis following heroin overdose.[18] Bronchiectasis causes

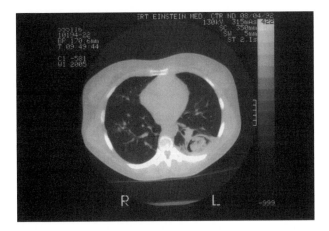

Figure 13B.1 *Computed tomographic scan showing aspergillosis of left lung.*

hemoptysis by rupture of the wall of tortuous enlarged bronchial arteries supplying the inflamed bronchi. As the pressures are systemic, the bleeding tends to be massive.

Hemoptysis caused by neoplasms is rarely massive. The most frequent type of neoplasm associated with hemoptysis is lung cancer. The most common cell types associated with hemoptysis are squamous cell and small cell carcinoma.[1,19] Carcinoid tumors have a higher tendency to produce hemoptysis. It may be as high as 50 percent of cases.[14] They produce hemoptysis by invading blood vessel walls. Metastatic disease to the lung is an infrequent cause of hemoptysis; however, when present it is usually due to endobronchial implants. Some metastatic tumors associated with hemoptysis include breast cancer,[15] colon cancer,[16] melanoma,[20] renal cell carcinoma,[21] hepatocellular carcinoma,[22] and uterine cancer.[23]

Immunologic disorders are another important cause of hemoptysis. They include such entities as the pulmonary renal syndromes, Behçet disease, Henoch–Schönlein purpura, microscopic polyarteritis, and the antiphospholipid syndrome. The more common pulmonary renal syndromes include Wegener's disease, SLE, and anti-GBM diseases such as Goodpasture syndrome. The mechanisms by which these entities produce hemoptysis vary. Wegener's disease is a pauci-immune necrotizing vasculitis; SLE is an immune complex disease and causes an autoimmune pneumonitis, and the anti-GBM antibodies in Goodpasture syndrome react with the alveolar basement membrane.

A number of medications have been associated with hemoptysis. Some of the more widely used medications include quinidine and phenytoin. Other important medications include anticoagulants, thrombolytics, and antiplatelet agents. The use of antiplatelet agents such as abciximab,[24] aspirin,[25] and tirofiban[26] has been associated with numerous reports of hemoptysis. Thrombolytics such as tissue plasminogen activator,[27] streptokinase,[28] and urokinase are widely used for acute myocardial infarctions and massive pulmonary embolism. They are well known to produce bleeding diatheses including hemoptysis; however, the reported incidence is less than 1 percent.[29] The literature is replete with reports of cocaine-induced hemoptysis.[30,31] The incidence is reported to be between 6 percent and 26 percent.[32,33] The mechanism of bleeding may be the rupture of bronchial or tracheal submucosal blood vessels or at the alveolar-capillary membrane. The membrane may be damaged directly or through vasoconstriction-induced epithelial damage.[30] Symptoms typically resolve within 36 hours, and treatment is supportive. The antiplatelet agents abciximab, eptifibatide, and tirofiban are glycoprotein IIb/IIIa inhibitors, widely used in acute coronary syndromes. All three agents have been associated with alveolar hemorrhage; abciximab has been the most frequently cited drug. The incidence appears to be 0.27 percent.[34] Risk factors for developing alveolar hemorrhage include acute myocardial infarction, low body weight, advanced age, prolonged and repeat percutaneous transluminal coronary angioplasty, chronic obstructive pulmonary disease, pulmonary hypertension, and an elevated pulmonary artery occlusion pressure.[35,36]

Vascular disorders comprise another entity that have the potential to cause hemoptysis. The vascular entities include abdominal and thoracic aneurysms,[37] AV malformations,[38] pulmonary sequestration,[39] tracheal enteric fistulae, pulmonary hypertension from any cause,[40] Ehlers–Danlos syndrome, and Dieulafoy disease.[41,42] A more recently described vascular entity is hemoptysis following catheter ablation of atrial fibrillation. Radiofrequency ablation is known to cause pulmonary vein stenosis, and the incidence ranges from less than 2 percent to 42 percent.[43,44] Foci from the pulmonary veins can cause atrial fibrillation, and ablation of these can eliminate the arrhythmia. The mean time to detection of severe pulmonary vein stenosis is 5.2 months. It is frequently asymptomatic (>50 percent), and when symptoms develop, they are often misdiagnosed. Common diagnoses include pneumonia, bronchogenic carcinoma, and venothromboembolic disease. The exact incidence of hemoptysis is not known.

Iatrogenic causes of hemoptysis have become an important cause. The list of causes includes mechanical interventions and medications. The mechanical causes include bronchoscopy and pulmonary artery catheters. A review of bronchoscopy-induced bleeding revealed that the incidence is between 0.5 percent and 1.3 percent.[45] There was a higher incidence in those undergoing transbronchial biopsy compared with endobronchial biopsy. The bleeding did not result in any deaths and was relatively easy to control with tamponade or topical epinephrine.[45] Risk factors for bleeding included immunosuppression, end-stage renal disease, and malignancy. Although the use of pulmonary artery catheters has declined, it remains an important cause in the differential diagnosis in the intensive care unit (ICU). Several large series have indicated that the incidence of pulmonary artery rupture is between 0.13 percent and 0.03 percent.[46,47] In a large series of 3500 patients, three sustained a pulmonary artery rupture and hemorrhage.[48] The exact incidence may be higher. There are autopsy series identifying unsuspected pulmonary artery rupture.[49] The overall mortality is approximately 70 percent.[50] Risk factors for pulmonary artery rupture include age greater than 60 years, pulmonary hypertension, anticoagulation, cardiopulmonary bypass, chronic steroid use,[51] distal migration of the catheter tip, pseudoaneurysm formation, catheter flushing in a wedged position, and overdistension of the balloon.[50] Hemoptysis occurs when endobronchial rupture occurs and the amount can be minimal to massive.

With the widespread prevalence of patients with HIV infection, a brief discussion of HIV and hemoptysis is essential. In one of the few studies published, the causative agents were in descending order: infectious, Kaposi sarcoma, pulmonary embolism, and lung cancer. The most common infectious causes were bacterial, mycobacterium, *P. carinii* pneumonia, bronchitis, bronchiectasis, and endocarditis.

The hemoptysis was defined as moderate to massive in 23 percent of the cases. In 92 percent of the patients the chest radiograph revealed abnormal findings, whereas 49 percent had a localizing film. When CT was used, only one patient had a normal radiographic exam.[52]

MANAGEMENT AND TREATMENT

General principles: diagnostic approach using the bronchoscope

As asphyxiation is the major life-threatening complication of massive hemoptysis, maintenance of an airway and adequate ventilation is crucial. The airway should be intubated with the largest endotracheal tube available – preferably a #8 or larger in an ICU setting. Of course, a large-bore intravenous line should be inserted and the patient should be typed and cross-matched for at least 6 units of blood.

The bleeding should be localized without delay. Although there is a debate regarding timing of bronchoscopy, most authorities favor early (within 48 hours) bronchoscopy. This approach is associated with the best success of identifying the bleeding site. In most cases, fiberoptic bronchoscopy via an existing endotracheal tube is the easiest and safest approach. In fact, the bronchoscope may be used to facilitate the intubation.[53] If fiberoptic bronchoscopy fails to identify the bleeding site, an experienced endoscopist can perform rigid bronchoscopy if time permits. Simultaneous use of both the rigid bronchoscope to achieve adequate ventilation and suctioning and the fiberoptic instrument to visualize the upper lobe orifices is an approach advocated by many. We have rarely resorted to the use of rigid bronchoscopy as in our hands bleeding will be localized in over 95 percent of patients between the chest radiograph, CT scan, and flexible bronchoscopy exam.[3,7] In McGuinness et al.'s study, which evaluated CT and fiberoptic bronchoscopy in 57 consecutive patients with hemoptysis, the diagnosis was suggested in 63 percent by CT scan and was most accurate in those with bronchiectasis or aspergillomas. Specific diagnoses were found at bronchoscopy in 49 percent and consisted of mucosal lesions, tumors or Kaposi sarcoma. Bronchoscopy localized the bleeding in only 40 percent of cases. However, the combined yield of CT and fiberoptic bronchoscopy in localizing the bleeding site was 81 percent. In a survey of pulmonologists, most favored the initial use of the fiberoptic bronchoscope to localize the bleeding site.[54] In our judgment, patient-described localization of bleeding (pain or sensation of gurgling on one side) or simply a radiographic abnormality are not reliable methods of localization. As many studies describe better outcomes in patients treated surgically versus medically, a thoracic surgeon should be notified.

Initial temporizing measures include: reversal of any coagulation disorders and protecting the nonbleeding lung from aspiration by placing the bleeding side down and selectively intubating the good lung. Regarding this latter approach, if bleeding is coming from the left lung, selective right main intubation is fairly easy with particular attention in avoiding blocking the right upper lobe bronchus resulting in atelectasis of that lobe. Should bleeding be coming from the right side, an experienced endoscopist can perform selective left mainstem intubation. In general, the placement of double-lumen endotracheal tubes is difficult in these emergent situations. This and their limited diameter make suctioning of clots difficult, making this option less attractive.[55,56]

Other acute temporizing measures administered bronchoscopically include: iced saline lavage,[9] topical epinephrine (1:20 000),[1] vasopressin, and fibrinogen-thrombin glues. In one series of patients with severe hemoptysis (defined as 150 mL in 12 hours), fibrin-thrombin was instilled endoscopically in 11 patients who could not undergo bronchial arterial embolization (BAE). Immediate control was achieved in all, but three had a relapse over a 39-month period. It was recommended that such glues be used only as temporizing measures.[57] Although there are reports of success with these glues, our experience has been disappointing. Intravenous desmopressin (DDVAP) has recently been used in an epidemic of leptospirosis associated with massive hemoptysis. Cessation of the hemoptysis occurred in five of the six patients in whom it was used.[58] One must be judicious in the administration of intravenous vasopressin as it may be associated with cardiac ischemia, fluid overload, and hyponatremia.[59,60]

Another approach to protect the nonbleeding lung is to introduce a Fogarty balloon through the working channel of the bronchoscope, which is then guided into the bleeding orifice. With some of the new balloons the bronchoscope can then be withdrawn and the balloon left in place.[61,62] Periodic deflations of the balloon by the bronchoscopist can then determine if the bleeding has ceased. Care should be taken to avoid prolonged use of such catheters to prevent mucosal ischemic injury.[63] The pulmonary artery catheter has been used in a similar fashion by placing it alongside the flexible bronchoscope and guiding it into the bleeding site.[64] In a similar vein, there is a recent description of an endobronchial balloon catheter[65] inserted alongside a bronchoscope to guide it to the bleeding site. This may be a promising technique. However, there are no data on the efficacy and outcome in patients with massive hemoptysis.[66] In general, these measures should be undertaken while awaiting more definitive therapy of the hemoptysis whether by surgery or BAE. Naturally, patients with alveolar hemorrhage syndromes, blood dyscrasias, or those on anticoagulant or antiplatelet therapy should receive appropriate medical therapy rather than invasive interventions. The use of cough suppressants containing codeine has been controversial as they have the potential to alter the level of consciousness and hence lead to the risk of aspiration. However, judicious use and careful titration should avoid this problem.

Medical therapy still has a role in the conservative management of major hemoptysis with bleeding ceasing in over 87 percent of patients managed medically in one large retrospective series.[67] As demonstrated in one study of 38 cases in which there were no deaths, patients with cystic fibrosis represent a group that can be managed conservatively without surgical intervention.[68] In one series of patients with cystic fibrosis, a Fogarty balloon was able to successfully tamponade the bleeding in all four patients.[69] In the rare patient who presents with hemoptysis and a normal chest radiograph (overall incidence 5 percent), fiberoptic bronchoscopy appears to be more cost effective as the initial diagnostic test as compared with CT scan.[70] However, in patients presenting with renal insufficiency and hemoptysis, bronchoscopy played a limited role in defining the bleeding site and had no impact on survival in one retrospective series of 34 patients. Other comorbidities played a more significant role and in no patient was the hemoptysis massive.[71] The use of Nd-Yag laser photocoagulation therapy is advocated only for bleeding endobronchial lesions.[72] In a recent series from MD Anderson Cancer Center, Morice *et al.* described the use of endobronchial argon plasma coagulation in 60 patients principally with bronchogenic carcinoma.[73] The volume of hemoptysis was greater than 50 mL/day in 50 percent of patients. Obstructions were documented in almost all patients with 24 having multiple obstructions. All procedures were performed with the fiberoptic bronchoscope with conscious sedation. Four patients were on mechanical ventilators at the time. All patients had complete cessation of hemoptysis with a mean follow-up of 97 days. It is evident that this technique is a viable option in those with airway lesions as the cause of their hemoptysis, provided that the proper equipment and training are available.[73] A rare but reported complication of massive hemoptysis is the formation of a large blood clot producing atelectasis and worsening ventilatory failure. Judicious use of the fiberoptic bronchoscope to remove the clot usually through an endotracheal tube and supportive measures which may include topical thrombolysis, usually results in resolution.[74,75]

Bronchial arterial embolization

As most bleeding originates from the systemic circulation via the bronchial arteries that originate from the aorta, embolization with various materials (steel coils, gelfoam, polyvinyl alcohol foam, gelatin pledgets) into feeding vessels appears reasonable as a therapeutic approach.[63] Bronchial artery embolization was first introduced by Remy, and in his largest series, the immediate success rate was 84 percent in 104 embolizations. Rebleeding only occurred in six patients.[76] It requires that the angiographer have thorough knowledge of the bronchial anatomy and its many variations particularly with regard to the take off of the spinal arteries. Inadvertent embolization into the anterior spinal artery can

result in ischemic injury to the spinal cord and permanent paralysis. Thus, visualization of the anterior spinal artery originating from a bronchial artery is a contraindication to embolization because of the risk of infarction and paraperesis.[77] In addition, embolized material can occasionally migrate to other vessels such as the popliteal or mesenteric systems. Other complications include pleuritic chest pain, fever, vessel perforation, and dissection.[78] Bronchial arterial embolization is clearly the treatment of choice in the nonsurgical candidate and may postpone definitive surgery in patients who are otherwise able to under resection. This would allow time to stabilize the patient.

Most reported series utilizing BAE have been in patients with postinflammatory conditions, principally bronchiectasis, tuberculosis, aspergillomas. and cystic fibrosis (Table 13B.1). It may be successful in the initial stemming of bleeding in 77–95 percent of patients with these disorders.[80–83] Only one small series has focused on patients with cancer with similarly described success and failure rates.[83] Frequently the identification of tortuous vessels or aneurysmal dilatation may be sufficient to identify a bleeding site rather than frank dye extravasation[77] (Fig. 13B.2). Recurrent bleeding has been reported in 16 percent to over

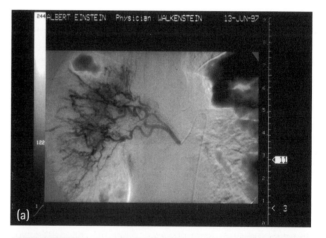

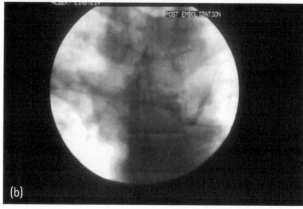

Figure 13B.2   *Angiograms: (a) pre-embolization and (b) post-embolization.*

Table 13B.1 *Current experience with bronchial artery embolization*

Study	Patients	Principal diagnoses	Initial success (%)	Recurrence rate (%)	Complications (n)
Remy et al.[76] 1977	49	TBC Bronchiectasis Aspergillosis	84	15	Bowel embolization Dysphagia (10) Fever
Uflacker et al.[79] 1983	33	TBC	82	18	Systemic embolization (2) Intimal tear (1)
Uflacker et al.[77] 1985	64	TBC	77	21	Systemic embolization(2) Intimal tear (1)
Fernando et al.[83] 1998	26	Inflammatory cancer	85	42	Splenic infarct (1)
Mal et al.[80] 1999	46	TBC	93	16	Neuro deficits (3)
Swanson et al.[81] 2002	54	Bronchiectasis PHBP	86	24	Intimal tear (2) Arterial perforation (1)
Barben et al.[82] 2002	20	Cystic fibrosis	95	55	None
Brinson et al.[84] 1998	18	Cystic fibrosis	93	46	Neuro deficits (3)
Katoh et al.[86] 1990	33	TBC Bronchiectasis	79	21	Intimal tear (2)
Osaki et al.[89] 2000	22	Bronchiectasis Aspergillosis	50	50	None
Swanson et al.[90] 1999	48	AVM	91	4	Hemothorax (1) Hemiparesis (1)
Wong et al.[88] 2002	16	TBC	100	25	Hemiparesis (1)
Cremaschi et al.[87] 1993	209	Bronchiectasis TBC	100	16	None
Kato et al.[85] 2000	101	Bronchiectasis TBC	94	38	Focal tear (5)

AVM, arteriovenous malformation; TBC, tuberculosis; PHBP, pulmonary hypertension.

50 percent[80,82–84,91] and may be due to recanalization of vessels or revascularization by collaterals.[86] In the largest study to date of 209 patients, the success rate 24 hours post-procedure was 98 percent, but recurrent bleeding occurred within a year in 16 percent.[87] In a recent report of its use in 16 patients with massive hemoptysis mainly from posttuberculous bronchiectasis, the procedure was successful in all.[88] Only two patients required further intervention – one requiring surgical resection and the other radiotherapy. An interesting observation in this study is the association of pleural disease and the presence of nonbronchial systemic collateral vessels.[88] The incidence of bleeding is highest in those with old or chronic tuberculosis and patients with mycetomas. Recurrent hemoptysis almost always occurs within the first 3 years after BAE.[89] The two peak periods of rebleeding are 1–2 months after embolotherapy and 1–2 years following the procedure.[81] Failure is often due to collaterals originating from nonbronchial sites such as the phrenic, intercostal, mammary, and subclavian arteries.[91,92] Patients with bronchogenic carcinomas as the reason for the bleeding have the highest failure rates.[81,93] The right lung was the source of the bleeding approximately 62 percent of the time in two large series of a total of 174 patients.[81,94]

The development of newer, selective catheter systems may reduce the complications of this procedure.[95] The use of post-procedure aortography may enhance the identification of bleeding from other systemic sites.[96] This technique has also been successful in patients with cystic fibrosis with bleeding cessation in almost all patients in one study.[97] In a more recent study of 18 patients with cystic fibrosis from a large cystic fibrosis center undergoing 36 BAE procedures, initial control of the hemoptysis ranged from 75 percent after one session to 93 percent after three. The overall recurrence in this population was 46 percent with a mean time to recurrence of about a year.[84] Embolization remains the treatment of choice for the management of pulmonary AV malformations particularly if there are multiple AV malformations. In a Mayo clinic series, 48 patients were treated with coil embolization utilizing 78 sessions for a total of over 200 lesions. Of these, 91 percent responded to therapy with either improvement in symptoms (only 14 patients had presented with hemoptysis) or gas exchange.[90] A recent survey of pulmonary physicians indicated that 50 percent favored the use of BAE even in operable patients compared with only 23 percent in a survey performed 15 years earlier.[98] Thus, it appears that with greater experience and acquired expertise of angiographers, BAE will be used earlier and may avoid surgery in selected patients.

Surgery

Surgery remains the definitive therapy of choice in those whose pulmonary physiology and overall general health including comorbidities allow. Often, estimates must be made of the patient's pulmonary function, as time and the critical nature of the illness may not allow for adequate assessment. As most surgery is emergent, mortality approaches 20 percent with a range of 1–50 percent in some series,[78] and postoperative morbidities occur frequently. In medically managed patients, mortality ranges a bit higher, generally from 11 to 80 percent. Crocco *et al.* were among the first to demonstrate a superior outcome in surgically managed patients (19 percent mortality) compared with medically treated patients (78 percent mortality).[99] The rate of bleeding played a role in outcome with those who had hemoptysis of 600 mL in 4 hours having a mortality of 71 percent as compared with those with the same amount in 48 hours with a mortality of only 5 percent. Gourin described similar findings with 37 percent mortality in those with active bleeding at the time of surgery compared with just 8 percent in those in whom the bleeding had ceased. Mortality was 58 percent when hemoptysis exceeded 1000 mL in 24 hours compared with 9 percent if less than 100 mL in 24 hours.[100]

The problems with studies comparing outcome in surgically and medically managed patients are that they are generally observational, nonrandomized and biased in the decision about how to manage these patients. In addition, almost all reported series on treatment were published prior to the advent and perfection of BAE. Surgery should not be considered in those with diffuse bilateral disease, inadequate pulmonary reserve including known baseline hypercapnia, inoperable carcinoma, inability to localize the bleeding site, multiple AV malformations, and diffuse alveolar hemorrhage syndromes. Surgery remains an important therapeutic option, particularly when BAE fails or is not available or when the hemoptysis is so massive that there is imminent threat to life, provided that adequate localization of the bleeding can be accomplished. In our two recently reported cases of massive hemoptysis associated with actinomycosis, one patient had a BAE that did not reveal a bleeding site. Both patients had successful emergent thoracotomies to control their bleeding.[101]

The definitive surgical management of a pulmonary artery rupture from an overinflated and peripherally located Swan–Ganz catheter may be delayed by withdrawing and reinflating the balloon. This compresses the bleeding site more proximally.[102] Distal embolization with steel coils or Gelfoam can then be considered in the definitive management of bleeding particularly in those with pseudoaneurysm formation who are not surgical candidates.[103]

Since the advent of newer angiographic and bronchoscopic techniques, survival rates with the use of medical therapy have improved, approaching that of surgically treated patients. This is particularly true when emergent surgery is required. When available, these techniques should be attempted as first-line therapy when available. A special group of patients is those with fungus balls or aspergillomas occupying cavities in patients with chronic pulmonary diseases such as tuberculosis, sarcoidosis, and more recently described cavities from *P. carinii* infections in those infected with HIV.[104] In the patients whose pulmonary physiology allows, surgery remains the most viable option with acceptable mortalities and complication rates in carefully selected populations.[105–108] However, in more compromised medical populations, intracavitary instillation of a regimen consisting of amphotericin B has been effective.[109–111] In addition there are isolated case reports advocating radiotherapy[112] or oral itraconazole in the treatment of inoperable patients with aspergillomas.[113] Occasionally fungus balls can undergo spontaneous lysis so a period of observation is recommended.[114] An algorithmic approach to the management of massive hemoptysis is outlined in Figure 13B.3. It must be stressed, however, that the management of each case is to be individualized, and there is no uniform approach to the care of these severely ill patients.

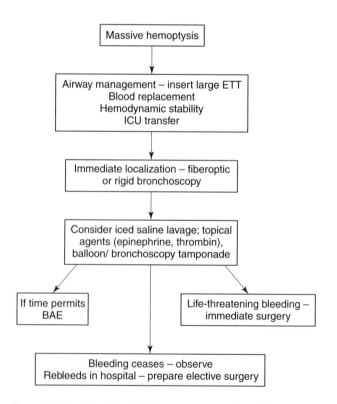

Figure 13B.3 *Algorithm for the management of massive hemoptysis. ETT, endotracheal tube; ICU, intensive care unit; BAE, bronchial arterial embolization.*

Key learning points

- The amount and rate of bleeding and overall medical condition are important factors in the management of hemoptysis.

- The history and physical exam are often normal, but the presence of certain signs and symptoms can offer insight into potential causes.

- A patient may experience pain or a warm feeling on the side of the hemoptysis, thus allowing self-localization of the bleeding. This, however, must always be confirmed by objective testing.

- In the patient with massive hemoptysis, localization of the bleeding site is of the utmost importance.

- The chest radiograph is the most readily available diagnostic tool. Bronchoscopy should probably be the next step in the management of massive hemoptysis. It provides several initial advantages over CT.

- The differential diagnosis of hemoptysis is extensive; however, it can be compartmentalized into the following etiologies: infectious, neoplastic, immunologic, vascular, and miscellaneous, including iatrogenic.

- Many medications have been associated with hemoptysis, including quinidine, phenytoin, anticoagulants, thrombolytics, and antiplatelet agents.

- As asphyxiation is the major life-threatening complication of massive hemoptysis, maintenance of an airway and adequate ventilation is crucial.

- Early (within 48 hours) bronchoscopy is associated with the best success of identifying the bleeding site.

- Initial temporizing measures include: reversal of any coagulation disorders and protecting the nonbleeding lung from aspiration by placing the bleeding side down and selectively intubating the good lung.

- Bronchial arterial embolization is clearly the treatment of choice in the nonsurgical candidate and may postpone definitive surgery in patients who are otherwise able to under resection.

- Surgery remains the definitive therapy of choice in those whose pulmonary physiology and overall general health including comorbidities allow.

REFERENCES

1. Jean-Baptiste E. Clinical assessment of massive hemoptysis. *Crit Care Med* 2000; **28**: 1642–7.

2. Deffebach ME, Charan NB, Lakshminarayan S, Butler J. The bronchial circulation. *Am Rev Respir Dis* 1987; **135**: 463–41.

3. Hirshberg B, Biran I, Glazer M, Kramer MR. Hemoptysis: etiology, evaluation, and outcome in a tertiary hospital. *Chest* 1997; **112**: 440–4.

4. Abal AT, Nair PC, Cherian J. Haemoptysis: aetiology, evaluation, and outcome. *Respir Med* 2001; **95**: 548–52.

5. Ong TH, Eng P. Massive hemoptysis requiring intensive care. *Intensive Care Med* 2003; **29**: 317–20.

6. Revel MP, Fournier LS, Hennebicque AS, *et al.* Can CT replace bronchoscopy in the detection of the site and cause of bleeding in patients with large or massive hemoptysis? *AJR Am J Roentgenol* 2002; **179**: 1217–24.

7. McGuinness G, Beacher JR, Harkin TJ, *et al.* Hemoptysis: prospective high resolution CT/bronchoscopic correlation. *Chest* 1994; **105**: 1155–62.

8. Gong H, Salvatierra C. Clinical efficacy of early and delayed fiberoptic bronchoscopy in patients with hemoptysis. *Am Rev Respir Dis* 1981; **124**: 221–5.

9. Conlan A, Hurwitz S, Krige L, *et al.* Massive hemoptysis. *J Thorac Cardiovasc Surg* 1983; **85**: 120–4.

10. Fidan A, Ozdogan S, Oruc O, Salepci B, Ocal Z, Caglayan B. Hemoptysis: a retrospective analysis of 108 cases. *Respiratory Medicine* 2002; **96**: 677–80.

11. Johnston H, Reisz G. Changing spectrum of hemoptysis. *Arch Intern Med* 1989; **149**: 1666–8.

12. Rafferty P, Biggs B, Crompton GK, *et al.* What happens to patients with pulmonary aspergilloma? Analysis of 23 cases. *Thorax* 1983; **38**: 579–83.

13. Barker AF. Bronchiectasis. *N Engl J Med* 2002; **346**: 1383–93.

14. Rosado de Christenson ML, Abbott GF, Kirejczyk WM, *et al.* Thoracic carcinoids: radiologic-pathologic correlation. *Radiographics* 1999; **19**: 707–36.

15. Ohno T, Nakayama Y, Kurihara T, *et al.* Endobronchial metastasis of breast cancer 5 years after breast-conserving therapy. *Int J Clin Oncol* 2001; **6**: 101–4.

16. Berg HK, Petrelli NJ, Herrera L, *et al.* Endobronchial metastasis from colorectal carcinoma. *Dis Colon Rectum* 1984; **27**: 745–8.

17. Glimp RA, Bayer AS. Pulmonary aspergilloma: diagnostic and therapeutic considerations. *Arch Intern Med* 1983; **143**: 303–8.

18. Schachter EN, Basta WB. Bronchiectasis following heroin overdose. *Chest* 1973; **63**: 363–6.

19. Miller RR, McGregor DH. Hemorrhage from carcinoma of the lung. *Cancer* 1980; **46**: 200–5.

20. Castro DJ, Saxton RE, Ward PH, *et al.* Flexible Nd:YAG laser palliation of obstructive tracheal metastatic lesions. *Laryngoscope* 1990; **100**: 1208–14.

21. Sakumoto N, Inafuku S, Shimoji H, *et al.* Endobronchial metastasis from renal cell carcinoma: report of a case. *Surg Today* 2000; **30**: 744–6.

22. Kawaguchi T, Tanaka M, Itano S. Successful treatment for bronchial bleeding from invasive pulmonary metastasis of hepatocellular carcinoma: a case report. *Hepatogastroenterology* 2001; **48**: 851–3.

23. Bouros D, Papadakis K, Siafakas N, Fuller AF Jr. Natural history of patients with pulmonary metastases from uterine cancer. *Cancer* 1996; **78**: 441–7.

● 24. Khalou H, Eiger G, Yazdanfar S. Abciximab and alveolar hemorrhage. *N Engl J Med* 1998; **339**: 1861–2.

25. Khanlou J. Hemoptysis during lung biopsy after aspirin. *AJR Am J Roentgenol* 1998; **171**: 261.

26. Ali M, Paul S, Grady KJ, Schreiber TL. Diffuse alveolar hemorrhage following administration of tirofiban or abciximab: a nemesis of platelet glycoprotein IIb/IIIa inhibitors. *Catheter Cardiovasc Interven* 2000; **49**: 181–4.

27. Masip J, Vecilla F, Paez J. Diffuse pulmonary hemorrhage after fibrinolytic therapy for acute myocardial infarction. *Int J Cardiol* 1998; **63**: 95–7.

28. Disler L J, Rosendorff A. Pulmonary hemorrhage following intravenous streptokinase for acute myocardial infarction. *Int J Cardiol* 1990; **29**: 387–90.

29. Chang Y, Patz EF, Goodman PC, Granger CB. Significance of hemoptysis following thrombolytic therapy for acute myocardial infarction. *Chest* 1996; **109**: 727–9.

● 30. Haim DY, Lippmann ML, Goldberg SK, Walkenstein, MD. The pulmonary complications of crack cocaine. *Chest* 1995; **107**: 233–40.

● 31. Forrester JM, Steele AW, Waldron JA, Parsons PE. Crack lung: an acute pulmonary syndrome with a spectrum of clinical and histopathologic findings. *Am Rev Respir Dis* 1990; **142**: 462–7.

◆ 32. Tashkin DP, Khalsa ME, Gorelick D, *et al.* Pulmonary status of habitual cocaine smokers. *Am Rev Respir Dis* 1992; **145**: 92–100.

33. Suhl J, Gorelick DA. Pulmonary function in male freebase cocaine smokers. *Am Rev Respir Dis* 1988; **137**(Suppl A): 188.

34. Kalra S, Bell MR, Rihal CS. Alveolar hemorrhage as a complication of treatment with abciximab. *Chest* 2001; **120**: 126–31.

35. Aguirre FV, Topol EJ, Ferguson JJ, *et al.* Bleeding complications with the chimeric antibody to platelet glycoprotein IIb/IIIa integrin in patients undergoing percutaneous coronary intervention. *Circulation* 1995; **91**: 2882–90.

36. Khanlou H, Tsiodras S, Eiger G. Fatal alveolar hemorrhage and Abciximab (ReoPro) therapy for acute myocardial infarction. *Cathet Cardiovasc Diagn* 1998; **44**: 313–16.

37. Liu SF, Chen YC, Lin MC, Kao CL. Thoracic aortic aneurysm with aortobronchial fistula: a thirteen-year experience. *Heart Lung.* 2004; **33**: 119–23.

38. Marchesani F, Cecarini L, Pela R, *et al.* Pulmonary arteriovenous fistula in a patient with Rendu-Osler-Weber syndrome. *Respiration* 1997; **64**: 367–70.

39. Dyer JD, Anderson JM, John PR. A familial case of pulmonary arterial sequestration. *Arch Dis Child* 2000; **82**: 148–9.

40. Koerner SK. Pulmonary hypertension: etiology and clinical evaluation. *J Thorac Imaging* 1988; **3**: 25–31.

41. Bhatia P, Hendy MS, Li-Kam-Wa E, Bowyer PK Recurrent embolotherapy in Dieulafoy's disease of the bronchus. *Can Respir J* 2003; **10**: 331–3.

42. BA Yost, JP Vogelsang, Lie JT. Fatal hemoptysis in Ehlers–Danlos syndrome. Old malady with a new curse. *Chest* 1995; **107**: 1465–7.

● 43. Saad EB, Marrouche NF, Saad CP, *et al.* Pulmonary vein stenosis after ablation of atrial fibrillation: emergence of a new clinical syndrome. *Ann Intern Med* 2003; **138**: 634–8.

44. Purerfellner H, Aichinger J, Martinek, *et al.* Incidence, management, and outcome in significant pulmonary vein stenosis complicating ablation for atrial fibrillation. *Am J Cardiol* 2004; **93**: 1428–31.

● 45. Cordasco EM Jr, Mehta AC, Ahmad M Bronchoscopically induced bleeding. A summary of nine years' Cleveland clinic experience and review of the literature. *Chest* 1991; **100**: 1141–7.

46. Kearney TJ, Shabot MM. Pulmonary artery rupture associated with the Swan-Ganz catheter. *Chest* 1995; **108**: 1349–52.

◆ 47. Boyd KD, Thomas SJ, Gold J, *et al.* A prospective study of complications of pulmonary artery catheterizations in 500 consecutive patients. *Chest* 1983; **84**: 245–9.

48. Pellegrini RV, Marcelli G, Di Marco RF. Swan-Ganz catheter induced pulmonary hemorrhage. *J Cardiovasc Surg* 1987; **28**: 646–9.

49. Fraser RS Catheter-induced pulmonary artery perforation: Pathologic and pathogenic features. *Hum Pathol* 1987; **18**: 1246–51.

50. Coulter TD, Wiedemann HP. Complications of hemodynamic monitoring. *Clin Chest Med* 1999; **20**: 249–67.

51. Lois JF, Takiff H, Schechter MS, *et al.* Vessel rupture by balloon catheters complicating chronic steroid therapy. *Am J Roentgenol* 1985; **144**: 1073–4.

52. Nelson JE, Forman M. Hemoptysis in HIV-infected patients. *Chest* 1996; **110**: 737–43.

53. Imgrund SP, Goldberg SK, Walkenstein MD, *et al.* Clinical diagnosis of massive hemoptysis using the fiberoptic bronchoscope. *Crit Care Med* 1985; **13**: 438–43.

54. Haponik EF, Chin R. Hemoptysis: clinicians' perspectives. *Chest* 1990; **97**: 469–75.

55. Strange C. Double lumen endotracheal tubes. *Clin Chest Med* 1991; **12**: 497–506.

● 56. Gourin A, Garzon A. Operative management of massive hemoptysis. *Ann Thorac Surg* 1974; **18**: 52–60.

57. Javier de Gracia, David de la Rosa, Edelia Catalán, *et al.* Use of endoscopic fibrinogen–thrombin in the treatment of severe hemoptysis. *Respir Med* 2003; **97**: 790–5.

58. Pea L, Roda L, Boussaud V, Lonjon B. Desmopressin therapy for massive hemoptysis associated with severe leptospirosis. *Am J Respir Crit Care Med* 2003; **167**: 726–8.

59. Bilton D, Webb AK, Foster H, Mulvenna P, Dodd M. Life threatening haemoptysis in cystic fibrosis: an alternative therapeutic approach. *Thorax* 1990; **45**: 975–6.

60. Magee G, Williams MH, Jr. Treatment of massive hemoptysis with intravenous pitressin. *Lung* 1982; **160**: 165–9.

61. Freitag L, Tekolf E, Stamatis G, *et al.* Three years experience with a new balloon catheter for the management of haemoptysis. *Eur Respir J* 1994; **7**: 2033–7.

62. Freitag L. Development of a new balloon catheter for management of hemoptysis with bronchofiberscopes. *Chest* 1993; **103**: 593.

63. Lordan JL, Gascoigne A, Corris PA The pulmonary physician in critical care. Illustrative case 7: Assessment and management of massive haemoptysis. *Thorax* 2003; **58**: 814–19.

64. Jolliet P, Soccal P, Chevrolet JC. Control of massive hemoptysis by endobronchial tamponade with a pulmonary artery balloon catheter *Crit Care Med* 1992; **20**: 1730–2.

65. Arndt endobronchial blocker; Cook Critical Care.

66. Susanto I. Managing a patient with hemoptysis. *J Bronchol* 2002; **9**: 40–5.

● 67. Bobrowitz ID, Ramakrishna S, Shim YS. Comparison of medical v surgical treatment of major hemoptysis. *Arch Intern Med* 1983; **143**: 1343–6.

◆ 68. Stern RC, Wood RE, Boat TF, *et al.* Treatment and prognosis of massive hemoptysis in cystic fibrosis. *Am Rev Respir Dis* 1978; **117**: 825–8.

69. Swersky RB, Chang JB, Wisoff BG, Gorvoy J. Endobronchial balloon tamponade of hemoptysis in patients with cystic fibrosis. *Ann Thorac Surg* 1979; **27**: 262–4.

70. Colice GL. Detecting lung cancer as a cause of hemoptysis in patients with a normal chest radiograph: bronchoscopy vs CT. *Chest* 1997; **111**: 877–84.

71. Kallay N, Dunagan DP, Adair N, *et al.* Hemoptysis in patients with renal insufficiency: the role of flexible bronchoscopy. *Chest* 2001; **119**: 788–94.

72. Dweik RA Mehta AC Bronchoscopic management of malignant airway disease. *Clin Pulm Med* 1996; **3**: 43–51.

73. Morice RC, Ece T, Ece F, Keus L. Endobronchial argon plasma coagulation for treatment of hemoptysis and neoplastic airway obstruction. *Chest* 2001; **119**: 781–7.

74. Arney KL, Judson MA, Sahn SA. Airway obstruction arising from blood clot: three reports and a review of the literature. *Chest* 1999; **115**: 293–300.

75. Vajo Z, Parish JM. Endobronchial thrombolysis with streptokinase for airway obstruction due to blood clots. *Mayo Clin Proc* 1996; **71**: 595–6.

76. Remy J, Arnaud A, Fardou H, *et al.* Treatment of hemoptysis by embolization of bronchial arteries. *Radiology* 1977; **122**: 33–7.

● 77. Uflacker R, Kaemmerer A, Picon PD, *et al.* Bronchial artery embolization in the management of hemoptysis: technical aspects and long-term results. *Radiology* 1985; **157**: 637–44.

78. Dweik RA. Role of bronchoscopy in massive hemoptysis. *Clin Chest Med* 1999; **20**: 89–105.

79. Uflacker R, Kaemmerer A, Neves C, *et al.* Management of massive hemoptysis by bronchial artery embolization. *Radiology* 1983; **146**: 627–34.

80. Mal H, Rullon I, Mellot F, *et al.* Immediate and long-term results of bronchial artery embolization for life-threatening hemoptysis. *Chest* 1999; **115**: 996–1001.

● 81. Swanson KL, Johnson CM, Prakash UB, *et al.* Bronchial artery embolization: experience with 54 patients. *Chest* 2002; **121**: 789–95.

82. Barben J, Robertson D, Olinsky A, Ditchfield M. Bronchial artery embolization for hemoptysis in young patients with cystic fibrosis. *Radiology* 2002; **224**: 124–30.

83. Fernando HC, Stein M, Benfield JR, Link DP. Role of bronchial artery embolization in the management of hemoptysis. *Arch Surg* 1998; **133**: 862–6.

84. Brinson GM, Noone PG, Mauro MA, *et al.* Bronchial artery embolization for the treatment of hemoptysis in patients with cystic fibrosis. *Am J Respir Crit Care Med* 1998; **157**: 1951–8.

85. Kato, Kudo S, Matsumoto K, *et al.* Bronchial artery embolization for hemoptysis due to benign disease: immediate and long term results. *Cardiovasc Intervent Radiol* 2000; **23**: 351–7.

● 86. Katoh O, Kishikawa T, Yamada H, *et al.* Recurrent bleeding after arterial embolization in patients with hemoptysis. *Chest* 1990; **97**: 541–6.

87. Cremaschi P, Nascimbene C, Vitulo P, *et al.* Therapeutic embolization of bronchial artery: a successful treatment in 209 cases of relapse hemoptysis. *Angiology* 1993; **44**: 295–9.

88. Wong ML, Szkup P, Hopley MJ. Percutaneous embolotherapy for life-threatening hemoptysis. *Chest* 2002; **121**: 95–102.

89. Osaki S, Nakanishi Y, Wataya H, Takayama K, Prognosis of bronchial artery embolization in the management of hemoptysis. *Respiration* 2000; **67**: 412–16.

◆ 90. Swanson KL, Prakash UB, Stanson AW. Pulmonary arteriovenous fistulas: Mayo Clinic experience, 1982–1997. *Mayo Clin Proc* 1999; **74**: 671–80.

91. Keller FS, Rosch J, Loflin TG, *et al.* Nonbronchial systemic collateral arteries: significance in percutaneous embolotherapy for hemoptysis. *Radiology* 1987; **164**: 687–92.

92. Cowling MG, Belli AM. A potential pitfall in bronchial artery embolization. *Clin Radiol* 1995; **50**: 105–7.

93. Hayakawa K, Tanaka F, Torizuka T, *et al.* Bronchial artery embolization for hemoptysis: immediate and long-term results. *Cardiovasc Interv Radiol* 1992; **15**: 154–8.

◆ 94. Knott-Craig CJ, Oostuizen JG, Rossouw G, *et al.* Management and prognosis of massive hemoptysis. Recent experience with 120 patients. *J Thorac Cardiovasc Surg* 1993; **105**: 394–7.

95. Tanaka N, Yamakado K, Murashima S, *et al.* Superselective bronchial artery embolization for hemoptysis with a coaxial microcatheter system. *J Vasc Interven Radiol* 1997; **8**: 65–70.

96. Chun HJ, Byun JY, Seung-Schik Y, *et al.* Added benefit of thoracic aortography after transarterial embolization in patients with hemoptysis. *AJR Am J Roentgenol* 2003; **180**: 1577–81.

97. Fellows KE, Stigol L, Shuster S, *et al.* Selective bronchial arteriography in patients with cystic fibrosis and massive hemoptysis. *Radiology* 1975; **114**: 551–6.

98. Haponik EF, Fein A, Chin R. Managing life-threatening hemoptysis: has anything really changed? *Chest* 2000; **118**: 1431–5.

99. Crocco J, Rooney J, Fankuschen D. Massive hemoptysis. *Arch Int Med* 1968; **121**: 495–501.

100. Corey R, Hla KM. Major and massive hemoptysis: reassessment of conservative management. *Am J Med Sci* 1987; **294**: 301–9.

101. Murali G, Selcer U, Lippmann M. Life-threatening hemoptysis with thoracic actinomycosis: two case reports and review of the literature. *Clin Pulm Med* 2004; **11**: 112–16.

102. Thomas R, Siproudhis L, Laurent JF, *et al.* Massive hemoptysis from iatrogenic balloon catheter rupture of pulmonary artery: successful early management by balloon tamponade. *Crit Care Med* 1987; **15**: 272–3.

103. Guttentag AR, Shepard JA, McLoud TC. Catheter-induced pulmonary artery pseudoaneurysm: the halo sign on CT. *AJR Am J Roentgenol* 1992; **158**: 637–9.

104. Addrizzo-Harris DJ, Harkin TJ, McGuinness G, *et al.* Pulmonary aspergilloma and AIDS. A comparison of HIV-infected and HIV-negative individuals. *Chest* 1997; **111**: 612–18.

105. Chen JC, Chang YL, Luh SP, *et al.* Surgical treatment for pulmonary aspergilloma: a 28 year experience. *Thorax* 1997; **52**: 810–13.

◆ 106. Karas A, Hankins JR, Attar S, *et al.* Pulmonary aspergillosis: an analysis of 41 patients. *Ann Thorac Surg* 1976; **22**: 1–7.

107. Jewkes J, Kay PH, Paneth M, Citron KM. Pulmonary aspergilloma: analysis of prognosis in relation to haemoptysis and survey of treatment. *Thorax* 1983; **38**: 572–8.

108. Butz RO, Zvetina JR, Leininger BJ. Ten-year experience with mycetomas in patients with pulmonary tuberculosis. *Chest* 1985; **87**: 356–8.

109. Rumbak M, Kohler G, Eastrige C, Winer-Muram H. Topical treatment of life threatening haemoptysis from aspergillomas. *Thorax* 1996; **51**: 253–5.

● 110. Shapiro MJ, Albelda SM, Mayock RL, McLean GK. Severe hemoptysis associated with pulmonary aspergilloma. Percutaneous intracavitary treatment. *Chest* 1988; **94**: 1225–31.

111. Hargis JL, Bone RC, Stewart J, *et al.* Intracavitary amphotericin B in the treatment of symptomatic pulmonary aspergillomas. *Am J Med* 1980; **68**: 389–94.

112. Shneerson JM, Emerson PA, Phillips RH. Radiotherapy for massive haemoptysis from an aspergilloma. *Thorax* 1980; **35**: 953–4.

113. Campbell JH, Winter JH, Richardson MD, *et al.* Treatment of pulmonary aspergilloma with itraconazole. *Thorax* 1991; **46**: 839–41.

114. Fahey PJ, Utell MJ, Hyde RW. Spontaneous lysis of mycetomas after acute cavitating lung disease. *Am Rev Respir Dis* 1981; **123**: 336–9.

115. Keller FS, Rosch J, Loflin TG, *et al.* Nonbronchial systemic collateral arteries: significance in percutaneous embolotherapy for hemoptysis. *Radiology* 1987; **164**: 687–92.

Pulmonary vasculitis and diffuse alveolar hemorrhage

JOHN E FITZGERALD, MARVIN I SCHWARTZ

INTRODUCTION

The hallmark of vasculitis is inflammation of blood vessels and surrounding tissues.[1,2] This process results in stenosis and necrosis of vascular structures, and may produce bleeding, ischemia, or infarction of affected organs. Vasculitis should be considered whenever a patient presents with persistent constitutional complaints, a multisystem disease, and/or elevated serum markers of systemic inflammation. Some patients have months of prodromal symptoms, whereas others experience a fulminant, life-threatening disease course.

The clinical presentation of vasculitis in the lung includes the development of pulmonary arterial aneurysms, pulmonary hypertension, diffuse alveolar hemorrhage, and focal nodules or infiltrates. Most vasculitides involving the lungs are systemic in nature. These include the small-vessel vasculitides associated with antineutrophil cytoplasmic antibodies (ANCAs), Takayasu arteritis, Behçet disease, and vasculitis complicating collagen vascular disease. On occasion, the vasculitic process is limited to the lungs, as in most cases of necrotizing sarcoid granulomatosis, or the condition known as isolated pulmonary capillaritis.[3,4] Diffuse alveolar hemorrhage is a well recognized complication of vasculitis, but also develops as a result of antibody or immune-complex-mediated lung injury, inhalation of toxins, and exposure to certain drugs. The most common causes of alveolar hemorrhage also produce glomerulonephritis, and are known collectively as the pulmonary–renal syndromes.

SMALL-VESSEL VASCULITIS

Wegener granulomatosis, microscopic polyangiitis, and Churg–Strauss syndrome are a group of closely related, idiopathic, and pauci-immune forms of small vessel vasculitis that mainly affect arterioles, capillaries, and venules.[5,6] These are the most commonly recognized forms of vasculitis involving the lungs. Wegener granulomatosis and microscopic polyangiitis develop in approximately 1–3 per 100 000 individuals, and Churg–Strauss syndrome is much less common.[7] Each of these conditions is associated with a characteristic set of clinical, laboratory, and histopathologic patterns, but there is significant overlap.[5,8] As a result, these disorders are best considered variations of a single disease entity, ANCA-associated small vessel vasculitis.

The ANCAs are autoantibodies that react with various proteins contained in the cytoplasmic granules of neutrophils and monocytes.[9] Indirect immunofluorescence testing reveals two major ANCA staining patterns (Fig. 13C.1). The perinuclear (p-ANCA) pattern is classically associated with microscopic polyangiitis and Churg–Strauss syndrome. Enzyme-linked immunosorbent assay (ELISA) usually confirms the target antigen in these cases to be myeloperoxidase (MPO). The cytoplasmic (c-ANCA) pattern is most commonly seen in Wegener granulomatosis.[10] These antibodies typically react with the proteinase 3 (PR3) antigen. The diagnostic specificity for idiopathic small vessel vasculitis is 99 percent when the combination of c-ANCA/anti-PR3 or p-ANCA/anti-MPO is present.[11] This abrogates the need for biopsy confirmation in the appropriate clinical setting.[12] As an isolated test for confirming the presence of a small-vessel vasculitis, p-ANCA is less specific than c-ANCA (81 percent vs. 95 percent). Perinuclear ANCA may be identified in patients with inflammatory bowel disease, autoimmune hepatitis, primary biliary cirrhosis, and collagen vascular disease. Cytoplasmic ANCA are sometimes detected in association with chronic infections including hepatitis C virus, paracoccidioido-mycosis, and tuberculosis. These autoantibodies are also rarely detected in patients with collagen vascular disease and ulcerative colitis. In about 20 percent of Wegener granulomatosis patients, a perinuclear staining pattern is seen, and a similar number of Churg–Strauss and microscopic polyangiitis patients demonstrate a c-ANCA pattern.[11]

Antineutrophil cytoplasmic antibodies are thought to be directly involved in the pathogenesis of small-vessel vasculitis.[13–15] These antibodies bind to and activate neutrophils and endothelial cells. They trigger a respiratory burst in neutrophils, and promote the release of a variety of proinflammatory cytokines including interleukin (IL)-1, IL-8, and monocyte chemoattractant protein-1.[16] Autoreactive T lymphocyte clones specific for MPO and PR3 are also present in ANCA-associated vasculitis patients.[17] These cells play a key role in the development of vascular injury by assisting B cells with ANCA production, and through direct cell-mediated cytotoxicity. Also, the elaboration of interferon-γ and tumor necrosis factor-α contributes to T cell activation and granuloma formation.[18,19] In some patients, ANCA titers correlate with disease activity. However, these autoantibodies are not always detectable in patients with active disease, and some patients have persistent antibody positivity despite clinical remission.

Some interesting clinical differences have been noted between patients who express PR3-ANCA with those expressing MPO-ANCA.[20] Patients demonstrating anti-PR3 antibodies are more likely to have eye, ear, and upper respiratory tract involvement, granuloma formation, and a higher risk of disease relapse.[21,22] These patients also tend to have active renal lesions resulting in faster declines in renal function, although the long-term renal outcome is not different.[23] Distinguishing small-vessel vasculitis on the basis on their ANCA specificity rather than clinical features may be the most rational approach.

Many patients can be diagnosed with ANCA-associated small vessel vasculitis on the basis of clinical, radiologic, and serologic parameters. If serologic tests are negative or inconclusive, or if clinical features are atypical, then tissue biopsy is indicated. A diagnosis of Wegener granulomatosis, microscopic polyangiitis, and Churg–Strauss syndrome may require histologic examination, but that information has little impact on treatment. In patients with small-vessel vasculitis, therapeutic decisions are not based on diagnostic labels but rather on the type and severity of organ dysfunction encountered.

Clinical presentation of Wegener granulomatosis

Wegener granulomatosis is characterized by a triad of upper and lower respiratory tract and renal involvement.[24,25] The small-vessel vasculitides may also feature prominent constitutional complaints such as fever, weight loss, chronic fatigue, myalgias, and arthralgias. Common laboratory abnormalities include an elevated erythrocyte sedimentation rate, C-reactive protein and rheumatoid factor level, normochromic normocytic anemia, mild leukocytosis, thrombocytosis, and polyclonal gammopathy. Anti-cardiolipin antibodies are present in 25 percent.

Upper airway disease develops in 90 percent of Wegener granulomatosis patients and manifests as recurrent or persistent sinus infections, chronic nasal congestion, or epistaxis.[26] Physical findings include nasal crusting, mucosal ulceration, perforation of the nasal septum, and saddle-nose deformity. There are several other relatively common head and neck manifestations of Wegener granulomatosis that are

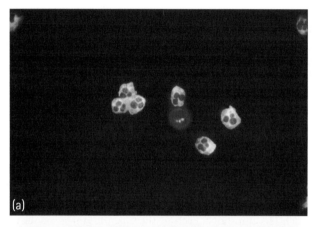

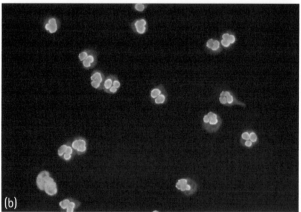

Figure 13C.1 *Indirect immunofluorescence patterns caused by antineutrophil cytoplasmic antibodies. (a) Cytoplasmic (c-ANCA) staining pattern after incubation of patient serum with alcohol-fixed neutrophils. (b) Perinuclear (p-ANCA) pattern. (Courtesy of Qasim Ansari, MD.)*

less appreciated. Ocular disease, occurring in up to a quarter of these patients, may take the form of scleritis, uveitis, optic neuritis, occlusion of the central retinal vessels, or proptosis due to retroorbital inflammatory pseudotumors.[27] Some patients develop or present with serous otitis or sensorineural hearing loss.[28] Oral ulceration and localized or diffuse gingivitis may also be observed.

Pulmonary disease is seen in 65–85 percent of patients with Wegener granulomatosis.[24,25,29] Symptoms include cough, chest pain, and hemoptysis, but respiratory symptoms may be absent. Pulmonary nodules, masses, or focal infiltrates represent the most common radiographic abnormalities (Fig. 13C.2).[30,31] They may be single, but are often multiple, and cavitation is frequent. Pleural effusions are occasionally seen. Diffuse alveolar hemorrhage may produce widespread alveolar opacities, often with respiratory failure. This complication develops in 5–10 percent of patients with Wegener granulomatosis and carries a 25 percent risk of death (see section on Alveolar hemorrhage syndromes).[24,32]

Lower airway involvement is underappreciated. Inflammation and scarring within the trachea and bronchi may lead to airway stenosis and lobar atelectasis. Subglottic stenosis is particularly common, occurring in 15 percent, and must be excluded in any Wegener granulomatosis patient who complains of hoarseness or dyspnea.[33] Spirometry may reveal flattening of the inspiratory flow-volume loop in such cases, consistent with a variable extrathoracic airway obstruction. In patients with symptoms, management may include mechanical dilatation of the stricture with intralesional glucocorticoid injection, or sometimes tracheostomy.

Renal disease is usually asymptomatic until severe functional impairment occurs. Serum chemistries may reveal an elevation in creatinine and blood urea nitrogen levels. The urinalysis shows proteinuria, hematuria, and erythrocyte casts. The kidneys are eventually affected in 50–90 percent of Wegener granulomatosis patients, but only 20 percent have glomerulonephritis at the time of presentation.[24,25,29] Because patients frequently do not have a classic pulmonary–renal syndrome when they first present to medical attention, lengthy diagnostic and treatment delays often ensue. This contributes to the long-term morbidity faced by these individuals, and reinforces the importance of recognizing the other systemic clues to the presence of a vasculitis.

Up to a half of Wegener granulomatosis patients will develop cutaneous involvement during the course of their disease.[34,35] Most often, this takes the form of palpable purpura due to a leukocytoclastic vasculitis. Other manifestations include signs of digital ischemia, skin nodules or lesions resembling pyoderma gangrenosum. Gastrointestinal symptoms including abdominal pain, diarrhea, and bleeding from colonic or small bowel ulcerations are the result of mesenteric vasculitis, and are seen in less than 15 percent of patients.[29,36] In severe cases, bowel perforation or infarction may develop. Neurologic complications are also underappreciated in Wegener granulomatosis, yet occur in 20–50 percent of patients.[37,38] The most common abnormality is a mononeuritis multiplex. Cranial neuropathies, stroke, seizures, and cerebritis may also be seen.

Clinical presentation of microscopic polyangiitis

Many of the features of Wegener granulomatosis also occur in microscopic polyangiitis, with the exception of cavitating pulmonary lesions and granuloma formation.[39] Renal involvement is more common (80–100 percent), and is usually evident at the initial presentation.[40] Diffuse alveolar hemorrhage is also more frequent, being identified in 10–40 percent of polyangiitis patients.[41,42] Palpable purpura is seen in half (Fig. 13C.3). Ocular involvement, sinusitis, epistaxis, and oral ulceration occur, but less frequently (30 percent overall). Absent are the destructive, granulomatous lesions seen in Wegener granulomatosis that lead to nasal septum perforation, saddle nose deformity, and retroorbital pseudotumors. Mesenteric vasculitis is more common in microscopic polyangiitis (30 percent), and there is probably a similar frequency of nervous system involvement.[42] Although, traditionally, they have been considered separate entities, patients presenting with only cutaneous leukocytoclastic vasculitis, or isolated pulmonary capillaritis, or idiopathic, pauci-immune glomerulonephritis may simply represent skin, lung and kidney-limited forms of microscopic polyangiitis.

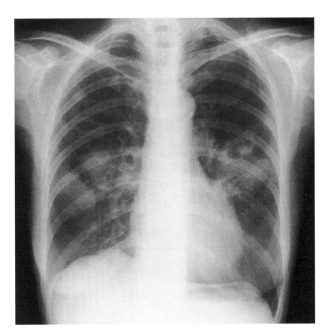

Figure 13C.2 *Wegener granulomatosis. The chest radiograph demonstrates multiple bilateral pulmonary masses, some of which are cavitating.*

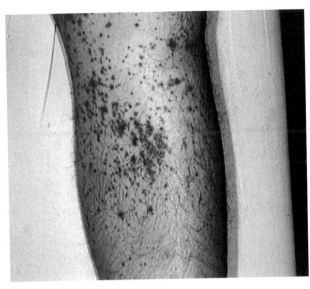

Figure 13C.3 *Palpable purpura in a patient with microscopic polyangiitis. This is the most common skin lesion associated with vasculitis. (Courtesy of Melissa Costner, MD.)*

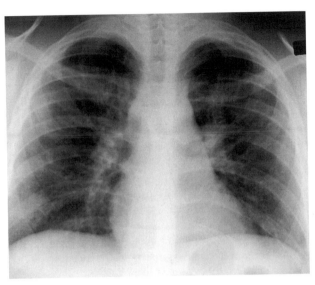

Figure 13C.4 *Churg–Strauss syndrome. The chest radiograph demonstrates patchy, bilateral ground glass opacities. This patient had a history of asthma and chronic rhinosinusitis, and presented with eosinophilia, a peripheral neuropathy, and a nodular skin rash. Serologic evaluation revealed p-ANCA and antimyeloperoxidase antibodies.*

Clinical presentation of Churg–Strauss syndrome

The hallmark of Churg–Strauss syndrome is the presence of asthma and eosinophilia in association with a necrotizing vasculitis.[43,44] Most frequently involved sites include the lungs, nervous system, skin, heart, and gastrointestinal tract. Kidney involvement is less severe in comparison with the other small-vessel vasculitides, but renal failure can still occur. Chronic allergic rhinosinusitis and nasal polyposis are often seen with asthma in the prodromal phase of Churg–Strauss syndrome, which may last for years. Simple tissue eosinophilia follows, commonly involving the lung or gastrointestinal tract.[45] Control of asthma worsens during this phase of the illness, and marked elevations in serum IgE levels may be seen. If not suppressed with systemic corticosteroid therapy, patients then enter the vasculitic phase of the illness. Constitutional symptoms develop at this point, but the asthmatic complaints may actually remit. Skin disease in the form of palpable purpura or subcutaneous nodules develops in two-thirds of the patients with Churg-Strauss syndrome.[46] When abnormal, lung imaging studies reveal nodular lesions, patchy ground glass opacities, or frank alveolar infiltrates (Fig. 13C.4).

Gastrointestinal involvement occurs in 50 percent during the course of the disease, and manifests as either eosinophilic gastroenteritis or mesenteric ischemia (bowel ulceration, abdominal pain, diarrhea, gastrointestinal hemorrhage). Among the ANCA-associated vasculitides, intestinal involvement is most common in Churg–Strauss syndrome. The same is true for neurologic impairment. Peripheral neuropathies, typically in the form of mononeuritis multiplex, are seen in at least two-thirds.[47] Involvement of the heart can be expected in 40 percent, and is the leading cause of death.[43,48,49] It may manifest as congestive heart failure due to eosinophilic myocarditis, or myocardial infarction due to coronary vasculitis. Pericardial effusions are common. Renal failure and cerebral hemorrhage are each responsible for approximately 15 percent of deaths associated with Churg–Strauss syndrome.[48]

Histopathology of small-vessel vasculitis

Histopathologically, Wegener granulomatosis features a triad of vasculitis, granulomatous inflammation, and tissue necrosis. The upper airway is commonly involved, and sinonasal biopsies are easily obtained. Unfortunately, these specimens often reveal only nonspecific, chronic inflammation. The 'diagnostic' combination of vasculitis and granulomas is seen in only 20 percent of sinonasal biopies.[50] Renal biopsies typically demonstrate a segmental, necrotizing, and crescentic glomerulonephritis, without vasculitis or granulomas.[51] Immunofluorescence techniques can confirm the presence of a pauci-immune glomerulonephritis, but that will not distinguish Wegener granulomatosis from microscopic polyangiitis or Churg–Strauss syndrome. Lung biopsies are much more likely to reveal necrotizing granulomatous vasculitis (Fig. 13C.5), particularly when focal nodules, infiltrates or cavities are identified on the chest radiograph.[51] Patients with Wegener granulomatosis who present with diffuse alveolar hemorrhage typically have pulmonary capillaritis, with or

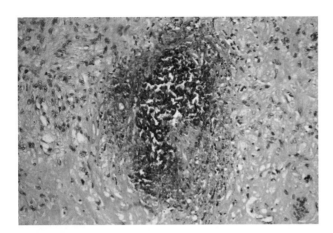

Figure 13C.5 *Wegener granulomatosis. This lung biopsy demonstrates vasculitis with fibrinoid necrosis of portions of the vascular wall. A multinucleated giant cell can be seen in the lower right hand corner, confirming an underlying granulomatous process.*

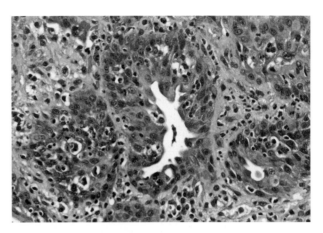

Figure 13C.7 *Churg–Strauss syndrome. Numerous eosinophils are seen infiltrating the vessel wall in this lung biopsy specimen. (Courtesy of Carlyne Cool, MD.)*

without giant cells or granulomas. Pulmonary capillaritis is not specific for small-vessel vasculitis. It is also seen in patients with collagen vascular disease, isolated pulmonary capillaritis, certain drug-induced lung injuries, and a subset of patients with Goodpasture syndrome. Capillaritis is characterized by the presence of neutrophils within alveolar septae and surrounding alveolar capillaries (Fig. 13C.6). Evidence of leukocytoclasis (nuclear dust and pyknotic nuclei associated with neutrophil apoptosis) can usually be seen. The release of proteolytic enzymes and toxic oxygen species from neutrophils results in fibrinoid necrosis of the alveolar wall, and erythrocytes spill into the alveolar lumen.[52]

Microscopic polyangiitis is not associated with granulomatous inflammation, but the histopathology is otherwise indistinguishable from Wegener granulomatosis.[39,42] The inflammatory process is focused on small vessels, but medium-sized arteries can be involved. Pulmonary capillaritis, leukocytoclastic vasculitis in the skin,

and rapidly progressive crescentic glomerulonephritis are the common features.[42,53]

When fully developed, Churg–Strauss syndrome is characterized by necrotizing vasculitis involving small- and medium-sized arteries, granulomatous inflammation, and eosinophilic infiltration of vessel walls and tissues (Fig. 13C.7).[54,55] However, more subtle presentations are now commonplace due to partial disease suppression by exogenous steroids used to control severe asthma.[45] In one series of 23 patients, only four demonstrated all of the classic histopathologic findings.[56] Eosinophilic organ infiltration (e.g. eosinophilic pneumonia or gastroenteritis) is enough to raise suspicion for Churg–Strauss syndrome. In the appropriate clinical setting, a positive ANCA and eosinophilia can be considered strong evidence of the disease without biopsy. Renal disease may result from interstitial nephritis or pauci-immune crescentic glomerulonephritis.[43,57] Diffuse alveolar hemorrhage is unusual in Churg–Strauss syndrome.[58] However, subclinical alveolar bleeding may be very common in all of the ANCA-associated vasculitides. In one study, bronchoalveolar lavage demonstrated hemosiderin-laden macrophages (indicating prior extravasation of red blood cells) in 53 percent of Wegener granulomatosis and Churg–Strauss syndrome patients, compared with only a small percentage of those with collagen vascular disease.[59]

Treatment of small-vessel vasculitis

Without treatment, the ANCA-associated vasculitides are fatal. Treatment with cytotoxic agents and corticosteroids significantly reduces mortality and allows recovery of organ function in patients with pauci-immune small vessel vasculitis.[60] Patients survive longer, but some must contend with considerable disease and treatment-related morbidity. Relapse is common despite lengthy courses of immunosuppressive therapy.[61] The intensity of initial

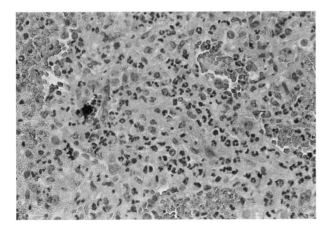

Figure 13C.6 *Pulmonary capillaritis. This lung biopsy shows marked thickening of the alveolar walls by infiltrating neutrophils. Hemorrhage is seen within alveolar lumens.*

treatment is determined by the severity of the clinical presentation. Patients with generalized vasculitis or serious organ dysfunction (including alveolar hemorrhage, severe glomerulonephritis, central nervous system, cardiac or gastrointestinal involvement) should receive 3–6 months of induction therapy with daily oral cyclophosphamide (2 mg/kg per day) in addition to corticosteroids.[62] Prednisone is initiated at a dose of 1 mg/kg per day and can usually be tapered to 20 mg/day within 2–3 months, and off by 6–12 months. For patients with diffuse alveolar hemorrhage or rapidly progressive glomerulonephritis 3 days of pulse methylprednisolone, 250 mg intravenously every 6 hours, is often utilized. Steroids alone may control acute alveolar hemorrhage, upper airway disease, and systemic symptoms, but will not prevent progression of other pulmonary or renal manifestations.[24,42]

The combination of methotrexate (20–25 mg/week) and prednisone has also demonstrated an ability to induce remission in most Wegener granulomatosis patients who present without life-threatening complications.[63] Methotrexate is effective in patients with active glomerulonephritis, but should not be used in patients with a serum creatinine level above 176.8 µmol/L (2 mg/dL), or in those with other serious organ dysfunction. Corticosteroid monotherapy is capable of inducing disease remission in patients with Churg–Strauss syndrome. However, up to 60 percent of these patients will require combination therapy.[64] Cyclophosphamide should be employed in patients who respond poorly to steroids alone, and in those with cardiac or central nervous system involvement, rapidly progressive glomerulonephritis, or significant mesenteric ischemia.[64,65]

Plasma exchange may improve outcomes in subsets of patients with diffuse alveolar hemorrhage or dialysis-dependent renal failure.[6,66] An additive benefit to drug therapy has not been demonstrated, however, when plasmapheresis is applied to unselected populations of small-vessel vasculitis patients.[67] Intravenous infusions of immunoglobulin have resulted in clinical improvement, and even in complete disease remissions, in patients with ANCA-associated vasculitis.[68–70] Unfortunately, there are few prospective, randomized, and controlled data available to clearly define a role for this treatment. Presently, it is used mostly as adjunctive therapy in patients with refractory disease or poor tolerance of conventional therapies.

ALVEOLAR HEMORRHAGE SYNDROMES

Diffuse alveolar hemorrhage (DAH) is a life-threatening condition associated with several immunologic and nonimmunologic disorders that affect the integrity of the alveolar capillary interface.[71–73] Injury at this site allows for the accumulation of erythrocytes within air spaces. The clinical presentation of DAH consists of cough, hemoptysis, dyspnea, and bilateral alveolar infiltrates.[32,74] However, hemoptysis may be scant or absent in up to a third at the time of presentation. All subjects with significant alveolar hemorrhage will demonstrate anemia or a falling hematocrit, and many patients present with acute hypoxemic respiratory failure.[71] Mortality is approximately 25 percent per episode, and the syndrome may recur.[24,32,75] Fever is common. Chest radiographs typically reveal symmetric, bilateral airspace disease or ground glass opacification, sometimes with a 'batwing' distribution (Fig. 13C.8).[74] Asymmetric and, rarely, unilateral patterns can also be seen, and are likely to be mistaken for infectious pneumonias.

The differential diagnosis includes systemic vasculitis, isolated pulmonary capillaritis, collagen vascular disease, Goodpasture syndrome, drug or toxin exposure, severe coagulation disorders (including thrombocytopenia, anticoagulant overdose, and the antiphospholipid antibody syndrome), mitral stenosis, diffuse alveolar damage, and rare entities such as lymphangioleiomyomatosis, pulmonary veno-occlusive disease, and idiopathic pulmonary hemosiderosis.[72] The focus of the medical history should be on systemic symptoms associated with vasculitis and connective tissue disease, symptoms of a bleeding or clotting diathesis, a history of rheumatic fever or mitral valve disease, and a history of bone marrow transplantation. Other important factors include a history of cigarette or crack cocaine use, and occupational exposure to hydrocarbons, isocyanates, or trimellitic anhydride. A complete list of recent medication use must be obtained. Drugs implicated in the development of DAH include D-penicillamine, amiodarone, abciximab, all-*trans* retinoic acid, mitomycin C, phenytoin, hydralazine, anticoagulants, and propylthiouracil. Lymphangiography contrast dye is another potential offender.

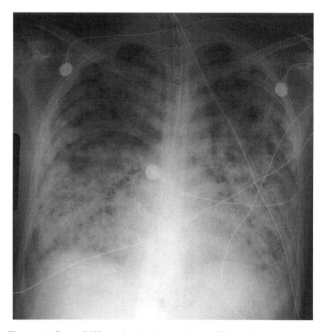

Figure 13C.8 *Diffuse alveolar hemorrhage. This patient presented with renal failure, hemoptysis, diffuse alveolar infiltrates, and hypoxemic respiratory failure due to microscopic polyangiitis.*

Physical examination may be useful if signs of a systemic vasculitis or collagen vascular disease are detected. Careful attention should be paid to the eyes, nose, oral mucosa, skin, joints, and neurologic exam. The chest exam may reveal inspiratory crackles, but is sometimes normal, even with diffuse infiltrates on the chest radiograph. The presence of an opening snap or diastolic rumble on cardiac auscultation suggests mitral stenosis. Bronchoscopy should be performed early when alveolar hemorrhage is suspected. Serial aliquots of normal saline instilled during bronchoalveolar lavage will return an increasingly bloody effluent. Cytologic review reveals abundant hemosiderin-laden macrophages, unless the lavage is completed very soon after the onset of bleeding. Stains and cultures for microorganisms should be performed since lower respiratory tract infection is sometimes a precipitating factor in alveolar hemorrhage.

Laboratory analysis in cases of known or suspected alveolar hemorrhage should include measurement of antinuclear antibodies, rheumatoid factor, serum complement, cryoglobulins, antibasement membrane antibodies, ANCAs, and antiphospholipid antibodies. A urinalysis, including microscopic examination, and measurement of blood urea nitrogen and serum creatinine levels are essential due to the frequent association between lung hemorrhage and nephritis. When the diagnosis remains in question, a surgical biopsy is required. Immunofluorescence staining can be done of lung or kidney specimens. Patients with Goodpasture syndrome have linear deposition of immunoglobulin (IgG) along the basement membrane. In Henoch–Schönlein purpura and IgA nephropathy, occasional causes of DAH, IgA will be deposited in alveolar walls and glomeruli. Coarse, granular deposits of immune complexes are present in patients with systemic lupus erythematosus, but in patients with vasculitides, immune deposits are absent or limited (pauci-immune).

The pulmonary–renal syndromes are responsible for most cases of DAH. These syndromes include the small-vessel vasculitides, Goodpasture syndrome, collagen vascular disease, Henoch–Schönlein purpura, and IgA nephropathy. Depending on the specific disorder, lung involvement in the pulmonary–renal syndromes may include the development of nodules, cavities, focal consolidation, or interstitial lung disease in addition to diffuse alveolar hemorrhage. The clinical presentation of renal disease is similar in all cases, but immunofluorescence patterns can vary. Glomerulonephritis is the usual lesion, often with crescent formation. It manifests as proteinuria and/or hematuria, with or without clinically significant impairment in renal function. Examination of the urinary sediment often reveals the presence of red blood cell casts, which are characteristic of glomerular injury.

Alveolar hemorrhage is often an ANCA-associated condition, and is more frequently caused by microscopic polyangiitis than Wegener granulomatosis.[75] Perinuclear ANCA may be detected in a third of patients with antibasement membrane antibody disease (Goodpasture syndrome) as well, usually with MPO specificity.[76–79] Patients with both types of autoantibody may be prone to develop

fulminant alveolar hemorrhage. Among those with collagen vascular disease, DAH is most common in patients with systemic lupus erythematosus. There are only a handful of reports in patients with polymyositis, rheumatoid arthritis, and mixed connective tissue disease.

Diffuse alveolar hemorrhage related to Wegener granulomatosis, microscopic polyangiitis and most cases of collagen vascular disease is associated with pulmonary capillaritis.[72,80] Significant bleeding occasionally occurs in the setting of diffuse alveolar damage (e.g. acute lupus pneumonitis). When capillaritis is not present, the histology of alveolar hemorrhage is usually 'bland', with no overt abnormalities on routine hematoxylin/eosin stains. Common causes of bland alveolar hemorrhage include most drug or toxin-mediated cases, most cases of antiglomerular basement membrane antibody disease, and idiopathic pulmonary hemosiderosis.

Idiopathic pulmonary hemosiderosis, also known as idiopathic pulmonary hemorrhage, is a rare disorder of unknown etiology. It is characterized by repeated episodes of hemoptysis, transient alveolar infiltrates, and iron deficiency anemia.[81] It is more common in children, and is a diagnosis of exclusion. Histologically, an abundance of hemosiderin-laden macrophages is seen in the absence of capillaritis or immune deposits. Eosinophilia is seen in 10 percent, and some patients have cold agglutinins or increased serum IgA levels.[82] Complications include the development of pulmonary fibrosis and cor pulmonale. Azathioprine or corticosteroids are beneficial in some cases, but treatment response and prognosis is highly variable.[81,83,84]

Diffuse alveolar hemorrhage sometimes occurs in the setting of isolated pulmonary capillaritis. When ANCAs are identified, this simply represents a 'lung limited' form of microscopic polyangiitis. Some cases, however, occur in the absence of serologic or histopathologic evidence of an associated systemic disorder.[85] Whether this represents a separate clinical entity is unclear, but even when there is overt systemic involvement by a small-vessel vasculitis, some patients do not have detectable ANCA.

For patients with capillaritis, treatment usually consists of a combination of cyclophosphamide and corticosteroids. In the setting of systemic lupus erythematosus, azathioprine may be used in place of cyclophosphamide. Goodpasture syndrome requires a combination of cyclophosphamide or azathioprine, corticosteroids, and plasmapheresis.[86] Early initiation of plasma exchange is reasonable in patients with severe pulmonary–renal syndromes while awaiting laboratory and biopsy results. Plasmapheresis has not been shown to be helpful in lupus-related nephritis, but may be useful in ANCA-associated vasculitis.[87,88]

TAKAYASU ARTERITIS

Takayasu arteritis is a large-vessel vasculitis involving the aorta and its major branches.[89] The disease is most prevalent among women from southeast Asia, India, and Mexico. Women account for roughly 85 percent of all reported cases. In North America and Europe, there are 1–3 new cases/million/year.[90,91] In Japan, the incidence is 50 times higher. Symptoms typically develop during the second or third decade of life.[89] During the early inflammatory phase of the disease, nonspecific constitutional symptoms predominate. These include fever, night sweats, weight loss, fatigue, malaise, anorexia, and musculoskeletal complaints.[92] Most patients during this phase have an elevated erythrocyte sedimentation rate and C-reactive protein. Anemia of chronic disease is also common. Ultimately, inflammation subsides and remodeling of the vascular wall leads to stenosis or aneurysm formation (Fig 13C.9).[92]

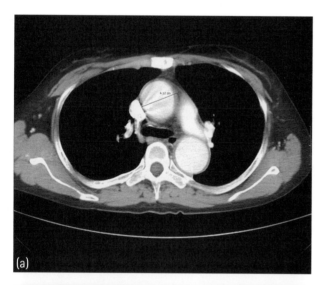

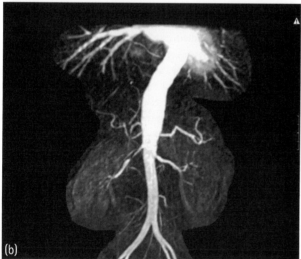

Figure 13C.9 *(a) Chest computed tomography scan of a 31-year-old woman with Takayasu arteritis showing aneurysmal dilatation of the ascending and descending thoracic aorta. (b) Abdominal magnetic resonance angiogram on the same patient. A suprarenal abdominal aortic aneurysm is seen, along with a high-grade right renal artery stenosis with poststenotic dilatation.*

In many patients, the disease is not identified until the late 'occlusive' phase of the illness, which most often features limb claudication or symptoms of cerebral ischemia.[93] Patients may complain of headache, vertigo, memory loss, orthostasis, or frank syncope. Visual disturbances related either to Takayasu retinopathy or decreased cerebral perfusion are seen in a third of patients. Although the disease classically involves the aortic arch and its branches, involvement of the abdominal aorta and iliac arteries also occurs.[94] Abdominal pain, diarrhea, or gastrointestinal bleeding may result from mesenteric ischemia.[95] Over 50 percent develop hypertension, usually as a result of renal artery stenosis.[95] Aneurysmal dilatation of the ascending aorta often leads to aortic valve insufficiency. Hypertension and aortic regurgitation may combine to produce congestive heart failure. Up to 15 percent of patients have disease involving their coronary arteries which may cause angina pectoris, myocardial infarction, and acute pulmonary edema.[96] Autopsy evidence suggests that the pulmonary arteries are affected in up to 50 percent of Takayasu arteritis patients, but it is usually clinically silent.[97,98] Chest radiographs may demonstrate focal oligemia, enlarged central vessels or localized aneurismal dilatation.

Symptoms include chest pain, dyspnea, and hemoptysis. The differential diagnosis of dyspnea in a patient with Takayasu arteritis includes direct involvement of the pulmonary vasculature, coronary arteritis (angina equivalent), and congestive heart failure. Less than 10 percent of patients develop symptomatic pulmonary hypertension, although more have echocardiographic evidence of elevated right-sided pressures. Life-threatening hemorrhage from ruptured pulmonary artery aneurysms may occur, but is uncommon. Physical findings in Takayasu's arteritis may include diminished or absent pulses (hence, the moniker 'pulseless disease'), a blood pressure differential of 10 mm Hg or more between the arms, vascular bruits in various locations, carotid artery tenderness, or a blowing diastolic heart murmur.

Histologically, Takayasu arteritis presents as a focal panarteritis with a mixed cellular infiltrate including giant cells and granulomas during the active phase of the disease (Fig. 13C.10).[99] The inflammatory process results in degeneration of the internal elastic lamina and the development of adventitial fibrosis. When the muscular media is destroyed, aneurysms may develop. Natural killer cells, cytotoxic and gamma delta T lymphocytes may play a key role in the pathogenesis of this disease through the elaboration of a potent cytolytic factor, perforin, directly onto the surface of arterial vascular cells.[100] Lymphocytes from aortic tissue also demonstrate a restricted T cell receptor repertoire suggesting that the cellular immune system is responding to a specific, but as yet unidentified, antigen within the vessel wall.[101] A high percentage of patients also demonstrate the presence of anti-endothelial cell antibodies.[102]

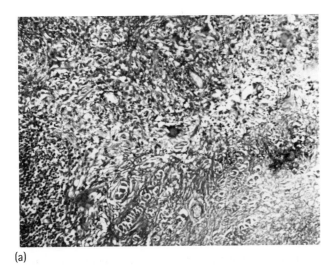

(a)

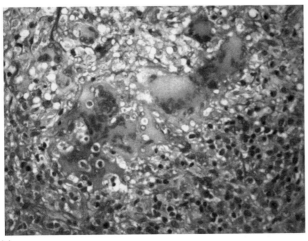

(b)

Figure 13C.10 *(a) Section of the aortic wall in a patient with Takayasu arteritis. An intense vasculitis is seen involving the entire thickness of the vessel wall. (b) High-power view showing a mixed cellular infiltrate with lymphocytes, histiocytes, and multinucleated giant cells.*

Biopsy of involved vessels is technically difficult, fraught with complications, and not required to make the diagnosis. When Takayasu arteritis is suspected, complete aortography and pulmonary angiography should be employed to assess the extent of disease.[103] Magnetic resonance (MR) and computed tomographic (CT) angiography offer the advantage of demonstrating both luminal and mural pathology, while avoiding the risks associated with arterial puncture.[103,104] Involved vessel walls may be thickened and exhibit high attenuation before contrast is administered, or may enhance after contrast delivery. Such early inflammatory changes may be present without luminal abnormalities, and would be missed by conventional angiography. Positron emission tomography (PET) is also useful for identifying active vascular inflammatory changes.[105,106] This technique may help determine the likelihood of a favorable response to medical therapy for specific vascular lesions.

Most patients with Takayasu arteritis require treatment with immunosuppressive agents, although 20 percent may have a self-limiting condition.[95] Corticosteroids are the initial drugs of choice. Patients with early stage lesions and active inflammation are much more likely to respond to immunomodulating therapy when compared with those with established vascular stenosis. Disease activity is improved by glucocorticoid treatment in about 50 percent of cases.[90,107] Another 25 percent may achieve remission with the addition of a cytotoxic agent including cyclophosphamide, methotrexate, azathioprine, or mycophenolate.[95,108] A quarter of affected individuals have disease refractory to these measures, and half of those who achieve remission will later relapse.[95] Surgical bypass, or angioplasty and vascular stenting, may be required in cases of persistent upper extremity claudication, hypertension due to renal artery stenosis, and cardiac, mesenteric, or cerebral ischemia.[109,110] Vascular repair of aortic or pulmonary artery aneurysms may also be required.

In follow-up studies of Takayasu arteritis, 80–85 percent overall 5-year and 15-year survival rates have been identified.[111,112] Some patients exhibit a pattern of periodic exacerbation and remission, while others have a progressive disease course. The latter is associated with a worse prognosis.[112] Major complications that also adversely affect prognosis include the development of hypertension, aneurysm formation, aortic regurgitation, and Takayasu retinopathy. The presence of both a progressive course and a major complication predicts higher mortality (43 percent at 15 years), and the absence of both is associated with prolonged survival.[112]

BEHÇET DISEASE

Behçet disease is an idiopathic vasculitic disorder affecting all types and sizes of vessels, and numerous organ systems. It is characterized by recurrent bouts of acute inflammation rather than chronic, persistent disease.[113] Distinctive features include orogenital ulceration, skin lesions, ocular disease, joint pain, and neurologic and large-vessel involvement.[114] The disease is most common in individuals of Middle Eastern or Far Eastern descent, with the highest prevalence being noted in Turkey. It typically affects young adults between 20 and 40 years of age.

All layers of the vessel wall are involved with an inflammatory infiltrate consisting of activated neutrophils and lymphocytes. Destruction of the elastic lamina, intimal thickening, and luminal thrombosis are typical. A hypercoaguable state exists in this condition due to platelet and endothelial cell activation. As a result, both venous and arterial thrombosis may occur, including thrombosis of the superior or inferior vena cava.

The diagnosis requires the presence of recurrent aphthous oral ulceration plus two of the following: recurrent genital ulcers, uveitis or retinal vasculitis, compatible skin lesions, or a positive pathergy test.[115] A positive pathergy test is indicated by development of an erythematous papule or pustule 24–48 hours after the oblique insertion of a sterile needle into the skin. Cutaneous findings consistent with Behçet disease include erythema nodosum, papulopustular lesions, palpable purpura, and pseudofolliculitis.[116] Neurologic manifestations are seen in 10–20 percent. The presentation may include chronic meningoencephalitis, mononeuritis multiplex, bulbar dysfunction, dementia, or psychiatric symptoms.[117] Oligoarthritis occurs in approximately half of patients. Intestinal tract involvement may cause abdominal pain, vomiting, diarrhea, or gastrointestinal hemorrhage, and has a predilection for the ileocecal region. As a result, confusion with Crohn disease may occur, but granulomatous inflammation is not seen in Behçet disease. Microscopic hematuria or proteinuria are sometimes noted, but without an active urinary sediment or associated renal insufficiency.[118] Thoracic involvement classically occurs in the form of aortic or pulmonary artery aneurysms (Fig. 13C.11).[119] Such large-vessel disease is seen in up to 25 percent of patients, and is especially common in young men.[120] Behçet disease is the most common vasculitic cause of pulmonary artery aneurysms, and rupture of these lesions is often fatal.[121,122] A third of patients with

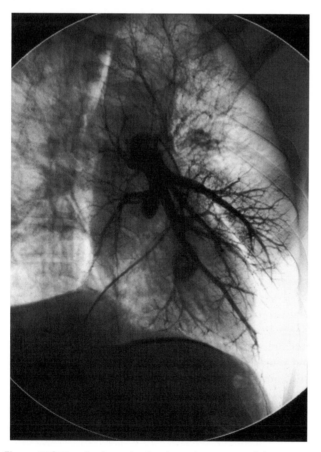

Figure 13C.11 *Angiography showing pulmonary arterial aneurysms in a patient with Behçet disease and hemoptysis.*

pulmonary artery aneurysms will die within 2 years. The average survival after developing hemoptysis was less than a year in one study.[123] A small number of patients have been reported with DAH secondary to pulmonary capillaritis.

For the diagnosis of vascular lesions, MR angiography is preferred.[124] Procedures involving arterial or venous puncture carry a substantial risk of thrombophlebitis and pseudoaneurysm formation. Deep vein thrombosis is common, but pulmonary thromboembolism is not. Thrombi usually adhere tightly to the inflamed veins.[123] Still, ventilation/perfusion lung scans are frequently abnormal.[125] *In situ* thrombosis may produce a patchy distribution of blood flow with zones of focal oligemia. In some cases, pulmonary infarction occurs accompanied by Hampton humps (pleural-based triangular opacities radiating toward the hilum), regions of atelectasis, subpleural nodules, or reticular opacities on the plain film. Recurrent pneumonia, bronchiolitis obliterans with organizing pneumonia, mediastinal adenopathy, DAH, and pleurisy have all been described in Behçet disease.[119] Pleural effusions may result from pleural vasculitis or superior vena cava thrombosis. Rarely, obstructive airways disease may develop as a complication of Behçet disease.[119,126]

As with many autoimmune disorders, both genetic and environmental factors appear to play a role in the pathogenesis of this disease. Behçet disease has an association with the HLA-B51 allele, as well as viral, streptococcal, and mycobacterial infections.[113] It has been suggested that ubiquitous antigens such as microbial heat shock proteins may trigger a cross-reactive immune response in genetically susceptible individuals.[127] Various autoantibodies and autoreactive T cell populations have been identified in these patients. Excessive production of T helper (Th)1 cytokines (IL-1 and interferon-γ) is seen during the active phase of the disease.[128]

Treatment of Behçet disease varies depending on the site of involvement. Mucocutaneous lesions may respond to topical steroids, colchicine, or dapsone. Refractory lesions and systemic disease require oral corticosteroids, thalidomide, or cytotoxic agents.[113] Interferon-α and infliximab are other options.[114] Sulfasalazine is often useful in patients with gastrointestinal involvement. There are no controlled trials demonstrating superiority of any particular regimen. Aneurysm formation suggests a poor prognosis, and these patients are usually treated aggressively with a combination of cyclophosphamide and corticosteroids.[122] Azathioprine is a less toxic alternative that may be used as maintenance therapy once remission is achieved. Interestingly, medical therapy may result in complete regression of aneurysmal lesions.[129] Surgical intervention is sometimes required, especially with massive bleeding related to bronchoarterial fistulas, but there is a tendency for aneurysms to recur at anastomotic sites.[130] Anticoagulation is appropriate for patients with deep vein thrombosis in conjunction with short-term corticosteroid administration. Involvement of the pulmonary arteries, however, substantially increases the risk of anticoagulation. In this case, anticoagulation may be carefully applied in patients with substantial clot burdens only after initial immunosuppressive treatment. If the extent of thrombosis is not great in these patients, aspirin is a reasonable alternative.

NECROTIZING SARCOID GRANULOMATOSIS

Necrotizing sarcoid granulomatosis is a rare form of vasculitis that is usually isolated to the lungs. The peak incidence occurs among middle-aged people, and women are affected twice as often as men. The presentation is usually subacute, and not associated with respiratory failure. It features respiratory and constitutional complaints including cough, dyspnea, chest pain, fever, weight loss, and general malaise.[131,132] Twenty percent report no symptoms. Histologically, necrotizing sarcoid granulomatosis is characterized by nodules or masses comprised of confluent, well-formed epithelioid granulomas.[133] Necrosis occurs at the center of these conglomerate masses, but is noncaseous in nature. A lymphoplasmacytic infiltrate, giant cells or granulomas can be identified in and around vessel walls. The vasculitis chiefly involves muscular arteries and veins, disrupting the elastic laminae and causing fibrinoid necrosis.[134] Extrapulmonary involvement appears to be rare. When it occurs, there is a tendency to involve the eye and central nervous system.[133,135]

Radiographically, necrotizing sarcoid granulomatosis usually presents as multiple, bilateral pulmonary nodules that vary in size from a few millimeters to a few centimeters (Fig. 13C.12).[136] They may be sharply demarcated, or have ill-defined margins. Lesions tend to concentrate within the lower lung zones. Some patients have solitary nodules or masses.[132] Confluent parenchymal opacification with a peribronchovascular and subpleural distribution resembling bronchiolitis obliterans organizing pneumonia may also be

seen.[137] Cavitation may occur, and CT may reveal low attenuation centers within some lesions reflecting prominent necrosis. Hilar or mediastinal lymphadenopathy can develop, but is frequently absent. Bilateral pleural thickening is reported in some cases.

Definitive diagnosis requires a surgical lung biopsy to confirm the presence of necrosis and vasculitis in association with granulomas. Necrotizing sarcoid granulomatosis is a diagnosis of exclusion, and infection with fungal and mycobacterial agents must be carefully ruled out.[133] Such infections can also be associated with a vasculitis.[138] Nodular sarcoidosis, Wegener granulomatosis, bronchocentric granulomatosis, and lymphomatoid granulomatosis are the other major differential diagnoses. An elevated erythrocyte sedimentation rate is common in necrotizing sarcoid granulomatosis, but ANCAs have not been reported.

Necrotizing sarcoid granulomatosis generally has a benign course, and may remit spontaneously. The response to corticosteroid therapy is generally excellent, and clinical relapses are uncommon.[132,139] Cytotoxic agents should be avoided, as the only deaths associated with this disorder stem from infectious complications of overly aggressive immune suppression.[132] The localized form of the disease may be cured by resection.

The relation between sarcoidosis and necrotizing sarcoid granulomatosis remains unclear. Major differences in necrotizing sarcoid granulomatosis include the prominent necrosis and vasculitis, isolation to the lung in most cases, and the usual lack of mediastinal lymphadenopathy.[135] Serum calcium and angiotensin-converting enzyme levels are normal in patients with necrotizing sarcoid granulomatosis, and progression to advanced lung fibrosis has not been reported. In classic sarcoidosis, incidental granulomatous involvement of blood vessels is not uncommon, and appears related to the extent of parenchymal granulomas.[140] Rarely, however, a systemic angiitis affecting large or small vessels is seen that may mimic Takayasu arteritis, polyarteritis nodosa, or hypersensitivity vasculitis.[141]

POLYARTERITIS NODOSA

Polyarteritis nodosa is a necrotizing medium- and small-vessel vasculitis affecting many organ systems, but rarely the lung. Common features include constitutional symptoms, renal involvement (hypertension or renal insufficiency), mononeuritis multiplex, skin lesions, orchitis, myalgias, and gastrointestinal complaints. The coronary arteries are sometimes affected causing myocardial ischemia. The lungs are almost never involved in a clinically significant way, but autopsies reveal that the bronchial arteries are not uncommonly affected.[142,143] It is likely that most previously reported cases citing pulmonary involvement were actually examples of small-vessel vasculitis (Churg–Strauss syndrome or microscopic polyangiitis).[144] One case of

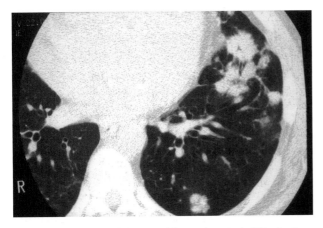

Figure 13C.12 *Necrotizing sarcoid granulomatosis. This chest computed tomography image indicates a typical finding of multiple, irregular pulmonary nodules and masses.*

treatment responsive vasculitis involving the medium-sized pulmonary arteries has been reported.[145] Histopathologic evidence of diffuse alveolar damage and interstitial fibrosis has also been reported in polyarteritis nodosa, but a causative relation has not been established.[143]

SECONDARY VASCULITIS

Collagen vascular disease is associated with a wide range of pleural and parenchymal lung pathology. Pulmonary vasculitis is a relatively rare complication of these disorders. It was identified in roughly 8 percent of polymyositis patients, and 2 percent of systemic lupus erythematosus patients in two large autopsy studies.[146,147] It is well documented to occur in patients with rheumatoid arthritis as well.[148,149] Pulmonary vasculitis in this patient population usually involves large- or medium-sized arteries, and presents as pulmonary hypertension. Plexogenic pulmonary arteriopathy and advanced interstitial lung disease are other important causes of pulmonary hypertension in these patients, and more than one lesion may be present. Pulmonary hypertension caused primarily by large-vessel vasculitis is more likely to respond to therapy, however, and should always be considered. This is particularly true when pulmonary hypertension develops rapidly, or in association with an elevated erythrocyte sedimentation rate. Small-vessel vasculitis (pulmonary capillaritis) also occurs in association with collagen vascular disease, and is the major cause of alveolar hemorrhage in this group.[4]

A variety of bacteria including *Staphylococcus*, *Pseudomonas*, and *Legionella* are known to invade and destroy blood vessels in the lung.[150,151] Necrotizing granulomatous inflammation due to fungal or mycobacterial pathogens may also produce a secondary vasculitis.[138] In immunocompromised patients, angioinvasive organisms such as *Aspergillus* and *Mucor* may cause mycotic pulmonary artery aneurysms, or vascular occlusion with tissue infarction.[152] Parasitic infections and *Pneumocystis carinii* are other rare causes of pulmonary vasculitis.[153]

Key learning points

- Manifestations of pulmonary vasculitis include DAH, pulmonary arterial aneurysms, pulmonary arterial hypertension, nodules, cavities, infiltrates, and infarction.

- The most common pulmonary vasculitides, Wegener granulomatosis and microscopic polyangiitis, are associated with ANCAs.

- The pulmonary–renal syndromes feature DAH and glomerulonephritis. Pauci-immune small-vessel vasculitis, Goodpasture syndrome, and collagen vascular disease may present in this manner.

- Takayasu arteritis classically involves the aorta and its major vessels. Pulmonary artery stenoses and aneurysms also occur.

- Behçet disease is the most common vasculitic cause of pulmonary artery aneurysms, and is reported to cause DAH.

- Necrotizing sarcoid granulomatosis causes nodules or masses in the lung. The histopathology features prominent necrosis and vasculitis, and extrapulmonary involvement is rare.

- Pulmonary vasculitis is a treatable cause of pulmonary hypertension in patients with collagen vascular disease.

REFERENCES

◆ 1. Langford CA. 15. Vasculitis. *J Allergy Clin Immunol* 2003; **111**(2 Suppl): S602–12.

◆ 2. Gatenby PA. Vasculitis – diagnosis and treatment. *Aust N Z J Med* 1999; **29**: 662–77.

● 3. Rolfes DB, Weiss MA, Sanders MA. Necrotizing sarcoid granulomatosis with suppurative features. *Am J Clin Pathol* 1984; **82**: 602–7.

4. Franks TJ, Koss MN. Pulmonary capillaritis. *Curr Opin Pulm Med* 2000; **6**: 430–5.

5. Frankel SK, Sullivan EJ, Brown KK. Vasculitis: Wegener granulomatosis, Churg-Strauss syndrome, microscopic polyangiitis, polyarteritis nodosa, and Takayasu arteritis. *Crit Care Clin* 2002; **18**: 855–79.

◆ 6. Falk RJ, Nachman PH, Hogan SL, Jennette JC. ANCA glomerulonephritis and vasculitis: a Chapel Hill perspective. *Semin Nephrol* 2000; **20**: 233–43.

7. Watts RA, Scott DG. Epidemiology of the vasculitides. *Curr Opin Rheumatol* 2003; **15**: 11–16.

8. Lie JT. Histopathologic specificity of systemic vasculitis. *Rheum Dis Clin North Am* 1995; **21**: 883–909.

9. Gross WL, Schmitt WH, Csernok E. ANCA and associated diseases: immunodiagnostic and pathogenetic aspects. *Clin Exp Immunol* 1993; **91**: 1–12.

10. Rao JK, Weinberger M, Oddone EZ, *et al.* The role of antineutrophil cytoplasmic antibody (c-ANCA) testing in the diagnosis of Wegener granulomatosis. A literature review and meta-analysis. *Ann Intern Med* 1995; **123**: 925–32.

● 11. Hagen EC, Daha MR, Hermans J, *et al.* Diagnostic value of standardized assays for anti-neutrophil cytoplasmic antibodies in idiopathic systemic vasculitis. EC/BCR Project for ANCA Assay Standardization. *Kidney Int* 1998; **53**: 743–53.

12. Niles JL. A renal biopsy is essential for the management of ANCA-positive patients with glomerulonephritis: the contra-view. *Sarcoidosis Vasc Diffuse Lung Dis* 1996; **13**: 232–4.

13. Harper L, Savage CO. Pathogenesis of ANCA-associated systemic vasculitis. *J Pathol* 2000; **190**: 349–59.

◆ 14. Kallenberg CG, Rarok A, Stegeman CA, Limburg PC. New insights into the pathogenesis of antineutrophil cytoplasmic autoantibody-associated vasculitis. *Autoimmun Rev* 2002; **1**(1–2): 61–6.

15. Falk RJ, Jennette JC. ANCA are pathogenic – oh yes they are! *J Am Soc Nephrol* 2002; **13**: 1977–9.

16. Kallenberg CG, Heeringa P. Pathogenesis of vasculitis. *Lupus* 1998; **7**: 280–4.

● 17. King WJ, Brooks CJ, Holder R, Hughes P, Adu D, Savage CO. T lymphocyte responses to anti-neutrophil cytoplasmic autoantibody (ANCA) antigens are present in patients with ANCA-associated systemic vasculitis and persist during disease remission. *Clin Exp Immunol* 1998; **112**: 539–46.

18. Griffith ME, Coulthart A, Pusey CD. T cell responses to myeloperoxidase (MPO) and proteinase 3 (PR3) in patients with systemic vasculitis. *Clin Exp Immunol* 1996; **103**: 253–8.

19. Ballieux BE, van der Burg SH, Hagen EC, *et al*. Cell-mediated autoimmunity in patients with Wegener's granulomatosis (WG). *Clin Exp Immunol* 1995; **100**: 186–93.

20. Specks U. ANCA subsets: influence on disease phenotype. *Cleve Clin J Med* 2002; **69** (Suppl 2): SII56–9.

● 21. Franssen C, Gans R, Kallenberg C, *et al*. Disease spectrum of patients with antineutrophil cytoplasmic autoantibodies of defined specificity: distinct differences between patients with anti-proteinase 3 and anti-myeloperoxidase autoantibodies. *J Intern Med* 1998; **244**: 209–16.

● 22. Geffriaud-Ricouard C, Noel LH, Chauveau D, *et al*. Clinical spectrum associated with ANCA of defined antigen specificities in 98 selected patients. *Clin Nephrol* 1993; **39**: 125–36.

● 23. Franssen CF, Gans RO, Arends B, *et al*. Differences between anti-myeloperoxidase- and anti-proteinase 3-associated renal disease. *Kidney Int* 1995; **47**: 193–9.

● 24. Hoffman GS, Kerr GS, Leavitt RY, *et al*. Wegener granulomatosis: an analysis of 158 patients. *Ann Intern Med* 1992; **116**: 488–98.

● 25. Anderson G, Coles ET, Crane M, *et al*. Wegener's granuloma. A series of 265 British cases seen between 1975 and 1985. A report by a sub-committee of the British Thoracic Society Research Committee. *Q J Med* 1992; **83**: 427–38.

26. Murty GE. Wegener's granulomatosis: otorhinolaryngological manifestations. *Clin Otolaryngol* 1990; **15**: 385–93.

27. Bullen CL, Liesegang TJ, McDonald TJ, DeRemee RA. Ocular complications of Wegener's granulomatosis. *Ophthalmology* 1983; **90**: 279–90.

28. Guyot JP, Baud C, Montandon P. Wegener's granulomatosis with otological disorders as primary symptoms. *ORL J Otorhinolaryngol Relat Spec* 1990; **52**: 327–34.

29. Lie JT. Wegener's granulomatosis: histological documentation of common and uncommon manifestations in 216 patients. *Vasa* 1997; **26**: 261–70.

● 30. Cordier JF, Valeyre D, Guillevin L, *et al*. Pulmonary Wegener's granulomatosis. A clinical and imaging study of 77 cases. *Chest* 1990; **97**: 906–12.

◆ 31. Seo JB, Im JG, Chung JW, *et al*. Pulmonary vasculitis: the spectrum of radiological findings. *Br J Radiol* 2000; **73**: 1224–31.

◆ 32. Schwarz MI, Brown KK. Small vessel vasculitis of the lung. *Thorax* 2000; **55**: 502–10.

33. Langford CA, Sneller MC, Hallahan CW, *et al*. Clinical features and therapeutic management of subglottic stenosis in patients with Wegener's granulomatosis. *Arthritis Rheum* 1996; **39**: 1754–60.

34. Irvine AD, Bruce IN, Walsh M, *et al*. Dermatological presentation of disease associated with antineutrophil cytoplasmic antibodies: a report of two contrasting cases and a review of the literature. *Br J Dermatol* 1996; **134**: 924–8.

35. Daoud MS, Gibson LE, DeRemee RA, *et al*. Cutaneous Wegener's granulomatosis: clinical, histopathologic, and immunopathologic features of thirty patients. *J Am Acad Dermatol* 1994; **31**: 605–12.

36. Tupler RH, McCuskey WH. Wegener granulomatosis of the colon: CT and histologic correlation. *J Comput Assist Tomogr* 1991; **15**: 314–16.

● 37. Nishino H, Rubino FA, DeRemee RA, Swanson JW, Parisi JE. Neurological involvement in Wegener's granulomatosis: an analysis of 324 consecutive patients at the Mayo Clinic. *Ann Neurol* 1993; **33**: 4–9.

◆ 38. Moore PM, Calabrese LH. Neurologic manifestations of systemic vasculitides. *Semin Neurol* 1994; **14**: 300–6.

◆ 39. Jennette JC, Thomas DB, Falk RJ. Microscopic polyangiitis (microscopic polyarteritis). *Semin Diagn Pathol* 2001; **18**: 3–13.

● 40. Guillevin L, Durand-Gasselin B, Cevallos R, *et al.* Microscopic polyangiitis: clinical and laboratory findings in eighty-five patients. *Arthritis Rheum* 1999; **42**: 421–30.

● 41. Lauque D, Cadranel J, Lazor R, *et al.* Microscopic polyangiitis with alveolar hemorrhage. A study of 29 cases and review of the literature. Groupe d'Etudes et de Recherche sur les Maladies 'Orphelines' Pulmonaires (GERM'O'P). *Medicine (Baltimore)* 2000; **79**: 222–33.

● 42. Savage CO, Winearls CG, Evans DJ, *et al.* Microscopic polyarteritis: presentation, pathology and prognosis. *Q J Med* 1985; **56**: 467–83.

● 43. Guillevin L, Cohen P, Gayraud M, *et al.* Churg-Strauss syndrome. Clinical study and long-term follow-up of 96 patients. *Medicine (Baltimore)* 1999; **78**: 26–37.

44. Conron M, Beynon HL. Churg-Strauss syndrome. *Thorax* 2000; **55**: 870–7.

45. Churg A. Recent advances in the diagnosis of Churg-Strauss syndrome. *Mod Pathol* 2001; **14**: 1284–93.

46. Davis MD, Daoud MS, McEvoy MT, Su WP. Cutaneous manifestations of Churg-Strauss syndrome: a clinicopathologic correlation. *J Am Acad Dermatol* 1997; **37**(2 Pt 1): 199–203.

◆ 47. Guillevin L, Lhote F, Gherardi R. Polyarteritis nodosa, microscopic polyangiitis, and Churg-Strauss syndrome: clinical aspects, neurologic manifestations, and treatment. *Neurol Clin* 1997; **15**: 865–86.

48. Lanham JG, Elkon KB, Pusey CD, Hughes GR. Systemic vasculitis with asthma and eosinophilia: a clinical approach to the Churg-Strauss syndrome. *Medicine (Baltimore)* 1984; **63**: 65–81.

● 49. Guillevin L, Lhote F, Gayraud M, *et al.* Prognostic factors in polyarteritis nodosa and Churg-Strauss syndrome. A prospective study in 342 patients. *Medicine (Baltimore)* 1996; **75**: 17–28.

50. Devaney KO, Travis WD, Hoffman G, *et al.* Interpretation of head and neck biopsies in Wegener's granulomatosis. A pathologic study of 126

biopsies in 70 patients. *Am J Surg Pathol* 1990; **14**: 555–64.

● 51. Travis WD, Hoffman GS, Leavitt RY, *et al.* Surgical pathology of the lung in Wegener's granulomatosis. Review of 87 open lung biopsies from 67 patients. *Am J Surg Pathol* 1991; **15**: 315–33.

● 52. Travis WD, Colby TV, Lombard C, Carpenter HA. A clinicopathologic study of 34 cases of diffuse pulmonary hemorrhage with lung biopsy confirmation. *Am J Surg Pathol* 1990; **14**: 1112–25.

53. Jennette JC, Falk RJ. The pathology of vasculitis involving the kidney. *Am J Kidney Dis* 1994; **24**: 130–41.

54. Travis WD. Pathology of pulmonary granulomatous vasculitis. *Sarcoidosis Vasc Diffuse Lung Dis* 1996; **13**: 14–27.

● 55. Churg J, Strauss L. Allergic granulomatosis, allergic angiitis and periarteritis nodosa. *Am J Pathol* 1951; **27**: 27–301.

56. Reid AJ, Harrison BD, Watts RA, Watkin SW, McCann BG, Scott DG. Churg-Strauss syndrome in a district hospital. *Q J Med* 1998; **91**: 219–29.

57. Gaskin G, Clutterbuck EJ, Pusey CD. Renal disease in the Churg-Strauss syndrome. Diagnosis, management and outcome. *Contrib Nephrol* 1991; **94**: 58–65.

58. Clutterbuck EJ, Pusey CD. Severe alveolar haemorrhage in Churg-Strauss syndrome. *Eur J Respir Dis* 1987; **71**: 158–63.

59. Schnabel A, Reuter M, Csernok E, *et al.* Subclinical alveolar bleeding in pulmonary vasculitides: correlation with indices of disease activity. *Eur Respir J* 1999; **14**: 118–24.

◆ 60. Jayne DR. Conventional treatment and outcome of Wegener's granulomatosis and microscopic polyangiitis. *Cleve Clin J Med* 2002; **69**(Suppl 2): SII110–15.

61. Carruthers D, Bacon P. Activity, damage and outcome in systemic vasculitis. *Best Pract Res Clin Rheumatol* 2001; **15**: 225–38.

● 62. Jayne D, Rasmussen N, Andrassy K, *et al.* A randomized trial of maintenance therapy for vasculitis associated with antineutrophil cytoplasmic autoantibodies. *N Engl J Med* 2003; **349**: 36–44.

63. Stone JH, Tun W, Hellman DB. Treatment of non-life threatening Wegener's granulomatosis with methotrexate and daily prednisone as the initial therapy of choice. *J Rheumatol* 1999; **26**: 1134–9.

● 64. Solans R, Bosch JA, Perez-Bocanegra C, *et al.* Churg-

Strauss syndrome: outcome and long-term follow-up of 32 patients. *Rheumatology (Oxford)* 2001; **40**: 763–71.

◆ 65. Stone JH, Calabrese LH, Hoffman GS, *et al.* Vasculitis. A collection of pearls and myths. *Rheum Dis Clin North Am* 2001; **27**: 677–728, v.

66. Lhote F, Guillevin L. Indications of plasma exchanges in the treatment of polyarteritis nodosa and other systemic vasculitides. *Transfus Sci* 1996; **17**: 211–13.

● 67. Guillevin L, Cevallos R, Durand-Gasselin B, *et al.* Treatment of glomerulonephritis in microscopic polyangiitis and Churg-Strauss syndrome. Indications of plasma exchanges, Meta-analysis of 2 randomized studies on 140 patients, 32 with glomerulonephritis. *Ann Med Interne (Paris)* 1997; **148**: 198–204.

68. Jayne DR, Lockwood CM. Pooled intravenous immunoglobulin in the management of systemic vasculitis. *Adv Exp Med Biol* 1993; **336**: 469–72.

69. Jayne DR, Lockwood CM. Intravenous immunoglobulin as sole therapy for systemic vasculitis. *Br J Rheumatol* 1996; **35**: 1150–3.

70. Jayne DR, Chapel H, Adu D, *et al.* Intravenous immunoglobulin for ANCA-associated systemic vasculitis with persistent disease activity. *Q J Med* 2000; **93**: 433–9.

71. Leatherman JW, Davies SF, Hoidal JR. Alveolar hemorrhage syndromes: diffuse microvascular lung hemorrhage in immune and idiopathic disorders. *Medicine (Baltimore)* 1984; **63**: 343–61.

72. Specks U. Diffuse alveolar hemorrhage syndromes. *Curr Opin Rheumatol* 2001; **13**: 12–17.

73. Schwarz MI, Fontenot AP. Drug-induced diffuse alveolar hemorrhage syndromes and vasculitis. *Clin Chest Med* 2004; **25**: 133–40.

74. Primack SL, Miller RR, Muller NL. Diffuse pulmonary hemorrhage: clinical, pathologic, and imaging features. *AJR Am J Roentgenol* 1995; **164**: 295–300.

● 75. Niles JL, Bottinger EP, Saurina GR, *et al.* The syndrome of lung hemorrhage and nephritis is usually an ANCA-associated condition. *Arch Intern Med* 1996; **156**: 440–5.

76. Hellmark T, Niles JL, Collins AB, *et al.* Comparison of anti-GBM antibodies in sera with or without ANCA. *J Am Soc Nephrol* 1997; **8**: 376–85.

77. Short AK, Esnault VL, Lockwood CM. Anti-neutrophil cytoplasm antibodies and anti-glomerular basement membrane antibodies: two coexisting distinct autoreactivities detectable in patients with rapidly progressive glomerulonephritis. *Am J Kidney Dis* 1995; **26**: 439–45.

78. Bosch X, Mirapeix E, Font J, *et al.* Prognostic implication of anti-neutrophil cytoplasmic autoantibodies with myeloperoxidase specificity in anti-glomerular basement membrane disease. *Clin Nephrol* 1991; **36**: 107–13.

79. Bonsib SM, Goeken JA, Kemp JD, *et al.* Coexistent anti-neutrophil cytoplasmic antibody and antiglomerular basement membrane antibody associated disease = report of six cases. *Mod Pathol* 1993; **6**: 526–30.

● 80. Zamora MR, Warner ML, Tuder R, Schwarz MI. Diffuse alveolar hemorrhage and systemic lupus erythematosus. Clinical presentation, histology, survival, and outcome. *Medicine (Baltimore)* 1997; **76**: 192–202.

81. Milman N, Pedersen FM. Idiopathic pulmonary haemosiderosis. Epidemiology, pathogenic aspects and diagnosis. *Respir Med* 1998; **92**: 902–7.

82. Valassi-Adam H, Rouska A, Karpouzas J, Matsaniotis N. Raised IgA in idiopathic pulmonary haemosiderosis. Arch Dis Child 1975; **50**: 320–2.

83. Airaghi L, Ciceri L, Giannini S, *et al.* Idiopathic pulmonary hemosiderosis in an adult. Favourable response to azathioprine. *Monaldi Arch Chest Dis* 2001; **56**: 211–13.

84. Byrd RB, Gracey DR. Immunosuppressive treatment of idiopathic pulmonary hemosiderosis. *JAMA* 1973; **226**: 458–9.

85. Jennings CA, King TE, Jr, Tuder R, *et al.* Diffuse alveolar hemorrhage with underlying isolated, pauciimmune pulmonary capillaritis. *Am J Respir Crit Care Med* 1997; **155**: 1101–9.

86. Levy JB, Turner AN, Rees AJ, Pusey CD. Long-term outcome of anti-glomerular basement membrane antibody disease treated with plasma exchange and immunosuppression. *Ann Intern Med* 2001; **134**: 1033–42.

87. Lewis EJ, Hunsicker LG, Lan SP, *et al.* A controlled trial of plasmapheresis therapy in severe lupus nephritis. The Lupus Nephritis Collaborative Study Group. *N Engl J Med* 1992; **326**: 1373–9.

88. Pusey CD, Rees AJ, Evans DJ, *et al.* Plasma exchange in focal necrotizing glomerulonephritis without anti-GBM antibodies. *Kidney Int* 1991; **40**: 757–63.

● 89. Lupi-Herrera E, Sanchez-Torres G, Marcushamer J, *et al.* Takayasu's arteritis. Clinical study of 107 cases. *Am Heart J* 1977; **93**: 94–103.

● 90. Hall S, Barr W, Lie JT, *et al.* Takayasu arteritis. A study of 32 North American patients. *Medicine (Baltimore)* 1985; **64**: 89–99.

91. Arend WP, Michel BA, Bloch DA, *et al.* The American College of Rheumatology 1990 criteria for the classification of Takayasu arteritis. *Arthritis Rheum* 1990; **33**: 1129–34.

92. Johnston SL, Lock RJ, Gompels MM. Takayasu arteritis: a review. *J Clin Pathol* 2002; **55**: 481–6.

93. Subramanyan R, Joy J, Balakrishnan KG. Natural history of aortoarteritis (Takayasu's disease). *Circulation* 1989; **80**: 429–37.

94. Sharma BK, Sagar S, Singh AP, Suri S. Takayasu arteritis in India. *Heart Vessels Suppl* 1992; **7**: 37–43.

95. Kerr GS, Hallahan CW, Giordano J, *et al.* Takayasu arteritis. *Ann Intern Med* 1994; **120**: 919–29.

96. Park JH, Han MC, Kim SH, *et al.* Takayasu arteritis: angiographic findings and results of angioplasty. *AJR Am J Roentgenol* 1989; **153**: 1069–74.

97. Haque U, Hellmann D, Traill T, *et al.* Takayasu's arteritis involving proximal pulmonary arteries and mimicking thromboembolic disease. *J Rheumatol* 1999; **26**: 450–3.

98. Nasu T. Takayasu's truncoarteritis in Japan. A statistical observation of 76 autopsy cases. *Pathol Microbiol (Basel)* 1975; **43**(2-O): 140–6.

99. Hotchi M. Pathological studies on Takayasu arteritis. *Heart Vessels Suppl* 1992; **7**: 11–17.

100. Seko Y, Minota S, Kawasaki A, *et al.* Perforin-secreting killer cell infiltration and expression of a 65-kD heat-shock protein in aortic tissue of patients with Takayasu's arteritis. *J Clin Invest* 1994; **93**: 750–8.

101. Seko Y, Sato O, Takagi A, *et al.* Restricted usage of T-cell receptor Valpha-Vbeta genes in infiltrating cells in aortic tissue of patients with Takayasu's arteritis. *Circulation* 1996; **93**: 1788–90.

102. Eichhorn J, Sima D, Thiele B, *et al.* Anti-endothelial cell antibodies in Takayasu arteritis. *Circulation* 1996; **94**: 2396–401.

103. Park JH. Conventional and CT angiographic diagnosis of Takayasu arteritis. *Int J Cardiol* 1996; **54**(Suppl): S165–71.

104. Tanigawa K, Eguchi K, Kitamura Y, *et al.* Magnetic resonance imaging detection of aortic and pulmonary artery wall thickening in the acute stage of Takayasu arteritis. Improvement of clinical and radiologic findings after steroid therapy. *Arthritis Rheum* 1992; **35**: 476–80.

◆ 105. Kissin EY, Merkel PA. Diagnostic imaging in Takayasu arteritis. *Curr Opin Rheumatol* 2004; **16**: 31–7.

106. Meller J, Strutz F, Siefker U, *et al.* Early diagnosis and follow-up of aortitis with [F]FDG PET and MRI. *Eur J Nucl Med Mol Imaging* 2003; **30**: 730–6.

107. Shelhamer JH, Volkman DJ, Parrillo JE, *et al.* Takayasu's arteritis and its therapy. *Ann Intern Med* 1985; **103**: 121–6.

108. Hoffman GS, Leavitt RY, Kerr GS, *et al.* Treatment of glucocorticoid-resistant or relapsing Takayasu arteritis with methotrexate. *Arthritis Rheum* 1994; **37**: 578–82.

109. Sharma BK, Jain S, Bali HK, *et al.* A follow-up study of balloon angioplasty and de-novo stenting in Takayasu arteritis. *Int J Cardiol* 2000; **75**(Suppl 1): S147–52.

110. Giordano JM. Surgical treatment of Takayasu's arteritis. *Int J Cardiol* 2000; **75**(Suppl 1): S123–8.

111. Ishikawa K. Natural history and classification of occlusive thromboaortopathy (Takayasu's disease). *Circulation* 1978; **57**: 27–35.

● 112. Ishikawa K, Maetani S. Long-term outcome for 120 Japanese patients with Takayasu's disease. Clinical and statistical analyses of related prognostic factors. *Circulation* 1994; **90**: 1855–60.

◆ 113. Sakane T, Takeno M, Suzuki N, Inaba G. Behcet's disease. *N Engl J Med* 1999; **341**: 1284–91.

◆ 114. Yurdakul S, Hamuryudan V, Yazici H. Behcet syndrome. *Curr Opin Rheumatol* 2004; **16**: 38–42.

115. Criteria for diagnosis of Behcet's disease. International Study Group for Behcet's Disease. *Lancet* 1990; **335**: 1078–80.

116. Magro CM, Crowson AN. Cutaneous manifestations of Behcet's disease. *Int J Dermatol* 1995; **34**: 159–65.

117. Stratigos AJ, Laskaris G, Stratigos JD. Behcet's disease. *Semin Neurol* 1992; **12**: 346–57.

118. Rosenthal T, Weiss P, Gafni J. Renal involvement in Behcet's syndrome. *Arch Intern Med* 1978; **138**: 1122–4.

◆ 119. Tunaci A, Berkmen YM, Gokmen E. Thoracic involvement in Behcet's disease: pathologic, clinical, and imaging features. *AJR Am J Roentgenol* 1995; **164**: 51–6.

120. Koc Y, Gullu I, Akpek G, Akpolat T, Kansu E, Kiraz S, *et al.* Vascular involvement in Behcet's disease. *J Rheumatol* 1992; **19**: 402–10.

121. Grenier P, Bletry O, Cornud F, *et al.* Pulmonary

involvement in Behcet disease. *AJR Am J Roentgenol* 1981; **137**: 565–9.

◆ 122. Erkan F, Gul A, Tasali E. Pulmonary manifestations of Behcet's disease. *Thorax* 2001; **56**: 572–8.

● 123. Hamuryudan V, Yurdakul S, Moral F, *et al.* Pulmonary arterial aneurysms in Behcet's syndrome: a report of 24 cases. Br *J Rheumatol* 1994; **33**: 48–51.

124. Berkmen T. MR angiography of aneurysms in Behcet disease: a report of four cases. *J Comput Assist Tomogr* 1998; **22**: 202–6.

125. Raz I, Okon E, Chajek-Shaul T. Pulmonary manifestations in Behcet's syndrome. *Chest* 1989; **95**: 585–9.

126. Ahonen AV, Stenius-Aarniala BS, Viljanen BC, *et al.* Obstructive lung disease in Behcet's syndrome. *Scand J Respir Dis* 1978; **59**: 44–50.

◆ 127. Gul A. Behcet's disease: an update on the pathogenesis. *Clin Exp Rheumatol* 2001; **19**(5 Suppl 24): S6–12.

128. Frassanito MA, Dammacco R, Cafforio P, Dammacco F. Th1 polarization of the immune response in Behcet's disease: a putative pathogenetic role of interleukin-12. *Arthritis Rheum* 1999; **42**: 1967–74.

129. Park JH, Chung JW, Joh JH, *et al.* Aortic and arterial aneurysms in behcet disease: management with stent-grafts – initial experience. *Radiology* 2001; **220**: 745–50.

130. Tuzun H, Besirli K, Sayin A, *et al.* Management of aneurysms in Behcet's syndrome: an analysis of 24 patients. *Surgery* 1997; **121**: 150–6.

131. Stephen JG, Braimbridge MV, Corrin B, *et al.* Necrotizing 'sarcoidal' angiitis and granulomatosis of the lung. *Thorax* 1976; **31**: 356–60.

● 132. Churg A, Carrington CB, Gupta R. Necrotizing sarcoid granulomatosis. *Chest* 1979; **76**: 406–13.

133. Le Gall F, Loeuillet L, Delaval P, *et al.* Necrotizing sarcoid granulomatosis with and without extrapulmonary involvement. *Pathol Res Pract* 1996; **192**: 306–13; discussion 314.

134. Warren J, Pitchenik AE, Saldana MJ. Granulomatous vasculitides of the lung: a clinicopathologic approach to diagnosis and treatment. *South Med J* 1989; **82**: 481–91.

135. Dykhuizen RS, Smith CC, Kennedy MM, *et al.* Necrotizing sarcoid granulomatosis with extrapulmonary involvement. *Eur Respir J* 1997; **10**: 245–7.

136. Niimi H, Hartman TE, Muller NL. Necrotizing sarcoid granulomatosis: computed tomography and pathologic findings. *J Comput Assist Tomogr* 1995; **19**: 920–3.

137. Fisher MR, Christ ML, Bernstein JR. Necrotizing sarcoid-like granulomatosis: radiologic-pathologic correlation. *J Can Assoc Radiol* 1984; **35**: 313–15.

138. Ulbright TM, Katzenstein AL. Solitary necrotizing granulomas of the lung: differentiating features and etiology. *Am J Surg Pathol* 1980; **4**: 13–28.

139. Koss MN, Hochholzer L, Feigin DS, *et al.* Necrotizing sarcoid-like granulomatosis: clinical, pathologic, and immunopathologic findings. *Hum Pathol* 1980; **11**(5 Suppl): 510–19.

140. Takemura T, Matsui Y, Saiki S, Mikami R. Pulmonary vascular involvement in sarcoidosis: a report of 40 autopsy cases. *Hum Pathol* 1992; **23**: 1216–23.

141. Fernandes SR, Singsen BH, Hoffman GS. Sarcoidosis and systemic vasculitis. *Semin Arthritis Rheum* 2000; **30**: 33–46.

142. Bonsib SM. Polyarteritis nodosa. *Semin Diagn Pathol* 2001; **18**: 14–23.

143. Matsumoto T, Homma S, Okada M, *et al.* The lung in polyarteritis nodosa: a pathologic study of 10 cases. *Hum Pathol* 1993; **24**: 717–24.

144. Leavitt RY, Fauci AS. Pulmonary vasculitis. *Am Rev Respir Dis* 1986; **134**: 149–66.

145. Nick J, Tuder R, May R, Fisher J. Polyarteritis nodosa with pulmonary vasculitis. *Am J Respir Crit Care Med* 1996; **153**: 450–3.

146. Haupt HM, Moore GW, Hutchins GM. The lung in systemic lupus erythematosus. Analysis of the pathologic changes in 120 patients. *Am J Med* 1981; **71**: 791–8.

147. Lakhanpal S, Lie JT, Conn DL, Martin WJ, 2nd. Pulmonary disease in polymyositis/dermatomyositis: a clinicopathological analysis of 65 autopsy cases. *Ann Rheum Dis* 1987; **46**: 23–9.

148. Young ID, Ford SE, Ford PM. The association of pulmonary hypertension with rheumatoid arthritis. *J Rheumatol* 1989; **16**: 1266–9.

149. Baydur A, Mongan ES, Slager UT. Acute respiratory failure and pulmonary arteritis without parenchymal involvement: demonstration in a patient with rheumatoid arthritis. *Chest* 1979; **75**: 518–20.

150. Winn WC, Jr, Myerowitz RL. The pathology of the Legionella pneumonias. A review of 74 cases and the literature. *Hum Pathol* 1981; **12**: 401–22.

151. Soave R, Murray HW, Litrenta MM. Bacterial invasion of pulmonary vessels. Pseudomonas bacteremia mimicking pulmonary thromboembolism with infarction. *Am J Med* 1978; **65**: 864–7.

152. Jamadar DA, Kazerooni EA, Daly BD, *et al.* Pulmonary zygomycosis: CT appearance. *J Comput Assist Tomogr* 1995; **19**: 733–8.

153. Travis WD, Pittaluga S, Lipschik GY, *et al.* Atypical pathologic manifestations of *Pneumocystis carinii* pneumonia in the acquired immune deficiency syndrome. Review of 123 lung biopsies from 76 patients with emphasis on cysts, vascular invasion, vasculitis, and granulomas. *Am J Surg Pathol* 1990; **14**: 615–25.

Cardiogenic pulmonary edema

HAL A SKOPICKI, JONATHAN SACKNER-BERNSTEIN

INTRODUCTION

During the era of Hippocrates (460–370 BC), heart failure was believed to be caused

> when the [cold humor] phlegm descends cold to the lungs and heart, the blood is chilled; and the veins beat forcefully against the lungs and heart and the heart palpates so that under this compulsion difficulty of breathing and orthopnea result.[1]

Several hundred years later, descriptions of the clinical state of pulmonary congestion applicable today were noted by Celsus in *De Medicina* (25–50 BC)

> [Difficulty in breathing] when moderate is called dyspnea … when in addition the patient can hardly draw in his breath unless the neck is elevated and outstretched, orthopnea.

> [Blood-letting was the remedy] as the body becomes depleted … the patient begins to draw his breath more readily. Moreover, even in bed the head is to be raised.

At the turn of the twentieth century, the 'effusion of pleurisy' was treated by agents in an attempt to try to reabsorb the fluid, including the iodine painted upon the surface of the thorax, sodium chloride, and potassium or sodium iodide administered internally.

> Common salt is occasionally given – in as large amounts and as frequently as the patient can bear it. It is believed that if the blood can be made strongly saline a demand on the part of the system will be created for water, which will be satisfied by the absorption of the exudates if water is not drunk. The good effect of the iodides probably results from their increasing diuresis. They are not, however, as efficient as the acetate of potash or ammonia.[2]

Patients hospitalized with worsening heart failure face a 5–8 percent risk of inhospital death, a rehospitalization rate as high as 50 percent over the next 6 months, and a mortality up to 30 percent within the year (references 3–10 and the American Heart Association. *2002 Heart and Stroke Statistical Update.* Dallas, TX: American Heart Association, 2001). Therefore, a thorough understanding of the clinical pathophysiology is critical to deliver both efficacious and timely acute treatment of cardiogenic pulmonary edema in addition to determining the optimum paradigm to assess the reversibility of the cardiomyopathy and its long-term management.

ANATOMY AND PHYSIOLOGY OF CARDIOGENIC PULMONARY EDEMA

The edematous lungs of cardiogenic pulmonary edema contain a frothy sputum that may result in lungs that weigh nearly two to three times normal. As is the case with all biologic membranes, fluid flux across the alveolar wall is dynamic and controlled by Starling forces,[11] consisting of competing vascular hydrostatic pressure, capillary permeability, and plasma and interstitial oncotic pressure.

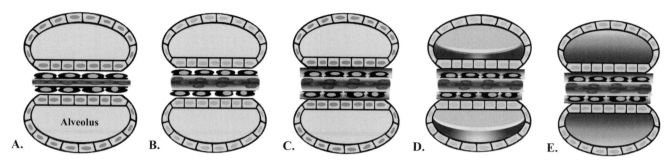

Figure 13D.1 *Progression of pulmonary edema. A. Capillary alveolar membrane at normal hydrostatic pressures. B. Increased hydrostatic pressure is initially countered by the permeability of the endothelial membrane and the plasma oncotic forces; C. Increasing hydrostatic pressure results in an increase in interstitial fluid. The degree of transudation is determined by the ability of the lymphatic system to bilge the transudate. D. Initial appearance of alveolar fluid resulting clinically in significant dyspnea on exertion. E. Representation of frank pulmonary edema with shortness of breath at rest.*

Together with surfactant, these factors are primarily responsible for keeping fluid out of the alveoli and within the pulmonary vascular tree.

When the plasma oncotic pressure is higher (approximately 25 mm Hg) than the pulmonary hydrostatic pressure (about 7–12 mm Hg), the air–blood cellular barrier is fairly impermeable to plasma proteins and the alveoli are kept dry (Fig. 13D.1). Whether through increased hydrostatic pressure, decreased oncotic pressure, or increased capillary permeability, the initial presence of fluid in the pericapillary interstitial space results in enhanced absorption by the lymphatic system.[12] When the production of pericapillary fluid exceeds the absorptive capacity of the lymphatic system (the lung's interstitial spaces can only accommodate a few hundred milliliters of excess fluid[13]), this gives way to edema fluid in the alveoli in the presence of intact[14] or compromised[15] alveolar membranes. As pulmonary septal capillaries become engorged, alveoli eventually fill with protein-poor edema fluid (specific gravity <1.012). Initially, fluid within the alveoli is crescentic but eventually floods the entire alveolus. There is an abundance of macrophages in the edema fluid, many of which contain hemosiderin pigment from erythrocyte egress across the alveolar-capillary membrane, accounting for the fluid's pink color (Fig. 13D.2).

Although the alveolar type II cell has been thought to be primarily responsible for the transport of ions and fluid from the airspaces of the lungs,[16] there is increasing evidence that the type I cell is also capable of active fluid transport.[17,18] Moreover, distal airway epithelial cells such as the Clara cell, may also participate.[19] Once alveolar edema develops, movement of fluid out of the airspace is accomplished by active ion transport, predominantly by the alveolar epithelium to establish an osmotic gradient across the epithelium. Ion transport is predominantly due to amiloride-sensitive epithelial sodium (Na^+) and amiloride-insensitive sodium channels, with a lesser role of chloride[20–22] channels. Amiloride can block 40–90 percent of fluid clearance in the lung, whereas the less well-understood amiloride insensitive channels depends on cyclic nucleotide

gating. Fluid clearance from the airspaces involves sodium pumping through channels located on the luminal surfaces of alveolar epithelial cells down a sodium concentration gradient created by the continuous cellular extrusion of sodium by Na^+/K^+ ATPase pumps on the basolateral membrane of the alveolar epithelial cell. As the Na^+/K^+ ATPase pumps sodium out of the alveolar epithelial cell into the blood, a gradient is created that drives sodium movement through channels on the apical membrane into the cell. Sodium is then passively transported from the alveolar edema fluid in the airspace into the epithelial cell and then into the blood. The ion channels are also regulated by both catecholamine (β1- and β2-adrenergic[18–26] receptors) and noncatecholamine receptors. Noncatecholamine regulation of pulmonary fluid clearance occurs through aldosterone,[23,24] epidermal growth factor,[25,26] transforming growth factor-α,[27] keratinocyte growth factor,[28–30] and hepatocyte growth factor. Negative regulators of alveolar fluid clearance include β-blockers,[31,32] atrial natriuretic

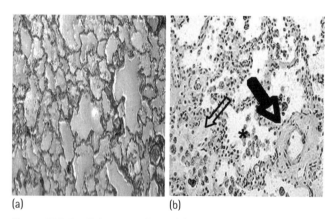

(a)   (b)

Figure 13D.2 *Pulmonary edema. (a) Acute pulmonary edema demonstrating diffuse passive congestion in pulmonary alveoli. (b) Chronic passive congestion where a fibrosed pulmonary vessel (closed arrow) appears resistant to surrounding edema while other areas of the lung show passive congestion (open arrow) and hemosiderin-laden macrophages (asterisk).*

peptide,[33] and nitric oxide,[34] although the clinical significance of each remains undetermined.[35]

ETIOLOGY OF CARDIOGENIC PULMONARY EDEMA

Cardiogenic pulmonary edema most often results from increases in pulmonary capillary hydrostatic pressures that may be clinically modified by increases in alveolar capillary permeability, although decreased plasma oncotic pressure and reduced lymphatic clearance can play an additive role (Box. 13D.1). Causes of increased vascular hydrostatic pressure include disorders involving the systemic circulation, aortic valve, left ventricle, mitral valve, or pulmonary venous system.

Box 13D.1 Causes of pulmonary edema

Increased pulmonary capillary transmural pressure

- Left ventricular failure, acute or chronic
- Severe hypertension
- Aortic stenosis
- Hypertophic cardiomyopathy
- Aortic insufficiency
- Myocarditis
- Acute myocardial infarction/ischemia
- Mitral valve stenosis
- Severe mitral regurgitation
- Pulmonary veno-occlusive disease

Decreased plasma colloid osmotic pressure

- Hypoalbuminemia (nephrotic syndrome, hepatic failure)

Reduced lymphatic clearance

- Lymphangitic carcinoma
- Following lung transplant

Increased pulmonary capillary endothelial permeability

- Infectious (bacteremia, viremia, fungemia, sepsis)
- Inflammation
- Disseminated intravascular coagulation
- High-altitude pulmonary edema
- Following cardiopulmonary bypass, cardioversion
- Acute respiratory distress syndrome

Increased alveolar epithelial permeability

- Toxins
- Aspiration
- Drowning
- Depletion of surfactant through high tidal volume positive-pressure mechanical ventilation
- Surfactant deficiency

Severe hypertension, end-stage aortic stenosis, or obstructive hypertrophic cardiomyopathy can result in abrupt limitations to cardiac emptying. This leads to increases in pulmonary vascular hydrostatic pressure and acute pulmonary edema.[36,37] Sudden cardiogenic pulmonary edema can also manifest with abrupt aortic or mitral valvular insufficiency, myocarditis, acute myocardial infarction, or myocardial ischemia, the last most often in the presence of severe three-vessel or left main disease.

Over a more prolonged period of time, chronic valvular aortic stenosis and less severe systemic hypertension can transmit a diastolic pressure load from the left ventricle to the left atrium leading to elevations in pulmonary hydrostatic pressure. Similarly, chronic aortic regurgitation and left ventricular dilatation (remodeling) transmit the pressure of increasing volume loads into the pulmonary circulation, which may be exacerbated in the presence of mitral regurgitation. With more chronic systolic or diastolic dysfunction, exercise studies indicate the presence of decreased conductance across the alveolar-capillary barrier.[38]

Chronic ischemic or nonischemic mitral regurgitation is produced by systolic displacement of the mitral leaflets apically and outwardly, which is caused by annular dilatation and outward bulging of the inferoposterior wall and the papillary muscles.[39] The resulting ineffective closure of the tethered leaflets leads to increases in pulmonary vascular hydrostatic pressure that can be demonstrated with exercise testing.[40] Chronic mitral stenosis, which progressively leads to increased pulmonary vascular hydrostatic pressure, can present acutely in the setting of new-onset atrial fibrillation or supraventricular tachycardias due to decreased atrial diastolic emptying times.

Although cardiogenic pulmonary edema most often presents in isolation, it may be accompanied by clinical scenarios that contribute to altered capillary permeability or decreased intravascular oncotic pressure. Potentially important confounding causes of increased capillary permeability are seen with uremia, sepsis, infection (viral or bacterial), acute respiratory distress syndrome (ARDS), the release of inflammatory vasoactive substances (i.e. histamine and kinins), and disseminated intravascular coagulopathy. Likewise, decreased oncotic pressure can be due to hypoalbuminemia from a variety of causes (renal, hepatic, nutritional, or protein-losing enteropathy) or lymphatic insufficiency.[41] Neurogenic pulmonary edema can occur secondary to central nervous system trauma or subarachnoid bleeding. The mechanisms by which pulmonary embolism, cardioversion, and the postanesthesia, postextubation and postcardiopulmonary bypass states cause noncardiogenic pulmonary edema are unknown.

Pulmonary edema is most often due to cardiogenic and/or noncardiogenic causes, but diseases that affect the pulmonary venous system, such as sarcoidosis, pulmonary venoocclusive disease, and venous thrombosis, can also increase pulmonary vascular pressures. This diagnosis warrants consideration when pulmonary capillary wedge pressure is elevated in the absence of mitral valvular disease, but at the same time a low left ventricular end-diastolic pressure is recorded, that latter which is unchanged by exercise. Finally, the presence of chronic pulmonary edema is exacerbated by any condition that results in decreased cardiac output thus causing increased preload via stimulation of antidiuretic hormone (free water retention) and activation of the renin–angiotensin aldosterone system (sodium reabsorption).

CLINICAL PRESENTATION AND DIAGNOSIS OF CARDIOGENIC PULMONARY EDEMA

The presentation of cardiogenic pulmonary edema can be acute or preceded by subtle herald signs, but in either case it is dominated by the decrease in oxygen absorption and carbon dioxide release across the pulmonary capillary membrane and compounded by alveoli that cannot completely expand due to volume excess (Box 13D.2). Acute cardiogenic pulmonary edema may be associated with chest pain, palpitations, and a suffocating feeling ('air hunger'). When pulmonary edema is the result of a chronic process, the patient generally describes a progression from dyspnea on exertion to paroxysmal nocturnal dyspnea and orthopnea, culminating in dyspnea at rest and cough. This clinical scenario represents the progression of fluid extravasation into the pulmonary interstitium during the early phase to extensive fluid within the alveoli during the later phases. A cough productive of pink, frothy sputum is highly suggestive for pulmonary edema.

Longstanding peripheral edema results in a history of leg swelling that usually worsens at the end of day when the patient is not confined to the recumbent position. Symptoms of ischemia or palpitations consistent with arrhythmias must be sought. Systemic processes can precipitate pulmonary edema and symptoms of anemia and both hypo- and hyperthyroidism should be elicited. Moreover, patients should be investigated for noncompliance issues including sodium and fluid restriction and uncontrolled hypertension. Past medical problems that may predispose to pulmonary edema include the history of a cardiomyopathy, prior myocardial infarction, angina, valvular heart disease, alcohol use, hypertension, angina, or familial heart disease.

Physical exam

Physical findings in cardiogenic pulmonary edema are based on the degree of edema and the amount of myocardial dysfunction present. Generally, cardiogenic pulmonary edema is associated with tachypnea, an S3,[42] an elevated jugular venous pressure, hepatojugular reflux,[42] extensive use of accessory muscles of respiration, moist rales with or without wheezing,[43] and peripheral edema.

In the chronic setting, rales appear when pulmonary fluid is approximately three times the normal level and may be absent in over 80 percent of patients due to chronic compensation by the lymphatic system.[44,45] It is reasonable to postulate that the scalability of lymphatic absorption, up to a 10-fold increase over time, is probably responsible for an individual's ability to tolerate chronic pulmonary edema,[46] in addition to alveolar fibrosis with thickening of the capillary endothelial and alveolar epithelial cell membranes.[47,48] It is also important to note that even the heart failure specialist can underappreciate the presence of volume excess, as measured by circulating blood volume.[49] Cardiac auscultation may reveal aortic or mitral valvular abnormalities. In addition, the presence of an S4 may suggest the presence of coronary artery disease, hypertension, or aortic stenosis. Peripheral hypoperfusion can manifest with cold, cyanotic, or diaphoretic skin.

Diagnostic testing

B–TYPE NATRIURETIC PEPTIDE AND OTHER SERUM MARKERS

Recent studies have demonstrated that serum B-type natriuretic peptide (BNP) levels correlate with elevations in left and/or right ventricular wall stress, both with systolic and diastolic dysfunction. BNP levels are especially useful due to their ability to rapidly assist with the triage of patients to cardiogenic or noncardiogenic causes of dyspnea. With BNP levels greater than 500 ng/L, the diagnosis of heart failure

---

Box 13D.2 Clinical presentations

Acute pulmonary edema

- Acute onset dyspnea
- Chest pain
- Palpitations/tachycardia
- Tachypnea
- Hypotension/hypertension
- Elevated jugular venous pressure (JVP)

Chronic pulmonary edema

- Dyspnea on exertion
- Paroxysmal nocturnal dyspnea
- Orthopnea
- Hypotension/hypertension
- Elevated JVP
- Peripheral edema

Markers of severity

- Pallor/Hypotension
- Dyspnea at rest
- Central/peripheral cyanosis
- Active chest pain

decompensation in the setting of dyspnea on presentation is relatively certain. In one study in an emergency room setting, serum BNP levels were 90 percent sensitive and 76 percent specific for the detection of heart failure with a positive predictive value of 79 percent and a negative predictive value of 89 percent.[50] In patients with left ventricular heart failure, serum BNP levels closely correlate with an elevated pulmonary capillary wedge pressure. In addition, conditions that elevate right filling pressures, such as pulmonary embolus and primary pulmonary hypertension, may cause elevated BNP levels in the 100–500 ng/L range.

However, in patients with obesity and chronic kidney disease, the utility of BNP as a screening biomarker may be more limited. One analysis showed that as the creatinine goes up to approximately 177 μmol/L (2 mg/dL) the optimal BNP value for the diagnosis of congestive heart failure may go from 100 ng/L to about 200 ng/L.[51] This may be further complicated by the recent introduction of N-terminal pro-BNP, which is excreted almost exclusively through the kidney. Therefore, it is important to ascertain the baseline BNP level in a patient with renal dysfunction to differentiate how much of the elevation is from left ventricular dysfunction and how much is from not clearing BNP. Falsely low levels of BNP can be seen in flash pulmonary edema with acute papillary muscle rupture or in cases of extreme obesity. In the Breathing Not Properly trial the BNP level was greater than 1000 ng/L in half of the nonobese patients compared with only about 10–20 percent of patients whose body mass index was above 35 kg/m^2.[50]

In addition, the clinical relevance of BNP levels may extend beyond its diagnostic use. Preliminary data suggest that serial measurement of BNP levels may be useful to direct therapy with one strategy showing that only 27 percent of patients admitted in heart failure managed by BNP levels had a cardiovascular event compared with 53 percent managed independent of BNP levels ($P = 0.034$).[52] BNP levels independently predict the risk of rehospitalization and death in patients with heart failure[53] and values at 80 percent or above of population norms for healthy adults without cardiac disease predict increased risk for heart failure.[54] Future studies will determine the optimum means of utilizing BNP measurements in clinical practice.

Recently, plasma surfactant peptide B as marker of cardiogenic pulmonary edema.[55,56] Surfactant peptide B is necessary for the normal functioning of pulmonary surfactant and is synthesized by type II alveolar epithelial cells. It is secreted through the apical surface into alveoli, reaching the plasma by moving down its concentration gradient from the alveoli into the blood when the alveolar-capillary barrier is damaged.[57,58] Although promising, levels may also be elevated in ARDS and with pulmonary disease that affects the integrity of the pulmonary capillary membrane. Moreover, whereas BNP reflects left ventricular wall stress and the cause of elevated hydrostatic pressure, surfactant protein B reflects the *effects* of elevated plasma hydrostatic pressure on the lung. Whether circulating levels provide additional information to serum BNP levels has not been determined.

SERUM CREATININE

Renal dysfunction is a strong predictor of outcome in patients with heart failure.[59–63] Worsening of serum creatinine levels by as little as 8.8 μmol/L (0.1 mg/dL) in patients hospitalized for acutely decompensated heart failure is predictive of increased risk.[64–67] With acute cardiogenic pulmonary edema, creatinine levels may be elevated due to the hypoperfusion secondary to decreased cardiac output, intrinsic renal disease, or postrenal obstruction. A urinalysis to assess whether proteinuria is present to determine the role diabetes may also be indicated. Whether a renal duplex ultrasound is indicated depends on the response of renal function to diuresis and improved cardiac output.

OTHER SERUM MARKERS

Dilutional hyponatremia is also present in patients with chronic heart failure due to enforced sodium diuresis and its replacement, in many cases, with free water. For many years, the presence of hyponatremia was considered an especially poor prognostic sign. This finding needs to be confirmed in the light of current use of β-blockers and aldosterone antagonists. Elevated serum aspartate aminotransferase and alanine aminotransferase levels and hyperbilirubinemia are suggestive of hepatic congestion. Total creatine kinase enzyme and percentage MB fractionation, in addition to serum troponin levels, should be assessed for the loss of myocytes or clinical myocardial infarction. D-dimer levels should be assessed to assist in the diagnosis of acute pulmonary embolism whereas serum thyroid stimulating hormone levels (for hypothyroidism or hyperthyroidism) and Lyme titers should also be assessed for reversible causes of myocardial dysfunction.

An arterial blood gas should be ascertained to assess the degree of acidosis, hypoxemia, or acidosis. Pulse oximetry can be misleading in patients who have peripheral vasoconstriction. In cardiogenic pulmonary edema, P_{O_2} is reduced due to impaired oxygen transport across the alveolar membrane, and the associated tachypnea leads to the classic drop in P_{CO_2} as is seen in any hyperventilation syndrome. As respiratory reserve is exhausted, P_{O_2} remains reduced while carbon dioxide retention results in a drop in pH. This finding suggests that the optimal moment for intubation may have passed.

CHEST RADIOGRAPHY

Chest radiography is useful in cardiogenic pulmonary edema during staging and to determine underlying etiologies.[68,69] First the radiograph should be assessed for cardiomegaly – a cardiothoracic ratio greater than 50 percent of the chest. Early signs of pulmonary edema are associated with the presence of interstitial edema and include cephalization of pulmonary vessels (reflecting a pulmonary capillary wedge pressure ~12–18 mm Hg) and Kerley B lines (~2 cm horizontal lines extending to the lateral edge of the lung image itself) seen laterally in the lower zones when the pulmonary capillary wedge pressure ~18–25 mm Hg). As the edema progresses to the alveoli, a 'butterfly' pattern is seen, indicative of a pulmonary capillary wedge pressure greater than 25 mm Hg. It is characterized by central shadows and clear peripheral zones presenting along with pleural effusions. Although most common bilaterally, when the effusion is unilateral the pattern is almost always observed on the right. It deserves to be mentioned that although most of these effusions are transudates, up to 20 percent may be exudates, principally in patients receiving diuretic therapy.[70,71] A cardiac source is also suggested by a pleural fluid/serum albumin gradient of more than 12 g/L.

Although useful, a radiographic lag from onset of symptoms may occur. In addition, radiographic findings may persist for several days despite clinical improvement and therefore serial chest radiographs are of little utility to assess short-term responses. Lastly, since chronically elevated pressures may induce alveolar-capillary fibrosis, which protects the lung from alveolar edema, a high-resolution chest computed tomography (CT) scan may occasionally be useful to support the diagnosis of heart failure.

ELECTROCARDIOGRAM

The electrocardiogram (EKG), although nonspecific, is useful in detecting precipitating arrhythmias or myocardial ischemia, or underlying old myocardial infarctions and the presence of left ventricular hypertrophy cardiac dysrhythmias.

ECHOCARDIOGRAPHY

Echocardiography is critical for the effective evaluation of acute cardiogenic pulmonary edema and should be performed as soon as is feasible. In addition to determining the presence and severity of acute or chronic valvular diseases, echocardiography is also important in establishing whether the cardiomyopathy is systolic or diastolic in nature. Regional wall motion abnormalities may establish the presence of ischemic heart disease. Echocardiography can also be used to determine pulmonary artery systolic pressure as well as establishing the chronicity of elevated pulmonary pressures with secondary right ventricular failure. Echocardiography may also help exclude cardiac tamponade, pericardial constriction, and pulmonary embolus.

MANAGEMENT OF ACUTE PULMONARY EDEMA

Patients with pulmonary edema require expeditious assessment of the degree of respiratory and hemodynamic instability (Fig. 13D.3). Initial management involves the administration of 100 percent oxygen via a non-rebreather facemask (8–10 L). If intubation is not indicated and noncardiac causes of pulmonary edema have been excluded,

---

Box 13D.3 Common etiologies for provocation of acute pulmonary edema

- Myocardial ischemia or infarct
- Arrhythmias (tachy or bradyarrhythmias)
- Insufficiency (mitral) or stenosis (mitral or aortic)
- Hypertension
- Embolism
- Myocarditis
- Tachycardia
- Infection (concomitant)
- Renal failure
- Anemia
- Dietary indiscretion (salt or fluid intake)
- Endocrine (thyrotoxicosis)

- 100% FiO$_2$ by facemask
- Cardiac monitor
- Start IV
- If atrial fibrillation, atrial flutter or ventricular tachycardia: treat arrhythmia
- Sublingual nitroglycerin 0.4–0.8 mg or nitropaste 2.5 cm to chest wall
- Furosemide 80 mg IV push
- Morphine 1–2 mg IV; assess further dosing
- Arterial blood gas
- 12-lead electrocardiogram
- Foley catheter
- Consider nitroglycerine 10–20 µg/min IV with increases until blood pressure maximum or >100 mm Hg

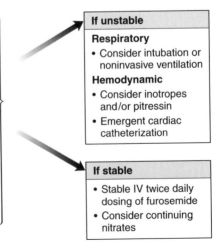

If unstable

Respiratory
- Consider intubation or noninvasive ventilation

Hemodynamic
- Consider inotropes and/or pitressin
- Emergent cardiac catheterization

If stable
- Stable IV twice daily dosing of furosemide
- Consider continuing nitrates

Figure 13D.3 *Management of acute cardiogenic pulmonary edema. IV, intravenous.*

temporizing measures to reduce venous return should be initiated, such as elevating the head of the bed or allowing the patient to sit with legs dangling over the side of the bed. The EKG must be monitored continuously for the onset of arrhythmias and a Foley catheter inserted to assess fluid balance, in addition to relieving the most common form of urinary obstruction. Also a search for underlying or exacerbating disease must be pursued concomitantly (Box 13D.3).

Ventilation

If the arterial PO_2 cannot be maintained at 60 mm Hg or more during facemask ventilation or if the PCO_2 rises with ventilatory fatigue (in the presence of a declining arterial pH), the patient should be intubated. It is important to remember that pulmonary alveolar edema may be further compromised by the presence of large pleural effusions and shunting may also be present with concomitant atelectasis, pneumonia, pulmonary hemorrhage, or ARDS.

Noninvasive continuous positive airway pressure (CPAP), where a single airway pressure is present throughout the respiratory phases, may promote early clinical stabilization and thereby permit introduction of more definitive therapy to reverse the problem without resorting to intubation. Although probably efficacious as far as avoidance of intubation is concerned, CPAP does not appear to affect overall outcome as measured by short-term mortality and length of hospital stay.[72–81] Bilevel positive airway pressure (BiPAP) therapy, where higher pressures can be applied during inspiration and lower pressures during expiration, may improve ventilation and vital signs more rapidly then CPAP and be preferred over nasal cannula. An earlier study suggested an increased incidence of myocardial infarction with BiPAP,[82] but this was not seen in two later studies.[83,84] However, no large trials have yet been performed so the clinical scenario should dictate whether BiPAP is considered.

Diuresis and perfusion

Once ventilatory control has been established, hemodynamic stability must be ensured. One study showed that in patients with cardiogenic pulmonary edema requiring mechanical intubation, 24-hour mortality was highest when systolic blood pressure was less than 130 mm Hg or vasopressor medications were required.[85] In patients with preserved systolic function, acute cardiogenic pulmonary edema is most likely due to left main coronary artery disease, severe three-vessel (left main equivalent) disease, or severe hypertension. In addition to diuretics, prompt treatment of the blood pressure with vasodilators and heart rate (with β-blockers) usually results in immediate clinical improvement. However, administration of β-blockers should not be considered if there is any possibility of acute cardiogenic pulmonary edema with left ventricular systolic dysfunction.

In such a setting, the negative hemodynamic effects of even small doses could prove catastrophic. All patients should be evaluated for coronary artery disease and, in those presenting with severe hypertension, a search for secondary causes, such as renal artery stenosis, should be pursued.

For the hemodynamic management of patients who present with acute cardiogenic pulmonary edema secondary to systolic dysfunction, a useful schemata involves a direct assessment of perfusion and congestion, resulting in a 2×2 treatment box (Fig. 13D.4).[45] Clinical indicators of congestion include orthopnea, paroxysmal nocturnal dyspnea, jugular venous distension, rales, hepatic tenderness, hepatojugular reflex, and/or peripheral edema. Indicators of low perfusion are hypotension, low pulse pressure, decreased alertness, renal dysfunction, and/or cool extremities. Patients admitted with pulmonary edema but still showing evidence of good end-organ perfusion (wet-warm) have appropriate extreme increases in their systemic vascular resistance and generally respond to diuretics alone or diuretics with vasodilators. Those who have volume overload but insufficient increases in systemic vascular resistance to atone for low cardiac output demonstrate compromised end-organ perfusion (wet-cold) and typically require increasing doses of inotropes in addition to diuretics. In some cases, ultrafiltration and right heart catheterization, the latter to optimize hemodynamics, should be considered. Those patients who do not have volume overload but nonetheless have severe inotropic insufficiency (the 'dry-cold' patient) require inotropes, consideration of mechanical device

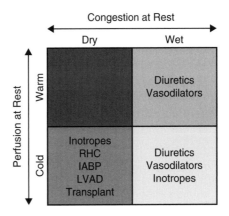

Figure 13D.4 *Symptomatic management of pulmonary edema. Patients who are 'warm-wet' require diuretics and may also benefit from concomitant use of vasodilators like nitroglycerin. Patients who are 'cold-wet' require enhanced end-organ perfusion via increased cardiac output that can be obtained with vasodilators such as nitroprusside or inotropes such as dobutamine or milrinone. Those who are 'cold-dry' suffer from severe contractile dysfunction requiring use of inotropes with catheter-based guidance (RHC) to optimize stroke volume. Acutely, intraaortic balloon counterpulsation (IABP) may be beneficial but the need for heart replacement therapies, in appropriate patients, is almost always required. LVAD, left ventricular assist device.*

support, and evaluation for transplant. A subset of patients admitted with decompensated heart failure who have adequate perfusion and have no volume overload (warm-dry) do not require intense medical therapy. However, it is interesting to note that a 16 percent mortality at 18 months has been shown in these 'compensated' patients.[86]

In general, the goal of pharmacotherapy is to optimize stroke volume while reducing pulmonary capillary wedge pressure. This is achieved by approximating a pulmonary capillary wedge pressure of 15–18 mm Hg and a cardiac index >2.2 L/min/m^2, adjusting for optimization of blood pressure and end-organ perfusion.

DIURETICS

Diuretics are a critical part of therapy for acute cardiogenic pulmonary edema. The primary goal is the reduction in pulmonary capillary wedge pressure with attendant increases in stroke volume, and diuretics act rapidly (intravenously 5–10 minutes; orally 1–2 hours), with an increase in urine output via the intravenous route often within 30 minutes and a peak in their natriuretic effect at 1 hour.[87] In addition to their effect on volume, loop diuretics can cause immediate venodilation (and improvement in dyspnea) prior to diuresis.[88] Most loop diuretics have a duration of action of 4–6 hours and patients should be redosed according to the clinical scenario. Surprisingly, few controlled trials have studied the optimum use of diuretics in acute pulmonary edema.[89]

Via the intravenous route, all loop diuretics act in a dose-dependent manner by inhibiting the Na$^+$/K$^+$/2Cl$^-$ cotransporter in the thick ascending limb of Henle, the site where approximately 20 percent of all filtered sodium is reabsorbed. All loop diuretics require filtration at the glomerular level and, therefore, increasing doses must be used with decreasing glomerular filtration rate (GFR). As a general rule of thumb, we usually initiate furosemide calculated at a dose of 40 multiplied by the creatinine level, given twice daily via the intravenous route as a starting dose, increasing or decreasing as needed based on the urine output over the following 2 hours. In chronic loop diuretic use, the distal tubule increases in the activity and number of Na$^+$/Cl$^-$ cotransporters. Therefore, in these cases if the patient is still 'warm-wet' without appreciable diuresis, the dose of furosemide is doubled and/or a thiazidelike diuretic (i.e. metolazone 5–10 mg orally) designed to block the distal tubule (the site of approximately 7 percent of sodium reabsorption) in series, is then added.[90–92] Thiazidelike diuretics, unlike thiazides, remain effective even if the GFR is less than 30 mL/min. The potential utility of continuous infusion of furosemide has been demonstrated in a few small clinical trials[93–95] and may be considered when bolus dosing may not be adequate.

Although useful, diuretics have many undesirable actions, including promotion of potassium and magnesium loss that can provoke arrhythmias, exacerbation of glucose intolerance, and activation of the renin–angiotensin system.

Caution is also warranted since some studies have shown a significant increase in adverse events among patients treated with high-dose diuretics.[96] Overdiuresis can be reversed by a bolus of saline solution but should be avoided through the close monitoring of fluid input and output as therapy proceeds.

Ultrafiltration

Patients with cardiogenic pulmonary edema, who prove refractory to diuretic therapy despite adequate renal perfusion enhanced by vasodilators and/or inotropes (see below), may require dialysis. Historically, arteriovenous ultrafiltration was the only consideration, but its use requires adequate blood pressures (i.e. SBP >130 mm Hg). However, by removing blood via a venous catheter and passing it through a porous filter where fluid is removed prior to return to the venous system, continuous veno-venous hemodialysis (ultrafiltration) effectively removes volume while avoiding the hemodynamic instability associated with arteriovenous hemodialysis.[97] While previously performed using central venous access, a system using one antecubital venous catheter (similar to a peripherally inserted central catheter) for blood withdrawal can be coupled with a second short, large-bore intravenous catheter placed in the opposite arm to effectively remove up to 500 mL of ultrafiltrate per hour. A recent study of 21 patients with severe volume overload who underwent treatments for up to 8 hours showed an average fluid removal of 3725 mL with improvement in symptoms and little change in serum electrolytes.[98] Further studies are required to determine whether veno-venous ultrafiltration can be used safely in patients with volume overload and pulmonary edema as routine therapy.

Morphine

Morphine is administered in acute cardiogenic pulmonary edema as an anxiolytic, to decrease the work of breathing and to cause venodilation, resulting in decreased preload. There is little evidence that it can improve morbidity or mortality in this clinical setting[99] and may, in some circumstances be deleterious.[100] However, like nitrates and nesiritide, morphine can also cause arterial dilatation, which reduces systemic vascular resistance and increases cardiac output,[101,102] so its careful use as an adjunctive medicine may be beneficial. Morphine should be given as a 2–5 mg intravenous bolus, which may be repeated every 10–15 minutes as needed in the absence of respiratory (<20 breaths/min) or blood pressure (<100 mm Hg systolic) compromise. It should be rarely used in patients with decreased sensorium or respiratory drive, and if respiratory compromise occurs, the specific antidote naloxone (Narcan; 0.8–2.0 mg intravenous bolus) should be administered. Morphine has mild vagolytic effects and should be carefully used in the presence of supraventricular tachycardias.

Vasodilators

Vasodilators such as nitroglycerin are potent nitric oxide donors and induce prompt venodilation. Nitroglycerin is used in cardiogenic pulmonary edema to abruptly lower the pulmonary capillary wedge pressure/preload in an attempt to increase stroke volume and cardiac output according to the Starling curve. In addition, they can also dilate epicardial coronary arteries facilitating improved myocardial perfusion which, in addition to the systemic effects, can lead to hemodynamic stability, enhanced renal perfusion, increased filtration of diuretics, and concomitant diuresis.[103–105] Compared with inotropes, they are much less likely to cause ventricular arrhythmias.

Nitroglycerin may be given as a sublingual tablet 0.4–0.8 mg or spray, transdermal nitropaste (2.5–5 cm to chest wall; variable absorption may be present in diaphoretic patients) or preferentially intravenously. If given sublingually, nitroglycerin tablets or spray can be repeated twice at 5-minute intervals, as long as there is no major fall in blood pressure. If given to someone with a systolic blood pressure <120 mm Hg, an intravenous line for volume resuscitation must first be in place. Typical intravenous doses employed in clinical practice start at 5 μg/min with gradual up-titration into the 50–100 μg/min range, but clinical studies that support the role of intravenous nitroglycerin for acutely decompensated heart failure used doses that started at 10–20 μg/min with up-titration every 5–10 minutes to target doses often in excess of 500 μg/min.[104] This dosing regimen demonstrated significant improvements in hemodynamic status. However, tolerance does occur, limiting the effectiveness of intravenous nitroglycerin to approximately 16–48 hours.

Vasodilators should not be used with severe hypotension or shock unless the shock is of known ischemic etiology with an elevation in pulmonary capillary wedge pressure. In addition, vasodilators should also be avoided in conditions that are dependent on venous return, such as significant valvular stenosis, restrictive or obstructive cardiomyopathy, constrictive pericarditis, and pericardial tamponade. Nitrates are also contraindicated in patients who have taken the phosphodiesterase type 5 inhibitors such as sildenafil or vardenafil within the past 1–2 days.[106]

Recombinant BNPs can also decrease preload and be used in patients with decompensated pulmonary edema. They are believed to act via binding to the guanylate cyclase receptor of vascular smooth muscle and endothelial cells causing increased cyclic GMP, which is a second messenger in the vasodilatory pathway. Agents such as the recombinant form of BNP (nesiritide) have been used in patients with decompensated pulmonary edema with results similar to those of low-dose intravenous nitroglycerin.[7,8,107] Initiation of nesiritide is usually begun with a bolus of 2 μg/kg intravenously over 1 minute, followed by a maintenance dose of 0.01 μg/kg per minute continuous infusion. However, the use of nesiritide has not been studied in acute pulmonary edema. Moreover, the persistence of excessive hypotension is significantly longer with recombinant BNP than intravenous nitroglycerin, so it is better avoided in this clinical scenario.[7] All other contraindications for the use of vasodilators are germane to the BNPs. Additional controversy exists regarding the impact of nesiritide on renal function. In patients with worsening renal function and volume overload, nesiritide infusion produced no benefit on GFR or volume status relative to placebo.[108,109] A metaanalysis investigating the association of nesiritide therapy with worsening renal function demonstrated a significantly higher likelihood for this adverse effect than control. Despite these concerns preliminary data suggest that it remains a safer choice than dobutamine[99] in more stable situations.

Afterload agents and inotropes

When reductions in wedge pressure result in a stroke volume that is still inadequate to maintain sufficient perfusion pressures, the use of arterial dilators and inotropes should be considered (Fig. 13D.5). However, it is worth noting that changes in cardiac index have not been shown to be predictive of subsequent outcome.[110]

INTRAVENOUS NITROPRUSSIDE

Intravenous nitroprusside is an arterial vasodilator (activates guanylate cyclase to increase the level of cyclic GMP in smooth muscle resulting in vasodilation) that results in rapid reduction in left ventricular end-diastolic pressure, causing an increase in stroke volume and cardiac output without increasing heart rate. It is easily titratable and is usually started in patients with cardiogenic pulmonary edema whose systolic blood pressure is at least 90 mm Hg at 0.5 μg/kg per minute and increase to 3–5 μg/kg per minute. In addition to severe hypotension, nitroprusside should be avoided in patients with rate-dependent arrhythmias, hypertrophic cardiomyopathy, hypothyroidism, or optic atrophy. However, a small study suggests it may be used safely in patients with severe aortic stenosis and heart failure.[111] In addition, its use in patients with hepatic or renal failure must be closely monitored as nitroprusside levels may increase and can cause cyanide toxicity.

INOTROPES

Although inotropes play an undeniably important role in the management of patients with decompensated pulmonary edema and cardiogenic shock, it is important to note that prospective, randomized controlled trials of inotropes have not been performed. A variety of agents and mechanisms are involved in agents that act as inotropes. Inotropic effects, through the use of dobutamine and milrinone, a β-adrenergic agonist and phosphodiesterase inhibitor, respectively, and newer agents such as levosimendan, act to enhance cardiac contractility. However, it is important to

Agent	Dobutamine	Milrinone	Dopamine			Nitroprusside	Levosimendan
			Dopamine agonist	β-receptor agonist	α-receptor agonist		
Mechanism of Action	β-receptor agonist	PDE III inhibitor				NO donor	Troponin C agonist
Hemodynamic Effects — PCWP	↓	↓	↔	↔	↔	↓↓	↓↓
HR	↑	↑	↔	↑	↑↑	↔↑	↑
CO	↑↑↑	↑↑	↔	↑↑	↑	↑↑	↑↑↑
SVR	↓	↓↓	↔	↑	↑↑↑	↓↓↓	↓↓
mABP	↔↓	↔↓	↔	↑	↑↑	↔	↓
Common Dosage	2.5 µg/kg/min titrate as necesssary up to 20 µg/kg/min	0.22 µg/kg/min titrate up to 0.75 µg/kg/min	2 µg/kg/min and uptitrate to 10 µg for desired effects			0.1 µg/kg/min up-titrate to effect	2 µg/min with up-titration to 10 µg/min for optimum effect
	↑ "Increase"		↔ "No change"		↓ "Decrease"		

Figure 13D.5 *Pharmacology of positive inotropes and nitroprusside. Multiple mechanisms of action may result in improvements in cardiac output. The choice of the 'best' agent is usually dependent on the desired vascular effects.*

reiterate that before using any inotrope, extreme caution should accompany the care of patients with a potentially septic picture or hypovolemia complicating cardiogenic pulmonary edema. In cases where it is suspected and consideration of inotropes is still contemplated, invasive hemodynamic monitoring may be helpful.

Dobutamine

Dobutamine is the classic inotrope, enjoying the benefit of a short half-life (~5 minutes) that allows tight control. Dobutamine acts via β1 and β2 receptors to increase intracellular calcium in cardiomyocytes and enhance inotropic effects. However, activation of β2 receptors on the vascular tree can result in systemic hypotension, especially if the increase in stroke volume/cardiac output is insufficient to compensate for the decrease in systemic vascular resistance. Although at low doses it may provoke rate-independent arrhythmias, at high doses dobutamine can increase heart rate and thus exacerbate myocardial ischemia.

Dobutamine is usually initiated at 2.5 µg/kg per minute intravenously and then up-titrated for desired effects to generally less than 10 µg/kg per minute but may be higher. Titration in patients who do not have a pulmonary catheter can be achieved by monitoring heart rate since the chronotropic effects generally occur at higher doses than the inotropic effects. Extreme caution should be employed with contraindications where tachycardia or arrhythmia may be deleterious, such as with hypertrophic cardiomyopathy, atrial fibrillation, or flutter. Since dobutamine works through β receptors, higher doses may be necessary to overcome the competitive inhibition of β-blocking agents. However, a strategy of using a β-agonist and β-antagonist simultaneously is unlikely to achieve optimal effects of either drug. However, the risks associated with acute β-blocker withdrawal would argue strongly against a strategy of stopping a β-antagonist at the time of initiating this inotrope.

Milrinone

Milrinone inhibits phosphodiesterase, resulting in an increase in intracellular cyclic adeno monophosphate (AMP) and calcium, resulting in its inotropic effect. Although dobutamine may be more effective as a positive inotrope than milrinone, the latter decreases pulmonary capillary wedge pressure more consistently,[112,113] resulting in similar clinical effects. The vasodilation of phosphodiesterase inhibition appears to be due to smooth muscle increases in cyclic AMP.[114] Compared with nitroglycerin in early studies, intravenous milrinone has been shown to be more efficacious at reaching and maintaining desired hemodynamic parameters in patients with advanced heart failure.[115] When vasodilators are ineffective (or contraindicated) the addition of an inotrope is warranted. As noted above, dobutamine is a first choice because of its shorter half-life compared with milrinone. However, milrinone may be more effective with low-output heart failure and pulmonary hypertension, in patients with chronic heart failure in whom β-receptor down-regulation or desensitization has occurred (making them less responsive to dobutamine), and in patients receiving chronic β-receptor blockade.[116] Some have also argued that the use of milrinone and dobutamine in combination may have a greater positive inotropic effect with a greater decrease in the pulmonary capillary wedge pressure compared with treatment by either medication.[117]

However, in the OPTIME (Outcomes of a Prospective Trial of Intravenous Milrinone) study, involving the intravenous infusion of milrinone for 48 hours during hospitalization for stable heart failure in patients requiring diuresis, an increased risk of atrial arrhythmias and hypotension was seen without a benefit of symptomatic dyspnea.[118] Use of milrinone was not associated with a reduction in hospital mortality (3.8 percent for milrinone, 2.3 percent for placebo), 60-day mortality (10.3 percent vs. 8.9 percent), or the combined incidence of death or readmission (35.0 percent vs. 35.3 percent). Both groups showed similar improvements in heart failure scores on study day 3 and at discharge although patients given milrinone reported feeling better on day 30 than those who received placebo. However, inotropic therapy is associated with a high 6-month mortality of about 25 percent and so patients chosen for inotropic therapy must be carefully assessed and followed.[8]

Dopamine, norepinephrine, and vasopressin

In patients with marked systolic hypotension (<90 mm Hg) that does not respond to nitroprusside with or without inotropes, stopping the nitroprusside and initiating dopamine at α-receptor stimulating doses (>10 µg/kg per minute), norepinephrine (Levophed; titrated to effect) and/or vasopressin 1–4 U/h may be helpful. Dopamine is an effective yet complicated inotrope with both adrenergic and dopaminergic effects and hemodynamic effects, depending on the dose. Lower doses (1–5 µg/kg per minute) stimulate mainly dopaminergic receptors that produce renal and mesenteric vasodilation of unknown significance whereas higher doses (3–7 µg/kg per minute) stimulate β receptors and even higher doses 5–10 µg/kg per minute cause peripheral constriction. Due to its inotropic effects, dopamine can cause tachycardia and dysrhythmias. It may also provoke ischemia by increasing the double product (heart rate multiplied by blood pressure). As a vasoconstrictor, it is useful for mixed cardiogenic and vascular shock. Dopamine is usually begun at 5 µg/kg per minute intravenously and increased at 1–2 µg/kg per minute increments every 15 minutes. Contraindications include pheochromocytoma and extreme caution should be used in patients with ventricular fibrillation. One study evaluated the effects of low-dose dopamine on renal function in heart failure patients admitted with volume excess, and, although the addition of dopamine to diuretics was associated with marked improvement in renal function after 5 days, studied patients were not refractory to diuretics.[119] The widespread use of renal dopamine should not be advocated until definitive data can support its safety and efficacy. Norepinephrine and vasopressin both increase afterload, but in conditions where systemic vascular resistance may be lowered (i.e. concomitant sepsis or system inflammation), these vasoconstrictors may be useful to acutely manage a refractory patient until vascular tone returns.

LEVOSIMENDAN

Levosimendan is a new calcium sensitizer that binds to sarcomeric troponin C to enhance myocardial contractility.[120–123] Early studies showed the ability of levosimendan to cause rapid dose-related improvement with significant reductions in pulmonary capillary wedge pressure, improvement in cardiac contractility and the symptoms of dyspnea and fatigue.[124] In one study, in patients admitted with cardiogenic pulmonary edema (intolerant of outpatient β-blockers and without signs of myocardial ischemia) refractory to high-dose dobutamine and diuretics, levosimendan was able to reduce pulmonary capillary wedge pressure at least 25 percent and raise cardiac index at least 40 percent in 39 percent of patients (pigmented = 0.008) treated when dobutamine alone could not. More recently, levosimendan treatment led to better survival over 6 months of follow-up compared with dobutamine.[125]

Right heart catheterization

Pulmonary artery catheterization is performed in 3–5 percent of heart failure hospitalizations and is capable of providing information on wedge, pulmonary artery, right ventricular and central venous pressures, in addition to providing a continuous determination of oxygen saturation.[117] In addition to providing information to help distinguish cardiogenic from non-cardiogenic or complex pulmonary edema, right heart catheterization may be useful in some cases to optimize therapy.

However, observational studies examining the 30-day survival rate with and without the use of a pulmonary artery catheter in patients with multiorgan failure, demonstrated a significant increase in intensive care unit stay, and morbidity and mortality in those with pulmonary artery catheterization, compared with similar individuals who did not have right heart catheterization.[126] Moreover, recent studies of acutely decompensated heart failure patients do not support the routine need for right heart catheterization for the management of pulmonary edema, even if the patient has been placed on mechanical ventilation.

The ESCAPE (Evaluation Study of Congestive Heart Failure and Pulmonary Artery Catheterization Effectiveness) trial is a recently completed randomized, multicenter (26 sites in the United States and Canada) study that evaluated the long-term efficacy of treatment guided by hemodynamic monitoring and clinical assessment (n = 215 patients) versus that guided by clinical assessment alone (n = 218 patients) in hospitalized patients with class IV heart failure (mean age 56 years, mean left ventricular ejection fraction 40 percent, mean creatinine 132.6 µmol/L (1.5 mg/dL) and mean blood pressure 105.6 mm Hg systolic pressure) (results presented at the American Heart Association's Scientific Sessions 2004). Data awaiting publication demonstrated that pulmonary artery catheterization did not impact the composite primary endpoints of time to death, death plus hospitalization, or days hospitalized over 6 months (hazard ratio 1.00). Whether or not therapy was guided by pulmonary artery catheter (PAC)measurements, patients were hospitalized for a median of 11 days. The 30-day mortality was similar in the two groups (4.7 percent for the PAC group and 5.0 percent in the clinical assessment) as was the 6-month mortality (20.9 percent vs. 17.4 percent). Rehospitalization at 6 months was identical (2.1 percent vs. 2.1 percent). Exercise improved in both groups with the PAC group showing slightly greater improvement. Although safe (PAC-associated complications occurred in nine patients randomized to PAC and one patient randomized to clinical assessment alone [P = 0.01], with no PAC-related deaths occurring), it is reasonable to conclude preliminarily that catheterization for cardiogenic pulmonary edema should not be performed routinely. Individualization of care should be considered for patients with persistent symptoms of heart failure or those with cardiogenic shock with pulmonary edema and concomitant renal dysfunction when the need to optimize medical therapy using inotropes and vasopressor therapy might be more pressing. Results not yet available include secondary endpoints of BNP levels, heart remodeling, resource use, distance walked in 6 minutes, and survival adjusted for patient preferences.

In addition to 'hard endpoints', the ESCAPE trial also offered a glimpse into patient wishes with the question 'If you had 24 months to live in your current state of health, how many months would you trade to feel better?'. At the beginning, the average patient was willing to trade 9 months away. By the trial's end, patients who had been managed with the PAC asked for 6 months more time in their current state of health than before treatment, compared with only 1.5 months of improvement in the clinical assessment group.

Mechanical devices

Cardiogenic shock occurs when a severe reduction in cardiac output is not compensated for by an adequate increase in peripheral vascular resistance after optimization of filling pressures. Therefore when the addition of inotropic support and vasoconstrictors is inadequate, cardiogenic shock requires consideration of intraaortic balloon pump counterpulsation, immediate revascularization, and mechanical ventricular support device implantation.

The intraaortic balloon pump can increasing mean diastolic and decrease peak systolic pressures resulting in decreased left ventricular end-diastolic pressure, increased stroke volume, and an increased cardiac output. In addition, it improves coronary blood flow and myocardial perfusion, increases collateral coronary blood flow, improves subendocardial oxygenation, and decreases myocardial oxygen consumption. Intraaortic balloon pumps are most often used for patients in cardiogenic shock after acute myocardial infarction or in those who have developed

sudden and severe mitral insufficiency.[127] It is contra-indicated in the presence of significant aortic regurgitation.

In patients with cardiogenic shock/pulmonary edema unresponsive to intraaortic balloon counterpulsation and intravenous inotropes, mechanical circulatory support with a left ventricular or biventricular support device should be considered in those who are appropriate transplant candidates or in whom myocardial recovery is deemed likely.[128] The only left ventricular assist device (LVAD) currently approved as an alternative to transplant and the first to be approved as a bridge consists of an inflow cannula to the apex of the left ventricle and an outflow cannula to the aorta. Complications following LVAD implantation are common and involve infection, stroke, coagulopathy, and bleeding.[129] However, in parallel to the significant risk, LVAD placement increases the likelihood that patients will survive to reach transplantation and yields significantly prolonged life in those patients who undergo implantation as an alternative to transplant.[129]

Miscellaneous

- When vasodilators or diuretics are unavailable, alternating tourniquets and phlebotomy (500 mL) may provide a respite to decrease preload. If these measures are not enough, tourniquets may be used in the limbs (three at a time for 15–20 minutes) if there is no arterial obstructions. With the potency of available pharmacologic and mechanical therapies, this strategy is rarely required.
- Oral or intravenous angiotensin converting enzyme (ACE) inhibitors (i.e. intravenous enalapril 1 mg over 2 hours) have been studied as a rapid means to reduce afterload in acute pulmonary edema.[130–132] Although promising, adequately powered randomized controlled trials are required and caution is advised. When the strategy of intravenous ACE inhibition with enalapril was tested as therapy for acute myocardial infarction, the only trends apparent suggested the possibility of increased risk.[133]
- Acutely decompensated patients should not be routinely given β-blockers unless supraventricular tachycardia is present until euvolemia is reached. However, maintenance of patients already on β-blockers on their present dose (or half their present dose) is reasonable unless profound cardiogenic shock is present.
- Even with significant left ventricular dysfunction, a revascularization procedure or correction of underlying structural cardiac pathology may stabilize or reverse significant left ventricular dysfunction.[134] In patients with chronic coronary disease and ventricular dysfunction, the safety and efficacy will be determined by the ongoing STICH (Surgical Treatment for Ischemic Heart Failure) trial.

Key learning points

- Cardiogenic pulmonary edema most often results from increases in pulmonary capillary hydrostatic pressures that may be clinically modified by increases in alveolar capillary permeability although decreased plasma oncotic pressure and reduced lymphatic clearance can play an additive role.

- Acute cardiogenic pulmonary edema may be associated with chest pain, palpitations, and a suffocating feeling ('air hunger').

- When pulmonary edema is the result of a chronic process, the patient generally describes a progression from dyspnea on exertion to paroxysmal nocturnal dyspnea and orthopnea, culminating in dyspnea at rest and cough.

- BNP levels assist with the triage of patients to cardiogenic or noncardiogenic causes of dyspnea. However, it is important to ascertain the baseline BNP level in a patient with renal dysfunction to differentiate how much of the elevation is from left ventricular dysfunction and how much is from not clearing BNP.

- Worsening of serum creatinine levels by as little as 8.8 µmol/L (0.1 mg/dL) in patients hospitalized for acutely decompensated heart failure is predictive of increased risk.

- Chest radiography is useful in cardiogenic pulmonary edema during staging and to determine underlying etiologies.

- Echocardiography is critical for the effective evaluation of acute cardiogenic pulmonary edema. In addition to determining the presence and severity of acute or chronic valvular diseases, echocardiography is also important in establishing whether the cardiomyopathy is systolic or diastolic in nature.

- Patients with pulmonary edema require expeditious assessment of the degree of respiratory and hemodynamic instability.

- Noninvasive continuous positive airway pressure, where a single airway pressure is present throughout the respiratory phases, may promote early clinical stabilization and thereby permit introduction of more definitive therapy to reverse the problem without resorting to intubation.

- Once ventilatory control has been established, hemodynamic stability must be ensured.

- The goal of pharmacotherapy is to optimize stroke volume while reducing pulmonary capillary wedge pressure.

- Diuretics are a critical part of therapy for acute cardiogenic pulmonary edema. The primary goal is the reduction in pulmonary capillary wedge pressure with attendant increases in stroke volume, and diuretics act rapidly.

- Patients with cardiogenic pulmonary edema, who prove refractory to diuretic therapy despite adequate renal perfusion enhanced by vasodilators and/or inotropes may require dialysis.

- Before using any inotrope, extreme caution should accompany the care of patients with a potentially septic picture or hypovolemia complicating cardiogenic pulmonary edema.

ACKNOWLEDGMENT

The authors gratefully acknowledge the expert work of Elizabeth Maas in the production of all figures in this chapter and her careful editing.

REFERENCES

1. Katz A. *Heart Failure.* Philadelphia: Lippincott, Williams & Wilkins, 2000: 381.

2. Davis NSJ. *Diseases of the Lungs, Heart, and Kidneys,* 1st ed. London: The FA Davis Company, 1894: 359.

3. Levy D, Kenchaiah S, Larson MG, *et al.* Long-term trends in the incidence of and survival with heart failure. *N Engl J Med* 2002; **347**: 1397–402.

4. Senni M, Tribouilloy CM, Rodeheffer RJ, *et al.* Congestive heart failure in the community: trends in incidence and survival in a 10-year period. *Arch Intern Med* 1999; **159**: 29–34.

5. Hunt SA, *et al.* ACC/AHA guidelines for the evaluation and management of chronic heart failure in the adult: executive summary. *J Heart Lung Transplant* 2002; **21**: 189–203.

6. Ofili EO, Mayberry R, Alema-Mensah E, *et al.* Gender differences and practice implications of risk factors for frequent hospitalization for heart failure in an urban center serving predominantly African-American patients. *Am J Cardiol* 1999; **83**: 1350–5.

7. Publication Committee for the VMAC Investigators (Vasodilatation in the Management of Acute CHF). Intravenous nesiritide vs nitroglycerin for treatment of decompensated congestive heart failure: a randomized controlled trial. *JAMA* 2002; **287**: 1531–40.

8. Burger AJ, Horton DP, LeJemtel T, *et al.* Effect of nesiritide (B-type natriuretic peptide) and dobutamine on ventricular arrhythmias in the treatment of patients with acutely decompensated congestive heart failure: the PRECEDENT study. *Am Heart J* 2002; **144**: 1102–8.

9. Brophy JM, Deslauriers G, Boucher B, Rouleau JL. The hospital course and short term prognosis of patients presenting to the emergency room with decompensated congestive heart failure. *Can J Cardiol* 1993; **9**: 219–24.

10. Vinson JM, Rich MW, Sperry JC, *et al.* Early readmission of elderly patients with congestive heart failure. *J Am Geriatr Soc* 1990; **38**: 1290–5.

11. Starling E. On the absorption of fluids from the connective tissue spaces. *J Physiol* 1896; **19**: 312–26.

12. Allen SJ, Drake RE, Laine GA, Gabel JC. Effect of thoracic duct drainage on hydrostatic pulmonary edema and pleural effusion in sheep. *J Appl Physiol* 1991; **71**: 314–16.

13. Staub NC. Pulmonary edema. *Physiol Rev* 1974; **54**: 678–811.

14. Bachofen H, Schurch S, Weibel ER. Experimental hydrostatic pulmonary edema in rabbit lungs. Barrier lesions. *Am Rev Respir Dis* 1993; **147**: 997–1004.

15. Costello ML, Mathieu-Costello O, West JB. Stress failure of alveolar epithelial cells studied by scanning electron microscopy. *Am Rev Respir Dis* 1992; **145**: 1446–55.

16. Matthay MA, Folkesson HG, Clerici C. Lung epithelial fluid transport and the resolution of pulmonary edema. *Physiol Rev* 2002; **82**: 569–600.

17. Borok Z, Liebler JM, Lubman RL, *et al.* Na transport proteins are expressed by rat alveolar epithelial type I cells. *Am J Physiol Lung Cell Mol Physiol* 2002; **282**: L599–608.

18. Dobbs LG, Gonzalez R, Matthay MA, *et al.* Highly water-permeable type I alveolar epithelial cells confer high water permeability between the airspace and vasculature in rat lung. *Proc Natl Acad Sci USA* 1998; **95**: 2991–6.

19. Van Scott MR, Davis CW, Boucher RC. Na$^+$ and Cl$^-$ transport across rabbit nonciliated bronchiolar epithelial (Clara) cells. *Am J Physiol* 1989; **256**(4 Pt 1): C893–901.

20. Fang X, Fukuda N, Barbry P, *et al.* Novel role for CFTR in fluid absorption from the distal airspaces of the lung. *J Gen Physiol* 2002; **119**: 199–207.

21. Jiang X, Ingbar DH, O'Grady SM. Adrenergic regulation of ion transport across adult alveolar epithelial cells: effects on Cl$^-$ channel activation and transport function in cultures with an apical air interface. *J Membr Biol* 2001; **181**: 195–204.

22. Reddy MM, Light MJ, Quinton PM. Activation of the epithelial Na$^+$ channel (ENaC) requires CFTR Cl$^-$ channel function. *Nature* 1999; **402**: 301–4.

23. Olivera WG, *et al.* Aldosterone regulates Na,K-ATPase and increases lung edema clearance in rats. *Am J Respir Crit Care Med* 2000; **161**(2 Pt 1): 567–73.

24. Jain L, Chen XJ, Ramosevac S, *et al.* Expression of highly selective sodium channels in alveolar type II cells is determined by culture conditions. *Am J Physiol Lung Cell Mol Physiol* 2001; **280**: L646–58.

25. Sznajder JI, Ridge KM, Yeates DB, *et al.* Epidermal growth factor increases lung liquid clearance in rat lungs. *J Appl Physiol* 1998; **85**: 1004–10.

26. Borok Z, Hami A, Danto SI, *et al.* Effects of EGF on alveolar epithelial junctional permeability and active sodium transport. *Am J Physiol* 1996; **270**(4 Pt 1): L559–65.

27. Folkesson HG, Pittet JF, Nitenberg G, Matthay MA. Transforming growth factor-alpha increases alveolar liquid clearance in anesthetized ventilated rats. *Am J Physiol* 1996; **271**(2 Pt 1): L236–44.

28. Wang Y, Folkesson HG, Jayr C, *et al.* Alveolar epithelial fluid transport can be simultaneously upregulated by both KGF and beta-agonist therapy. *J Appl Physiol* 1999; **87**: 1852–60.

29. Guery BP, Mason CM, Dobard EP, *et al.* Keratinocyte growth factor increases transalveolar sodium reabsorption in normal and injured rat lungs. *Am J Respir Crit Care Med* 1997; **155**: 1777–84.

30. Borok Z, Danto SI, Dimen LL, *et al.* Na$^+$-K$^+$-ATPase expression in alveolar epithelial cells: upregulation of active ion transport by KGF. *Am J Physiol* 1998; **274**(1 Pt 1): L149–58.

31. Sakuma T, Okaniwa G, Nakada T, *et al.* Alveolar fluid clearance in the resected human lung. *Am J Respir Crit Care Med* 1994; **150**: 305–10.

32. Norlin A, Finley N, Abedinpour P, Folkesson HG, *et al.* Alveolar liquid clearance in the anesthetized ventilated guinea pig. *Am J Physiol* 1998; **274**(2 Pt 1): L235–43.

33. Olivera W, Ridge K, Wood LD, Sznajder JI. ANF decreases active sodium transport and increases alveolar epithelial permeability in rats. *J Appl Physiol* 1993; **75**: 1581–6.

34. Guo Y, DuVall MD, Crow JP, Matalon S. Nitric oxide inhibits Na$^+$ absorption across cultured alveolar type II monolayers. *Am J Physiol* 1998; **274**(3 Pt 1): L369–77.

35. Mutlu GM, Sznajder JI. [beta]2-agonists for treatment of pulmonary edema: Ready for clinical studies? *Crit Care Med* 2004; **32**: 1607–8.

36. Gandhi S, *et al.* The pathogenesis of acute pulmonary edema associated with hypertension. *N Engl J Med* 2001; **344**: 17–22.

37. Kitzman DW. Diastolic heart failure in the elderly. *Heart Fail Rev* 2002; **7**: 17–27.

38. Agostoni P, Cattadori G, Bianchi M, Wasserman K. Exercise-induced pulmonary edema in heart failure. *Circulation* 2003; **108**: 2666–71.

39. Otsuji Y, Handschumacher MD, Schwammenthal E, Jiang L, *et al.* Insights from three-dimensional echocardiography into the mechanism of functional mitral regurgitation: direct in vivo demonstration of altered leaflet tethering geometry. *Circulation* 1997; **96**: 1999–2008.

40. Pierard LA, Lancellotti P. The role of ischemic mitral regurgitation in the pathogenesis of acute pulmonary edema. *N Engl J Med* 2004; **351**: 1627–34.

41. Arques S, Ambrosi P, Gelisse R, *et al.* Hypoalbuminemia in elderly patients with acute diastolic heart failure. *J Am Coll Cardiol* 2003; **42**: 712–16.

42. Marantz PR, Kaplan MC, Alderman MH. Clinical diagnosis of congestive heart failure in patients with acute dyspnea. *Chest* 1990; **97**: 776–81.

43. Peacock, WFT. The B-type natriuretic peptide assay: a rapid test for heart failure. Cleve *Clin J Med* 2002; **69**: 243–51.

44. Stevenson LW, Perloff JK. The limited reliability of physical signs for estimating hemodynamics in chronic heart failure. *JAMA* 1989; **261**: 884–8.

45. Nohria A, Lewis E, Stevenson LW. Medical management of advanced heart failure. *JAMA* 2002; **287**: 628–40.

46. Uhley HN, Leeds SE, Sampson JJ, Friedman M. Role of pulmonary lymphatics in chronic pulmonary edema. *Circ Res* 1962; **11**: 966–70.

47. Kay JM, Edwards FR. Ultrastructure of the alveolar-capillary wall in mitral stenosis. *J Pathol* 1973; **111**: 239–45.

48. Heard BE, Steiner RE, Herdan A, Gleason D. Oedema and fibrosis of the lungs in left ventricular failure. *Br J Radiol* 1968; **41**: 161–71.

49. Androne AS, Hryniewicz K, Hudaihed A, *et al.* Relation of unrecognized hypervolemia in chronic heart failure to clinical status, hemodynamics, and patient outcomes. *Am J Cardiol* 2004; **93**: 1254–9.

50. Maisel AS, Krishnaswamy P, Nowak RM, *et al.* Rapid measurement of B-type natriuretic peptide in the emergency diagnosis of heart failure. *N Engl J Med* 2002; **347**: 161–7.

51. McCullough PA, *et al.* B-type natriuretic peptide and renal function in the diagnosis of heart failure: an analysis from the Breathing Not Properly Multinational Study. *Am J Kidney Dis* 2003; **41**: 571–9.

52. Troughton RW, Frampton CM, Yandle TG, *et al.* Treatment of heart failure guided by plasma aminoterminal brain natriuretic peptide (N-BNP) concentrations. *Lancet* 2000; **355**: 1126–30.

53. Cheng V, Kazanagra R, Garcia A, *et al.* A rapid bedside test for B-type peptide predicts treatment outcomes in patients admitted for decompensated heart failure: a pilot study. *J Am Coll Cardiol* 2001; **37**: 386–91.

54. Wang TJ, *et al.* Plasma natriuretic peptide levels and the risk of cardiovascular events and death. *N Engl J Med* 2004; **350**: 655–63.

55. De Pasquale CG, Arnolda LF, Doyle IR, *et al.* Plasma surfactant protein-B: a novel biomarker in chronic heart failure. *Circulation* 2004; **110**: 1091–6.

56. De Pasquale CG, Arnolda LF, Doyle IR, *et al.* Prolonged alveolocapillary barrier damage after acute cardiogenic pulmonary edema. *Crit Care Med* 2003; **31**: 1060–7.

57. Hermans C, Bernard A. Lung epithelium-specific proteins: characteristics and potential applications as markers. *Am J Respir Crit Care Med* 1999; **159**: 646–78.

58. Doyle IR, Nicholas TE, Bersten AD. Partitioning lung and plasma proteins: circulating surfactant proteins as biomarkers of alveolocapillary permeability. *Clin Exp Pharmacol Physiol* 1999; **26**: 185–97.

59. Hillege HL, Girbes AR, de Kam PJ, *et al.* Renal function, neurohormonal activation, and survival in patients with chronic heart failure. *Circulation* 2000; **102**: 203–10.

60. Al-Ahmad A, Rand WM, Manjunath G, *et al.* Reduced kidney function and anemia as risk factors for mortality in patients with left ventricular dysfunction. *J Am Coll Cardiol* 2001; **38**: 955–62.

61. McAlister FA, *et al.* Renal insufficiency and heart failure: prognostic and therapeutic implications from a prospective cohort study. *Circulation* 2004; **109**: 1004–9.

62. Mahon NG, Blackstone EH, Francis GS, *et al.* The prognostic value of estimated creatinine clearance alongside functional capacity in ambulatory patients with chronic congestive heart failure. *J Am Coll Cardiol* 2002; **40**: 1106–13.

63. Dries DL, Exner DV, Domanski MJ, *et al.* The prognostic implications of renal insufficiency in asymptomatic and symptomatic patients with left ventricular systolic dysfunction. *J Am Coll Cardiol* 2000; **35**: 681–9.

64. Krumholz HM, Chen YT, Vaccarino V, *et al.* Correlates and impact on outcomes of worsening renal function in patients > or = 65 years of age with heart failure. *Am J Cardiol* 2000; **85**: 1110–13.

65. Butler J, Forman DE, Abraham WT, *et al.* Relationship between heart failure treatment and development of worsening renal function among hospitalized patients. *Am Heart J* 2004; **147**: 331–8.

66. Smith GL, Vaccarino V, Kosiborod M, *et al.* Worsening renal function: what is a clinically meaningful change in creatinine during hospitalization with heart failure? *J Card Fail* 2003; **9**: 13–25.

67. Gottlieb SS, Abraham W, Butler J, *et al.* The prognostic importance of different definitions of worsening renal function in congestive heart failure. *J Card Fail* 2002; **8**: 136–41.

68. Milne EN, Pistolesi M, Miniati M, Giuntini C. The radiologic distinction of cardiogenic and noncardiogenic edema. *AJR Am J Roentgenol* 1985; **144**: 879–94.

69. Miniati M, Pistolesi M, Paoletti P, *et al.* Objective radiographic criteria to differentiate cardiac, renal, and injury lung edema. *Invest Radiol* 1988; **23**: 433–40.

70. Chakko SC, Caldwell SH, Sforza PP. Treatment of congestive heart failure. Its effect on pleural fluid chemistry. *Chest* 1989; **95**: 798–802.

71. Burgess LJ, Maritz FJ, Taljaard JJ. Comparative analysis of the biochemical parameters used to distinguish between pleural transudates and exudates. *Chest* 1995; **107**: 1604–9.

72. Rasanen J, Heikkila J, Downs J, *et al.* Continuous positive airway pressure by face mask in acute cardiogenic pulmonary edema. *Am J Cardiol* 1985; **55**: 296–300.

73. Lin M, Yang YF, Chiang HT, *et al.* Reappraisal of continuous positive airway pressure therapy in acute cardiogenic pulmonary edema. Short-term results and long-term follow-up. *Chest* 1995; **107**: 1379–86.

74. Lin M, Chiang HT. The efficacy of early continuous positive airway pressure therapy in patients with acute cardiogenic pulmonary edema. *J Formos Med Assoc* 1991; **90**: 736–43.

75. Bersten AD, Holt AW, Vedig AE, *et al.* Treatment of severe cardiogenic pulmonary edema with continuous positive airway pressure delivered by face mask. *N Engl J Med* 1991; **325**: 1825–30.

76. Yan AT, Bradley TD, Liu PP. The role of continuous positive airway pressure in the treatment of congestive heart failure. *Chest* 2001; **120**: 1675–85.

77. Giacomini M, Iapichino G, Cigada M, *et al.* Short-term noninvasive pressure support ventilation prevents ICU admittance in patients with acute cardiogenic pulmonary edema. *Chest* 2003; **123**: 2057–61.

78. Nava S, Carbone G, DiBattista N, *et al.* Noninvasive ventilation in cardiogenic pulmonary edema: a multicenter randomized trial. *Am J Respir Crit Care Med* 2003; **168**: 1432–7.

79. L'Her E, Duquesne F, Girou E, *et al.* Noninvasive continuous positive airway pressure in elderly cardiogenic pulmonary edema patients. *Intensive Care Med* 2004; **30**: 882–8.

80. Masip J, *et al.* Risk factors for intubation as a guide for noninvasive ventilation in patients with severe acute cardiogenic pulmonary edema. *Intensive Care Med* 2003; **29**: 1921–8.

81. Pang D, Keenan SP, Cook DJ, Sibbald WJ. The effect of positive pressure airway support on mortality and the need for intubation in cardiogenic pulmonary edema: a systematic review. *Chest* 1998; **114**: 1185–92.

82. Mehta S, Jay GD, Woolard RH, *et al.* Randomized, prospective trial of bilevel versus continuous positive airway pressure in acute pulmonary edema. *Crit Care Med* 1997; **25**: 620–8.

83. Levitt MA. A prospective, randomized trial of BiPAP in severe acute congestive heart failure. *J Emerg Med* 2001; **21**: 363–9.

84. Masip J, Betbese AJ, Paez J, *et al.* Non-invasive pressure support ventilation versus conventional oxygen therapy in acute cardiogenic pulmonary oedema: a randomised trial. *Lancet* 2000; **356**: 2126–32.

85. Fedullo AJ, Swinburne AJ, Wahl GW, Bixby K. Acute cardiogenic pulmonary edema treated with mechanical ventilation. Factors determining in-hospital mortality. *Chest* 1991; **99**: 1220–6.

86. Nohria A, Tsang SW, Fang JC, *et al.* Clinical assessment identifies hemodynamic profiles that predict outcomes in patients admitted with heart failure. *J Am Coll Cardiol* 2003; **41**: 1797–804.

87. Brater DC. Diuretic therapy. *N Engl J Med* 1998; **339**: 387–95.

88. Dikshit K, Vyden JK, Forrester JS, *et al.* Renal and extrarenal hemodynamic effects of furosemide in congestive heart failure after acute myocardial infarction. *N Engl J Med* 1973; **288**: 1087–90.

89. Cody RJ. Clinical trials of diuretic therapy in heart failure: research directions and clinical considerations. *J Am Coll Cardiol* 1993; **22**(4 Suppl A): 165A–171A.

90. Kiyingi A, Field MJ, Pawsey CC, *et al.* Metolazone in treatment of severe refractory congestive cardiac failure. *Lancet* 1990; **335**: 29–31.

91. Channer KS, McLean KA, Lawson-Matthew P, Richardson M, *et al.* Combination diuretic treatment in severe heart failure: a randomised controlled trial. *Br Heart J* 1994; **71**: 146–50.

92. Dormans TP, Gerlag PG. Combination of high-dose furosemide and hydrochlorothiazide in the treatment of refractory congestive heart failure. *Eur Heart J* 1996; **17**: 1867–74.

93. Vasko MR, Cartwright DB, Knochel JP, *et al.* Furosemide absorption altered in decompensated congestive heart failure. *Ann Intern Med* 1985; **102**: 314–18.

94. Dormans TP, van Meyel JJ, Gerlag PG, *et al.* Diuretic efficacy of high dose furosemide in severe heart failure: bolus injection versus continuous infusion. *J Am Coll Cardiol* 1996; **28**: 376–82.

95. van Meyel JJ, Smits P, Dormans T, *et al.* Continuous infusion of furosemide in the treatment of patients with congestive heart failure and diuretic resistance. *J Intern Med* 1994; **235**: 329–34.

96. Cotter G, Weissgarten J, Metzkor E, *et al.* Increased toxicity of high-dose furosemide versus low-dose dopamine in the treatment of refractory congestive heart failure. *Clin Pharmacol Ther* 1997; **62**: 187–93.

97. Sackner-Bernstein JD, Obeleniene R. How should diuretic-refractory, volume-overloaded heart failure patients be managed? *J Invasive Cardiol* 2003; **15**: 585–90.

98. Jaski BE, Ha J, Denys BG, *et al.* Peripherally inserted veno-venous ultrafiltration for rapid treatment of volume overloaded patients. *J Card Fail* 2003; **9**: 227–31.

99. Hoffman JR, Reynolds S. Comparison of nitroglycerin, morphine and furosemide in treatment of presumed pre-hospital pulmonary edema. *Chest* 1987; **92**: 586–93.

100. Sacchetti A, *et al.* Effect of ED management on ICU use in acute pulmonary edema. *Am J Emerg Med* 1999; **17**: 571–4.

101. Vasko JS, Henney RP, Oldham HN, *et al.* Mechanisms of action of morphine in the treatment of experimental pulmonary edema. *Am J Cardiol* 1966; **18**: 876–83.

102. Vismara LA, Leaman DM, Zelis R. The effects of morphine on venous tone in patients with acute pulmonary edema. *Circulation* 1976; **54**: 335–7.

103. Beltrame JF, Zeitz CJ, Unger SA, *et al.* Nitrate therapy is an alternative to furosemide/morphine therapy in the management of acute cardiogenic pulmonary edema. *J Card Fail* 1998; **4**: 271–9.

104. Cotter G, Metzkor E, Kaluski E, *et al.* Randomised trial of high-dose isosorbide dinitrate plus low-dose furosemide versus high-dose furosemide plus low-dose isosorbide dinitrate in severe pulmonary oedema. *Lancet* 1998; **351**: 389–93.

105. Nelson GI, Silke B, Ahuja RC, *et al.* Haemodynamic advantages of isosorbide dinitrate over frusemide in acute heart-failure following myocardial infarction. *Lancet* 1983; **1**: 730–3.

106. Brindis RG, Kloner RA. Sildenafil in patients with cardiovascular disease. *Am J Cardiol* 2003; **92**(9A): 26M–36M.

107. Colucci WS, *et al.* Intravenous nesiritide, a natriuretic peptide, in the treatment of decompensated congestive heart failure. Nesiritide Study Group. *N Engl J Med* 2000; **343**: 246–53.

108. Wang DJ, *et al.* Nesiritide does not improve renal function in patients with chronic heart failure and worsening serum creatinine. *Circulation* 2004; **110**: 1620–5.

109. Butler J, Emerman C, Peacock WF, *et al.* The efficacy and safety of B-type natriuretic peptide (nesiritide) in patients with renal insufficiency and acutely decompensated congestive heart failure. *Nephrol Dial Transplant* 2004; **19**: 391–9.

110. Stevenson LW, *et al.* Importance of hemodynamic response to therapy in predicting survival with ejection fraction less than or equal to 20% secondary to ischemic or nonischemic dilated cardiomyopathy. *Am J Cardiol* 1990; **66**: 1348–54.

111. Khot UN, Novaro GM, Popovic ZB, *et al.* Nitroprusside in critically ill patients with left ventricular dysfunction and aortic stenosis. *N Engl J Med* 2003; **348**: 1756–63.

112. Colucci WS, Wright RF, Jaski BE, *et al.* Milrinone and dobutamine in severe heart failure: differing hemodynamic effects and individual patient responsiveness. *Circulation* 1986; **73**(3 Pt 2): III175–83.

113. Monrad ES, Baim DS, Smith HS, Lanoue AS. Milrinone, dobutamine, and nitroprusside: comparative effects on hemodynamics and myocardial energetics in patients with severe congestive heart failure. *Circulation* 1986; **73**(3 Pt 2): III168–74.

114. Karlsberg RP, *et al.* Comparative efficacy of short-term intravenous infusions of milrinone and

dobutamine in acute congestive heart failure following acute myocardial infarction. Milrinone-Dobutamine Study Group. *Clin Cardiol* 1996; **19**: 21–30.

115. Loh E, Elkayam U, Cody R, *et al.* A randomized multicenter study comparing the efficacy and safety of intravenous milrinone and intravenous nitroglycerin in patients with advanced heart failure. *J Card Fail* 2001; **7**: 114–21.

116. Lowes BD, Tsvetkova T, Eichhorn EJ, *et al.* Milrinone versus dobutamine in heart failure subjects treated chronically with carvedilol. *Int J Cardiol* 2001; **81**(2–3): 141–9.

117. Sharkey SW. Beyond the wedge: clinical physiology and the Swan-Ganz catheter. *Am J Med* 1987; **83**: 111–22.

118. Cuffe MS, Califf RM, Adams KF Jr, *et al.* Outcomes of a Prospective Trial of Intravenous Milrinone for Exacerbations of Chronic Heart Failure (OPTIME-CHF) Investigators. Short-term intravenous milrinone for acute exacerbation of chronic heart failure: a randomized controlled trial. *JAMA* 2002; **287**: 1541–7.

119. Varriale P, Mossavi A. The benefit of low-dose dopamine during vigorous diuresis for congestive heart failure associated with renal insufficiency: does it protect renal function? *Clin Cardiol* 1997; **20**: 627–30.

120. Edes I, Kiss E, Kitada Y, *et al.* Effects of Levosimendan, a cardiotonic agent targeted to troponin C, on cardiac function and on phosphorylation and Ca^{2+} sensitivity of cardiac myofibrils and sarcoplasmic reticulum in guinea pig heart. *Circ Res* 1995; **77**: 107–13.

121. Pollesello P, Ovaska M, Kaivola J, *et al.* Binding of a new Ca^{2+} sensitizer, levosimendan, to recombinant human cardiac troponin C. A molecular modelling, fluorescence probe, and proton nuclear magnetic resonance study. *J Biol Chem* 1994; **269**: 28584–90.

122. Haikala H, *et al.* Cardiac troponin C as a target protein for a novel calcium sensitizing drug, levosimendan. *J Mol Cell Cardiol* 1995; **27**: 1859–66.

123. Levijoki J, Pollesello P, Kaivola J, *et al.* Further evidence for the cardiac troponin C mediated calcium sensitization by levosimendan: structure-response and binding analysis with analogs of levosimendan. *J Mol Cell Cardiol* 2000; **32**: 479–91.

124. Slawsky MT, Colucci WS, Gottlieb SS, *et al.* Acute hemodynamic and clinical effects of levosimendan in patients with severe heart failure. Study Investigators. *Circulation* 2000; **102**: 2222–7.

125. Follath F, Cleland JG, Just H, *et al.* Efficacy and safety of intravenous levosimendan compared with dobutamine in severe low-output heart failure (the LIDO study): a randomised double-blind trial. *Lancet* 2002; **360**: 196–202.

126. Connors AF, Jr, Speroff T, Dawson NV, *et al.* The effectiveness of right heart catheterization in the initial care of critically ill patients. SUPPORT Investigators. *JAMA* 1996; **276**: 889–97.

127. Sanborn TA, Feldman T. Management strategies for cardiogenic shock. *Curr Opin Cardiol* 2004; **19**: 608–12.

128. Deng MC, Young JB, Stevenson LW, *et al.* Board of Directors of the International Society for Heart and Lung Transplantation. Destination mechanical circulatory support: proposal for clinical standards. *J Heart Lung Transplant* 2003; **22**: 365–9.

129. Rose EA, Gelijns AC, Moskowitz AJ, *et al.* Randomized Evaluation of Mechanical Assistance for the Treatment of Congestive Heart Failure (REMATCH) Study Group. Long-term mechanical left ventricular assistance for end-stage heart failure. *N Engl J Med* 2001; **345**: 1435–43.

130. Adigun AQ, Ajayi OE, Sofowora GG, Ajayi AA. Vasodilator therapy of hypertensive acute left ventricular failure: comparison of captopril-prazosin with hydralazine-isosorbide dinitrate. *Int J Cardiol* 1998; **67**: 81–6.

131. Annane D, Bellissant E, Pussard E, *et al.* Placebo-controlled, randomized, double-blind study of intravenous enalaprilat efficacy and safety in acute cardiogenic pulmonary edema. *Circulation* 1996; **94**: 1316–24.

132. Hamilton RJ, Carter WA, Gallagher EJ. Rapid improvement of acute pulmonary edema with sublingual captopril. *Acad Emerg Med* 1996; **3**: 205–12.

133. Swedberg K, Held P, Kjekshus J, *et al.* Effects of the early administration of enalapril on mortality in patients with acute myocardial infarction. Results of the Cooperative New Scandinavian Enalapril Survival Study II (CONSENSUS II). *N Engl J Med* 1992; **327**: 678–84.

134. Castro PF, Bourge RC, Foster RE. Evaluation of hibernating myocardium in patients with ischemic heart disease. *Am J Med* 1998; **104**: 69–77.

Pulmonary hypertension and acute right heart failure

SHOAIB ALAM, HAROLD I PALEVSKY

INTRODUCTION

Pulmonary hypertension (PH) and acute right heart failure are relatively frequently encountered, but are less commonly recognized clinical entities for most clinicians. Hence the first few pages of this chapter are dedicated to a brief introduction of PH in general, with a relevant account of the disease and its management in non-acute setting. Knowledge of this basic background is important to clearly understand the disease process in the acute care setting. The primary difference between acute and non-acute care settings is that in the non-acute setting the main stress is on establishing the diagnosis of PH and, whenever possible, determining its etiology. Once the diagnosis has been established, instituting the right therapy is relatively straightforward. On the other hand, in the acute care setting PH may not always be the primary focus of management especially if other acute issues warrant immediate attention. In the absence of overt right heart failure (RHF) manifested by profound hypotension, life-threatening hypoxemia or signs of shock, mild to moderate PH may not need to be addressed while the patient is hospitalized for an unrelated acute issue.

PULMONARY HYPERTENSION: BASIC CONCEPTS

The resistance of the normal pulmonary circulation is one-eighth of the total peripheral vascular resistance. Cardiac output being equal for both left and right sides of heart, the pressure difference between the pulmonary artery (PA) and left atrium is also about one-eighth of the pressure difference between the systemic blood pressure and the right atrium (normally a pressure drop of 5–10 mm Hg between the PA and left atrium is enough to bring about the pulmonary blood flow). Cardiac output in young men at rest is about 5.5 L/min. In a trained individual it can be as high as 40 L/min during exercise. Despite this seven- to eightfold increase in cardiac output, in normal individuals the mean PA pressures do not go more than 20 mm Hg above the normal resting baseline of 14–18 mm Hg (Table 13E.1).[1] This is because of the ability of the pulmonary circulation to accommodate increased blood flow by recruiting blood vessels that are not perfused during normal resting circumstances and by distension of the vascular bed. This is virtually analogous to the addition of parallel resistances to an electric circuit, which results in decrease of overall impedance of the circuit. Moreover, the endothelial cells lining the pulmonary blood vessels play an important role in dynamic control of overall pulmonary vascular resistance (PVR). In certain pathologic situations the mechanisms that effectively decrease the PVR in response to increased cardiac output fail. This results in an abnormal increase of pulmonary arterial pressure with exercise or in states such as severe critical illness in which cardiac output is increased due to high metabolic demand. An abnormal increase in PA pressure with increased physical activity may be the first sign of pulmonary vascular disease. Later, as the PVR increases, even resting cardiac output results in elevated PA pressures (Table 13E.2).[1]

Work performed by the ventricles to pump out the blood is equal to the product of blood volume pumped and the pressure against which this volume is pumped out of the

Table 13E.1 *Normal hemodynamics values at rest and with exercise*

Hemodynamic parameters	At rest	With moderate exercise
Cardiac output (L/min)	6	16
Heart rate (beats/min)	80	130
Right atrial pressure (mm Hg)	4–6	6–8
Pulmonary arterial pressures (mm Hg)		
Systolic	20–25	30–35
Diastolic	10–12	11–14
Mean	14–18	20–25
Pulmonary wedge pressure (mm Hg)	6–10	10–14
Systemic arterial pressure (mm Hg)	120/80	150/95
Mean	90–100	110–120
Pulmonary vascular resistance (Wood's units)	0.7–1.0	0.6–0.9

From references 1, 2.

Table 13E.2 *Definition of pulmonary hypertension*

Hemodynamic parameters	At rest	With moderate exercise
Mean PAP	Above 25 mm Hg*	Above 30 mm Hg
Increase in mean PAP	–	More than
compared with resting value		20 mm Hg rise

The values are from right heart catheterization and not echocardiogram. Pulmonary capillary wedge pressure should be below 15 mm Hg for pulmonary arterial hypertension. There is no formally accepted definition; however, most experts in the field accept this criterion.

From references 1, 2.

PAP, pulmonary artery pressure.*

heart (work = pressure × volume). In normal individuals the pressure in PA is much less (one-eighth) than in the aorta so work performed by the right ventricle is much less than that of the left heart. In situations in which the pulmonary pressure is raised, the workload of the right ventricle is also increased. Sometimes because of its smaller muscle mass the right ventricle is unable to generate a work output sufficient to pump the whole venous return, resulting in RHF. This in turn results in increased hydrostatic pressure at the right atrium and consequently peripheral edema, hepatomegaly and hepatic congestion, splenomegaly, pleural effusion, pericardial effusion, and raised jugular venous pulse.

As the left heart preload is dependent on the right heart, there is a relative inability to increase the cardiac output with demand. An abrupt attempt to increase physical activity may result in dizziness, syncope, or chest pain. On formal cardiopulmonary exercise testing, these patients show a rapid increase in heart rate with only small increase in workload or oxygen consumption. Over time, a persistently raised PVR results in hypertrophy of the right ventricle. This enables the

Box 13E.1 Diagnostic classification

Pulmonary arterial hypertension (PAH)

- Idiopathic PAH (IPAH)
- Familial PAH

  Related to:
  - Collagen vascular disease
  - Congenital systemic-to-pulmonary shunt
  - Portal hypertension
  - Human immunodeficiency virus infection
  - Drugs and toxins
  - Other (glycogen storage disease, Gaucher disease, hereditary hemorrhagic telangiectasia, hemoglobinopathies, myeloproliferative disorders, splenectomy)

  Associated with significant venous or capillary involvement:
  - Pulmonary venoocclusive disease
  - Pulmonary capillary hemangiomatosis

Pulmonary venous hypertension

- Left-sided atrial or ventricular heart disease
- Left-sided valvular heart disease

Pulmonary hypertension associated with hypoxemia

- Chronic obstructive pulmonary disease
- Interstitial lung disease
- Sleep-disordered breathing
- Alveolar hypoventilation disorders
- Chronic exposure to high altitude
- Neonatal lung disease
- Alveolar-capillary dysplasia

Pulmonary hypertension due to chronic thrombotic and/or embolic disease

- Thromboembolic obstruction of proximal pulmonary arteries
- Thromboembolic obstruction of distal pulmonary arteries
- *Pulmonary embolism* (tumor, parasites, foreign material, amniotic fluid)

Miscellaneous

- Sarcoidosis, histiocytosis X, lymphangiomatosis
- Compression of pulmonary vessels (adenopathy, tumor, fibrosing mediastinitis)

right ventricle to maintain quite high PA pressures to drive the cardiac output through a restricted pulmonary vascular bed (Box 13E.1[1] and Table 13E.3).[1] A non-hypertrophied heart is not able to generate or maintain very high pulmonary pressures (i.e. mean PA pressure above 50 mm Hg). Thus presence of very high PA pressure points against an acute cause for the process and is thus a clinically useful observation. Cor pulmonale is the term used for hypertrophy and/or dilation of the right ventricle in the setting of acute or

Table 13E.3 *Risk factors for primary pulmonary hypertension*

Drugs and toxins	Demographics and medical conditions	Diseases
Definite casual relation Aminorex Fenfluramine Dexfenfluramine Toxic rapeseed oil	Sex (female)	Human immunodeficiency virus infection
Very likely casual relation Amphetamine L-tryptophan		Portal hypertension Collagen vascular diseases Congenital systemic–pulmonary cardiac shunts (Eisenmenger's syndrome)
Possible casual relation Meta-amphetamines Cocaine Chemotherapeutic drugs	Pregnancy Systemic hypertension Splenectomy	Thyroid disorders Hemoglobinopathies (sickle cell disease, thalassemia, spherocytosis, etc.) Type-1a glycogen storage disease (von Gierke disease) Lipid storage disorders (Gaucher disease) Hereditary hemorrhagic telangiectasia (Osler–Rendu–Weber disease)
Unlikely casual relation Antidepressants Oral contraceptives Estrogen therapy Cigarette smoking	Obesity	

From reference 1.

chronic respiratory (or more precisely 'noncardiac') disease. Presence of RHF, which is a late manifestation of PH, is not necessary to make a diagnosis of cor pulmonale.

Epidemiology

Approximately 300–1000 new cases of IPAH are identified in the United States every year giving rise to an approximate incidence rate of 1–2 cases per million population per year.[1–4] The US National Institutes of Health registry of patients with primary pulmonary hypertension (PPH) (1981–85)[1,2] found an overall male to female ratio of 1:1.7.[1,2] (PPH is an old term for IPAH. In this chapter the term PPH is used when referring to older studies conducted when the term IPAH was not yet coined.) Among the older populations men and women are equally affected.[1,2] In the registry the median age at presentation was 36 years, 10 percent of patients presented after the age of 60, and the age ranged from 1 to 81 years.[1,2] About 5–15 percent of the cases of IPAH are familial.[1,2]

The overall prevalence and demographics of secondary PH vary depending on the cause. Prevalence of secondary PH in specific disease conditions is shown in Table 13E.4.

The estimation of prevalence of PH in acute care or critical care setting is extremely difficult and no accurate estimates are agreed upon.

Table 13E.4 *Estimated prevalence of PAH in various diseases*

Disease	Prevalence PAH (%)
Connective tissue diseases	2
CREST syndrome	50
Congenital heart disease	5
Portal hypertension	2
HIV infection	0.5–1.5
Pulmonary thromboembolic disease	3.8% have PAH at the end of 1 year after PE diagnosis

PAH, pulmonary arterial hypertension; CREST, Calcinosis, Raynaud phenomenon, Esophageal dysmotility, Sclerodactyly, Telangiectasia; HIV, human immunodeficiency virus; PE, pulmonary embolism.

From references: 1–3.

Clinical presentation

Almost all patients with PH experience dyspnea on exertion as their initial symptom.[1,5–8] The mean interval from the onset of symptoms to diagnosis was 2 years in US National Institutes of Health PPH registry.[2] Definitive diagnostic testing is often delayed secondary to low index of suspicion. This is because in secondary PH dyspnea is often blamed on the underlying lung or heart disease and sometimes to deconditioning, obesity, or smoking. Not uncommonly, young females with PPH are treated for anxiety or reactive airways disease until the symptoms become quite overt. Symptoms attributable to PH are shown in Table 13E.5.

Pulmonary hypertension should always be suspected in the presence of appropriate risk factors or predisposing conditions or in the following circumstances:

Table 13E.5 *Symptoms attributable to PAH*

Symptoms	Comments
Dyspnea	Most frequent presenting symptom. Present in almost all patients
Fatigue	May occur in the absence of reported dyspnea
Chest pain	Occurs in up to 50% of patients with severe PH, often resembles angina
Dizziness and syncope	Mostly with abrupt onset of activity, occurs in advanced disease with high resting pressures; poor prognostic sign; may be associated with bradyarrhythmia
Leg edema	Sign of right heart failure; poor prognostic sign
Palpitations	Sinus tachycardia or multifocal atrial tachycardia; atrial fibrillation uncommon in the absence of left heart disease
Hemoptysis	Related to dilated submucosal veins, bronchial collateral circulation hypertrophy and aneurysms of alveolar capillaries in postcapillary, precapillary and CHD associated-PH, respectively; cause of 11% deaths in patients with PAH associated with CHD
Hoarseness	Due to compression of left recurrent laryngeal nerve between aorta and left pulmonary artery (Ortner's syndrome)

PH, pulmonary hypertension; PAH, pulmonary atrial hypertension; CHD, congenital heart disease.

- an isolated decreased diffusion capacity on otherwise normal pulmonary function testing or a diffusion capacity reduced to a greater degree than other pulmonary function abnormalities
- dsypnea out of proportion to the severity of underlying lung or heart disease as estimated by forced expiratory volume in 1 second (FEV_1), total lung capacity (TLC) or parameters such as ejection fraction or history of heart disease
- loud P2 (pulmonic component of second heart sound) on physical examination
- signs of RHF without history of heart, liver or kidney disease
- prominent PA on an erect posteroanterior chest radiograph with no signs of heart failure
- a pulmonary artery larger than the aorta or an interventricular septum with a convexity into the left ventricle on a computed tomography (CT) scan of chest with contrast
- rapid, steep rise of heart rate on small increments in exercise workload, elevated dead space to tidal volume (VD/VT) ratio at rest with only small decrement with exercise along with worsening of PaO_2 and $P(A\text{-}a)O_2$ on increasing exercise on cardiopulmonary exercise testing for dyspnea evaluation.

Many of the symptoms of the PH can be explained on the basis of inability of the right ventricle to adequately increase the cardiac output during activities secondary to the impedance posed by elevated PVR and PA pressure. Symptoms suggesting RHF result from either rapid development of high pulmonary arterial pressure without enough time for right ventricle to become hypertrophied or pulmonary resistance high enough that even the hypertrophied heart cannot sufficiently overcome the outflow resistance. Significant tricuspid regurgitation worsens RHF symptoms because it decreases the output of the right ventricle.

Signs of PH may be used to assess the severity of disease or to determine the presence of heart failure; however, they lack objectivity and standardization, and hence have poor interobserver agreement. Diseases in which manifestations of PH may be the initial presentation are listed in Box 13E.2. Diseases which are almost always advanced if secondary PH is present are listed in Box 13E.3.

The disease conditions where an alternative or concurrent diagnosis should be sought if mean PA pressure is above 50 mm Hg are listed in Box 13E.4. However, contrary to the traditional view, such search is frequently not productive. Prevalence of such cases is probably higher than what can be expected based on prevalence of PPH in general population.

Box 13E.2 Diseases in which manifestations of PAH or RHF may be the initial presentation

- Scleroderma/CREST (*C*alcinosis, *R*aynaud phenomenon, *E*sophageal dysmotility, *S*clerodactyly, *T*elangiectasia)
- Obesity hypoventilation syndrome (OHS)
- Obstructive sleep apnea with OHS
- Human immunodeficiency virus (HIV) infection
- PAH associated with drug abuse
- Systemic lupus erythematosus

Box 13E.3 Diseases which are almost always advanced if associated with secondary PAH

- Chronic obstructive pulmonary disease (COPD)
- Interstitial lung disease (ILD)
- Obstructive sleep apnea
- Rheumatoid arthritis

Box 13E.4 Diseases where an alternative or concurrent diagnosis should be sought if mean PA pressure is above 50 mm Hg

- COPD without hypoxemia
- ILD without hypoxemia
- Obstructive sleep apnea without OHS
- Lung disease without hypoxemia

Natural history of disease

The natural history of PH varies, depending upon the underlying etiology. However, generally mortality is higher among patients with PH compared with patients without PH (e.g. in COPD, ILD, congenital heart disease). The natural history of PPH prior to the onset of symptoms is not known. Survival varies widely among various subgroups (Table 13E.6). Furthermore, with the advent of prostacyclin and its analogs, endothelin receptor inhibitors and phosphodiestrase-5 inhibitors, the natural history of disease has dramatically changed.[35–46]

Table 13E.6 *Survival in patients with primary pulmonary hypertension*

	Survival/Prognosis
Overall survival without treatment from NIH registry	2.8 years
NYHA 2, 3, and 4 (untreated)	58.6, 31.5, and 6 months, respectively
NYHA 3 and 4 treated with intravenous prostacyclin	Survival is twice that of matched control
Responders to CCB	95% 5-year survival
RA pressure above 15 mm Hg	Poor prognostic indicator
Cardiac index below 2 L/min/m²	Poor prognostic indicator

NIH, National Institutes of Health; NYHA, New York Heart Association; CCB, calcium channel blockers; RA, right atrium.

The cause of death in most patients with PPH is progressive RHF or sudden death. Right heart failure is marked by metabolic acidosis, worsening renal failure, metabolic derangements and death in weeks to months. Sudden death is a feature of late disease. Terminal bradyarrhythmias are common. The practice of routine prophylactic anticoagulation appears to have decreased incidence of pulmonary embolism as a cause of death in patients with PH.

Management

In patients in whom PH is clinically suspected, transthoracic echocardiography or stress echocardiography is generally utilized as the first test for noninvasive documentation of PH and right ventricular dysfunction. However, echocardiography has poor specificity and sensitivity, especially in borderline PH. The next task is determining the etiology of PH (Figs 13E.1[10–17] and 13E.2) and initiating specific therapies,[152–60] wherever possible, for secondary pulmonary hypertension (an old term for PH with identifiable underlying cause) (Tables 13E.7,[9] 13E.8,[152] 13E.9,[18–30] 13E.10[31–36] and Box 13E.5[18–30]). Right heart catheterization (RHC) is performed in most patients with WHO[157–60] class II, III, or IV symptoms for confirming the diagnosis of PAH by documenting high mean PA pressure along with high PVR and a pulmonary capillary wedge pressure less than 11 mm Hg. Right atrial pressure and cardiac index can also be measured by RHC, and have been found to have prognostic significance. Similarly, clinically significant left-to-right shunt can be detected if there is a step-up in oxygen saturation along the right side of the heart.

If PAH is confirmed then acute vasoreactivity testing (Table 13E.9[18–30] and Box 13E.5[18–30]) is performed primarily to determine whether calcium-channel blockers will be an acceptable therapeutic choice. After acute vasoreactivity testing, the PA catheter may be left in place and patients who are responders (have positive vasoreactivity) are started on a low dose of CCBs. The dose of the CCB is increased relatively rapidly to maximal beneficial effect or to tolerance while the PA catheter is in place, with close monitoring. In patients with class III or IV symptoms who are to be treated with intravenous prostacyclin or subcutaneous treprostinil (Figs 13E.1 and 13E.2,[31–58] Table 13E.10), the drug is started while the patient is still in the hospital and at least initially with the PA catheter in place, as the dose escalation is done relatively rapidly. The patient and preferably one of the patient's caregivers are trained to administer the therapy. The patient is discharged when either of them feels capable of independently managing the therapy at home.

ACUTE VASOREACTIVITY TESTING

Acute vasoreactivity testing is performed by the administration of inhaled nitric oxide (iNO), intravenous prostacyclin, intravenous adenosine, inhaled prostacyclin, or other short-acting vasodilators, while monitoring hemodynamics with a PA catheter in place. The primary purpose of acute vasoreactivity testing is to determine usefulness of CCBs (Table 13E.8[18–30] and Box 13E.5[18–30]). Five-year survival is 95 percent in responders with PPH (old name for IPAH). Empiric trial of CCB without acute vasoreactivity testing is not recommended. Use of CCBs in nonresponders may be unsafe and fatal on rare occasions.

Nonresponders to acute vasoreactivity testing are not likely to respond to long-term CCB therapy, hence this therapy should not be administered to this patient population. Conversely it has been shown in several independent studies that failure to respond during acute

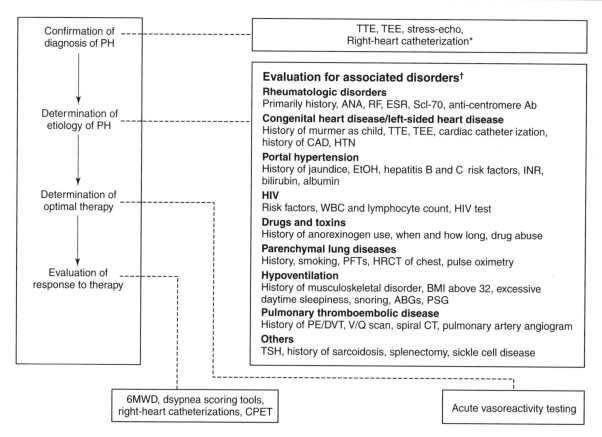

Figure 13E.1 *The four major steps in the management of PH. Diagnostic workup of PH should be individualized. *Use of routine annual right heart catheterization (RHC) as part of ongoing care of patients with PAH is controversial. Many centers do not do routine RHC. There are no data to support the use of routine RHC. †No test is absolutely necessary as routine. The choice of test depends upon the clinical suspicions based on history, physical examination, and the results of the available workup. PH, pulmonary hypertension; TTE, transthoracic echocardiogram; TEE, transesophageal echocardiogram; Echo, echocardiogram; ANA, antinuclear antigen; RF, rheumatoid factor; Ab, antibody; CAD, coronary artery disease; HTN, hypertension; EtOH, alcohol; INR, international normalized ratio; HIV, human immunodeficiency virus; WBC, white blood cells; PFTs, pulmonary function testing; HRCT, high-resolution computed tomography; BMI, body mass index (kg/m²); ABGs, arterial blood gases analysis; PSG, polysomnogram; PE, pulmonary embolism; DVT, deep venous thrombosis; V̇/Q, ventilation/perfusion; CT, computed tomography; TSH, thyroid stimulating hormone; 6MWD, 6 minutes walk distance; CPET, cardiopulmonary exercise testing.*

Box 13E.5 Criteria for a significant response

1   – Drop in mean PA pressure by more than 10 mm Hg

    OR – Attaining a mean PA pressure of less than 40 mm Hg

    OR – Decrease in PVR by 20 percent or more

    OR – Attaining a PVR less than 8 Wood units

2   – **AND** – No decrease in cardiac output

3   – **AND** – None or clinically acceptable drop in systemic blood pressure

Note: There are no uniformly acceptable criteria, and 10–15 percent of patients with IPAH are acute responders. However, as a general principle the choice of more stringent criteria translates into more likelihood of response to calcium-channel blockers (CCBs) and better prognosis (5-year survival is 95 percent in patients with PPH who had a decrease in PVR of 50 percent and a mean PA pressure of less than 30 mm Hg)

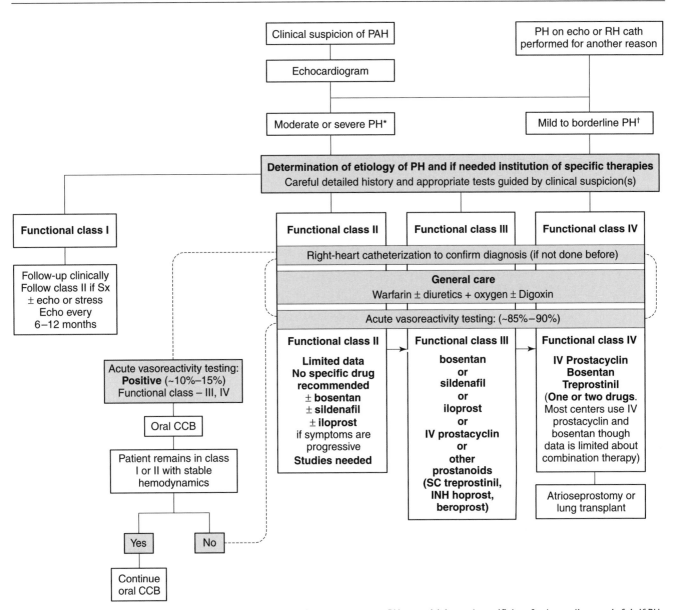

Figure 13E.2 *Management of PAH in the nonacute setting. *Moderate or severe PH – sensitivity and specificity of echocardiogram is fair if PH is moderate to severe; †mild to borderline PH – sensitivity and specificity of echocardiogram is fair if PH is moderate to severe. Right heart catheterization may be required to confirm the diagnosis in most but not all symptomatic patients who are likely candidates for some form of PH therapy. PH, pulmonary hypertension; Echo, echocardiogram; RH cath, right heart catheterization; Sx, symptom; CCB, calcium-channel blocker; IV, intravenous; SC, subcutaneous.*

vasoreactivity testing does not exclude the possibility of response to long-term intravenous subcutaneous or inhaled prostacyclin endothilin receptor inhibitors or phosphodiesterase-5 inhibitors or therapy in terms of hemodynamics, functional improvement, and mortality. Similarly, retrospective data show that a vast majority of acute responders progress to nonresponder over the follow up period of several years. Restoration of vasoreactivity has been

shown to occur in some patients after long-term (greater than 2 years) prostacyclin therapy. Patients with PH associated with thromboembolic disease and parenchymal lung disease are much less likely to respond to CCBs; the clinician may choose not to perform acute vasoreactivity testing in these patients. As CCBs are not used with severely depressed cardiac output, acute vasoreactivity testing has no role in the management of acute RHF.

Table 13E.7 *Disease-specific management of pulmonary hypertension*

Disease	Therapy	Comments
Collagen vascular diseases	Prospective controlled studies to show significant benefit from IV prostacyclin[32], bosentan[33,34] and SC treprostinil[35] in scleroderma	Limited data are available for other forms of rheumatologic diseases
Portal hypertension	Supplemental oxygen to keep Sao_2 above 90%; diuretics to control volume overload; may precipitate liver failure by overaggressive diuresis Avoid anticoagulation if significant coagulopathy Caution in using CCB to avoid hypotension Avoid Bosentan secondary to potential liver toxicity; IV prostacyclin may be used but no controlled data to support the use Most but not all liver transplant centers consider moderate to severe PH as a contraindication to liver transplant. There are reports of improvement of PH after liver transplant	Two types, hepatopulmonary syndrome (hypoxemia, intrapulmonary shunting, increased calculated shunt fraction upon oxygen supplementation, orthodeoxia – may improve with liver transplant in some patients) and portopulmonary hypertension (associated with pulmonary hypertension with or without cirrhosis, lower diastolic and mean PA pressures, higher cardiac output, lower PVR and SVR), some patients have features of both
HIV	Antiretroviral therapy also improves PAH in most but not all cases Prostacyclin and Bosentan have been shown to be very effective in improving symptoms and hemodynamics in uncontrolled studies. No data about use of sildenafil	Therapeutic options often limited due to concurrent complications of HIV or HAART Anticoagulation contraindicated if significant hemostasis abnormalities or thrombocytopenia Adjust HAART doses if on bosentan, though recent uncontrolled study did not show any significant concerns[152]
Left-sided heart disease	Treatment of congenital/left-sided atrial, ventricular, or valve disease generally (but not always) decreases, not only the PAP but also improves the PVR	This is the most common cause of PH If despite appropriate treatment PVR remains high, specific PAH therapies are used
Extrinsic compression of central pulmonary vessels, e.g. in fibrosing mediastinitis	Several case reports of marked reduction in PA pressures and symptomatic improvement by endovascular stent placement	Vascular bypass surgery has been successfully tried
Pulmonary venoocclusive disease	No controlled studies Several case reports of use of IV prostacyclin and/or bosentan Several reports of acute cardiogenic pulmonary edema in some patients on IV protacyclin and bosentan	Radiographic appearance resembles left heart failure
COPD/interstitial lung disease	Oxygen is mainstay of treatment if associated with hypoxemia No controlled studies to support the use of prostacyclin or bosentan	Worsening of hypoxemia may be seen in patients on IV prostacyclin possibly due to alteration of V/Q ratio
Sleep disorder breathing, OSA/OHS	CPAP for OSA, and NIPPV or BiPAP for OHS Mortality of untreated OHS is very high and patients unable to tolerate NIPPV or BiPAP should be treated with tracheostomy Treatment benefit is generally dramatic in OHS: expect only modest decrease in PAP in OSA PAP may not normalize after CPAP in OSA patients with severe PAH	Sleep study is only recommended in patients with PAH who have high clinical suspicion for OSA; similarly in patients with OSA routine screening for PH is not recommended
Neuromuscular disorders with hypercapnia	NIPPV or BiPAP even with mild hypercapnia	Consider long-term use of portable mechanical ventilators in younger patients with otherwise good health
Chronic exposure to high altitude	Oxygen supplementation, phlebotomies if high hematocrit, migration to lower altitude IV prostacyclin has been used successfully in refractory case, though no controlled data	Presence of other risk factors for PAH may compound the problem
Pulmonary thromboembolic disease	Anticoagulation; thromboendarterectomy in patients who have persistent proximal pulmonary artery clots even after several months of acute embolic event and class 3 or 4 symptoms IV prostacyclin or bosentan improve dyspnea and hemodynamics in PAH associated with distal CPTED	Surgery carries a high risk of mortality (6–20%); 3.8% of patients who are diagnosed with PE have PAH after 2 years of their PE event

HIV, human immunodeficiency virus; COPD, chronic obstructive pulmonary disease; OSA, obstructive sleep apnea; OHS, obesity hypoventilation syndrome; IV, intravenous; SC, subcutaneous, Sao_2, oxyhemoglobin saturation; CCB, calcium-channel blockers; PH, pulmonary hypertension; PAH, pulmonary arterial hypertension; PAP, pulmonary artery pressure; PVR, pulmonary vascular resistance; PA, pulmonary artery; CPAP, continuous positive airway pressure; NIPPV, noninvasive positive pressure ventilation; BiPAP, bilevel positive airway pressure; HAART, highly active antiretroviral therapy; V/Q: ventilation/perfusion; PE, pulmonary embolism.

Table 13E.8 *Conventional therapies*

Therapy	Rationale	Level of evidence	Comments
Oxygen	Relieves hypoxic pulmonary vasoconstriction in patients with hypoxemia	Well-established mortality benefit in COPD, two large prospective trials Expert opinion in other disease conditions with hypoxemia, no trials	PAH patients with hypoxemia should be treated with oxygen to maintain oxygen saturation above 90% at all times Oxygen is mainstay of treatment in PAH associated with advanced lung disease
Diuretics	Used in patients with edema and ascites secondary to right heart failure	Expert opinion, no controlled trials to show mortality benefit	Use with caution to avoid a drop in cardiac output due to decreased left ventricular preload Monitor serum electrolytes Consider restriction of dietary sodium and fluid intake
Anticoagulation	Prevention of intrapulmonary thrombosis in patients with already compromised pulmonary vascular bed, low cardiopulmonary reserves and a sedentary lifestyle	Retrospective data and uncontrolled prospective study of PPH (old name for idiopathic PAH) and anorectics-associated PAH showed mortality benefit Expert opinion (controversial) for PAH associated with conditions such as scleroderma, CHD	Target INR: PAH alone: 1.5–2.5 PE/DVT : 2.0–3.0 Prosthetic valve: 2.5–3.5 Contraindicated if significant coagulopathy or thrombocytopenia in patients with advanced liver disease or HIV Relative contraindication in patients with CHD with history of significant hemoptysis IV prostacyclin has antiplatelet properties but there is high risk of catheter-associated thrombosis. No data to evaluate need for anticoagulation in patients on IV prostacyclin. However, most experts use warfarin if no signs of bleeding
Digoxin	Positive inotropic and negative chronotropic effect	No controlled trials to support the benefit One short-term study demonstrating transient increase in cardiac output with single administration of 1 mg digoxin	May be used in patients with right ventricular failure and/or atrial dysarrhythmias Close monitoring of drug levels required
Calcium-channel blockers	Pulmonary vasodilation	Prospective trials with historic controls, survival benefit in 'responders'* only 5-year survival is 95% in responders with PPH Empiric trial of CCB without acute vasoreactivity testing[†] is not recommended Use of CCB in nonresponders is unsafe, may be fatal on rare occasions Contraindicated if acute RHF with compromised hemodynamics	The primary purpose of acute vasoreactivity testing[†] is to determine usefulness of CCBs Nifedipine (preferred if relative bradycardia), diltiazem (preferred if relative tachycardia) or amlodipine may be used (not verapamil secondary to profound negative inotropic effect) The vasoreactivity may be lost in a significant proportion of patients on long term follow-up There are reports of conversion of nonresponders to responders on prolonged IV prostacyclin therapy
ACE inhibitors, α-adrenergic blockers, hydralazine	Reduction of preload and/or afterload	No well controlled trial, mostly case reports	No proved benefit in PPH
Prevention and prompt treatment of respiratory tract infections	May cause worsening of hypoxemia and hypoxic pulmonary vasoconstriction	Expert opinion	PH patients should receive influenza vaccination every fall and pneumonia vaccine every 5–10 years Respiratory tract infections should be promptly treated Pneumonia is one of the major causes of death in patients with PAH

* 'Responders': patients who manifest a significant (usually more than 20%) reduction in pulmonary artery pressure and pulmonary vascular resistance with an increased or unchanged cardiac output, and a minimally reduced or unchanged systemic blood pressure upon acute vasoreactivity testing.

[†]Acute vasoreactivity testing: acute administration of inhaled nitric oxide, intravenous prostacyclin, inhaled prostacyclin, intravenous adenosine or other vasodilators and simultaneous hemodynamic monitoring with PA catheter in place.

COPD: chronic obstructive pulmonary disease; PAH, pulmonary artery hypertension; PPH, primary pulmonary hypertension; INR, international normalization ratio; PE, pulmonary embolism; DVT, deep venous thrombosis; HIV, human immunodeficiency virus; CHD, congenital heart disease; IV, intravenous; CCB, calcium-channel blocker; RHF, right heart failure; ACE, angiotensin-converting enzyme.
References:

Table 13E.9 *Agents used in acute vasoreactivity testing*

Agent	Administration and dosing
Inhaled nitric oxide	Inhalation of low concentration (20 parts per million) for 6–10 minutes by facemask
Intravenous prostacyclin	1 ng/kg/min, increased by 1–2 ng/kg/min every 5–15 minutes to a maximum dose of 12 ng/kg/min
	Or 2.5 ng/kg/min, increase by 2.5 ng/kg/min every 10 minutes to maximum of 12 ng/kg/min*
Inhaled prostacyclin	Inhalation of 50 ng/kg/min by nebulizer for 15 minutes
Intravenous adenosine	Fast intravenous bolus of 50 µg/kg/min, increased by 50 µg/kg/min every 2 minutes to a maximum dose of 500 µg/kg/min

*The dose escalation is stopped before maximum dose if patient experience discomfort such as headache, flushing, heat or thoracic oppression. The mean tolerated dose is 8.0 ng/kg/min during acute dosing.

†There is no proved advantage of testing reactivity with more than one agent typically used.

RIGHT VENTRICULAR DYSFUNCTION AND PULMONARY HYPERTENSION IN ACUTE CARE SETTINGS

Peripheral edema or elevated neck veins in the absence of overt pulmonary edema on chest radiograph should raise the suspicion for RHF. Similarly, hypotension with signs of inadequate tissue perfusion such as low urine output or decreased mentation, when accompanied with marked peripheral edema and jugular venous distension, the differential diagnosis includes RHF. As left heart failure is far more common in acute care settings, use of all available clinical and laboratory data is pivotal in making decisions about further testing and management. It is important to make the distinction between left and right heart failure, as the differential diagnosis and management of these two conditions are different.

Not all clinical situations in which there is suspicion of RHF warrant further testing to confirm the presence of RHF and quantification of PAH (Box 13E.6).

Right heart catheterization has the advantage of being the most accurate and reproducible technique for the determination of PA pressure. It is also able to evaluate PVR and can be used to rule out elevated pulmonary pressures due to left heart disease (valvular or myocardial), and to exclude clinically significant left-to-right shunt by serial measurements of oxyhemoglobin saturations along the right heart blood flow. Echocardiography, however, due to its noninvasive nature is often an extremely useful initial test to evaluate estimated PA pressure, right ventricle and right atrium wall thickness and chamber size, as well as right ventricular systolic function and valvular function, left ventricle size and function, presence or absence of regional wall motion abnormalities, or pericardial effusion. In the right clinical setting it may be reasonable to give an empiric trial of diuretics or volume challenge to achieve certain physiologic goals and defer any further testing. The decision to initiate workup for pulmonary thromboembolic disease, which is often a common concern in such situations, should be guided by pretest probability and presence or absence of

plausible alternative explanation of presentation. An effort to 'rule out pulmonary embolism' in patients with low pretest probability may result in delay in definite diagnosis and management, and difficulty interpreting test results.

Finding of elevated PA pressure or signs of RHF in the acute care setting deserve slightly different consideration compared with outpatient settings. Left heart failure (LHF) is extremely common in acutely ill patients. Some elevation of PA pressure and PVR can be commonly seen in patients with ARDS or sepsis, or in those on positive pressure ventilation; this may not require special treatment. It may be noted that some elevation of PVR may be seen in most patients with LHF. One study[59] found that only 28 percent of the patients undergoing RHC for LHF had normal PVR (<1.5 Wood units).

It is the difference in epidemiology, along with differences in priorities in acute care, which makes approach and management of PH and RHF in acute care setting somewhat different from that in outpatient care. Extreme caution should be observed while drawing conclusions from studies

---

Box 13E.6 Situations where RHF is suspected but clinicians may choose to defer any further workup to confirm RHF or to quantify PA pressure or PVR

- Absence of significant hypoxia and hemodynamic compromise where further testing is not likely to alter acute management
- When it is evident that even if mild to moderate PAH is present, management would still consist of routine management of underlying condition such as mild to moderate acute respiratory distress syndrome (ARDS), moderate to severe exacerbation of COPD
- Patient is a known case of PAH and the acute management does not require further investigation to make immediate treatment decisions
- Futility of care is evident

Table 13E.10 Summary of trials of prostacyclin analogs, endothelin receptor inhibitors and phosphodiestrase-5 inhibitors in pulmonary hypertension

Study	Year	n	Design	Diagnoses (n)	Duration of follow-up	WHO class (n)	Drugs	6MWD change (m)	PVR change (mm Hg/L/m)	mPAP change (mm Hg)	CI change (L/min/m²)	Survival impact	Symptoms change
Epoprostinol IV Rubin et al.[31]	1990	24	NB, R for 8 wk then NR for up to 18 mo, C	PPH (24)	8 wk		10 on Epo and conventional, 9 on conventional (anticoagulation, diuretics, oral vasodilators)		-7.9 vs none in controls				38% in treated improved NYHA class vs none in controls
Epoprostinol IV Badesch et al.[32]	2000	111	NB, R, C, MC	Scleroderma spectrum PAH (111)	12 wk	II (5), III (87), IV (19)	56 on Epo and conventional, 55 on conventional	+46 m vs -48 m in controls	-4.6 vs +0.9 in controls	-5 vs +0.9 in controls	+0.5 vs -0.1 in controls	No statistical difference in 12 wk	
Bosentan oral Channick et al.[33]	2001	32	DB, R, PC, MC, for 12 wk then open-label up to 28 wk	PPH (27), Scleroderma Spectrum PAH (5)	12 wk	III (32), IV(excluded)	21 on bosentan, 11 on placebo, both groups on conventional, none on any form of prostacyclins	+70 m vs -6 m in placebo	-2.8 vs +2.4 in controls	-1.6 vs +5.1 in controls	+0.5 vs -0.5 in controls	No deaths occurred during 12 wk	Bosentan significantly better, functional class improved in 43% and remained same in 57% (vs 9% and 73% on placebo, respectively)
Bosentan oral Rubin et al.[34]	2002	213	DB, R, PC, MC for 16 wk then only 45 patients on DB treatment for up to 28 wk	PPH (150), Scleroderma (47) PAH, SLE (16)	16 wk	III (195), I V (18)	74 on bosentan 125 BID, 70 on bosentan 250 BID, 69 on placebo, all groups on conventional, none on any form of prostacyclins	+54 on 250 mg BID, +35m on 125 BID vs -8m on placebo	NA	NA	NA	During 16 wk study 2 on placebo, 1 on 125 mg BID died, ***3 on 250 BID died within 4 wk of withdrawal (2/3) from or completion (1/3) of study	On bosentan 250 BID and 125 BID: functional class improved in 41% and 34% respectively, vs 30 in placebo after 16 wk
Treprostinil SC Simonneau et al.[35]	2002	470	DB, R, PC, MC, (as local and systemic side effects are common with drug, the blinding of physician may not be effective)	PPH (270), Connective tissue disorder-PAH (90) Congenital systemic to pulmonary shunt (109)	12 wk	II (53), III (382), V (34)	233 on treprostinil, 236 on placebo. All groups on conventional, none on any other form of prostacyclins	+10 m vs 0 m on placebo	-3.5 vs +1.2 in controls	-2.3 vs +0.7 in controls	+0.12 vs -0.06 in controls	During 12 wk study 7 on drug and 7 on placebo died ***2 on placebo 3 on drug died within 12 wk after study drug withdrawl##	Signs and symptoms composite score improved by 1.1 from baseline of 7.6 in treprostinil group vs a decrease of 0.1 from baseline of 7.5 in placebo group
Iloprost aerosolized Hoeper et al.[36]	2000	24	Retrospective review of consecutive patients	PPH (24)	1 year or more between 3/1997 and 6/1998	III (20) IV (4)	Aerosolized iloprost 50 µg/5NS inhaled over 10-15 min six to eight times/day. All groups on conventional, none on any other form of prostacyclins	+85 m	280 dyn. s/cm5	-7.0	0.60 L/min	Survival not evaluated (retrospective study)	Not reported
Sildenafil vs bosentan Wilkins et al.[154]	2005	26	DB, R, 16 wk, then all patients to open label bosentan	iPAH (23) Scleroderma-PAH(2), SLE(1)	16 wk	III (26)	14 on sildenafil 50 mg PO BID for 4 wk then 50 mg PO TID for total of 16 wk. 12 on bosentan 62.5 mg PO BID for 4 wk then 125 mg PO BID for total of 16 wk	+59 m on bosentan and +114 m on sildenafil	On sildenafil 8.8 gm reduction in RV mass vs 3 gm on bosentan		+0.3 in both groups	Survival was not the end point as the study was only 16 wk long. One patient on sildenafil had sudden death during wk 14	Kansas City Cardiomyopathy Quality of life questionnaire score +27 on sildenafil, +6 on bosentan

Abbreviations: n, total number of patients in the study; Diagnosis (n), number of patients with the specified diagnosis; WHO (n), number of patients with the specified World Health Organization functional class; 6MWD (m), 6 minutes walk distance in meters; PVR, pulmonary vascular resistance; mPAP, mean pulmonary artery pressure; CI, cardiac index; IV, intravenous; SC, subcutaneous; NB, nonblinded; R, randomized; NR, nonrandomized; wk, weeks; C, controlled; MC, multicenter; DB, double-blinded; PC, placebo-controlled; PPH, primary pulmonary hypertension (old name for idiopathic PAH); PAH, pulmonary arterial hypertension; Epo, epoprostinol or prostacyclin; SLE, systemic lupus erythematosis; BID, twice daily; NYHA, New York Heart Association.

on PAH done in outpatients settings. Prevalence of various disorders, variables influencing the pathophysiology, or course of disease and prognosis may be entirely different and diverse when these patients are acutely ill.

Understanding the factors influencing the pulmonary circulation

Shock is recognized by the presence of hypotension and signs of inadequacy of tissue perfusion such as decreased urine output, altered mentation or cyanosis. Significantly decreased cardiac output relative to metabolic demand is a hallmark of cardiogenic shock. Left ventricle failure is far more common as a cause of cardiogenic shock than right ventricle failure. Although right ventricle dysfunction is less common, it still constitutes a substantial minority of patients presenting with compromised systemic blood pressure and signs of tissue hypoperfusion. Failure to include RHF in the differential diagnosis of cardiogenic shock may result in insufficient or inappropriate treatment.

The circulation can be viewed as a one-way closed circuit, containing two pumps connected in series, separated by two resistances. A weak pump (right ventricle) is meant to force the blood through a small resistance, and a stronger pump (left ventricle) is meant to pump the same amount of blood through the higher resistance. The same amount of blood is pumped through the larger resistance by generation of higher pressures by the bulkier muscle mass of left ventricle, thus performing more work than the right ventricle. 'The chain is as strong as the weakest link': the overall effectiveness of this pumping system depends upon the integrity of each individual component of the system. If one of the pumps is unable to effectively force the blood through the given resistance, because of an increased resistance (increased systemic vascular resistance or PVR), decreased pump strength (systolic dysfunction), or inability to properly load the ventricle for pumping (diastolic dysfunction), the overall ability of the system is affected resulting in decreased circulating volumes (diminished cardiac output).

If there is a large disparity between the pumping ability of one pump–resistance set compared with the other, the overall efficiency of the whole system will depend on one pump–resistance set and not both. It is extremely important to determine whether the right ventricle–PVR or left ventricle–systemic vascular resistance is the limiting element in the generation of cardiac output in a given patient with a compromised cardiac output.

The performance of both ventricles also depends upon the preload, which in turn determines the end-diastolic volume and hence strength of each systolic contraction. Therefore, there is a definite mutual dependence between right ventricle function, left ventricle function, PVR, and systemic vascular resistance. Preload for right ventricle not only depends upon right ventricle compliance and right-sided valvular function but also on systemic vascular

resistance and left ventricle performance. Similarly, left ventricle performance also depends on right ventricle function and PVR. The left ventricle output is more sensitive to preload and the right ventricle output is more sensitive to after-load (PVR). Furthermore, although strength of myocardial contraction increases with increasing preload, the relation is not linear for most physiologic and pathologic states. The interdependence of various components, the influence of sympathetic, myogenic, and other regulatory mechanisms as well as the nonlinear nature of most interactions, the effect of on board vasoactive drugs and devices such as mechanical ventilators, makes the whole system immensely complex. So in a given patient, it is almost impossible to predict the response to a certain intervention. The most practical solution to this complexity is to monitor clinical and hemodynamic trends after an intervention (such as a fluid bolus or changing the rate of infusion of a vasoactive drug) to evaluate its usefulness in a given patient. In the setting of cardiogenic shock with RHF it is important that in evaluating the effect of interventions we:

- assess the effect on systemic and pulmonary circulations separately
- obtain serial observations as they are particularly valuable to see the effectiveness of interventions
- monitor gas exchange as it is not uncommon to find that despite increase in cardiac output, hypoxemia gets worse, probably secondary to worsening of overall ventilation/perfusion mismatch and shunting.

Specific acute care situations associated with pulmonary arterial hypertension

HIGH PA PRESSURES AND PVR IN ACUTE LUNG INJURY AND ARDS

Elevated PA pressure and PVR has been observed in a significant proportion of patients with ARDS and severe hypoxemia.[60] In patients with severe ARDS, correction of hypoxemia results in significant decrease in PAP.[60] However, despite correction of hypoxemia elevated PA pressures persist in almost all patients. Similar observations have been made in ARDS in postsurgical patients. High pulmonary pressures in ARDS have been attributed to hypoxic pulmonary vasoconstriction, positive pressure ventilation and mediators released as a result of lung injury. In addition, fibroproliferative changes in severe ARDS may involve or entrap small pulmonary arterioles resulting in an increase in PVR.

Uncontrolled trials have demonstrated that use of iNO in a subset of ARDS patients with life-threatening hypoxemia, PAH, and RHF results in improvement in hypoxemia, and hemodynamics. However, several randomized controlled trials (RCTs) of iNO have failed to show any survival benefit for patients with ARDS. Inhaled prostacyclin has also been shown to have pulmonary vasodilator properties. However, its survival benefit has not been evaluated. No RCTs have been done to evaluate the survival benefit of selective pulmonary vasodilators in ARDS patients with less severe hypoxemia along with elevated PVR and RHF.

The prevalence of clinically significant PH in ARDS is not known. Similarly, incidence of PH in survivors of ARDS is not known. Nevertheless, currently a history of ARDS is not considered as a risk factor for subsequent development of PAH. Just like in COPD, the presence of PH with ARDS is a poor prognostic indicator.

HIGH PA PRESSURES AND PVR IN SEPSIS

Sepsis has been associated with PH and right ventricle dysfunction in animal[61] and in a few human[62] studies. However in the absence of other factors such as ARDS or mechanical ventilation, PH of any clinical significance is only rarely observed. Evidence for or against the hypothesis that sepsis causes clinically significant PH is sparse. Theoretically speaking, elevated PA pressure may be observed in high cardiac output states without elevated PVR, and in the setting of depressed left ventricle function secondary to hypotension and sepsis. There is a component of postcapillary pulmonary hypertension.

HIGH PA PRESSURES AND PVR AFTER CARDIOTHORACIC SURGERY

Pulmonary hypertension is common after coronary artery bypass graft surgery (CABG), valvular repair or replacement, heart transplantation, lung transplantation, heart-lung transplantation, significant lung resection surgery or pneumonectomy.[63] Right ventricle failure is among the leading causes of death during the first week after heart transplantation.[63] Significantly elevated PVR after CABG is a rule rather than exception. A proportion of patients with longstanding mitral valve disease continue to have elevated PVR and right ventricle dysfunction after surgical correction of a valve. Right ventricle dysfunction is more pronounced if surgical procedure involved incision of the ventricular myocardium as well as procedures involving intraoperative ischemia, such as with aortic cross-clamping. The evidence of right ventricle dysfunction on preoperative echo-cardiogram, e.g. in certain congenital heart diseases, chronic PAH due to any cause, is a significant risk factor for postcardiothoracic surgical right ventricle failure. In such patients any hemodynamic compromise as indicated by hypotension, decreased cardiac output, or signs of poor tissue perfusion should raise the possibility of RVF while considering further diagnostic and therapeutic inter-ventions. Evidence of preexisting PAH and preoperative evidence of right ventricle dysfunction on echocardiogram should lead to more aggressive monitoring and anticipation of postsurgical right ventricle failure. High right atrial pressure with normal or slightly elevated pulmonary capillary wedge pressure with elevated PVR should be regarded as right ventricle failure if accompanied with

decreased cardiac output, hypotension and signs of poor tissue perfusion, such as decreased urine output. In such cases the therapy should be directed towards RHF as described in the section on management of RHF below.

HIGH PA PRESSURES AND PVR IN COPD PATIENTS DURING AN ACUTE EXACERBATION OR AN INTERCURRENT CRITICAL ILLNESS

Many COPD patients with normal resting PA pressures show evidence of significantly elevated PA pressures after moderate exercise along with elevated right ventricle end-diastolic pressure. Intercurrent critical illness with increased cardiac output secondary to high metabolic demand may similarly unmask PH.[64] Worsening of hypercapnia and acidosis in severe obstructive disease with either disease exacerbation or critical-illness-associated high metabolic state and higher rate of carbon dioxide production may result in hypoxemia and exaggerated hypoxic pulmonary vasoconstriction, high PVR, and right ventricle dysfunction. Acidosis acts synergistically with hypoxemia to cause pulmonary vasoconstriction. Presence of PH with COPD is a poor prognostic indicator.[65,66]

The subset of COPD patients with cor pulmonale who show improvement in hemodynamics with oxygen supplementation have better prognosis on long-term oxygen therapy (LTOT) compared with those who do not show improvement in hemodynamics with oxygen supple-mentation.[70] Most hypoxemic COPD patients show improvement in PVR, PA pressures and stroke volume index[67] with low-flow LTOT. A study on LTOT showed arrest of progression of PVR in the study group whereas the control group (without LTOT) had 25 percent increase in PVR after 500 days.[68] The subset of COPD patients who develop marked peripheral edema during acute exacerbations have more marked right ventricular failure (increased right ventricular end-diastolic pressure) compared with patients with normal end-diastolic pressure. In another study patients with RHF had more marked increase in PAP as well as more severe hypoxemia and hypercapnia.[69] Similarly worsening of the RHF may be seen in other advanced lung diseases during exacerbations of pulmonary disease with worsened hypoxemia.

RIGHT HEART FAILURE, HIGH PA PRESSURES AND PVR IN MORBIDLY OBESE HOSPITALIZED PATIENTS OR IN PATIENTS WITH NEUROMUSCULAR OR SKELETAL DISORDERS ASSOCIATED WITH HYPOVENTILATION

Morbidly obese patients and patients with severe neuromuscular or skeletal disorders often present to the hospital with worsening hypoxemia, hypercapnia, increased edema, somnolence, and often hypotension and full-blown cardiogenic shock. These patients may or may not be known to have daytime hypoventilation and hypercapnia. Their ability to increase their minute ventilation is limited. Similarly their ability to respond to hypercapnia is also limited due to impaired sensitivity of their central nervous system (CNS) to hypercapnic stimulus. Key to their management is correction of hypoventilation by noninvasive positive pressure ventilation (NIPPV) or, when necessary, intubation and mechanical ventilation in addition to identification and correction of cause of their deterioration. There is a theoretical concern of worsening of hypercapnia by excessive oxygen supplementation as hypoxemic ventilatory drive is thought to be the primary mechanism used by the CNS in such patients for respiratory homeostasis.

Several options have been described for long-term treatment of hypoventilation. However, at most US centers the practical option is to use NIPPV or bilevel positive airway pressure (BiPAP), and if the mask is not tolerated by the patient secondary to claustrophobia, tracheostomy, to institute positive pressure ventilation. A dramatic clinical improvement within a few days is the rule. Over the period of several weeks, reversal of polycythemia, pulmonary hypertension and peripheral edema as well as lowering of the awake P_{CO_2} occurs in most patients with no other underlying reason for pulmonary hypertension. Improvement may not be as drastic in patients with musculoskeletal abnormalities or accompanying congenital heart disease.

Patients with known pulmonary arterial hypertension presenting to acute care settings

Acute hospitalization is not uncommon among patients with moderate to severe PAH. This poses a dilemma, as most physicians are not comfortable taking care of such patients. These patients may present with worsening RHF, worsening of underlying etiology of secondary pulmonary hypertension, complication of therapy, or an unrelated intercurrent illness. Similarly they may be hospitalized for a surgery which may or may not be related to PH. Box 13E.7 summarizes key points for management of these patients.

Pregnancy and pulmonary arterial hypertension

Pregnancy in women with moderate to severe PAH is associated with high maternal mortality (30–56 percent).[71,72] Due to the high risk, primarily of maternal mortality and also increased neonatal mortality (12 percent), most experts strongly recommend effective contraception and in the event of pregnancy, early termination.[73] A review[72] of reports published between 1978 and 1996 on (i) Eisenmenger syndrome (n = 73), (ii) PPH (n = 27), and (iii) secondary PAH (n = 25) complicating late pregnancy found that maternal mortality was 36 percent, 30 percent, and 56 percent respectively, in these groups. Of the deaths, 94 percent occurred during or after the delivery. Neonatal survival was also decreased (87–89 percent) and was similar in three groups. Late diagnosis of PAH and delayed start of formal medical care were significant risk factors for maternal mortality.

Box 13E.7 Patients with known PAH presenting to acute care settings with an issue not directly linked to PAH: important points in management

Indicators of disease severity

- Worse pre-admission World Health Organization (WHO) class of symptoms
- Low cardiac index
- High right atrial pressure

Use of PA catheter

- There is no evidence to support routine use of PA catheter, even in patients with severe PAH and it should be avoided unless it is likely to affect the management
- Insertion may require fluoroscopic guidance in patients with severe tricuspid regurgitation
- The Fick method should be used for cardiac output determination as thermodilution method becomes inaccurate in the presence of severe tricuspid regurgitation. Note that the Fick method involves certain assumptions in the assessment of the patient's rate of oxygen consumption – which may result in inaccurate results, especially in high metabolic states as well as in the presence of shunt

General care

Oxygenation and ventilators

- Avoid hypoxemia
- Avoid high positive end-expiratory pressure (PEEP)
- Avoid hypercapnia or respiratory acidosis
- Hypoxemia is common
- Significant worsening of hypoxemia may be seen without major change in patient's lung pathology

Fluids and diuretics

- Cautious use of fluids and diuretics to avoid sudden large volume fluctuations
- Monitor daily weights and fluid intake and output
- RHF should be considered as a possibility if there is hypotension, hypoxemia or signs of decreased tissue perfusion such as decreased urine output, cool extremities, or altered mentation

Acid–base and electrolytes

- Avoid acidosis as it may cause increase in PA pressure

PAH-related medications

Warfarin and anticoagulation

- If PAH is the only indication for anticoagulation (i.e. there is no history of pulmonary embolism, deep vein thrombosis (DVT), prosthetic valves, atrial fibrillation or severe cardiomyopathy, etc.) and there is a need for holding anticoagulation, e.g. for surgical procedure or line placement, warfarin may be held a few days prior to the procedure and be restarted after the procedure without any overlap with intravenous heparin or subcutaneous low-molecular-weight heparin

- If the patient is immobilized, DVT prophylaxis should be instituted similarly to the patients with left heart failure (if patient is not on warfarin or if warfarin is on hold for some procedure)

Bosentan

- The outpatient dose should be continued. If patient is nil by mouth, the drug can be held, as no parenteral form of drug is available. Restart as soon as possible, preferably within 24–36 hours

Intravenous prostacyclin (epoprostenol)

- No other drug should be administered through the port being used for prostacyclin
- Prostacyclin should not be interrupted for more than a few minutes, as this may be fatal on rare occasions
- If for some reason, central access is transiently unavailable, the drug can be given through a peripheral intravenous line for up to a few days. Erythema along the vein and more frequent loss of intravenous access is the rule

Anesthesia

- Preferably should be managed by a doctor experienced in PH

Cesarean section delivery is associated with higher mortality than vaginal delivery.[74] However, this observation may be due to the selection bias for the patients in whom vaginal delivery fails or there is a need to perform an emergency cesarean section. Currently, reliable data are lacking to infer whether planning an elective cesarean section poses an additional risk for mothers with PAH.

Under normal circumstances a pregnancy causes significantly increased hemodynamic stress,[75] which is maximum during the second and third stages of labor and in the immediate postpartum period.[75] This is primarily due to large fluid shifts and, in certain cases, use of vasoactive medications. The increased maternal mortality is thought to be secondary to inability of the right ventricle to meet the need for high cardiac output during pregnancy in the face of high PVR.[76]

Women may be first diagnosed with PAH (i.e. elevated PA pressure as well as elevated PVR) with no known etiology during pregnancy. This PAH has been found to persist after pregnancy.[77] Similarly, women with known mild PAH who become pregnant may have escalation of disease severity during pregnancy which persists even after the delivery.[78] Also, women with history of congenital heart disease, who are not known to have PAH and are completely asymptomatic prior to the pregnancy, may develop severe PAH with significant signs and symptoms, resulting in poor maternal and fetal outcomes.[79] There are reports of pregnancy-associated transformation of vasoreactive, well-controlled disease to non-vasoreactive disease, requiring more aggressive therapy in addition to CCBs. The underlying mechanisms for these observations are unknown. Pregnancy is listed as a possible risk factor for PAH. In one series 10 percent of women with PPH referred for transplant evaluation were diagnosed as having PPH during the third trimester of pregnancy or the first 6 months postpartum. On the other hand estrogen therapy or use of oral contraceptives is considered unlikely to be a risk factor for PAH.

Role of echocardiography in diagnosing PAH in pregnancy

Echocardiography tends to overestimate PA pressure in pregnant women with suspected PAH. Similarly, like any physiologic state with high cardiac output, in pregnancy, the PVR may still be normal, even though the PA pressure may be elevated. A retrospective study[80] of 25 pregnant women with suspected PH, who underwent echocardiography and catheterization, showed (using definition of PH as systolic PA pressure of above 30 mm Hg on catheterization) that 32 percent of women who were labeled as having PH by echocardiography did not have PH on catheterization. Discrepancy between echocardiography and catheterization estimates of systolic PA pressure is even more pronounced in patients with congenital heart disease.

PREGNANCY AND PAH DRUGS

Warfarin and bosentan are considered category X (highly unsafe), whereas prostacyclin is classified as category B (only animal data to suggest possible safety) drug for pregnancy. Warfarin is known to cause congenital defects in the fetus. Women who need to be on anticoagulation during pregnancy should be on some form of heparin, preferably low-molecular-weight heparin, as it can be self-administered by the subcutaneous route and there is no need for partial thromboplastin time monitoring. However, use of heparin for several months may be associated with increased risk of developing osteoporosis in mothers.

Bosentan is known to have severe teratogenic effects. It also decreases effectiveness of hormonal contraception, both the oral and depot forms. It is highly recommended that women on bosentan should use an effective barrier contraception in addition to the hormonal method if they are at risk to become pregnant. If pregnancy occurs while on bosentan, the woman should be advised for termination of pregnancy secondary to the teratogenic potential of bosentan alone, even if she has controlled PAH and the risk to her due to the PAH itself are considered modest.

There are several reports of completing pregnancy with the use of prostacyclin during the last trimester with no reported fetal abnormalities.[81] However, the data are limited and nonconclusive about safety for the fetus if the drug is used during the first or second trimester.

Management of pregnant women with PAH who decide against termination of pregnancy

Some women may decide to continue the pregnancy. The physician should be very clear and frank in explaining the risks so that the woman's decision is actually an informed decision. Women who have received more than a year of intravenous epoprostenol therapy and have normalized their right ventricular function are more likely to have successful completion of pregnancy.[82]

If a woman chooses to continue the pregnancy, early initiation of care with a multidisciplinary team, including obstetrician, cardiologist or pulmonologist experienced in PAH, and anesthetist, has been shown to positively impact the outcome.[83] Hospitalization as early as late second or early third trimester may be necessary. Hemodynamic monitoring during intrapartum and immediate postpartum should be done in all unstable patients. Routine use of PA catheter is considered unnecessary by many experts but is still used in many US and Western European centers. Elective induction and stable epidural anesthesia for labor and vaginal delivery should be the first choice.

There are several reports of use of epoprostenol with successful completion of pregnancy and no fetal malformation. Similarly iNO[84,85] or inhaled iloprost, and in some cases, both inhaled iloprost and intravenous epoprostenol have been used in the peripartum period.[86] However, there have been no formal controlled studies to support these observations. The successful use of emergency cardiopulmonary bypass has been reported for cesarean section in women with PAH and deteriorating status.[76]

It should be realized that pregnancy in PAH carries a risk of mortality (30–56 percent)[71,72] which is several times greater than the risk in pulmonary thromboendarterectomy (6–15 percent). Hence it is not unreasonable that these women should be managed in centers which specialize in care of PAH.

Oncology patients and pulmonary arterial hypertension

The differential diagnosis of dyspnea and hypoxemia in acutely ill oncology patients is broad, ranging from infectious etiologies to drug-related pulmonary toxicity. Peripheral edema with elevated PA pressure on echocardiography or PA catheter are not uncommon in these patients. This could be a result of left ventricle failure due to fluid overload (secondary to aggressive fluid administration, high output failure due to severe anemia or worsening of renal function), cardiac or pulmonary toxicity of chemotherapeutic agents, or myocardial infarction. Mechanical ventilation, ARDS, or any other cause of increased PA pressure can result in acute RHF.

In oncology patients a mean PA pressure above 50 mm Hg and normal or near-normal pulmonary capillary wedge pressure, in the absence of right ventricle hypertrophy and history of congenital heart disease, should always raise suspicion of pulmonary thromboembolic disease or less commonly of tumor emboli syndrome (no infiltrates on high-resolution CT), or of pulmonary venoocclusive disease (chest radiograph and high-resolution CT findings similar to those of heart failure). Pulmonary thromboembolic disease is especially common in patients with adenocarcinomas, pelvic cancers, and in bedridden patients. However, no group can be considered immune.

Patients with mediastinal tumors or tumors with mediastinal lymphadenopathy may have elevated neck veins and edema secondary to the involvement of central pulmonary veins, pericardial infiltration, or direct compression of major pulmonary vessels. A magnetic resonance (MR) image/angiogram or CT with contrast may be extremely helpful in identifying proximal pulmonary emboli and mediastinal masses. External compression of the PA may be interpreted as a filling defect and mistaken as pulmonary embolism, resulting in unnecessary treatment for pulmonary embolism and inappropriate management of malignancy due to failure to register mediastinal involvement by tumor. Rarely, tumors of the pulmonary arteries (sarcomas) may present with pulmonary hypertension. Because of the intravascular filling defects present, these are frequently initially diagnosed as pulmonary thromboembolic disease.

TUMOR MICROEMBOLI SYNDROME AND PAH IN ONCOLOGY PATIENTS

Tumor microemboli syndrome is a relatively rare diagnosis.[87] Patients usually present with a history of present malignancy, worsening dyspnea, and hypoxemia over a course of a few days or weeks, and eventually cor pulmonale and death. There are reports of occult gastric[88] and hepatocellular[89] carcinoma, in which the finding of cor pulmonale was the initial presenting feature. This diagnosis is extremely difficult to make. Workup for pulmonary embolism (spiral CT, $\dot{V}/Q$ scan, or pulmonary angiogram) is nonrevealing as the obstructing tumor emboli are in vessels too small to be visualized. As opposed to bronchoalveolar carcinoma of the lung or lymphangitic spread of cancers, the CT scan does not show any interstitial infiltrates or thickening of interlobular septae. Lung fields are typically clear on chest radiograph or CT scan. Definite diagnosis can only be made by biopsy. Transbroncheal bronchoscopic biopsy may be sufficient to make a diagnosis. However, there is significantly high risk of bleeding with transbronchial biopsy secondary to high PA pressure and frequently accompanying thrombocytopenia and coagulopathy. There are reports of the diagnosis being made on cytologic evaluation of blood aspirated from a wedged right heart catheter, but the diagnosis is most often made at autopsy.

PULMONARY VENOOCCLUSIVE DISEASE AND PAH IN ONCOLOGY PATIENTS

Pulmonary venoocclusive disease is an infrequent subtype of IPAH (PPH) with involvement of the small veins and venules and, in 50 percent of patients, concurrent involvement of the pulmonary arterioles as well. Pulmonary venoocclusive disease has been reported after mitomycin use in nonsmall cell carcinoma of lung[90] and after use of bleomycin, mitomycin, and cisplatin in carcinoma of liver.[95] Similarly, it has been described after bone marrow transplantation,[91,93] in Hodgkin lymphoma,[92] and after radiotherapy of the chest.[94] It is important to know if the patient with PAH has PVOD, as massive pulmonary edema and death may occur with IV prostacyclin therapy and such therapy should be instituted with extreme caution in such patients.

DRUG–RELATED VASCULITIS AND PAH IN ONCOLOGY PATIENTS

Use of interferon α in chronic myelogenous leukemia, malignant melanoma,[97] and metastatic renal cell carcinoma[98] has been associated with PAH with other concurrent vascular manifestations, such as Raynaud phenomenon, pulmonary vasculitis, thrombotic thrombocytopenic purpura and hemolytic uremic syndrome.[97] Such reactions have occurred after 3 months to 3 years of interferon therapy at a daily dose in the range 3–10 million units. Discontinuation of interferon and immunosuppressive treatment has resulted in complete resolution or arrested progression of these reactions.[97]

Management of acute right heart failure

The management of acute RHF demands early recognition. This is only possible if there is a high index of suspicion in appropriate clinical settings. This is extremely important, as interventions aimed at treatment of left ventricle failure may actually be detrimental for RHF. The principal goals for therapy are the same as those for any form of shock, i.e. to improve tissue oxygen delivery and minimize oxygen consumption. Similarly, the aim is to maintain adequate organ circulation to allow removal of toxic wastes and mediators by optimal volume or fluid status, and appropriate use of vasopressor and inotropic agents. An additional important variable in the case of RHF is PVR. In patients with compromised right ventricle function or in whom the PVR is significantly elevated, decreasing PVR becomes one of the most important determinant for successfully improving overall cardiac output. As most pulmonary vasodilators are also systemic vasodilators, administration of these agents by parenteral route is frequently associated with a fall in systemic blood pressure, which may be unacceptable in patients who are already compromised. Inhaled pulmonary vasodilators that have a short half-life or are extensively metabolized by the lung during the first-pass, such as iNO or inhaled prostacyclins, have been used to overcome this problem.

FLUIDS AND DIURETICS

One of the key points in understanding the management of RHF is that in many patients with elevated PVR and RHF, administration of intravenous fluids and withholding of diuretics may worsen left ventricle function by resulting in dilation of the right ventricle, further displacing the interventricular septum into the left ventricle, and thus impeding left ventricle diastolic filling. Similarly, the dilated right ventricle may be operating at a portion of the Frank–Starling curve that further fluid loading may cause only increased right-sided pressures, with further dilatation of the right ventricle and displacement of interventricular septum and no significant improvement in force of right ventricle myocardial contraction. Thus it may decrease cardiac output by impeding left ventricle diastolic filling through displacement of interventricular septum and increase in peripheral edema through elevated right-sided pressures. As many variables which ultimately determine overall cardiac output are involved, it is practically impossible, in most circumstances, to predict the impact of fluid administration unless a fluid challenge is actually given optimally during hemodynamic monitoring with a PA catheter.

In patients with hypotension and shock even with suspected elevated PVR and RHF, it is reasonable to give a fluid bolus while withholding diuretics to watch the response. Indications of impaired perfusion may be seen in systemic blood pressure, heart rate, cardiac output, mixed venous oxygen saturation (SvO_2), pulse oximetry, urine output, and blood urea nitrogen (BUN) to creatinine ratio trends. If no benefit is seen, similar trials of vasoactive drugs should be considered with or without concurrent fluid administration depending upon presence and severity of hypotension.

In the absence of significantly low systemic blood pressure but prominent peripheral edema and signs of decreased tissue perfusion in patients with severe PAH and RHF when one of the goals of treatment is achieving a negative fluid balance, fluid restriction (1200–1800 ml/day) and dietary salt restriction (no added salt diet) should be considered. Such patients often require very high doses of intravenous diuretics (sometimes as high as furoesemide 200 mg IV BID along with a potassium sparing diuretiuc such as spironolactone with or without thiazide diuretic). A reasonable approach could be to start intravenous loop diuretics at a dose which is half of the patient's routine oral dose at home and titrating upward relatively quickly depending upon the diuretic response and tolerance as evaluated primarily by systemic blood pressure, oxygen requirement and symptomatic improvement. In the situations where even with high doses of diuretics, a desired negative fluid balance is not achieved or there is a two to three fold rise in serum creatinine (or a creatinine value above 3–4 mg/dl), low dose vasoactive agents (such as dopamine 1–2 μg/Kg/min through a separate central venous access) may be used with caution (watching the effects on fluid balance, systemic blood pressure, heart rate, oxygen requirement, signs of tissue perfusion, and if available hemodynamic parameters). In such situations intravascular fluid status should be re-evaluated by appropriate means (which may involve an echocardiogram to look at the left ventricular and valvular functions, possibly of large shunts as well as assessment of intravascualr fluid status such as looking for diastolic collapse of inferior venacava. Pulmonary artery catheter can be used in selected situations; however, it is not necessary in most situations without significant and sustained haemodynamic instability that is not responsive to current therapeutic interventions. Wherever clinically relevant, other causes of rising creatinine such as drug reaction, sepsis, infection or obstructive uropathy etc. should be considered in the differential diagnosis. Vasodilators may also be used with caution in patients with left ventricle dysfunction and high systemic vascular resistance to decrease the afterload.

TRADITIONAL VASOACTIVE AGENTS

A large number of uncontrolled studies are available, both in animal models and in patients with acute RHF (with acute pulmonary embolism, ARDS, or acute right ventricle infarction), in which various vasoactive agents were used with variable success to demonstrate improved hemo-dynamics. Such studies have used inotropes (dopamine,[99] dobutamine,[100] epinephrine, isoproterenol, amrinone), vasoconstrictors (norepinephrine,[101] dopamine, phenyl-ephrine) and nonspecific vasodilators (hydralazine, nitroprusside).[102] However, controlled studies aimed at assessing survival impact are lacking due to the difficulty of designing such studies and the fact that it is practically impossible to recruit patients in numbers large enough to show survival benefit and at the same time take into account a large number of confounding variables.

SPECIFIC PULMONARY VASODILATORS IN ACUTE RHF

Inhaled pulmonary vasodilators (iNO and prostacyclins)

Nitric oxide (NO), inhaled aerosolized prostacyclin (Flolan) and inhaled aerosolized iloprost (a stable analog of prostacyclin) have been shown to decrease PVR without significantly decreasing systemic blood pressure.[103–106] Noncontrolled nitric oxide studies have demonstrated that it can improve physiologic parameters in a subset of patients with PAH and RHF with hypoxemia.[107] However, at least three large RCTs[108–113] of nitric oxide have failed to show any survival benefit for patients with ARDS. These results are contrary to three large trials of PPH of the newborn[114–116] which showed decreased need for extracorporeal membrane oxygenation with use of iNO. It can be speculated that like most trials with critically ill adult patients heterogeneity of patient population and presence of multiple comorbid conditions make it almost impossible to detect a benefit of small magnitude because of practical limitations of having a sample size large enough to perform a satisfactory multivariate analysis. No RCT has evaluated clinical impact of NO or other selective pulmonary vasodilators in acutely ill patients with PAH and acute RHF. In the short-term studies inhaled aerosolized prostacyclin (Flolan) was as effective as iloprost. Hemodynamic effects of

---

Box 13E.8 Aerosolized prostacyclin

Carefully review indications (diagnostic certainty, severely depressed cardiac index <2.5 L/min/m^2 with high PVR, failure of conventional measures, etc.) and contraindications (significant active bleeding, thrombocytopenia <50 000/mm^2, left ventricle failure)

Administration

Aerosolized 30 000 ng/mL solution, starting at the maximum dose, i.e. 50 ng/kg per minute and titrate down to minimum effective dose needed for the desired effect

Dose minimization

Initiated after 4 hours of administration. Decrease the dose by half every 15 minutes to minimum effective dose needed for clinician-defined effects or until one of the following is observed:

- 15 percent decrease in cardiac output or 20 percent increase in PVR (or 10 percent increase in PA pressure)

OR

- 10 mm Hg decrease in P_{O_2} (or >4 percent decrease in Sa_{O_2})

Monitoring response

- Record physiologic parameters every 15 minutes following dose change and every 2–4 hours thereafter
- If any change in drug dose results in ≥10 percent decrease in mean arterial pressure within 10 minutes of start of that dose, without any other attributable cause, decrease the dose by half immediately
- If any change in drug dose results in significant (as defined above) decrease in cardiac output, increase in PVR or decrease in P_{O_2}, the dose should be doubled immediately

Duration of therapy

Once the lowest effective dose is established, the drug may be continued even for several days at the same dose, until the patient's condition improves

Discontinuation

Once the patient's condition is improved the drug should be slowly weaned off while closely monitoring hemodynamics

---

inhaled prostacyclin (Flolan) last for 10–30 minutes, of inhaled iloprost for 60–120 minutes, and of iNO for 2–5 minutes. Nitric oxide and 100 percent oxygen were less potent pulmonary vascular vasodilators than inhaled prostacyclin and iloprost[117] (Box 13E.8).

Currently only inhaled nitric oxide and aerosolized prostacyclin is used in the clinical practice in the management of acute RHF. Aerosolized iloprost may have a role in management of acute RHF in future. Currently the drug delivery systems for iloprost delivery are patient specific and are programmed in a way that they can be used to administer the drug doses suitable for stable outpatients only.

Role of intravenous prostacyclin, bosentan and sildenafil in the acute care setting

Although intravenous prostacyclin has been use in clinical trials of acute care setting, this has been associated with more significant fall in systemic blood pressure compared with inhaled prostacyclin. Moreover, dose escalation cannot be done rapidly as it is limited by the appearance of significant side effects, such as flushing, headaches, diarrhea, and hypotension, with rapidly increasing dose. Hence its utility in acutely ill patients is limited. It takes several weeks

to months for bosentan to have any significant effect on hemodynamics, so it is not appropriate for and not used to treat acute RHF.

Multiple studies have shown improvement in hemodynamics in clinically stable patients with PAH after acute administration of intravenous or oral sildenafil (25–50 mg every 6–8 hours).[153] However, studies are lacking in the patients who are acutely ill with acute RHF. Currently, oral or intravenous sildenafil may be used with caution (starting at a dose 12.5 mg, once and if tolerated in terms of systemic blood pressure, oxygen requirement, and if available, hemodynamics, may be increased to 25–50 mg every 8 hours). However, there are no controlled studies available 'for or

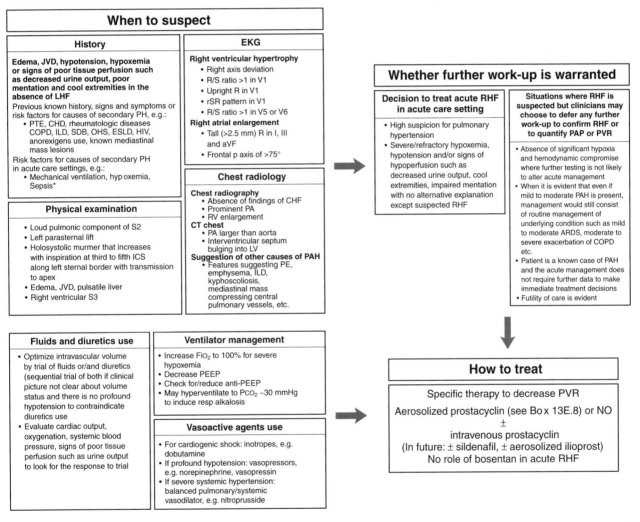

Figure 13E.3 *Management of pulmonary hypertension and acute right heart failure in acute care settings. JVD, jugular venous distension; LHF, left heart failure; secondary PH, secondary pulmonary hypertension (an old term used for pulmonary hypertension associated with identifiable cause or etiology); PTE, pulmonary thromboembolic disease; CHD, congenital heart disease; COPD, chronic obstructive pulmonary disease; ILD, interstitial lung disease; SDB, sleep disorder breathing; OHS, obesity-hypoventilation syndrome; ESLD, end-stage liver disease; HIV, human immunodeficiency virus; S2, second heart sound; ICS, intercostal space; S3, third heart sound; CHF, congestive heart failure; PA, pulmonary artery; LV, left ventricle; PE, pulmonary embolism; Fio$_2$, fractional inspired oxygen; PEEP, positive end-expiratory pressure; RHF, right heart failure; PAP, pulmonary artery pressure; PVR, pulmonary vascular resistance; PAH, pulmonary arterial hypertension; ARDS, acute respiratory distress syndrome; NO, nitric oxide; PH, pulmonary hypertension; Echo, echocardiography; RH cath, right heart catheterization; Sx, symptoms; CCB, calcium-channel blockers; IV, intravenous; SC, subcutaneous.*

Box 13E.9 Ventilator strategies in acute RHF

- High Fio_2 to maintain sufficient Pao_2 to minimize hypoxic vasoconstriction
- Minimize PEEP and auto-PEEP
- Consider hyperventilation to $Paco_2$ ~30 mm Hg to induce respiratory alkalosis
- Use of lowest possible tidal volume, sufficient to meet ventilation goals as monitored by $Paco_2$ and pH
- Vigilant and continued assessment of impact of an intervention or change and modification of strategy accordingly
- Recognize that effect of change in ventilator settings such as PEEP may be highly variable among patients

against' evaluating the safety and effectiveness of use of sildenafil in acutely ill patients with acute RHF.

If the patient is on prostacyclin or bosentan as an outpatient and is hospitalized due to an acute illness or elective surgical procedure, they should be continued on their same outpatient dose. Abrupt discontinuation of prostacyclin may result in significant hemodynamic compromise or even death. If for some reason central venous access is transiently unavailable, prostacyclin may be administered through a peripheral vein. This may cause a moderately severe local erythema and tenderness along with phlebitis and a frequent need for changing intravenous access site. Patients on bosentan who are nil by mouth for surgery or any other reason, will have to hold their bosentan as there is no parenteral form of bosentan available. The oral bosentan should be restarted as soon as possible, preferably within 12–36 hours.

VENTILATOR MANAGEMENT IN ACUTE RHF

Small changes in ventilator settings may have profound effect on cardiac output.[118] The changes are even more pronounced in patients with elevated PVR and acute RHF.[119] Positive pressure ventilation, especially with high PEEP, increases PVR, and thus causes an acute increase in afterload for the right ventricle.[120] On the other hand the venous return, which is the primary determinant of right ventricle contractility,[121] is decreased during inspiration of positive pressure ventilation. This effect is more pronounced in hypovolemic patients. The conventional belief that the PEEP decreases venous return by decreased pressure gradient between systemic circulation and right atrium has been challenged by more recent studies.[122–124] Currently the effect of change in PEEP on right ventricle function is thought to be more complex and highly variable from patient to patient[125,126] (Box 13E.9).

In patients where increased PEEP improves hypoxemia and lung compliance such as in certain ARDS patients, the increased PEEP has no deleterious effects on right ventricle function when used in an amount which was associated with improving respiratory system compliance.

In summary, practically the effect of changes in PPV settings and PEEP may vary from patient to patient depending upon underlying disease, volume status, hypoxemia, hypercarbia, and effects of ventilator-related interventions on these and on lung compliance. Hence the reasonable approach would be to attempt to keep PEEP, auto-PEEP, plateau pressure, and tidal volume to a minimum as long as these are not compromising lung compliance, alveolar ventilation, and oxygenation. Vigilant and continued assessment of the impact of the given intervention on hemodynamics and parameters of tissue perfusion in individual patients should be carried out and decisions made depending upon priorities of acute care in the individual patient (see Fig. 13E.3).

PROGNOSTIC SIGNIFICANCE OF PULMONARY ARTERIAL HYPERTENSION IN CRITICALLY ILL PATIENTS

Generally for the outpatient population, PH is associated with higher mortality compared with patients without PAH, such as in COPD, ILD, congenital heart disease, liver disease, and scleroderma. However, data are limited and sparse to confirm or negate the impact of mild to moderate PH on survival in critically ill patients with the exception of PH associated with ARDS. It has been known for a long time that the recovery of pulmonary circulation is a highly likely outcome in certain clinical situations such as correction of mitral valve disease, PA banding in congenital PH, closure of cardiac septal defects, and treatment of OHS by NIPPV or BiPAP and, in some patients by weight loss through gastric bypass surgery. It may take months to years for the vessels to restructure and PA pressure to normalize. Disease processes which result in destruction of vascular bed or pulmonary parenchyma, for example in parenchymal lung diseases such as ILD and COPD, are relatively irreversible. Nevertheless, there are reports of restoration of reversibility on acute vasoreactivity testing after long-term intravenous prostacyclin use.

OUTCOME OF CARDIOPULMONARY RESUSCITATION IN PULMONARY ARTERIAL HYPERTENSION

Outcome of cardiopulmonary resuscitation (CPR) in patients with PAH is poor. The single most important factor that appears to determine the success of CPR is the presence of an identifiable, correctable cause of cardiac arrest and its prompt correction. In a retrospective multicenter international study[152] on frequency and results of CPR in patients with PAH (3130 patients treated in participating centers between 1997 and 2002), CPR was attempted in one quarter of the patients (26 percent) who had cardiopulmonary arrests. Although 21 percent of patients had primary successful CPR, survival rates were 11 percent at 24 hours and 8 percent at day 7. Only 6 percent survived for more than 3 months. Review of hemodynamic parameters within the 3 months prior to the CPR did not reveal any significant difference between survivors and nonsurvivors. Seven out of eight survivors had a readily identifiable and correctable cause for cardiopulmonary arrest such as vasovagal reaction, digitalis toxicity, or pericardial tamponade. Thus in the absence of identifiable and correctable causes of cardiopulmonary arrest patients with PAH who need CPR rarely survive beyond 1 week without significant neurologic deficits. In the multicenter study there was no significant difference between survivors and nonsurvivors with respect to age, sex, underlying condition, and initial rhythm.

LUNG TRANSPLANTATION IN PULMONARY ARTERIAL HYPERTENSION

Lung transplantation in PAH is associated with higher mortality than is seen in other conditions. For PPH, 1, 3, and 5-year mortality is 65 percent, 55 percent, and 44 percent, respectively,[127] which is significantly higher (77 percent, 58 percent, and 44 percent, respectively for overall lung transplantation) compared with most other groups.

Decision analysis regarding listing for lung transplantation and the timing of transplant has been significantly affected by advances in the treatment of PAH in past decade.[128] Use of intravenous prostacyclin has improved median survival of PPH from 2.8 years to approximately 6 years or even more. Up to 60–70 percent of patients who were placed on the transplant list and who were on intravenous prostacyclin therapy were de-listed secondary to clinical improvement.[38,128–130] This has resulted in a decrease in the percentage of transplants performed for PPH out of total lung transplants from 12.5 percent in 1991 to 3.8 percent in 2000.[127] Recently, an assessment of the response to 3 months of prostacyclin therapy has been used to determine which patients to list immediately and which patients to defer.[44]

Higher posttransplant mortality in pulmonary arterial hypertension

Primary pulmonary hypertension and Eisenmenger syndrome have the highest perioperative mortality and lowest overall survival rates compared with any other conditions after lung transplantation.[131–133] This is thought to be primarily due to:

- complexity of the surgery including routine need for cardiopulmonary bypass[132]
- frequently encountering postoperative right ventricle dysfunction and resulting hemodynamic instability and frequent need for prolonged hemodynamic monitoring.

Mortality among patient with PPH or Eisenmenger syndrome, who survive beyond 1 month after lung transplantation, is comparable with that of other transplant recipients.[131] The presence of secondary PAH does not seem to adversely affect the outcome after single lung transplantation.[134]

CRITERIA FOR LISTING ON LUNG TRANSPLANT LIST AND TIMING OF LUNG TRANSPLANTATION

The criteria for the priority in lung transplant listing in US centers has recently been revised. The current system assigns the priority based on anticipated benefit that involves consideration of anticipated mortality without transplant and expected survival with transplant in a given patient. This comprises using a complex mathematical equation that considers a number of variables to generate a score. These variables include but are not limited to age, primary diagnosis, lung functions, functional status and concurrent co-morbid conditions. Before this revision the priority in the lung transplant list was based on seniority (time) on the list and not on the acuity of clinical need or expected magnitude of benefit. Hence most US centers were initiating the process of transplant listing without waiting to see the response to therapy. As a substantial number of PH patients improve on currently available therapies and up to 60–70% are de-listed down the road,[38] the previous system of listing and prioritizing on the list was subjecting many patients to unnecessary risk, cost and inconvenience of transplant evaluation and related testing at an inappropriate time. The current system for the assignment of priority is expected to change the practice of routine referral of all PAH patients for lung transplant evaluation regardless of the extent and severity of their disease.

Some form of exercise testing such as cardiopulmonary exercise testing or exercise testing (6-minute walk test) and echocardiography are widely used to access the functional status and to screen the patients for need for transplant

---

Box 13E.10 Criteria for lung transplant listing*

Exercise testing

- 6-minute walk distance – <332 m
- Cardiopulmonary exercise testing – VO$_2$ maximum <10 mL/kg per minute

Echocardiography

Evidence of even severe right ventricle dysfunction is not an indication of heart-lung transplantation instead of lung transplantation

*Criteria vary from center to center and many centers use a subset of these parameters

listing. About 40 percent of centers use one or more hemodynamic criteria such as right atrial pressure above 15 mm Hg, PVR 4–15 Wood units, SvO_2 below 63 percent, cardiac index below 2 L/min/m². Cardiopulmonary exercise testing is used in 26 percent of centers with a peak oxygen consumption less than 10 mL/kg/min as cut-off for transplant listing (Box 13E.10).

CHOICE OF PROCEDURE FOR LUNG TRANSPLANT

Single, bilateral or heart-lung transplants have been used for patients with PAH.[136–138] No prospective randomized studies are available to support the current practice regarding the choice of procedure for lung transplantation. Patients with PAH do not require heart-lung transplant if there is no significant left ventricular problem in addition to cor pulmonale. Severe right ventricle dysfunction has been found to be reversible after isolated lung transplantation.[139–144] Hence even severe right ventricle dysfunction and cor pulmonale is not an indication for heart-lung transplantation instead of lung transplantation alone.

Contrary to early impressions,[142,144,147,148] more recent reports[140,145,146,149] indicate that there is no difference in median duration of intubation; length of stay in the intensive care unit; hospital stay; 1-month, 12-month, and 4-year survival; and ultimate late functional status in single versus bilateral lung transplantation for most indications. Other recent reports suggest that bilateral lung transplant may be superior for IPAH but there is no difference in outcome between single and bilateral lung transplantation for secondary pulmonary hypertension.[150,151] Hence, currently, there is no universal agreement on the choice of procedure. At present the choice of type of procedure is largely determined by the experience and preference of local teams as well as local donor situation. The choice is made between single or bilateral transplantation. Heart-lung transplantation is rarely necessary. Details of indications and choice of various surgical procedures for congenital heart diseases and thromboendarterectomy for persistent proximal pulmonary emboli is beyond the scope of this chapter.

Key learning points

- The normal pulmonary circulation is a low-resistance and high-compliance system.

- The hallmark of PAH is elevated PVR, which results in increased workload for right ventricle and eventually RHF if left untreated.

- There is paucity of data regarding PH and RHF in the acute care setting. Extreme caution should be observed while extrapolating the results of studies of PH in the outpatient population to PH and RHF in acute care settings.

- Right heart failure should be a part of differential diagnosis of hypotension, hypoxemia or shock especially when accompanying peripheral edema and raised jugular venous pressure that is not fully explained by left ventricle failure.

- Mild to moderate PAH can be caused by factors such as hypoxemia, ARDS, mechanical ventilation and perhaps sepsis. The clinical significance of such PAH remains unknown.

- Pregnancy in patients with moderate to severe pulmonary hypertension is associated with extremely high maternal mortality (30–56 percent), acceleration of disease progression in many survivors as well as increased fetal risk. Effective contraception, and, in the event of contraception failure, termination of pregnancy should be strongly recommended.

- PH is a relatively underrecognized cause of hypoxemia and dyspnea in oncology patients. In addition to echocardiography, CT of the chest to evaluate lung parenchyma, as well as to rule out pulmonary embolism and any mediastinal compression, may be valuable in such cases.

- When patients with known PAH present to acute care settings for a reason unrelated to PH, their outpatient PH medications (prostacyclin and bosentan) should be continued in the same doses without interruption. An interruption in IV prostacyclin for more than a few minutes may be fatal. Bosentan can be held if patient is nil by mouth; however, it should be restarted as soon as possible (within 24–36 hours).

- Management of acute RHF comprises at least two immensely important decisions: (i) whether further workup of PH will have any impact on acute management, and (ii) if PH requires acute management, whether conventional management will suffice, or specific pulmonary vasodilator treatment (e.g. inhaled prostacyclin or nitric oxide) is needed.

- There is no evidence to support routine use of PA catheterization in patients with PH or acute RHF presenting to acute care settings.

- Hypoxia, acidosis, hypercapnia, high PEEP, sudden large volume changes in a PAH patient who is currently hemodynamically stable, should be avoided.

- Modern therapy has significantly decreased the lung transplant requirement in patients with PAH. As the current criteria for lung transplant list priority depends solely upon seniority in the list and not on the acuity of need or projected magnitude of benefit, most US centers refer all the patients with moderate to severe PAH to lung transplantation programs.

- In the absence of a readily identifiable reversible cause of cardiopulmonary arrest in PH patients, CPR is unlikely to yield any meaningful outcome.

REFERENCES

✱ 1. Rich S, Rubin LJ, Abenhaim L, *et al.* Executive summary from the World Symposium on Primary Pulmonary Hypertension. Evian, France, September 6–10, 1998. Geneva: World Health Organization, 1998.

✱ 2. Rich S, Dantzker DR, Ayres SM, *et al.* Primary pulmonary hypertension. A national prospective study. *Ann Intern Med* 1987; **107**: 216–23.

3. Delcroix M, *et al.* Pulmonary arterial hypertension: genetics, reversibility testing and follow-up. *European Respiratory Monograph on Pulmonary Vascular Pathology: A Clinical Update.* 9: 33–56, Monograph 27, January 2004.Publisher.

4. Goodale F, Jr, Thomas WA. Primary pulmonary arterial disease; observations with special reference to medial thickening of small arteries and arterioles. *AMA Arch Pathol* 1954; **58**: 568–75.

✱ 5. Hatano S, Strasser T, *et al. World Health Organization: Primary Pulmonary Hypertension. Report on a WHO meeting.* Geneva: World Health Organization, 1975.

6. Chapman DW, Abbot JP, Latson J. Primary pulmonary hypertension: Review of literature and results of cardiac catheterization in ten patients. *Circulation* 1957; **12**: 35–46.

7. Yu PN. Primary pulmonary hypertension. *Ann Intern Med* 1958; **49**: 1138–61.

8. Walcott G, Burchell HB, Brown AL. Primary pulmonary hypertension. *Am J Med* 1970; **49**: 70–9.

9. D'Alonzo G, Barst RJ, Ayres SM, *et al.* Survival in patients with primary pulmonary hypertension. *Ann Intern Med* 1991; **115**: 343–9.

10. McGoon MD. The assessment of pulmonary hypertension. *Clin Chest Med* 2001; **22**: 493–508.

11. Hinderliter AL, Willis PW, Barst RJ, *et al.* Effects of long term infusion of prostacyclin (epoprostenol) on echocardiographic measures of right ventricular structure and function in primary pulmonary hypertension. *Circulation* 1997; **95**: 1479–86.

12. Galie N, Hinderliter AL, Torbicki A, *et al.* Effects of the oral endothelin receptor antagonist Bosentan on echocardiographic and Doppler measures in patients with pulmonary arterial hypertension. *J Am Coll Cardiol* 2002; **39**: 224A.

13. Sun XG, Hansen JE, Oudiz RJ, Wasserman K. Exercise pathophysiology in patients with primary pulmonary hypertension. *Circulation* 2001; **104**: 429–35.

14. Raeside DA, Smith A, Brown A, *et al.* Pulmonary artery pressure measurement during exercise testing in patients with suspected pulmonary hypertension. *Eur Respir J* 2000; **16**: 282–7.

15. Wax D, Garofano R, Barst RJ. Effects of long-term infusion of prostacyclin on exercise performance in patients with primary pulmonary hypertension. *Chest* 1999; **116**: 914–20.

16. Wensel R, Opitz CF, Anker SD, *et al.* Assessment of survival in patients with primary pulmonary hypertension: importance of cardiopulmonary exercise testing. *Circulation* 2002; **106**: 319–24.

17. Miyamoto S, Nagaya N, Satoh T, *et al.* Clinical correlates and prognostic significance of six-minute walk test in patients with primary pulmonary hypertension. Comparison with cardiopulmonary exercise testing. *Am J Respir Crit Care Med* 2000; **161**: 487–92.

18. Palevsky HI, Schloo BL, Pietra GG, *et al.* Primary pulmonary hypertension. Vascular structure, morphometry, and responsiveness to vasodilator agents. *Circulation* 1989; **80**: 1207–21.

19. Raffy O, Azarian R, Brenot F, *et al.* Clinical significance of the pulmonary vasodilator response during short-term infusion of prostacyclin in primary pulmonary hypertension. *Circulation* 1996; **93**: 484–8.

● 20. Sitbon O, Humbert M, Jagot JL, *et al.* Inhaled nitric oxide as a screening agent for safely identifying responders to oral calcium-channel blockers in primary pulmonary hypertension. *Eur Respir J* 1998; **12**: 265–70.

21. Ricciardi MJ, Knight BP, Martinez FJ, Rubenfire M. Inhaled nitric oxide in primary pulmonary hypertension: a safe and effective agent for predicting response to nifedipine. *J Am Coll Cardiol* 1998; **32**: 1068–73.

22. Palevsky HI, Long W, Crow J, Fishman AP. Prostacyclin and acetylcholine as screening agents for acute pulmonary vasodilator responsiveness in primary pulmonary hypertension. *Circulation* 1990; **82**: 2018–26.

23. Rubin LJ, Groves BM, Reeves JT, *et al.* Prostacyclin-induced acute pulmonary vasodilation in primary pulmonary hypertension. *Circulation* 1982; **66**: 334–8.

24. Morgan JM, McCormack DG, Griffiths MJ, *et al.* Adenosine as a vasodilator in primary pulmonary hypertension. *Circulation* 1991; **84**: 1145–9.

25. Nootens M, Schrader B, Kaufmann E, *et al.*

Comparative acute effects of adenosine and prostacyclin in primary pulmonary hypertension. *Chest* 1995; **107**: 54–7.

26. Schrader BJ, Inbar S, Kaufmann L, *et al.* Comparison of the effects of adenosine and nifedipine in pulmonary hypertension. *J Am Coll Cardiol* 1992; **19**: 1060–4.

27. Sitbon O, Brenot F, Denjean A, *et al.* Inhaled nitric oxide as a screening vasodilator agent in primary pulmonary hypertension. A dose-response study and comparison with prostacyclin. *Am J Respir Crit Care Med* 1995; **151**: 384–9.

28. Jolliet P, Bulpa P, Thorens JB, *et al.* Nitric oxide and prostacyclin as test agents of vasoreactivity in severe precapillary pulmonary hypertension: predictive ability and consequences on haemodynamics and gas exchange. *Thorax* 1997; **52**: 369–72.

29. Ziesche R, Petkov V, Wittmann K, *et al.* Treatment with epoprostenol reverts nitric oxide non-responsiveness in patients with primary pulmonary hypertension. *Heart* 2000; **83**: 406–9.

30. Rich S. Seidlitz M. Dodin E, *et al.* The short-term effects of digoxin in patients with right ventricular dysfunction from pulmonary hypertension. *Chest* 1998; **114**: 787–92.

31. Rubin LJ, Mendoza J, Hood M, *et al.* Treatment of primary pulmonary hypertension with continuous intravenous prostacyclin (epoprostenol). Results of a randomized trial. *Ann Intern Med* 1990; **112**: 485–91.

32. Badesch DB, Tapson VF, McGoon MD, *et al.* Continuous intravenous epoprostenol for pulmonary hypertension due to the scleroderma spectrum of disease. A randomized, controlled trial. *Ann Intern Med* 2000; **132**: 425–34.

33. Channick RN, Simonneau G, Sitbon O, *et al.* Effects of the dual endothelin-receptor antagonist bosentan in patients with pulmonary hypertension: a randomised placebo-controlled study. *Lancet* 2001; **358**: 1119–23.

34. Rubin LJ, Badesch DB, Barst RJ, *et al.* Bosentan therapy for pulmonary arterial hypertension. *N Engl J Med* 2002; **346**: 896–903.

35. Simonneau G, Barst RJ, Galie N, *et al.* Treprostinil Study Group. Continuous subcutaneous infusion of treprostinil, a prostacyclin analogue, in patients with pulmonary arterial hypertension: a double-blind, randomized, placebo-controlled trial. *Am J Respir Crit Care Med* 2002; **165**: 800–4.

36. Hoeper MM, Schwarze M, Ehlerding S, *et al.* Long-term treatment of primary pulmonary hypertension with aerosolized iloprost, a prostacyclin analogue. *N Engl J Med* 2000; **342**: 1866–70.

37. Barst RJ, Rubin LJ, McGoon MD, *et al.* Survival in primary pulmonary hypertension with long-term continuous intravenous prostacyclin. *Ann Intern Med* 1994; **121**: 409–15.

38. Robbins IM, Christman BW, Newman JH, *et al.* A survey of diagnostic practices and the use of epoprostenol in patients with primary pulmonary hypertension. *Chest* 1998; **114**: 1269–75.

39. Castelain V, Chemla D, Humbert M, *et al.* Pulmonary artery pressure-flow relations after prostacyclin in primary pulmonary hypertension. *Am J Respir Crit Care Med* 2002; **165**: 338–40.

40. McLaughlin VV, Genthner DE, Panella MM, *et al.* Compassionate use of continuous prostacyclin in the management of secondary hypertension: a case series. *Ann Intern Med* 1999; **130**: 740–3.

41. Kuo PC, Johnson LB, Plotkin JS, *et al.* Continuous intravenous infusion of epoprostenol for the treatment of portopulmonary hypertension. *Transplantation* 1997; **63**: 604–6.

42. Aguilar RV, Farber HW. Epoprostenol (prostacyclin) therapy in HIV-associated pulmonary hypertension. *Am J Respir Crit Care Med* 2000; **162**: 1846–50.

43. Higenbottam T, Butt AY, McMahon A, *et al.* Long-term intravenous prostaglandin (epoprostenol or iloprost) for treatment of severe pulmonary hypertension. *Heart* 1998; **80**: 151–5.

44. Sitbon O, Humbert M, Nunes H, *et al.* Long-term intravenous epoprostenol infusion in primary pulmonary hypertension: prognostic factors and survival. *J Am Coll Cardiol* 2002; **40**: 780–8.

45. McLaughlin VV, Shillington A, Rich S. Survival in primary pulmonary hypertension: the impact of epoprostenol therapy. *Circulation* 2002; **106**: 1477–82.

46. Rich S, McLaughlin VV. The effects of chronic prostacyclin therapy on cardiac output and symptoms in primary pulmonary hypertension. *J Am Coll Cardiol* 1999; **34**: 1184–7.

47. Barst RJ, Rubin LJ, Long WA, *et al.* A comparison of continuous intravenous epoprostenol (prostacyclin) with conventional therapy for primary pulmonary hypertension. *N Engl J Med* 1996; **334**: 296–301.

48. Vachiery JL, Hill N, Zwicke D, *et al.* Transitioning from IV epoprostenol to subcutaneous treprostinil in pulmonary arterial hypertension. *Chest* 2002; **121**: 1561–5.

49. Opitz CF, Wensel R, Winkler J, *et al.* Clinical efficacy and survival with first-line inhaled iloprost therapy in patients with idiopathic pulmonary arterial hypertension. *Eur Heart Journal* 2005; **26**: 1895–902.

50. Olschewski H, Ghofrani HA, Schmehl T, *et al.* Inhaled iloprost to treat severe pulmonary hypertension. An uncontrolled trial. German PPH Study Group. *Ann Intern Med* 2000; **132**: 435–43.

51. Olschewski H, Simonneau G, Galie N, *et al.* Inhaled iloprost for severe pulmonary hypertension. *N Engl J Med* 2002; **347**: 322–9.

52. Wilkens H, Guth A, König J, *et al.* Effect of inhaled iloprost plus oral sildenafil in patients with primary pulmonary hypertension. *Circulation* 2001; **104**: 1218–22.

53. Ghofrani HA, Wiedemann R, Rose F, *et al.* Combination therapy with oral sildenafil and inhaled iloprost for severe pulmonary hypertension. *Ann Intern Med* 2002; **136**: 515–22.

54. Petkov V, Ziesche R, Mosgoeller W, *et al.* Aerosolised iloprost improves pulmonary hemodynamics in patients with primary pulmonary hypertension receiving continuous epoprostenol treatment. *Thorax* 2001; **56**: 734–6.

55. Nagaya N, Uematsu M, Okano Y, *et al.* Effect of orally active prostacyclin analogue on survival of outpatients with primary pulmonary hypertension. *J Am Coll Cardiol* 1999; **34**: 1188–92.

56. Vizza CD, Sciomer S, Morelli S, *et al.* Long term treatment of pulmonary arterial hypertension with beraprost, an oral prostacyclin analogue. *Heart* 2001; **86**: 661–5.

57. Barst RJ, Rich S, Widlitz A, Horn EM, *et al.* Clinical efficacy of sitaxsentan, an endothelin-A receptor antagonist, in patients with pulmonary arterial hypertension: open-label pilot study. *Chest* 2002; **121**: 1860–8.

58. Higenbottam T, Wheeldon D, Wells F, Wallwork J. Long-term treatment of primary pulmonary hypertension with continuous intravenous epoprostenol (prostacyclin). *Lancet* 1984; **1**: 1046–7.

59. Butler J, Chomsky DB, Davis SF, Wilson JR. Prevalence of pulmonary hypertension in patients with chronic heart failure. *Circulation.* 1997; **96**(8 Suppl): 321-I.

60. Zapol WA, Snider MT. Pulmonary hypertension in severe acute respiratory failure. *N Engl J Med* 1977; **296**: 476.

61. Dehring DJ, Fader RC, Traber LD, Traber DL. Cardiopulmonary changes occurring with pulmonary intravascular clearance of live bacteria in sheep. *Circ Shock* 1989; **29**: 245–56.

62. Reuse C, Frank N, Contempre B, Vincent JL. Right ventricular function in septic shock. *Intensive Care Med* 1988; **14** (Suppl 2): 486–7.

63. Civetta JM, Taylor RW, Kirby RR. *Critical Care*, 3rd ed. Philadelphia: Lippincott Williams and Wilkins, 1997.

64. Barbera JA, Peinado VI, Santos S. Pulmonary hypertension in chronic obstructive pulmonary disease. *Eur Respir J* 2003; **21**: 892–905.

65. Bishop JM. Role of hypoxia in the pulmonary hypertension of chronic bronchitis and emphysema. *Scand J Respir Dis Suppl* 1971; **77**: 61–5.

66. Dallari R, Barozzi G, Pinelli G, *et al.* Predictors of survival in subjects with chronic obstructive pulmonary disease treated with long-term oxygen therapy. *Respiration* 1994; **61**: 8–13.

67. Nocturnal Oxygen Therapy Trial Group. Continuous or nocturnal oxygen therapy in hypoxemic chronic obstructive lung disease: a clinical trial. *Ann Intern Med* 1980; **93**: 391–8.

68. Report of the Medical Research Council Working Party. Long term domiciliary oxygen therapy in chronic hypoxic cor pulmonale complicating chronic bronchitis and emphysema. *Lancet* 1981; **1**: 681–6.

69. Weitzenblum E, Apprill M, Oswald M, *et al.* Pulmonary hemodynamics in patients with chronic obstructive pulmonary disease before and during an episode of peripheral edema. *Chest* 1994; **105**: 1377–82.

70. Weitzenblum E, Sautegeau A, Ehrhart M, *et al.* Long-term oxygen therapy can reverse the progression of pulmonary hypertension in patients with chronic obstructive pulmonary disease. *Am Rev Respir Dis* 1985; **131**: 493–8.

71. McCaffrey RN, Dunn LJ. Primary pulmonary hypertension in pregnancy. *Obstet Gynecol Surv* 1964; **19**: 567–91.

72. Weiss BM, Zemp L, Seifert B, Hess OM. Outcome of pulmonary vascular disease in pregnancy: a systematic overview from 1978 through 1996. *J Am Coll Cardiol* 1998; **31**: 1650–7.

73. Elkayam, U, Dave, R, Bokhari. Primary pulmonary hypertension and pregnancy. In: Elkayam, U Gleicher, N eds. *Cardiac Problems in Pregnancy*. New York: Wiley-Liss, 183–90.

74. Penning S, Thomas N, Atwal D, *et al.* Cardiopulmonary bypass support for emergency

cesarean delivery in a patient with severe pulmonary hypertension. *Am J Obstet Gynecol* 2001; **184**: 225–6.

75. Ueland K. Pregnancy and cardiovascular disease. *Med Clin North Am* 1977; **61**: 17–41.

76. Weiss BM, Hess OM. Pulmonary vascular disease and pregnancy: current controversies, management strategies, and perspectives. *Eur Heart J* 2000; **21**: 104–115.

77. Takeuchi K, Yokota H, Moriyama T, *et al.* Two cases of primary pulmonary hypertension diagnosed during pregnancy. *J Perinat Med* 1998; **26**: 248–51.

78. Tampakoudis P, Grimbizis G, Chatzinicolaou K, Mantalenakis S. Successful pregnancy in a patient with severe pulmonary hypertension. *Gynecol Obstet Invest* 1996; **42**: 63–5.

79. Jackson GM, Dildy GA, Varner MW, Clark SL. Severe pulmonary hypertension in pregnancy following successful repair of ventricular septal defect in childhood. *Obstet Gynecol* 1993; **82** (4 Pt 2 Suppl): 680–2.

80. Kiss Z, Galuska L, Timar S. Multiplane transesophageal echocardiographic detection and differential diagnosis of isolated right pulmonary artery agenesis. *Echocardiography* 1996; **13**: 411–14.

81. Badalian SS, Silverman RK, Aubry RH, Longo J. Twin pregnancy in a woman on long-term epoprostenol therapy for primary pulmonary hypertension. A case report. *J Reprod Med* 2000; **45**: 149–52.

82. Easterling TR, Ralph DD, Schmucker BC. Pulmonary hypertension in pregnancy: treatment with pulmonary vasodilators. *Obstet Gynecol* 1999; **93**: 494–8.

83. Smedstad KG, Cramb R, Morison DH. Pulmonary hypertension and pregnancy: a series of eight cases. *Can J Anaesth* 1994; **41**: 502–12.

84. Lam GK, Stafford RE, Thorp J, *et al.* Inhaled nitric oxide for primary pulmonary hypertension in pregnancy. *Obstet Gynecol* 2001; **98** (5 Pt 2): 895–8.

85. Decoene C, Bourzoufi K, Moreau D, *et al.* Use of inhaled nitric oxide for emergency Cesarean section in a woman with unexpected primary pulmonary hypertension. *Can J Anaesth* 2001; **48**: 584–7.

86. Monnery L, Nanson J, Charlton G. Primary pulmonary hypertension in pregnancy; a role for novel vasodilators. *Br J Anaesth* 2001; **87**: 295–8.

87. Roberts KE, Hamele-Bena D, Saqi A, *et al.* Pulmonary tumor embolism: a review of the literature. *Am J Med* 2003; **115**: 228–32.

88. Matsuda H, Chida K, Miwa S, *et al.* An autopsy case of cor pulmonale due to a pulmonary tumor embolism as the first clinical manifestation of occult gastric cancer. *Nihon Kokyuki Gakkai Zasshi* 2002; **40**: 910–14.

89. Gutierrez-Macias A, Barandiaran KE, Ercoreca FJ, De Zarate MM. Acute cor pulmonale due to microscopic tumour embolism as the first manifestation of hepatocellular carcinoma. *Eur J Gastroenterol Hepatol* 2002; **14**: 775–7.

90. Gagnadoux F, Capron F, Lebeau B. Pulmonary veno-occlusive disease after neoadjuvant mitomycin chemotherapy and surgery for lung carcinoma. *Lung Cancer* 2002; **36**: 213–15.

91. Williams LM, Fussell S, Veith RW, *et al.* Pulmonary veno-occlusive disease in an adult following bone marrow transplantation. Case report and review of the literature. *Chest* 1996; **109**: 1388–91.

92. Swift GL, Gibbs A, Campbell IA, *et al.* Pulmonary veno-occlusive disease and Hodgkin's lymphoma. *Eur Respir J* 1993; **6**: 596–8.

93. Salzman D, Adkins DR, Craig F, *et al.* Malignancy-associated pulmonary veno-occlusive disease: report of a case following autologous bone marrow transplantation and review. *Bone Marrow Transplant* 1996; **18**: 755–60.

94. Kramer MR, Estenne M, Berkman N, *et al.* Radiation-induced pulmonary veno-occlusive disease. *Chest* 1993; **104**: 1282–4.

95. Joselson R, Warnock M. Pulmonary veno-occlusive disease after chemotherapy. *Hum Pathol* 1983; **14**: 88–91.

96. Palmer SM, Robinson LJ, Wang A, *et al.* Massive pulmonary edema and death after prostacyclin infusion in a patient with pulmonary veno-occlusive disease. *Chest* 1998; **113**: 237–40.

97. Al-Zahrani H, Gupta V, Minden MD, *et al.* Vascular events associated with alpha interferon therapy. *Leuk Lymphoma* 2003; **44**: 471–5.

98. Kramers C, de Mulder PH, Barth JD, Wagener DJ. Acute right ventricular heart failure in a patient with renal cell carcinoma after interferon therapy. *Neth J Med* 1993; **42**: 65–8.

● 99. Holloway EL, Polumbo RA, Harrison DC. Acute circulatory effects of dopamine in patients with pulmonary hypertension. *Br Heart J* 1975; **37**: 482–5.

100. Dell'Italia LJ, Starling MR, Blumhardt R, *et al.* Comparative effects of volume loading, dobutamine and nitroprusside in patients with predominant right ventricular infarction. *Circulation* 1985; **72**: 1327.

101. Molloy WD, Lee KY, Girling L, *et al.* Treatment of shock in canine model of pulmonary embolism. *Am Rev Respir Dis* 1984; **130**: 870.

102. Cockrill BA, Kacmarek RM, Fifer MA, *et al.* Comparison of the effects of nitric oxide, nitroprusside, and nifedipine on hemodynamics and right ventricular contractility in patients with chronic pulmonary hypertension. *Chest* 2001; **119**: 128–36.

103. Pepke-Zaba J, Higenbottam TW, Dinh-Xuan AT, *et al.* Inhaled nitric oxide as a cause of selective pulmonary vasodilatation in pulmonary hypertension. *Lancet* 1991; **338**: 1173–4.

104. Opitz CF, Wensel R, Bettmann M, *et al.* Assessment of the vasodilator response in primary pulmonary hypertension: comparing prostacyclin and iloprost administered by either infusion or inhalation. *Eur Heart J* 2003; **24**: 356–65.

105. Haraldsson A, Kieler-Jensen N, Nathorst-Westfelt U, *et al.* Comparison of inhaled nitric oxide and inhaled aerosolized prostacyclin in the evaluation of heart transplant candidates with elevated pulmonary vascular resistance. *Chest* 1998; **114**: 780–6.

106. Hoeper MM, Olschewski H, Ghofrani HA, *et al.* A comparison of the acute hemodynamic effects of inhaled nitric oxide and aerosolized iloprost in primary pulmonary hypertension. German PPH study group. *J Am Coll Cardiol* 2000; **35**: 176–82.

107. Frostell CG, Blomqvist H, Hedenstierna G, *et al.* Inhaled nitric oxide selectively reverses human hypoxic pulmonary vasoconstriction without causing systemic vasodilation. *Anesthesiology* 1993; **78**: 427–35.

108. Girard C, Lehot JJ, Pannetier JC, *et al.* Inhaled nitric oxide after mitral valve replacement in patients with chronic pulmonary artery hypertension. *Anesthesiology* 1992; **77**: 880–3.

109. Rossaint R, Falke KJ, Lopez F, *et al.* Inhaled nitric oxide for the adult respiratory distress syndrome. *N Engl J Med* 1993; **328**: 399–405.

110. Sokol J, Jacobs SE, Bohn D. Inhaled nitric oxide for acute hypoxemic respiratory failure in children and adults. *Cochrane Database Syst Rev* 2003:CD002787.

111. Dellinger RP, Zimmerman JL, Taylor RW, *et al.* Effects of inhaled nitric oxide in patients with acute respiratory distress syndrome: results of a randomized phase II trial. Inhaled Nitric Oxide in ARDS Study group. *Crit Care Med* 1998; **26**: 15–23.

112. Lundin S, Mang H, Smithies M, *et al.* Inhalation of nitric oxide in acute lung injury: results of a European multicentre study. *Intensive Care Med* 1999; **25**: 911–19.

113. Payen D, Vallet B. Results of the French prospective multicentric randomized double blind placebo controlled trial on inhaled nitric oxide in ARDS *Intensive Care Med* 1999; **25**: S166.

114. Roberts J, Jr, Fineman JR, Morin FR, *et al.* Inhaled nitric oxide and persistent pulmonary hypertension of the newborn. The Inhaled Nitric Oxide Study group. *N Engl J Med* 1997; **336**: 605–10.

115. Wessel DL, Adatia I, Van Marter LJ, *et al.* Improved oxygenation in a randomized trial of inhaled nitric oxide for persistent pulmonary hypertension of the newborn. *Pediatrics* 1997; **100**: E7.

116. The Neonatal Inhaled Nitric Oxide Study Group. Inhaled nitric oxide in full-term and nearly full-term infants with hypoxic respiratory failure. *N Engl J Med* 1997; **336**: 597–604.

117. Olschewski H, Walmrath D, Schermuly R, *et al.* Aerosolized prostacyclin and iloprost in severe pulmonary hypertension. *Ann Intern Med* 1996; **124**: 820–4.

118. Pinsky MR. The effects of mechanical ventilation on the cardiovascular system. *Crit Care Clin* 1990; **6**: 663–78.

119. Versprille A. The pulmonary circulation during mechanical ventilation. *Acta Anaesthesiol Scand Suppl* 1990; **94**: 51–62.

120. Pick RA, Handler JB, Murata GH, Friedman AS. The cardiovascular effect of positive end-expiratory pressure. *Chest* 1982; **82**: 345–50.

121. Biondi JW, Schulman DS, Wiedemann HP, Matthay RA. Mechanical heart-lung interaction in the adult respiratory distress syndrome. *Clin Chest Med* 1990; **11**: 691–714.

122. Fessler HE, Brower RG, Wise RA, Permutt S. Effects of positive end-expiratory pressure on the gradient for venous return. *Am Rev Respir Dis.* 1991; **143**: 19–24.

123. Jellinek H, Krenn H, Oczenski W, *et al.* Influence of positive airway pressure on the pressure gradient for venous return in humans. *J Appl Physiol* 2000; **88**: 926–32.

124. Van den Berg PC, Jansen JR, Pinsky MR. Effect of positive pressure on venous return in volume-loaded cardiac surgical patients. *J Appl Physiol* 2002; **92**: 1223–31.

125. Jardin F, Brun-Ney D, Hardy A, *et al.* Combined thermodilution and two-dimensional

echocardiographic evaluation of right ventricular function during respiratory support with PEEP. *Chest* 1991; **99**: 162–8.

126. Pinsky MR, Desmet JM, Vincent JL. Effect of positive end-expiratory pressure on right ventricular function in humans. *Am Rev Respir Dis* 1992; **146**: 681–7.

127. United Network for Organ Sharing. *US scientific registry for transplant recipients and the organ procurement and transplantation network: transplant data: 1990–2000. Annual report.* Washington, DC: US Department of Health and Human Services, 2002.

● 128. Conte JV, Gaine SP, Orens JB, *et al.* The influence of continuous intravenous prostacyclin therapy for primary pulmonary hypertension on the timing and outcome of transplantation. *J Heart Lung Transplant* 1998; **17**: 679–85.

129. Hoeper MM, Markevych I, Spiekerkoetter E, Welte T, Niedermeyer J. Goal-oriented treatment and combination therapy for pulmonary arterial hypertension. *Eur Heart J* 2005; **26**(5): 858–63.

130. Lipson DA, Edelman JD, Palewsky HI. Alternatives to lung transportation: lung volume reduction surgery and continuous prostacyclin. *Transplant Proc* 2002; **34**(4): 1283–6.

131. The US Organ Procurement and Transplantation Network and the Scientific Registry of Transplant Recipients. http://www.ustransplant.org Last accessed: April 31, 2006.

132. Bando K, Keenan RJ, Paradis IL, *et al.* Impact of pulmonary hypertension on outcome after single-lung transplantation. *Ann Thorac Surg* 1994; **58**: 1336–42.

133. Aeba R, Griffith BP, Kormos RL, *et al.* Effect of cardiopulmonary bypass on early graft dysfunction in clinical lung transplantation. *Ann Thorac Surg* 1994; **57**: 715–22.

134. Huerd SS, Hodges TN, Grover FL, *et al.* Secondary pulmonary hypertension does not adversely affect outcome after single lung transplantation. *J Thorac Cardiovasc Surg* 2000; **119**: 458–65.

135. Sitbon O, Humbert M, Nunes H, *et al.* Long-term intravenous epoprostenol infusion in primary pulmonary hypertension: prognostic factors and survival. *J Am Coll Cardiol* 2002; **40**: 780–8.

136. Glanville AR, Burke CM, Theodore J, Robin ED. Primary pulmonary hypertension. Length of survival in patients referred for heart-lung transplantation. *Chest* 1987; **91**: 675–81.

137. Reitz BA, Wallwork JL, Hunt SA, *et al.* Heart-lung transplantation: successful therapy for patients with pulmonary vascular disease. *N Engl J Med* 1982; **306**: 557–64.

138. Pielsticker EJ, Martinez FJ, Rubenfire M. Lung and heart-lung transplant practice patterns in pulmonary hypertension centers. *J Heart Lung Transplant* 2001; **20**: 1297–304.

139. Bando K, Armitage JM, Paradis IL, *et al.* Indications for and results of single, bilateral, and heart-lung transplantation for pulmonary hypertension. *J Thorac Cardiovasc Surg* 1994; **108**: 1056–65.

140. Kramer MR, Valantine HA, Marshall SE, *et al.* Recovery of the right ventricle after single-lung transplantation in pulmonary hypertension. *Am J Cardiol* 1994; **73**: 494–500.

141. Pasque MK, Trulock EP, Cooper JD, *et al.* Single lung transplantation for pulmonary hypertension: Single institution experience in 34 patients. *Circulation* 1995; **92**: 2252–8.

142. Pasque MK, Trulock EP, Kaiser LR, *et al.* Single-lung transplantation for pulmonary hypertension: Three-month hemodynamic follow-up. *Circulation* 1991; **84**: 2275–9.

143. Ritchie M, Waggoner AD, Davila-Roman VG, *et al.* Echocardiographic characterization of the improvement in right ventricular function in patients with severe pulmonary hypertension after single-lung transplantation. *J Am Coll Cardiol* 1993; **22**: 1170–4.

144. Kramer MR, Valantine HA, Marshall SE, *et al.* Recovery of the right ventricle after single-lung transplantation in pulmonary hypertension *Am J Cardiol* 1994; **73**: 494–500.

145. Bando K, Armitage JM, Paradis IL, *et al.* Indications for and results of single, bilateral, and heart-lung transplantation for pulmonary hypertension. *J Thorac Cardiovasc Surg* 1994; **108**: 1056–65.

146. Bando K, Keenan RJ, Paradis IL, *et al.* Impact of pulmonary hypertension on outcome after single-lung transplantation. *Ann Thorac Surg* 1994; **58**: 1336–42.

147. Levine SM, Gibbons WJ, Bryan CL, *et al.* Single lung transplantation for primary pulmonary hypertension *Chest* 1990; **98**: 1107–15.

148. McCarthy PM, Rosenkranz ER, White RD, *et al.* Single-lung transplantation with atrial septal defect repair for Eisenmenger's syndrome. *Ann Thorac Surg* 1991; **52**: 300–3.

149. Gammie JS, Keenan RJ, Pham SM, *et al.* Single- *versus* double-lung transplantation for pulmonary hypertension. *J Thorac Cardiovasc Surg* 1998; **115**: 397–402.

150. Conte JV, Borja MJ, Patel CB, *et al.* Lung transplantation for primary and secondary pulmonary hypertension. *Ann Thorac Surg* 2001; **72**: 1673–9.

151. Mendeloff EN, Meyers BF, Sundt TM, *et al.* Lung transplantation for pulmonary vascular disease. *Ann Thorac Surg* 2002; **73**: 209–19.

● 152. Sitbon O, Gressin V, Speich R, *et al.* Bosentan for the treatment of human immunodeficiency virus-associated pulmonary arterial hypertension. *Am J Respir Crit Care Med* 2004; **170**: 1212–17.

● 153. Mikhail GW, Prasad SK, Li W, *et al.* Clinical and hemodynamic effects of sildenafil in pulmonary hypertension: acute and mid-term effects. *Eur Heart J* 2004; **25**: 431–6.

● 154. Wilkins MR, Paul GA, Strange JW, *et al.* Sildenafil versus endothelin receptor antagonist for pulmonary hypertension (SERAPH) study. *Am J Respir Crit Care Med* 2005; **171**: 1292–7.

● 155. McLaughlin VV, Sitbon O, Badesch DB, *et al.* Survival with first-line bosentan in patients with pulmonary hypertension. *Eur Respir J* 2005; **25**: 244–9.

● 156. Galie N, Ghofrani HA, Torbicki A, *et al.* Sildenafil citrate therapy for pulmonary arterial hypertension. *N Eng J Med* 2005; **17L** 353(20): 2148–57.

◆ 157. Badesch DB, Abman SH, Ahearn GS, *et al.* Medical therapy for pulmonary arterial hypertension: ACCP evidence-based clinical practice guidelines. *Chest* 2004; **126**(1): 35S–62S.

◆ 158. Galie N, Torbicki A, Barst R, *et al.* Guidelines on diagnosis and treatment of pulmonary arterial hypertension: The Task Force on Diagnosis and Treatment of Pulmonary Arterial Hypertension of the European Society of Cardiology. *Eur Heart J* 2004; **25**(24): 2243–78.

159. Humbert M, Sitbon O, Simmoneau G. Treatment of pulmonary arterial hypertension. *N Eng J Med* 2004; **351**: 1425–36.

160. Farber HW, Loscalzo J. Pulmonary arterial hypertension. *N Eng J Med* 2004; **351**: 1655–65.

Status asthmaticus

LAWRENCE SHULMAN, MARIO SOLOMITA, JILL P KARPEL

INTRODUCTION

The prevalence of asthma has been increasing over the past 20 years.[1] A recent report from the Centers for Disease Control approximated that 16 million adults in the United States, or 7.5 percent of the American population, have asthma.[2] The number of emergency room visits for asthma has also been increasing. In the 1990s, there were approximately 2 million annual emergency room visits listing asthma as the first diagnosis. Most of these patients are between 5 and 14 years old, African American, and female. However, since 1995 asthma-related rates of hospitalization and death have decreased. Yet, approximately 5000 patients still die from asthma each year.[3]

PATHOPHYSIOLOGY

Pathology of the asthmatic airway

Asthma, by definition, is a disorder of the airways in which many cells play a role. In particular, mast cells, eosinophils, T lymphocytes, macrophages, neutrophils, and epithelial cells are all working together to create inflammation that causes variable airflow obstruction.[4]

Asthma is believed to be caused by a balance between nature and nurture. There is increasing evidence of a genetic predisposition toward having asthma. When these predisposed people are exposed to a variety of environmental factors during early life they develop a unique inflammatory response to airway stimulants, which results in abnormal airway inflammation and obstruction. The initiation of the inflammatory cascade begins when the CD4 cells respond to the presentation of airway antigens by dendritic cells. The CD4 cells initiate the T helper (Th)2-mediated cytokine cascade, which produces airway inflammation. It is hypothesized that Th2 cells produce interleukin (IL)-4 and -13 which act through effector cells, stimulating B cells, mast cells, and eosinophils to produce the obstruction that typifies asthma. Epithelial-derived cytokines may also be responsible for attracting circulating leukocytes, producing increased mucus in the airways, and may have a role in the control of airway tone.

Eosinophils within the airways are also a major contributor to the asthmatic response and may be one of the targets of successful steroid use in people with asthma.[5,6] Eosinophil counts increase in airways after exposure to allergen challenges.[7–11] The role of the neutrophil is more controversial. Neutrophilic infiltration is seen in acute and fatal asthma, but is not seen in all chronic asthmatic airways. Neutrophils, which are steroid unresponsive, have been linked to severe asthma and are believed to cause epithelial damage, extensive mucus plugging, and abnormalities in epithelial and endothelial permeability.[12] Interestingly, subtypes of neutrophils found in the airways of patients with chronic asthma have been noted to be instrumental in the development of airway remodeling.[13]

New research is beginning to elucidate the role of other inflammatory cells and markers in asthma. Leukocyte adhesion and migration is a large component of the asthmatic airway. Macrophages are involved in the uptake and presentation of antigens to surrounding cells. The smooth muscle tension in the airways contributes to bronchoconstriction. Additionally, goblet cells and gland cells within the bronchial epithelium are involved both in the hypersecretion of mucus and in the leak of plasma proteins into the airways.

Chronic asthma is the result of structural changes in the epithelium and submucosa of the airways. Epithelial desquamation of the airways continues to be a controversial finding. A review of pathology in the 1980s by Laitinen et al. described desquamation as a hallmark of asthma.[14] More recent studies have debated that the initial desquamation of the epithelium seen is actually a result of drying artifact and not truly unique to people with asthma.[15] In the epithelium, goblet cells and mucin production have been found to be increased in people with asthma and have been linked to patients with fatal asthma.[16] Eosinophilic infiltration of the epithelium and submucosa is a hallmark of asthmatic airways. In addition, myofibroblast proliferation in the subepithelium causes an increase in collagen and fibronectin deposition.

In people with asthma there is disruption of mucus production and clearance. The quantity and quality of mucus produced accounts for a large part of the obstruction of the airways and has been associated with the development of fatal asthma attacks.[17] Autopsy studies in cases of fatal asthma describe increased thickness of all layers of the airway wall in comparison with the airways of patients who died from nonrespiratory diseases but with a definite history of asthma.[18]

Physiology of an asthma attack

An asthma attack is initiated by a trigger. The specific trigger varies from patient to patient. Most commonly, an allergen is inhaled and starts the inflammatory and broncho-constriction cascade. Triggers can also be air pollutants, upper respiratory tract infections, food allergies, smoke inhalation, cold air, and exercise. During the initial phases of the attack the large and small airways constrict and the epithelial lining becomes inflamed and edematous. The end result is progressive airway narrowing causing airflow limitation and progressive ventilation/perfusion mis-matching. The patient become increasingly dyspneic, hypoxemic, and eventually has muscle fatigue and respiratory failure.

There are two types of asthma exacerbation.[19] Type I asthma attack is slowly progressive. It is most commonly initiated by upper respiratory tract infections, primarily viral in nature. The symptoms develop slowly over hours to weeks. In general, type I asthma attacks are more resistant to therapy and result in a greater percentage of hospital admissions. Sudden progressive or type II asthma attacks only account for 10–20 percent of asthma exacerbations. The trigger is most commonly inhaled allergens, exercise, and stress. Though more acute, this type is generally more responsive to

early, aggressive therapy with a lower hospitalization rate (Table 14A.1).

The cardiopulmonary sequelae of airflow limitation manifest secondary to hyperinflation. Hyperinflation occurs as the work of breathing increases and the patient begins to take in larger tidal volumes to keep the constricted bronchi open.[20] This results in greater elastic recoil pressure in the lungs which increases the positive end-expiratory alveolar pressure. This is the phenomenon of auto or intrinsic PEEP (PEEPi). Intrinsic PEEP causes increases in intrathoracic pressure, which decreases venous return and right ventricular filling. At other times, increased work of breathing causes increased venous return and right ventricular filling. Afterload can also become increased by the high intrathoracic and pleural pressures which are generated by hyperinflation. The increased afterload causes a drop in cardiac output. The exaggeration of the difference in blood pressure during inspiration and expiration, or pulsus paradoxus, is a clinical manifestation of large swings in pleural pressure during an acute asthma attack. There has also been described direct mechanical compression of the heart and surrounding coronary arteries due to the increased intrathoracic pressure. This can lead directly to myocardial ischemia and constricted cardiac function.[21]

Most asthma attacks are not associated with profound hypoxemia. The average PaO_2 has been studied to be 69 mm Hg on room air.[20] The hypoxemia seen is a result of ventilation/perfusion mismatching, as the lungs are unable to fully compensate for the nonuniform distribution of obstruction throughout the bronchi. Shunt physiology seems to be much less of a physiologic consequence and most patients with asthma are able to be oxygenated with lower concentrations of oxygen.[19] If the patients begin to demonstrate higher oxygen demands, other causes of shunt, such as pneumonia or patent foramen ovale, need to be explored.

Arterial blood gases during an asthma attack can be used to denote clinical stages. In the early stage of an exacerbation, asthma patients increase their respiratory rate and minute ventilation. A large majority of patients with acute asthma are hypocapneic primarily due to tachypnea. As the severity of the obstruction increases, the arterial partial pressure of

Table 14A.1 *Types of asthma exacerbation*

Type I (Slow)	Type II (Acute)
80–90% of patients	10–20% of patients
Progressive worsening over days to weeks	Rapid onset in less than 6 hours
Female predominance	Male predominance
Triggered by infection	Triggered by inhalation of allergens, exercise, and stress
Less severe	More severe
Less responsive to therapy	More responsive to therapy

Adapted from Rodrigo *et al.*[19]

carbon dioxide (Pa_{CO_2}) begins to approach normal even in the face of deteriorating oxygenation. Decreased cardiac output and increased work of the respiratory musculature can cause lactic acidosis. The lungs' inability to compensate for the concomitant metabolic acidosis also contributes to increased carbon dioxide levels. This 'pseudonormalization' of Pa_{CO_2} indicates that gas exchange has deteriorated and the patient's respiratory muscles are dangerously close to fatigue. The arterial pH level falls as both metabolic acidosis and respiratory acidosis develop. The presence of metabolic acidosis heralds a poor prognosis.[22] When Pa_{CO_2} measurements exceed normal values, respiratory muscle fatigue develops and acute respiratory failure ensues. Hypercapnia, by itself, can cause muscle fatigue and decreased respiratory drive. 'Carbon dioxide narcosis' is a hallmark for impending respiratory failure.[23]

Physiology of the fatal asthma attack

Mortality for asthma, in comparison with other chronic diseases, is low. Out of 16–17 million people with asthma in the United States, the most recent statistics reveal 5438 deaths.[24] The vast majority of these deaths are thought to be avoidable with appropriate patient and physician education. In addition, 15–30 percent of the asthma deaths occur in patients with only mild disease.[23] Risk factors for death from asthma include age greater than 70, smoking history of more than 20 pack years, reduced forced expiratory volume in 1 second (FEV_1), history of psychosocial problems, family dysfunction, low education, and unemployment.[23] Autopsy studies of the airways from patients who died of an acute asthma attack demonstrated greater obstruction and thicker walls.[25] The airways of patients experiencing fatal attacks contained a greater percentage of neutrophils and eosinophils.[26–28] The combination of pathologic changes causes severe limitation of airflow, hypoxemia, and marked hyperinflation.[29] Death is usually from asphyxia due to extensive mucus plugging.[23]

Asthmatic deaths have also been linked to the use of β-agonists.[30] Whether this is a direct drug effect or failure of patients to seek medical assistance when experiencing asthma exacerbations is not known. However, high doses of β-agonists have been shown to cause hypokalemia and prolong the QTc interval.[31] Cardiac arrhythmias could potentially result from these electrolyte abnormalities. However, studies have failed to confirm these findings.[32]

EVALUATION AND MANAGEMENT IN THE EMERGENCY ROOM

In 1995, there were 1.8 million emergency room visits listing asthma as the primary diagnosis. There were over 400 000 admissions and approximately 5000 fatalities.[1] Appropriate evaluation and treatment of an asthma patient in the emergency room is essential to reduce asthma morbidity and mortality.

History

A thorough medical history is the cornerstone of the initial evaluation of an asthma patient in the emergency room. Criteria have been developed to identify patients at risk for potentially fatal episodes of asthma. These include:

- history of intubation for respiratory failure or arrest
- respiratory acidosis without intubation
- two or more hospitalizations for status asthmaticus despite long-term administration of oral corticosteroids
- two episodes of acute pneumomediastinum or pneumothorax associated with severe asthma.[33]

History of anxiety and/or depression has also been linked to higher hospitalization rates for asthma[34] (Table 14A.2).

Table 14A.2 *Impending respiratory failure*

Asthma history	Demographic history	Signs and symptoms
History of intubation for respiratory failure	Age >70 years	'Pseudonormalization' of arterial blood gas
History of respiratory acidosis without intubation	Smoking history greater than 20 pack years	High doses of β-agonists
	Reduced FEV_1	– Hypokalemia – Prolonged QTc
Two or more hospitalizations for status asthmaticus despite long term administration of oral corticosteroids	History of psychosocial problems	Increased pulsus paradoxus
	Family dysfunction	Hypoxemia
Two or more episodes of acute mediastinum or pneumothorax associated with severe asthma	Low education	PEFR <120 L or FEV_1 <1 L
	Unemployment	Persistent PEFR <40% of predicted despite treatment

FEV_1, forced expiratory volume in 1 second; PEFR, peak expiratory flow rate.

In addition one should obtain a detailed history of maintenance medications and interventions prior to arrival in the emergency room. Exposure history and identification of asthmatic triggers may also be useful, particularly in preventing future exacerbations.

The history will also assist with the formation of a differential diagnosis. Asthma mimics may include acute myocardial infarction, congestive heart failure, chronic obstructive pulmonary disease (COPD) exacerbations, pulmonary embolism, and vocal cord dysfunction. Diseases of the upper airway such as epiglottitis and foreign body obstruction should also be considered. Coincidental infections of the respiratory tract, such as pneumonia or sinusitis, may also be diagnosed.

Vital signs

The vital signs of an asthma patient are important in the emergency setting. Respiratory rate, blood pressure, and pulse oximetry need to be monitored frequently. A respiratory rate of greater than 30 breaths/min has been demonstrated to predict the need for hospitalization.[35] In contrast, Hardern failed to show any relation between pulse oximetry and rate of hospitalization and length of stay.[36] Pulsus paradoxus, as a measure of the change in blood pressure during inspiration and expiration, can be found in severe obstruction.[37,38] However, pulsus paradoxus measurements are extremely difficult to perform and should not be solely relied upon as a measure of improvement or failure.

Measurement of airflow obstruction

The pathophysiologic hallmark of an acute asthma attack is airflow obstruction. Peak expiratory flow rate (PEFR) or FEV_1 is used to quantify the degree of obstruction. The PEFR and FEV_1 have been shown to correlate with each other and either can be used as an assessment tool.[39] Patients with a PEFR below 120 L/min or an FEV_1 below 1 L are in danger of retaining carbon dioxide.[22] Serial measurements of airflow obstruction are essential in determining if a patient is responding to therapy or if the patient's clinical status is deteriorating.[40,41] Failure to improve PEFR following bronchodilator therapy is also a predictor of the need for hospitalization.[41,42]

Additional assessment

Most patients presenting with asthma exacerbations do not require arterial blood gas measurements. However, some patients may benefit from them. For example, patients with PEFR <120 L/min; those unable to speak in complete sentences or exhibiting extreme dyspnea; the presence of pulsus paradoxus; or other clinical signs of impending respiratory failure. Uses of arterial blood gas measurements include determining the degree of hypoxemia and trending pH and carbon dioxide levels. It is imperative to find which patients are in dangerous stages of an asthma exacerbation and may demonstrate pseudonormalization of the arterial blood gas, as these are the patients with impending respiratory failure. However, one should not wait for the results of an arterial blood gas before initiating therapy or intubating a patient if clinically indicated.[43] Chest radiographs should be obtained to rule out pneumonia, pneumothorax, or pneumomediastinum. A 12-lead electrocardiogram (EKG) will demonstrate any ischemic changes, arrhythmias, right ventricular strain patterns, and alterations in QTc intervals related to medications.[44] Continuous telemetry monitoring is important in older patients and those with coexisting heart disease, but is not needed for all patients.[19]

Bronchodilators

The use of a short-acting β-agonist is the cornerstone of acute asthma therapy. The onset of action is rapid and the medication is generally well tolerated. β-Agonists reduce the acute bronchospasm associated with an asthma attack, but have no effect on the inflammatory component of airway obstruction and do not affect the late-phase response. The common side effects of albuterol are tachycardia, tremors, and hypokalemia. It has also been shown to cause lactic acidosis and transient ventilation/perfusion mismatching with clinically insignificant falls in Pa_{O_2}.[19] Long-acting β-agonists have not been recommended in the treatment of acute asthma because of their slow onset of action. However, formoterol is a long-acting β-agonist which has an onset of action of approximately 15 minutes. It has been shown to have potential in the emergency treatment of acute asthma.[45] Recently in a large multicenter trial the combination of budesonide and formoterol in a single inhaler device was shown to decrease severe asthma exacerbations when patients took additional inhalations upon experiencing worsening asthma symptoms.[46]

Albuterol, 2.5 mg per dose, is most commonly given via a nebulizer. The optimal total dose required to treat acute bronchoconstriction is between 5 mg and 10 mg.[47] Cydulka et al. demonstrated that three 2.5 mg nebulized doses of albuterol were as efficacious as a single 7.5 mg nebulized dose, but there was a trend for the 7.5 mg dosage group to experience more side effects.[48] In another study, a comparison of a total of 15 mg of albuterol conferred no advantage over the 7.5 mg cumulative dose.[49]

Levalbuterol, the pure (R)-isomer of racemic albuterol has shown some promise in the treatment of acute asthma. Clinical studies have demonstrated that the 0.63 mg dose of levalbuterol has similar efficacy with decreased side effects when compared to the 1.25 mg dose of racemic albuterol.[50] Another study in patients treated with racemic albuterol, compared with those treated with levalbuterol, required less medication, had shorter lengths of hospital stay, had decreased costs for nebulizer therapy and hospitalization, and appeared to have a more prolonged therapeutic benefit.[51] The precise role of levalbuterol in both asthma and COPD awaits further investigation.

The use of a metered-dose inhaler (MDI) with a spacer has been proved to be as efficacious as jet nebulizer therapy. The MDI takes approximately 2 minutes to deliver a dose, while a jet nebulizer takes approximately 20 minutes. Idris et al. demonstrated that 4 MDI inhalations of albuterol given with a spacer produced equivalent bronchodilation compared with 2.5 mg of nebulized albuterol.[52] A metaanalysis of 1076 children and 444 adults, in 22 emergency room studies confirmed that there was no difference in response between nebulizers and MDIs. In addition, in children, there was a trend toward lower hospitalization rates and significantly lower side effect profiles.[53]

Initial studies of intermittent β-agonist therapy versus continuous nebulization showed some benefit of using continuous regimens.[54] Recently Rodrigo and Rodrigo's metaanalysis of six studies involving 393 patients demonstrated equivalence of continuous and intermittent nebulizers in the emergency treatment of acute asthma.[55] However, there was a lower heart rate response and less hypokalemia observed in the continuous nebulizer group.[55]

The dosing frequency for inhaled β-agonists continues to remain controversial. The 1997 Expert Panel Report II suggested giving three treatments at 20–30-minute intervals as initial therapy in the emergency room.[56] A study done at Montefiore Medical Center compared MDI treatments (six puffs) given at either 30, 60, or 120-minute intervals. Patients, who had less than 15 percent improvement in FEV_1 15 minutes after therapy had begun, achieved four times the improvement in FEV_1 with albuterol given at 30-minute intervals as did those given the drug at 60- or 120-minute intervals. Among patients who demonstrated greater than 15 percent improvement in FEV_1 at 15 minutes, responses were similar in the 30- and 60-minute groups.[57] Therefore, dosing regimens need to be tailored to individual patients. Those who are responding well to therapy (based on monitoring of PEFR or FEV_1) can have the intervals lengthened to 1 hour during emergency room therapy. Patients who are not responding may benefit from much more rapid dosing. High-dose β-agonists can be given as four puffs of albuterol by MDI every 10 minutes or 2.5 mg by nebulizer every 20 minutes. In patients with extremely severe conditions, one or more puffs can be given by MDI every 10–20 seconds.[19]

Intravenous β-agonists are generally not recommended. A metaanalysis by Travers et al. demonstrated that there was no statistically significant difference in vital signs, pulmonary functions, laboratory measures, adverse effects, or clinical success between intravenous and inhaled β-agonists.[58] Those receiving intravenous β-agonist demonstrated a trend toward more autonomic side effects and tachycardia.[58] Intravenous β-agonists should be reserved for patients who

have become moribund and unable to receive nebulized or inhaled β-agonists.

Subcutaneous epinephrine can be given to patients who are not responding to inhaled β-agonists. In a study by Karpel et al. a significant number of patients who did not respond to nebulized β-agonist did respond to subcutaneous epinephrine. In contrast, if a patient did not respond to epinephrine, they were unlikely to respond to β-agonists. Lack of response also predicted the need for hospitalization.[42] There was no difference in PEFR response between the 0.1 mg, 0.3 mg, or 0.5 mg dose of epinephrine.[59] Epinephrine needs to be used cautiously in patients with known cardiac disease and hypertension. It has also been demonstrated to cause severe lactic acidosis.[60]

Anticholinergic medications

Anticholinergic medications, such as ipratropium bromide, decrease the airway tone and bronchoconstriction by relaxing the smooth muscles of the bronchi and bronchioles. In general, anticholinergics alone are inferior to β-agonists as initial treatment for acute asthma, but their use in an emergency setting may still be beneficial. Two metaanalyses in 1999 demonstrated a modest statistical improvement with the use of ipratropium in the acute asthmatic.[61,62] A recent review of the literature also supports the use of anticholinergics and provides a set of guidelines.[63] Ipratropium bromide in combination with albuterol is indicated in initial treatment of adults and children with severe acute asthma as it was associated with improved FEV_1 and PEFR and a lower hospitalization rate. Ipratropium can be used as a nebulizer or MDI. Nebulizers are given at 250 μg or 500 μg dose every 20 minutes. A metered-dose inhaler with spacer can be given as four puffs every 10–20 minutes. Single-dose regimens also improve pulmonary function and decrease hospitalization rates. The FEV_1 response to ipratropium has been found to be independent of previous use of β-agonists.[63] In summary, anticholinergic medications can be recommended to be used, along with β-agonists, in the emergency treatment of a severe asthma exacerbation. Subgroup analysis showed increased benefit in those patients with FEV_1 <30 percent and long duration of symptoms prior to emergency department presentation.[64] No benefit of anticholinergic use during hospitalization has been demonstrated.

Ipratropium has no systemic side effects. Its onset of action is 60–90 minutes and increases PEFR by approximately 15 percent.[65] The use of long-acting anticholinergics, such as tiotropium, in the emergency setting, has not been studied.

Corticosteroids

Treatment of airway inflammation is essential in the management of the acute asthmatic patient. Steroids act by suppressing cytokines, inhibiting eosinophil recruitment in the airway, inhibiting inflammatory mediator production, and preventing airway remodeling. Clinically, they prevent and relieve acute exacerbations and reduce the severity of asthma symptoms. Steroids have been shown to improve lung function, reduce admissions, and decrease asthma mortality.[66,67]

The route of administration of steroids has been widely debated. McFadden demonstrated no statistically significant differences between oral and intravenous steroid administration.[68] However, all of the studies addressing this issue studied small numbers of patients and the results may have been affected by statistical error (underpowering the studies).

Although the literature does not provide good evidence as to how much steroid to give, we would recommend either intravenous doses of 20–40 mg of solumedrol (or its equivalent) every 6 hours or comparable doses of oral steroids given in divided doses. Administering one single dose of oral steroid during acute exacerbations may result in poorer pulmonary function response as oral prednisone (Medrol) has a duration of action of about 6–8 hours, therefore, patients may require more frequent dosing. The National Institutes of Health (NIH) daily recommendation is for 60–80 mg of methylprednisolone, 300–400 mg of hydrocortisone, or an equivalent dose of glucocorticoids.[69] There is a theoretical benefit with higher doses of corticosteroids for more severe asthma, but no controlled studies have been completed. There is no consensus on the duration of steroid therapy or how to taper. Often, knowing the patient's previous history of steroid use is helpful in guiding these decisions. The PEFR can be monitored to guide the steroid-tapering regimen.

A metaanalysis conducted by Rowe in 2001 reviewed 12 studies involving 863 patients receiving systemic steroids.[66] The study concluded that systemic steroids given within an hour of arrival to the emergency room reduced the hospitalization rate for patients with acute asthma. The side effects were no different from placebo. Increased benefit was seen in those patients with severe asthma and those who were not already taking steroids. In addition, the use of systemic steroids on discharge from the hospital prevented future asthma relapses.[66] One should also prescribe inhaled corticosteroids at the time of discharge and provide appropriate education for the patient.

The role of inhaled corticosteroids in acute asthma is controversial. Systemic steroids exert effects by gene transcription and protein synthesis, often requiring 6–24 hours to improve pulmonary function. Inhaled corticosteroids work earlier, often in less than 3 hours. It has been postulated that the inhaled corticosteroids cause local vasoconstriction and reduce mucosal edema thereby reducing airflow limitation. In comparison with prednisone, one study of high-dose inhaled flunisolide showed a decrease in hospitalization rate and in lung function greater than 24 hours after emergency room discharge.[70] A Cochrane analysis by Edmonds concluded that inhaled corticosteroids

were effective in reducing the hospitalization rate when used in the emergency room for acute asthma.[71] It was unclear as to whether the inhaled corticosteroids are better, worse, or the same as systemic steroids. The utility of adding inhaled corticosteroids to systemic steroids also needs further studying.[71]

Theophylline

The use of theophylline in the acute asthmatic patient has been in and out of popularity since its inception. Initially theophylline was thought to be a potent bronchodilator, but is much less effective than β-agonists.[72] A series of metaanalyses has failed to show any benefit for the use of theophylline, instead of, or in addition to, any other treatment.[69,73] In addition, studies have not been able to demonstrate any improvement in pulmonary function testing or hospitalization rates with the use of theophylline. Interestingly, it has been shown recently that theophylline has some anti-inflammatory effects when used in low concentrations.[74]

The methylated xanthines should be reserved for patients who are refractory to any other therapy. A recommended theophylline loading dose is 6 mg /kg over 30 minutes followed by an infusion of 0.5 mL/kg per hour. Theophylline levels need to be monitored and close attention needs to be paid to a long list of medication interactions. Current recommendations are to maintain serum levels between 33.3 μmol/L and 66.6 μmol/L (6 μg/mL and 12 μg/mL).

Oxygen

Profound hypoxemia is not common in patients with acute asthma. In a report by McFadden and Lyons, only 5 percent of patients with acute asthma had arterial oxygen tension of 55 mm Hg or less.[75] Additionally, as asthma physiology is primarily ventilation/perfusion mismatch, any desaturation is usually correctable with low amounts of supplemental oxygen. Oxygen saturation should be continuously monitored by pulse oximetry. A recent study showed that hypoxemia itself could alter the perceptions of asthmatic patient with regard to their respiratory difficulty.[76] Patients should receive oxygen to keep the pulse oximetry greater than 92 percent. Hyperoxia does not appear to be beneficial, and may actually be detrimental. A study comparing acute asthmatic patients receiving 28 percent oxygen versus 100 percent oxygen demonstrated that those receiving hyperoxia actually have an increase in the P_{CO_2} and a decrease in the PEFR.[77]

Heliox

The helium–oxygen mixture, heliox, theoretically can assist an asthmatic patient by changing airflow dynamics in the bronchi. The balance between the two major types of airflow through the bronchi, laminar and turbulent, is altered in patients with asthma. During regular, non-stressed, breathing the majority of airflow is laminar. But, at high velocities with airway narrowing, there is a large component of turbulent flow. Heliox mixture has a lower density and a higher viscosity than air and improves laminar flow. Increased laminar flow can then ensure better oxygen and better medication delivery to the peripheral and distal airways.

A small emergency room study concluded that heliox, when mixed with albuterol, resulted in an improvement in spirometry when compared with albuterol delivered with oxygen.[78] There have also been studies demonstrating improvement in pulsus paradoxus and in peak flow using heliox.[79,80] A recent review of the literature included six randomized controlled studies involving 369 acute asthmatic patients. When measuring improvement in PEFR or FEV_1 as the outcome, there was no benefit of heliox in the initial treatment of acute asthma. The NIH guidelines recommend avoiding heliox for the moderate acute asthmatic patient and only using it in the severe asthmatic patient.[69]

Magnesium

In people with asthma magnesium sulfate functions by causing smooth muscle relaxation. Multiple studies and reviews have concluded that the use of magnesium sulfate should be reserved for the severe, acute asthmatic patient. An early study by Rolla et al. demonstrated a small, but transient, improvement in FEV_1 following 2 g of intravenous magnesium.[81] A study in 1989 demonstrated that 1.2 g of magnesium trended toward lower hospitalization rates for those patients who did not improve with β-agonists.[82] In two studies, by Green and Rothrock and then by Tiffany et al., magnesium sulfate failed to show any benefit in acute asthma exacerbations.[83,84] A more recent study by Bloch et al. demonstrated benefit from magnesium when given to the severely asthmatic patient, defined as FEV_1 <25 percent on admission. No benefit was seen in the patient with moderate asthma (FEV_1 25–75 percent).[85] Silverman et al. also demonstrated improvement in FEV_1 with the most severely affected patients.[86]

The use of magnesium has also been studied in the nebulized form. An early study involving methacholine-induced bronchospasm failed to show any reversal of bronchospasm with inhaled magnesium.[87] Hill demonstrated that inhalation of magnesium prior to the inhalation of histamine did not protect the patient from bronchospasm. In fact, it was shown that the inhaled magnesium may increase the airway reactivity to histamine.[88] When nebulized magnesium is mixed with nebulized albuterol there is also no improvement in lung function.[89]

Reviews of the literature have concluded that magnesium sulfate, either intravenous or nebulized, does not benefit the

moderate to severe acute asthmatic patient.[90,91] Magnesium should be reserved for patients who are refractory to other therapy and may benefit the subset of patients who present with an FEV_1 less than 25 percent of predicted. It should be given as a single 2 g infusion over 20 minutes. Possible side effects are hypotension, loss of deep tendon reflexes, flushing, and mild sedation. However, the drug is generally well tolerated and can be given without need for additional monitoring.

Leukotriene antagonists

Leukotriene antagonists may have some role in the treatment of the acute asthmatic patient. A large study was conducted of zafirlukast given as adjunctive therapy for acute asthma. Patients received either 20 mg or 160 mg of zafirlukast or placebo in addition to standard asthma therapy. There was a decrease in the 28-day relapse period in those patients who received the 160 mg dose of zafirlukast.[92] In another study, Camargo et al. randomized two groups of acute asthmatic patients to receive either 7 mg or 14 mg of intravenous montelukast or placebo. The patients receiving montelukast had a greater improvement in FEV_1 and tended to receive less β-agonists. There was no difference observed between the 7 mg and 14 mg group.[93] Oral montelukast has also been shown to yield additive improvement in lung function when added to oral or intravenous steroids in acute asthma.[94] Additional studies are necessary to determine where leukotriene antagonists fit into the algorithm for the treatment of the acute asthmatic patient.

Other therapy

The use of antibiotics for acute asthma exacerbations is not recommended.[69] However, if a patient exhibits clinical signs of bacterial infection such as purulent sputum or nasal drainage, fever, or radiographic signs of pneumonia or sinusitis, antibiotics should be administered.[69]

Acetylcysteine, as a mucolytic, has not been shown to improve pulmonary function in acute asthma. In fact, the use has been shown to worsen cough, increase airflow limitation, and, when combined with β-agonists, it can worsen the exacerbation.[95]

Inhaled furosemide had been shown to prevent or diminish airway responses to certain provocation challenges as well as to exercise. However, when inhaled furosemide, albuterol, or the combination of the two was administered to emergency department patients with acute asthma, no significant improvement in pulmonary function could be demonstrated for furosemide, alone or in combination, compared with albuterol. Inhaled furosemide probably has no role in the treatment of acute asthma.[96]

Sedatives should be strictly avoided in the treatment of acute asthma. Sedatives and antipsychotic medications have been shown to decrease the respiratory drive and increase the mortality associated with acute asthma.[97]

Home versus admission versus intensive care

The response to therapy during the first hours of emergency department care dictates the disposition of the acute asthmatic patient. One should have a lower threshold for admission to the hospital when the patient has risk factors for fatal asthma. These include a history of intubation for respiratory failure or arrest, respiratory acidosis without intubation, two or more hospitalizations for status asthmaticus despite long-term administration of oral corticosteroids, and two episodes of acute pneumomediastinum or pneumothorax associated with severe asthma[33] (Table 14A.2).

Quantification of the response to therapy can be measured with PEFR or FEV$_1$. Response at 30 minutes has been proved to be highly predictive of outcome.[98] Patients who have a PEFR greater than 60 percent of predicted after 2–3 hours of therapy in the emergency room can usually be discharged as long as they are asymptomatic. If the PEFR is persistently under 40 percent of predicted the patient should remain in the hospital. Those with PEFT between 40 percent and 60 percent may require additional therapy in the emergency room and may be able to be discharged.[99]

Patients who are discharged should receive a 7–14-day course of oral steroid taper. They should have a β-agonist MDI with spacer available for their use at home. They should also have follow-up with their primary provider shortly after discharge from the hospital. Those patients who have a history of frequent emergency department visits or hospitalizations should be considered for referral to an asthma specialist.

Patients who show clinical deterioration despite therapy should be admitted to the intensive care unit (ICU). Those patients who are persistently hypoxemic (SaO$_2$ <90 percent) or demonstrate a widening pulsus paradoxus should also be monitored in the ICU.[19] Hypercapnia or normocapnia is a sign of poor response to therapy. In addition, admission to the ICU is mandatory in patients with altered mental status, profound fatigue, or impending respiratory failure (Box 14A.1).

MANAGEMENT AND VENTILATORY SUPPORT IN THE INTENSIVE CARE UNIT

Ventilatory assistance can be life saving in acute asthma exacerbations when medical therapy alone has failed. It can also provide an opportunity to allow medical therapy to take effect, and reverse the airway inflammation and bronchospasm. Both invasive ventilation and noninvasive positive pressure ventilation (NIPPV) can be used to provide short-term support. The goal of this support is to provide the longest possible expiratory time to minimize dynamic hyperinflation and increased intrinsic or auto PEEP. Dynamic hyperinflation is the direct result of airway inflammation and obstruction, which leads to the collapse of small airways during exhalation and air trapping. This phenomenon can lead to increased intrathoracic pressure, increase in the work of breathing, impairment of cardiac filling, and eventually, hemodynamic collapse. These complications can be avoided with the prompt administration of medical therapy, and the use of invasive and noninvasive ventilatory support as an adjunct to medical treatment when clinically indicated.

Noninvasive positive pressure ventilation

Noninvasive positive pressure ventilation should be used first as an attempt to avoid endotracheal intubation. It can decrease the work of breathing by relieving dynamic hyperinflation, preserving respiratory muscle function, and allowing additional time for medications to relieve obstruction during the period of impending respiratory failure.[100] By improving inspiratory muscle function, patients may be able to reach their total lung capacity more effectively, and can start forced expiration at higher lung volumes leading to improvements in FEV$_1$.[101] Other possible effects include a direct bronchodilating effect which decreases airway resistance, reexpansion of atelectasis and promotion of secretion clearance, offsetting of iPEEP, and recruitment of collapsed alveoli which can improve ventilation/perfusion mismatch.[102]

Noninvasive positive pressure ventilation can be administered via a nasal mask or full facemask, and by two types of ventilation device, continuous positive airway pressure (CPAP) or bilevel positive airway pressure (BIPAP). Nasal masks are often preferred, as full facemasks can increase the risk of aspiration, gastric distension, and cause sensations of claustrophobia in patients who are already under tremendous stress.[100] However, full facemasks can provide better ventilatory support, especially in patients who

---

Box 14A.1 Evidence supporting admission to the ICU for potentially fatal asthma

- Respiratory distress, with any alteration in consciousness
- Patient unable to speak in full sentences
- Central cyanosis
- Thoracic overdistension, with decreased or absent breath sounds
- Significant pulsus paradoxus and retraction of sternocleidomastoid muscles
- Metabolic or respiratory acidosis
- 'Pseudonormal' arterial blood gases
- Potential need for intubation and mechanical ventilation

mouth breathe, and improve delivery of inhaled, nebulized medications. Patients must be alert and oriented enough to cooperate with NIPPV in order to protect their airway. It should not be used on any patient who is obtunded.

Initial NIPPV settings should start with low inspiratory pressures and should be titrated up to achieve tidal volumes of 7–8 mL/kg and a respiratory rate fewer than 25 breaths/min.[100] When using CPAP, an initial setting of 5 cm H_2O can provide enough support. With BIPAP, an initial expiratory pressure of 5 cm H_2O and an inspiratory pressure of approximately 8 cm H_2O are recommended.[19] Expiratory pressure can be gradually increased if the patient has difficulty triggering breaths during inspiration, and inspiratory pressure can be increased if tidal volumes are shallow (less than 7 mL/kg).[19]

Evidence of the efficacy of BIPAP in acute asthmatic emergencies was demonstrated by Soroksky and colleagues in a randomized, placebo control trial.[101] They took 30 patients with severe asthma attacks with FEV_1 <60 percent of predicted, respiratory rate >30 breaths/min, a 1-year history of asthma, and current asthma symptoms for at least 7 days, and randomly assigned 15 patients to receive BIPAP plus conventional therapy, and 15 patients to receive conventional therapy alone. Patients in the BIPAP group were treated with inspiratory pressures initially set at 8 cm H_2O, which were increased by 2 cm H_2O every 15 minutes to a maximum of 15 cm H_2O or until the respiratory rate was <25 breaths/min. Expiratory pressure was initially set at 3 cm H_2O, and was increased by 1 cm H_2O every 15 minutes to a maximum of 5 cm H_2O, or when patient comfort was achieved. The primary endpoint was an increase in FEV_1 of at least 50 percent from baseline. Eighty percent of the patients in the BIPAP group reached this endpoint, as compared with only 20 percent in the control group. Hospitalization was required in 17.6 percent of the BIPAP patients and 62.5 percent of the control group patients.[101]

Clinical improvement is usually seen within a few hours of treatment with NIPPV. When clinical improvement is sustained for several hours, reduction in support pressures can be attempted, as well as interval mask removal to allow the patient break periods. These breaks can improve circulation to facial skin, allow the patient to expectorate secretions, and enable them to appreciate the benefit of NIPPV.[100] Intolerance of the face mask, hypoxia, hypercarbia, and somnolence all indicate failure of therapy and may necessitate endotracheal intubation.

Invasive ventilation

In the face of clinical deterioration, intubation may be an unavoidable consequence of an acute asthma exacerbation. Indications for intubation include obtundation, apnea or near apnea, and impending cardiopulmonary collapse. Hypercapnia alone is not considered an absolute indication for intubation unless other clinical criteria for mechanical ventilation are present. Nasal intubation should be avoided because of the higher incidence of nasal polyps and sinusitis in asthma patients. The largest endotracheal tube possible should be used to allow for mobilization of large secretions and mucus plugs, and to provide the lowest amount of airway resistance possible.[19] The ultimate goal of invasive ventilation is to facilitate gas exchange, maximize expiratory time, and decrease end-inspiratory lung volumes and intrinsic PEEP.

Immediately following intubation, increased vagal tone, low intravascular volume, and high levels of air trapping with auto PEEP can combine to cause bradycardia, hypotension, and possible cardiac arrest.[100] Catecholamine release associated with patient distress, metabolic acidosis, respiratory alkalosis, hypoxia, hypokalemia, hypo-magnesemia, and toxicity from inhaled β-agonists or theophylline can all contribute to the development of arrhythmias.[100] Mortality associated with intubation ranges from 6 percent to 8 percent, and cardiopulmonary collapse can occur in approximately 20 percent of patients.[19,100] It is important to take these factors into account, and enact measures to prevent them from causing negative outcomes. Improving oxygenation with bag masking and intravenous fluid resuscitation should be started immediately during the peri-intubation period. In the immediate post-intubation period, it is common to see patients being hyperventilated with bag mask devices in an attempt to reduce carbon dioxide levels; however, this is incorrect and can be dangerous. Hyperventilation can lead to hyperinflation and air trapping which increases intrathoracic pressure, and reduces venous return and cardiac output. Depression of cardiac output can worsen hypoxia and metabolic acidosis and trigger cardiac arrest. Manual ventilation with a bag device should be slow and gradual with a goal of maintaining an adequate arterial oxygen saturation which can be accomplished with as little as 2–3 breaths/min.[19] If hypotension is present, manual ventilation should be discontinued. If the patient does not improve, pneumothorax should be considered which is usually manifested by decreased or absent breath sounds, tracheal deviation, and difficulty with manual bag ventilation.

The main goal of mechanical ventilation is to maintain adequate oxygenation while preventing iatrogenic lung injury long enough for medical therapy to take effect and allow for the withdrawal of ventilatory assistance. No one ventilator mode has been shown to be more beneficial, but generally volume cycled, assist control mode is used most frequently. Ventilator strategies are designed to minimize dynamic hyperinflation by allowing for optimal exhalation time. Expiratory time can be prolonged by decreasing minute ventilation, either by reducing tidal volume or respiratory rate, or by decreasing inspiratory time by increasing the inspiratory flow rate.[19] Inspiratory flow rates should be increased to 60–100 L/min to allow for greater expiration time for each breath. The use of high inspiratory flow rates can minimize end-inspiratory lung volume and intrinsic

PEEP, but it can cause higher peak airway pressures. Although peak airway pressures generated with high inspiratory flow rates do not correlate with either barotrauma or plateau pressure, the amount of pressure that is transmitted to the alveolus which can cause barotrauma is difficult to judge.[103] Minute ventilation should be between 6 L/min and 8 L/min and can usually be achieved with a tidal volume of 5–7 mL/kg and a respiratory rate of 11–14 breaths/min. The use of low minute ventilation can cause hypercapnia, which is an accepted side effect. This 'permissive hypercapnia' is generally well tolerated as long as it develops slowly, and the $Pa{CO_2}$ remains at or below 90 mm Hg.[19] Bicarbonate can be used to correct the pH if necessary but is generally used only if the pH falls below 7.2. The main contraindication to permissive hypercapnia is elevated intracranial pressure, and should be avoided in patients with anoxic brain injury and cerebral edema following cardiopulmonary arrest.[104] External PEEP from the ventilator may worsen hyperinflation. It has also been postulated to have a beneficial effect by keeping small airways open during exhalation and decreasing intrinsic PEEP. It is not routinely recommended to add PEEP in the initial management of an acute asthma flare unless the patient remains difficult to oxygenate or has high levels of auto PEEP (>10 cm H_2O).[100]

Response to therapy and risk for hyperinflation can be monitored through the use of end-inspiratory peak and plateau pressures. It is recommended to maintain plateau pressure <35 cm H_2O to avoid the complications of barotrauma.[103] Accurate measurement of plateau pressures does require adequate sedation and paralysis, which can be difficult in some patients. There have also been efforts to target end-inspiratory lung volume as a marker for treatment efficacy. Tuxen et al. measured end-inspiratory lung volumes and used these to adjust minute ventilation regardless of $Pa{CO_2}$. A safe minute ventilation was defined as the minute ventilation necessary to maintain an end-inspiratory volume of 20 mL/kg. When the safe minute ventilation resulted in a $Pa{CO_2}$ of 40 mm Hg or less, the patients were considered to be at the weaning point, and were taken off mechanical ventilation. In the study, 9 of 10 patients were successfully weaned from mechanical ventilation within 24 hours of reaching the weaning point, showing that end-inspiratory lung volumes could be used to accurately guide the extent of hypoventilation and the duration of mechanical ventilation.[105] Williams and colleagues[106] also looked at end-inspiratory volumes and complication rates in patients with severe asthma exacerbations who were being mechanically ventilated. In this retrospective study of 22 ICU patients, it was found that there was a higher incidence of pulmonary barotrauma and hypotension in patients with higher minute ventilation volumes and end-inspiratory volumes. For patients with an end-inspiratory volume of <1.4 L, none of the five patients had complications. In comparison, 11 of the 17 patients with an end-inspiratory volume >1.4 L had complications. End-inspiratory volume is felt to be a more sensitive indicator of a safe level of hypoventilation and when weaning can begin.[106]

Medication use during mechanical ventilation is a continuum of what was begun prior to intubation. Albuterol should be continued and should be administered in whatever delivery system is compatible with the specific ventilator. Systemic steroids should be continued and slowly tapered as the patient improves. The addition of heliox to the ventilatory cycle may be beneficial in reducing the required concentration of oxygen as demonstrated by Schaeffer et al.[107] However, heliox should be reserved for those patients who do not respond to conventional therapy.[69,108]

Sedative agents with a rapid onset of action can be used in the peri- and postintubation period for patient comfort and to enhance compliance with ventilation. Midazolam is a benzodiazepine with rapid onset of action within 1–2 minutes, and is generally the agent of choice. Diazepam and lorazepam can also be used effectively. Ketamine is a nonbarbiturate, rapid-acting dissociative anesthetic which can be used for intubation and then administered long term by infusion for ongoing sedation. It can have bronchodilatory effects, but can also increase heart rate and blood pressure and cause delirium in adults. Its use is generally limited to children. Propofol is an intravenous, sedative-hypnotic agent belonging to the alkylphenol family, which is also an excellent choice for sedation. It has a rapid onset of action and can be used in a continuous infusion. It should not be used in patients with documented egg allergies, and it may cause elevations of liver transaminases and triglyceride levels. The majority of patients will also require administration of an opioid such as fentanyl. Morphine, as it has been associated with histamine release, should be avoided, if possible. All of these sedative agents and opioids have the potential to lower blood pressure and precipitate cardiac events. Daily cessation of continuous drug infusions has been associated with avoidance of drug accumulation, and decreased duration of mechanical ventilation[19] (Table 14A.3).

Paralytic agents are also administered to facilitate synchronization of the patient with the ventilator, to avoid hyperinflation, to allow permissive hypercapnia, and to decrease respiratory muscle activity.[19] By decreasing respiratory muscle activity, the amount of carbon dioxide generated by the work of breathing can be reduced and can lead to improvements in acidosis and hypercarbia. The agents used are usually depolarizing paralytic agents such as pancuronium, vecuronium, and cis-atracurium. All paralytic agents are associated with the risk of muscle weakness. Myopathy can be worse if paralytics are coadministered corticosteroids and aminoglycoside antibiotics. When paralytics are being used, a bedside nerve stimulator should be available to monitor the level of paralysis. The drug infusion should also be held every 4–6 hours to prevent drug accumulation and prolonged paralysis.[19]

Intubated patients should have daily decrease of paralytics and sedation and undergo a daily assessment as to their

Table 14A.3 *Sedatives in acute asthma*

Drug	Dose	Side effects
Midazolam	Loading: 1 mg IV repeat every 2–3 minutes PRN Maintenance: 1–10 mg per hour	Hypotension
Ketamine	Loading: 1-2 mg/kg IV Maintenance: 0.5 mg/kg per minute	Sympatheticomimetic effects
Propofol	Loading: 60-80 mg/min, up to 2 mg/kg Maintenance: 1–4.5 mg/kg per hour	Respiratory depression, lactic acidosis, hypertriglyceridemia
Morphine sulfate	Maintenance: 1-5 mg/hr	Nausea, vomiting, ileus
Lorazepam	Maintenance: 1-5 mg/hr or IV bolus as needed	Drug accumulation

IV, intravenous; PRN, as needed.

potential for extubation. No specific criteria have been developed to determine the patient's readiness for extubation. In general, when the patient is alert, airway pressures are reduced, and arterial blood gases improved extubation should be considered. After weaning and extubation, most asthmatic patients should be observed in the ICU for 24–48 hours, depending on the clinical situation. The peak flow meter can be used to monitor treatment efficacy. Medical therapy with inhaled bronchodilators and corticosteroids should be continued. Patients can be taught to effectively use MDIs for their β-agonist treatments and nebulizers may be discontinued, resulting in cost savings for the hospital.

In summary, NIPPV should be utilized as an early adjunct to treatment in acute asthmatic emergencies. If patients fail to respond, mechanical ventilation should be started. Although there is a significant morbidity and mortality associated with mechanical ventilation, it is a life-saving measure when the appropriate ventilatory strategies are employed.

GET OUT AND STAY OUT!

When a patient who has recovered from status asthmaticus is discharged from the hospital a detailed and individualized plan must be in place. The patient should have an 'action plan' which includes a complete list of medications and what to do if their asthma symptoms worsen. Medications may include 'controller' medications, such as inhaled steroids,

appropriate oral steroid tapers, and other necessary medications such as long-acting β-agonists, as well as 'rescue' medications (albuterol). Every patient should have a peak flow meter at home and should be instructed on the proper use and interpretation of results. An expedited follow up with a primary care physician or referral to a specialist should also be coordinated prior to discharge. Patients should be counseled on the proper care and use of their previous and new medications. If appropriate, patients should also be informed of newer medications that are available for people with asthma, such as anti-IgE therapy (omalizumab). Hopefully, with proper education and follow-up, patients will not experience the morbidity and mortality associated with uncontrolled asthma.

Key learning points

- The prevalence of asthma has been increasing over the past 20 years.

- There is increasing evidence of a genetic predisposition toward having asthma.

- Eosinophils within the airways are also a major contributor to the asthmatic response and may be one of the targets of successful steroid use in people with asthma.

- An asthma attack is initiated by a trigger, which varies from patient to patient. Most commonly, an allergen is inhaled and starts the inflammatory and bronchoconstriction cascade.

- The pathophysiologic hallmark of an acute asthma attack is airflow obstruction with primarily ventilation/perfusion mismatch and most asthma attacks are not associated with profound hypoxemia. If the patients begin to demonstrate higher oxygen demands, other causes of shunt, such as pneumonia or patent foramen ovale, need to be explored.

- The vital signs of an asthma patient are important in the emergency setting. Respiratory rate, blood pressure, and pulse oximetry need to be monitored frequently.

- The use of a short-acting β-agonist is the cornerstone of acute asthma therapy.

- A metered-dose inhaler with a spacer has been proved to be as efficacious as jet nebulizer therapy.

- Anticholinergic medications can be recommended to be used, along with β-agonists, in the emergency treatment of a severe asthma exacerbation but not during hospitalization.

- Steroids have been shown to improve lung function, reduce admissions, and decrease asthma mortality but the role of inhaled corticosteroids in acute asthma is controversial.

- Magnesium sulfate should be reserved for the severe, acute asthmatic patient.

- Ventilatory assistance can be life saving in acute asthma exacerbations when medical therapy alone has failed. The main goal of mechanical ventilation is to maintain adequate oxygenation while preventing iatrogenic lung injury long enough for medical therapy to take effect and allow for the withdrawal of ventilatory assistance.

- Noninvasive positive pressure ventilation should be used first as an attempt to avoid endotracheal intubation. Indications for intubation include obtundation, apnea or near apnea, and impending cardiopulmonary collapse.

- Sedative agents with a rapid onset of action can be used in the peri- and post-intubation period for patient comfort and to enhance compliance with ventilation.

- When a patient who has recovered from status asthmaticus is discharged from the hospital a detailed and individualized 'action plan' must be in place.

REFERENCES

1. Mannino DM, Homa DM, Pertowski CA, *et al.* Surveillance for asthma – United States, 1960–1995. *MMWR CDC Surveill Summ* 1998; **47**: 1–27.

2. Asthma prevalence and control characteristics by race/ethnicity – United States, 2002. *MMWR Weekly* 2004; **53**: 145–8.

3. Mannino DM, Homa DM, Akinbami LJ, *et al.* Surveillance for asthma – United States, 1980–1999. *MMWR Surveill Summ* 2002; **51**: 1–13.

4. *NHLBI/WHO Workshop Report: Global Strategy for Asthma Diagnosis and Management.* Washington, DC: US Department of Health and Human Services; 1995. NIH Publication No 95–3659.

5. Schleimer RP. An overview of glucocorticoid anti-inflammatory actions. *Eur J Clin Pharmacol* 1993; **45**(Suppl 1): S3–7; discussion S43–4.

6. Barnes PJ. Inhaled glucocorticoids for asthma. *N Engl J Med* 1995; **332**: 868–75.

7. Montefort S, Gratziou C, Goulding D, *et al.* Bronchial biopsy evidence for leukocyte infiltration and upregulation of leukocyte-endothelial cell adhesion molecules 6 hours after local allergen challenge of sensitized asthmatic airways. *J Clin Invest* 1994; **93**: 1411–21.

8. Woolley KL, Adelroth E, Woolley MJ, *et al.* Effects of allergen challenge on eosinophils, eosinophil cationic protein, and granulocyte-macrophage colony-stimulating factor in mild asthma. *Am J Respir Crit Care Med* 1995; **151**: 1915–24.

9. Fahy JV, Liu J, Wong H, Boushey HA. Analysis of cellular and biochemical constituents of induced sputum after allergen challenge: a method for studying allergic airway inflammation. *J Allergy Clin Immunol* 1994; **93**: 1031–9.

10. Kroegel C, Julius P, Matthys H, *et al.* Endobronchial secretion of interleukin-13 following local allergen challenge in atopic asthma: relationship to interleukin-4 and eosinophil counts. *Eur Respir J* 1996; **9**: 899–904.

11. Beasley R, Roche WR, Roberts JA, Holgate ST. Cellular events in the bronchi in mild asthma and after bronchial provocation. *Am Rev Respir Dis* 1989; **139**: 806–17.

12. Tillie-Leblond I, Gosset P, Tonnel AB. Inflammatory events in severe acute asthma. *Allergy* 2005; **60**: 23–9.

13. Maestrelli P, Saetta M, Mapp CE, Fabbri LM. Remodeling in response to infection and injury. Airway inflammation and hypersecretion of mucus in smoking subjects with chronic obstructive pulmonary disease. *Am J Respir Crit Care Med* 2001; **164**(10 Pt 2): S76–80.

14. Laitinen LA, Heino M, Laitinen A, *et al.* Damage of the airway epithelium and bronchial reactivity in patients with asthma. *Am Rev Respir Dis* 1985; **131**: 599–606.

15. Ordonez C, Ferrando R, Hyde DM, *et al.* Epithelial desquamation in asthma: artifact or pathology? *Am J Respir Crit Care Med* 2000; **162**: 2324–9.

16. Aikawa T, Shimura S, Sasaki H, *et al.* Marked goblet cell hyperplasia with mucus accumulation in the airways of patients who died of severe acute asthma attack. *Chest* 1992; **101**: 916–21.

17. Houston JC, De Navasquez S, Trounce JR. A clinical and pathological study of fatal cases of status asthmaticus. *Thorax* 1953; **8**: 207–13.

18. Carroll N, Elliot J, Morton A, James A. The structure of large and small airways in nonfatal and fatal asthma. *Am Rev Respir Dis* 1993; **147**: 405–10.

19. Rodrigo GJ, Rodrigo C, Hall JB. Acute asthma in adults: a review. *Chest* 2004; **125**: 1081–102.

20. McFadden ER, Jr. Acute severe asthma. *Am J Respir Crit Care Med* 2003; **168**: 740–59.

21. Pinsky M. Cardiopulmonary interactions associated with airflow obstruction. In: Hall J, Corbridge T, Rodrigo C, *et al.*, eds. *Acute Asthma: Assessment and Management.* New York: McGraw-Hill; **2000**: 105–23.

22. Karpel J. When to hospitalize your patient with asthma. *J Crit Illn* 1995; **10**: 235–44.

23. Boushey HA, Corry DB, Fahy JV. Asthma. In: Murray JF, ed. *Textbook of Respiratory Medicine*, 3rd edition. New York: WB Saunders Company, 2000: 1247–90.

24. Services. DoD. *New asthma estimates: tracking prevalence, health care, and mortality.* Hyattsville, MD: National Center for Health Statistics, 2001.

25. Saetta M, Di Stefano A, Rosina C, et al. Quantitative structural analysis of peripheral airways and arteries in sudden fatal asthma. *Am Rev Respir Dis* 1991; **143**: 138–43.

26. Roe PF. Sudden death in asthma. *Br J Dis Chest* 1965; **59**: 158–63.

27. Sur S, Hunt LW, Crotty TB, Gleich GJ. Sudden-onset fatal asthma. *Mayo Clin Proc* 1994; **69**: 495–6.

28. Carroll N, Carello S, Cooke C, James A. Airway structure and inflammatory cells in fatal attacks of asthma. *Eur Respir J* 1996; **9**: 709–15.

29. Bai TR, Cooper J, Koelmeyer T, et al. The effect of age and duration of disease on airway structure in fatal asthma. *Am J Respir Crit Care Med* 2000; **162** (2 Pt 1): 663–9.

30. Sears MR. Asthma treatment: inhaled β-agonists. *Can Respir J* 1998; **5**(Suppl A): 54A–9A.

31. Crane J, Burgess CD, Graham AN, Maling TJ. Hypokalaemic and electrocardiographic effects of aminophylline and salbutamol in obstructive airways disease. *N Z Med J* 1987; **100**: 309–11.

32. Turner MO, Noertjojo K, Vedal S, et al. Risk factors for near-fatal asthma. A case-control study in hospitalized patients with asthma. *Am J Respir Crit Care Med* 1998; **157**(6 Pt 1): 1804–9.

33. Greenberger P. Potentially fatal asthma. *Chest* 1992; **101**: S401–2.

34. Dahlen I, Janson C. Anxiety and depression are related to the outcome of emergency treatment in patients with obstructive pulmonary disease. *Chest* 2002; **122**: 1633–7.

35. Fischl MA, Pitchenik A, Gardner LB. An index predicting relapse and need for hospitalization in patients with acute bronchial asthma. *N Engl J Med* 1981; **305**: 783–9.

36. Hardern R. Oxygen saturation in adults with acute asthma. *J Accid Emerg Med* 1996; **13**: 28–30.

37. Rebuck AS, Pengelly LD. Development of pulsus paradoxus in the presence of airways obstruction. *N Engl J Med* 1973; **288**: 66–9.

38. Knowles GK, Clark TJ. Pulsus paradoxus as a valuable sign indicating severity of asthma. *Lancet* 1973; **2**: 1356–9.

39. Nowak RM, Pensler MI, Sarkar DD, et al. Comparison of peak expiratory flow and FEV$_1$ admission criteria for acute bronchial asthma. *Ann Emerg Med* 1982; **11**: 64–9.

40. Grunfeld AF, Ho K. Emergency management of acute adult asthma. *Can Fam Physician* 1995; **41**: 1909–16.

41. Rodrigo G, Rodrigo C. Early prediction of poor response in acute asthma patients in the emergency department. *Chest* 1998; **114**: 1016–21.

42. Karpel JP, Appel D, Breidbart D, Fusco MJ. A comparison of atropine sulfate and metaproterenol sulfate in the emergency treatment of asthma. *Am Rev Respir Dis* 1986; **133**: 727–9.

43. Nowak RM, Tomlanovich MC, Sarkar DD, et al. Arterial blood gases and pulmonary function testing in acute bronchial asthma. Predicting patient outcomes. *JAMA* 1983; **249**: 2043–6.

44. Rosero SZ, Zareba W, Moss AJ, et al. Asthma and the risk of cardiac events in the Long QT syndrome. Long QT Syndrome Investigative Group. *Am J Cardiol* 1999; **84**: 1406–11.

45. Hospenthal MA, Peters JI. Long-acting β-agonists in the management of asthma exacerbations. *Curr Opin Pulm Med* 2005; **11**: 69–73.

46. O'Byrne PM, Bisgaard H, Godard PP, et al. Budesonide/formoterol combination therapy as both maintenance and reliever medication in asthma. *Am J Respir Crit Care Med* 2005; **171**: 129–36.

47. Ciccolella DE, Brennan K, Kelsen SG, Criner GJ. Dose-response characteristics of nebulized albuterol in the treatment of acutely ill, hospitalized asthmatics. *J Asthma* 1999; **36**: 539–46.

48. Cydulka RK, McFadden ER, Sarver JH, Emerman CL. Comparison of single 7.5-mg dose treatment vs sequential multidose 2.5-mg treatments with nebulized albuterol in the treatment of acute asthma. *Chest* 2002; **122**: 1982–7.

49. Stein J, Levitt MA. A randomized, controlled double-blind trial of usual-dose versus high-dose albuterol via continuous nebulization in patients with acute bronchospasm. *Acad Emerg Med* 2003; **10**: 31–6.

50. Nowak RM, Emerman CL, Schaefer K, et al. Levalbuterol compared with racemic albuterol in the treatment of acute asthma: results of a pilot study. *Am J Emerg Med* 2004; **22**: 29–36.

51. Truitt T, Witko J, Halpern M. Levalbuterol compared to racemic albuterol: efficacy and outcomes in

patients hospitalized with COPD or asthma. *Chest* 2003; **123**: 128–35.

52. Idris AH, McDermott MF, Raucci JC, *et al.* Emergency department treatment of severe asthma. Metered-dose inhaler plus holding chamber is equivalent in effectiveness to nebulizer. *Chest* 1993; **103**: 665–72.

53. Cates CC, Bara A, Crilly JA, Rowe BH. Holding chambers versus nebulisers for β-agonist treatment of acute asthma. *Cochrane Database Syst Rev* 2003: CD000052.

54. Shrestha M, Bidadi K, Gourlay S, Hayes J. Continuous vs intermittent albuterol, at high and low doses, in the treatment of severe acute asthma in adults. *Chest* 1996; **110**: 42–7.

55. Rodrigo GJ, Rodrigo C. Continuous vs intermittent β-agonists in the treatment of acute adult asthma: a systematic review with meta-analysis. *Chest* 2002; **122**: 160–5.

56. *Guidelines for the Diagnosis and Management of Asthma: Expert Panel Report II*. Bethesda, MD: National Institutes of Health, 1997. Report No. 97–4051.

57. Karpel JP, Aldrich TK, Prezant DJ, *et al.* Emergency treatment of acute asthma with albuterol metered-dose inhaler plus holding chamber: how often should treatments be administered? *Chest* 1997; **112**: 348–56.

58. Travers AH, Rowe BH, Barker S, *et al.* The effectiveness of IV β-agonists in treating patients with acute asthma in the emergency department: a meta-analysis. *Chest* 2002; **122**: 1200–7.

59. Gotz VP, Brandstetter RD, Mar DD. Bronchodilatory effect of subcutaneous epinephrine in acute asthma. *Ann Emerg Med* 1981; **10**: 518–20.

60. Murphy FT, Manown TJ, Knutson SW, Eliasson AH. Epinephrine-induced lactic acidosis in the setting of status asthmaticus. *South Med J* 1995; **88**: 577–9.

61. Stoodley RG, Aaron SD, Dales RE. The role of ipratropium bromide in the emergency management of acute asthma exacerbation: a metaanalysis of randomized clinical trials. *Ann Emerg Med* 1999; **34**: 8–18.

62. Rodrigo G, Rodrigo C, Burschtin O. A meta-analysis of the effects of ipratropium bromide in adults with acute asthma. *Am J Med* 1999; **107**: 363–70.

63. Rodrigo GJ, Rodrigo C. The role of anticholinergics in acute asthma treatment: an evidence-based evaluation. *Chest* 2002; **121**: 1977–87.

64. Rodrigo GJ, Rodrigo C. First-line therapy for adult patients with acute asthma receiving a multiple-dose protocol of ipratropium bromide plus albuterol in the emergency department. *Am J Respir Crit Care Med* 2000; **161**: 1862–8.

65. Gross NJ, Skorodin MS. Anticholinergic, antimuscarinic bronchodilators. *Am Rev Respir Dis* 1984; **129**: 856–70.

66. Rowe BH, Spooner C, Ducharme FM, *et al.* Early emergency department treatment of acute asthma with systemic corticosteroids. *Cochrane Database Syst Rev* 2001: CD002178.

67. Benatar SR. Fatal asthma. *N Engl J Med* 1986; **314**: 423–9.

68. McFadden ER, Jr. Dosages of corticosteroids in asthma. *Am Rev Respir Dis* 1993; **147**: 1306–10.

69. Global Strategy for Asthma Prevention and Management. In: National Institutes of Health: National Heart L, and Blood Institute, editor. 2002.

70. Lee-Wong M, Dayrit FM, Kohli AR, *et al.* Comparison of high-dose inhaled flunisolide to systemic corticosteroids in severe adult asthma. *Chest* 2002; **122**: 1208–13.

71. Edmonds ML. Evidence-based emergency medicine/systematic review abstract. Are corticosteroids effective in acute exacerbations of chronic obstructive pulmonary disease? *Ann Emerg Med* 2003; **42**: 426–8.

72. Rossing TH, Fanta CH, Goldstein DH, *et al.* Emergency therapy of asthma: comparison of the acute effects of parenteral and inhaled sympathomimetics and infused aminophylline. *Am Rev Respir Dis* 1980; **122**: 365–71.

73. Littenberg B. Aminophylline treatment in severe, acute asthma. A meta-analysis. *JAMA* 1988; **259**: 1678–84.

74. Kobayashi M, Nasuhara Y, Betsuyaku T, *et al.* Effect of low-dose theophylline on airway inflammation in COPD. *Respirology* 2004; **9**: 249–54.

75. McFadden ER, Jr, Lyons HA. Arterial-blood gas tension in asthma. *N Engl J Med* 1968; **278**: 1027–32.

76. Eckert DJ, Catcheside PG, Smith JH, *et al.* Hypoxia suppresses symptom perception in asthma. *Am J Respir Crit Care Med* 2004; **169**: 1224–30.

77. Rodrigo GJ, Rodriquez Verde M, Peregalli V, Rodrigo C. Effects of short-term 28% and 100% oxygen on $PaCO_2$ and peak expiratory flow rate in acute asthma: a randomized trial. *Chest* 2003; **124**: 1312–17.

78. Kress JP, Noth I, Gehlbach BK, *et al.* The utility of

albuterol nebulized with heliox during acute asthma exacerbations. *Am J Respir Crit Care Med* 2002; **165**: 1317–21.

79. Manthous CA, Hall JB, Caputo MA, *et al.* Heliox improves pulsus paradoxus and peak expiratory flow in nonintubated patients with severe asthma. *Am J Respir Crit Care Med* 1995; **151**(2 Pt 1): 310–14.

80. Kudukis TM, Manthous CA, Schmidt GA, *et al.* Inhaled helium-oxygen revisited: effect of inhaled helium-oxygen during the treatment of status asthmaticus in children. *J Pediatr* 1997; **130**: 217–24.

81. Rolla G, Bucca C, Caria E, *et al.* Acute effect of intravenous magnesium sulfate on airway obstruction of asthmatic patients. *Ann Allergy* 1988; **61**: 388–91.

82. Skobeloff EM, Spivey WH, McNamara RM, Greenspon L. Intravenous magnesium sulfate for the treatment of acute asthma in the emergency department. *JAMA* 1989; **262**: 1210–13.

83. Green SM, Rothrock SG. Intravenous magnesium for acute asthma: failure to decrease emergency treatment duration or need for hospitalization. *Ann Emerg Med* 1992; **21**: 260–5.

84. Tiffany BR, Berk WA, Todd IK, White SR. Magnesium bolus or infusion fails to improve expiratory flow in acute asthma exacerbations. *Chest* 1993; **104**: 831–4.

85. Bloch H, Silverman R, Mancherje N, *et al.* Intravenous magnesium sulfate as an adjunct in the treatment of acute asthma. *Chest* 1995; **107**: 1576–81.

86. Silverman RA, Osborn H, Runge J, *et al.* IV magnesium sulfate in the treatment of acute severe asthma: a multicenter randomized controlled trial. *Chest* 2002; **122**: 489–97.

87. Chande VT, Skoner DP. A trial of nebulized magnesium sulfate to reverse bronchospasm in asthmatic patients. *Ann Emerg Med* 1992; **21**: 1111–15.

88. Hill J, Lewis S, Britton J. Studies of the effects of inhaled magnesium on airway reactivity to histamine and adenosine monophosphate in asthmatic subjects. *Clin Exp Allergy* 1997; **27**: 546–51.

89. Bessmertny O, DiGregorio RV, Cohen H, *et al.* A randomized clinical trial of nebulized magnesium sulfate in addition to albuterol in the treatment of acute mild-to-moderate asthma exacerbations in adults. *Ann Emerg Med* 2002; **39**: 585–91.

90. Rowe BH, Bretzlaff JA, Bourdon C, *et al.* Intravenous magnesium sulfate treatment for acute asthma in the emergency department: a systematic review of the literature. *Ann Emerg Med* 2000; **36**: 181–90.

91. Rodrigo G, Rodrigo C, Burschtin O. Efficacy of magnesium sulfate in acute adult asthma: a meta-analysis of randomized trials. *Am J Emerg Med* 2000; **18**: 216–21.

92. Silverman RA, Nowak RM, Korenblat PE, *et al.* Zafirlukast treatment for acute asthma: evaluation in a randomized, double-blind, multicenter trial. *Chest* 2004; **126**: 1480–9.

93. Camargo CA, Jr, Smithline HA, Malice MP, *et al.* A randomized controlled trial of intravenous montelukast in acute asthma. *Am J Respir Crit Care Med* 2003; **167**: 528–33.

94. Cylly A, Kara A, Ozdemir T, *et al.* Effects of oral montelukast on airway function in acute asthma. *Respir Med* 2003; **97**: 533–6.

95. Bernstein IL, Ausdenmoore RW. Iatrogenic bronchospasm occurring during clinical trials of a new mucolytic agent, acetylcysteine. *Dis Chest* 1964; **46**: 469–73.

96. Karpel JP, Dworkin F, Hager D, *et al.* Inhaled furosemide is not effective in acute asthma. *Chest* 1994; **106**: 1396–400.

97. Joseph KS. Asthma mortality and antipsychotic or sedative use. What is the link? *Drug Saf* 1997; **16**: 351–4.

98. Rodrigo G, Rodrigo C. Corticosteroids in the emergency department therapy of acute adult asthma: an evidence-based evaluation. *Chest* 1999; **116**: 285–95.

99. Beveridge RC, Grunfeld AF, Hodder RV, Verbeek PR. Guidelines for the emergency management of asthma in adults. CAEP/CTS Asthma Advisory Committee. Canadian Association of Emergency Physicians and the Canadian Thoracic Society. *CMAJ* 1996; **155**: 25–37.

100. Wait JL K, JP. Managing acute respiratory failure in asthma: mechanical ventilation. *J Crit Illn* 1998; **13**: 347–55.

101. Soroksky A, Stav D, Shpirer I. A pilot prospective, randomized, placebo-controlled trial of bilevel positive airway pressure in acute asthmatic attack. *Chest* 2003; **123**: 1018–25.

102. Meduri GU, Cook TR, Turner RE, *et al.* Noninvasive positive pressure ventilation in status asthmaticus. *Chest* 1996; **110**: 767–74.

103. Slutsky AS. Mechanical ventilation. American College of Chest Physicians' Consensus Conference. *Chest* 1993; **104**: 1833–59.

104. Shapiro JM. Intensive care management of status asthmaticus. *Chest* 2001; **120**: 1439–41.

105. Tuxen DV, Williams TJ, Scheinkestel CD, *et al.* Use of a measurement of pulmonary hyperinflation to control the level of mechanical ventilation in patients with acute severe asthma. *Am Rev Respir Dis* 1992; **146** (5 Pt 1): 1136–42.

106. Williams TJ, Tuxen DV, Scheinkestel CD, *et al.* Risk factors for morbidity in mechanically ventilated patients with acute severe asthma. *Am Rev Respir Dis* 1992; **146**: 607–15.

107. Schaeffer EM, Pohlman A, Morgan S, Hall JB. Oxygenation in status asthmaticus improves during ventilation with helium-oxygen. *Crit Care Med* 1999; **27**: 2666–70.

108. Gluck EH, Onorato DJ, Castriotta R. Helium-oxygen mixtures in intubated patients with status asthmaticus and respiratory acidosis. *Chest* 1990; **98**: 693–8..

Emergency diagnoses and treatment of acute exacerbations of chronic obstructive pulmonary disease

ANTONIO ANZUETO, SANDRA G ADAMS

INTRODUCTION

The American Thoracic Society(ATS)/European Respiratory Society (ERS) has proposed defining exacerbations of chronic obstructive pulmonary disease (COPD) as an event in the natural course of the disease characterized by a change in the patient's baseline dyspnea, cough, and/or sputum beyond day-to-day variability sufficient to warrant a change in management.[1] This chapter reviews the emergency treatment of acute exacerbations of COPD (AECOPD). We will discuss the epidemiology, etiology (many patients with AECOPD are thought to have an infectious condition [viral and or bacterial] which contributes to the exacerbation), diagnostic procedures, therapies (including bronchodilators, corticosteroids, antibiotics), clinical parameters to stratify patients' severity, need for hospitalization, and ventilatory support (invasive and noninvasive).

EPIDEMIOLOGY

Chronic obstructive pulmonary disease comprises several clinical conditions including chronic bronchitis, emphysema, and asthma, which often coexist. Patients are prone to exacerbations under conditions that are usually associated with increased breathlessness. Often there is increase in cough, which may be productive of mucoid or purulent sputum, and malaise. These symptoms may produce significant decrement in quality of life. Acute exacerbations result in significant morbidity and mortality in this patient population.[1–4] The cost to treat AECOPD is high, not only because of the economic impact, but also because of increase in morbidity and early mortality.[5] In the United States, COPD annually accounts for 16 000 367 office visits, 500 000 hospitalizations, and 18 billion in direct healthcare cost.[6–8] Despite treatment with antibiotics, bronchodilators, and corticosteroids, up to 28 percent of patients with acute exacerbations discharged from emergency departments have recurrent symptoms within 14 days[9] and 17 percent relapse and require hospitalization.[10] Significant numbers of hospitalized patients with acute exacerbations have modifiable risk factors including influenza vaccination, oxygen supplementations, active smoking, and occupational exposures.

Identification of patients with AECOPD who are at risk for relapse should improve decisions about hospital admissions and follow-up visits. Several investigators have confirmed that relapse is more likely among patients who have lower pre-treatment or post-treatment forced expiratory volume in 1 second (FEV_1); those who receive more bronchodilator treatments or corticosteroids during visits; and those who have higher rates of previous relapse.[11] These factors can provide clinical guidance on the basis of identifying predictors of failure, but they have poor sensitivity and specificity.

Prospective studies have identified the risk factors associated with mortality during AECOPD. The Study to Understand Prognosis and Preferences for Outcomes and Rates of Treatment (SUPPORT)[12] enrolled 1016 patients who had severe AECOPD at hospital admissions due to respiratory infections, including pneumonia (48 percent), congestive heart failure (26 percent), worsening respiratory failure due to lung cancer (3.3 percent), pulmonary emboli (1.4 percent), and pneumothorax (1 percent). The 180-day mortality was 33 percent and the 2-year mortality was 49 percent. Significant predictors of mortality include acute physiology and chronic health evaluation (APACHE III) score,[13] body mass index, age, functional status 2 weeks prior to admission, lower ratio of Po_2 to Fio_2, congestive heart failure, serum albumen level, cor pulmonale, lower activities of daily living scores, and lower scores on the Duke Activity Status Index. This study also reported that only 25 percent of patients were both alive and able to report a good, very good, or excellent quality of life 6 months after discharge.

Another large prospective cohort study included patients who were admitted to intensive care units with COPD-related respiratory failure.[11] The inhospital mortality (23.8 percent) was predicted by number of hospital days before transfer to intensive care unit, and the nonrespiratory component of the APACHE III score. A separate analysis to identify true predictors of 180-day mortality included acute physiological score, age, and hospital days before transfer to intensive care unit. Activities of daily living were also significant predictors in the univariate analysis.

In another cohort of 101 patients with moderate to severe COPD (mean FEV_1 41.9 percent predicted), which was closely followed up for 2.5 years, increased dyspnea and colds at onset of exacerbation were associated with prolonged recovery times. Recovery was incomplete in a significant proportion of COPD exacerbations.[14] Patients with frequent exacerbations (median 3–8/year) experience significantly worse quality of life, as measured by the St George Respiratory Questionnaire. Factors that predicted frequent exacerbations were the number of exacerbations in the previous year and a history of bronchitic symptoms (cough and sputum production), but lung function was not related.[15]

ETIOLOGY

Although respiratory infections are assumed to be an important factor for AECOPD, other noninfectious conditions have to be considered. These include congestive heart failure, pulmonary embolism, and seasonal allergies[16] (Box 14B.1).

Box 14B.1 Risk factors for AECOPD

Infections

- Bacteria (Gram-positive and Gram-negative)
- Virus

Environmental factors

- Cigarette smoking
- Passive smoking
- Ambient air pollution
- Occupational factors

A variety of microorganisms have been shown to be associated with AECOPD. The bacteria most frequently isolated are *Haemophilus influenzae*, *Haemophilus parainfluenzae*, *Moraxella catarrhalis*, and *Streptococcus pneumoniae* (Fig. 14B.1).[16] Recently it has been recognized that patients can be infected by atypical pathogens such as *Mycoplasma pneumoniae* and *Chlamydia pneumoniae*, but because of limitations with the diagnosis, the true prevalence of these organisms is not known. We also have to recognize that viruses are also important pathogens that precipitate this condition.[17]

Several studies have shown that patients with severe COPD have a significantly higher prevalence of Gram-negative organisms such as Enterobacteriaceae and *Pseudomonas* species.[18–20] One of the first groups of investigators to report these findings were Eller *et al.*[18] who evaluated sputum cultures from 112 inpatients with AECOPD. Sixty-four percent of patients with an FEV_1 ≤35 percent predicted versus only 30 percent of those with FEV_1 ≥50 percent ($P = 0.016$) had evidence of Gram-negative organisms. The most commonly isolated organisms included Enterobacteriaceae, *Pseudomonas* species, *Proteus vulgaris*,

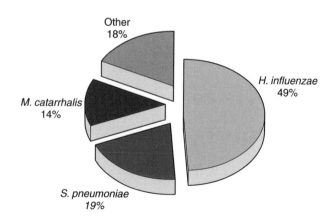

Figure 14B.1 *Most frequently isolated bacteria in acute exacerbation of chronic obstructive pulmonary disease.*

Serratia marcescens, Stenotrophomonas maltophilia, and *Escherichia coli.* Miravitlles *et al.*[19] found similar results. These investigators evaluated the relation between FEV_1 and the isolation of diverse pathogens in the sputum of 91 patients with COPD who presented with type 1 (severe) or type 2 (moderate) symptoms of AECOPD. Patients were separated into groups by FEV_1 (≥ 50 percent versus <50 percent predicted). There were significantly larger numbers of *H. influenzae* and *P. aeruginosa* in the group with $FEV_1 < 50$ percent predicted ($P < 0.05$). In contrast, there were significantly larger numbers of nonpotentially pathogenic microorganisms in the group with $FEV_1 \leq 50$ percent ($P < 0.05$). These authors also performed a multivariate analysis with logistic regression and found that *H. influenzae* was cultured significantly more often in patients who were active smokers (odds ratio [OR] 8.2, confidence interval [CI] 1.9 to 43) and whose FEV_1 was <50 percent predicted (OR 6.85, CI 1.6 to 52). *P. aeruginosa* was also cultured significantly more frequently in those with poor lung function, $FEV_1 < 50$ percent (OR 6.6, CI 1.2 to 124).

DIAGNOSTIC PROCEDURES

Recent reviews on the evidence base summarized the available information related to the use of diagnostic tests in AECOPD.[21,22] These reviews concluded that data on the utility of most diagnostic tests are limited. However, chest radiography and arterial blood gas sampling seem useful whereas acute spirometry does not. On the basis of observational studies, for patients with AECOPD treated in emergency departments or hospitals the chest radiograph is a useful diagnostic test. In a study that evaluated 685 patients, chest radiographs showed a 16 percent abnormality rate, mainly the presence of infiltrates consistent with pneumonia.[23] In another prospective cohort of 128 hospital admissions for asthma or COPD, 21 percent of patients had a change in management prompted by the findings of the chest radiograph. Most patients had new pulmonary infiltrate or evidence of congestive heart failure.[24] We recommend that in those patients with AECOPD who are evaluated in an emergency room and/or required hospitalization a chest radiograph be obtained to rule out any other abnormalities. Although chest tomography is more sensitive, and therefore, potentially valuable in evaluation of patients with AECOPD, there are no clinical studies on it use.

Spirometric assessment at presentation or during treatment of acute exacerbation is not useful in judging the severity or guiding the management of the patient. Although peak expiratory flow rate and FEV_1 are correlated ($r = 0.84$; $P < 0.001$), the FEV_1 showed no significant correlation with Po_2 and only weak correlation with Pco_2.[10] At this time, there are no data to support the routine use of peak flow meters or FEV_1 assessment in the management of COPD exacerbations. Therefore, we do not recommend it.

TREATMENT

The ATS/ERS recommendation for the diagnoses and treatment of AECOPD proposed an operational classification of severity related to the 'site' that the patient received their care.[1] These guidelines proposed that AECOPD be classified as (Table 14B.1):

- Level I – treated at home
- Level II – requires hospitalization
- Level III – leads to respiratory failure.

Bronchodilator therapy

Bronchodilator drugs are the primary therapeutic intervention in patients with AECOPD (Table 14B.2). There are no clearly defined objective endpoints that can routinely be use to assess the patient's improvement. The endpoints that most investigators use are improvement in symptoms. Other parameters such as improvement in physical findings or pulmonary functions tests are more variable. The bronchodilators used to treat AECOPD are: short-acting β_2-agonists, long-acting β_2-agonists, and anticholinergic agents.[25–28] Clinical studies have shown that short-acting β_2-agonists and ipratropium bromide are equally efficacious in AECOPD. Furthermore, adding ipratropium bromide to a short- or long-acting β_2-agonist will improve the patient's spirometry and clinical response.[27,29,30] Thus, the current clinical practice is to use both drugs together.

The inhaled route for delivering these drugs has been shown to result in fewer adverse events and maximum efficacy. Patients can receive metered-dose inhalers (MDIs) in combination with devices such as large-volume attachments (spacers), breath-attenuated MDIs, and dry-powdered inhalers. The techniques to use MDI and their attachments must be taught to the patients and reinforced. Drug deposition may vary among delivery systems. Nebulization has been the preferred mode to deliver bronchodilators during acute exacerbation mainly because patients have difficulty in using MDIs. The safety and value of continued drug nebulization delivery has not been established in COPD. Randomized controlled trials using MDI versus nebulization have not shown the superiority of continuous nebulization therapy.[31,32] In patients being mechanically ventilated, bronchodilator delivery via MDI with a spacer results in higher particle deposition as compared with nebulization.[33,34] The dose schedule for the β_2-agonists and ipratropium bromide during an acute exacerbation has not been established. In most patients these drugs are giving every 4–6 hours to avoid side effects.

There is no evidence that oral or intravenous β_2-agonists improve bronchodilator response; therefore these routes of administration are not recommended. High doses of β_2-agonists are known to be associated with increased side effects, including tachyrhythmias, tremors, and morbidity.

Table 14B.1   *Guidelines of the American Thoracic Society/European Respriatory Society classification and treatment recommendations based on the site of care*[1]

Level I – treatment for the ambulatory patient	Patient education
	   Inhalation techniques
	   Use of spacers
	Bronchodilators
	   Short acting β_2–agonist (albuterol, salbutamol) and/or ipratropium MDI with spacer or handheld nebulizer as needed
	   Consider add long-acting bronchodilator if patient is not using it
	Consider – corticosteroids
	   Dose not well defined
	   Prednisone 30–40 mg orally daily for 5–7 days
	   Consider using an inhaled corticosteroid
	Antibiotics – may be initiated in patients who have a change in their sputum characteristics (purulence and/or volume) choice should be based on local bacteria resistance patterns

Level II – treatment for hospitalized patient	Bronchodilators
	   Short acting β_2–agonist (albuterol, salbutamol) and/or ipratropium MDI with spacer or handheld nebulizer as needed
	Supplemental oxygen (if saturation <90%)
	Corticosteroids
	   Dose not well defined
	   If patient tolerates per oral - prednisone 30–40 mg orally daily for 5–7 days
	   If patient can not tolerate per oral, give the equivalent dose intravenously for up to 14 days
	   Consider use of inhaled corticosteroids by MDI or handheld nebulizer
	   Antibiotics (based on local bacteria resistance patterns)

Level III – treatment for the special care and/or intensive care unit patient	Supplemental oxygen
	Ventilatory support
	Bronchodilators
	   Short acting β_2–agonist (albuterol, salbutamol) and ipratropium MDI with spacer, 2 puffs every 2–4 h
	   If the patient is on the ventilator, consider MDI administration
	   Consider long-acting β-agonist
	Corticosteroids
	   Dose not well defined.
	   If patient tolerates per oral – prednisone 30–40 orally daily for 5–7 days
	   If patient can not tolerate per oral, give the equivalent dose intravenously for up to 14 days
	   Consider use of inhaled corticosteroids by MDI or handheld nebulizer
	Antibiotics (based on local bacteria resistance patterns)

MDI, metered-dose inhaler.

Table 14B.2   *Pharmacotherapy for acute exacerbations of chronic obstructive pulmonary disease: onset of action and dosing frequency of commonly use inhalers*

Drug	Inhaler dose (μg)	Dosing frequency
Short-acting β_2–agonists		
Albuterol (Ventolin®, Proventil®)	100–200 MDI, DPI	Q 4–6 hours
Pirbuterol (Maxair®)	100 MDI	Q 4–hours
Short-acting anticholinergics		
Ipratropium bromide (Atrovent®)	20–40 MDI	Q 4–6 hours
Long-acting β_2–agonists		
Salmeterol (Serevent®)	4.5–12 MDI, DPI	Q 12 hours
Formoterol (Foradil®)	25–50 MDI, DPI	Q 12 hours
Short-acting anticholinergics		
Tiotropium (Spiriva®)	18 DPI	Q 24 hours
Inhaled corticosteroids		
Budesonide (Pulmicort®)	100, 200, 400 DPI	Q 12 hours
Fluticasone (Flovent®)	50–500 MDI, DPI	Q 12 hours
Combination therapy		
Salmeterol + Fluticasone (Advir®)	50/100, 250, 500 DPI 25/50, 125, 250 MDI	Q 12 hours

MDI, metered dose inhaler; DPI, dry power inhaler; Q, every.

Recent studies have described the increased rate of cardiac events associated with use of β_2-agonists in patients with COPD,[35] and they failed to show a benefit of regular use of albuterol in stable patients.[36]

Short-acting β_2-agonists may be associated with an idiosyncratic bronchoconstriction response and tachyphylaxis with a decrease in the patient's clinical response.[37] Ipratropium bromide has been demonstrated to have minimal side effects, mainly unpleasant taste, and cough. There is no evidence that patients on ipratropium bromide can develop tolerance to chronic therapy.[38]

Methylxanthines, theophylline, and/or aminophylline

Methylxanthines, theophylline, and/or aminophylline have been shown to have comparable or less bronchodilator effect than β_2-agonists or anticholinergic agents.[38] The major limitations of these drugs include the need for continuous blood level monitoring.[39] Their side effects include cardiac arrhythmias, electrolyte imbalances, and extensive drug interactions.[40] Because of the potential for fatal adverse effects and the need for serum level monitoring, we do not recommend the use of methylxanthines in the treatment of AECOPD.

Corticosteroids

Corticosteroids are recommended in most cases of AECOPD. There is consensus that patients with significant bronchodilator response are more likely to benefit from this therapy. Corticosteroids can be administered intravenously, orally, and by inhalation. There are few data on the use of inhaled corticosteroids during an acute exacerbation of COPD.

Albert *et al.*[41] published the first randomized, double-blind, placebo-controlled trial of systemic corticosteroids in the treatment of AECOPD. A regimen of intravenous methylprednisolone four times daily for 3 days produced an early improvement in FEV$_1$ during the treatment period. Other studies have suggested that a short course of oral prednisone therapy can be useful.[42,43] A 2-week course of 30 mg daily oral prednisone in patients with severe airflow obstruction resulted in a significantly lower rate of treatment failure, a decreased length of hospital stay and a more rapid improvement in FEV$_1$.[43] In the largest study published to date – the Systemic Corticosteroids in Chronic Obstructive Pulmonary Disease Exacerbations (SCCOPE) study – 271 patients with AECOPD were enrolled.[44] Patients received placebo or a two-dose regimen of corticosteroids therapy for 2 or 8 weeks. For the combined glucocorticoid group, the risk for treatment failure as compared with placebo was reduced by 10 percentage points (33 percent vs. 23 percent respectively) and FEV$_1$ significantly improved during the first 3 days of therapy. There was no difference in FEV$_1$ after

2 weeks. The SCCOPE trial demonstrated equivalent outcome between 2-week and 8-week corticosteroid regimens (Figure 14B.2).

The role of inhaled corticosteroids in AECOPD is not well defined. Although some studies have failed to show a role for inhaled corticosteroids in speeding up symptom resolution, these trials were not designed to answer this question. A recently published prospective randomized trial comparing high-dose nebulized budesonide (2 mg every 6 hours × 72 hours) with prednisone (30 mg twice daily × 72 hours), demonstrated no difference between active treatments, with both being superior to placebo in terms of recovery of FEV$_1$.[45] In patients with moderate to severe lung disease and frequent exacerbations of COPD, ongoing treatment with inhaled corticosteroids has been shown to reduce the numbers of yearly exacerbation.

Well-known side effects of systemic corticosteroids are the major limiting factors of this therapy. The SCCOPE trial showed that hyperglycemia was significantly more frequent in patients who received corticosteroids compared with placebo.[44] In patients with COPD, corticosteroid-induced myopathy may be more common than was initially appreciated. Histologically, both myopathic changes and generalized muscle fiber atrophy have been reported.[46] In one study, survival of patients with steroid-induced myopathy was significantly lower compared to those without myopathy, but with similar airflow obstruction.[47] However, these studies showed that systemic corticosteroids lead to a faster improvement in FEV$_1$, more rapid recovery of partial arterial oxygen tension (PaO$_2$), fewer treatment failures, and lower hospitalization rates.

The exact dose and duration of therapy should be individualized, and more specific recommendations must await further evidence. It appears that 7–10 days of therapy

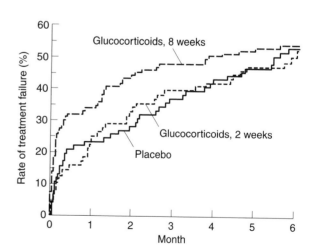

Figure 14B.2   *FEV$_1$ response to corticosteroids and placebo. (Redrawn with permission from Thompson WH, Nielson CP, Carvalho P, et al. Controlled trial of oral prednisone I outpatients with acute COPD exacerbation. Am J Respir Crit Care Med 1996;* **154:** *407–12.[44]) PERMISSION PENDING*

are more effective than longer periods of time. The oral studies have demonstrated that the peak effect is seen around day 5. A patient who responds to corticosteroids therapy during an AECOPD will not, however, necessarily benefit from long-term use of these drugs. Therefore, patients should be carefully selected for their suitability for these drugs.

Mucus-clearing strategies: expectorants, mucolytics, and mucokinetic agents

In COPD, mucus is generally copious and tenacious and is a major feature both during the stable condition and exacerbations. Current data suggest that pharmacologic mucus-clearing strategies do not shorten the disease course of patients with acute exacerbation or improve FEV_1.[48] We cannot recommend the use of any currently available mucolytic agents during acute exacerbations of AECOPD.

Antibiotics

The specific etiology of AECOPD is difficult to determine in an outpatient office setting on the basis of symptoms and signs. Sputum studies, although potentially useful, have significant limitations. Their routine use is mainly limited by the delay in obtaining the results, cost, and lack of sensitivity and specificity. Recent treatment guidelines for AECOPD reflect the lack of an evidence base to provide specific recommendations for the use of antibiotics.[22,23] The Global Initiative for Chronic Obstructive Pulmonary Disease (GOLD) guideline, a joint initiative of the National Heart, Lung, and Blood Institute and the World Health Organization for COPD recommends antibiotic choices on the basis of local sensitivity patterns of the most common pathogens associated with AECOPD, but does not provide any specific reccomendations.[1–3]

A number of clinical trials have examined the use of antibiotics in the treatment of AECOPD.[49–55] Many of the earlier studies showed no or minimal benefit when antibiotics were prescribed. More recent publications, including a metaanalysis,[49] demonstrated a benefit of antibiotics during an acute exacerbation, but not in preventing exacerbations. In 1987, Anthonisen et al.[50] reported the results of a large-scale placebo-controlled trial designed to determine the effectiveness of antibiotics in the treatment of AECOPD. In this study, 173 patients with chronic bronchitis were followed for 3.5 years, during which time they had 362 exacerbations. This study finally brought some conformity to the definition of AECOPD and gave the first widely accepted classification for the severity of presenting symptoms. Patients who are classified as 'severe' AECOPD include those with all three clinical symptoms (increased shortness of breath, increased sputum production, and a change in sputum purulence) at initial presentation. The study patients were randomized to either

antibiotics or placebo in a double-blind, crossover fashion. Three oral antibiotics were used (chosen by the primary physician) for 10 days: amoxicillin, trimethoprim-sulfamethoxazole (co-trimoxazole), and doxycycline. Patients with the most severe exacerbations (type 1) received a significant benefit from antibiotics, whereas there was no significant difference between antibiotic and placebo in patients who had only one of the defined symptoms (type 3). Overall, the antibiotic-treated patients showed a more rapid improvement in peak flow, a greater percentage of clinical successes, and a smaller percentage of clinical failures than those who received placebo. In addition, the length of illness was 2 days shorter for the antibiotic-treated group. The major criticisms of this study were that no microbiologic investigations were done and that all antibiotics were assumed to be equivalent.

Allegra et al.[51] found significant benefit with the use of amoxicillin-clavulanate acid (Augmentin®) therapy compared with placebo in patients with severe disease. Patients who received this antibiotic exhibited a higher success rate (86.4 percent vs. 50.3 percent in the placebo group, P <0.01) and a lower frequency of recurrent exacerbations. In 1995 Saint et al.[49] published the results of a metaanalysis examining the role of antibiotics in the treatment of AECOPD (Fig. 14B.3). These investigators analyzed nine randomized, placebo-controlled trials published between 1957 and 1992. There was an overall, statistically significant benefit for the antibiotic-treated

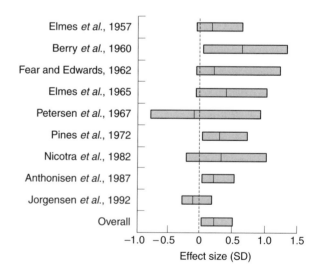

Figure 14B.3 *Effect sizes (mean differences in outcome divided by the pooled standard deviation) in nine studies of the use of antibiotics for exacerbations of chronic obstructive pulmonary disease. Horizontal lines denote 95 percent confidence intervals. The data indicate a significant improvement due to antibiotic therapy. (Redrawn with permission from 49 Saint S, Bent S, Vittinghoff E, et al. Antibiotics in chronic obstructive pulmonary disease exacerbations: a meta-analysis. JAMA 1995;273: 957–60.[49]) PERMISSION PENDING*

patients. Analysis of the studies that provided data on expiratory flow rates showed an improvement of 10.75 L/min in the antibiotic-treated groups. The authors conclude that this antibiotic-associated improvement is likely to be clinically significant, particularly in patients with low baseline peak flow rates and limited respiratory reserve.

There are additional potential benefits of antibiotic therapy for patients with AECOPD. Antibiotics can reduce the burden of bacteria in the airway.[52] Bronchoscopic studies, using sterile protected specimen brush, have demonstrated that approximately 25 percent of stable COPD patients show colonization (usually $\leq 10^3$ organisms) with potentially pathogenic bacteria.[53,54] However, during an acute exacerbation, a much larger percentage (50–75 percent) of patients have potentially pathogenic microorganisms in addition to significantly higher concentrations (frequently $\geq 10^4$ organisms) of bacteria.[20,54–56] Treatment with appropriate antibiotics will significantly decrease the bacterial burden (and frequently eradicate the organisms that are sensitive) and reduce the risk of progression to more severe infections such as pneumonia.[57] A prospective, randomized, double-blind, placebo-controlled trial, evaluating the use of ofloxacin in 90 consecutive patients with AECOPD who required mechanical ventilation, showed that the antibiotic-treated group had a significantly lower inhospital mortality rate (4 percent vs. 22 percent, $P = 0.01$) and significantly reduced length of stay in the hospital (14.9 vs. 24.5, $P = 0.01$) compared with the placebo group. In addition, the patients receiving ofloxacin were less likely to develop pneumonia than those on placebo, especially during the first week of mechanical ventilation (mean ± standard deviation: 7.2 ± 2.2 days [range 4–11] vs. 10.6 ± 2.9 days [range 9–14], $P = 0.04$ by log-rank test).

Relapse or no improvement after initial therapy in patients with AECOPD has recently being associated with significant risk for hospitalization and increased cost. The published relapse rates for patients with AECOPD range from 17 percent to 32 percent.[10,58,59] A retrospective study of outpatients with documented COPD conducted at our institution evaluated the risk factors for therapy failure at 14 days after an acute exacerbation.[58] The participating patients had a total of 362 exacerbations over an 18-month period. One group received antibiotics (270 visits) and the second group (92 visits) did not. The overall relapse rate (defined as a return visit with persistent or worsening symptoms within 14 days) was 22 percent. After an extensive multivariate analysis, the major risk factor for relapse was lack of antibiotic therapy (32 percent vs.19 percent compared with the antibiotic-treated group, $P < 0.001$). The type of antibiotic used was also an important variable associated with the 14-day treatment failure. Patients treated with amoxicillin had a 54 percent relapse rate compared with only 13 percent for the other antibiotics ($P < 0.01$). Furthermore, treatment with amoxicillin resulted in a higher incidence of failure, even when compared with those who did not receive

antibiotics ($P = 0.006$) (Fig. 14B.4). Other variables, such as COPD severity, types of exacerbation, prior or concomitant use of corticosteroids, and current use of chronic oxygen therapy were not significantly associated with the 14-day relapse. This study showed that the use of antibiotics was associated with a significantly lower rate of therapy failure. In contrast with Anthonisen's data,[50] our data show that antibiotics are beneficial regardless of the severity of AECOPD (i.e. those with mild AECOPD still benefit from treatment with antibiotics). Furthermore, patients who received antibiotics, but the treatment failed within 14 days, had a significantly higher rate of hospital admissions than those who did not receive antibiotics. Although there may be many explanations for these treatment failures, the most likely is that the pathogens were resistant to amoxicillin.

Destache et al. reported the impact of antibiotic selection, antimicrobial efficacy, and related cost in AECOPD.[59] The participating patients had a total of 224 episodes of AECOPD requiring antibiotic treatment. The antibiotics were arbitrarily divided into three groups: 'first-line' (amoxicillin, co-trimoxazole, erythromycin, and tetracycline), 'second-line' (cephradine, cefuroxime, cefaclor, cefprozil), and 'third-line' (amoxicillin-clavulanate, azithromycin, and ciprofloxacin). The failure rates were significantly higher (at 14 days) for the first-line compared with the third-line agents (19 percent vs. 7 percent, $P < 0.05$). When compared with those who received the first-line agents, the patients treated with the third-line agents had significantly longer time between exacerbations (17 weeks vs. 34 weeks, $P < 0.02$), overall fewer hospitalizations (18/26 [69 percent] vs. 3/26 [12 percent] patients, $P < 0.02$), and considerably lower total cost ($942 vs. $542, $P < 0.0001$) (Table 14B.3).

Based on the results of these studies, in addition to widespread reports of increasing antimicrobial resistance to

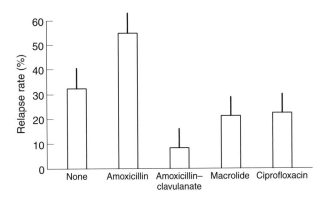

Figure 14B.4 *Acute exacerbations of chronic obstructive pulmonary disease: 14-day relapse rates after treatment with or without antibiotics. (Redrawn with permission from Adams S, Melo J, Luther M, et al. Antibiotics are associated with lower relapse rates in outpatients with acute exacerbations of chronic obstructive pulmonary disease. Chest 2000; 117: 1345–52.[58]) PERMISSION PENDING*

Table 14B.3 *Differences in clinical outcomes based on antibiotic selection**

	First-line	Second-line	Third-line
Days of therapy	8.9 ± 3.3	8.3 ± 2.3	7.5 ± 2.5[†]
Weeks between AECOPD	17.1 ± 22	22.7 ± 30	34.3 ± 35.5[†]
14-day failure rate (n = 36) (%)	19	16	7
Hospitalizations (% of total failures)	53	14	8
Cost per episode (US$)	942 ± 2173	563 ± 2296	542 ± 1946

*First-line – amoxicillin, co-trimoxazole, erythromycin, and tetracycline; second-line – cephradine, cefuroxime, cefaclor, cefprozil; and third-line–amoxicillin-clavulanate, azithromycin, and ciprofloxacin.

Data are presented in percentages (as indicated) and otherwise in mean ± SD.

[†]$P < 0.05$ third-line versus first-line.

Adapted with permission from Destache *et al.*[59]

the common pathogens isolated in patients with AECOPD, appropriate antibiotic selection is extremely important. Therefore, it is not only essential to treat these patients with antibiotics, but also critical to choose the appropriate one.

CLINICAL PARAMETERS TO STRATIFY PATIENTS INTO RISK GROUPS

Since AECOPD is associated with high morbidity and mortality, many investigators have attempted to describe characteristics that could be used to risk stratify patients with AECOPD. Based on the concept of risk stratification of patients by clinical parameters, a target approach for the treatment of AECOPD has been proposed by the Canadian Respiratory Society[60](Table 13B.4 and Box 14B.2).

This group developed a classification for patients presenting with symptoms of acute bronchitis taking into consideration the following variables: (i) number and severity of acute symptoms; (ii) age; (iii) severity of airflow obstruction (measured by FEV_1); (iv) frequency of exacerbations; and (v) history of comorbid conditions. Patients can be stratified into the following categories (see Table 14B.4):

- acute bronchitis (group 1) – healthy patients without previous respiratory problems
- 'simple' AECOPD (group 2) – patients younger than 65 years, have ≤4 exacerbations per year, with minimal or no impairment in lung function (by pulmonary function tests), AND without any comorbid conditions

Box 14B.2 Indications for hospitalization for patients with COPD exacerbation[1]

- Presence of high-risk comorbid conditions including pneumonia, cardiac arrhythmia, congestive heart failure, diabetes mellitus, renal or liver failure
- Inadequate response of symptoms to outpatient management
- Marked increase in dyspnea
- Inability to eat or sleep due to symptoms
- Worsening hypoxemia
- Worsening hypercapnia
- Changes in mental status
- Inability of patients to care for themselves (lack of home support)
- Uncertain diagnosis

Table 14B.4 *Treatment recommendations for antibiotic therapy for acute excerbations of chronic obstructive lung disease (AECOPD) based on the Canadian Lung Association classification of severity*

Category	Probable pathogen	Oral therapy
Acute bronchitis (group 1)	Viral	Symptomatic
'Simple' AECOPD (group 2)	*Haemophilus* spp. (*H. influenzae*) *M. catarrhalis*, *S. pneumoniae*, atypical organisms (possibly)	Doxycycline *or* newer macrolide (azithromycin/clarithromycin) *or* newer cephalosporins
'Complicated' AECOPD (groups 3 and 4)	As above, with the possible addition of *Pseudomonas* spp, Enterobacteriaceae, and other Gram-negative organisms	Fluoroquinolones* Amoxicillin–clavulanate

*If at risk for *Pseudomonas* infection, use ciprofloxacin.

Adapted from Balter *et al.*[60]

- 'complicated' AECOPD (group 3) – patients older than 65 years, with FEV_1 <50 percent predicted, and/OR with ≥4 exacerbations per year
- 'complicated' AECOPD with associated comorbid illnesses (group 4) – patients with congestive heart failure, liver disease, diabetes, or chronic renal failure.

CRITERIA FOR HOSPITAL ADMISSION AND DISCHARGE

The objective for hospitalization in patients with AECOPD is to manage the patient's acute decompensation and comorbid condition, and to prevent further deterioration. Increased age and severe hypoxemia have been the two major factors identified in predicting mortality in patients who have been hospitalized.[61] The criteria for hospitalization suggested by the ATS/ERS guidelines are summarized in Box 14B.2 above.

Length of stay has been a challenge in these patients. Longer hospital stays have being reported in patients with worse baseline lung function and multiple comorbid conditions.[62] Insufficient clinical data exist to further elucidate the factor that may influence the duration of hospitalization and the therapies that may help reduce it. In a randomized controlled trial of 184 patients referred to a hospital for admission for an AECOPD, it was shown that home-supported discharge is an alternative to a selected group of patients.[63] Home-supported therapy was a well tolerated, safe, and economic alternative to hospital admission. Since large numbers of patients could not be included in the trial due to the severity of their disease, comorbidities or social circumstances, the conclusions of this study apply only to a relative small proportion of patients presenting to the hospital with AECOPD (26 percent).[63] A study by Cotton and Bucknall[64] in 81 patients with acute respiratory failure that was uncomplicated by acidosis showed no differences in readmission rates in patients receiving either conventional inpatient care or early discharge with home treatment by respiratory nurses. Emergent data suggest that prolonged hospitalization in patients with AECOPD can be avoided and good clinical outcome assured, even in patients with severe disease, when effective discharge planning is combined with coordination of multidisciplinary care. Additional studies are required to determine precisely which patients with AECOPD are more likely to benefit from hospital admission, as well as their duration of hospitalization.

VENTILATORY SUPPORT

In patients with AECOPD and acute respiratory failure ventilator support should be considered when, despite 'optimal' medical therapy and oxygen administration, one of the followings persists:

- moderate to severe dyspnea with respiratory frequency >25 breaths/min
- use of respiratory accessory muscles and abdominal paradox
- moderate to severe acidosis (pH <7.35) and hypercapnia ($Paco_2$ >45–60 mm Hg).

Mechanical ventilation can be delivered through an endotracheal, i.e. 'conventional' or 'invasive' mechanical ventilation; or noninvasive positive pressure ventilation (NIPPV) via nasal or face masks. In such patients NIPPV should be considered as a first line of therapy.[65,66] It is important to identify any contraindication that the patients may have for NIPPV (Box 14B.3) prior to its use. A reduction in mortality, and decrease in the need for endotracheal intubation and invasive mechanical ventilation have been shown with the use of NIPPV.[67] Figure 14B.5 provides the flow chart recommended by the ATS/ERS guidelines for the use of NIPPV.[1]

With NIPPV, an improvement in alveolar ventilation without significant modifications in the lung ventilation/perfusion mismatch and gas exchange capability had been shown,[68] and it also provides a greater reduction of the work of breathing by decreasing intrinsic end-expiratory pressure and improving lung mechanics.[69] It has also the advantage that it can be used in different clinical settings including medical wards, intermediate or step down units and the intensive care unit.

Several factors that have been shown to predict NIPPV success include good level of consciousness at the start of the trial, higher pH, lower $Paco_2$, and improvements in pH and $Paco_2$ within an hour of NIPPV initiation. The most frequent complications of NIPPV include facial skin erythema, nasal congestion, nasal bridge ulceration, sinus/ear pain, nasal/oral dryness, eye irritation, gastric irritation, aspiration pneumonia, and poor control of secretions. Most of these complications can be prevented and the clinical team should be aware of them.[66–68]

Box 14B.3 Contraindications for NIPPV[1]

Contraindications for NIPPV include the following:

- Respiratory arrest
- Cardiovascular instability (hypotension, arrhythmias, myocardial infarction)
- Impaired mental status, somnolence, inability to cooperate
- Copious and/or viscous secretions with high aspiration risk
- Recent facial or gastroesophageal surgery
- Craniofacial trauma and/or fixed nasopharyngeal abnormality
- Burns
- Extreme obesity

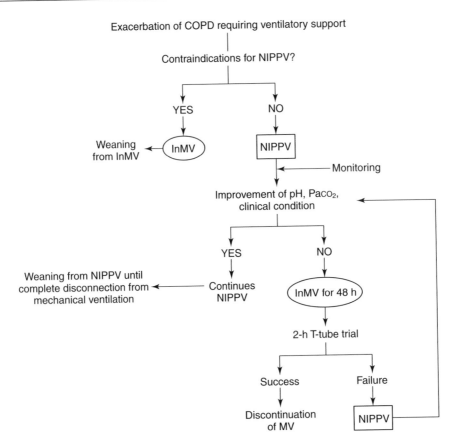

Figure 14B.5 *Flow chart for the use of noninvasive positive pressure ventilation (NIPPV) in exacerbation of chronic obstructive pulmonary disease (COPD) complicated by acute respiratory failure. InMV, invasive mechanical ventilation. (Redrawn with permission from Celli BR, MacNeed W for the ATS/ERS COPD Committee. Standard for the diagnoses and treatment of patients with COPD: A summary of the ATS/ERS position paper.* Eur Respir J *2004;* **23***: 932–46.[1]) PERMISSION PENDING*

Endotracheal intubation should be considered in patients who do not improve with NIPPV, manifested as worsening of arterial blood gases and /or pH within 1–2 hours or lack of improvement in arterial blood gases and/or pH after 4 hours of NIPPV; severe acidosis (pH <7.25) and hypercapnia ($Paco_2$ >60 mm Hg); life-threatening hypoxemia ($Paco_2$/Fio_2 <200 mm Hg); tachypnea >35 breaths/min; other complications such as metabolic abnormalities, sepsis, pneumonia, pulmonary embolism, barotrauma, massive pleural effusion. In patients who required endotracheal intubated, NIPPV can be considered as a potential successful strategy for weaning.[67,70,71]

SUMMARY

Morbidity and mortality related to AECOPD remain significantly elevated. Acute exacerbation of COPD occurs in an heterogeneous patient population and continues to be associated with a unacceptably high rate of treatment failures. Emergency treatment of AECOPD requires the identification of the patients who are more severely ill and therapy should include appropriate use of antibiotics when indicated, bronchodilators, corticosteroids, and ventilatory support.

Key learning points

- Patients are prone to exacerbations under conditions that are usually associated with increased breathlessness.

- Acute exacerbations result in significant morbidity and mortality in this patient population.

- Significant numbers of hospitalized patients with acute exacerbations have modifiable risk factors including influenza vaccination, oxygen supplementations, active smoking, and occupational exposures.

- Patients with severe COPD have a significantly higher prevalence of Gram-negative organisms such as Enterobacteriaceae and *Pseudomonas* species.

- In patients with AECOPD who are evaluated in an emergency room and/or required hospitalization a chest radiograph should be obtained to rule out any other abnormalities.

- There are no data to support the routine use of peak flow meters or FEV_1 assessment in the management of COPD exacerbations.

- Bronchodilator drugs are the primary therapeutic intervention in patients with AECOPD.

- There is consensus that patients with significant bronchodilator response are more likely to benefit from corticosteroid therapy. However, a patient who responds to corticosteroids therapy during an AECOPD will not, however, necessarily benefit from long-term use of these drugs. Therefore, patients should be carefully selected for their suitability for these drugs.

- Although it is essential to treat these patients with antibiotics, it is also critical to choose the appropriate one.

- Emergent data suggest that prolonged hospitalization in patients with AECOPD can be avoided and good clinical outcome assured, even in patients with severe disease, when effective discharge planning is combined with coordination of multidisciplinary care.

- In patients with AECOPD and acute respiratory failure ventilator support should be considered.

REFERENCES

1. Celli BR, MacNeed W for the ATS/ERS COPD Committee. Standard for the diagnoses and treatment of patients with COPD: A summary of the ATS/ERS position paper. *Eur Respir J* 2004; **23**: 932–46.

2. Fabbri L, Pauwels RA, Hurd S on behalf of the GOLD Scientific Committee. Global Strategy for the Diagnosis, Management and Prevention of Chronic Obstructive Pulmonary Disease: GOLD Executive Summary Updated 2003. *COPD* 2004; **1**: 105–41.

3. Pauwels RA, Buist S, Calvery PMA, *et al.* on behalf of the GOLD Scientific Committee. Global Strategy for the diagnosis, management, and prevention of Chronic Obstructive Pulmonary Disease. NHLBI/WHO Global Initiative for Chronic Obstructive Pulmonary Disease (GOLD) Workshop Summary. *Am J Respir Crit Care Med* 2001; **163**: 1256–76.

4. Peters DK, Kochanek DK, Murphy SL. Deaths: final data for 1996. *U S Nationalortl Vital Statistics Rep* 1998; **47**: 1–100.

5. Higgins MW, Thom T. Incidence, prevalence and mortality: Intra- and inter-country difference. In: Hensley MJ, Saunders NA, eds. *Clinical Epidemiology of Chronic Obstructive Pulmonary Disease.* New York: Marcel Dekker, 1990: 23–43.

6. *Statistical Abstract of the United States 1997.* US Department of Commerce, Bureau of the Census. Washington, DC: US Department of Commerce, 1997.

7. Healthcare Cost and Utilization Project. 1997 Nationwide Inpatient Sample. Agency for Healthcare Research and Policy. Available at: www.ahcpr.gov/data/hcup/hcupnet.htm (accessed September 2004).

8. Feinleib M, Rosenberg HM, Collins JG, *et al.* Trends in COPD morbidity and mortality in the United States. *Am Rev Respir Dis* 1989; **140**: S9–18.

9. Emerman CL, Effron D, Lukens TW. Spirometric criteria for hospital admission of patients with acute exacerbations of COPD. *Chest* 1991; **99**: 595–9.

10. Murata GH, Gorby MS, Kapsner CO, *et al.* A multivariate model for the prediction of relapse after outpatient treatment of decompensated chronic obstructive pulmonary disease. *Arch Intern Med* 1992; **152**: 73–7.

11. Seneff MG, Wagner DP, Wagner RP, *et al.* Hospital and 1-year survival of patients admitted to intensive care units with acute exacerbation of chronic obstructive pulmonary disease. *JAMA* 1995; **274**: 1852–7.

12. Connors AF Jr, Dawson NV, Tomas C, *et al.* Outcomes following acute exacerbation of severe chronic obstructive lung disease. The SUPPORT investigators (Study to Understand Prognoses and Preferences for Outcomes and Risks of Treatment). *Am J Respir Crit Care Med* 1996; **154**: 959–67.

13. Knaus WA, Wagner DP, Draper EA, *et al.* The APACHE III prognostic system. Risk prediction of hospital mortality for critically ill hospitalized adults. *Chest* 1991; **100**: 1619–36.

14. Seemungal TAR, Donaldson GC, Bhowmik A, *et al.* Time course and recovery of exacerbations in patients with chronic obstructive pulmonary disease. *Am J Respir Crit Care Med* 2000; **161**: 1608–13.

15. Seemungal TAR, Donaldson GC, Paul EA, *et al.* Effect of exacerbation on quality of life in patients with chronic obstructive pulmonary disease. *Am J Respir Crit Care Med* 1998; **157**: 1418–22.

16. Ball P. Epidemiology and treatment of chronic bronchitis and is exacerbations. *Chest* 1995; **108**(Suppl 2): S43–52.

✱ 17. Seemugal T, Harper-Owen R, Bhowmik A, *et al.* Respiratory viruses, symptoms and inflammatory markers in acute exacerbations and stable chronic obstructive pulmonary disease. *Am J Respir Crit Care Med* 2001; **164**: 1618–23.

✱ 18. Eller J, Ede A, Schaberg T, *et al.* Infective exacerbations of chronic bronchitis. Relation between bacteriologic etiology and lung function. *Chest* 1998; **13**: 1542–8.

✱ 19. Miravitlles M, Espinosa C, Fernandez-Laso E, *et al.* Relationship between bacterial flora in sputum and functional impairment in patients with acute exacerbations of COPD. *Chest* 1999; **116**: 40–6.

✱ 20. Soler N, Torres A, Ewig S, *et al.* Bronchial microbial patterns in severe exacerbations of chronic obstructive pulmonary disease (COPD) requiring mechanical ventilation. *Am J Respir Crit Care Med* 1998; **157**: 1498–505.

● 21. Snow V, Lascher S, Mottur-Pilson for the Joint Expert Panel of Chronic Obstructive Pulmonary Disease of the American College of Chest Physicians and the American College of Physicians-American Society of Internal Medicine. Evidence base for management of acute exacerbations of chronic obstructive pulmonary disease. *Ann Intern Med* 2001; **134**: 595–9.

● 22. Bach BB, Brown C, Gelfand SE, McCrory DC. Management of acute exacerbations of chronic obstructive pulmonary disease: A summary and appraisal of published evidence. *Ann Intern Med* 2001; **134**: 600–20.

✱ 23. Emerman CL, Cydulka RK. Evaluation of high-yield criteria for chest radiography in acute exacerbation of chronic obstructive pulmonary disease. *Ann Emerg Med* 1993; **22**: 680–84.

✱ 24. Tsay TW, Gallagher EJ, Lombardi G, *et al.* Guidelines for the selective ordering of admission chest radiography in adult obstructive airway disease. *Ann Emerg Med* 1993; **22**: 1854–8.

✱ 25. O'Driscoll BR, Taylor RJ, Horsley MG, *et al.* Nebulised salbutamol with and without ipratropium with and without ipratropium bromide in acute airflow obstruction. *Lancet* 1989; **1**: 1418–20.

✱ 26. Turner MO, Patel A, Ginsburg S, *et al.* Bronchodilator delivery in acute airflow obstruction. A meta-analysis. *Arch Intern Med* 1997; **157**: 1736–44.

✱ 27. Emerman CL, Cydulka RK. Effect of different albuterol dosing regimens in the treatment of acute exacerbation of chronic obstructive pulmonary disease. *Ann Emerg Med* 1997; **29**: 474–8.

✱ 28. Shretha M, O'Brien T, Haddox R, *et al.* Decreased duration of emergency department treatment of chronic obstructive pulmonary disease exacerbations with the addition of ipratropium bromide to beta-agonist therapy. *Ann Emerg Med* 1991; **20**: 1206–9.

✱ 29. Moayyedi P, Congleton J, Page RI, *et al.* Comparison of nebulized salbutamol and ipratropium bromide with salbutamol alone in the treatment of chronic obstructive pulmonary disease. *Thorax* 1995; **50**: 834–7.

✱ 30. Karpel JF. Bronchodilator response to anticholinergic and beta-adrenergic agents in acute and stable COPD. *Chest* 1991; **99**: 871–6.

✱ 31. Mestitz H, Copland JM, McDonald CF. Comparison of outpatient nebulized vs. metered dose inhaler terbutaline in chronic airflow obstruction. *Chest* 1989; **96**: 1017–20.

✱ 32. Turner JR, Corkery KJ, Eckman D, *et al.* Equivalence of continuous flow nebulizer and metered-dose inhaler with reservoir bag for treatment of acute airflow obstruction. *Chest* 1988; **93**: 476–81.

✱ 33. Dhand R, Jubran A, Tobin MJ. Bronchodilator delivery by metered-dose inhaler in ventilator-supported patients. *Am J Respir Crit Care Med* 1995; **151**: 1827–33.

✱ 34. Duarte AG, Dhand R, Reid R, *et al.* Serum albuterol levels in mechanically ventilated patients and healthy subjects after metered-dose inhaler administration. *Am J Respir Crit Care Med* 1996; **154**: 1658–63.

✱ 35. Au DH, Crutis JR, Every MB, *et al.* Inhaled beta-agonists and risk of myocardial ischemia. *Am J Respir Crit Care Med* 2000; A489.

✱ 36. Cook D, Guyatt G, Wong E, *et al.* Regular versus as-needed short-acting inhaled β-agonist therapy for chronic obstructive pulmonary disease. *Am J Respir Crit Care Med* 2001; **163**: 85–90.

✱ 37. Tashkin DP, Ashutosh K, Bleeker ER, *et al.* Comparison of the anticholinergic bronchodilator ipratropium bromide with metaproterenol in chronic obstructive pulmonary disease: a 90 day multicenter study. *Am J Med* 1986; **8**(Suppl 5A): 81–9.

✱ 38. Rice KL, Leatherman JW, Duane PG, *et al.* Aminophylline for acute exacerbations of chronic obstructive pulmonary disease. A controlled trial. *Ann Intern Med* 1987; **107**: 305–9.

✱ 39. Emerman CL, Connors AF, Lukens TW, *et al.* Theophylline concentrations in patients with acute exacerbations of COPD. *Am J Emerg Med* 1990; **8**: 289–92.

✱ 40. Emerman CL, Devlin C, Connors AF. Risk of toxicity in patients with elevated theophylline levels. *Ann Emerg Med* 1990; **19**: 643–8.

◆✱41.   Albert RK, Martin TR, Lewis SW. Controlled clinical trial of methylprednisolone in patients with chronic bronchitis and acute respiratory insufficiency. *Ann Intern Med* 1980; **92**: 753–8.

✱ 42. Davies L, Angus RM, Calverley PM. Oral corticosteroids in patients admitted to hospital with exacerbations of chronic obstructive pulmonary disease: a prospective randomized controlled trial. *Lancet* 1999; **354**: 456–60.

✱ 43. Niewoehner DE, Erbland ML, Deupree RH, *et al.* Effect of systemic glucocorticoids on exacerbations of chronic obstructive pulmonary disease. Department of Veterans Affairs Cooperative Study Group. *N Engl J Med* 1999; **340**: 1941–7.

◆ 44. Thompson WH, Nielson CP, Carvalho P, *et al.* Controlled trial of oral prednisone in outpatients with acute COPD exacerbation. *Am J Respir Crit Care Med* 1996; **154**: 407–12.

✱ 45. Maltais F, Ostinelli J, Bourbeau J, *et al.* Comparison of nebulized budesonide and oral prednisolone with placebo in the treatment of acute exacerbations of chronic obstructive pulmonary disease: a randomized controlled trial. *Am J Respir Crit Care Med* 2002; **1654**: 698–703.

✱ 46. Decramer M, de Bock V, Dom R. Functional and histologic picture of steroid-induced myopathy in chronic obstructive pulmonary disease. *Am J Respir Crit Care Med* 1996; **153**: 1958–64.

✱ 47. Decramer M, Lacquet LM, Fagard R, *et al.* Corticosteroids contribute to muscle weakness in chronic airflow obstruction. *Am J Respir Crit Care Med* 1994; **150**: 11–16.

✱ 48. Langlands JH. Double-blind clinical trial of bromhexine as a mucolytic drug in chronic bronchitis. *Lancet* 1970; **1**: 448–50.

◆ 49. Saint S, Bent S, Vittinghoff E, *et al.* Antibiotics in chronic obstructive pulmonary disease exacerbations: a meta-analysis. *JAMA* 1995; **273**: 957–60.

● 50. Anthonisen NR, Manfreda J, Warren CP, *et al.* Antibiotic therapy in acute exacerbation of chronic obstructive pulmonary disease. *Ann Intern Med* 1987; **106**: 196–204.

✱ 51. Allegra L, Grassi C. Ruolo degli antibiotici nel trattamento delle riacutizza della bronchite cronica. *Ital J Chest* Dis 1991; **45**: 138–48.

✱ 52. Sonnesyn SW, Gerdin DN. Antimicrobials for the treatment of respiratory infection. In: Niederman MS, Sarosi GA, Glassroth J, eds. *Respiratory Infections: A Scientific Basis For Management.* Philadelphia: WB Saunders, 1994: 511–37.

✱ 53. Cabello H, Torres A, Celis R, *et al.* Bacterial colonization of distal airways in healthy subjects and chronic lung disease: a bronchoscopic study. *Eur Respir J* 1997; **10**: 1137–44.

◆ 54. Mansó JR, Rosell A, Manterola J, *et al.* Bacterial infection in chronic obstructive pulmonary disease. Study of stable and exacerbated outpatients using the protected specimen brush. *Am J Respir Crit Care Med* 1995; **152**: 1316–20.

✱ 55. Fagon JY, Chastre J, Trouillet JL, *et al.* Characterization of distal bronchial microflora during acute exacerbation of chronic bronchitis. *Am Rev Respir Dis* 1990; **142**: 1004–8.

✱ 56. Martinez JA, Rodriguez E, Bastida T, *et al.* Quantitative study of the bronchial bacterial flora in acute exacerbations of chronic bronchitis. *Chest* 1994; **105**: 976.

✱ 57. Nouira S, Marghli S, Belghith M, *et al.* Once daily oral ofloxacin in chronic obstructive pulmonary disease exacerbation requiring mechanical ventilation: a randomized placebo-controlled trial. *Lancet* 2001; **358**: 2020–5.

✱ 58. Adams S, Melo J, Luther M, *et al.* Antibiotics are associated with lower relapse rates in outpatients with acute exacerbations of chronic obstructive pulmonary disease. *Chest* 2000; **117**: 1345–52.

✱ 59. Destache CJ, Dewan N, O'Donohue WJ, *et al.* Clinical and economic considerations in the treatment of acute exacerbations of chronic bronchitis. *J Antimicrob Chemother* 1999; **43**(Suppl A):107–13.

● 60. Balter MS, Hyland RH, Low DE, *et al.* Recommendations on the management of chronic bronchitis: A practical guide for Canadian physicians. *Can Respir J* 2003; **110**(Suppl A): 10A.

✱ 61. Fuso L, Incalzi RA, Pistelli R, *et al.* Predicting mortality of patients hospitalized for acutely exacerbated chronic obstructive pulmonary disease. *Am J Med* 1995; **98**: 272–7.

✱ 62. Mushlin AI, Black ER, Connolly CA, *et al.* The necessary length of hospital stay for chronic pulmonary disease. *JAMA* 1991; **266**: 80–3.

✱ 63. Skwarska E, Cohen G, Skwarski KM, *et al.* Randomized controlled trial of supported discharge in patients with exacerbations of COPD. *Thorax* 2000; **55**: 907–12.

✳ 64. Cotton MM, Bucknall CE. Early discharge for patients with exacerbations COPD: a randomized controlled trial. *Thorax* 2000; **55**: 902–6.

● 65. International consensus conference in intensive care medicine: noninvasive positive pressure ventilation in acute respiratory failure. *Am J Respir Crit Care Med* 2001; **163**: 283–91.

● 66. British Thoracic Society Guideline. Non invasive ventilation in acute respiratory failure. British Thoracic Society Standaeds of Care Committee. *Thorax* 2002; **57**: 192–211.

◆ 67. Mehta S, Hill NS. Non invasive ventilation. State of the Art. *Am J Respir Crit Care Med.* 2001; **163**: 540–77.

✳ 68. Lightower JV, Wedzicha JA, Elliot M, Ram SF. Non invasive positive pressure ventilation to treat respiratory failure resulting from exacerbations of chronic obstructive pulmonary disease: Cochrane systematic review and meta-analysis. *BMJ* 2003; **326**: 185–9.

✳ 69. Rossi A, Appendini L, Roca J. Physiological aspects of non invasive positive pressure ventilation. *Eur Respir Mon* 2001; **16**: 1–10.

✳ 70. Diaz O, Iglesias R, Ferrer M, *et al.* Effects of non invasive ventilation on pulmonary gas exchange and hemodynamics during acute exacerbations of chronic obstructive pulmolnary disease. *Am J Respir Crit Care Med* 1997; **156**: 1840–5.

✳ 71. Contin G, Antonelli M, Navalesi P, *et al.* Noninvasive vs conventional mechanical ventilation in patients with chronic obstructive pulmonary disease after failure of medical management in the ward: a randomized trial. *Intensive Care Med* 2002; **28**: 1701–7.

Large airway tumors and obstruction

MARK E LUND, ARMIN ERNST

INTRODUCTION

Central airway obstruction (CAO) may be caused by both benign and malignant disease. Thirty percent of lung cancers will present with or develop CAO.[1] Palliative care will be required in 90 percent of all patients diagnosed with lung cancer.[2] Based upon Poiseuille's law, small changes in lumen can greatly impair tracheobronchial flow. Untreated CAO leads to profound morbidity and eventually to death by suffocation. Conversely, moderate increases in luminal diameter can have significant impact upon ventilation and dyspnea.

In light of the prevalence of CAO there has been an interest in developing minimally invasive techniques to manage these patients. The field of interventional pulmonology has developed over the past 20 years. Interventional bronchoscopy should be an early and integral therapy in the management paradigm of lung cancer and other thoracic malignancies. Bronchoscopic therapy should be utilized early to allow improvement in functional status, quality of life and reduced risk of infectious complications. A multidisciplinary team ideally constitutes an interventional pulmonologist, thoracic surgeon, thoracic radiologist, an anesthesiologist, and radiation oncologist. Although interventional bronchology is frequently palliative, initial endobronchial therapies should be utilized as a bridge to subsequent definitive chemotherapeutic, radiotherapeutic or surgical therapy. It can be a curative option in many benign disorders. Interventional bronchoscopy techniques have been demonstrated to improve functional status, opening further treatment options.

The bronchoscopist evaluating a patient for CAO should have the training and equipment to proceed with a therapy. If either equipment or operator experience is limited, the patient should be referred to a multidisciplinary center. Rigid bronchoscopy should be the core therapy for life-threatening CAO.

DEFINITIONS

Central airways

The central airways include the trachea and carina bifurcation as well as the right and left mainstem bronchi, and the intermediate bronchus. Based upon the volume of impacted lung and the discrepancy in results of interventions for lesions at the lobar and segmental levels, we do not consider these central airways.

Stenosis

Stenosis is defined as a narrowing of the tracheobronchial luminal diameter. A generic system divides stenosis into four severity categories and defines the length, consistency, type and location. This system is most beneficial to interventional bronchoscopy. Grade I is defined as less than 50 percent stenosis, grade II from 51 percent to 70 percent, grade III any detectable lumen above 70 percent. An airway obstruction is assigned to grade IV. When no lumen is present an obstruction is present.

Extrinsic compression occurs when an external force causes a reduction in the lumen by distorting the intact bronchial wall. Intrinsic obstruction is caused by endobronchial growth of tumor.

INCIDENCE/EPIDEMIOLOGY

Historically, 50 percent of lung cancer patients developed endobronchial disease; currently the incidence is approximately 30 percent. The possibility of central airway obstruction should be considered in any cancer patient with respiratory failure. Up to 5 percent of nonpulmonary malignancies directly metastasize to tracheobronchial structures.[3–6] The average time from primary diagnosis to the localization of endobronchial disease is 5 years.

Primary tracheal neoplasms are rare, accounting for less than 0.1 percent of tracheal malignancies. Benign tracheal stenosis or obstructing granulation/inflammatory tissue is not uncommon. This occurs in 10 percent of patients requiring prolonged mechanical ventilator support and is not eliminated by tracheostomy. Five percent of patients admitted for failure to wean have tracheal obstruction.[7]

ETIOLOGY OF ENDOBRONCHIAL MASSES AND OBSTRUCTION

Primary bronchogenic carcinoma

A variety of processes are known to cause CAO (Box 14C.1). The most common cause of CAO is primary bronchogenic carcinoma. Unusual lung primaries have been the subject of recent reviews.[8,9] Carcinoid constitute 1–5 percent of all lung tumors.[9,10] Carcinoid syndrome is uncommon but bronchoscopy has been reported to cause 'carcinoid crisis', manifesting as tachycardia, flushing, hypertension or hypotension and possibly coronary spasm.[11] Symptoms and 5- hydroxyindoleacetic acid (5-HIAA) levels do not predict its development. Somatostatin has been used to control this complication. Adenoid cystic carcinoma (cylindroma) is the most common of the salivary gland tumors in the tracheobronchial tree. In contradistinction to the carcinoid tumor, most arise in the trachea.

Airway metastasis

The most common nonpulmonary malignancies that metastasize to the airways are breast, colorectal, and renal cell carcinomas as well as melanoma. The frequency of breast cancer airway metastasis has been reported with an incidence of 14–63 percent, making it the most common cause of endobronchial metastasis.[6,12–15] It may be less frequent in younger patients.[16] Colon carcinoma frequently metastasizes

---

Box 14C.1 Causes of CAO

Bronchogenic carcinoma

- Nonsmall cell carcinoma
- Small cell carcinoma
- Carcinoid
- Adenoid cystic carcinoma
- Mucoepidermoid
- Kaposi sarcoma
- Rhabdomyosarcoma
- Chondrosarcoma

Endobronchial metastatic disease

- Breast carcinoma
- Colon carcinoma
- Renal cell carcinoma
- Melanoma
- Uterine/cervix
- Lymphoma
  - Posttransplant lymphoproliferative
- Ovarian
- Endometrial
- Thyroid
- Testicular
- Choriocarcinoma
- Prostate
- Stomach
- Adrenal
- Transitional cell
- Parotid
- Nasopharyngeal carcinoma
- Pancreas
- Penis
- Laryngeal
- Neuroblastoma (olfactory)
- Basal cell carcinoma
- Chronic lymphocytic leukemia – Richter transformation
- Hepatocellular carcinoma
- Plasmacytoma
- Waldenström macroglobuinemia
- Fibrous histiocytoma
- Sacromas – angiosarcoma, osteogenic, fibrosarcoma, leiomyosarcoma, fibrous histiosarcoma, liposarcoma
- Esophageal metastasis

Mediastinal malignancies

- Lymphoma (extrinsic compression)
- Thyroid
- Esophageal carcinoma

Benign causes of endobronchial obstruction

- Postintubation tracheal stenosis
- Relapsing polychondritis
- Inflammatory polyps

- Amyloidosis
- Plasma cell granuloma
- Granular cell myoblastoma
- Squamous papilloma
- Fibroma
- Lipoma
- Chondroma
- Hemangioma
- Hamartoma
- Achalasia
- Mega aorta syndrome
- Intrathoracic goiter

Infectious processes

- Bacterial tracheitis
- Bacillary angiomatosis
- Nocardiosis
- Mycobacterial disease (tuberculosis and nontuberculosis)
- Aspergillosis
- *Actinomycosis* infections
- *Pneumocystis carinii* infection
- Cytomegalovirus tracheitis
- Recurrent respiratory papillomatosis
- Ebstein–Barr virus infections

Miscellaneous

- Organized thrombus
- Broncholithiasis
- Fibromucinous cast
- Tracheobronchopathia osteochondroplastica
- Crohn disease
- Launois–Bensaude syndrome

to the lung, it has been shown to cause a third of airway metastasis.[6,12–14] The most frequent site of metastasis in renal cell carcinoma is the lung. An endobronchial location occurs in 12–17 percent.[5,14,17,18] In a pattern reminiscent of its renal vasculature invasion, renal cell carcinoma has a propensity to extend up the airways. Endobronchial melanoma metastasis is not uncommon, with a range from 4.3 percent to 6.3 percent.[6,12,17,19,20] Benign and malignant mediastinal processes may cause obstruction by direct extension of tumors or by extrinsic compression. Airway involvement of the trachea and left mainstem bronchus occurs in a third of patients with esophageal cancer. After esophageal stenting, the incidence of central airway obstruction is 25 percent.[21] Placement of esophageal stents can precipitate airway compromise.

Benign causes of endobronchial masses or obstruction

Endobronchial tumors are accountable for virtually all the deaths from benign tumors of the lung. The most common

benign lung tumor is a hamartoma. Chondroma, lipoma, fibroma, granular cell myoblastoma, and leiomyoma all can occur in the airway. Most granular cell myoblastomas occur in the endobronchial location, whereas half of leiomyomas occur in proximal endobronchial locations. Approximately half of patients with relapsing polychondritis have tracheobronchial involvement, frequently with diffuse stenosis. Biopsy may lead to an acute inflammatory response with acute loss of the airway. Glottic stenosis and rapid loss of airway support makes intubation difficult and bronchoscopy potentially hazardous.

Worldwide, mycobacterial disease is the most prevalent infectious cause of CAO. Clinically significant endobronchial disease occurs in up to a third. The occlusive tumorous type is frequently mistaken for lung cancer. Obstructing lesions have been described in infections caused by *Mycobacterium avium complex*, *M. fortuitum*, and *M. kansasii*.

Clinical presentation

The various clinical presentations are related to the location of the obstruction, rapidity of onset, and comorbid illnesses. Comorbidities may be preexistent (chronic obstructive pulmonary disease, coronary artery disease) or secondary to the obstruction (pneumonia, abscess, fistula). Early symptoms may be variable due to the borderline nature of an obstruction. Symptoms develop when sufficient narrowing of the airway is caused by edema, swelling, or increased secretions. Patients are frequently misdiagnosed with asthma or an exacerbation of chronic lung disease.

The routine presentation is with dyspnea, cough, wheeze or stridor, and hemoptysis. Up to 54 percent of patients may present in respiratory distress or extremis with little premonitory signs or symptoms.[22] In high-grade central obstruction hypoxemic, hypercapneic respiratory failure is common. Dyspnea is the most prevalent symptom. The severity of dyspnea is related to the extent of the luminal obstruction, volume of obstructed lung, and coexistent cardiopulmonary disease. A consistent sign of CAO is exacerbation with positional changes. A persistent, focal wheeze should always be investigated with bronchoscopy. A tracheal syndrome present in 85 percent of tracheal stenosis, consists of cough, wheeze, dyspnea, and stridor.[23] Hemoptysis occurs in roughly half of CAOs. Hemoptysis is more common in bronchogenic carcinoma than metastatic disease.

Analysis of the flow volume loop is required. Analysis may show the classic plateau in flow when tracheal lumen is compromised 80 percent (<8 mm^2). In patients with no underlying pulmonary disease, this coincides with the onset of dyspnea on exertion. Dyspnea develops at rest when the tracheal lumen is <5 mm^2. Changes in the forced expiratory volume in 1 second (FEV$_1$), forced vital capacity (FVC), and the FEV$_1$/FVC commonly appear later in CAO. Four distinguishable expiratory flow patterns have been shown to be indicative of specific regional stenosis.[24] Patients with high-grade obstruction or respiratory distress should not have spirometry for concern of inducing respiratory failure.

The standard radiograph is an inadequate study on which to base therapy. Pleural effusion may develop in central bronchial obstruction. Drainage of this effusion will leave a pneumothorax *ex-vacuo*. A sign of trapped lung is significant pain during the completion of pleural drainage.

INVESTIGATIONS (DIAGNOSTIC STUDIES)

Computed tomography

A routine computed tomography (CT) scan provides information for routine diagnostic purposes. Discriminating tumor from atelectasis or postobstructive consolidation is problematic. Unfortunately, the sensitivity for tracheobronchial disease with standard CT remains 59 percent with a specificity of 85 percent.[25] The sensitivity to detect endoluminal disease is only 50 percent, and increases modestly to 72 percent for obstructing lesions. Three-dimensional volume rendering now allows the interventional bronchoscopist to more easily understand the complex relations of endoluminal surfaces, mediastinal vessels, adjacent structures, and their interaction or proximity to an obstruction. Three-dimensional rendering provides important supplemental information (50 percent) or corrects interpretive errors (10 percent).[26] Internal three-dimensional rendering is also referred to as virtual bronchoscopy (VB). Central airway regions VB had a sensitivity of 83–90 percent, specificity 95.6–100 percent, and accuracy of 95.5 percent. The positive predictive value is 84.4 percent.[25,27] The length, width, shape, and contour all correlate very well.

External three-dimensional rendering or surface/volume rendering is the reconstruction of data to provide an 'airway cast'.[28] Subtle stenosis is more easily seen and complex airways are more accurately assessed (Fig. 14C.1). In addition, the cephalocaudal positioning and extent of disease are more accurately evaluated using external rendering.[26] The external renderings provide supplemental information, improve confidence, or corrected interpretive errors.

Bronchoscopy

Bronchoscopy is a required study in any patient with CAO. Bronchoscopy allows the only direct visualization of the airway. It is complemented by advanced imaging techniques but cannot be replaced by them. The only caveat to the requirement of diagnostic/evaluative bronchoscopy is in high-grade obstruction. Flexible bronchoscopy and the sedation required to perform it may be overly risky or contraindicated in some patients. The flexible bronchoscope would further obliterate a small lumen. The use of conscious sedation or induction of anesthesia may produce an unstable airway. Once problems develop, securing the airway may be problematic. Rigid bronchoscopy is the procedure of choice in any suspected high-grade or proximal tracheal obstruction. In situations where the anatomy is less certain, the bronchoscopist should be able to switch rapidly to rigid bronchoscopy or have a multidisciplinary team available for advanced airway management.

Endobronchial ultrasound

Endobronchial ultrasound determines depth of tumor penetration and correlates well with histopathology (95.8

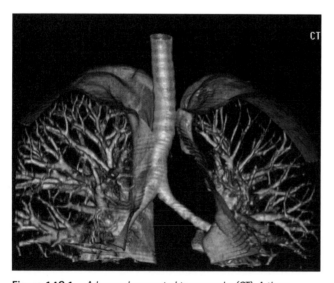

Figure 14C.1 *Advanced computed tomography (CT). A three-dimensional CT rendering of a patient with a long high-grade stenosis of the left mainstem bronchus after tuberculosis as a child.*

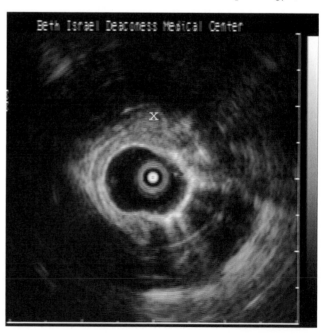

Figure 14C.2 *Endobronchial ultrasound image of a mucosal lesion found on conventional bronchoscopy. The lesion (x) is not confined to the bronchial wall and is too large for endobronchial curative intervention.*

percent).[29] In an assessment of tumor infiltration into the bronchial wall, endobronchial ultrasound is more accurate than CT and improved the accuracy of determining invasion by 55 percent.[30] An interruption of the outer hyperechoic line indicates invasion of the extraluminal surface (Fig. 14C.2). Tumor invasion can be differentiated from extrinsic compression with high accuracy.[30,31] In the management of airway obstruction endobronchial ultrasound can provide additional valuable information as it can be used to assess patent distal airways and bronchial size to select appropriate stent size and facilitate stent placement as well as direct other interventions.[32,33]

TREATMENT/MANAGEMENT

Management of patients with CAO is complex. The initial management involves immediately evaluating and stabilizing the airway, typically under difficult and tenuous circumstances. The management complexities continue during evaluation and provision of endobronchial therapy. Acute loss of the airway can be irreversible. Planning must include initial stabilization of the airway and managing complications. Patients with CAO may present in extremis, requiring immediate stabilization of the airway. Therapy begins with supplemental, humidified oxygen. Patients with significant airway compromise benefit from a seated position.

Initial therapy

Helium–oxygen mixtures (heliox) may be required in the initial stabilization of severe CAO. The viscosity of helium is greater than air but it is less dense, altering Reynolds number and improving laminar flow. Heliox effectively reduces work of breathing. Heliox should be administered through a mask and with a high flow rate. The concentration should be based upon the predominant issue. Hypercarbia is best treated with increasing helium whereas hypoxemia is best approached with less helium, tolerating some increased work of breathing. When no effect is demonstrated with increasing heliox, there may be a need for increasing fractional inspired oxygen (FiO_2). Heliox can be administered through a laryngeal mask airway and does not prohibit the use of interventional therapies.

Securing the airway

Any patient with a critical, proximal CAO should be managed in a location that enables rapid definitive intervention if needed. The first decision is intubation with a rigid bronchoscope or endotracheal tube. Regardless, the interventional bronchoscopist must be present throughout induction. Patients with obstruction in the mid or lower

trachea who have a large anterior mediastinal mass or very tight stenosis may have profound decompensation with supine or recumbent positioning. An awake, seated intubation does not eliminate the possibility of an acute loss of airway. The use of the rigid bronchoscope enables the bronchoscopist to quickly move past the obstruction, debulking tissue, and immediately restoring and securing the airway. 'Target controlled total intravenous anesthesia' is used by many centers for rigid bronchoscopy. The use of neuromuscular blockade is beneficial and safe after intravenous induction. Once the airway is secured, oxygenation and ventilation may be maintained using any standard modality. High peak airway pressures are to be expected and tolerated.

Therapeutic interventions

External beam radiation therapy (EBRT) has been the standard therapy for malignant airway obstruction. However, there has been a variable efficacy in resolution of atelectasis and improving airway obstruction or lumen diameter, and EBRT is only 25–30 percent efficacious. There is a significant therapeutic delay, limiting the utility of external radiotherapy in high-grade CAO.

Rigid versus flexible bronchoscopy

Many interventionalists clearly favor a rigid bronchoscope. Advantages include better airway control, ability to immediately restore patency, ability to ventilate and oxygenate, sufficient ability to control hemorrhage, more efficient debridement, larger biopsy sampling, shorter duration of intervention reducing anesthesia time and cost.[34,35]

There is little doubt that if maximal control of an airway is indicated, rigid bronchoscopy is the method of choice. Hemorrhage is always possible in interventional bronchoscopy and is best managed with a rigid scope. Rigid bronchoscopy should be the core therapy for life-threatening CAO. Contraindications to rigid bronchoscopy are few and include lack of adequate training, hypoxemia or cardiovascular instability unrelated to airway obstruction, unstable cervical spine, cervical spine fixations, and severe arthritis.

Tumor ablation

When endoluminal tumor is the principal cause of CAO ablation of tumor is indicated. There are three general approaches to destruction of tumor: contact and noncontact methods of destruction, and excision of tumor ('coring out'). Most contact and noncontact methods are similar, utilizing high energy to destroy tissue. This high energy may be electrical current (argon plasma coagulation [APC], electrocautery) or photons (laser, photodynamic therapy [PDT]). The one different modality is cryotherapy, utilizing repeated freeze-thaw cycles. The choice of method in general is dictated by the operator's experience, available modalities, and urgency to establish airway patency. The most rapid relief is obtained by coring out a tumor with the rigid bronchoscope. The differences between contact and noncontact methods are probably inconsequential.

Neodymium:yttrium aluminum garnet laser

Neodymium:yttrium aluminum garnet (Nd:YAG) laser is rapidly effective in reestablishing a patent airway and in controlling vascular tumors. Laser light has three unique properties: (i) it is composed of a single wavelength of (ii) parallel light rays (iii) that are in synchronous phase. The tissue absorption is determined by the wavelength, and tissue effects are mediated by the power density. The Nd:YAG laser emits an invisible beam (1064 nm) that is applied continuously or is pulsed. The depth of penetration may be as deep as 10 mm and is not initially evident. Many experienced interventionalists use the rigid bronchoscope to allow general anesthesia, superior airway control, debulking and rigid dilation concurrent with laser therapy. Although tumor destruction will take longer with flexible bronchoscopy, it is an alternative in low-risk patients. Complications of laser bronchoscopy include airway perforation and fistula formation, hemorrhage, air embolism, and airway fire.

The overall efficacy of Nd:YAG photoablation has been reported in the range of 68–97 percent. The efficacy of bronchoscopic intervention in the trachea, and right mainstem, left mainstem, and right bronchus intermedius has been shown to be 97 percent, 95 percent, 92 percent, and 90, percent respectively.[36] The lesions most responsive include central, endobronchial, and small (<4 cm) lesions with patent distal airways. There is little doubt about the rapidity of response and overall efficacy of this therapy in relieving dyspnea. Locoregional recurrence of tumor is likely unless sequential or concurrent stenting, PDT or brachytherapy is utilized.

Argon plasma coagulation

In APC ionized argon gas flowing through a rigid or flexible conduit is exposed to high voltage at a tungsten tip. The highly charged argon gas exits the probe carrying the current to the tissue. Appropriate grounding is required. The desiccation of the endoluminal tissues limits the depth of coagulation to 2–4 mm. Argon plasma coagulation elicits good hemostasis and desiccation, but no vaporization. Hemostasis is particularly good and can quickly cover large areas. A unique property of APC is its ability to bend around corners. This allows coagulation in bronchi which are

difficult to approach or on the distal aspect of endobronchial tumors.

Argon plasma coagulation is used effectively in malignant or benign obstruction <4 cm and hemoptysis of central origin. Stent-induced granulation tissue and respiratory papillomatosis are effectively reduced. Small spurting arterial bleeding is controllable. Complications, including wall perforation, pneumothorax, subcutaneous emphysema, flash fire or bronchoscope damage can occur.

Photodynamic therapy

Photodynamic therapy is a relatively tumor-selective process that employs cold laser activation of a cellular sensitizer. The most commonly used sensitizer is porfimer sodium. The photosensitizer reacts with resident oxygen species primarily in a type II reaction. The most prevalent tumoricidal effects of PDT are vascular destruction. The effective treatment depth extends to 5–10 mm (Fig. 14C.3).

Endobronchial PDT has been used for endobronchial carcinoma, metastatic disease, and papillomatosis. Stump recurrence is an excellent indication. After infusion, the patients are considered photosensitive for 4–6 weeks. They return 48–72 hours after infusion for laser application. The 630 nm laser light is applied with a quartz fiber with a 360° cylindrical diffuser or a linear fiber with a microlens. Bulky endobronchial tumors are best treated with interstitial therapy. The patients return again for a toilet bronchoscopy at 48 hours to remove necrotic tumor and tissue slough. Laser may be reutilized if any visible tumor or bleeding base is present. Treatment may be readminstered with sequential injections of photosensitizer.

Although Nd:YAG laser provides immediate efficacy, PDT provides greater symptom relief of longer duration. A potential benefit exists for sequential staged therapy. The role of PDT in acute respiratory failure is complementary to more rapid techniques.

Electrocautery

The primary contact form of endobronchial resection is electrocautery. The application of high frequency alternating current across resistant tissues produces heat while avoiding neuromuscular side effects. The generated heat causes tissue destruction and coagulation. Increasing the current increases heat and can produce tissue water vaporization and cutting. Most bronchoscopic electrocautery is monopolar. Bipolar, coagulation-only probes are now available. The most common indication for electrocautery is nonlife-threatening endobronchial obstruction, granulation tissue, and tracheal webs. Electrocautery may be used via a flexible or rigid bronchoscope. Use of the snare utilizes electrical cutting and not mechanical severing by the wire loop. A spatula knife can be used to debulk lesions or cut radial incisions in web

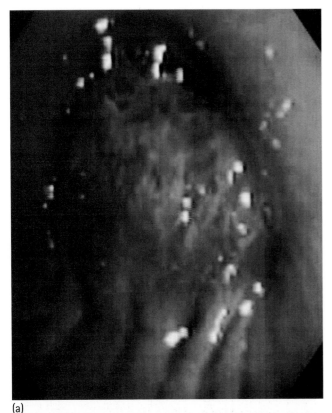

(a)

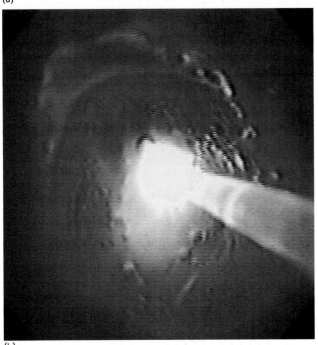

(b)

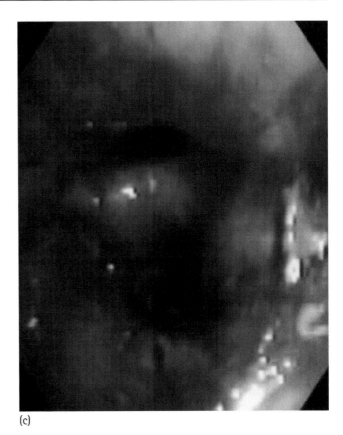

(c)

Figure 14C.3 *Photodynamic therapy. (a) A complete right mainstem obstruction from nonsmall cell lung cancer. (b) Light application for photodynamic therapy. (c) The result 1 week later after debridement is clearly visible.*

strictures. The probe tip must be kept clean or build-up of char will decrease the tissue effects.

Complications of electrocautery include airway perforation, airway stenosis, endobronchial fire, bronchoscope damage, or electrical shock.

In a fully equipped interventional pulmonology program, both laser and electrocautery should be available as complementary therapies. In smaller centers where a laser is not available or start-up costs are prohibitive, an electrocautery unit can be used for many endobronchial therapies.

Cryotherapy

Cryotherapy is another contact method of tumor ablation. The most common cryogen is nitrous oxide, which can be easily stored and has a boiling point of −89 °C. Common endobronchial probes rely upon the Joule–Thompson principle. The pressure change results in a decrease in temperature to the boiling point of the cryogen. Cryotherapy relies upon immediate tissue and delayed vascular damage dependent upon the rapidity of freezing, the end temperature, a slow thaw rate, the number of cycles, and the tissue water content.

Rigid and flexible cryoprobes are available. The flexible probes are passable through the working channel of a flexible bronchoscope. The rigid probes are larger and require rigid bronchoscopy. The probe is advanced into or onto the mass for freezing. Discontinuation of the cryogen allows thawing. The main difficulty with cryotherapy in life-threatening CAO has been the delayed effects required for recanalization.

Other therapeutic uses of cryotherapy include extraction of organized fibrinous blood clot and viscous mucus plugs. These airway casts can be frozen and then fractured with the probe in place. While still frozen they may be withdrawn proximally, allowing removal. Foreign bodies and large volume necrotic tissue slough following PDT can be approached in a similar fashion.

Rigid bronchoscopic coring

One of the principal advantages to the rigid bronchoscope is the ability to debulk large volumes of tumor and rapidly reestablish a patent airway. In fact the preferred method of establishing airway recanalization in critical CAO is rigid debulking. The rigid bronchoscope is advanced cutting an 'apple-core' of tumor that is removed. The rigid bronchoscope is then left in place tamponading the tumor base and providing a stable airway. The rigid bronchoscope can be slowly withdrawn allowing coagulation with argon plasma, Nd: YAG laser, or electrocautery. The use of rigid coring-out saves valuable procedure time (Fig. 14C.4).

High dose rate brachytherapy

External beam radiotherapy is modestly effective for malignant CAO, with roughly 50 percent of patients responding. The average time to palliation is 2–3 weeks. The use of brachytherapy allows endobronchial delivery of intense radiation doses at short radius (5–10 mm) limiting collateral tissue damage. The most commonly used source is iridium-192 (^{192}Ir) which is delivered by an afterloading device via an endobronchial catheter. Brachytherapy can be delivered in varying doses. The delivered dose in centigray (cGy) per hour is arbitrarily divided. Delivered doses of over 1000–1200 cGy/hour define high dose rate (HDR) brachytherapy. The low dose rate delivers 75–200 cGy/h over 20–60 hours. When using HDR brachytherapy the exposure time is typically less than 30 minutes. Low dose rate and HDR brachytherapy have similar efficacy.

Fatal hemoptysis is a concern with brachytherapy. The incidence of fatal hemorrhage is up to 50 percent and can be delayed in onset. Fraction size and bronchial contact are most predictive. A significant survival advantage has been demonstrated with combined therapy. In a retrospective analysis comparing Nd:YAG laser and brachytherapy the combination produced significantly longer survival (264 days) compared with either therapy alone (111–115 days).[37]

Extrinsic compression

The absence of bulky endoluminal disease does not allow consideration of ablative therapies as first-line therapy. The use of tumor ablation will destroy the integrity of the tracheobronchial wall creating a fistula. The primary therapy in recanalizing the stenotic airway is airway dilation and stent placement.

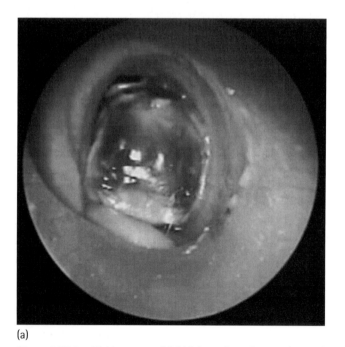

(a)

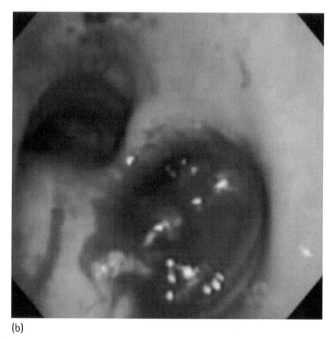

(b)

Figure 14C.4   *Rigid core-out. (a) A high-grade malignant obstruction of the distal trachea in a patient with severe respiratory distress. Rigid bronchoscopy was performed and the tumor cored. (b) Immediate result in a patient with a patent airway and normalizing oxygenation and ventilation.*

Bronchoplasty/tracheoplasty

Bronchoplasty or tracheoplasty is the dilation of stenotic airway. Indications for bronchoplasty include:

- preparation of stenosis for stenting or placement of a HDR brachytherapy catheter
- assisting in stent opening after deployment
- treatment of a CAO when other interventional therapies are not possible or desired.

In an emergent situation, the rigid bronchoscope can be used to dilate the central airways. In nonemergent settings, the use of balloon catheters or semirigid bougies is indicated. Using balloon bronchoplasty decreases the shearing forces and induces less mucosal and submucosal trauma, potentially decreasing the likelihood of granulation tissue and restenosis. The use of balloon bronchoplasty allows implementation of bronchoplasty with flexible bronchoscopes. The results are not sustained and need to be followed with a lasting therapy. The primary risks of balloon bronchoplasty are tracheobronchial rupture causing pneumomediastinum, pneumothorax, mediastinitis, or hemorrhage.

Stent placement

Jean-Francois Dumon developed the silicone stent that became the standard in bronchial stenting. Stents have been manufactured from various metals, silicone, polyester, and mixed (hybrid) materials. More recently, stainless steel has been used in metallic stents (e.g. Wallstent®). Nitinol, a superelastic alloy developed by the US Navy, has replaced stainless in virtually all stent applications.

Silicone stents, which are placed with rigid bronchoscopy, are available in straight tracheobronchial varieties as well as Y. The Montgomery T stent and the Westaby T-Y are still available. Hybrid stents, such as the Dynamic Stent® include metallic supports and a silicone body. This is meant to more appropriately match the natural structure of the trachea and carinal bifurcation. The dynamic stent requires specially designed forceps and suspension laryngoscopy to place. The Gianturco® and Palmaz® stents are considered unsafe by many interventional bronchoscopists (Fig. 14C.5).

Metallic stents have gained popularity because of their safe and relatively simple deployment with flexible bronchoscopy. Metallic stents are prone to granulation tissue formation, are problematic to remove and are known to fracture (Fig. 14C.6). The only appropriate stent for malignant disease is covered metal or silicone to impair tumor ingrowth. A review of several published studies using airway stenting is presented in Table 14C.1. Stents are very effective in relieving dyspnea. In extrinsic compression, they are the best alternative.

Carinal obstruction is a special and generally difficult problem to manage. Several methods may be utilized to stent the carina. The anatomic changes and bronchoscopist experience dictate the method employed. Bilateral mainstem or distal tracheal disease at the carina can be approached with a Dumon Y Stent® or a Dynamic® stent. Each stent protects and stents the distal trachea, carinal bifurcation, and

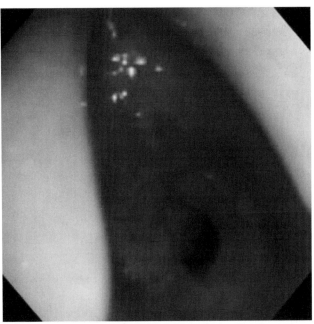

(a)

(b)

Figure 14C.5 *Airway stenting. (a) Endoscopic image from a patient with stridor and high-grade subglottic obstruction. After gentle dilation, a silicone stent was placed (b) with normalized tracheal lumen and complete symptom relief. A silicone stent was chosen because of the benign nature of the lesion, as the patient may still need to undergo surgical resection.*

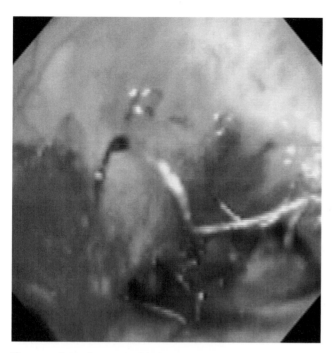

Figure 14C.6   *Stent complication. A completely fractured and embedded metal stent. The stent disintegrated 9 months after placement, requiring complicated removal.*

the proximal mainstem bronchi. Care must be taken when placing a Y stent so that the right upper lobe take-off remains patent. Recurrence of disease at a pneumonectomy stump allows deployment of a simple tubular stent across the carina into the remaining mainstem.

Stents are effective in emergency management of respiratory failure from CAO. Surveillance bronchoscopy is not required. Bacterial colonization is frequent after stenting but is not associated with clinical disease. Overall, roughly 20 percent of stents develop complications, most commonly, mucus impaction, granulation, tumor growth, or migration.

Adjunctive methods

ENDOBRONCHIAL INJECTIONS

The use of an endoscope for intraluminal injections is well known in gastroenterology. In the field of bronchology, it is still in its formative stage. A growing body of evidence is suggesting endobronchial application of pharmacotherapy may be beneficial. Intratumoral injection of ethanol has been used for endobronchial tumor causing necrosis allowing forceps debridement. Intralesional injection of epinephrine has been used for acute hemorrhage. Endoscopic injections of steroids have been used to treat recurrent granulation tissue.

The use of intralesional cidofovir has been described for respiratory papillomatosis. Celikoglu and colleagues have published a study on the use of direct intratumoral injection of chemotherapeutic drugs.[38,39] Eighty-seven percent of their

patients had relief of the obstruction with no systemic effects or serious complications. This interesting approach appears to hold some promise. However, it requires further study of its primary and potential adjunctive use before it can be recommended.

ADJUNCTIVE MEDICAL THERAPY

Systemic corticosteroids are used empirically by many interventionalists after tracheal therapies. There are no data to suggest a reduction in granulation tissue after stenting when patients are empirically started on systemic corticosteroids. Empiric antibiotics are unnecessary in most patients after interventional bronchoscopy.

MULTIMODALITY THERAPY

Substantial data have been published supporting a multimodality approach.[2,36,40–43] There appears to be a survival advantage with multiple therapies.[44] Interventional bronchoscopic therapies should be performed before radiotherapy to allow optimal patient physiology when combining therapies. Figure 14C.7 shows an algorithm on how to approach CAO using all described modalities.

BRIDGE TO DEFINITIVE SURGICAL/ONCOLOGIC THERAPY

Bronchoscopic therapies should be approached in a broader sense than simply palliative. There is an important role for interventional bronchology in bridging to definitive surgical or chemo-radiotherapy and enhancing the ability to receive salvage therapy. The improvement in functional status provided makes previously excluded patients candidates for surgical or medical oncology therapies. It allows staging that is more appropriate and treats or prevents infectious complications, allowing safer and more appropriate definitive therapy. Temporary stenting can be utilized with removal of stents after tumor specific therapy. Those patients who undergo resection after endobronchial therapy usually have no anastomotic complications following the resection. Endobronchial therapy may improve operability and surgical results in select patients.

EVALUATION OF OUTCOME/FUNCTIONAL STATUS

A review of functional status and spirometry after interventional bronchoscopy is presented in Table 14C.2. Dyspnea is almost universally improved or relieved immediately. In the largest published series of 2008 patients, overall 93 percent of patients had immediate relief of dyspnea.[36] The location of the obstruction was important. When tracheal obstruction was relieved, 97 percent of patients had immediate benefit. The immediate benefit remained 90–95 percent for the mainstem bronchi and the bronchus intermedius. Only 50–77 percent obtained relief of dyspnea when a lobar or segmental bronchus was involved.

Table 14C.1   *Airway stenting for central airway obstruction (CAO)*

Study	N	Indication	Therapy	Stent type	Complications	Remarks
Noppen et al. 1997[49]	58	Malignant and benign tracheo-bronchial stenosis	93 patients in total received stent or laser or dilation	Metallic, silicone	Retained secretions 17%, stent infection 5%, migration 14%	89% of malignant CAO had symptomatic and/ or spirometric improvement, 87% with benign CAO had symptomatic and/ or spirometric improvement
Miyazawa & Arita 1998[50]	35	Malignant tracheobronchial obstruction	Stent, laser, coring out, dilation	Silicone	Migration 5%, retained secretions 11.5%, granulation 18%, tumor overgrowth 3%	89% had immediate relief of respiratory symptoms, increased FEV_1, VC, PEFR, Pao_2, improved performance status
Dumon et al. 2000[51]	50	Malignant carinal obstruction or TE fistula	Stenting	Silicone Y	No migration	Survival 109 days in malignancy, 71 days with TE fistula, good quality of life
Hautmann et al. 2000[52]	51	Malignant and benign airway obstruction	Stent	Metallic	Migration 12%, initial displacement of stent 11%, stent/airway diameter mismatch 5%	80% immediate relief of respiratory symptoms improved FEV_1, FEV_1/ FVC, PEFR
Matsuo & Colt 2000[53]	88	Malignant and benign airway obstruction	Stent	Silicone		Asymptomatic stent complication in 10%, 5% required intervention. The routine use of surveillance bronchoscopy is not needed. New respiratory symptoms should prompt re-evaluation
Miyazawa et al. 2000[54]	34	Malignant CAO	Stent, laser, argon plasma, or coring out if needed	Metallic	No migration, no retained secretions, tumor ingrowth 24%, tumor overgrowth 21%	56% placed emergently. Immediate relief in dyspnea in 82%. Significant improvement in VC, FEV_1, PEFR
Tanigawa et al. 2000[55]	44	Malignant CAO	Stent after dilation	Metallic	Restenosis in 27.3%, 58% of these required reintervention	95% improved dyspnea
Madden et al. 2002[56]	28	Malignant and benign tracheo-bronchial stenosis, obstruction, or fistula	Stent	Metallic	Late complications: halitosis, retained secretions, granulation tissue; no migration	100% of tracheomalacia weaned from mechanical ventilator, 20 had symptomatic improvement
Stockton et al. 2003[57]	162	Malignant CAO	Stent	Metallic	No mortality	Survival for lung cancer 103 days vs. metastatic EBL 431days ($P < 0.001$)
Bolliger et al. 2004[58]	26	Malignant CAO	Stent	Studded woven silastic	Retained secretions 14.8%, migration 3.8%	Statistically increased KPS, WHO activity index, dyspnea index, FEV_1 and FVC at 1 month, FEV_1 at 3 months
Miyazawa 2004	64	Malignant CAO	Stent placement after precise localization of 'choke point'	Metallic, silicone	Retained secretions 31%, tumor growth 28%, granulation tissue 22%, migration 8%	Significant improvement in WHO dyspnea from III / IV to 0/I poststent. Significant improvement in FEV_1, FVC, PEFR in tracheal and bronchial stenting, Significant improvement in FEV_1 and PEFR in both carinal and extensive stenosis post-stenting. Choke point may move after stenting requiring secondary stenting

TE, tracheoesophegeal; FEV_1, forced expiratory volume in 1 second; VC, viral capacity; PEFR, peak expiratory flow rate; FVC, forced vital capicity; KPS, Karnofsky Performance Score; WHO, World Health Organization.

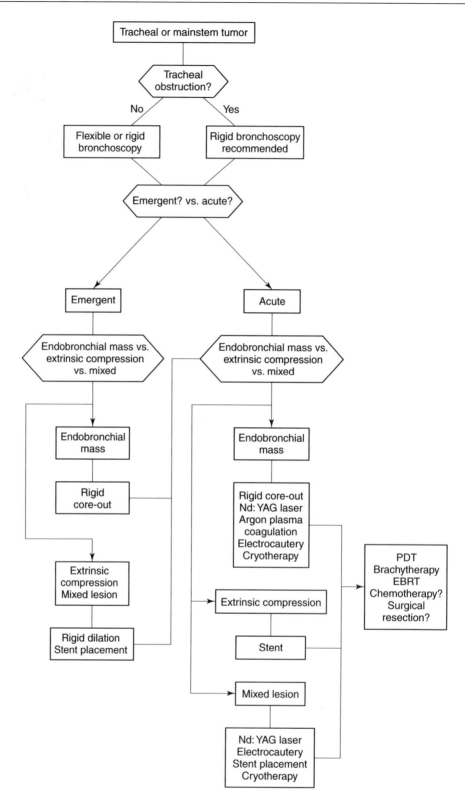

Figure 14C.7 *Algorithm for the management of central airway obstruction. PDT, photodynamic therapy; EBRT, external beam radiotherapy.*

Table 14C.2 *Changes in performance status and spirometry after interventional pulmonary recanalization*

	Study	N	Therapy	Result
Performance status	McCaughan et al. 1988[59]	31	PDT	KPS: 57 improved to 65
	Ross et al. 1990[60]	69	Nd:YAG	KPS: Successful recanalization: 41 ± 13 improved to 60 ± 17; unsuccessful: 45 ± 8 improved to 54 ± 5
	Monnier et al. 1996[61]	40	Laser, stent	KPS: 40 improved to 70
	McCaughan 1999[62]	13	PDT	KPS: 53.8 improved to 73.07 $(P = 0.02)$
	Maiwand et al. 2004[1]	476	Cryotherapy	KPS: 59.6 improved to 75.2, WHO: 3.04 improved to 2.20
	Moghissi et al. 1997[42]	17	Nd:YAG, PDT	WHO: 2.23 (2–3) improved to 0.71 (0–2)
	Moghissi et al. 1999[63]	100	PDT	WHO 43% <2 improved to 87% <2 post PDT
	Bolliger et al. 2004[58]	26	Stent	WHO: 2.7 improved to 1.5 at 1 month, changed to 1.6 at 3 months, KPS: 44 improved to 72 at 1 month, stable at 71 at 3 months
	Miyazawa 1998[50]	35	Stent	ECOG 86% 3–4 improved to 86% 0–2
FEV$_1$	Miyazawa 1998[50]	35	Stent	1.67 improved to 2.05 $(P < 0.01)$
	Moghissi et al. 1999[42]	100	PDT	1.38 ± 0.56 improved to $1.66 + 0.57$
	Noppen et al. 1999[64]	14	Stent	1.17 ± 0.81 improved to $1.83 \pm 0.74 (P < 0.006)$
	Miyazawa et al. 2000[54]	34	Stent	1.40 ± 0.51 improved to 1.74 ± 0.52 $(P < 0.001)$
	Hautman et al. 2000[52]	51	Stent	1.57 ± 0.49 improved to 1.99 ± 0.62 $(P\ 0.019)$
	Gotway et al. 2002[66]	22	Stent	1.33 improved to 1.75 $(p < 0.001)$
	Bolliger et al. 2004[63]	26	Stent	1.2 improved to 1.9 at 1 month, changed to 1.5 at 3 months
	Maiwand et al. 2004[1]	476	Cryotherapy	1.38 improved to 1.41 $(p \leqslant 0.0001)$
	Miyazawa et al. 2004[24]	64	Stent	Tracheal 1.67 ± 0.60 improved to $2.32 \pm 0.57 (p < 0.001)$, carinal 1.56 ± 0.68 improved to 2.04 ± 0.55 $(p < 0.001)$, bronchial 1.46 ± 0.40 improved to 1.79 ± 0.55 $(p < 0.01)$, extensive stenosis 1.06 ± 0.36 improved to 1.33 ± 0.50 improved to 1.91 ± 0.41 after second stent $(p < 0.01)$
FVC	Moghissi et al. 1997[42]	17	Nd:YAG, PDT	Improved 28%
	Maiwand et al. 1997[67]	21	Cryotherapy, dilation, stent	25% improved $(p < 0.001)$
	Moghissi et al. 1999[63]	100	PDT	2.07 ± 0.78 improved to 2.5 ± 0.74
	Noppen et al. 1999[64]	14	Stent	2.00 ± 0.81 improved to $2.81 \pm 1 (p\ 0.048)$
	Gotway et al. 2002[66]	22	Stent	2.92 improved to 2.98 $(p = 0.555)$
	Maiwand et al. 2004[1]	476	Cryotherapy	1.91 improved to 2.04 $(p < 0.0001)$
	Miyazawa et al. 2004[24]	64	Stent	Tracheal 2.94 ± 0.95 improved to 3.15 ± 1.87 $(p < 0.05)$, bronchial 2.04 ± 0.55 improved to 2.50 ± 0.79 $(p < 0.01)$
	Bolliger et al. 2004[66]	26	Stent	2.1 improved to 2.8 at 1 month, changed to 2.5 at 3 months

KPS, Karnofsky Performance Score; WHO, World Health Organization; PDT, photodynamic therapy.

Removal of mechanical ventilation

Mortality of lung cancer patients requiring ventilatory support in the intensive care unit (ICU) is dismal, ranging from 54.5 percent to 91.1 percent.[45] Lin et al. retrospectively studied 95 episodes of respiratory failure in 81 patients with lung cancer.[45] Successful weaning occurred in 27.4 percent. Interventional bronchoscopy has shown significant improvements in liberation from mechanical ventilation. After stent placement, 87.5 percent could be weaned.[46] Colt and Harrell evaluated 32 ICU patients admitted with CAO, of which 19 were being mechanically ventilated.[47] After rigid bronchoscopy, 52.6 percent had immediate removal of ventilatory support.

Life expectancy

In an evaluation of patients with respiratory failure who were successfully removed from mechanical ventilation immediately after therapy survival was improved.[48] The average survival in those extubated on day 1 was 98 days as compared with 8.5 days in those extubated an average 6 days after therapy. Multimodality treatment increases 3-year survival. Patients treated with single therapy experienced a 2.3 percent survival at 3 years as compared with a 22 percent survival in those undergoing complementary therapies.[44]

Key learning points

- Bronchoscopic therapeutic procedures are safe with an overall mortality of less than 1 percent.

- The utility of interventional bronchoscopy is applicable to any cause of central airway obstruction.

- Interventional pulmonology is best viewed as a bridge to definitive tumor specific therapy or as a palliative modality in CAO. Select processes are amenable to definitive interventional bronchoscopic therapy.

- The use of advanced imaging, internal and external three-dimensional reconstructions and endobronchial ultrasonography, significantly enhances the planning and determination of appropriate endobronchial therapy.

- An interventional bronchoscopist must be familiar with all aspects of minimally invasive therapy including the use of rigid bronchoscopy.

- Referral should be considered to a center of excellence with a multidisciplinary team with experience and availability of technology that allow multiple modalities to be utilized.

REFERENCES

1. Maiwand MO, Evans JM, Beeson JE. The application of cryosurgery in the treatment of lung cancer. *Cryobiology* 2004; **48**: 55–61.

2. Cavaliere S, Dumon J-F. Laser bronchoscopy. In: Bolliger CT, Mathur PN, eds. *Interventional Bronchoscopy*. Basel: Karger, 2000: 108–19.

3. Froudarakis ME, Bouros D, Siafakas NM. Endoluminal metastases of the tracheobronchial tree. Is there any way out? *Chest* 2001; **119**: 679–81.

4. Katsimbri PP, Bamias AT, Froudarakis ME, *et al.* Endobronchial metastases secondary to solid tumors: report of eight cases and review of the literature. *Lung Cancer* 2000; **28**: 163–70.

5. Braman SS, Whitcomb ME. Endobronchial metastasis. *Arch Intern Med* 1975; **135**: 543–7.

6. Ormerod LP, Horsfield N, Alani FSS. How frequently do endobronchial secondaries occur in an unselected series? *Respir Med* 1998; **92**: 599–600.

7. Rumbak MJ, Walsh FW, Anderson WM, *et al.* Significant tracheal obstruction causing failure to wean in patients requiring prolonged mechanical ventilation. *Chest* 2004; **115**: 1092–5.

8. Sterman DH, Sztejman E, Rodriguez E, Friedberg J. Diagnosis and staging of 'other bronchial tumors'. *Chest Surg Clin North Am* 2003; **13**: 79–94.

9. Litzky L. Epithelial and soft tissue tumors of the tracheobronchial tree. *Chest Surg Clin North Am* 2003; **13**: 1–40.

10. Hage R, Brutel de la Riviere A, Seldenrijk A, van den Bosch JMM. Update in pulmonary carcinoid tumors: a review article. *Ann Surg Oncol* 2003; **10**: 697–704.

11. Mehta AC, Rafanan AL, Bulkey R, *et al.* Coronary spasm and cardiac arrest from carcinoid crisis during laser bronchoscopy. *Chest* 1999; **115**: 598–600.

12. Salud A, Porcel JM, Rovirosa A, Bellmunt J. Endobronchial metastatic disease: analysis of 32 cases. *J Clin Oncol* 1996; **62**: 249–52.

13. Shepherd MP. Endobronchial metastatic disease. *Thorax* 1982; **37**: 362–5.

14. Heitmiller RF, Marasco WJ, Hruban RH, Marsh BR. Endobronchial metastasis. *J Thorac Cardiovasc Surg* 1993; **106**: 537–42.

15. Ohno T, Nakayama Y, Kurihara T, *et al.* Endobronchial metastasis of breast cancer 5 years after breast-conserving therapy. *Int J Clin Oncol* 2001; **6**: 101–4.

16. Ettensohn DB, Bennett JM, Hyde RW. Endobronchial metastasis from carcinoma of the breast. *Med Pediatr Oncol* 1985; **13**: 9–13.

17. Fitzgerald RHJ. Endobronchial metastases. *South Med J* 1977; **70**: 440–1.

18. Lim DJ, Carter MF. Computerized tomography in preoperative staging for pulmonary metastases in patients with renal cell carcinoma. *J Urol* 1993; **150**: 1112–14.

19. Ondo K, Sugio K, Yamazaki K, *et al.* Pulmonary metastasis with an endobronchial growth pattern: report of a case. *Ann Thorac Cardiovasc Surg* 2000; **6**: 326–8.

20. Casino AR, Bellmunt J, Salud A, *et al.* Endobronchial metastases in colorectal adenocarcinoma. *Tumori* 1992; **78**: 270–3.

21. Colt HG, Meric B, Dumon J-F. Double stents for carcinoma of the esophagus invading the tracheo-bronchial tree. *Gastrointest Endosc* 1992; **38**: 485–9.

22. Brichet A, Verkindre C, Dupont J, *et al.* Multidisciplinary approach to management of postintubation tracheal stenoses. *Eur Respir J* 1999; **13**: 888–93.

23. Chen K, Varon J, Wenker OC. Malignant airway obstruction: recognition and management. *J Emerg Med* 1998; **16**: 83–92.

24. Miyazawa T, Miyazu Y, Iwamoto Y, *et al.* Stenting at the flow-limiting segment in tracheobronchial stenosis due to Lung cancer. *Am J Respir Crit Care Med* 2004; **169**: 1096–102.

25. Finkelsteiin SE, Schrump DS, Nguyen DM, *et al.* Comparative evaluation of super high-resolution CT scan and virtual bronchoscopy for the detection of tracheobronchial malignancies. *Chest* 2003; **124**: 1834–40.

26. Remy-Jardin M, Remy J, Artaud D, *et al.* Volume rendering of the tracheobronchial tree: clinincal evaluation of bronchographic images. *Radiology* 1998; **208**: 761–70.

27. Hoppe H, Dinkel H-P, Walder B, *et al.* Grading airway stenosis down to the segmental level using virtual bronchoscopy. *Chest* 2004; **125**: 704–11.

28. Remy-Jardin M, Remy J, Artaud D, *et al.* Tracheobronchial tree: assessment with volume rendering – technical aspects. *Radiology* 1998; **208**: 393–8.

29. Kurimoto N, Murayama M, Yoshioka S, *et al.* Assessment of the usefulness of endobronchial ultrasonography in determination of depth of tracheobronchial tumor invasion. *Chest* 1999; **115**: 1500–6.

30. Takemoto Y, Kawahara M, Ogawara M, *et al.* Ultrasound-guided flexible bronchoscopy for the diagnosis of tumor invasion to the bronchial wall and mediastinum. *J Bronchol* 2000; **7**: 127–32.

31. Herth F, Ernst A, Schulz M, Becker HD. Endobronchial ultrasound reliably differentiates between airway infiltration and compression by tumor. *Chest* 2003; **123**: 458–62.

32. Herth F, Becker HD, LoCicero JI, Ernst A. Endobronchial ultrasound in therapeutic bronchoscopy. *Eur Respir J* 2002; **20**: 118–21.

33. Shirakawa T, Imamura F, Hamamoto J, Shirkakusa T. A case of successful airway stent placement guided by endobronchial ultrasonography. *J Bronchol* 2004; **11**: 45–8.

34. Beamis JFJ. Modern use of rigid bronchoscopy. In: Bolliger CT, Mathur PN, eds. *Interventional Bronchoscopy*. Basel: Karger, 2000: 22–30.

35. Turner JF, Ernst A, Becker HD. Rigid bronchoscopy. *J Bronchol* 2000; **7**: 171–6.

36. Cavaliere S, Venuta F, Foccoli P, *et al.* Endoscopic treatment of malignant obstructions in 2,008 patients. *Chest* 1996; **110**: 1536–42.

37. Jang TW, Blackman G, George JJ. Survival benefits of lung cancer patients undergoing laser and brachytherapy. *J Korean Med Sci* 2002; **17**: 341–7.

38. Celikoglu SI, Karayel T, Demirci S, *et al.* Direct injection of anti-cancer drugs into endobronchial tumors for palliation of major airway obstruction. *Postgrad Med J* 1997; **73**: 159–62.

39. Celikoglu F, Celikoglu SI. Intratumoral chemotherapy with 5-fluorouracil for palliation of bronchial cancer in patients with severe airway obstruction. *J Pharm Pharmacol* 2003; **55**: 1441–8.

40. Desai SJ, Mehta AC, Vanderbrug Medendorp S, *et al.* Survival experience following Nd:YAG laser photoresection for primary bronchogenic carcinoma. *Chest* 1988; **94**: 939–44.

41. Shea JM, Allen RP, Tharratt RS, *et al.* Survival of patients undergoing Nd:YAG laser therapy compared with Nd:YAG laser therapy and brachytherapy for malignant airway disease. *Chest* 1993; **103**: 1028–31.

42. Moghissi K, Dixon K, Hudson E, *et al.* Endoscopic laser therapy in malignant tracheobronchial obstruction using sequential NdYAG laser and photodynamic therapy. *Thorax* 1997; **52**: 281–3.

43. Stephens KE, Wood DE. Bronchoscopic management of central airway obstruction. *J Thorac Cardiovasc Surg* 2000; **119**: 289–96.

44. Santos RS, Raftopoulos Y, Keenan RJ, *et al.* Bronchoscopic palliation of primary lung cancer: Single or multimodality therapy? *Surg Endosc* 2004; **18**: 931–6.

45. Lin Y-C, Tsai Y-H, Huang C-C, *et al.* Outcome of lung cancer patients with acute respiratory failure requiring mechanical ventilation. *Respir Med* 2004; **98**: 43–51.

46. Saad CP, Murthy S, Krizmanich G, Mehta AC. Self-expandable metallic airway stents and flexible bronchoscopy long term outcomes analysis. *Chest* 2003; **124**: 1993–9.

47. Colt HG, Harrell JHI. Therapeutic rigid bronchoscopy allows level of care changes in patients with acute respiratory failure from central airways obstruction. *Chest* 1997; **112**: 202–6.

48. Stanopoulos IT, Beamis JFJ, Martinez FJ, *et al.* Laser bronchoscopy in respiratory failure from malignant airway obstruction. *Crit Care Med* 1993; **21**: 386–91.

49. Noppen M, Meysman M, D'Haese J, *et al.* Interventional bronchoscopy: 5-year experience at

the Academic Hospital of the Vrije Universiteit Brussel (AZ-VUB). *Acta Clin Bel* 1997; **52**: 371–80.

50. Miyazawa T, Arita K. Airway stenting in Japan. *Respirology* 1998; **3**: 229–34.

51. Dumon J-F, Dumon MC. Dumon-Novatech Y-Stents: A four-year experience with 50 tracheobronchial tumors involving the carina. *J Bronchol* 2000; **7**: 26–32.

52. Hautman H, Bauer M, Pfeifer KJ, Huber R. Flexible bronchoscopy: a safe method for metal stent implantation in bronchial disease. *Ann Thorac Surg* 2000; **69**: 398–401.

53. Matsuo T, Colt HG. Evidence against routine scheduling of surveillance bronchoscopy after stent insertion. *Chest* 2000; **118**: 51–5.

54. Miyazawa T, Yamakido M, Ikeda S, *et al.* Implantation of ultraflex nitinol stents in malignant tracheobronchial stenoses. *Chest* 2000; **118**: 959–65.

55. Tanigawa N, Sawada S, Okuda Y, *et al.* Symptomatic improvement in dyspnea following tracheobronchial metallic stenting for malignant airway obstruction. *Acta Radiol* 2000; **41**: 425–8.

56. Madden BP, Datta S, Charokopos N. Experience with ultraflex expandable metallic stents in the management of endobronchial pathology. *Ann Thorac Surg* 2002; **73**: 938–44.

57. Stockton PA, Ledson MJ, Hind CRK, Walshaw MJ. Bronchoscopic insertion of Gianturco stents for the palliation of malignant lung disease: 10 year experience. *Lung Cancer* 2003; **42**: 113–17.

58. Bolliger CT, Breitenbuecher A, Brutsche M, *et al.* Use of studded polyflex stents in patients with neoplastic obstructions of the central airways. respiration 2004; **71**: 83–7.

59. McCaughan JSJ, Hawley PC, Bethel BH, Walker J. Photodynamic therapy of endobronchial malignancies. *Cancer* 1988; **62**: 691–701.

60. Ross DJ, Mohsenifar Z, Koerner SK. Survival characteristics after neodymium:YAG laser photoresection in advanced stage lung cancer. *Chest* 1990; **98**: 581–5.

61. Monnier P, Mudry A, Stanzel F, *et al.* The use of the covered wallstent for the palliative treatment of inoperable tracheobronchial cancers. *Chest* 1996; **110**: 1161–8.

62. McCaughan JSJ. Survival after photodynamic therapy to non-pulmonary metastatic endobronchial tumors. *Laser Surg Med* 1999; **24**: 194–201.

63. Moghissi K, Dixon K, Stringer M, *et al.* The place of bronchoscopic photodynamic therapy in advanced unresectable lung cancer: experience of 100 cases. *Eur J Cardiothorac Surg* 1999; **15**: 1–6.

64. Noppen M, Pierard D, Meysman M, *et al.* Bacterial colonization of central airways after stenting. *Am J Respir Crit Care Med* 1999; **160**: 672–7.

65. Vergnon J-M, Costes F, Polio J-C. Efficacy and tolerance of a new silicone stent for the treatment of benign tracheal stenosis. *Chest* 2000; **118**: 422–6.

66. Gotway MB, Golden JA, LaBerge JM, *et al.* Benign tracheobronchial stenoses: changes in short-term and long-term pulmonary function testing after expandable metallic stent placement. *J Comput Assist Tomogr* 2002; **26**: 564–72.

67. Maiwand MO, Zehr KJ, Dyke CM, *et al.* The role of cryotherapy for airway complications after lung and heart-lung transplantation. *Eur J Cardiothorac Surg* 1997; **12**: 549–54.

Aspiration syndromes

ALI A EL SOLH

INTRODUCTION

The complications of pulmonary aspiration have been recognized since Hippocrates warned in 400 BC 'for drinking to provoke a slight cough, or for swallowing to be forced is bad'.[1] However it was not until 1946 when Mendelson reported on the outcome of 66 obstetric patients who aspirated gastric contents that a scientific account of aspiration syndromes has been recognized.[2]

Aspiration is broadly defined as inhalation of endogenous contents or exogenous substances into the lower airways.[3] An assortment of pulmonary syndromes associated with the inhalation of these substances has been described depending on the frequency of aspiration, the nature of the aspirated material, as well as the underlying host response.[4] Three pathologic entities, each displaying a characteristic but not exclusive pattern of pulmonary injury, are reported: the irritant-toxic, the inert-nontoxic, and the infectious type. These can be further categorized as acute or chronic in nature depending on the clinical presentation and the progression of the disease. A complete discussion of these aspiration syndromes is, however, beyond the scope of this chapter. This chapter focuses on non-gaseous aspirations that are implicated in adult respiratory emergencies. The discussion summarizes the phenomenon of gastric content aspiration (aspiration pneumonitis), oropharyngeal aspiration (aspiration pneumonia), aspiration of solid materials, and near-drowning.

EPIDEMIOLOGY

In the absence of reliable markers for the diagnosis of aspiration, an accurate estimate of the incidence of aspiration syndromes is not available. The frequency rate of this syndrome is further complicated by the fact that up to 37 percent of aspiration episodes are occult in nature.[5] Furthermore, most clinical investigations do not distinguish between aspiration pneumonia and aspiration pneumonitis.

Based on literature review, aspiration pneumonitis is reported to occur in 10–25 percent of patients hospitalized because of overdose[6] and in about 1 in 3000 patients following anesthesia.[7] Aspiration of gastric contents is considered to be the second or the third most frequent cause of the adult respiratory distress syndrome.[8] Alternatively, aspiration pneumonia affects some 300 000 to 600 000 Americans each year.[9] Aspiration pneumonia has been reported to be the second most frequent diagnosis among hospitalizations of Medicare patients.[10] The discharges of patients hospitalized for aspiration pneumonia has doubled over the period of 1991–1998 whereas those of older Medicare beneficiaries have increased by only 11.1 percent.[11] The yearly increases in the number of hospitalizations for aspiration pneumonia per 100 000 persons are mostly reported in the very old and are expected to rise even more in the decades to come.

GASTRIC CONTENTS ASPIRATION (ASPIRATION PNEUMONITIS OR MENDELSON SYNDROME)

Aspiration pneumonitis is defined as the occurrence of an acute lung injury following the aspiration of toxic substances into the lower airways. The qualities of the aspirate – pH, volume, and the presence of particulate matter – are all deemed major determinants of lung injury after aspiration.

Gastric acid aspiration represents the prototype of aspiration pneumonitis in what is commonly referred to as the Mendelson syndrome. Mendelson showed that the introduction of acid gastric contents into the lungs of rabbits induced severe pneumonitis similar to that caused by an equivalent amount of 0.1 N hydrochloric acid. However, the injury can be minimized if the pH of the gastric contents was neutralized prior to aspiration.[12] In these experimental animals, the critical pH for lung injury was determined at 2.4 with no permanent injury noted above this threshold. Conversely, an incremental increase in inflammation was observed as the pH value was lowered to 1.5. Below this level, no incremental inflammatory reaction occurred. Similar critical care pH thresholds have been identified in other species including rats (pH 2.5),[13] dogs (pH 3.8),[14] and mice (pH 5.9).[15] The threshold pH for humans is quoted at 2.5.

Acute lung injury becomes independent of gastric pH as the volume of the aspirate is increased[16] or particulate matter is added.[17,18] Whereas volume as small as 0.2 mL/kg could induce lung injury if the pH was 1.0, the addition of fecally contaminated gastric contents could lead to pneumonitis and death in dogs despite a pH of 6.4 and treatment with antibiotics.[19] Bacterial infection plays no substantial role in the early phase of aspiration pneumonitis. The acidity of the gastric contents renders the medium sterile, but as the pH increases above 7.0, the bacterial density in the gastric aspirates may approach the bacterial density of the mouth and the pharynx at 10^8 colony-forming units per milliliter

(CFU/mL).[20] If host defense is not impaired, these concentrations are unlikely to cause a lower respiratory tract infection.[21] However, conditions that promote oropharyngeal or gastric colonization (poor dental hygiene,[22] bowel obstruction,[14] enteral tube feeding,[23] suppressed acid production[24]) elevate the bacterial count to more than 10^{20} CFU/mL increasing the likelihood of bacterial infection (Fig. 14D.1).

Pathophysiology

Massive aspiration of gastric contents produces a dramatic pathophysiologic picture that manifests in two stages. The early stage is characterized by a rapid development of atelectasis which is thought to be the result of acid denaturation of pulmonary surfactant. In the later stage, there is outpouring of fluid into the alveolar space resulting in hemoconcentration, elevation of pulmonary artery pressure, and depressed cardiac output.[25] These pathologic changes lead to inflammatory reactions manifested as capillary leak, release of inflammatory cytokines and chemokines especially tumor necrosis factor-α and interleukin-8,[26] cellular infiltration, and oxidative injury of a greater magnitude than those resulting from the aspiration of acid or gastric particles alone.

Clinical features

The clinical picture is dominated by symptoms of dyspnea, cough, and wheezing. Abrupt onset of tachypnea, low-grade fever, cyanosis, and diffuse rales are almost universal.[27] Severe hypoxemia is immediate and is attributed to worsening ventilation/perfusion mismatching caused by reflex-mediated small-airway closure.[28]

Evaluation of chest radiographs of patients with chemical pneumonitis reveals no typical or characteristic appearance. However, three basic patterns of disease can be identified:[27]

- extensive airspace disease (confluent acinar opacities)
- widespread acinar opacities (5–6 mm nodularlike opacities)
- irregular shadows including indistinct vascular markings.

Pleural abnormalities are considered unusual on initial radiographic films and should raise the possibility on of an alternative diagnosis. Although the extent of infiltrate on the first chest radiograph does not necessarily correlate with outcome, the subsequent clinical course takes one of three pathways:

- The majority (62 percent) show rapid clinical and radiographic improvement. Radiographic resolution is expected to occur within 2–16 days.
- A minority (12 percent) demonstrate a rapid progression with worsening clinical and radiographic picture. Death ensues within 24–48 hours.

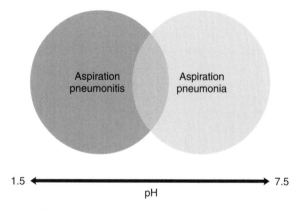

1.5 ⟷ 7.5
pH

Figure 14D.1 *In the presence of predisposing factors, aspiration syndromes represent a spectrum of diseases ranging from aspiration pneumonitis at a low pH to aspiration pneumonia at normal or near normal level.*

- The remainder (26 percent) exhibit rapid improvement from the initial insult followed by clinical deterioration associated with new or expanding radiographic infiltrates indicative of superimposed nosocomial infection.

Diagnosis

Despite extensive investigation, there is no reliable marker for diagnosing pulmonary aspiration of gastric contents. This lack of a sensitive and specific marker makes accurate epidemiologic study of this syndrome difficult and the design of prospective treatment protocol problematic. Post-aspiration tracheobronchial fluid pH has proved an insensitive test for the diagnosis of silent pulmonary aspiration. The mechanical dispersion of the aspirate bolus into the distal airways and the buffering of acid contents within minutes of aspiration make any reliable measurement inconclusive.[29,30] Lipid-laden macrophages have been identified as useful markers for chronic aspiration[31] but such methods are of limited use for the detection of acute aspiration. It has been postulated that the gastric proteolytic enzyme, pepsin, could be used as a biochemical marker since pepsin concentrations in the lung are nondetectable.[32] Assay of peptic activity in bronchoalveolar lavage of rabbits following intratracheal installation of gastric juice has been reported to be highly sensitive.[33] Because the test (Anson method) relies on the presence of proteolytically active pepsin to digest a hemoglobin substrate, a time-dependent decrease in peptic activity is observed in the alkaline medium in the lung limiting the utility of the test to less than 1 hour for highly suspected cases of aspiration. An immunoassay with polyclonal antibodies to purified human pepsin has been developed with improved sensitivity and specificity compared with other available techniques.[34] The immunoassay was proved to detect human tracheal secretion in suspected cases of gastric juice but its validity has not been confirmed in clinical trials.

Treatment

Treatment is designed to support the patient during the acute lung injury and to prevent complications (Box 14D.1). Hypoxemia is treated with supplemental oxygen. Aerosolized bronchodilators may be beneficial in the presence of wheezing or air trapping. These can be administered every 20 minutes if necessary to treat bronchospasm. Noninvasive positive pressure ventilation with an inspiratory pressure to not exceed 19 cm H_2O should be considered in patients who are alert and cooperative. Otherwise, intubation and mechanical ventilation would be needed to sustain adequate oxygenation and improve arterial blood gas values. Ventilatory management of acute lung injury is detailed in a Chapter 10C and will not be discussed here.

There are no randomized controlled trials assessing the role of empiric antimicrobial therapy in the treatment of aspiration pneumonitis. Evidence accumulated from retrospective studies has indicated that prophylactic antibiotic therapy does not decrease the incidence of lung infection or improve clinical outcome. It might, however, promote the selection of drug-resistant pathogens.[35] Most experts agree that antibiotics should be withheld initially with the exception of aspiration associated with intestinal obstruction or conditions associated with gastric colonization. Nevertheless, antimicrobial agents are frequently prescribed because of the difficulty in excluding bacterial infection.

Several human and animal studies have reached conflicting results regarding the use of adjunct systemic corticosteroids for the management of aspiration pneumonitis ranging from beneficial to ineffective to harmful.[36–38] The only randomized, placebo-controlled trial that showed decreased length of intubation, mechanical ventilation, and length of stay in the intensive care unit, using methylprednisolone (15 mg/kg per day) administered for 3 days, had no impact on the incidence of complications or outcome.[39] In a subsequent study of follow-up pulmonary function tests conducted 1 year following aspiration, improvements in lung volumes were similar irrespective of whether steroids or placebo were administered during the acute phase.[40] Given the failure of corticosteroids in two multicenter randomized controlled trials to alter the outcome of acute respiratory distress syndrome,[41,42] the use of corticosteroids in the management of aspiration pneumonitis is currently not recommended.

Prevention

Since the description of the syndrome, important therapeutic strategies intended to minimize the risks of aspiration have evolved. Because 50 percent of patients undergoing emergency surgery[43] and all pregnant women are considered at risk, much of the work on prevention of aspiration pneumonitis has emanated from trials conducted on these patients. The preventive strategies which have been adopted include:

- fasting prior to anesthesia
- measures which may increase gastric pH

> ## Box 14D.1 Initial management of aspiration syndromes
>
> - Establishment of airway patency
> - Ensuring adequate ventilation
> - Administration of supplemental oxygen
> - Airways suctioning
> - Nebulized bronchodilators
> - Fluid therapy to maintain normovolemic state

- measures which may reduce the volume of gastric secretions
- application of cricoid pressure prior to intubation
- elevation of head of the bed.

It has been clearly demonstrated that both the intake of food and the drinking of dextrose-containing solutions can significantly delay gastric emptying. Keeping patients nil per os is intended to decrease gastric volume. However, despite overnight fasting, 33 percent of patients have gastric volumes greater than 25 mL, and 64–85 percent have a gastric pH of 2.5 or less.[44] Two techniques intended to raise the gastric pH before the administration of an anesthetic in *highly-at-risk* patients have gained widespread acceptance:

- The administration of 30 mL of 0.3 M sodium citrate 15–60 minutes before anesthesia has been shown to raise gastric pH above 2.5 in about 90 percent of patients.[45] This antacid is preferable to the particulate antacids because the solution mixes more effectively with the gastric contents and carries a lesser risk of lung injury if aspirated inadvertently.
- The administration of an H_2-antagonist is even more effective than sodium citrate at raising gastric pH and reducing gastric volume.[46] If used prior to elective surgery, two oral doses of ranitidine or cimetidine should be given with one dose given the night before surgery and one on the morning of surgery.

When given intravenously for an emergency surgery, these agents should be administered at least 45 minutes before anesthetic induction is given to assure effectiveness.[47] Famotidine offers the potential advantages of longer duration and fewer drug interactions. With a duration of action of 12 hours, a single dose on the night before surgery increases the gastric pH to low-risk values.[48] Proton-pump inhibitors are considered more potent than H_2-antagonists in reducing gastric acid secretion. A single oral dose of 40 mg of omeprazole on the night before surgery increased gastric pH to greater than 2.5.[49] When metoclopramide (10 mg given intramuscularly at least 20 minutes before induction of anesthesia) was used concomitantly, the efficacy of omeprazole was enhanced.[50]

For healthy patients who are undergoing elective procedures (exclusive of women in labor), the American Society of Anesthesiologists Task Force on Preoperative Fasting has indicated that the minimum recommended fasting period for clear liquids is 2 hours prior to the induction of anesthesia.[51] A light meal is permitted up to 6 hours before the induction of anesthesia. Routine use of gastrointestinal stimulants, gastric acid secretion inhibitors, antacids, and antiemetics in these patients is not recommended for the purpose of reducing the risk of aspiration.

Other preventive measures that have been advocated include application of cricoid pressure (Sellick maneuver) to prevent regurgitation during tracheal intubation.[52] The technique involves applying firm pressure over the cricoid cartilage to occlude the upper end of the esophagus. Effective and safe use of the technique requires adequate training and experience. The technique is contraindicated in patients with suspected cricotracheal injury, active vomiting, or unstable cervical spine injuries. Reported complications of cricoid pressure during intubation include esophageal rupture and exacerbation of unsuspected airway injuries.

Premature postoperative extubation should be avoided as laryngeal incompetence could persist for several hours after anesthesia.[53] Patients intubated or those fed by nasogastric tubes should be maintained in a semirecumbent position because it has been shown to be associated with a lower incidence of aspiration than those in a supine one.[54] Moreover, radiographic confirmation of nasogastric tube placement should be performed routinely to avoid inadvertent endobronchial intubation and massive aspiration.

OROPHARYNGEAL ASPIRATION (ASPIRATION PNEUMONIA)

Aspiration pneumonia refers to the inhalation of oropharyngeal material in patients with radiographically evident infiltrate who are at increased risk of aspiration.[55] Oropharyngeal aspiration occurs in approximately 50 percent of healthy adults[56] during sleep, but aspiration pneumonia is an uncommon event in these subjects. The low bacterial burden, the preserved ciliary motility, and the intact humoral and cellular immunity result in clearance of the inoculum without sequelae. However, in the presence of an impaired swallowing reflex, enhanced oropharyngeal colonization, or a large inoculum, these protective defense mechanisms can be overwhelmed and pneumonia may ensue.

Risk factors

Risk factors for the development of aspiration pneumonia are broadly classified into those that alter host defenses and others that increase exposure to bacteria. Although aging might not be recognized as an independent risk factor, it is well established that pulmonary function deteriorates with age.[57] Some of the anatomic changes implicated in the loss of function include:

- decreased mean bronchiolar diameter
- increased diameter of the alveolar sac
- decrease in elastic fibers.

These anatomic changes result in loss of elastic recoil of the lung and a decrease in the exhalation force generated by the respiratory muscles.[58] The net effect is an increased probability of pathogenic bacteria entering the lungs. Among the established mechanical host factors that have been implicated in increased risk for aspiration include stroke, endotracheal, and naso-oral gastric tube feedings, gastroesophageal motility disorders, supine position, bolus feeds, and postgastrectomy state[59,60] (Box 14D.2). Aspiration pneumonia has been estimated to occur in about a third of patients with stroke.[61] The risk has been shown to be significantly higher in patients with basal ganglia infarcts than in patients with cerebral hemispheric strokes.[62] The most recognized factor contributing to the increased risk of aspiration pneumonia is dysphagia. Not surprisingly, the prevalence of swallowing dysfunction in these patients ranges from 40 percent to 70 percent.[63] Moreover, the oral cavity has long been suspected to be a reservoir for respiratory pathogens responsible for aspiration pneumonia. Normally, saliva lubricates the oral cavity and maintains a bacterial level of less than 7×10^8 bacteria/mL. In conditions of poor oral hygiene such as the case in severe periodontal disease or gingivitis, the bacterial count can rise up to 10^{11} organisms/mL. Xerostomia, mostly drug related, induces a similar pathologic milieu so that when patients with these oral disorders aspirate, the lower respiratory tract is exposed to a large inoculum of bacteria and aspiration pneumonia can result.[64]

Box 14D.2 Predisposing factors for aspiration pneumonia

Decreased level of consciousness

- Sedation

Neurologic and neuromuscular diseases

- Cerebrovascular accident
- Guillain–Barrè
- Myasthenia gravis
- Parkinson's disease
- Multiple sclerosis
- Pseudobulbar palsy
- Botulism
- Poliomyelitis
- Polymyositis

Gastrointestinal diseases

- Esophageal and gastric dysmotility
- Diverticular disease of the hypopharynx and esophagus
- Stricture
- Tracheoesophageal fistula
- Sphincter incompetency
- Scleroderma
- Bowel obstruction
- Tumor

Mechanical factors

- Endotracheal tubes
- Nasoenteric tubes

Conditions that weaken the host response to aspirated material include diabetes mellitus, congestive heart failure, malnutrition, chronic obstructive pulmonary disease (COPD), renal failure, and malignancy. Diabetes mellitus is associated with neutrophil dysfunction, including diminished chemotaxis and impaired phagocytosis.[65] Decreased pulmonary clearance of pneumococci and staphylococci secondary to pulmonary edema has been noted in patients with congestive heart failure.[66] Atelectasis from pleural effusions and/or ascites can result in stagnation of secretions and increased risk of infection whereas cirrhosis has been associated with diminished leukocyte chemotaxis in response to inflammation, depressed complement levels, and defects in cellular immunity.[67] Renal failure increases the rate of Gram-negative and *Staphylococcus aureus* colonization of the oropharynx. It has also been linked to a decreased clearance of staphylococci and *Pseudomonas aeruginosa* along with an increase in buccal cell binding capacity for Gram-negative bacteria.[68]

Clinical features

Clinical manifestations of aspiration pneumonia comprise a spectrum ranging from minimally symptomatic episode to necrotizing lung infections, abscess formation, and empyema. Typical symptoms consist of cough, dyspnea, increased sputum production, fever, and altered mental status particularly in older people.[69] Because the right main bronchus offers the most direct accessible path for aspirated material, the right lower lobe is the most frequently affected site in the upright or semirecumbent position. The left lower lobe comes second followed by the right middle lobe. In the supine position, the posterior segments of the upper lobes and the posterior segments of the lower lobes are usually involved. Overall, more than one segment is commonly affected.

Microbiology

The causative pathogen is determined by whether the aspiration syndrome occurred in the community, in a long-term care facility, or was acquired in a hospital. A number of investigations dating back to the 1970s have pointed to a mixed infection including aerobic and anaerobic bacteria in community-acquired aspiration pneumonia.[70–72] The most commonly encountered anaerobes were pigmented *Prevotella* species, *Fusobacterium nucleatum*, *Peptostreptococcus* species, and *Bacteroides* species. In all these studies, the microbiologic specimens were collected later in the course of the illness, the participants had necrotizing pneumonia, or empyema had developed. Moreover the techniques used for recovery of these pathogens relied on transtracheal aspirates which may have been contaminated with oropharyngeal flora. With the widespread use of protected brush and bronchoalveolar samplings, contemporary investigations of aspiration pneumonia have yielded common isolates including enteric Gram-negative bacilli, *Streptococcus pneumoniae*, *Staph. aureus*, and *Haemophilus influenzae*.[73,74] None of these studies recovered anaerobic organisms. A recent study involving nursing home patients at risk for aspiration found that anaerobic isolates were present in 20 percent of those with microbiologically proved pneumonia.[69] Institutionalized patients can also harbor drug-resistant pathogens such as methicillin-resistant *Staph. aureus* (MRSA). These organisms usually colonize the nares and the oropharyngeal cavity and if aspirated they can lead to severe aspiration pneumonia.

The spectrum of pathogens recovered from nosocomial aspiration pneumonia reflects oropharyngeal colonization by pathogens acquired during hospitalization. In these patients, Gram-negative bacilli including *P. aeruginosa* and MRSA represent the majority of isolates. Anaerobes have not been reported consistently and their role in the pathogenesis of nosocomial aspiration pneumonia remains controversial.[75]

Treatment

The selection of antimicrobial agents is guided by the patient's age and history, physical and radiographic findings, the setting in which the aspiration event occurred (community versus hospital versus long-term care facility), and recovery of an organism from the blood, lungs, or pleural space (Table 14D.1). The initial treatment in most patients with aspiration pneumonia is empiric. Few controlled clinical trials comparing treatment regimens for aspiration pneumonia have been performed. Recommended antibiotic regimens for community-acquired aspiration pneumonia include clindamycin, β-lactam and β-lactamase

Table 14D.1 *Empiric antimicrobial coverage for suspected aspiration pneumonia*

	Suggested antimicrobial coverage
Community-acquired aspiration pneumonia	Ampicillin–clavulanate (1.5 g q 6 h) or clindamycin (600 mg q 8 h) + ceftriaxone (1 g qd)
Nursing-home-acquired aspiration pneumonia	Ampicillin–clavulanate (1.5 g q 6 h) or clindamycin (600 mg q 8 h) + ceftriaxone (1 g qd) Piperacillin–tazobactam (3.375 g q 6 h) ± vancomycin (1–2 g qd) depending on prior history of antibiotic use and colonization with drug-resistant pathogens
Hospital-acquired aspiration pneumonia	Piperacillin–tazobactam (3.375 g q 6 h) or ceftazidime (2 g q 8 h) or imipenem (500 mg q 8 h) ± vancomycin (1–2 g qd)

q, every; qd, daily.

inhibitor combinations such as ampicillin sodium and sulbactam sodium, or penicillin plus metronidazole. Despite good *in vitro* activity against most anaerobes, monotherapy with metronidazole has been associated with a 50 percent failure rate, and metronidazole should not be used alone to treat aspiration pneumonia.[76] The newer fluoroquinolones (e.g. gatifloxacin, moxifloxacin) have reasonable anaerobic activity[77] and achieve high concentrations in lung tissue and endobronchial secretions. However, no randomized clinical trials have evaluated these agents in the treatment of aspiration pneumonia.

Antimicrobial coverage for Gram-negative enteric bacilli and methicillin resistant staphylococci must be considered in nosocomial aspiration pneumonia or in those admitted from long-term care facilities. The risk of drug-resistant pathogens, such as *P. aeruginosa* and *Acinetobacter* species, is more prevalent in these patients[78] and should be entertained when a patient fails to respond to initial empiric treatment.[79] Patients with coma, head trauma, diabetes mellitus, or end-stage renal disease are at high risk for *Staph. aureus* pneumonia and antistaphylococcal coverage should be considered.

Patients with hospital-acquired aspiration pneumonia may be treated with cefepime plus clindamycin; a β-lactam and β-lactamase inhibitor combination such as piperacillin and tazobactam, or ticarcillin and clavulanate. For patients who are allergic to penicillin, ciprofloxacin or a combination of clindamycin plus aztreonam may be considered. Antistaphylococcal coverage (vancomycin, linezolid) may be added for patients known to have nasopharyngeal colonization with staphylococci or other active staphylococcal infections. Once the microbiologic results are available, antimicrobial therapy should be streamed down to match the susceptibility profile of recovered pathogens.

When the decision is made to treat with antibiotics from the outset, the patient's clinical course should be monitored. In one study,[80] resolution of fever in patients treated for aspiration pneumonia was comparable with that in patients with pneumococcal pneumonia. Defervescence occurred in half of the patients with aspiration pneumonia within 2 days of initiation of antibiotic therapy, and 80 percent became afebrile within 5 days. Prolonged fever should raise suspicion of a lung abscess or an infection due to drug-resistant pathogens. No controlled studies have addressed the duration of antibiotic therapy for aspiration pneumonia. Treatment for 7–10 days appears reasonable for patients who respond promptly. Patients with cavitary pneumonia or lung abscess require long-term treatment for 4–8 weeks or more.

Prevention

Preventing aspiration pneumonia entails identifying at-risk patients and implementing protective measures. These can be categorized as pharmacologic or nonpharmacologic interventions.

PHARMACOLOGIC AGENTS

In a number of observational studies, the use of angiotensin-converting enzyme (ACE) inhibitors has been associated with a reduced risk of pneumonia in patients with previous strokes.[81,82] The mechanism is thought to be related to the increased levels of substance P, a neurotransmitter for primary sensory afferent nerves that is normally degraded by ACE. Elevated levels of substance P in the upper respiratory tract improve the swallowing reflex and increase the sensitivity of the cough reflex[83] thus providing a reasonable basis for the decreased incidence of aspiration pneumonia among patients treated with ACE inhibitors. However not all studies have shown a positive reduction with the use of ACE inhibitors. In a recent analysis of the participants of the Perindopril Protection Against Recurrent Stroke Study, treatment with ACE inhibitors showed no reduction of fatal or nonfatal pneumonia whether the event was preceded by stroke or not.[84] Of interest, only participants of Asian ethnicity showed significant reduction in the risk of pneumonia compared with placebo.

Amantadine has been associated with a 20 percent absolute reduction in pneumonia in patients with cerebral infarctions.[85] By increasing the release of dopamine from dopaminergic nerve terminals, it is thought that amantadine might improve the swallowing reflex thus reducing the risk of aspiration. Other mechanisms that have been entertained included reduction of the lower esophageal sphincter and prophylaxis against influenza infection. Amantadine is known however to cause gastrointestinal and neurologic side effects and has propensity to interact with psychotropic medications.

Cilostazol, a phosphodiesterase inhibitor, was shown also to reduce aspiration in a randomized trial compared with no active treatment but 18 percent who received the drug developed side effects including 7 percent who experienced bleeding.[86] At present, there are no approved pharmacologic agents indicated for the prevention of aspiration pneumonia.

NONPHARMACOLOGIC MEASURES

The management plan for patients at risk for oropharyngeal aspiration varies according to history, physical findings, and prognosis. A multidisciplinary approach is essential for the success of any strategy. A clinical swallowing assessment performed either via a fiberoptic endoscopic evaluation or videofluoroscopic swallowing study should be performed to determine the need for and type of dietary modification and therapy. Modified diets are graded according to the dynamic changes of the swallowing ability of the patient in relation to the physical properties of the food bolus. In fact, many patients with neurologically related dysphagia will have better ability to handle thickened bolus of food than fluids. A new technology has been developed using the 'Brix' value to assess dietary formula concentration. The technology based on measuring the refractory index of fructose content is a promising tool for bedside monitoring of tolerance and gastric emptying in patients receiving tube enteral feedings.[87] However, there are few clinical trial data to support the use of changes in diet consistency for reducing aspiration pneumonia. Swallowing rehabilitation is complementary to an improved outcome and involves educating the patient and the healthcare provider in safe swallowing methods. These include upright posture, keeping the chin tucked, and the head turned while eating. Few data exist to support any of these strategies but they are inexpensive and potentially feasible.

Small-bore (3 mm) feeding tubes have been advocated in lieu of traditional large-bore nasogastric tubes for improved patient comfort and reduced risk for aspiration. However, there is no difference in the timing and amount of gastroesophageal reflux and tracheal aspiration between large-bore and small-bore nasogastric feeding tubes.[88] Similarly, no difference in the rate of aspiration pneumonia has been shown in patients with nasogastric feeding tubes compared with percutaneous endoscopic gastrostomy tubes.[89,90]

Improving oral hygiene has been suggested as a mean to reduce the risk of pneumonia among subjects who are at risk for aspiration. The association seems most notably to occur in critically ill intubated patients and in frail institutionalized elderly people.[91] Unfortunately, little is known about the effects of oral care interventions in critically ill patients on the incidence of hospital-acquired pneumonia. Routine oral care is a low priority throughout the stay in the intensive care unit and is highly unlikely to be addressed in the initial days of critical illness when changes to the oral flora occur and risk of colonization with respiratory pathogens is significant.

Among the pharmacologic interventions that have been studied in critical care settings is chlorhexidine. Chlorhexidine is a broad-spectrum bactericidal agent used to prevent gingivitis. Oral rinse with 0.12 percent chlorhexidine gluconate twice daily has been shown to reduce the rate of nosocomial pneumonia in patients undergoing elective cardiovascular surgery.[92] Application of these findings to other critical settings is limited due to lack of randomized trials. The outcome of mechanical (toothbrushing) plus pharmacologic interventions has been suggested but its efficacy in reducing aspiration pneumonia has not been demonstrated.

In the elderly population, controlling plaque accumulation on the teeth and dentures of nursing home residents is challenging because healthcare providers in residential homes give little assistance with tooth and denture cleaning[93] even if training and education are provided. Yet there is enough evidence pointing to a decrease in the relative risk of death attributable to pneumonia in those patients who received oral care compared with the no oral care group.[94] Additional research is needed to determine optimal frequency, procedures, and materials for oral care interventions in these at-high risk patients.

SOLID PARTICLE ASPIRATION

More than 3000 deaths are attributed to the aspiration of foreign bodies each year in the United States.[95] The majority of cases are reported in young children under 1 year of age. In adults, the incidence increases from the fourth decade onward and peaks in the seventh decade. Old age, alcoholism, sedative drugs, and depressed consciousness are common predisposing factors. The initial symptoms vary depending on the size of the aspirate and whether airway obstruction is complete or partial. Complete airway obstruction –referred to as the 'café coronary syndrome' – occurs in the upper airway at levels above the carina and results in acute respiratory distress, asphyxia, and may proceed to death if not removed emergently. The Heimlich maneuver is the recommended treatment for relieving airway obstruction.[96]

Partial obstruction presents invariably with cough followed by dyspnea, chest pain, or wheezing. The right side is more commonly involved because the diameter of the right main bronchus is larger than the left. A history consistent with foreign body aspiration is present in only 70 percent of cases.[97] Inspiratory radiographs often do not reveal any abnormalities. However, the expiratory film may reveal air trapping in 50 percent of the cases on the affected side. With complete bronchial obstruction, the chest films may show atelectasis and complete collapse of the involved segment. Current state-of-the-art helical multidetector-row computed tomography scanners may improve the sensitivity of the radiologic evaluation in patients who are unable to cooperate for inspiration and expiration radiography.

As a result of the limitations of radiographic studies, all patients in whom the clinical suspicion for aspirated foreign bodies is high should undergo a bronchoscopy for definitive diagnosis and treatment. Rigid bronchoscopy has been considered the procedure of choice for extracting foreign bodies because of the large lumen and the ability to introduce other instruments. The procedure is successful in 98 percent of the cases compared to 60 percent for fiberoptic bronchoscopy.[97] Fiberoptic bronchoscopy has the advantage of extracting peripherally located foreign bodies, and in certain cases of maxillofacial trauma or in patients being mechanically ventilated. Noncardiogenic pulmonary edema and persistent pneumonia represent the most common complications following extraction.[98,99] Recurrent pneumonias may warrant a repeat bronchoscopy to remove any remaining foreign bodies.[100]

NONTOXIC FLUID ASPIRATION

Blood

Blood aspiration occurs usually subsequent to massive hemoptysis. Mycetoma, abscess, bronchiectasis, vascular anomalies or fistulas, and carcinoma are among the most common causes. Early steps in management include securing the airway, cross-matching of several units of blood, and close monitoring of vital signs. Mortality occurs from asphyxia. Detailed discussion of this topic is provided in Chapter 13B.

Water (near-drowning)

For public health purposes, drowning is defined as unintentional death from asphyxia during or within 24 hours of submersion in water. Near-drowning is defined as survival for 24 hours or more after submersion, whether the victim ultimately survives or not.

At least 9000 drowning deaths occur annually in the United States.[101] The incidence follows a bimodal distribution, the first peak occurs in children between 2 and 4 years, and the second in adolescents and young adults. In Alaska, the risk of drowning is increased tenfold over the national mean among 20–29-year-old men, particularly native Alaskans involved in the fishing industry. In fact, drowning is the leading cause of death among native Alaskans.[102] In Mississippi, the highest mortality from drowning is found in 14–17-year-old Asian and native Americans, with a male to female ratio of 5:1. Alcohol intoxication accounts for a third of adult fatalities from drowning.[103] High-speed boating, in particular that involving personal watercraft, has increased in the past decade and has heightened the risk of drowning associated with head and neck injury. Even more alarming is the disproportionate number of drownings that occur among people who are developmentally delayed or neurologically impaired.

The medical literature has made a distinction between aspiration of seawater and fresh water. However, most victims of drowning fail to aspirate large quantities of fluid. In autopsy series, 7–10 percent of victims experience 'dry drowning' without actual aspiration of water.[104] In these cases, intense laryngospasm protects the lung from aspiration. When seawater is aspirated into the lung, it produces an osmotic pressure causing plasma to pour into the alveoli despite decreased intravascular volume.[105] The flooded alveoli cease to participate in gas exchange and intrapulmonary shunting ensues. Although the amount of surfactant in the hypertonic medium is decreased, its function remains largely unchanged.[106] In contrast, the hypotonic nature of freshwater interferes with the surface tension of pulmonary surfactant resulting in alveolar collapse and atelectasis. In addition, the presence of water in the alveoli may damage the type II pneumocytes thus preventing the production of surfactant for up to 24 hours.[107] Particulate matter such as mud, sewage, or vomitus aspirated along with water adds to the pulmonary insult. The net result is asphyxia with rapid decline in arterial oxygen saturation and concomitant metabolic and respiratory acidosis. Although electrolyte abnormalities can be detected experimentally in the event of massive aspiration of fresh or seawater in animals (more than 22 mL/kg), these changes are rarely detected in humans because the amount of fluid aspirated does not approach the volume observed in animal models.[108] The pathologic effects of drowning on other vital organs aside from the lung are those associated with anoxia. The two most important prognostic factors for survival with good neurologic function are the duration of the anoxic episode and the temperature of the water. Several factors have been identified as indicators of poor prognosis in warm water drowning: submersion for more than 5 minutes, delay of cardiopulmonary resuscitation (CPR) for more than 10 minutes, a continuing need for CPR or a pH <7.10 on arrival to the emergency room, and the persistence of fixed dilated pupils.[109] However, these factors may not apply to cases of submersion in cold water. Hypothermia may have a protective effect on brain tissue by slowing the biochemical reactions that require oxygen substrate. The protective effect is limited by the frequent occurrence of fatal dysrhythmias when the core temperature drops below 28 °C. Renal function remains intact in most drowning victims, but acute tubular necrosis, hemoglobinuria, and albuminuria have been reported.[110] A transient rise in central venous pressures and pulmonary artery balloon occlusion pressures is noted as a result of the decrease in cardiac output. These hemodynamic changes are independent of the tonicity and are postulated to be the consequences of anoxia.

Treatment

When faced with a near-drowning victim, the primary goal is to focus on keeping the airway open and stabilizing the neck in case of suspected cervical spine or head injury. Rescue breathing should begin while the victim is still in the water. The oral cavity should be cleared from any debris. Full CPR should be initiated on arrival to shore and conducted according to standard guidelines. The Heimlich maneuver is not routinely indicated unless there is a high suspicion of foreign body aspiration. One animal study did not show a survival advantage in applying abdominal thrusts or gravitational drainage compared with placebo when attempting to remove the water from the lung.[111]

In awake, cooperative victims, supplemental oxygen via venti-mask should be initiated to maintain oxygen saturation >90 percent. Nasal continuous positive airway pressure may be used for those patients with pulmonary edema.[112] Mechanical ventilation should be instituted for those who regained spontaneous respiration but have persistent low Glasgow coma scale, evidence of gross aspiration of particulate matter, new onset of seizure, or inability to maintain oxygen saturation on supplemental oxygen.

Cross-table films of the cervical spine should be obtained early in unconscious patients and those with suspected diving injury. When the patient's condition stabilizes, a full cervical spine series or CT scan should be taken. The initial chest film may show normal findings in up to 20 percent despite marked respiratory distress.[113] The remainder may show perihilar confluent alveolar densities or bilateral homogeneous nodular pattern.

A complete blood count, serum electrolytes, arterial blood gas analysis, and coagulation profile should be drawn on arrival although they are usually normal in the first few hours irrespective of whether the near-drowning occurred in freshwater or saltwater.[114] A blood alcohol level and a drug screen should always be sent also for analysis.

Nearly all near-drowning victims are hypothermic. Core temperature is difficult to determine accurately in the field, but in general, patients who underwent prolonged immersion in cold water are probably severely hypothermic (core temperature <30 °C [86 °F]). Per Advanced Cardiac Life Support (ACLS) protocol, cardiopulmonary arrest in the face of profound hypothermia deserves one or two series of attempts at defibrillation and administration of epinephrine and lidocaine hydrochloride. Cardiopulmonary bypass may be attempted if available particularly in those with circulatory collapse.[115] Otherwise, peritoneal lavage, hemodialysis, or warm, humidified oxygen by endotracheal tube could be used. For those near-drowning victims who have often swallowed large amounts of water, a nasogastric tube may be inserted to relieve gastric distention and prevent further aspiration.

Bronchodilators should be administered as needed to treat bronchospasm. Occasionally, sodium bicarbonate is given for profound metabolic acidosis, but its administration is controversial. Correction of hypoxemia and maintenance of tissue perfusion are the best treatment for systemic acidosis. Prophylactic therapy with antibiotics has not improved the outcome of near-drowning victims.[116] Similarly, the use of intravenous corticosteroids has not demonstrated a survival benefit in either near-drowning or acute respiratory distress syndrome.[117] Because of massive catecholamine release in near-drowning victims, hyperglycemia is common, even in nondiabetic people, and may worsen encephalopathy. Administering insulin by intravenous drip to keep the blood glucose level less than 11.1 mmol/L (200 mg/dL) is a reasonable treatment approach.

Seizures are best treated supportively. Intravenous lorazepam (0.1 mg/kg) is effective for prolonged seizures but further suppresses the level of consciousness and respiratory drive. Most victims have rapid improvement of neurologic status with resuscitation. If mental status worsens despite resuscitative efforts, underlying head injury should be suspected, and a CT scan should be done. Alternatively, positive results on blood alcohol or drug testing might explain a slow response to mental recovery. Other potential complications of near-drowning are summarized in Box 14D.3. In the absence of symptoms and preexisting neurologic, neurodevelopmental, or cardiopulmonary disease, young victims can be safely discharged. For those with minimal symptoms and normal oxygen saturation, a 24-hour observation in a hospital setting is recommended.

Box 14D.3 Early and late complications of near-drowning

Early (within 4 hours)

- Bronchospasm
- Vomiting with aspiration of gastric contents
- Hyperglycemia
- Hypothermia: mild (30–35 °C [86–95 °F]) to severe (<30 °C [86 °F])
- Seizures
- Hypovolemia (especially with saltwater)
- Fluid and electrolyte disturbances
- Metabolic and lactic acidosis

Late (4 hours or more)

- Adult respiratory distress syndrome (pulmonary edema)
- Anoxic-ischemic encephalopathy
- Aspiration pneumonia
- Lung abscess
- Pneumothorax
- Myoglobinuria
- Hemoglobinuria
- Renal failure
- Coagulopathy
- Sepsis
- Barotrauma

PROGNOSTIC INDICATORS

The prognosis of the near-drowning victim is good. Approximately 80 percent of these patients recover completely, and 2–9 percent survive with some degree of brain damage.[118] The best predictors of outcome are the victim's hemodynamic status at initial evaluation and level of consciousness after 3–4 hours of resuscitation efforts. However, if acidosis and coma persist after 4 hours of resuscitation attempts, the chance of recovering neurologically intact is small. A simple classification scale has been developed to guide the initial neurologic assessment of near-drowning victims:[119]

- Category A – Patients who are fully alert within 1 hour of presentation to the emergency room and uniformly have no neurologic complications.
- Category B – Patients who are obtunded but arousable at the time of evaluation and usually survive with minimal if any neurologic deficit.
- Category C – Patients who present with labored respiration and abnormal respiration to pain. They are further classified into:
  - C1 – those who exhibit decorticate posturing
  - C2 – those who exhibit decerebrate posturing
  - C3 – those who are flaccid.

Category C patients have much higher morbidity and mortality, and a higher rate of neurologic dysfunction.

SUMMARY AND CONCLUSION

The clinical presentation and course of aspiration syndromes ranges from mild self-limited disease to severe, life-threatening acute lung injury, depending on the nature of the aspirate and the underlying condition of the host. Unfortunately, most studies do not distinguish between aspiration pneumonitis and aspiration pneumonia. The assumption that all complications of aspiration are infectious in nature is partially to blame behind the overuse of antimicrobial agents and the rise in drug-resistant pathogens. Although antibiotics are considered the standard of care for cases with aspiration pneumonia, there is currently no evidence that antimicrobial therapy alters the outcome or the prognosis of patients with aspiration pneumonitis.

A mixed aerobic-anaerobic infection usually occurs after aspiration of oropharyngeal secretion into the dependent segment of the lung. If infection is not controlled, abscess formation and empyema may result within 10–14 days. Neither nasopharyngeal nor sputum aspirates can provide reliable specimens for the identification of pathogens because of oropharyngeal contamination. Sampling of the lower respiratory tract using protected bronchoalveolar lavage provides a more accurate diagnosis of the offending pathogens. In most instances, selection of antimicrobials can be made without any of these invasive procedures. However, in those patients who do not respond to therapy, or who are at risk of harboring unusual or resistant pathogens, obtaining culture through these techniques should be considered.

Optimal prehospital care of near-drowning victims requires bystanders and emergency-response personnel who are knowledgeable in CPR and proper rescue techniques. Rapid response and appropriate ventilation and airway protection can improve the condition of near-drowning victims on arrival in the emergency department and their chances for neurologically intact survival.

With knowledge of the local risks of drowning, proper emergency treatment, appropriate referral, and conscientious efforts at prevention conducted in the office and the community, primary care physicians can have maximum impact on this summertime killer.

Key learning points

- Inhalation of substrate with a pH less than 2.5 in combination with particulate matter is invariably responsible for lung injury in aspiration pneumonitis.

- Antibiotics are not recommended for aspiration pneumonitis and corticosteroid therapy has not been proven to be beneficial.

- Aspiration pneumonia should be suspected in the presence of dysphagia and radiographic infiltrates in the dependent segments.

- The choice of antimicrobial therapy in aspiration pneumonia should reflect the bacterial profile of the location where the aspiration occurred.

- A non-opaque aspirated foreign body may be a constant source for recurrent pneumonias, abscesses, and bronchiectasis.

- Prognosis of drowning victims is excellent for patients who are conscious on arrival to the emergency room but poor for those in coma.

REFERENCES

1. Chadwick J, Mann WN, eds. *Medical Works of Hippocrates*. Springfield: Charles Thomas, 1950.

2. Mendelson C. The aspiration of stomach contents into the lungs during obstetric anesthesia. *Am J Obstet Gynecol* 1946; **52**: 191–205.

3. Cassiere HA, Niederman MS. Aspiration pneumonia, lipoid pneumonia, and lung abscess. In: Baum GL, Crapo JD, Celli BR, Karlinsky JB, eds. *Textbook of Pulmonary Diseases*, 6th ed. Vol 1. Philadelphia: Lippincott-Raven, 1998: 645–55.

4. Bartlett JG, Gorbach SI. The triple threat of aspiration. *Chest* 1975; **68**: 560–6.

5. Goodwin RS. Prevention of aspiration pneumonia: a research-based protocol. *Dimens Crit Care Nurs* 1996; **15**: 58–71.

6. Roy TM, Ossorio MA, Cipolla LM, *et al.* Pulmonary complications after tricyclic antidepressant overdose. *Chest* 1989; **96**: 852–6.

7. Olsson GL, Hallen B, Hambraeus-Jonzon K. Aspiration during anaesthesia: a computer-aided study of 185,358 anaesthetics. *Acta Anaesthesiol Scand* 1986; **30**: 84–92.

8. Doyle R, Szaflaraski N, Modin G, *et al.* Identification of patients with acute lung injury. *Am J Respir Crit Care Med* 1995; **152**: 1818–24.

9. Anonymous. *Diagnosis and treatment of swallowing disorders in acute-care stroke: summary, evidence report/technology assessment*. No. 8. Rockville, MD: Agency for Health Care Policy and Research, March 1999.

10. Baine WB, Yu W, Summe JP. Epidemiologic trends in the hospitalization of elderly Medicare patients for pneumonia, 1991–1998. *Am J Public Health* 2001; **91**: 1121–3.

11. Baine WB, Yu W, Summe JP. The epidemiology of hospitalization of elderly Americans for septicemia or bacteremia in 1991–1998: application of Medicare claims data. *Ann Epidemiol* 2001; **11**: 118–26.

12. Teabeaut JR. Aspiration of gastric contents: an experimental study. *Am J Pathol* 1952; **28**: 51–67.

13. James CF, Modell JH, Gibbs CP, *et al.* Pulmonary aspiration: effects of volume and pH in the rat. *Anesth Analg* 1984; **63**: 665–8.

14. Bosomworth PP, Hamelberg W. Etiologic and therapeutic aspects of aspiration pneumonitis: an experimental study. *Surg Forum* 1962; **13**: 158–9.

15. Wynne J, Ramphal R, Hood C. Tracheal mucosal damage after aspiration. *Am Rev Respir Dis* 1981; **124**: 728–32.

16. Exharos ND, Logan WD, Abbott OA, *et al.* Importance of pH and volume in tracheobronchial aspiration. *Dis Chest* 1965; **47**: 167–9.

17. Schwartz DJ, Wynne JW, Gibbs CP, *et al.* The pulmonary consequences of aspiration of gastric contents at pH values greater than 2.5. *Am Rev Respir Dis* 1980; **121**: 119–26.

18. Knight PR, Rutter T, Tait AR, *et al.* Pathogenesis of gastric particulate lung injury: a comparison and interaction with acidic pneumonitis. *Anesth Analog* 1993; **77**: 754–60.

19. Hamelberg W, Bosomworth PP. Aspiration pneumonitis: experimental studies and clinical observations. *Anesth Analg* 1964; **43**: 699–705.

20. Finegold SM, Wexler HM. Minireview: therapeutic implications of bacteriologic findings in mixed aerobic-anaerobic infections. *Antimicrob Agents Chemother* 1988; **32**: 611–16.

21. Murray HW. Antimicrobial therapy in pulmonary aspiration. *Am J Med* 1979; **66**: 188–90.

22. El-Solh A, Pietrantoni C, Bhat A, *et al.* Colonization of dental plaques: a reservoir of respiratory pathogens for hospital acquired pneumonia in institutionalized elders. *Chest* 2004; **126**: 1575–82.

23. Pingleton SK, Hinthorn DR, Liu C. Enteral nutrition in patients receiving mechanical ventilation: multiple sources of tracheal colonization include the stomach. *Am J Med* 1986; **80**: 827–32.

24. Du Moulin GC, Hedley-Whyte J, Paterson DG, *et al.* Aspiration of gastric bacteria in antacid-treated

patients: a frequent cause of postoperative colonization of the airway. *Lancet* 1982; **1**: 242–6.

25. Lewis RT, Burgess JH, Hampson LG. Cardiorespiratory studies in critical illness: changes in aspiration pneumonitis. *Arch Surg* 1971; **103**: 335–40.

26. Folkesson HG, Matthay MA, Hebert CA, *et al.* Acid aspiration-induced lung injury in rabbits is mediated by interleukin-8-dependent mechanisms. *J Clin Invest* 1995; **96**: 107–16.

27. Landay MJ, Christensen EE, Bynum LJ. Pulmonary manifestations of acute aspiration of gastric contents. *Am J Roentgenol* 1978; **131**: 587–92.

28. Colebatch HJ, Halmagyi DF. Reflex airway reaction to fluid aspiration. *J Appl Physiol* 1962; **17**: 787–94.

29. Jorgenson NH, Byer DE, Gould AB. Aspiration pneumonitis: prevention and treatment. *Minn Med* 1989; **72**: 517–19.

30. Awe W, Fletcher W, Jacob S. The pathophysiology of aspiration pneumonitis. *Surgery* 1966; **60**: 232–9.

31. Moran JR, Block SM, Lyerly AD, *et al.* Lipid laden alveolar macrophage and lactose assay as markers of aspiration in neonates with lung disease. *J Pediatr* 1988; **112**: 643–5.

32. Samloff I, Liebman WM. Radioimmunoassay of group I pepsinogens in serum. *Gastroenterology* 1974; **66**: 494–502.

33. Badellino M, Buckman RF, Malaspina PJ, *et al.* Detection of pulmonary aspiration of gastric contents in an animal model by assay of peptic activity in bronchoalveolar fluid. *Crit Care Med* 1996; **24**: 1881–5.

34. Metheny N, Chang Y, Ye JS, *et al.* Pepsin as a marker for pulmonary aspiration. *Am J Crit Care* 2002; **11**: 150–4.

35. Bynum LJ, Pierce AK. Pulmonary aspiration of gastric contents. *Am Rev Respir Dis* 1976; **114**: 1129–36.

36. Downs JB, Chapman R, Modell J, *et al.* An evaluation of steroid therapy in aspiration pneumonitis. *Anesthesiology* 1974; **40**: 129–35.

37. Dudley WR, Marshall BE. Steroid treatment for acid aspiration pneumonitis. *Anesthesiology* 1974; **40**: 136–41.

38. Wynne J, Reynolds J, Hood I, *et al.* Steroid therapy for pneumonitis induced in rabbits by aspiration of foodstuff. *Anesthesiology* 1979; **51**: 11–19.

39. Sukumaran M, Granda MJ, Berger H, *et al.* Evaluation of corticosteroid treatment in aspiration of gastric contents. A controlled clinical trial. *Mt Sinai J Med* 1980; **47**: 335–40.

40. Lee M, Sukumaran M, Berger H, *et al.* Influence of corticosteroid treatment on pulmonary function after recovery from aspiration of gastric contents. *Mt Sinai J Med* 1980; **47**: 341–6.

41. Bernard G, Luce J, Sprung C, *et al.* High dose corticosteroids in patients with the adult respiratory distress syndrome. *N Engl J Med* 1987; **317**: 1565–70.

42. Bone R, Fisher C, Clemmer T, *et al.* Early methylprednisolone treatment for septic syndrome and the adult respiratory distress syndrome. *Chest* 1987; **92**: 1032–6.

43. Kinni M, Stout M. Aspiration pneumonitis: predisposing conditions and prevention. *J Oral Maxillofac Surg* 1986; **44**: 378–84.

44. Sutherland AD, Maltby JR, Sale JP, *et al.* The effect of pre-operative oral fluid and ranitidine on gastric fluid volume and pH. *Can J Anaesth* 1987; **34**: 117–21.

45. Dewan DM, Floyd AM, Thistlewood JM, *et al.* Sodium citrate pretreatment in elective cesarean section patients. *Anesth Analg* 1985; **64**: 34–7.

46. Manchikanti L, Collivier JA, Marrero T, *et al.* Ranitidine and metoclopramide for prophylaxis of aspiration pneumonitis in elective surgery. *Anesth Analg* 1984; **63**: 903–10.

47. Rout CC, Rocke DA, Gousw E. Intravenous ranitidine reduces the risk of acid aspiration of gastric contents at emergency cesarean section. *Anesth Analg* 1993; **76**: 156–61.

48. Gallagher EG, White M, Ward S, *et al.* Prophylaxis against acid aspiration syndrome. *Anesthesia* 1988; **43**: 1011–14.

49. Ng Wingtin L, Glomaud D, Hardy F, *et al.* Omeprazole for prophylaxis of acid aspiration in elective surgery. *Anaesthesia* 1990; **45**: 436–8.

50. Orr DA, Bill KM, Gillon KR, *et al.* Effects of omeprazole, with and without metoclopramide, in elective obstetric anesthesia. *Anaesthesia* 1993; **48**: 114–19.

✱ 51. Practice guidelines for preoperative fasting and the use of pharmacologic agents to reduce the risk of pulmonary aspiration: Application to healthy patients undergoing elective procedures. A report by the American Society of Anesthesiologists Task Force on Preoperative Fasting. *Anesthesiology* 1999; **90**: 896–905.

52. Sellick BA. Cricoid pressure to control regurgitation of stomach contents during induction of anesthesia. *Lancet* 1961; **2**: 404–6.

53. Burgess GE, Cooper JR, Marino RJ, *et al.* Laryngeal competence after tracheal extubation. *Anesthesiology* 1979; **51**: 73–7.

54. Orozco-Levi M, Torres A, Ferrer M, *et al.* Semirecumbent position protects from pulmonary aspiration but not completely from gastroesophageal reflux in mechanically ventilated patients. *Am J Respir Crit Care Med* 1995; **152**: 1387–90.

◆ 55. Marik P. Aspiration pneumonitis and aspiration pneumonia. *N Engl J Med* 2001; **344**: 665–71.

56. Gleeson K, Eggli D, Maxweel S. Quantitative aspiration during sleep in normal subjects. *Chest* 1997; **111**: 1266–72.

◆ 57. Chan ED, Welsh CH. Geriatric respiratory medicine. *Chest* 1998; **114**: 1704–33.

58. Pack AI, Millman RP. The lungs in later life. In: Fishman AP, ed. *Pulmonary Diseases and Disorders.* New York: McGraw-Hill, 1988; 79–90.

59. Kidd D, Lawson J, Nesbitt R, *et al.* Aspiration in acute stroke: a clinical study with videofluoroscopy. *Q J Med* 1993; **86**: 825–9.

60. Marumo K, Homma S, Fukuchi Y. Postgastrectomy aspiration pneumonia. *Chest* 1995; **107**: 453–6.

61. Kobayashi H, Hoshino M, Okayama K, *et al.* Swallowing and cough reflexes after onset of stroke. *Chest* 1994; **105**: 1623.

62. Nakagawa T, Sekizawa K, Arai H, *et al.* High incidence of pneumonia in elderly patients with basal ganglia infarction. *Arch Intern Med* 1997; **157**: 321–4.

63. Smithard DG, O'Neill PA, England RE, *et al.* The natural history of dysphagia following a stroke. *Dysphagia* 1997; **12**: 188–93.

64. Terpenning M, Bretz W, Lopatin D, *et al.* Bacterial colonization of saliva and plaque in the elderly. *Clin Infect Dis* 1993;**16**: S314–16.

65. Sima AA, O'Neill SJ, Naimark D, *et al.* Bacterial phagocytosis and intracellular killing by alveolar macrophages in BB rats. *Diabetes* 1988; **37**: 544–9.

✴ 66. Bartlett JG, Breiman RF, Mandell LA, *et al.* Community-acquired pneumonia in adults: guidelines for management. The Infectious Diseases Society of America. *Clin Infect Dis* 1998; **26**: 811–38.

67. Wyke RJ. Problems of bacterial infection in patients with liver disease. *Gut* 1987; **28**: 623–41.

68. Cardenosa Cendrero JA, Sole-Violan J, Bordes Benitez A, *et al.* Role of different routes of tracheal colonization in the development of pneumonia in patients receiving mechanical ventilation. *Chest* 1999; **116**: 462–70.

69. El-Solh A, Pietrantoni C, Bhat A, *et al.* Microbiology of severe aspiration pneumonia in institutionalized elderly. *Am J Respir Crit Care* 2003; **167**: 1650–4.

70. Lorber B, Swenson RM. Bacteriology of aspiration pneumonia: a prospective study of community- and hospital-acquired cases. *Ann Intern Med* 1974; **81**: 329–31.

71. Bartlett JG, Gorbach SL. Treatment of aspiration pneumonia and primary lung abscess: penicillin G vs clindamycin. *JAMA* 1975; **234**: 935–7.

72. Cesar L, Gonzalez C, Calia FM. Bacteriologic flora of aspiration-induced pulmonary infections. *Arch Intern Med* 1975; **135**: 711–14.

73. Mier L, Dreyfuss D, Darchy B, *et al.* Is penicillin G an adequate initial treatment for aspiration pneumonia? A prospective evaluation using a protected specimen brush and quantitative cultures. *Intensive Care Med* 1993; **19**: 279–84.

74. Leroy O, Vandenbussche C, Coffinier C, *et al.* Community-acquired aspiration pneumonia in intensive care units. *Am J Respir Crit Care Med* 1997; **156**: 1922–9.

75. Marik PE, Careau P. The role of anaerobes in patients with ventilator-associated pneumonia and aspiration pneumonia: a prospective study. *Chest* 1999; **115**: 178–83.

76. Sanders CV, Hanna BJ, Lewis AB. Metronidazole in the treatment of anaerobic infections. *Am Rev Respir Dis* 1979; **120**: 337–43.

77. Wexler HM. In vitro activity of gatifloxacin against 238 strains of anaerobic bacteria. *Anaerobe* 2001; **7**: 285.

✴ 78. American Thoracic Society. Hospital-acquired pneumonia in adults: diagnosis, assessment of severity, initial antimicrobial therapy, and preventive strategies. *Am J Respir Crit Care Med* 1996;**153**: 1711–25.

79. El-Solh A, Aquilina A, Dhillon R, *et al.* Impact of invasive strategy on management of antimicrobial treatment failure in institutionalized old people with severe pneumonia. *Am J Respir Crit Care Med* 2002; **166**: 1038–43.

80. Bartlett JG. Anaerobic bacterial infections of the lung. *Chest* 1987; **91**: 901–9.

81. Arai T, Yasuda Y, Takaya T, *et al.* Angiotensin-converting enzyme inhibitors, angiotensin-II receptor antagonists, and pneumonia in elderly

hypertensive patients with stroke. *Chest* 2001; **119**: 660–1.

82. Okaishi K, Morimoto S, Fukuo K, *et al.* Reduction of risk of pneumonia associated with use of angiotensin I converting enzyme inhibitors in elderly inpatients. *Am J Hypertens* 1999; **12**: 778–83.

83. Sekizawa K, Ebihara T, Sasaki H. Role of substance P in cough during bronchoconstriction in awake guinea pigs. *Am J Respir Crit Care Med* 1995; **151**: 815–21.

84. Ohkubo T, Chapman N, Neal B, *et al.* Effects of an angiotensin-converting enzyme inhibitor-based regimen on pneumonia risk. *Am J Respir Crit Care Med* 2004; **169**: 1041–5.

85. Nakagawa T, Wada H, Sekizawa K, *et al.* Amantadine and pneumonia. Lancet 1999; **353**: 1157.

86. Yamaya M, Yanai M, Ohrui T, *et al.* Antithrombotic therapy for prevention of pneumonia. *J Am Geriatr Soc* 2001; **49**: 687–8.

87. Chang WK, McClave SA, Lee MS, *et al.* Monitoring bolus nasogastric tube feeding by the Brix value determination and residual volume measurement of gastric contents. *J Parenter Enteral Nutr* 2004; **28**: 105–12.

88. Ferrer M, Bauer TT, Torres A, *et al.* Effect of nasogastric tube size on gastroesophageal reflux and microaspiration in intubated patients. *Ann Intern Med* 1999; **130**: 991–4.

89. Baeten C, Hoefnagels J. Feeding via nasogastric tube or percutaneous endoscopic gastrostomy: a comparison. *Scand J Gastroenterol Suppl* 1992; **194**: 95–8.

90. Park RH, Allison MC, Lang J, *et al.* Randomized comparison of percutaneous endoscopic gastrostomy and nasogastric tube feeding in patients with persisting neurological dysphagia. *BMJ* 1992; **304**: 1406–9.

91. Fourrier F, Duvivier B, Boutigny H, *et al.* Colonization of dental plaque: a source of nosocomial infections in intensive care unit patients. *Crit Care Med* 1998; **26**: 301–8.

92. DeRiso AJ, Ladowski JS, Dillon TA, *et al.* Chlorhexidine gluconate 0.12 percent oral rinse reduces the incidence of total nosocomial respiratory infection and nonprophylactic systemic antibiotic use in patients undergoing heart surgery. *Chest* 1996; **109**: 1556–61.

93. Simons D, Kidds EA, Beighton D. Oral health of elderly occupants in residential homes. *Lancet* 1999; **353**: 1761.

94. Yoneyama T, Yoshida M, Ohrui T, *et al.* Oral care reduces pneumonia in older patients in nursing homes. *J Am Geriat Soc* 2002; **50**: 430–3.

95. National Safety Council: Accident facts. Chicago, National Safety Council Press, 1987: 7.

✱ 96. Standards and guidelines for cardiopulmonary resuscitation and emergency cardiac care. *JAMA* 1986; **255**: 2979–84.

97. Limper AH, Prakash UB. Tracheobronchial foreign bodies in adults. *Ann Intern Med* 1990; **112**: 604–9.

98. Bernstein A. Re-expansion pulmonary edema. *Chest* 1980; **77**: 708–9.

99. McGuirt WF, Holmes KD, Feehs R, *et al.* Tracheobronchial foreign bodies. *Laryngoscope* 1988; **98**: 615–18.

100. Kim IG, Brummitt WM, Humphry A, *et al.* Foreign body in the airway: a review of 202 cases. *Laryngoscope* 1973; **83**: 347–54.

◆ 101. Kallas HJ. Drowning and near-drowning. In: Nelson WE, Behrman RE, Kliegman RM, *et al.*, eds. *Nelson Textbook of Pediatrics*, 15th ed. Philadelphia: Saunders, 1996: 264–7.

102. Lincoln JM, Perkins R, Melton F, *et al.* Drowning in Alaskan waters. *Public Health Rep* 1996;**111**: 531–5.

103. Dietz PE, Basker SP. Drowning epidemiology and prevention. *Am J Public Health* 1974; **64**: 303.

◆ 104. Modell JH. Drowning. *N Engl J Med* 1993; **328**: 253–6.

105. Orlowski JP, Abullicl MM, Phillips JM. Effects of toxicities of saline solutions on pulmonary injury in drowning. *Crit Care Med* 1987; **15**: 126–30.

106. Modell JH, Moya F, Newby EJ, *et al.* The effects of fluid volume in seawater drowning. *Ann Intern Med* 1967; **67**: 68–80.

107. Modell JH, Calderwood HW, Ruiz BC, *et al.* Effects of ventilatory patterns on arterial oxygenation after near drowning in sea water. *Anesthesiology* 1974; **40**: 376–84.

108. Modell JH, Davis JH. Electrolyte changes in human drowning victims. *Anesthesiology* 1969; **30**: 414–20.

109. Gross PL, Weber-Bornstein N, Castronovo FP, Baker AS. Environmental hazards. In: Wilkins E, ed. *Emergency Medicine*. Philadelphia: Williams and Wilkins, 1989: 168–208.

110. Grausz H, Amend WJ, Earley LE. Acute renal failure complicating submersion in seawater. *JAMA* 1971; **217**: 207–9.

111. Werner JZ, Safar P, Bircher NG, *et al.* No improvement in pulmonary status by gravity drainage or abdominal thrusts after sea water near drowning in dogs. *Anesthesiology* 1982; **57**: A81.

112. Dottorini M, Eslami A, Baglioni S, *et al.* Nasal continuous positive airway pressure in the treatment of near-drowning in fresh water. *Chest* 1996; **110**: 1122–4.

113. Hunter TB, Whitehouse WM. Freshwater near drowning: radiologic aspects. *Radiology* 1974; **112**: 51–6.

114. Sirik Z, Lev A, Ruach M, *et al.* Freshwater near-drowning: our experiment in life-supportive treatment. *Israel J Med Sci* 1984; **20**: 523–7.

115. Husby P, Anderson KS, Owen-Falkenberg A, *et al.* Accidental hypothermia with cardiac arrest: complete recovery after prolonged resuscitation and rewarming by extracorporeal circulation. *Intensive Care Med* 1990; **16**: 69–72.

116. Modell JH, Graves SA, Ketover A. Clinical course of 91 consecutive near-drowning victims. *Chest* 1976; **70**: 231–8.

117. Calderwood HW, Modell JH, Ruiz BC. The ineffectiveness of steroid therapy for treatment of fresh-water near-drowning. *Anesthesiology* 1975; **43**: 642–50.

118. Oakes DD, Sherck JP, Maloney JR, *et al.* Prognosis and management of victims of near-drowning. *J Trauma* 1982; **22**: 544–9.

119. Modell JH, Conn AW. Current neurological considerations in near-drowning. *Can Anaesth Soc* 1980; **3**: 197–8.

IV

Special Populations and Situations

15

Lung transplant emergencies

SEAN STUDER, JONATHAN B ORENS

INTRODUCTION

Lung transplantation is an acceptable treatment for patients with end-stage lung disease but this intervention is frequently complicated by a variety of problems over the short- and long-term, which may require urgent or emergent intervention. Patients will typically remain hospitalized or near their transplant center during the perioperative period. After the patient transitions from the hospital to home they are at risk for several complications including infection, allograft rejection, and adverse reactions to the medications used for immunosuppression. Indeed, patients may frequently present to their nontransplant physicians with any of these potential problems. Because of the complex nature of lung transplant care, and the fragility of transplanted lungs, it should be emphasized that most posttransplant problems should ideally be managed or guided by the patient's lung transplant center. However, because lung transplant recipients may live long distances from the transplant center, the primary care physician or nontransplant pulmonologist may be required to intervene or stabilize a patient prior to transfer.

This chapter reviews the major complications following lung transplantation and the appropriate approach to management, focusing on those that may require emergency care by the primary care physician or pulmonologist prior to intervention by the transplant center. Many critical care emergencies, for which transplant recipients are at high risk but are not specific to transplant, such as hypotension, pulmonary edema and sepsis, are beyond the scope of this chapter.

GENERAL CONSIDERATIONS

The problems that may occur in lung transplant recipients can be divided into several levels of urgency. Indeed some problems that would be considered nonemergent in other patients may truly be emergent in a lung transplant recipient. The transplanted lung is exquisitely sensitive to injury from both infection and rejection episodes and this injury may result in developing irreversible chronic allograft rejection (obliterative bronchiolitis/bronchiolitis obliterans syndrome). For this reason, complaints such as new-onset dyspnea may require urgent/emergent evaluation (Fig. 15.1). Other problems such as fever, radiographic infiltrates and hypoxemia warrant true emergent care since these signs may reflect either infection or rejection. The approach to managing these problems at the transplant center is somewhat prescribed in clinical pathways that usually include measurement of pulmonary function, radiographic imaging and ultimately bronchoscopy in most cases to exclude infection or rejection.

Spirometry is a simple and relatively sensitive method to detect acute rejection but is not specific in ruling out infection or other problems. When a significant fall in lung function occurs (with or without symptoms), a chest radiograph should be obtained to assess for any new findings, in particular, pulmonary infiltrates, volume loss, or native lung hyperinflation (in the case of single lung transplants for chronic obstructive pulmonary disease [COPD]). It should be stressed that any new pulmonary infiltrate, regardless of the extent or distribution, can represent infection or acute rejection and these complications may also occur in the setting of a normal chest

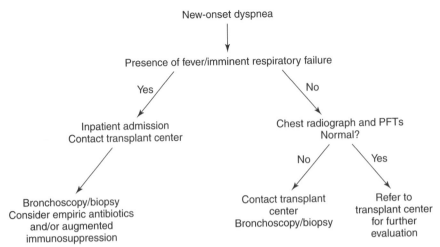

Figure 15.1 *Management of new onset dyspnea in lung transplant recipients. PFT, pulmonary function test.*

radiograph (or one that appears unchanged from a patient's baseline film). However, infiltrates associated with acute rejection tend to be diffuse and reticular in appearance (Fig. 15.2) and lobar infiltrates tend to suggest a bacterial process (Fig. 15.3). Viral and other opportunistic infections may result in radiographic patterns identical to those of acute rejection, hence invasive procedures such as bronchoscopy are often required to establish the correct diagnosis.

When a new pulmonary infiltrate is discovered in a symptomatic patient, urgent bronchoscopy is generally performed to obtain bronchoalveolar lavage (BAL) and transbronchial biopsies. Although BAL may be useful for cultures to diagnose infection, acute rejection can only be diagnosed with allograft biopsies.[1] It is also important to note that some patients may present with both infection and rejection. Therefore when bronchoscopy is performed it is desirable to perform both BAL and transbronchial biopsies. For patients with fever and pulmonary infiltrates, blood and urine cultures, as well as bronchoscopy are typically performed within 24 hours of presentation. Decisions regarding potential transfer to the transplant center must, therefore, be made early.

Initial therapy of suspected infection and rejection is discussed further in the respective sections in this chapter. As

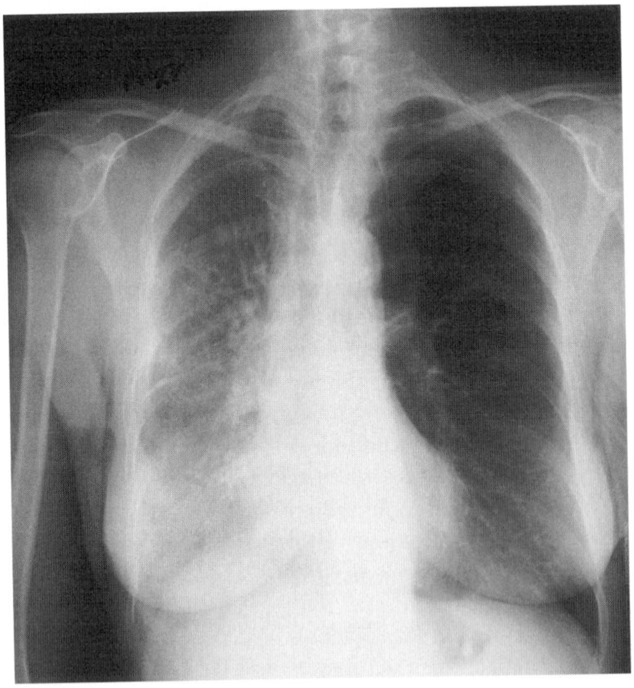

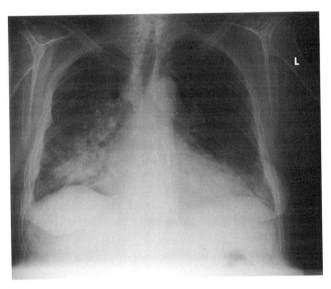

Figure 15.2 *Right lung transplant in a patient with chronic obstructive pulmonary disease with new diffuse pulmonary infiltrate. Bronchoscopy with transbronchial biopsy revealed mild to moderate acute cellular rejection (ISHLT grade A2–3). The infiltrate cleared rapidly with pulse intravenous steroids.*

Figure 15.3 *Chest radiograph of a 52-year-old man, status 6 years post double lung transplant for chronic obstructive pulmonary disease, who presented with fever, cough, chills, dyspnea, and hypoxemia. Bronchoscopic cultures grew heavy* Pseudomonas aeruginosa.

part of the treatment for new processes one must carefully consider the potential impact of adding or removing medications from the patient's often complicated maintenance regimen. Adverse effects of many of these medications may cause problems such as renal failure, metabolic derangements, bone marrow suppression, and acute neurologic changes, which may require urgent or emergent intervention.[2] These will be addressed in subsequent sections.

LUNG TRANSPLANT INFECTIONS

Following lung transplantation there is a marked increase in risk for infection due to a number of factors including the immunosuppression required to prevent allograft rejection, exposure of the transplanted lung to the outside world, and ineffective airway clearance mechanisms. The most recent International Society for Heart and Lung Transplantation (ISHLT) registry shows that nearly all lung transplant recipients are treated with triple-drug immunosuppression that includes steroids (usually prednisone), a calcineurin inhibitor (cyclosporine or tacrolimus), and either azathioprine or mycophenolate mofetil.[3] The use of sirolimus, a new immunosuppressive agent with potent antifibrotic properties, is also increasing for maintenance immunosuppression. In addition to this long-term 'maintenance' immunosuppression, almost half of the transplant centers in the United States use 'induction' immunosuppression perioperatively.[3] Such strategies create a state of profound immunosuppression, increasing the risk for infection. These drugs taken together greatly affect both the cell-mediated and antibody-mediated arms of the immune system.

Although such immunosuppression decreases the likelihood of allograft rejection, a price is paid by increasing the risk for bacterial, fungal, and viral infections. Furthermore, since lung allografts are exposed to the outside world, a direct portal of entry exists for infectious agents to reach the lower respiratory tract. Making the situation even worse, the transplanted lung is denervated resulting in a decreased sensation and reduced cough in response to airway irritants. There is also loss or dysfunction of mucociliary clearance mechanisms decreasing the ability to properly remove foreign substances that are deposited in the lower respiratory tract.[4–6] Taken together, it is not surprising that the most common infectious complication in lung transplant recipients is pneumonia.

When infections occur, the organism responsible may in large part be predicted by the time course from transplantation. Bacterial infections are most common perioperatively and then diminish somewhat by 3 months after transplantion.[7] During the early postoperative period, the bacterial pathogen is frequently similar to that carried with the donor at the time of transplant. In fact, at the time of transplantation bronchoscopic cultures are obtained from the donor lungs and antibiotic therapy is frequently directed at the pathogens grown from these cultures. Beyond the first few postoperative days, new infections are typically due to bacterial pathogens that are specific to the local hospital environment. Thus, the typical nosocomial pathogens such as *Staphylococcus aureus* and *Pseudomonas* are highly represented in this group. As the patient transitions from the hospital to the outpatient environment, community-acquired pathogens become more important.[7] Although the effects of corticosteroids and the other immunosuppressive agents may blunt typical symptoms of pneumonia in transplant recipients, the majority of patients still present with typical findings as in nontransplant patients. These include cough, sputum production, fever, and leukocytosis. It is however important to recognize that similar symptoms may be present with acute rejection; thus, symptoms alone should not be used as a diagnostic criteria for infection.[8] Chest radiographs typically show lobar infiltration with air bronchograms.

For serious infections, treatment should begin promptly with broad-spectrum antibacterial agents. A typical regimen would include a antipseudomonal β-lactam or cephalosporin together with a fluoroquinolone. This strategy provides adequate coverage for typical and atypical community-acquired organisms as well as Gram-negative pathogens. For less serious infections empiric therapy may be initiated with a fluoroquinolone alone. Aminoglycosides are avoided, if at all possible, to prevent the potential for nephrotoxicity that may compound the use of calcineurin immunosuppressive agents (cyclosporine or tacrolimus). Macrolide antibiotics are also avoided since these agents may dramatically increase the serum levels of the calcineurin inhibitors. Although the risk of bacterial infection is highest during the perioperative period, lung transplant recipients remain at increased risk for these infections throughout their life.[9–11] Pneumonia is also a major factor contributing to morbidity and mortality in those patients who develop chronic allograft rejection. Chronic allograft rejection, characterized histologically as bronchiolitis obliterans, is associated with colonization by organisms such as *Pseudomonas aeruginosa* and *Aspergillus* species. These colonizing organisms may ultimately become invasive leading to life-threatening pneumonia.[12]

From the second to the third month and extending throughout the first postoperative year, viral infection with cytomegalovirus (CMV) becomes an important problem.[9–11] Currently in most centers intravenous ganciclovir or oral valganciclovir is used for prophylaxis against CMV for a period of several weeks to several months following transplantation.[13] In addition to these agents, some centers give CMV hyperimmune globulin for high-risk individuals.[13] Although these strategies have dramatically reduced the incidence of CMV infection during the early postoperative period, CMV still remains a problem for posttransplant recipients. Despite the use of aggressive prophylactic regimens, CMV infection remains an important problem in lung transplant recipients and may present with acute or insidious onset of fever, chills, dyspnea, and interstitial pulmonary infiltrates. Pneumonia caused by CMV in lung transplant recipients is usually diagnosed by bronchoscopy with transbronchial biopsy confirming cytopathologic changes of CMV infection (Fig. 15.4). A positive culture for CMV from BAL fluid is usually not adequate to establish the diagnosis of invasive CMV disease since some patients may shed this organism without clinical significance. An elevated serum level of CMV by polymerase chain reaction (PCR) may indicate invasive disease or impending invasive infection.[14] Some centers now monitor serum PCR for CMV at regular intervals and initiate therapy with the rising levels, prior to the development of symptoms.

Aside from CMV infection, a number of other viruses have proved to be problematic after transplantion.[15] A common scenario for lung transplant recipients is to present with fever, rhinorrhea, nonproductive cough, and other symptoms suggestive of a 'flulike' illness associated with a sudden fall in pulmonary function studies. In some cases the condition is self-limited with a return of lung function back to baseline; however, sometimes the condition resolves with a persistent drop in lung function, qualifying the patient as having bronchiolitis obliterans syndrome, the spirometric correlate of histologic bronchiolitis obliterans or chronic allograft rejection.

The Washington University group recently examined the profile of these viruses and found that infection with influenza, parainfluenza, respiratory syncytial virus, and adenoviruses increased the risk for developing bronchiolitis obliterans syndrome and death.[16] The acute impact of these

viral infections warrants the use of uncommon therapies such as aerosolized ribavirin in some patients with community-acquired viral pathogens, particularly if respiratory syncytial virus is considered.[17] Finally, fungal and other opportunistic organisms such as *Nocardia* and atypical mycobacteria are of significant concern in the transplant population and may cause infection despite antimicrobial prophylaxis regimens.[18–21] Due to the widespread use of trimethoprim-sulfa or dapsone as prophylaxis for *Pneumocystis carinii* pneumonia, this entity is uncommonly encountered in adherent patients. Given the dizzying array of infectious possibilities, the early involvement of an infectious disease consultant is encouraged and the need for early bronchoscopy is emphasized.

When treatment decisions are formulated, it is important to be aware of drug interactions between some of the antimicrobials and immunosuppressive drugs. For instance, macrolide antibiotics (erythromycin and clarithromycin more than azithromycin) will markedly increase the levels of cyclosporine and tacrolimus, and aminoglycosides will compound the nephrotoxic potential of these agents. Transplant programs typically use an empiric regimen consisting of an antipseudomonal β-lactam or cephalosporin with/without a fluoroquinolone as empiric broad-spectrum therapy to cover for Gram-negative and community-acquired pathogens. Vancomycin or linezolid is also used if staphylococcal infection is a possibility (assuming a methicillin-resistant strain is present) pending culture results. Close communication with the patient's transplant center is essential to optimize therapy as decisions regarding reduction in immunosuppression and past infection history can be better addressed. It is worth noting that except in isolated cases, immunosuppression may be modified but is generally not completely withdrawn even for severe infection due to the possible risk for developing acute allograft rejection.

ACUTE LUNG TRANSPLANT REJECTION

Early experience with heart-lung transplant and subsequently single and double lung transplants has established that acute allograft rejection is exceedingly common with most lung transplant recipients experiencing at least one episode.[22] Unlike hyperacute allograft rejection that is rare and occurs in the operative or immediate postoperative period, and chronic allograft rejection, which is an indolent process that does not present as a transplant emergency, acute lung rejection is a commonly encountered emergency outside of the transplant center. Acute rejection occurs more commonly in lung recipients compared to heart or abdominal organ transplant recipients, perhaps in part, due to the lung's constant exposure to the environment. The pathophysiology of acute lung allograft rejection typically involves a perivascular, and often peribronchiolar,

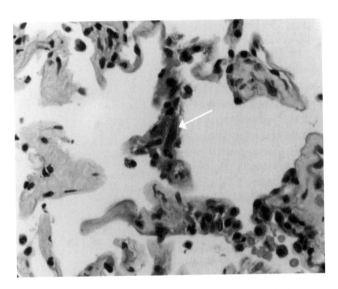

Figure 15.4 *Typical histologic appearance of cytomegalovirus (hematoxyin and eosin stain) from a patient who presented 9 months following lung transplantation with fever, dyspnea, and scant interstitial pulmonary infiltrates. The specimen was obtained by transbronchial biopsy. Arrow points to a 'cigar-shaped' cytomegalic cell.*

lymphocytic inflammation (Fig. 15.5). This manifests with nonspecific symptoms including dyspnea, fatigue, dry cough and low-grade fever, hypoxemia, and decline in spirometry.[8] This spirometric deterioration typically manifests as a fall in forced expiratory volume in 1 second (FEV_1), and, or the forced vital capacity (FVC).[23] A threshold of a 10 percent change from the patient's previous baseline (not necessarily a 10 percent decline in predicted value) in FEV_1 or FVC is considered significant since the average lung transplant patient is highly trained in performing the forced expiratory maneuver (most patients measure home spirometry daily).

The chest radiograph may also support the diagnosis of acute rejection when new interstitial diffuse or patchy reticular opacities are present. It is important to recognize that acute rejection may occur with a normal chest radiograph or computed tomography (CT) scan, particularly with mild forms of rejection.[24] However, more severe grades of acute rejection are typically associated with radiographic abnormalities (Fig. 15.6).[25] Although these clinical criteria have been used for the diagnosis of acute graft rejection, transbronchial lung biopsy is considered the gold standard and should be performed since augmented immunosuppressive therapy for treatment may exacerbate undiagnosed infection.

Transbronchial biopsies obtained during bronchoscopy are generally sufficient to diagnose acute rejection. The ISHLT recommends that a minimum of five pieces of alveolated lung parenchyma, each containing bronchioles and greater than 100 air sacs, be obtained in order to have enough tissue for adequate sensitivity to exclude acute rejection.[1] Often 8–10 biopsy pieces are obtained to secure a diagnostic specimen for interpretation by a pathologist experienced with evaluating lung transplant biopsies. If rejection is present, steroids or other forms of augmented immunosuppression are given, but the dose depends on the severity grade and varies widely between centers. Most centers treat only ISHLT grade A2 (mild) acute rejection or higher although recent evidence suggests that even minimal acute cellular rejection may be associated with adverse outcomes.[26] For grade A2, the majority of centers treat with oral prednisone with a dose of 1 mg/kg tapered over a 2-week period. For higher-grade rejection, intravenous solumedrol may be given at 1 g/day for 3 days followed by the same oral steroid taper given for grade A2 rejection. Other medications, such antithymocyte globulin or other T lymphocyte depletion, are sometimes used, particularly for higher grades of rejection that do not respond to corticosteroids. Follow-up bronchoscopy is performed to verify complete resolution even if signs and symptoms have abated. Under the direction of the transplant center the patient's maintenance immunosuppressive medication regimen may also be modified in an attempt to prevent recurrence of acute rejection. Close follow-up of the patient who has been treated for rejection is essential to ensure that the rejection resolves and to monitor for opportunistic infections during the period of extreme immune compromise. Infections

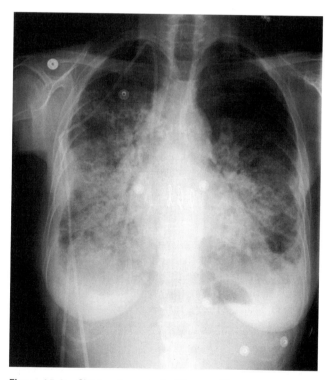

Figure 15.6 *Chest radiograph of a 54-year-old women, status post bilateral lung transplantation for sarcoidosis, who presented with 1 week of dyspnea and low-grade fever. Note diffuse bilateral pulmonary infiltrates. Transbronchial biopsy revealed severe acute rejection. Although the pulmonary infiltrates improved with high-dose pulse intravenous steroids, pulmonary function studies remained low and the patient died from chronic rejection 6 months after this event.*

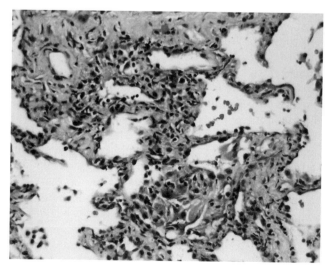

Figure 15.5 *Histologic specimen from a transbronchial biopsy showing moderate acute cellular rejection (ISHLT grade A3). Note mononuclear cells surrounding vessel and extending out into interstitium.*

in lung transplant recipients not only follow, but precede and/or occur concurrently with acute allograft rejection as discussed above. Since the ideal algorithms to evaluate transplant recipients at their nontransplant medical centers are not always feasible, the nontransplant clinician is forced to stabilize some patients without a definitive diagnosis of infection or rejection, a problem addressed in the following section.

MANAGEMENT OF RESPIRATORY COMPROMISE OF UNCLEAR ETIOLOGY

The most common cause for acute respiratory compromise in lung transplant recipients is either infection or acute rejection. For patients with acute respiratory deterioration following lung transplantation, circumstances may necessitate the initiation of treatment before the diagnosis of infection or rejection is established. Both allograft rejection and infection may present with a broad range of signs and symptoms, from an asymptomatic fall in home spirometry readings, to full blown respiratory failure with profound hypoxemia and pulmonary infiltrates. Empiric therapy is routinely initiated with broad-spectrum intravenous antibiotics (to cover both Gram-negative and positive infection) and intravenous solumedrol (1 g). Bronchoscopy is performed as soon as possible to help establish a diagnosis. A diagnosis of acute rejection requires continuing steroid treatment; however, if the results of bronchoscopy confirm infection alone then antibiotics are adjusted according to culture results. There are significant risks to treating empirically for prolonged periods of time with both augmented immunosuppression and antimicrobials such that this approach should not be considered adequate for most lung transplant recipients.

MANAGEMENT OF ACUTE RESPIRATORY FAILURE

Acute respiratory failure in the setting of lung transplantation may be due to either infection or severe forms of acute allograft rejection. Indeed lung transplant recipients are at increased risk for adult respiratory distress syndrome compared with normal hosts.[27] It is important to note that a picture similar to adult respiratory distress syndrome may be due to a variety of infectious stimuli (both bacterial and viral) but may also occur in association with allograft rejection.[27] Therefore, bronchoscopy with transbronchial biopsy is advisable when it can be safely performed based upon oxygenation and ventilatory parameters. Empiric broad-spectrum antibiotics and corticosteroids are administered pending results of bronchoscopy. Ventilatory support is provided in similar fashion to patients without lung transplants, although a

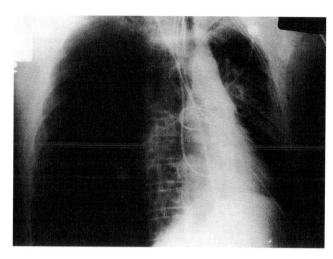

Figure 15.7 *Acute native lung hyperinflation. Chest radiograph of a patient who had a left single lung transplant for chronic obstructive pulmonary disease and presented with dyspnea, hypoxemia, and infiltrates in the allograft. Within hours of intubation, the patient became hypotensive and profoundly hypoxemic. The condition improved with independent ventilation to each lung through a double-lumen endotracheal tube.*

word of caution is necessary for patients with single lung transplants with underlying COPD. For these patients, close attention must be paid to the native lung which can become hyperinflated leading to mediastinal shift and compression of the transplanted lung (Fig. 15.7).[28] This scenario is best managed with a double-lumen endotracheal tube with independent lung ventilation.

MEDICATIONS AND SERIOUS ADVERSE EFFECTS

After considering infection and allograft rejection, complications attributable to the adverse effects of medications are the third broad category of posttransplant complications encountered both in and outside transplant centers. Medications are prescribed in this setting for both prophylaxis and treatment although the distinction between these indications may be difficult to make in some cases. The general classes of maintenance medications include immunosuppression (e.g. prednisone, cyclosporine, tacrolimus, azathioprine, mycophenolate mofetil, and sirolimus), infection prophylaxis (e.g. trimethoprim-sulfa, valganciclovir, itraconazole, voriconazole) and other (e.g. alendronate, HMG Co-A reductase inhibitors). Complications from these agents include metabolic derangements, bone marrow suppression, renal insufficiency, and acute neurologic changes (Box 15.1). Some require emergent therapy and consultation with the patient's lung transplant center is again advised to minimize potential problems that may result from modifying the maintenance medication regimen.

Box 15.1 Noninfectious adverse effects of transplant medications

- Anemia/pancytopenia
- Bowel perforation
- Gastoparesis
- Hypercoaguability
- Hyperkalemia
- Hypertension
- Hemolytic-uremic syndrome
- Lymphoproliferative disorders
- Myopathy
- Nephrotoxicity
- Neurotoxicity
- Peptic ulcer disease

Metabolic derangements

Emergent metabolic derangements associated with transplant-related medications include abnormal serum levels of glucose, potassium, and other electrolytes and the treatment is similar to the approach for the patient without a transplant. Although persistent elevation of serum potassium level may be due to relative mineralocorticoid insufficiency in patients taking prednisone, administration of low-dose fludrocortisone (0.1 mg/day) (after standard acute potassium-lowering medical therapy is successful) may ameliorate this problem. Other metabolic complications, such as rhabdomyolysis and hyperglycemia, are similar in presentation and management strategy to those in patients without transplants although they occur more commonly in this population given the prevalence of HMG Co-A reductase inhibitor and corticosteroid use, respectively. HMG Co-A reductase inhibitors are commonly used in solid-organ transplant recipients because of the elevated lipid levels induced by the immunosuppressive drug regimens, and there is an increased risk for myopathy and rhabdomyolysis when these agents are combined with ciclosporin.[29]

Bone marrow suppression

Bone marrow suppression may occur at any time following transplantation and a thorough evaluation for nonmedication-related causes is warranted to rule out such common explanations such as iron or folate deficiency and in cases of leukopenia infection with cytomegalovirus or parvovirus B-19. If no dietary or infectious cause is discovered in cases of pancytopenia, medication-related bone marrow suppression should be suspected and the approach will often depend on the nature and degree of the problem. Azathioprine, mycophenolate mofetil, and ganciclovir are common offenders and consideration must

be given to temporarily holding, replacing, or discontinuing these medications. Granulocyte colony-stimulating factor, recombinant erythropoietin, and/or transfusion may be necessary to treat neutropenia and anemia, respectively. It is extremely important to recognize that if blood transfusion is required then CMV seronegative blood should be used for patients who are naïve to this viral infection (patients who were CMV-negative prior to transplantation and received a lung from a donor who was also CMV-negative). This is necessary to prevent CMV infection.

Renal failure

Renal insufficiency occurs commonly in the lung transplant population primarily due to the use of the calcineurin inhibitors (cyclosporine and tacrolimus) which are innately nephrotoxic. Transplant recipients may also develop renal insufficiency for the same reasons as in patients without transplants: prerenal insufficiency, intrinsic renal injury (especially acute tubular necrosis), and postrenal urinary outflow tract obstruction. The nephrotoxicity associated with the calcineurin inhibitors may occur as acute or chronic renal failure. Acute renal failure is typically related to high serum levels of these agents, whereas chronic renal failure develops insidiously over years of drug exposure. Given the known nephrotoxicity of cyclosporine and tacrolimus, the serum levels of these drugs are monitored closely. In patients with oliguria, headaches, increased tremor, and elevated blood pressure, an elevated cyclosporine or tacrolimus level should immediately be suspected. Drawing a 12-hour trough level and holding further doses of these agents until it is verified the level is within therapeutic range is appropriate. It is important to note that the appropriate level for cyclosporine or tacrolimus may vary for an individual patient depending on the time course since transplantation, prior rejection history, and other factors such as underlying renal function. Acute renal failure associated with these agents is typically reversible and restarting these drugs at a lower dose with close monitoring of levels will usually allow for recovery of renal function to the previous baseline.

Neurologic abnormalities

Neurotoxicity related to medications may take a variety of forms and include severe headaches, delirium, seizures, and stroke. Although corticosteroids may cause delirium, the majority of these complications are ascribed to the calcineurin inhibitors, cyclosporine and tacrolimus.[30] Indeed, both cyclosporine and tacrolimus lower seizure threshold and this problem may be particularly worse with very high serum levels of these drugs.

A complete neurologic exam, head CT, and in some cases a lumbar puncture may be necessary to rule out nonmedication causes of neurologic dysfunction (i.e. infection). Brain magnetic resonance imaging (MRI) may demonstrate white matter loss in patients who have been exposed to either cyclosporine or tacrolimus for long periods of time.[31] The therapy is supportive with consideration of changing calcineurin inhibitor (i.e. cyclosporine substituted for tacrolimus or vice versa) since this often results in resolution of acute neurologic effects.

Although acute neurotoxicity is commonly associated with high serum levels of these agents, these same problems may occur with therapeutic levels. Therefore simply reducing the dosage of the offending agent does not reliably result in improvement.[30]

Posttransplant lymphoma

One of the most devastating noninfectious complications of immunosuppression therapy is posttransplant lymphoproliferative disorder. A variation of Epstein–Barr-related lymphoma, this entity presents often within the first posttransplant year. These patients may present with fever and infectiouslike symptoms and most commonly show either infiltrates or mass lesions in the allograft or mediastinum. Extranodal disease is common in posttransplant lymphoproliferative disorder with a higher tendency for central nervous system and allograft involvement observed.[32,33] While reduction or withdrawal of immunosuppression is often the first-line therapy, the risk of graft rejection will be increased at that time and consultation with an oncologist and the transplant center to assess the relative risk of these approaches is recommended.

Key learning points

- Lung transplant recipients may develop a wide variety of complications that present as medical emergencies.

- Most complications may be categorized as episodes of infection, acute allograft rejection, adverse medication effects, or a combination of these problems.

- These patients require a rapid and aggressive evaluation to prevent irreversible damage to the lung allograft.

- Due to the complexity for management of these patients, it is prudent to consult with the lung transplant center to discuss possible patient transfer or to coordinate further diagnostic evaluation and treatment.

REFERENCES

1. Yousem SA, Berry GJ, Cagle PT, et al. Revision of the 1990 working formulation for the classification of pulmonary allograft rejection: Lung Rejection Study Group. J Heart Lung Transplant 1996; 15 (1 Pt 1): 1–15.

2. Maurer JR, Tewari S. Nonpulmonary medical complications in the intermediate and long-term survivor. Clin Chest Med 1997; 18: 367–82.

3. Trulock EP, Edwards LB, Taylor DO, et al. The Registry of the International Society for Heart and Lung Transplantation: twenty-first official adult heart transplant report – 2004. J Heart Lung Transplant 2004; 23: 804–15.

4. Tomkiewicz RP, App EM, Shennib H, et al. Airway mucus and epithelial function in a canine model of single lung autotransplantation. Chest 1995; 107: 261–5.

5. Marelli D, Paul A, Nguyen DM, et al. The reversibility of impaired mucociliary function after lung transplantation. J Thorac Cardiovasc Surg 1991; 102: 908–12.

6. Shankar S, Fulsham L, Read RC, et al. Mucociliary function after lung transplantation. Transplant Proc 1991; 23(1 Pt 2): 1222–3.

7. Maurer JR, Tullis DE, Grossman RF, et al. Infectious complications following isolated lung transplantation. Chest 1992; 101: 1056–9.

8. De Vito DA, Hoffman LA, Iacono AT, et al. Are symptom reports useful for differentiating between acute rejection and pulmonary infection after lung transplantation? Heart Lung 2004; 33: 372–80.

9. Chan KM, Allen SA. Infectious pulmonary complications in lung transplant recipients. Semin Respir Infect 2002; 17: 291–302.

10. Fishman JA, Rubin RH. Infection in organ-transplant recipients. N Engl J Med 1998; 338: 1741–51.

11. Shreeniwas R, Schulman LL, Berkmen YM, McGregor CC, Austin JH. Opportunistic bronchopulmonary infections after lung transplantation: clinical and radiographic findings. Radiology 1996; 200: 349–56.

12. Reichenspurner H, Girgis RE, Robbins RC, et al. Stanford experience with obliterative bronchiolitis after lung and heart-lung transplantation. Ann Thorac Surg 1996; 62: 1467–72.

13. Zamora MR, Nicolls MR, Hodges TN, et al. Following universal prophylaxis with intravenous ganciclovir and cytomegalovirus immune globulin, valganciclovir is safe and effective for prevention of CMV infection following lung transplantation. Am J Transplant 2004; 4: 1635–42.

14. Weinberg A, Hodges TN, Li S, *et al.* Comparison of PCR, antigenemia assay, and rapid blood culture for detection and prevention of cytomegalovirus disease after lung transplantation. *J Clin Microbiol* 2000; **38**: 768–72.

15. Palmer SM, Jr, Henshaw NG, Howell DN, *et al.* Community respiratory viral infection in adult lung transplant recipients. *Chest* 1998; **113**: 944–50.

16. Khalifah AP, Hachem RR, Chakinala MM, *et al.* Respiratory viral infections are a distinct risk for bronchiolitis obliterans syndrome and death. *Am J Respir Crit Care Med* 2004; **170**: 181–7.

17. Krinzman S, Basgoz N, Kradin R, *et al.* Respiratory syncytial virus-associated infections in adult recipients of solid organ transplants. *J Heart Lung Transplant* 1998; **17**: 202–10.

18. Husain S, McCurry K, Dauber J, *et al.* Nocardia infection in lung transplant recipients. *J Heart Lung Transplant* 2002; **21**: 354–9.

19. Doucette K, Fishman JA. Nontuberculous mycobacterial infection in hematopoietic stem cell and solid organ transplant recipients. *Clin Infect Dis* 2004; **38**: 1428–39.

20. Gordon SM, Avery RK. Aspergillosis in lung transplantation: incidence, risk factors, and prophylactic strategies. *Transpl Infect Dis* 2001; **3**: 161–7.

21. Kesten S, Chaparro C. Mycobacterial infections in lung transplant recipients. *Chest* 1999; **115**: 741–5.

22. Frist WH, Loyd JE, Merrill WH, *et al.* Single lung transplantation: a temporal look at rejection, infection, and survival. *Am Surg* 1994; **60**: 94–102.

23. Otulana BA, Higenbottam T, Scott J, *et al.* Lung function associated with histologically diagnosed acute lung rejection and pulmonary infection in heart-lung transplant patients. *Am Rev Respir Dis* 1990; **142**: 329–32.

24. Gotway MB, Dawn SK, Sellami D, *et al.* Acute rejection following lung transplantation: limitations in accuracy of thin-section CT for diagnosis. *Radiology* 2001; **221**: 207–12.

25. Kundu S, Herman SJ, Larhs A, *et al.* Correlation of chest radiographic findings with biopsy-proven acute lung rejection. *J Thorac Imaging* 1999; **14**: 178–84.

26. Hopkins PM, Aboyoun CL, Chhajed PN, *et al.* Association of minimal rejection in lung transplant recipients with obliterative bronchiolitis. *Am J Respir Crit Care Med* 2004; **170**: 1022–6.

27. Paradis IL, Duncan SR, Dauber JH, *et al.* Distinguishing between infection, rejection, and the adult respiratory distress syndrome after human lung transplantation. *J Heart Lung Transplant* 1992; **11** (4 Pt 2): S232–6.

28. Weill D, Torres F, Hodges TN, *et al.* Acute native lung hyperinflation is not associated with poor outcomes after single lung transplant for emphysema. *J Heart Lung Transplant* 1999; **18**: 1080–7.

29. Ballantyne CM, Corsini A, Davidson MH, *et al.* Risk for myopathy with statin therapy in high-risk patients. *Arch Intern Med* 2003; **163**: 553–64.

30. Bechstein WO. Neurotoxicity of calcineurin inhibitors: impact and clinical management. *Transpl Int* 2000; **13**: 313–26.

31. Filley CM, Kleinschmidt-DeMasters BK. Toxic leukoencephalopathy. *N Engl J Med* 2001; **345**: 425–32.

32. Penn I. Incidence and treatment of neoplasia after transplantation. *J Heart Lung Transplant* 1993; **12** (6 Pt 2): S328–6.

33. Yousem SA, Randhawa P, Locker J, *et al.* Posttransplant lymphoproliferative disorders in heart-lung transplant recipients: primary presentation in the allograft. *Hum Pathol* 1989; **20**: 361–9.

16

Pulmonary complications in immunocompromised hosts following hematopoietic stem cell transplantation

VICKIE R SHANNON, GEORGE A EAPEN

INTRODUCTION

Over the past decade, the term 'bone marrow transplant' has been supplanted by the term 'hematopoietic stem cell transplant' (HSCT) to reflect the use of a broader range of donor stem cell sources (bone marrow, fetal blood, peripheral blood). Significant advances in HSCT-related basic research and clinical trials have led to an exponential growth in the numbers of HSCTs performed in the United States and elsewhere. Improved patient outcomes, owing in part to enhanced pretransplant preparative regimens and posttransplant supportive measures, have resulted in a growing list of disease states that are amenable to HSCT, which is now standard therapy for a variety of malignant and nonmalignant illnesses. Despite these advances, mortality rates following HSCT remain high. Lung injury occurs in 40–60 percent of HSCT recipients and accounts for a substantial number of deaths, especially during the first 3 months following transplantation.[1] Infectious and noninfectious sources of pulmonary complications may occur, both with potentially devastating outcomes. Pneumonia is the most frequent source of infection and the overall leading infectious cause of death following HSCT. The chronologic development of these often-recalcitrant infections is tightly linked to the patient's dynamically changing immunologic status subsequent to transplantation and may vary significantly depending on the rate of immune recovery and the presence of graft-versus-host disease (GVHD).[2–4]

In contrast with infection, which is more often seen following allogeneic transplantation, noninfectious acute lung injury syndromes, including idiopathic pneumonia syndrome (IPS) and diffuse alveolar hemorrhage (DAH) occur with similar frequency among the different transplant allotypes. Bronchiolitis obliterans, a form of chronic airways disease, occurs almost exclusively following allogeneic transplantation, presumably as a consequence of some poorly understood link to GVHD. The emergence of these noninfectious disease entities also bears a temporal relation to the rate of immune recovery. This chapter discusses the chronologic development of infectious and noninfectious pulmonary complications following HSCT.

DEFINITIONS AND RISK FACTORS FOR THE DEVELOPMENT OF LUNG INJURY FOLLOWING HSCT

The intent of HSCT is to induce marrow ablation while maximizing tumor cell kill. The severe immunosuppression that follows mitigates rejection of donor stem cells among allogeneic HSCT recipients. These objectives are achieved through intense chemotherapy conditioning regimens, given with or without radiation therapy, prior to stem cell infusion. Associated toxicities of the conditioning regimen are largely responsible for many of the pulmonary complications seen after transplantation. Transplant allotypes are defined by whether the donor source of stem cells is from the patient (autologous transplant), an identical twin (syngeneic transplant) or a nonidentical relative or unrelated donor (allogeneic transplant). Graft-versus-host disease represents a type of immunologic injury mediated by host-reactive donor T lymphocytes. Targeted tissues for GVHD-related injury include the mucosal surfaces, reticuloendothelial system, and the bone marrow. Thus, the appearance of this inherently immunosuppressive disorder may lead to additional pulmonary complications.

The predilection to infection in the transplant setting is best understood by examining the effects of HSCT on host defenses, including local, innate (neutrophil response) and adaptive (humoral and cellular) immunity (Table 16.1). Numerous factors, including the type of transplant, the timing and intensity of myeloablative therapies, underlying disease, stem cell source (cord blood, peripheral blood, bone marrow), degree of histocompatibility between the donor and recipient, use of T cell depleted donor cells, the emergence of GVHD, the use of prophylactic antimicrobial strategies, and the need for further immunosuppressive therapy following HSCT, strongly impact the duration of each of these periods and the rate of posttransplant infections. Consequently, allogeneic transplant recipients experience higher rates of pulmonary complications following transplantation than recipients of autologous transplants because of the more stringent preparative

Table 16.1   *Categories of depressed immunity and associated pneumonias following hematopoietic stem cell transplantation*

Predominant pathogen	Granulocytopenia	Depressed cellular immunity	Depressed humoral immunity/splenectomy	Mixed defects
Bacteria	*Staphylococcus aureus* *Streptococcus pneumoniae* *Streptococcus* species *Pseudomonas aeruginosa* Enterobacteriaceae *Escherichia coli* *Klebsiella* species *Stenotrophomonas maltophilia* *Acinetobacter* species	*Nocardia asteroids* complex *Salmonella typhimurium* *Salmonella enteritidis* *Rhodococcus equi* *Rhodococcus bronchialis* *Listeria monocytogenes* *Mycobacterium tuberculosis* Nontuberculous mycobacteria	*Streptococcus pneumoniae* *Haemophilus influenzae* *Neisseria meningitides* *Capnocytophaga canimorsus* *Campylobacter*	*Streptococcus pneumoniae* *Staphylococcus aureus* *Haemophilus influenzae* *Klebsiella pneumonia* *Pseudomonas aeruginosa* *Acinetobacter* species *Enterobacter* species *Stenotrophomonas maltophilia* *Nocardia asteroids* complex *Listeria monocytogenes* *Legionella* species
Fungi	*Aspergillus fumigatus;* nonfumigatus *Aspergillus* *Pseudallescheria boydii* *Fusarium solani* *Mucorales* (zygomycoses) Dematiaceous (black) fungi such as *Alternaria, Bipolaris, Curvularia, Scedosporium apiospermum Scedosporium prolificans*	*Aspergillus* and non-*Aspergillus* filamentous molds *Pneumocystis jiroveci* (*P. carini*) *Cryptococcus neoformans* Endemic mycoses due to *Histoplasma capsulatum, Coccidioides immitis, Blastomyces dermatitidis*	*Pneumocystis jiroveci* (*P. carini*)?	*Pneumocystis jiroveci* (*P. carini*) *Aspergillus* species *Candida* species *Cryptococcus neoformans* *Mucorales* (zygomycoses) Endemic mycoses (severe systemic dissemination)
Viruses	Herpes simplex virus I and II Varicella zoster virus	Human cytomegalovirus Respiratory viruses Influenza A and influenza B Parainfluenza type 3 Respiratory syncytial virus Adenovirus Varicella zoster virus HHV-6	Varicella zoster virus Echovirus Enterovirus	Respiratory viruses Influenza Parainfluenza Respiratory syncytial virus Adenovirus Varicella zoster virus
Parasites		*Toxoplasma gondii* *Microsporidium* species *Leishmania donovani* *Leishmania infantum* *Strongyloides stercoralis*	*Giardia lamblia* *Babesia microti*	*Toxoplasma gondii* *Strongyloides stercoralis*

chemotherapeutic regimens, delayed recovery of T and B cell functions, histoincompatible donor stem cells and the development of GVHD among this group of patients. Early susceptibility to infection is also strongly influenced by the duration of the period of engraftment (neutropenic period). Shortening this period through the administration of alternative hematopoietic precursor sources such as granulocyte colony-stimulating factors and mobilized peripheral blood stem cells effectively reduces the risk of infection. Increased rates of noninfectious, inflammatory pulmonary complications, such as DAH, idiopathic pneumonia, and engraftment syndromes are seen, however, ostensibly facilitated by the rapid reconstitution of the immune system. The augmented release of inflammatory cytokines during the period of rapid neutrophil recovery is postulated to play a key role.[5–7]

ALTERED HOST DEFENSES FOLLOWING HSCT

Impairments of local defense mechanisms

Breach of cutaneous and mucosal barriers caused by aggressive chemoradiation regimens as well as iatrogenic alterations in mechanical barriers that occur with the use of nasogastric catheters and endotracheal tubes following HSCT heightens infection risk. These catheters serve as conduits for chronic colonization of pathogenic organisms, which facilitate the development of infection.[8–10] Furthermore, nasogastric catheters hinder coordinated glottic activities and mucociliary function, thereby augmenting the risk for aspiration.

Impairment of local innate airway defense mechanisms: epithelial cells, mast cells, and macrophages

Some of the earliest derangements in local airway defense following HSCT include functional abnormalities of alveolar macrophage chemotaxis, phagocytosis, and killing. The effect of these disturbances is to significantly increase the risk of infection, particularly when other host defenses are compromised or overwhelmed, as by heavy inoculum, resistant or virulent organisms. Lung epithelial cells that line the airways and alveoli serve as the first point of contact of microbial pathogens entering the lungs and, hence, play an essential role in the early defense against airway pathogens. These cells respond to microbial exposure with an increased production of mediators such as chemokines, cytokines, and a variety of antimicrobial peptides.[11] Lung epithelial cells are relatively long lived and slowly dividing, and, as such, their susceptibility to the cytotoxic effects of chemoradiation is less that that seen with other types of more rapidly dividing epithelial cells, such as those lining the gut. Nonetheless, chemoradiation likely compromises the activity of key factors in epithelial host defense, although this concept is not well studied.

Mast cells have been most widely studied in the context of allergic disease. Their crucial role in host defense has only recently been recognized.[12,13] These cells reside along blood vessels within the surface epithelia and submucosa of the skin and mucosal surfaces where they act as sentinels of the immune system, sampling their environment and releasing cytokines, chemokines, and inflammatory mediators upon detection of microbial pathogens.[12,13] In addition, stimulated mast cells rapidly release vasoactive signaling molecules that allow extravasation of protective plasma proteins and recruitment of immune effector cells.[14]

Similarly, macrophages create a first line of defense with a unique armamentarium of mediators for responding to pathogen-associated signals. These resident cells of the skin and mucosa are professional phagocytes that play an essential role in the sensing and elimination of invasive microorganisms.[12,13] As nondividing, long-lived cells, macrophages are relatively protected against toxic effects of cytoablative chemotherapeutic regimens. Certain drugs, however, may profoundly alter macrophage cellular chemotaxis, phagocytosis, and killing, especially during the first 4 months following transplantation. Full recovery of these cellular activities typically occurs at 6–12 months following HSCT.[15]

Impairment of qualitative and quantitative neutrophil function (recruitable innate immunity)

Neutrophils are critical effector cells of innate immunity whose specialized functions, including chemotaxis, microbial killing, and phagocytosis, play a key role in host defense against microbial infections. Upon exposure to bacterial- or fungal-derived products or inflammatory mediators, these cells migrate to the site of infection where they bind to and kill the pathogen. These microbicidal activities occur in response to a series of complex, tightly regulated, and integrated cell signaling activities.[16] A growing list of gene products induced by neutrophils, including cytokines (tumor necrosis factor [TNF]-α), vascular endothelial growth factor, interleukin (IL)-1β, IL-IRα, IL-12), and chemokines (IL-8, macrophage inflammatory protein [MIP]-1α, MIP-1β, interferon-γ, have been identified.

Neutrophils are the central cellular defense against infections caused by bacterial and fungal organisms.[2,17,18] These organisms induce leukocyte migration from the circulation to the site of infection by the sequential activation of adhesive proteins and their ligands on leukocytes and endothelial cells. Lymphocytes and monocytes use similar sequential mechanisms for microvascular transmigration. However, they differ in their responses to chemotactic signals, as well as in the qualitative and quantitative expression of adhesion molecules. These discrepancies permit the sequential recruitment of discrete leukocyte subpopulations to the site of infection.[16] Unlike mast cells and macrophages, these cells are exquisitely sensitive to the cytotoxic effects of chemotherapy. Chemotherapy may induce absolute agranulocytosis by direct myelotoxicity as well as functional neutropenia by interfering with the phagocytic and chemotactic activity of neutrophils.[19,20] Altered neutrophil function is also a frequent sequela of other cancer-related treatment regimens, including radiation therapy and administration of glucocorticosteroids. In addition, neutrophil dysfunction owing to common cancer-related disorders, such as hypovolemia, prolonged hypoxemia, acidosis, and poorly controlled hyperglycemia is an underrecognized problem. Specific pathogens causing pneumonia that are commonly encountered in neutropenic patients are listed in Table 16.1.

IMPAIRMENT OF ADAPTIVE IMMUNITY

Altered humoral responses

Profound impairments in humoral immunity, occurring as a corollary of HSCT-induced B cell dysfunction, may persist for up to 12 months following transplantation. In addition to HSCT, underlying lymphoreticular malignancies, including multiple myeloma, chronic lymphocytic leukemia, and Waldenström macroglobulinemia may directly cause immunoglobulin dyscrasias and associated hypogammaglobulinemia.[21,22] Loss of proper B cell function is associated with impaired neutralization of toxins and disorders of immunoglobulin production, antibody-dependent cellular cytotoxicity and complement activation. Asplenism, either functional or anatomic, is a common problem among patients with lymphoreticular malignancies. Defects in opsonization, owing to asplenism, as well as qualitative and quantitative depression of the alternative complement pathway, which is housed in the spleen, may lead to unchecked proliferation of encapsulated organisms that require opsonization with complement (C_3, C_5) for elimination. Adding to this, defects in antibody-dependent lymphocyte cytolytic activity encourage the unbridled growth of recalcitrant parasitic organisms.

Altered cellular immune response

Interactions between macrophages and T lymphocytes subserve the cellular arm of adaptive immunity. Consequently, disorders that adversely affect the function and/or numbers of T lymphocytes and macrophages may severely depress this arm of the immune system. Many of these disorders, such as Hodgkin disease, hairy cell leukemia, adult T cell leukemia, lymphocytic leukemia, and GVHD, are unique to the cancer and posttransplant setting. In addition,

viral illnesses and multiple agents in the armamentarium of cancer therapy, including glucocorticosteroids, antineoplastic agents, and other immunosuppressive agents used for prophylaxis and/or treatment of established GVHD may depress the cellular arm of the immune system by inducing profound lymphopenia.

CLINICAL PRESENTATION AND EVALUATION OF THE HSCT RECIPIENT WITH PULMONARY INFILTRATES

The typical clinical presentation of pneumonia is often lacking in the posttransplant setting. Patients with severe neutropenia may present with only minimal cough and low-grade fever, and negligible radiographic change, despite fulminant infection. Furthermore, radiographic enhancement of pulmonary infiltrates despite appropriate therapy may occur coincident with neutrophil recovery. The classic radiographic appearance of lobar consolidations typical of bacterial pneumonias may be absent, and diffuse interstitial infiltrates or patchy areas of dense alveolar consolidation are seen instead. Although the clinical assessment of the cancer patient with pulmonary infiltrates is often ambiguous, the physical examination may yield critical clues to the diagnosis and is the final arbiter in determining the severity of the pneumonia.[23] Information regarding recent hospitalizations, treatment in a hospital or hemodialysis clinic, or residence in a nursing home or long-term care facility suggests hospital-acquired (HAP) or healthcare-associated (HCAP) pneumonia. These pneumonias are often multidrug resistant. Thus, the patient exposure history information provides an important framework for decisions regarding empiric therapy.

Antecedent infection, antibiotic history, and knowledge of cytomegalovirus (CMV) serologic status also have clinical relevance in this setting. For example, a history of recent travel to endemic areas for *Histoplasmosis* (Ohio-Mississippi river valley), *Coccidioidomycosis* (southwestern United States, Central and South America), multidrug resistant mycobacterial disease (inner-city New York), or *Babesiosis* (northeastern United States) may give important clues to the underlying pathogen. Antibiotic prophylaxis with trimethoprim-sulfamethoxazole or the fluoroquinolones following HSCT has been associated with increased rates of *Streptococcus viridans* pneumonia because of the variable coverage of these antibiotics against Gram-positive organisms. Accordingly, the differential diagnosis of unexplained pulmonary infiltrates in this group of patients should include *Strept. viridans* pneumonia.

The bedside assessment may be equally ambiguous. Nonspecific symptoms of productive cough, fever, dyspnea, and chest pain are variably present. Immunosuppressive therapy may mask fever and cough may be minimal in the debilitated cancer patient with severe pneumonia.

Furthermore, typical physical signs of lung consolidation, such as rales and egophony, may be absent. Fever and cough may be the presenting symptom of many comorbid illnesses that mimic pneumonia in patients with cancer, including radiation pneumonitis, drug toxicity, pulmonary embolic disease, alveolar hemorrhage, and thermoregulatory problems associated with polypharmacy, which add to the diagnostic challenge. Despite these limitations, the physical examination is a key component of the overall evaluation and offers important clues to the diagnoses. For example, patients with disseminated mycobacterial or fungal disease may present with extrathoracic manifestations of lung infection, such as nodular skin lesions, which may help with the diagnosis. Evidence of concomitant sinus disease offers support for *Mucormycosis* or *Legionella* species as potential etiologies of the pneumonia.

Although the chest radiograph alone cannot delineate with precision the underlying etiology of lung infiltrates, the classic morphologic patterns of infectious and noninfectious disorders and the anatomic localization of the radiographic abnormalities are often quite informative. Focal areas of consolidation, for instance, are more often associated with bacterial or fungal pneumonias, although some bacterial and fungal pathogens, such as *Pneumocystis jiroveci* (formally referred to as *P. carinii*), *Legionella*, *Mycoplasma*, disseminated *Histoplasma*, and *Strongyloides* may cause diffuse disease (Fig. 16.1). The appearance of nodular lesions or the presence of a predominant alveolar or interstitial process also helps to streamline the diagnosis (Figs 16.2 and 16.3). Infections caused by *Staphylococcus*, *Nocardia*,

Pseudomonas, and fungal pathogens may give rise to nodular lesions with or without cavitation. Alveolar filling processes broadly reflect the presence of water (pulmonary edema), blood (alveolar hemorrhage), pus (infection), or protein (alveolar proteinosis) within the distal airspaces. The differential diagnosis for interstitial disease is much broader and includes both infectious and noninfectious etiologies. Pleural effusions, hilar and mediastinal adenopathy are

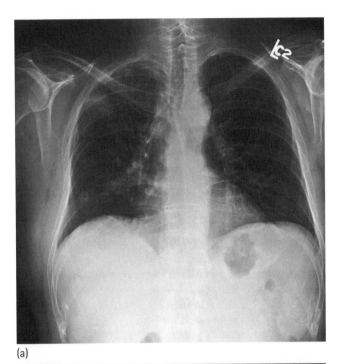

(a)

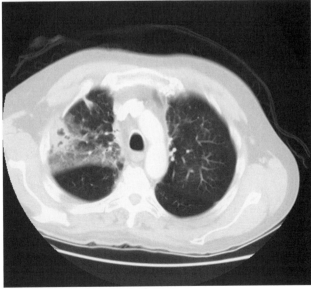

(b)

Figure 16.2 *Patient with respiratory failure and neutropenic fever 3 weeks following an allogeneic peripheral blood transplant for follicular lymphoma. Bilateral nodular infiltrates with cavitation were noted on the chest radiograph (a) and computed tomography scan (b) of the chest. Bronchioalveolar lavage fluid cultures were positive for* Aspergillus fumigatus.

Figure 16.1 *Chest radiograph of a 55-year-old patient with severe neutropenia and fever 6 days following an allogeneic transplant for non-Hodgkin lymphoma. There are bilateral areas of dense consolidation. Cultures of bronchioalveolar lavage samples were positive for* Strept. pneumophila.

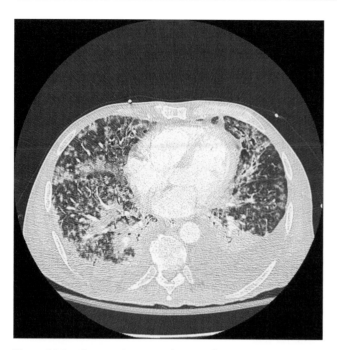

Figure 16.3 *Computed tomography scan of a 34-year-old patient with fever, sinus congestion and dry cough 10 weeks following a matched unrelated donor peripheral blood transplant for non-Hodgkin lymphoma. The scan of the chest showed diffuse nodular infiltrates with areas of consolidation and small bilateral effusion. Bronchioalveolar lavage fluid cultures were positive for mucormycosis.*

distinctive attributes of some infectious diagnoses, although overlapping features between infectious and noninfectious disease categories are common. The presence of a halo sign on computed tomography (CT) and ground glass attenuation surrounding segmental or nodular areas of consolidation in neutropenic patients is highly suggestive of pulmonary invasive aspergillosis.[24] Knowledge of the rapidity in which the infiltrates evolve is also helpful in narrowing the diagnosis. For example, blood or edema fluid commonly underlies infiltrates that resolve within 24–72 hours of their appearance, whereas inflammatory causes of pulmonary infiltrates typically resolve over days to weeks. The rapid doubling time of focal infiltrates of nonneoplastic origin (less than 3–4 weeks) also helps to exclude neoplastic processes as the underlying etiology of the infiltrate. Examination of expectorated sputum and endotracheal tube secretions has a limited role in the diagnosis of lung infiltrates in the cancer setting, although the recovery of certain pathogenic bacteria (*Legionella*, *Mycobacterium tuberculosis*, *Nocardia*) and endemic fungi (*Histoplasma*, *Coccidioidomycosis*, *Blastomycosis*) from the airway are felt to be diagnostic of lower tract disease.[25]

Emerging molecular markers may hold promise for the early detection of thoracic malignancies in the future; however, currently the utility of sputum analysis in the diagnosis of malignancy and other cancer-related noninfectious disorders, such as treatment-related lung

injury is negligible.[26] Culture-based analysis of lower respiratory tract samples is only able to identify an etiological diagnosis of pneumonia in approximately 50 percent of cases.[27,28] Recent advances in microbial detection using molecular diagnostic techniques, such as polymerase chain reaction (PCR) and new antigen and nucleic acid detection assays for *Legionella pneumophila*, *Streptococcus pneumonia*, *P. jiroveci*, and certain types of viral pneumonias offer promising adjuncts to culture-based technology in the detection of infection. Galactomannan assays have been successfully introduced into clinical practice for the early detection of invasive fungal infections,[29,30] although a high frequency of false positive results and, accordingly, low positive predictive values remain lingering challenges.[31,32]

The American Thoracic Society (ATS) and Infectious Disease Society of America (IDSA) recently published evidence-based guidelines advocating the use of semiquantitative or quantitative culture data obtained from bronchoscopically derived samples of the lower respiratory tract in the management of patients with HAP and HCAP.[33] Deescalation of antimicrobial therapy is recommended once the culture results are available, depending on the patient's clinical response to antibiotics. The diagnostic yield of bronchoalveolar lavage (BAL) among immunocompromised patients with HAP or HCAP ranges from 25 percent to 80 percent.[34–37] Fiberoptic bronchoscopy is felt to be a safe procedure, even among patients on mechanical ventilation, and in the setting of thrombocytopenia and coagulopathy.[35,38,39] The sensitivity of BAL in detecting organisms that have a high alveolar load (*P. carinii*, *Mycobacteria*, *Histoplasma*, CMV, and other viruses) exceeds 80 percent in published studies.[40] Prior antibiotic therapy may significantly diminish the sensitivity and specificity of bronchoscopically obtained quantitative cultures and diminish the yield of this procedure.[41,42]

Transbronchial biopsies have been found to be of only incremental value in the evaluation severely immunocompromised patients with suspected pneumonia over BAL alone.[43,44] This observation, coupled with the universal finding of posttransplant thrombocytopenia prohibit the performance of transbronchial biopsies in the posttransplant setting, especially when infection is suspected. On the other hand the utility of transbronchial biopsy in the assessment of patients with suspected pulmonary diseases that require histologic confirmation (bronchiolitis obliterans organizing pneumonia [BOOP]), diffuse alveolar damage, or interstitial pneumonitis is well established. Occasionally thoracotomy with open lung biopsy or thoracoscopic lung biopsy may be useful in select patients with hematologic malignancies and undiagnosed pulmonary infiltrates, although the yield of these procedures and their impact on therapeutic decision making have been variable (32–82 percent and 28–69 percent, respectively). The yield is lowest among patients with diffuse infiltrates, patients on mechanical ventilation, and those who have recently undergone pneumotoxic chemotherapy.[45,46]

Percutaneous transthoracic needle aspiration or biopsy is a useful tool in the diagnosis of focal lung lesions or pleural-based nodules or masses, especially when invasive fungal infections and malignancy is suspected.

Antimicrobial selections in the management of posttransplant pneumonia are based on the knowledge of the infecting pathogen, if available, pneumonia severity, underlying immune status, and the presence of comorbid conditions. General recommendations include the early use of broad-spectrum antibiotics with deescalation of empiric therapy based on clinical response and culture results. Antimicrobial therapy should not be withheld while diagnostic interventions are undertaken. Empiric antimicrobial selections should include agents that are from a different antibiotic class than those recently administered. The judicious use of combination therapy in the treatment of HAP or HCAP, including aminoglycoside therapy in combination with a β-lactam antibiotic in the treatment of pneumonias caused by *Pseudomonas aeruginosa* is also recommended.[33] Antipseudomonal coverage should be considered for all patients with suspected bacterial pneumonia and neutropenia.

PULMONARY INFECTIOUS COMPLICATIONS ASSOCIATED WITH STAGES OF IMMUNE RECOVERY FOLLOWING HSCT

Myeloablative pretransplant conditioning regimens used in the preparation of patients for HSCT result in severe decline of all three arms of the immune system. Immune suppression and the period of immune reconstitution that follows is roughly predictable and may be divided to reflect the three stages of major impairment of the specific arms of the host defense (pre-engraftment, immediate post-engraftment, late post-engraftment), which roughly correlate with the periods of highest vulnerability to specific types of infection. The stages of immune reconstitution following HSCT are also referred to as early (within the first 100 days) and late (greater than 100 days). The evaluation of the transplant recipient requires an understanding of specific host immune defects following transplantation and the temporal evolution of common, related infectious complications (Table 16.2).

Table 16.2   *Stages of immune deficiency post-HSCT and associated pulmonary disorders*

	Pre-engraftment	Immediate post-engraftment	Late post-engraftment
Infectious	Gram-positive cocci Gram-negative rods *Candida* species *Aspergillus* species *Zygomycetes* *Legionella* species *Stenotrophomonas maltophilia* Herpes simplex virus/HHV-6 RSV Influenza virus Parainfluenza virus	*Pneumococcus* *Nocardia* *Legionella* species *Aspergillus* *Histoplasma* *Coccidioides* *Cryptococcus* *Fusarium* *Zygomycetes* *Candida* *Pneumocystis jiroveci* *Pseudallaesceria boydii* *Mycobacteria tuberculosis* Nontuberculous mycobacteria *Salmonella* *Toxoplasma* Cytomegalovirus EBV Adenovirus RSV Rhinovirus	Staphylococci *Streptococcus pneumoniae* *Neisseria meningitides* *Haemophilus influenza* Gram-negative bacteria *Aspergillus* species EBV Varicellazoster virus *Pneumocystis jiroveci*
Noninfectious	Pulmonary edema DAH PERDS PVOD ARDS PAP	IPS Delayed pulmonary toxicity syndrome PVOD ARDS	Constrictive bronchiolitis BOOP PTLD ARDS
GVHD	Acute GVHD	Acute GVHD	Chronic GVHD

RSV, respiratory syncitial virus; EBV, Epstein-Barr virus; DAH, diffuse alveolar hemorrhage; IPS, idiopathic pneuomia syndrome; PERDS, peri-engraftment respiratory distress syndrome; ARDS, acute respiratory distress syndrome; PVOD, pulmonary veno-occlusive disease; PAP, pulmonary alveolar proteinosis; PTLD, posttransplant lymphoproliferative disorder; BOOP, bronchiolitis obliterans organizing pneumonia; GVHD, graft-versus-host disease.

Pre-engraftment stage

Severe neutropenia and lymphopenia herald the development of the pre-engraftment stage, which typically begins 1 week prior to stem cell infusion and may persist through the first 3 weeks following transplantation.[2,3,47,48] Predictably, bacterial infections caused by a variety of endogenous, extracellular, and pyogenic organisms are the predominant culprits of infection and may cause fatal pneumonias during this period. In one recent study, a 15 percent incidence of bacterial pneumonia was seen among allogeneic and autologous transplant recipients, most of which occurred within the first 100 days of transplantation and resulted in fatal pneumonia among 22 percent of the patients.[49] Recent reports document a decline in the prevalence of pre-engraftment infections, putatively due to the shortened period of neutropenia afforded by the use of hematopoietic growth factors and peripheral blood stem cell donation.[50] Both the duration and degree of neutropenia, defined as an absolute neutrophil count of $\leq 500/mm^3$, influence the risk of infection; as the neutrophil count drifts to less than 100/mL for 3 weeks or more, infection is virtually universal.[47,51] Methotrexate administration and T cell depletion of the donor marrow may prolong the period of neutropenia.

The most common bacterial pneumonias during the neutropenic period are caused by Gram-negative pathogens (*Pseudomonas*, *Enterobacteriaceae*, *Stenotrophomonas maltophilia*, *Legionella*, *Escherichia coli*, *Acinetobacter*). Simultaneous deficiencies in the humoral immune system during the pre-engraftment period increases the propensity for infections caused by Gram-negative rods, such as *Hemophilus influenzae*, *Neisseria meningitis*, and *Pseudomonas*, as well as encapsulated organisms such as *Streptococcus*. Pneumonias caused by Gram-positive organisms, such as *Strep. pneumoniae* and *Staphylococcus aureus* have been increasingly isolated over the past decade.[52] This shift is likely secondary to selection pressures induced by aggressive prophylactic strategies targeting Gram-negative organisms during periods of severe neutropenia. As neutropenia persists into the second and third week following transplantation, the selective pressure of antimicrobials targeting Gram-negative bacilli results in the emergence of pneumonias caused by resistant 'SPACE' organisms (*Serratia*, *Pseudomonas*, *Acinetobacter*, *Citrobacter*, *Enterobacter*) as well as molds. Monotherapy with antimicrobials, including ticarcillin-clavulanate, piperacillin-tazobactam, ceftazidime, and aztreonam may select for SPACE organisms owing to inducible β-lactamase production. Thus, empiric combination therapy against Gram-negative bacilli during the early neutropenic phase is recommended to prevent the emergence of SPACE pathogens. Fatal pneumonias caused by Gram-negative pathogens with *Legionella* and *S. maltophilia* have also been documented during the pre-engraftment period. Antimicrobial prophylaxis with trimethoprim-sulfamethoxazole or fluoroquinolones is commonly used in the immediate posttransplant setting. This regimen confers a higher risk for the development of *Strept. viridans* pneumonia and streptococcal toxic shock syndrome because of the less predictable coverage by these antibiotics against Gram-positive organisms.[53] Pneumonias caused by *Strept. viridans* are rapidly progressive. Palmar desquamation associated with a generalized rash is a clue to the diagnosis of this frequently fatal disease. Intravenous catheters and mucositis are dominant predisposing factors in the majority of Gram-positive infections during the period of neutropenia. Hence, the widespread use of indwelling central venous catheters and mucosal excoriation associated with pre-transplant high-dose chemotherapy also contribute to the shift in the microbial spectrum of pulmonary pathogens in this setting.[9,54]

The overall incidence of pre-engraftment fungal pneumonias has declined over the past two decades, coincident with the increased use of peripheral blood stem cell sources and the associated reduction in the duration of posttransplant neutropenia. Cord blood transplantation was associated with an increased risk of fungal pneumonia in one recent study, presumably as a result of delayed reconstitution of neutrophil and cellular immunity.[55,56] The dominant fungal infections encountered during the pre-engraftment period include the filamentous fungal pathogens (*Aspergillus*, *Fusarium*, and *Mucormycosis*) and the risk of infection caused by these organisms increases as the number of neutrophils falls below $100/mm^3$ and as the period of neutropenia extends beyond 7–14 days. The routine use of aggressive prophylactic therapy with azole derivatives after transplantation has successfully reduced the morbidity and mortality of pneumonias caused by *Candida albicans*, which are now rare. Unfortunately, these prophylactic strategies have promoted the emergence of triazole-resistant strains of nonalbicans candidal species, including *Candida glabrata* and *Candida kruseii*. The respiratory viruses (respiratory syncytial virus, parainfluenza virus, rhinovirus, influenza virus type A and B) have prominent seasonal presentations and may be particularly troublesome early on. In addition, infections caused by *Herpes simplex* virus may give rise to particularly fulminant pneumonias as a result of reactivation of latent infection or as primary disease.

Intermediate post-engraftment stage

In the intermediate post-engraftment stage, profound suppression of both the cellular and humoral arms of the host defense system encourages the development of unusual intracellular pathogens, including those caused by *Nocardia*, *Legionella*, *Mycobacteria*, and *Salmonella*. This period typically begins around week 3 and may persist for 3 months following transplantation. Reconstitution of lymphocyte numbers and partial recovery of nonspecific cytotoxic and proliferative activity of lymphocytes may be seen during this stage, although full lymphocyte activities may remain impaired for 12 months or more following transplantation.

Increased rates of infections caused by endemic fungi (*Histoplasmosis, Coccidioidomycosis*), as well as *Aspergillus, Fusarium, Zygomycetes* [*Mucorales, Rhizopus*], *Pseudallescheria boydii*, and resistant *Candida*, have also been reported during this time period. Pneumonias caused by *Fusarium* and *Zygomycetes* may closely mimic invasive aspergillosis clinically, frequently with fatal outcomes. Overall 1-year survival rates among patients infected with pathogenic molds following HSCT remain low (20 percent), although mortality rates caused by nonfumigatous *Aspergillus, Zygomycetes*, and *Fusarium* have improved slightly over the past decade.[57] The routine use of chemoprophylactic strategies through the immediate post-engraftment period that target *P. jiroveci* pneumonia has markedly reduced the incidence of this infection. Pneumonias owing to endemic fungi such as *Coccidioidomycosis, Cryptococcosis*, and *Histoplasmosis* may also be problematic during the immediate posttransplant period. Typical and atypical mycobacteria may rarely occur, usually as a consequence of reactivation or *de novo* disease.

The preponderance of viral infections in the post-engraftment period is due to reactivation of dormant viral organisms. Viral pneumonias caused by immunomodulating viruses (CMV, herpes simplex virus, Ebstein–Barr virus) are particularly prominent during this period and tend to occur at a higher frequency than in other types of organ transplants.[47,48] These viruses, as well as those typically found in the community (adenovirus, rhinovirus, respiratory syncytial virus) may be particularly troublesome during this time period. Pre-transplant donor CMV seropositivity is a dominant factor in the subsequent emergence of CMV infection in the seronegative transplant recipient. Seasonal fluctuations of enteric viruses (Norwalk virus, Coxsackie virus, echovirus, rotavirus) may also be seen.

Common viral pathogens during the immediate post-engraftment period include the immunomodulating viruses (CMV, herpes simplex virus) as well as those typically found in the community (adenovirus, rhinoviruses, and respiratory syncytial virus). Reactivation of endogenous latent infection caused by CMV or herpes simplex virus is typical although primary disease caused by the acquisition of infection from seropositive donors is seen in approximately 30 percent of patients.[47] Reactivated CMV infection is more commonly seen among allogeneic transplant recipients. Among the viral pathogens causing pneumonia following HSCT, reactivated CMV is the most common and the most virulent. The institution of aggressive strategies for the early detection of CMV coupled with early pre-emptive CMV therapy, has resulted in marked reductions in the incidence of transplant-related CMV pneumonia during the first 100 days following transplant. However, increased rates of late CMV disease (>100 days) have been noted, owing to delayed CMV-specific immune reconstitution.[58] Seasonal outbreaks caused by enteric viruses such as Norwalk, Coxsackie, echovirus, and rotavirus have also been reported.

Late post–engraftment stage

The late post-engraftment period characteristically occurs 3 months or more following transplantation. Severe, persistent dysfunction of the cellular and humoral immune arms of host defense coupled with mucocutaneous damage and hyposplenism highlight this stage of transplantation and facilitates the development of aggressive bacterial and fungal infections. Infectious complications during the late post-engraftment period are tightly linked to the appearance of chronic GVHD and, thus, are typically seen only among recipients of allogeneic transplants. The resurgence of recalcitrant, late bacterial infections caused by *Staphylococci, Strept. pneumoniae, N. meningitides, H. influenza*, and Gram-negative bacteria, including *Pseudomonas* species are common during this period. Functional and anatomic asplenia are common during this period of transplantation and may trigger the development of recalcitrant infections by encapsulated organisms. Viral infections caused by varicella zoster and Epstein–Barr virus occur with increased frequency, primarily as a result of reactivated disease. These viruses may occasionally widely disseminate, especially in the setting of intense antirejection immunosuppressive therapy, absolute lymphopenia, or a prior history of acute GVHD, resulting in fulminant and often fatal infections. Stringent antimicrobial prophylaxis against *P. jiroveci* during the early transplant period has markedly reduced the early occurrence of infection with this pathogen. These prophylactic strategies are relaxed during the late post-engraftment stage, resulting in a recrudescence of *P. jiroveci* pneumonia during this time period.

Over the past decade, the incidence of fungal infections following HSCT has increased, particularly following engraftment.[59] Post-engraftment invasive aspergillosis has increased among both allogeneic and autologous transplant recipients, although rates among allogeneic transplant recipients far outnumber those noted among recipients of autologous transplants.[59,60] The shift to late post-engraftment invasive aspergillosis appears coincident with the development of chronic GVHD and the attendant need for augmented immunosuppressive therapy.[57] In addition, neutrophil dysfunction, lymphopenia, corticosteroid therapy, and viral infections augment the risk of these late infections. Among the viral infections, CMV seropositivity and/or disease significantly increases the risk of subsequent invasive aspergillosis, independent of corticosteroid administration, neutropenia, and T cell engraftment.[59,61]

NONINFECTIOUS COMPLICATIONS OF HSCT

Early onset noninfectious complications

PULMONARY EDEMA

Pulmonary edema is a common complication that appears early after transplantation. The broad etiologic spectrum of post-transplant pulmonary edema includes conditions that occur as a consequence of alterations in hydrostatic pressure (large volume fluid resuscitation, chemoradiation-induced cardiac toxicity) and those caused by increased pulmonary capillary permeability (acute lung injury/acute respiratory distress syndrome associated with fat embolism or DMSO administration during stem cell infusion, chemoradiation-induced lung toxicity, sepsis, stem cell engraftment, aspiration, peri-engraftment respiratory distress syndrome).[4] Coexistent hydrostatic and permeability etiologies of pulmonary edema are common and may overlap with other early-onset pulmonary complications, which add to the diagnostic dilemma. Cough and dyspnea are usual presenting symptoms. Fever may be variably present, depending on the underlying disorder. Management includes the judicious use of diuretics coupled with measures aimed at treating the underlying disorder.

PERI-ENGRAFTMENT RESPIRATORY DISTRESS SYNDROME

Peri-engraftment respiratory distress syndrome (PERDS) is a capillary leak syndrome that occurs relatively early in the posttransplant course, usually within 5 days of engraftment. It was first described among recipients of autologous transplantation for breast cancer.[62,63] A virtually identical capillary leak syndrome has been reported following allogeneic HSCT; however, the vastly differing treatment outcomes may suggest a fundamental difference in underlying pathophysiology. The reported incidence of PERDS varies widely and most likely reflects the lack of consensus regarding diagnosis. Using clearly defined diagnostic criteria, PERDS is diagnosed in about 4.6 percent of patients following autologous HSCT.[64] The pathogenesis of PERDS is a subject of conjecture. Endothelial damage from the pretransplant conditioning regimens and cytokine release associated with neutrophil recovery at the time of engraftment are implicated mechanisms in the pathogenesis of this disorder. Various risk factors for the development of PERDS have been postulated, including underlying disease, stem cell dose, use of growth factors and amphotericin administration.[65] Patients typically present within the first 5 days of engraftment with symptoms of fever, dyspnea, hypoxia, and diffuse pulmonary infiltrates. This constellation of findings coupled with the absence of known or suspected cardiac dysfunction and pulmonary infections should heighten suspicion for PERDS. Dyspnea is a universal finding. Fever and diffuse pulmonary infiltrates are seen in 63 percent and 68 percent of patients, respectively.[64] The diagnosis is made on the basis of the clinical presentation and a reasonable exclusion of competing diagnoses, such as cardiac dysfunction, alveolar hemorrhage, and infection. Thus, a cardiac evaluation, including echocardiogram and bronchoscopic examination are usually standard components of the diagnostic workup. Common early posttransplant infections that may mimic PERDS include those caused by bacterial or fungal pathogens, herpes virus

and *Pneumocystis* organisms. Aggressive supportive measures, including assisted ventilation, broad-spectrum antibiotics and hemodynamic support are the mainstay of therapy. High-dose corticosteroids, given as 1–2 g/day of methylprednisolone for 3 days followed by a rapid taper, have been shown to be effective in patients with PERDS.[64] While the response to corticosteroids is usually good, the clinical course and prognosis are variable. Respiratory failure and the attendant need for mechanical ventilation are more often seen among allogeneic transplant recipients and portends a poor prognosis.[66]

DIFFUSE ALVEOLAR HEMORRHAGE

Post-transplant DAH was first recognized among autologous transplant recipients as an early complication of HSCT. DAH typically occurs within the first 30 days of transplantation, although late-onset DAH has been reported in 42 percent of cases.[57] This disorder is characterized by progressively bloodier return on bronchoalveolar lavage and widespread lung injury manifested as diffuse radiographic infiltrates that develop in the absence of an identifiable lower tract respiratory tract infection.[67] Later reports have documented DAH among allogeneic transplant recipients with a relative equal frequency to autologous allotypes.[57,68–71] Cytologic evidence of >20 percent hemosiderin-laden macrophages in BAL fluid, an increased alveolar-to-arterial oxygen gradient, and a restrictive ventilatory defect have been added to the diagnostic criteria for DAH. The validity of these diagnostic criteria has been challenged by recent studies that have shown disparities between autopsy-proven and BAL-derived diagnoses of DAH, and the absence of cytologic evidence of DAH in patients with bloody lavage fluid.[72] Although the presence of >20 percent hemosiderin-laden macrophages on BAL fluid is supportive, it may take 48–72 hours for this finding to appear, and thus their absence does not exclude an acute bleed. Furthermore, other disease entities associated with widespread lung injury in the posttransplant setting (PERDS, acute respiratory distress syndrome, IPS) may be associated alveolar hemorrhage, thus making the diagnostic and therapeutic implications of DAH as a distinct entity less clear. In post-mortem investigations, most patients with DAH have evidence of diffuse alveolar damage.[67,72] Thus, the presence of DAH may be a marker of severe acute lung injury rather than a separate disease entity. Interestingly, neither the presence nor severity of thrombocytopenia, a common problem in the early posttransplant setting, has been shown to be predictive of DAH. An abrupt onset of dyspnea, nonproductive cough, and low-grade fever are common presenting symptoms. Hemoptysis is unusual. High-dose corticosteroid therapy (0.5–1.0 g/day) given over 3–4 days with subsequent taper has shown favorable results in retrospective case reports, although no randomized studies supporting this practice have been done.[73] Mortality is high (80–100 percent) among patients who require mechanical ventilation for associated respiratory failure. Late-onset DAH and DAH following allogeneic transplantation confer worse prognoses.

IDIOPATHIC PNEUMONIA SYNDROME

Idiopathic pneumonia syndrome, defined in the 1993 National Heart Lung and Blood Institute consensus statement, describes a syndrome of widespread alveolar injury following HSCT that occurs in the absence of active lower respiratory tract infection or cardiac dysfunction.[74] Idiopathic pneumonia syndrome has been described following both allogeneic and autologous transplantation, with an incidence within the first 120 days of 7.6 percent and 5.7 percent, respectively.[75] Risk factors for the development of IPS include HSCT for a malignancy other than leukemia, high-intensity conditioning regimens, older patient age, total body irradiation, human leukocyte antigen (HLA) disparity, donor CMV seropositivity, and high-grade acute GVHD.[75] A multifactorial etiology is postulated, including occult infection, the release of inflammatory cytokines, and high-intensity myeloablative conditioning regimens. Reduced rates of IPS in patients undergoing nonmyeloablative conditioning regimens lends support to the belief that conditioning regimen toxicity underlies the development of this disorder.[76,77] Oxidative stress associated with the conditioning regimen may play a role in the development of IPS by triggering the release of chemokines associated with the recruitment of inflammatory cells. These events promote the release of cytokines such as TNF-α that perpetuate the inflammatory response. In addition, the association of IPS with GVHD among allogeneic transplant recipients implicates the involvement of alloreactive T lymphocytes in the pathogenesis of this disease.

The histopathologic correlates of IPS are variable but primarily include diffuse alveolar damage and interstitial pneumonitis. Diffuse alveolar injury related to IPS may be manifested radiographically as multilobar pulmonary infiltrates with ground glass opacities or frank consolidation. Negative cultures on BAL and a poor response to broad-spectrum antibiotics support the diagnosis. Transbronchial biopsies offer little additional information and typically are not feasible, owing to thrombocytopenia and/or prohibitive coagulopathy. Patients commonly present within 21–120 days of HSCT with fever, cough, and dyspnea. Many patients rapidly progress to frank respiratory failure requiring ventilatory support. Impaired gas exchange, manifested as hypoxia with hypo- or normocarbia is an early finding.[75] The management of IPS is mainly supportive. Although high-dose corticosteroid therapy is routinely used, the efficacy of this practice has not been evaluated in any randomized study. Murine models and individual case reports have suggested a promising role for novel anti-TNF-α agents, such as etanercept in the treatment of IPS. However, like corticosteroids, the efficacy of this therapy in humans has not been proved.[78] Patients may rapidly deteriorate and the development of respiratory failure signals a very poor outcome. Nearly two-thirds of mechanically ventilated patients with IPS-associated respiratory failure succumb to their disease.[75] Superimposed infectious complications and multiorgan failure among patients who require mechanical ventilation play a major role in increasing the overall mortality.

PULMONARY ALVEOLAR PROTEINOSIS

Rarely, HSCT recipients may present with pulmonary alveolar proteinosis (PAP), a diffuse lung disorder characterized by the excessive accumulation of lipoproteinaceous material into the alveoli with associated severe disturbance in gas exchange. Slowly progressive dyspnea and nonproductive cough are the usual presenting symptoms that typically occur within the first 3 months after HSCT.[1] Chest radiographic findings include bilateral diffuse alveolar densities and diffuse ground-glass attenuation with superimposed interlobular septal thickening and intralobular lines, suggesting a 'crazy paving' pattern. Evidence of a milky BAL effluent, which on cytologic examination contains foamy macrophages engorged with periodic acid-Schiff positive intracellular inclusions and granular, acellular eosinophilic proteinaceous material, suggests the diagnosis. Concentrically laminated phospholipid lamellar bodies seen on electron microscopy are confirmatory, but electron microscopy is rarely needed for diagnosis. Resolution of pulmonary alveolar proteinosis coincident with reconstitution of neutrophils following HSCT has been reported.

PULMONARY VENO-OCCLUSIVE DISEASE

Pulmonary veno-occlusive disease is a rare, but life-threatening cause of pulmonary hypertension that occasionally develops as an early complication of HSCT. Progressive occlusion of pulmonary veins and venules caused by intimal proliferation and fibrosis underlie the development of this disorder[79] The etiology of PVOD is not understood, although toxicity to the pulmonary endothelium following transplantation by chemotherapeutic agents such as mitomycin C, BCNU, and bleomycin or by viral infections has been postulated.[80,81] Nonspecific symptoms of progressive dyspnea and fatigue, occurring 6–8 weeks following HSCT, herald the development of this disease.[82,83] Anecdotal reports of successful treatment with high-dose steroids have been documented in the literature. Because pulmonary venous resistance is fixed, arterial vasodilation may result in marked increases in transcapillary hydrostatic pressure and precipitate fulminant pulmonary edema. Vasodilator therapy should be used with extreme caution.

Late noninfectious complications of HSCT

BRONCHIOLITIS OBLITERANS ORGANIZING PNEUMONIA

A recognized late noninfectious and relatively uncommon complication of HSCT is BOOP, with an incidence of only

1–2 percent among long-term survivors.[6,84] The predominant symptom complex is that of pneumonia rather than airflow obstruction. It can occur in a variety of settings, including viral and mycoplasma infections. The pathogenesis is poorly defined, although the nearly exclusive occurrence following allogeneic HSCT transplantation and the close association with GVHD lend credence to one hypothesis that alloimmunity plays a central role.

Patients typically present at 1–13 months following HSCT with fever, nonproductive cough, dyspnea, and multilobar, patchy, alveolar infiltrates (Fig. 16.4).[6,84] Arterial hypoxia and a restrictive defect on pulmonary function tests are commonly seen. The diagnosis is made by surgical or transbronchial lung biopsy showing intraluminal fibrosis in the small airways with chronic inflammation in the alveolar spaces. Management strategies for BOOP in the posttransplant setting are largely gleaned from experience gained in treating patients with BOOP in the non-HSCT setting. High-dose steroids (1–1.5 g/kg per day) are given initially for 1–3 months, followed by a slow steroid taper over the ensuing 6–12 months. Response to therapy is good with resolution of infiltrates reported in 80 percent of patients within 3 months of treatment initiation.[85] Case reports describing successful therapy with macrolides as steroid-sparing agents have been described.[86]

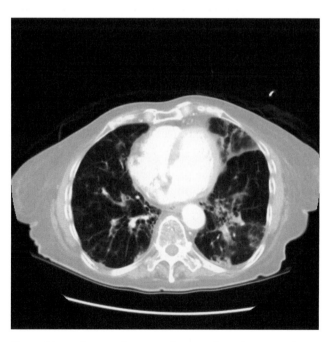

Figure 16.4 *Computed tomography scan of a patient 6 months after allogeneic stem cell transplantation for treatment of acute myeloid leukemia. This patient presented with progressive symptoms of dyspnea and a dry cough. Pathologic analysis of tissue obtained from a video-assisted thoracoscopic biopsy suggested bronchiolitis obliterans organizing pneumonia. The patient was receiving steroid therapy for treatment of chronic graft-versus-host disease at the time of diagnosis.*

CONSTRICTIVE BRONCHIOLITIS

Constrictive bronchiolitis, formally known as bronchiolitis obliterans, is an inflammatory disorder of the small airways that is clinically and pathologically distinct from BOOP. Constrictive bronchiolitis is one of the most common late complications of HSCT, typically emerging after the third transplant month. The lack of uniform diagnostic criteria and reporting requirements precludes precise estimates of the incidence of posttransplant constrictive bronchiolitis which vary widely from 10 percent to 26 percent. In the cancer setting, chronic GVHD, older age, methotrexate or busulfan administration, serum immunoglobulin deficiency, preexisting airflow limitation, and viral infections during the first 100 days after transplant are recognized risk factors for constrictive bronchiolitis.[6,87–89] The appearance of constrictive bronchiolitis is tightly linked to the appearance of chronic GVHD and thus occurs almost exclusively following allogeneic transplantation. Based on this observation an immune-mediated mechanism of constrictive bronchiolitis pathogenesis in which donor cytotoxic T lymphocytes target alloantigens on host bronchiolar epithelial and mesenchymal cells has been suggested. Unrecognized infection, recurrent aspiration associated with GVHD-related esophageal dysfunction, and abnormal local immunoglobulin secretory function within the lungs are also postulated pathogenic mechanisms.[90,91]

Clinically, CB is recognized by airflow obstruction, the hallmark of the disease, and histologically by periluminal fibrosis and narrowing of the small airways. Associated symptoms of nonproductive cough, dyspnea, and wheezing develop insidiously, usually 3 or more months following transplantation. Up to 20 percent of patients may be asymptomatic despite abnormalities noted on pulmonary function testing. The presence of fever is so rare that its occurrence should prompt the search for alternative diagnoses such as intercurrent infection.[92] Although the chest radiograph is usually unrevealing, high-resolution CT exams are typically abnormal and may demonstrate evidence of hypoattenuation, bronchial dilatation, mosaic perfusion, bronchiolectasis, or expiratory air trapping.[93]

The diagnosis of constrictive bronchiolitis is based on evidence of persistent airflow obstruction on pulmonary function testing coupled with the exclusion of alternative diagnoses. Bronchioalveolar lavage typically demonstrates neutrophilic and/or lymphocytic inflammation and is an important tool in ruling out infection.[94] Because of the patchy distribution of pulmonary infiltrates and the samples obtained, transbronchial biopsies offer little additional information over BAL alone and are not recommended. Open lung biopsy obtained either through video-assisted thoracic surgery or formal thoracotomy is the only viable option for histologic confirmation of constrictive bronchiolitis. Histologic evidence of intraluminal fibrosis in the small airways is the gold standard for diagnosis; however, surgical lung biopsy is rarely indicated. The diagnosis, instead, is usually made based on compatible clinical findings in an allogeneic HSCT recipient with a normal chest radiograph. The most reliable benchmark in identifying and quantifying the severity of airflow obstruction is thought to be FEV_1 expressed as a percent of predicted on pulmonary function testing. Disease severity is referred to as mild (FEV_1 of 66–80 percent), moderate (51–65 percent), and severe (FEV_1 < 50 percent).[95] Initial investigations should also include routine blood tests, including a complete blood count with differential, blood urea nitrogen, creatinine, total bilirubin, hepatic transaminases, γ-globulin levels, and urinalysis.[90] The distinction between constrictive bronchiolitis and preexisting obstructive lung disease poses as a difficult challenge. Other causes of respiratory dysfunction in the late posttransplant setting, such as infections, new-onset asthma, or interstitial lung diseases secondary to prior chemotherapy should also be considered.

The management of constrictive bronchiolitis has not been established in any prospective randomized trials. The mainstay of therapy is augmented immunosuppression aimed at controlling GVHD. Toward this end, various regimens are used. Stabilization of lung function has been variably reported with corticosteroid administration. Prednisone may be given at 1–2 mg/kg per day (not to exceed 100 mg/day) and slowly tapered after 4–6 weeks if a response is noted, over the ensuing 6–12 months.[90] Alternative regimens for corticosteroid failures include azathioprine, ciclosporin, macrolides, intravenous immunoglobulin, thalidomide, and photopheresis. However, the efficacy of these novel therapies remains unproved.[96,97] Some experts currently advocate the aggressive use of inhaled corticosteroids and bronchodilators early in the course of disease onset in an effort to limit progression, but empiric data are lacking thus far. The decline in pulmonary function is variable and rapid progression of airflow obstruction is associated with poor outcomes.[92] Response to therapy is poor. Improvement in pulmonary function is seen in less than 20 percent of patients.[84]

POSTTRANSPLANT LYMPHOPROLIFERATIVE DISORDER

Posttransplant lymphoproliferative disorder (PTLD) represents an uncommon, but serious late complication of allogeneic HSCT that occurs in approximately 1 percent of transplant recipients. This disorder arises as a result of dysfunction of cytotoxic T cells, which permits the uncontrolled expansion of B lymphocytes infected with the Ebstein–Barr virus.[98,99] Recipients of T cell depleted donor stem cells, antithymocyte globulin, and patients who received monoclonal anti-T-cell antibodies for prevention of GVHD are particularly vulnerable. Posttransplant lymphoproliferative disorder typically occurs as a multisystem disorder, with involvement of the lungs in 20 percent of the cases as well as other organ systems, including the liver, spleen, and lymph nodes.[100,101] Patients commonly present at 4–12 months following transplantation with dry cough, low-grade fever, and ill-defined pulmonary nodules. Treatment includes reduction of immunosuppressive therapy and infusion of anti-B cell monoclonal antibodies.[102] Potential benefits from infusion of Epstein–Barr-specific cytotoxic T cells have been reported,[103] although not proved in any prospective clinical trials.

LYMPHOCYTIC INTERSTITIAL PNEUMONITIS

Lymphocytic interstitial pneumonitis is a rare cause of late pulmonary complications following allogeneic HSCT that occurs coincident with GVHD.[84,104,105] Patients typically present with dry cough and progressive dyspnea, which may occur 1 or more years after transplantation. Prominent radiographic findings include diffuse, predominantly basilar, reticular, and reticulonodular infiltrates with infiltration of the interstitium. Concomitant infiltration of the airways, resulting in lymphocytic bronchiolitis may also be seen. Patients are frequently poorly steroid responsive. Additional immunosuppressive agents have been tried; however, their true therapeutic value has not been discerned.

FUTURE DIRECTIONS

Although advances in effective prophylactic strategies have reduced the lethal toll of pulmonary complications following HSCT, pulmonary complications remain the leading cause of morbidity and mortality in the posttransplant setting. Strategies such as the expanded use of peripheral blood sources for stem cells and nonmyeloablative preconditioning regimens mitigate the lung toxic effects of chemotherapy and reduce the period of neutropenia, thereby ameliorating the rates of infection, at least during the early peri-engraftment period. Further investigations aimed at curtailing the duration and severity of posttransplant neutropenia may significantly impact patient outcome. For example, pretransplant administration of cytokines or certain cytotoxic agents such as cyclophosphamide increases the number of circulating progenitor cells. These cells may be harvested and subsequently infused following myeloablative chemotherapy regimens, which may limit the duration and severity of posttransplant neutropenia.[106,107] The induction of donor T-lymphocyte hyporesponsiveness and other strategies that are designed to improve posttransplant immune tolerance may greatly diminish the risk of GVHD, obviate the need for prolonged immunosuppressive therapy and reduce the risk of infection as well as other noninfectious pulmonary complications that are mediated by alloimmunity.[108] Successful application of these therapeutic strategies may significantly diminish the rates of transplant-related infectious and noninfectious pulmonary complications in the future.

Key learning points

- Lung injury represents the most common source of morbidity and mortality in HSCT recipients and accounts for a substantial number of deaths, particularly during the first 3 months following transplantation.

- Pneumonia is the most frequent source of infection and the overall leading infectious cause of death following HSCT.

- Early susceptibility to infection is also strongly influenced by the duration of the period of engraftment (neutropenic period). Shortening this period through the administration of alternative hematopoietic precursor sources such as granulocyte colony-stimulating factors and mobilized peripheral blood stem cells effectively reduce the risk of infection.

- The chronologic development of infectious and noninfectious pulmonary complications is tightly linked to the patient's dynamically changing immunologic status subsequent to transplantation and may vary significantly depending on the type of transplant, degree of histocompatibility between the donor and recipient, intensity of myeloablative therapies, duration and severity of immunosuppression, stem cell source, underlying disease and the presence of GVHD, and the attendant need for further immunosuppressive therapy.

- The use of peripheral blood stem cell sources for HSCT has been associated with increased rates of noninfectious inflammatory pulmonary complications, such as DAH, idiopathic pneumonia, and engraftment syndromes which are ostensibly facilitated by the rapid reconstitution of the immune system.

- Atypical clinical and radiographic presentations of pneumonia in the post-transplant setting are common. Although early diagnosis may improve outcome, antimicrobial therapy should not be withheld while diagnostic interventions are undertaken.

- General recommendations in the management of transplant-related pneumonia include the early use of broad-spectrum antibiotics with deescalation of empiric therapy based on clinical response and culture results.

REFERENCES

◆ 1. Krowka MJ, Rosenow EC, Hoagland HC. Pulmonary complications of bone marrow transplantation. *Chest* 1985; **87**: 237–46.

◆ 2. Collin BA, Ramphal R. Lower respiratory tract infections. *Infect Dis Clin North Am* 1998; **12**: 781–805.

● 3. Reed E, Bowden R, Dandliker P, *et al.* Treatment of cytomegalovirus pneumonia with ganciclovir and intravenous cytomegalovirus immunoglobulin in patients with bone marrow transplants. *Ann Intern Med* 1988; **109**: 783–8.

◆ 4. Soubani A, Miller K, Hassoun P. Pulmonary complications of bone marrow transplantation. *Chest* 1996; **109**: 1066–77.

● 5. Weisdorf DJ. Diffuse alveolar hemorrhage: an evolving problem? *Leukemia* 2003; **17**: 1049–50.

◆ 6. Afessa B, Litzow MR, Tefferi A. Bronchiolitis obliterans and other late onset non-infectious pulmonary complications in hematopoietic stem cell transplantation. *Bone Marrow Transplant* 2001; **28**: 425–34.

● 7. Spitzer TR. Engraftment syndrome following hematopoietic stem cell transplantation. *Bone Marrow Transplant* 2001; **27**: 893–8.

● 8. Ibrahim EH, Tracy L, Hill C, *et al.* The occurrence of ventilator-associated pneumonia in a community hospital: risk factors and clinical outcomes. *Chest* 2001; **120**: 555–61.

● 9. Adair CG, Gorman SP, Feron BM, *et al.* Implications of endotracheal tube biofilm for ventilator-associated pneumonia. *Intensive Care Med* 1999; **25**: 1072–6.

✳ 10. Mermel LA, Farr BM, Sherertz RJ, *et al.* Guidelines for the management of intravascular catheter-related infections. *Clin Infect Dis* 2001; **32**: 1249–72.

● 11. Ganz T. Antimicrobial polypeptides in host defense of the respiratory tract. *J Clin Invest* 2002; **109**: 693–7.

● 12. Nathan C. Points of control in inflammation. *Nature* 2002; **420**: 846–52.

● 13. Bergqvist D, Agnelli G, Cohen AT, *et al.* Duration of prophylaxis against venous thromboembolism with enoxaparin after surgery for cancer. *N Engl J Med* 2002; **346**: 975–80.

● 14. Marshall JS. Mast-cell responses to pathogens. *Nat Rev Immunol* 2004; **4**: 787–99.

● 15. Winston D, Territo M, Ho W, *et al.* Alveolar macrophage dysfunction in human bone marrow transplant recipients. *Am J Med* 1982; **73**: 859–66.

● 16. Scapini P, Lapinet-Vera JA, Gasperini S, *et al.* The neutrophil as a cellular source of chemokines. *Immunol Rev* 2000; **177**: 195–203.

● 17. Lehrer R, Cline M. Leukocyte candidacidal activity and resistance to systemic candidiasis in patients with cancer. *Cancer* 1971; **27**: 1211–17.

◆ 18. Stossel T. Phagocytosis. *N Engl J Med* 1974; **290**: 717–23.

● 19. Hubel K, Hegener K, Schnell R, *et al.* Suppressed neutrophil function as a risk factor for severe infection after cytotoxic chemotherapy in patients with acute nonlymphocytic leukemia. *Ann Hematol* 1999; **78**: 73–7.

● 20. Pickering LK, Ericsson CD, Kohl S. Effect of chemotherapeutic agents on metabolic and bactericidal activity of polymorphonuclear leukocytes. *Cancer* 1978; **42**: 1741–6.

● 21. Fanger MW, Erbe DV. Fc gamma receptors in cancer and infectious disease. *Immunol Res* 1992; **11**: 203–16.

✱ 22. Hussein M. Multiple myeloma: an overview of diagnosis and management. *Cleve Clin J Med* 1994; **61**: 285–98.

● 23. Neill AM, Martin IR, Weir R, *et al.* Community acquired pneumonia: aetiology and usefulness of severity criteria on admission. *Thorax* 1996; **51**: 1010–16.

● 24. White DA, Wong PW, Downey R. The utility of open lung biopsy in patients with hematologic malignancies. *Am J Respir Crit Care Med* 2000; **161**(3 Pt 1): 723–9.

● 25. Ewig S, Schlochtermeier M, Goke N, Niederman MS. Applying sputum as a diagnostic tool in pneumonia: limited yield, minimal impact on treatment decisions. *Chest* 2002; **121**: 1486–92.

● 26. Crawford J, Foote M, Morstyn G. Hematopoietic growth factors in cancer chemotherapy. In: *Cancer Chemotherapy and Biological Modifiers Annual 18,* 1999: 250–67.

● 27. Reamer RH, Dey BP, White CA, Mageau RP. Comparison of monolayer and bilayer plates used in antibiotic assay. *J AOAC Int* 1998; **81**: 398–402.

● 28. Ewig S. Diagnosis of ventilator-associated pneumonia: nonroutine tools for routine practice. *Eur Respir J* 1996; **9**: 1339–41.

◆ 29. Hebart H, Loffler J, Meisner C, *et al.* Early detection of aspergillus infection after allogeneic stem cell transplantation by polymerase chain reaction screening. *J Infect Dis* 2000; **181**: 1713–19.

◆ 30. Erjavec Z, Verweij PE. Recent progress in the diagnosis of fungal infections in the immunocompromised host. *Drug Resist Updat* 2002; **5**: 3–10.

● 31. Verweij PE, Meis JF. Microbiological diagnosis of invasive fungal infections in transplant recipients. *Transpl Infect Dis* 2000; **2**: 80–7.

● 32. Verweij PE, Stynen D, Rijs AJ, *et al.* Sandwich enzyme-linked immunosorbent assay compared with Pastorex latex agglutination test for diagnosing invasive aspergillosis in immunocompromised patients. *J Clin Microbiol* 1995; **33**: 1912–14.

✱ 33. Guidelines for the management of adults with hospital-acquired, ventilator-associated, and healthcare-associated pneumonia. *Am J Respir Crit Care Med* 2005; **171**: 388–416.

● 34. Reichenberger F, Habicht J, Matt P, *et al.* Diagnostic yield of bronchoscopy in histologically proven invasive pulmonary aspergillosis. *Bone Marrow Transplant* 1999; **24**: 1195–9.

● 35. Duagan DP, Baker AM, Hurd DD. Bronchoscopic evaluation of pulmonary infiltrates following bone marrow transplantation. *Chest* 1997; **111**: 135–41.

● 36. Dharnidharka VR, Sullivan EK, Stablein DM, *et al.* Risk factors for posttransplant lymphoproliferative disorder (PTLD) in pediatric kidney transplantation: a report of the North American Pediatric Renal Transplant Cooperative Study (NAPRTCS). *Transplantation* 2001; **71**: 1065–8.

● 37. Glazer M, Breuer R, Berkman N, *et al.* Use of fiberoptic bronchoscopy in bone marrow transplant recipients. *Acta Haematol* 1998; **99**: 22–6.

● 38. Casetta M, Blot F, Antoun S, *et al.* Diagnosis of nosocomial pneumonia in cancer patients undergoing mechanicl ventilation. *Chest* 1999; **115**: 1641–5.

● 39. Weiss. Complications of fiberoptic bronchoscopy in thrombocytopenic patients. *Chest* 1993; **104**: 1025–8.

◆ 40. Pisani RJ, Wright AJ. Clinical utility of bronchoalveolar lavage in immunocompromised hosts. *Mayo Clin Proc* 1992; **67**: 221–7.

◆ 41. Torres A, el-Ebiary M, Padro L, *et al.* Validation of different techniques for the diagnosis of ventilator-associated pneumonia. Comparison with immediate postmortem pulmonary biopsy. *Am J Respir Crit Care Med* 1994; **149**: 324–31.

◆ 42. Rouby JJ, Martin De Lassale E, Poete P, *et al.* Nosocomial bronchopneumonia in the critically ill. Histologic and bacteriologic aspects. *Am Rev Respir Dis* 1992; **146**: 1059–66.

◆ 43. Alves C, Nicolas JM, Miro JM, *et al.* Reappraisal of the aetiology and prognostic factors of severe acute respiratory failure in HIV patients. *Eur Respir J* 2001; **17**: 87–93.

◆ 44. Hohenadel IA, Kiworr M, Genitsariotis R, *et al.* Role of bronchoalveolar lavage in immunocompromised patients with pneumonia treated with a broad spectrum antibiotic and antifungal regimen. *Thorax* 2001; **56**: 115–20.

● 45. Balajee SA, Weaver M, Imhof A, *et al. Aspergillus fumigatus* variant with decreased susceptibility to multiple antifungals. *Antimicrob Agents Chemother* 2004; **48**: 1197–203.

◆ 46. Crawford S, Schwartz D, Petersen F, *et al.* Mechanical ventilation after marrow transplantation: risk factors and clinical outcome. *Am Rev Respir Dis* 1988; **137**: 682.

✱ 47. Meyers JD, Thomas E. Infection complicating bone marrow transplantation. In: Rubin R, Young L, eds. *Clinical Approach to Infection in the Compromised Host* 1988: 525–55.

● 48. Clark J. The challenge of bone marrow transplantation [editorial]. *Mayo Clin Proc* 1990; **65**: 111–14.

● 49. Breuer R, Lossos IS, Or R, Krymsky M, *et al.* Abatement of bleomycin-induced pulmonary injury by cell-impermeable inhibitor of phospholipase A2. *Life Sci* 1995; **57**: PL237–40.

● 50. Grow WB, Moreb JS, Roque D, *et al.* Late onset of invasive aspergillus infection in bone marrow transplant patients at a university hospital. *Bone Marrow Transplant* 2002; **29**: 15–19.

● 51. Marschmeyer G, Link H, Hiddemann W, *et al.* Pulmonary infiltrations in febrile patients with neutropenia. *Cancer* 1994; **73**: 2296–304.

● 52. Spanik S, Kukuckova E, Pichna P, *et al.* Analysis of 553 episodes of monomicrobial bacteraemia in cancer patients: any association between risk factors and outcome to particular pathogen? *Support Care Cancer* 1997; **5**: 330–3.

● 53. Bochud P, Calandra T, Francioli P. Bacteremia due to viridans streptococci in neutropenic patients. A review. *Am J Med* 1997; **3**: 256–64.

● 54. Escande MC, Herbrecht R. Prospective study of bacteraemia in cancer patients. Results of a French multicentre study. *Support Care Cancer* 1998; **6**: 273–80.

◆ 55. Powles R, Mehta J, Kulkarni S, *et al.* Allogeneic blood and bone-marrow stem-cell transplantation in haematological malignant diseases: a randomised trial. *Lancet* 2000; **355**: 1231–7.

◆ 56. Storek J, Dawson MA, Storer B, *et al.* Immune reconstitution after allogeneic marrow transplantation compared with blood stem cell transplantation. *Blood* 2001; **97**: 3380–9.

◆ 57. Afessa B, Tefferi A, Litzow MR, *et al.* Diffuse alveolar hemorrhage in hematopoietic stem cell transplant recipients. *Am J Respir Crit Care Med* 2002; **166**: 641–5.

● 58. Li CR, Greenberg PD, Gilbert MJ, *et al.* Recovery of HLA-restricted cytomegalovirus (CMV)-specific T-cell responses after allogeneic bone marrow transplant: correlation with CMV disease and effect of ganciclovir prophylaxis. *Blood* 1994; **83**: 1971–9.

● 59. Marr KA, Carter RA, Boeckh M, *et al.* Invasive aspergillosis in allogeneic stem cell transplant recipients: changes in epidemiology and risk factors. *Blood* 2002; **100**: 4358–66.

● 60. Marr KA, Carter RA, Crippa F, *et al.* Epidemiology and outcome of mould infections in hematopoietic stem cell transplant recipients. *Clin Infect Dis* 2002; **34**: 909–17.

◆ 61. Clark RA, Johnson FL, Klebanoff SJ, Thomas ED. Defective neutrophil chemotaxis in bone marrow transplant patients. *J Clin Invest* 1976; **58**: 22–31.

◆ 62. Lee CK, Gingrich RD, Hohl RJ, Ajram KA. Engraftment syndrome in autologous bone marrow and peripheral stem cell transplantation. *Bone Marrow Transplant* 1995; **16**: 175–82.

● 63. Moreb JS, Kubilis PS, Mullins DL, *et al.* Increased frequency of autoaggression syndrome associated with autologous stem cell transplantation in breast cancer patients. *Bone Marrow Transplant* 1997; **19**: 101–6.

● 64. Capizzi SA, Kumar S, Huneke NE, *et al.* Peri-engraftment respiratory distress syndrome during autologous hematopoietic stem cell transplantation. *Bone Marrow Transplant* 2001; **27**: 1299–303.

● 65. Edenfield WJ, Moores LK, Goodwin G, Lee N. An engraftment syndrome in autologous stem cell transplantation related to mononuclear cell dose. *Bone Marrow Transplant* 2000; **25**: 405–9.

● 66. Cahill RA, Spitzer TR, Mazumder A. Marrow engraftment and clinical manifestations of capillary leak syndrome. *Bone Marrow Transplant* 1996; **18**: 177–84.

◆ 67. Robbins R, Linder J, Stahl M. Diffuse alveolar hemorrhage in autologous bone marrow transplant recipients. *Am J Med* 1989; **87**: 511–18.

● 68. Nevo S, Swan V, Enger C, *et al.* Acute bleeding after bone marrow transplantation (BMT)- incidence and effect on survival. A quantitative analysis in 1,402 patients. *Blood* 1998; **91**: 1469–77.

✱ 69. Metcalf J, Rennard S, Reed E, *et al.* Corticosteroids as adjunctive therapy for diffuse alveolar hemorrhage associated with bone marrow transplantation:

University of Nebraska Medical Center Bone Marrow Transplant Group. *Am J Med* 1994; **96**: 327–34.

70. Jules-Elysee K, Stover D, Yahalom J, *et al.* Pulmonary complications in lymphoma patients treated with high-dose therapy and autologous bone marrow transplantation. *Am Rev Respir Dis* 1992; **146**: 485.

71. Sisson J, Thompson A, Anderson J. Airway inflammation predicts diffuse alveolar hemorrhage during bone marrow transplantation in patients with Hodgkin disease. *Am Rev Respir Dis* 1992; **146**: 439–43.

72. Agusti C, Ramirez J, Picado C, *et al.* Diffuse alveolar hemorrhage in allogeneic bone marrow transplantation. A postmortem study. *Am J Respir Crit Care Med* 1995; **151**: 1006–10.

73. Raptis A, Mavroudis D, Suffredini A. High-dose corticosteroid therapy for diffuse alveolar hemorrhage in allogenic bone marrow stem cell transplant recipients. *Bone Marrow Transplant*ation 1999; **24**: 879–83.

74. Clark JG, Hansen JA, Hertz MI. Idiopathic pneumonia syndrome after bone marrow transplantation. *Am Rev Respir Dis* 1993; **147**: 1601–11.

75. Kantrow SP, Hackman RC, Boeckh M, *et al.* Idiopathic pneumonia syndrome: changing spectrum of lung injury after marrow transplantation. *Transplantation* 1997; **63**: 1079–86.

76. Bhalla KS, Folz RJ. Idiopathic pneumonia syndrome after syngeneic bone marrow transplant in mice. *Am J Respir Crit Care Med* 2002; **166**(12 Pt 1): 1579–89.

77. Fukuda T, Hackman RC, Guthrie KA, *et al.* Risks and outcomes of idiopathic pneumonia syndrome after nonmyeloablative and conventional conditioning regimens for allogeneic hematopoietic stem cell transplantation. *Blood* 2003; **102**: 2777–85.

78. Yanik G, Hellerstedt B, Custer J, *et al.* Etanercept (Enbrel) administration for idiopathic pneumonia syndrome after allogeneic hematopoietic stem cell transplantation. *Biol Blood Marrow Transplant* 2002; **8**: 395–400.

79. Salzman D, Adkins D, Freytes C, LeMaistre C. Malignancy-associated pulmonary veno-occlusive disease: report of a case following autologous bone marrow transplantation and review. *Bone Marrow Transplant* 1996; **18**: 755–60.

80. Mandel J, Mark EJ, Hales CA. Pulmonary veno-occlusive disease. *Am J Respir Crit Care Med* 2000; **162**: 1964–73.

81. Doll DC, Yarbro JW. Vascular toxicity associated with antineoplastic agents. *Semin Oncol* 1992; **19**: 580–96.

82. Crawford SW, Hackman RC, Clark JG. Biopsy diagnosis and clinical outcome of persistent focal pulmonary lesions after marrow transplantation. *Transplantation* 1989; **48**: 266–71.

83. Trobaugh-Lotrario AD, Greffe B, Deterding R, Deutsch G, Quinones R. Pulmonary veno-occlusive disease after autologous bone marrow transplant in a child with stage IV neuroblastoma: case report and literature review. *J Pediatr Hematol Oncol* 2003; **25**: 405–9.

84. Palmas A, Tefferi A, Myers JL, *et al.* Late-onset noninfectious pulmonary complications after allogeneic bone marrow transplantation. *Br J Haematol* 1998; **100**: 680–7.

85. Alasaly K, Muller N, Ostrow DN, *et al.* Cryptogenic organizing pneumonia. A report of 25 cases and a review of the literature. *Medicine (Baltimore)* 1995; **74**: 201–11.

86. Ishii T, Manabe A, Ebihara Y, *et al.* Improvement in bronchiolitis obliterans organizing pneumonia in a child after allogeneic bone marrow transplantation by a combination of oral prednisolone and low dose erythromycin. *Bone Marrow Transplant* 2000; **26**: 907–10.

87. Curtis DJ, Smale A, Thien F, *et al.* Chronic airflow obstruction in long-term survivors of allogeneic bone marrow transplantation. *Bone Marrow Transplant* 1995; **16**: 169–73.

88. Clark JG, Schwartz DA, Flournoy N, *et al.* Risk factors for airflow obstruction in recipients of bone marrow transplants. *Ann Intern Med* 1987; **107**: 648–56.

89. King TE, Jr. Overview of bronchiolitis. *Clin Chest Med* 1993; **14**: 607–10.

90. Crawford SW, Clark JG. Bronchiolitis associated with bone marrow transplantation. *Clin Chest Med* 1993; **14**: 741–9.

91. Holland HK, Wingard JR, Beschorner WE, *et al.* Bronchiolitis obliterans in bone marrow transplantation and its relationship to chronic graft-v-host disease and low serum IgG. *Blood* 1988; **72**: 621–7.

92. Clark J, Crawford S, Madtes D, *et al.* Obstructive lung disease after allogeneic marrow transplantation: clinical presentation and course. *Ann Intern Med* 1989; **111**: 368–76.

93. Philit F, Wiesendanger T, Archimbaud E, *et al.* Post-transplant obstructive lung disease ('bronchiolitis obliterans'): a clinical comparative study of bone marrow and lung transplant patients. *Eur Respir J* 1995; **8**: 551–8.

● 94. St John RC, Gadek JE, Tutschka PJ, *et al.* Analysis of airflow obstruction by bronchoalveolar lavage following bone marrow transplantation. Implications for pathogenesis and treatment. *Chest* 1990; **98**: 600–7.

✱ 95. Cooper JD, Billingham M, Egan T, *et al.* A working formulation for the standardization of nomenclature and for clinical staging of chronic dysfunction in lung allografts. International Society for Heart and Lung Transplantation. *J Heart Lung Transplant* 1993; **12**: 713–6.

◆ 96. Payne L, Chan CK, Fyles G, *et al.* Cyclosporine as possible prophylaxis for obstructive airways disease after allogeneic bone marrow transplantation. *Chest* 1993; **104**: 114–18.

◆ 97. Browne PV, Weisdorf DJ, DeFor T, *et al.* Response to thalidomide therapy in refractory chronic graft-versus-host disease. *Bone Marrow Transplant* 2000; **26**: 865–9.

● 98. Kotloff RM, Ahya VN, Crawford SW. Pulmonary complications of solid organ and hematopoietic stem cell transplantation. *Am J Respir Crit Care Med* 2004; **170**: 22–48.

◆ 99. Papadopoulos EB, Ladanyi M, Emanuel D, *et al.* Infusions of donor leukocytes to treat Epstein-Barr virus-associated lymphoproliferative disorders after allogeneic bone marrow transplantation. *N Engl J Med* 1994; **330**: 1185–91.

● 100. Stevens SJ, Verschuuren EA, Verkuujlen SA, *et al.* Role of Epstein-Barr virus DNA load monitoring in prevention and early detection of post-transplant lymphoproliferative disease. *Leuk Lymphoma* 2002; **43**: 831–40.

● 101. Curtis RE, Travis LB, Rowlings PA, *et al.* Risk of lymphoproliferative disorders after bone marrow transplantation: a multi-institutional study. *Blood* 1999; **94**: 2208–16.

◆ 102. Benkerrou M, Jais JP, Leblond V, *et al.* Anti-B-cell monoclonal antibody treatment of severe posttransplant B-lymphoproliferative disorder: prognostic factors and long-term outcome. *Blood* 1998; **92**: 3137–47.

◆ 103. Gottschalk S, Heslop HE, Roon CM. Treatment of Epstein-Barr virus-associated malignancies with specific T cells. *Adv Cancer Res* 2002; **84**: 175–201.

◆ 104. Yousem SA. The histological spectrum of pulmonary graft-versus-host disease in bone marrow transplant recipients. *Human Pathol* 1995; **26**: 668–75.

◆ 105. Perreault C, Cousineau S, D'Angelo G, *et al.* Lymphoid interstitial pneumonia after allogeneic bone marrow transplantation. A possible manifestation of chronic graft-versus-host disease. *Cancer* 1985; **55**: 1–9.

● 106. Duhrsen U, Villeval JL, Boyd J, *et al.* Effects of recombinant human granulocyte colony-stimulating factor on hematopoietic progenitor cells in cancer patients. *Blood* 1988; **72**: 2074–81.

● 107. Haas R, Ho AD, Bredthauer U, *et al.* Successful autologous transplantation of blood stem cells mobilized with recombinant human granulocyte-macrophage colony-stimulating factor. *Exp Hematol* 1990; **18**: 94–8.

● 108. Guinan EC, Boussiotis VA, Neuberg D, *et al.* Transplantation of anergic histoincompatible bone marrow allografts. *N Engl J Med* 1999; **340**: 1704–14.

17

Respiratory emergencies in human immunodeficiency virus infections

DEEPA G LAZAROUS, ANNE E O'DONNELL

INTRODUCTION

An estimated 362 827 persons are living with acquired immunodeficiency syndrome (AIDS) in the United States.[1] Since the advent of highly active antiretroviral therapy (HAART), survival of patients infected with human immunodeficiency virus (HIV) has improved, with decreased risk of immune suppression and a reduced incidence of opportunistic infections.[2–4] Despite this, there has been an increased utilization of intensive care units (ICUs) in the post-HAART era.[5] Respiratory emergencies triggered by infectious and noninfectious complications of HIV remain common and clinicians need to be vigilant, particularly if HIV has not been previously recognized. Unrecognized HIV is reported to be present in 2.1–4

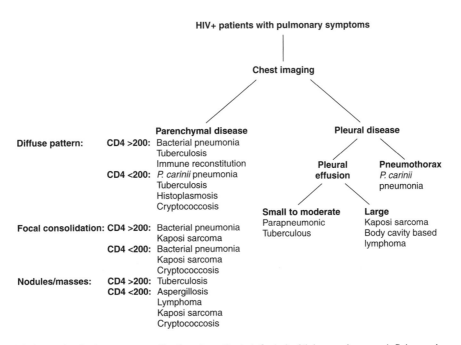

Figure 17.1 *Differential diagnosis of pulmonary complications in patients infected with human immunodeficiency virus.*

percent[6,7] of patients presenting to the emergency room. Of particular note, the prevalence of seropositivity for HIV in black men who have sex with men is as high as 16 percent in the United States,[8] so risk factor assessment is important in all patients presenting with respiratory emergencies.

Patients with HIV infection are at risk for developing many pulmonary complications, both infectious and noninfectious (Fig. 17.1). Infectious complications include bacterial and mycobacterial, fungal, and viral pneumonias. Noninfectious processes include acquired immune deficiency syndrome (AIDS)-related malignancies, inflammatory pneumonitis, pulmonary vascular disease, and pleural diseases. Special attention should also be given to the syndrome of immune reconstitution in patients admitted to the ICU.

INFECTIOUS RESPIRATORY EMERGENCIES

Pneumocystis carinii pneumonia

Pneumocystis carinii pneumonia (PCP) remains the most prevalent of opportunistic infection in AIDS and continues to be the most common cause of respiratory failure in HIV-infected patients admitted to the ICU. The ICU admission rate for PCP ranges from 11 percent to 22 percent.[9,10]

P. carinii pneumonia is often the AIDS-defining illness, particularly in HIV-infected patients with CD4 count <200 cells/mm³. Recently reclassified as a fungus and renamed as *Pneumocystis jiroveci*, this organism is ubiquitous in nature. Although PCP is usually a slowly progressive disorder with symptoms of cough, dyspnea, and low-grade fevers developing over weeks to months, it can occasionally present as an acute illness with rapid development of respiratory failure over a few days.[11] More often respiratory failure occurs when the treatment is postponed or delayed. Physical exam reveals tachypnea and tachycardia, but chest auscultatory findings are typically normal. When PCP leads to respiratory failure, the clinical and radiologic features resemble the acute respiratory distress syndrome (ARDS) with hypoxemia, intrapulmonary shunting, reduced pulmonary compliance, and diffuse alveolar opacities.[12] Diagnosis can be by sputum induction or by flexible bronchoscopy in spontaneously breathing patients or by endotracheal lavage in intubated patients.

Although empiric treatment can be undertaken in patients with a usual presentation of PCP, many physicians elect to proceed with bronchoscopy for definitive diagnosis. Karpel *et al.* found that a diagnosis of PCP was established in 95 percent of intubated patients by infusing 10 aliquots of sterile saline into the endotracheal tube, aspirating, and performing the appropriate tests.[13] There is still debate regarding the need for transbronchial biopsies to confirm the diagnosis of PCP. Given the high burden of organisms in this patient population, a diagnosis is usually established with bronchoalveolar lavage (BAL) in greater than 95 percent of cases.[14] Thus BAL can be performed as the first investigation. Transbronchial biopsies should be performed if a specific diagnosis is not established or if other coexisting conditions such as cytomegalovirus infection are suspected. Of note, patients receiving aerosolized pentamidine for PCP prophylaxis have a lower yield with sputum induction or BAL (60 percent)[15] and may need transbronchial biopsies.

There are at least six different regimens for treating active PCP. Trimethoprim-sulfamethoxazole is considered the drug of choice, and may be administered orally or intravenously. The usual dose is two double-strength tablets orally three times a day or 15 mg/kg per day (based on the trimethoprim component) intravenously in three to four divided doses. The optimal duration of treatment is 21 days. Adverse drug reactions related to treatment are skin rash (including the life-threatening Stevens–Johnson syndrome), neutropenia, hepatitis, and gastrointestinal toxicity. Occasionally trimethoprim-sulfamethoxazole can cause altered mental function with seizures, confusion, or agitation. Intravenous pentamidine is effective against active disease with PCP. The dose is 3–4 mg/kg per day intravenously for 21 days. The adverse drug reactions associated with pentamidine include renal toxicity, hypotension, hypoglycemia, neutropenia, and cardiac arrhythmias. Other regimens for PCP include dapsone-trimethoprim, clindamycin-primaquine, atovaquone, and trimetrexate-leucovorin. These agents are reserved for patients unable to tolerate trimethoprim-sulfamethoxazole or intravenous pentamidine.

Adjunctive corticosteroid therapy has improved survival and has decreased the occurrence of respiratory failure in patients with AIDS and severe PCP.[16,17] Currently corticosteroid therapy is recommended in moderate to severe PCP characterized by a Po_2 of less than 70 mm Hg or an alveolar arterial gradient greater than 35. Although no studies define the optimal dose of steroids, the commonly accepted regimen is prednisone 40 mg twice a day for 5 days, 40 mg once a day for 5 days and 20 mg once a day for 11 days. Respiratory failure requiring mechanical ventilation may ensue despite adequate therapy. In the 1980s a 25 percent incidence of respiratory failure was reported by Maxfield *et al.*[12] Several more recent studies showing a much lower incidence.[2,18] Once respiratory failure develops supportive measures including mechanical ventilation should be initiated. Noninvasive positive pressure ventilation avoided intubation in 67 percent of the studied population in a recent Italian study[19] and should be considered in patients with PCP. When patients with PCP do not improve with standard therapy, concurrent viral or bacterial infection should be ruled out in addition to noninfectious complications.

Bacterial infections

Although primarily a disorder of cell-mediated immunity, HIV infection is associated with substantial dysfunction of humoral immunity thereby increasing the host's susceptibility to bacterial infections.[20]

Bacterial pneumonia is the most common infection seen in HIV-positive patients. It occurs with increased frequency at all CD4 lymphocyte counts, but is much more frequent in those with counts less than 200 cells/mm^3. Other risk factors include smoking and injection drug use. The common etiological agents responsible for bacterial pneumonia include *Streptococcus pneumoniae*, *Haemophilus influenzae*, and *Staphylococcus aureus*.[20] Afessa and Green found that *Pseudomonas* was the most common cause of bacterial pneumonia requiring hospitalization.[21] *Pseudomonas* is an important pathogen in community-acquired pneumonia in the AIDS population especially when CD4 counts are less than 50 cells/mm^3.[22] In the HIV population, pneumonia due to atypical pathogens appears to be uncommon. Rimland *et al.* found that atypical organisms accounted only for 3.7 percent of all bacterial pneumonias.[23] The clinical presentation of bacterial pneumonia in HIV-infected patients is similar to that seen in immunocompetent patients. Patients presents with high fever, chills, and cough productive of purulent sputum. Chest radiographs may show localized areas of consolidation or diffuse disease. However, there are some notable differences between HIV-related bacterial pneumonia and pneumonia in HIV-negative patients. Patients infected with HIV have higher frequency of bacteremia regardless of the causative organism, unusual radiologic abnormalities, a higher incidence of pleural effusions and unusual pathogens such as *Rhodococcus equi* and *Nocardia*.[24] A case–control study by Gil Suay *et al.*[25] showed a twofold increase in the occurrence of pleural effusions associated with bacterial pneumonia in HIV patients. The yield of routine sputum cultures is similar to other invasive diagnostic tests.[26]

Empiric coverage for bacterial pneumonia in HIV patients should include treatment for *Strep. pneumoniae*, *H. influenzae*, and *Staph. aureus*.[20] Penicillin remains the drug of choice for sensitive pneumococcus, but the increased incidence of resistant pneumococcus should be kept in mind. There is geographic variation in the incidence of resistant pneumococcus, e.g. up to 44 percent in Spain compared with 7 to 9 percent in the United States.[21,27] Empiric antipseudomonal coverage should be considered in patients with CD4 counts less than 50 cells/mm^3. Mortality from bacterial pneumonia among HIV-infected patients is similar to the non-HIV population. However, compared with patients without bacterial pneumonia, those HIV-infected patients with bacterial pneumonia had a longer hospital stay, higher ICU admissions, and a higher case fatality rate.[21]

MYCOBACTERIAL INFECTIONS

Tuberculosis is an AIDS-defining illness and every year an estimated 1500–3000 cases are diagnosed in the United States. The risk of tuberculosis is about 50–100 times greater in the HIV-infected population compared with the general population.[28] The symptoms of tuberculosis in HIV-infected patients are similar to the non-HIV population and consist of weight loss, fevers, cough, dyspnea, and hemoptysis. The incidence of extrapulmonary involvement and pleural disease is higher in AIDS patients with tuberculosis.[29]

Chest radiographs typically show mediastinal adenopathy and consolidation with or without cavitation. However, atypical patterns such as interstitial infiltrates can also be seen. There is a relation between chest radiograph findings and CD4 count. In patients with mean CD4 counts greater than 200 cells/mm^3, the radiographic findings are similar to those seen in patients without HIV and include upper lobe infiltrates and cavitation. In patients with CD4 counts less than 200 cells/mm^3, mediastinal adenopathy is more common.[30] Approximately 5 percent of HIV-infected patients with pulmonary tuberculosis have positive results on acid-fast staining of sputum, despite normal findings in chest radiographs.[30] Patients with advanced HIV disease can be asymptomatic despite having abnormal findings in radiographs.

In one series, workup of asymptomatic patients with abnormal findings on chest films revealed tuberculosis to be the most common etiology.[31] The tuberculin skin test is not a reliable test in the setting of HIV, especially if the CD4 count is low. Three separate sputum samples should be collected in all patients suspected of having pulmonary tuberculosis. The reported yield for acid-fast staining of smears varies between 31 percent and 80 percent[32] and culture yield is 85–100 percent.[33] Rapid diagnostic tests are available and provide results within 24 hours. These tests have been approved by the US Food and Drug Administration only for respiratory tract secretions which are positive by acid-fast staining, and they help to differentiate tuberculous mycobacteria from nontuberculous mycobacteria.[34]

The treatment of tuberculosis in HIV-infected patients is similar to that in the non-HIV population. The most recent Centers for Disease Control and Prevention (CDC) guidelines state that the minimal duration of therapy is 6 months. If the clinical or bacteriologic response is slow, then treatment should be given for a total of 9 months.[35] Tuberculosis as a primary cause of respiratory failure requiring mechanical ventilation is uncommon. It occurs more often in miliary tuberculosis than in tuberculous bronchopneumonia.[36,37] Inhospital mortality among patients with tuberculous pneumonia requiring mechanical ventilation is significantly worse than for patients requiring mechanical ventilation for nontuberculous pneumonia. Despite the availability of effective antituberculous therapy, respiratory failure in tuberculosis is often associated with ARDS and is associated with high mortality.[37]

Atypical mycobacteria usually cause disseminated extrapulmonary infection in this patient population, and this rarely, if ever, presents as a respiratory emergency.

Viral infections

CYTOMEGALOVIRUS PNEUMONIA

Cytomegalovirus (CMV) virus is a beta herpes virus, which although commonly found in healthy patients, can cause pneumonia in immunosuppressed states. In HIV, a CD4 count of less than 50 cells/mm^3 is a risk factor for the development of CMV pneumonitis. Common clinical symptoms include cough, fever, and dyspnea with subacute onset. Physical exam may be normal or may show crackles or signs of effusion. Radiographic abnormalities range from ground glass or reticular infiltrates to nodules or effusions.

Establishing CMV as a cause of respiratory failure may be difficult. As CMV is often shed in respiratory secretions, the presence of CMV in bronchioalveolar lavage (BAL) fluid cannot be considered diagnostic of infection. Mann et al.[38] assessed the presence of CMV in HIV-infected patients and correlated its presence with clinical states during a 3-month follow-up period. They found that CMV was frequently detected in BAL fluid of HIV-infected patients regardless of pulmonary symptoms and its presence did not predict significant pulmonary morbidity or mortality. Cytomegalovirus was isolated from BAL fluid in more than 50 percent of HIV positive patients with pulmonary symptoms.[39] However no association was found between CMV and hypoxemia, abnormal chest radiographs, or increased mortality, nor did it significantly increase the severity of PCP. Despite this, the demonstration of CMV in BAL fluid by culture or cytopathic effects may indicate a poor outcome in terms of long-term survival.[40] The only precise criterion for the diagnosis of CMV pulmonary disease is the presence of widespread cytopathic changes in the lungs. Neither culture of BAL fluid nor the presence of cytopathic inclusions in transbronchial biopsy specimens are necessarily sufficient to make a diagnosis of CMV pneumonia.[40] Recently immunostaining of BAL fluid has been described as a helpful method for the diagnosis of CMV pneumonitis.[41]

Cytomegalovirus pneumonia is treated with intravenous ganciclovir or foscarnet. Treatment is divided into an induction phase and a subsequent maintenance phase. Ganciclovir is administered intravenously at 5 mg/kg twice a day for induction followed by 5 mg/kg per day for maintenance. The duration of the induction phase for CMV pneumonitis is not clearly defined, but it is common practice to continue the drug until clinical improvement occurs.[40] Foscarnet is given intravenously at 90 mg/kg twice daily for induction therapy and 120 mg once a day for maintenance therapy. Rapid infusion may cause seizures, the main adverse affect of foscarnet. Given the above data regarding CMV colonization versus infection, clinicians generally treat the underlying identified cause of pneumonia first. If there is no improvement or only partial improvement, then the addition of CMV therapy is indicated.

Other viruses

As in the general population, HIV-infected patients are at risk for developing other viral infections such as influenza, varicella, and zoster pneumonia. These should also be considered in the differential diagnosis of pneumonia, although they are uncommon.

Fungal infections

Although localized and systemic fungal infections are quite common in AIDS, isolated respiratory involvement is rare. In AIDS the most common fungal organism isolated from the respiratory tract is *Candida albicans*, but this usually represents oropharyngeal infection.[42] Candidal pneumonia is rare, except when associated with hematogenous dissemination. *Cryptococcus* is the most common cause of pulmonary fungal infection in AIDS patients. Although pulmonary cryptococcal infection is diagnosed less frequently than meningitis in patients with AIDS, the lung is the most frequent portal of entry.[43] Common presenting symptoms include fever, cough, dyspnea, weight loss, and pleuritic chest pain. Chest radiographic findings are varied and can show focal or diffuse disease including interstitial and alveolar infiltrates, mass lesions with or without cavitation, lymphadenopathy, and pleural effusions.[44] The diagnosis is established by identifying the organism in sputum, BAL, pleural fluid, or lung biopsy. Cryptococcal antigen titers can also be performed. A cryptococcal antigen titer of greater than 1:8 in BAL fluid is considered diagnostic of cryptococcal pneumonia.[45] Cryptococcal pneumonia is treated with amphotericin B or fluconazole. The combination of amphotericin and flucytosine is reserved for people with central nervous system involvement or multiorgan involvement. The natural history of untreated cryptococcosis in an immunocompromised host is that of dissemination.[46] Of note, acute respiratory failure due to cryptococcal pneumonia may be underestimated in the literature. Visnegarwala et al. reported that up to 13 percent of acute respiratory failure in AIDS patients was secondary to cryptococcal pneumonia.[47]

Aspergillus infection is relatively uncommon in AIDS and the incidence ranges from 0 percent to 12.5 percent.[48] However, a spectrum of pulmonary aspergillus involvement has been described, ranging from asymptomatic colonization to aspergillus empyema. Two forms, the invasive parenchymal disease and tracheobronchial disease, seem to be more common. Clinical symptoms vary depending on the form of disease. Invasive pulmonary aspergillosis, which accounts for more than 80 percent,[49] commonly presents with fever, cough, and dyspnea. Radiographs may show cavitary upper lobe disease, focal alveolar infiltrates, or diffuse nodular or reticulonodular disease. Tracheobronchial disease may take three forms:[50–52]

- obstructive bronchial disease – in which the airways are filled with thick mucus plugs
- ulcerative tracheobronchitis – in which there is fungal invasion of the mucosa or the cartilage
- pseudomembranous tracheobronchitis – in which there is extensive inflammation and invasion of the tracheobronchial tree with a pseudomembrane.

Patients with tracheobronchial disease predominantly have dyspnea and wheezing. Chest radiograph may be normal or may show atelectasis or infiltrates.[49] Invasive aspergillosis is exclusively seen in advanced AIDS with CD4 counts of less than 50 cells/mm³. Other risk factors for aspergillosis include marijuana use, neutropenia, broad-spectrum antibiotic use, prior PCP or prior opportunistic fungal infection. Diagnosis of *Aspergillus* infection is problematic, as even lower respiratory tract cultures are not considered reliable. Pisani and Wright noted that more than 60 percent of *Aspergillus* recovered from the lower respiratory tract represented colonization.[53] Hence culture of *Aspergillus*, even from the lower respiratory tract, should be interpreted on the basis of the clinical setting. Current antifungals used in the treatment of invasive aspergillosis include amphotericin and voriconazole. Despite newer modalities of treatment, mortality from invasive aspergillosis remains high.

Disseminated histoplasmosis is an AIDS-defining illness and is usually seen in advanced AIDS manifested by CD4 counts less than 75 cells/mm³. Disseminated histoplasmosis in AIDS can be due to acute infection, reactivation of latent disease or reinfection. Clinical symptoms include fever, hepatosplenomegaly, and lymphadenopathy. Chest radiographic findings are nonspecific and a normal chest radiograph does not exclude pulmonary involvement. *Histoplasmosis capsulatum* can be recovered from sputum, BAL, or lung tissue in up to 70 percent of patients. Disseminated histoplasmosis carries 50 percent mortality and amphotericin B is used to treat severe cases. For less severe disease, itraconazole can be used.

NONINFECTIOUS RESPIRATORY EMERGENCIES

Malignancies

KAPOSI SARCOMA

AIDS-related Kaposi sarcoma occurs primarily in those infected with human herpes virus 8, and is predominantly seen in homosexual and bisexual men. It is a multicentric tumor with mucocutaneous, gastrointestinal, lymph node, and sometimes, pulmonary involvement. Isolated pulmonary involvement in the absence of mucocutaneous involvement is rare.[54] The reported frequency of pulmonary Kaposi sarcoma ranges from 0 percent to 15.3 percent.[55–57] Kaposi sarcoma presents with nonspecific symptoms of dyspnea and cough. Fever and night sweats may be present,

but these symptoms usually suggest a concomitant infection. Hemoptysis may also be seen. Kaposi sarcoma can involve the trachea and the larynx causing hoarseness and stridor.[58]

The radiographic findings of pulmonary Kaposi sarcoma include reticulonodular infiltrates, diffuse interstitial infiltrates, focal airspace consolidation, pleural effusion, and lymphadenopathy.[59,60] Pulmonary Kaposi sarcoma presents some striking findings that provide important clues to the radiologist. The distinct pattern of Kaposi sarcoma following the bronchovascular pathways can result in poorly marginated nodular infiltrates radiating out from both the pulmonary hila along the bronchovascular structures into the surrounding interlobular structures. These are readily apparent on computed tomography (CT).[61] Direct inspection of lesions at bronchoscopy may be the most sensitive technique available for the diagnosis of pulmonary Kaposi sarcoma.[58] Kaposi sarcoma is the most common endobronchial lesion associated with HIV and has a characteristic red or purple macular or papular appearance often located at the airway bifurcations.[62] However, the diagnostic yield by bronchoscopy is only 45–73 percent. Bronchial biopsy is not usually done, as there is a 30 percent incidence of significant hemorrhage.[63]

Kaposi sarcoma is treated with combination chemotherapy, but the outcome is usually poor and relapses are common. Palliative radiation has also been employed to alleviate the dyspnea associated with parenchymal Kaposi sarcoma.

LYMPHOMA

Lymphoma is the second most common malignancy in AIDS. Although it is seen primarily in more advanced disease (CD4 count less than 100/mm³), it can occur at any stage of the disease. In fact, HIV seropositivity itself increases the risk of developing lymphoma by more than 60-fold compared with the general population.[64] Patients may present with typical constitutional symptoms as well as cough and dyspnea. Chest imaging may show multiple nodular densities or diffuse interstitial infiltrates.[65] Transbronchial biopsies are often nondiagnostic and open lung biopsies may be needed. Patients are treated with systemic chemotherapy. Prognosis of patients with AIDS-associated lymphoma is poor with a median survival of 4–6 months.

LUNG CANCER

Several case series have suggested an increased incidence of lung cancer in the HIV-positive population.[66,67] Lung cancer that occurs in association with HIV is seen in younger patients and may have a more aggressive course. The clinical presentation is similar to that in non-HIV patients: cough, dyspnea, and hemoptysis. However, systemic symptoms of fever and weight loss are more common in this patient population.[68] Lung cancer associated with HIV appears to have a more aggressive course with a much poorer survival.[69]

Interstitial pneumonias

LYMPHOID INTERSTITIAL PNEUMONIA

Lymphoid interstitial pneumonia is a rare disease seen in less than 1 percent of HIV-infected patients. It has an insidious onset and presents with dyspnea, cough, and fever. High-resolution CT is the radiographic procedure of choice to define pulmonary opacities in lymphoid interstitial pneumonia.[70] Nodules, ground glass opacities, and thickened bronchovascular bundles can be seen.[71] Thoracoscopic or open lung biopsies are necessary to confirm the diagnosis,[72] as the disease is patchy in nature. Lymphoid interstitial pneumonia is considered a steroid-responsive disease and oral corticosteroids remain the mainstay of therapy. The clinical course is variable; stabilization has been reported in some patients but in others there is progressive decline of pulmonary function and development of honeycomb lung.[71]

Pulmonary vascular disease

PULMONARY HYPERTENSION

It has been estimated that the incidence of pulmonary hypertension in HIV-infected patients is several thousand times greater when compared with the general population. In one series of HIV-infected patients, pulmonary hypertension was present in 0.5 percent overall and 8 percent of those with cardiopulmonary complaints.[73] In contrast with primary pulmonary hypertension, HIV-related pulmonary hypertension has a male predominance, with a male to female ratio of 1.6:1. There appears to be no correlation between either the CD4 count or the stage of the disease and the prevalence or the severity of pulmonary hypertension.[74] The exact mechanism of the development of pulmonary hypertension in HIV is not clear. It is unlikely to be secondary to direct viral action as attempts to locate evidence of HIV infection in human lung tissue have been unsuccessful.[75]

The histopathology of HIV-associated pulmonary vasculopathy is similar to that of primary pulmonary vascular disease and is predominantly a plexiform arteriopathy. Progressive shortness of breath is the most common presenting symptom, followed by pedal edema, nonproductive cough, fatigue, syncope or near-syncope, and chest pain.[76] Chest radiographs may show cardiomegaly, and pulmonary artery prominence and echocardiography shows right heart chamber enlargement and tricuspid regurgitation. Pulmonary vasodilators and antiretroviral therapy are the cornerstones of treatment. The prognosis is poor and the median survival is 1.3 years.[77]

Pleural disease

PLEURAL EFFUSIONS

The reported incidence of pleural effusion in hospitalized patients with HIV is quite variable. In a recent study by

Afessa the incidence was 14 percent.[78] In HIV-infected patients in the United States, bacterial pneumonia is the most common condition associated with pleural effusions.[79] The incidence of parapneumonic effusions is also high in HIV-positive patients when compared with HIV negative controls with community-acquired pneumonia.[25] Although *P. carinii* is a common cause of pneumonia in AIDS patients it rarely causes effusions. Joseph *et al.* found that 15 percent of PCP pneumonias were associated with pleural effusion.[79] However, the organism was rarely identified in the pleural fluid; Joseph *et al.* found organisms in two of nine cases.

Tuberculous pleural involvement is more common in HIV patients compared with patients with tuberculosis who do not have HIV. In a retrospective study by Joseph *et al.*, tuberculous effusions accounted for 10 percent of the total number of patients with pleural effusions and was the most common cause for large to massive effusions.[79] Among patients with AIDS, the percentage of tuberculosis cases with a pleural effusion is higher in patients with CD4 cell counts above 200 cells/mm^3 cells than in patients with CD4 counts less than 200. Tuberculosis-associated effusion is typically a lymphocyte predominant exudative effusion. However, pleural fluid adenosine deaminase levels appear to be less sensitive in identifying patients with tuberculosis in AIDS patients than in non-AIDS patients.[80] Diagnosis of tuberculosis pleuritis in HIV is made in the same way as it is in patients without HIV: by demonstrating acid-fast bacilli in the pleural fluid or in pleural biopsy material or by culturing mycobacterium from the fluid or biopsy specimen.[80]

It is unusual for AIDS-associated fungal infections to be accompanied by pleural effusions. The most common fungal effusions are secondary to *Cryptococcus neoformans* infection where an isolated pleural effusion may be the only manifestation.[81] Malignancy remains the second most common cause of pleural effusion in the HIV population and is frequently the cause of moderate to large effusions. Kaposi sarcoma and non-Hodgkin lymphomas are the most common malignancies in AIDS which cause effusions. About half of the patients with pulmonary Kaposi sarcoma will have pleural effusions. These are mostly hemorrhagic. The definitive diagnosis of pleural Kaposi sarcoma is difficult as the diagnosis cannot be established by cytology or needle biopsy but by thoracoscopy with the characteristic appearance of Kaposi sarcoma lesions on the visceral pleura.[80,82] Pleural effusions secondary to Kaposi sarcoma carry high morbidity and mortality. They respond poorly to chemical pleurodesis and systemic chemotherapy has little impact.

Malignant lymphomas cause pleural effusions due to pleural or mediastinal involvement. Lymphoma related to Kaposi sarcoma related herpes virus (KSHV), also called body cavity based lymphoma, is an uncommon malignancy found mainly in body cavities and presents as a lymphocyte-predominant effusion without an identifiable tumor mass.[83] The pleural fluid in these patients is an exudate with a high level of lactate dehydrogenase.[80] Among the other noninfectious causes of pleural effusion, hypoalbuminemia is the most common. Others include renal failure, congestive heart failure, pancreatitis, and atelectasis. Except in the case of malignancy, pleural effusion in HIV is not an independent predictor of increased mortality.

PNEUMOTHORAX

The incidence of pneumothorax in HIV-infected patients is about 2–6 percent.[84] Most patients with AIDS who develop spontaneous pneumothorax have *P. carinii* infection. All together, about 9 percent of patients with active PCP pneumonia will develop spontaneous pneumothorax.[84,85]

The high incidence of spontaneous pneumothorax in AIDS patients with *P. carinii* infection is due to the presence of multiple subpleural lung cavities, which are associated with subpleural necrosis.[86] There is also an association between spontaneous pneumothorax and aerosolized pentamidine use. Pulmonary tuberculosis[87] and bacterial pneumonias[78] can also cause pneumothorax in HIV. Other risk factors include cigarette smoking and injection drug use.

AIDS-related spontaneous pneumothorax may be difficult to treat; tube thoracostomy alone frequently fails.[84] Chemical pleurodesis, thoracoscopy, Heimlich valve placement, and surgery have all been advocated although none has emerged as the treatment of choice.[86] Metersky *et al.* recommend chest tube placement and empiric PCP therapy while other diagnostic evaluation is under way.[86] If there is complete reexpansion within 5 days, then chemical pleurodesis can be performed. If there is persistent air leak after pleurodesis or if there is incomplete reexpansion of the lungs at 5 days, surgical or thoracoscopic treatment is recommended as long as the patient can tolerate the procedure. If the patient is not a candidate for invasive therapy, then a Heimlich valve with an indwelling chest tube is the alternative treatment.[86] Corticosteroid therapy is associated with increased morbidity from pneumothorax. However, corticosteroids should not be withheld from patients with severe PCP.[86] The development of pneumothorax remains an independent risk factor for increased in hospital mortality.[78]

MISCELLANEOUS CONDITIONS

Immune reconstitution syndrome/immune restitution disease

Immune reconstitution syndrome (IRS) is defined as an acute symptomatic or paradoxical deterioration of a (presumably) preexisting infection that is temporally related to the recovery of the immune system.[88] In HIV-positive patients, IRS is associated with the initiation of HAART which enables sustained suppression of HIV replication and recovery of CD4 T cell counts.[89] The pathogenesis of this syndrome is incompletely defined. Two theories have been proposed: first, IRS represents unmasking of previously latent or incubating infection precipitated by HAART-induced immunologic changes; and second, IRS represents an augmented response to antigens present in low amounts in tissues.[90] The syndrome is estimated to occur in 10–25 percent of patients who receive highly active antiretroviral therapy.[91] It is characterized by paradoxical worsening of clinical or laboratory parameters despite favorable development of the HIV surrogate markers.[88,89] The interval between the start of HAART and the onset of IRS is highly variable, but most events occur within the first 8 weeks after initiation of therapy.[88–90]

Mycobacterial infections are the most common infections associated with IRS and account for about a third of all reported cases.[88] Other infectious agents associated with IRS are *C. neoformans*, cytomegalovirus, and hepatitis B and C virus.[88,89] Sarcoid and autoimmune disease can also rarely present as part of IRS. The clinical manifestations depend on the underlying disease process. Chest radiography and CT may reveal effusions, lymphadenopathy, and worsening parenchymal disease.[88] One of the dilemmas faced by physicians confronting a patient on HAART with an opportunistic infection is to discern immune restoration disease from HAART failure. The former is characterized by a sustained virologic and immunologic response with a rising CD4 count and falling or undetectable viral load.[92] With regard to the management of IRS, the question of whether the syndrome is elicited by an active infection or by persisting antigens arises. If active infection is suspected, antimicrobial therapy is warranted. Modification of treatment should be considered in patients already receiving antimicrobials.[89] Systemic steroids are often considered when inflammatory damage severely impairs organ function.[89]

Lactic acidosis

Lactic acidosis is a rare but often fatal complication in HIV-infected patients treated with nucleoside analog reverse transcriptase inhibitors. Mitochondrial toxicity secondary to this group of medication is thought to be the trigger. Patients present with nonspecific gastrointestinal symptoms: nausea, vomiting, and abdominal pain. Dyspnea and tachypnea secondary to metabolic acidosis are also present.[93] Since the symptoms are nonspecific a high level of clinical suspicion is required for diagnosis. Reported mortality ranges from 33 percent[94] to 60 percent.[95] Riboflavin and thiamine have been used successfully in the treatment of lactic acidosis.

SUMMARY

Despite highly active antiretroviral therapy, respiratory failure remains the most common reason for admission to the ICU among patients with HIV infection.[5,96–99] The ICU and inhospital mortality of HIV-infected patients admitted to the ICU for respiratory failure ranges from 17 percent to 67 percent.[96,99] Despite the decline of incidence of PCP in the era of HAART, PCP remains the most common cause of respiratory failure in patients admitted to the ICU.[97,100] Although overall mortality associated with respiratory failure in this patient population has improved, clinicians continue to see large numbers of these patients. Therefore, awareness of the multiple causes of respiratory emergencies in HIV-infected patients is essential.

Key learning points

- Highly active antiretroviral therapy has dramatically changed the spectrum and the outcome of AIDS.

- Despite this, respiratory emergencies triggered by infectious and noninfectious complications of HIV remain common and clinicians need to be vigilant.

- Pulmonary symptoms in HIV-infected patients may indicate parenchymal or pleural disease.

- *P. carinii* pneumonia continues to be the most common cause of respiratory failure in HIV-infected patients admitted to the ICU.

- Other common etiological agents responsible for bacterial pneumonia in HIV patients include *Strep. pneumoniae, H. influenzae,* and *Staph. aureus.*

- Compared with patients without bacterial pneumonia, HIV-infected patients with bacterial pneumonia have a longer hospital stay, higher ICU admissions, and a higher case fatality rate.

- The risk of tuberculosis is about 50–100 times greater in HIV-infected population compared with the general population.

- Fungal and viral infections also occur and may present as respiratory emergencies.

- Noninfectious causes include Kaposi sarcoma, lymphoma, and lung cancer.

- In HIV-positive patients the immune reconstitution syndrome, an acute symptomatic or paradoxical deterioration of a (presumably) preexisting infection, is associated with the initiation of HAART which enables sustained suppression of HIV replication and recovery of CD4 T cell counts.

REFERENCES

1. Centers for Disease Control and Prevention. HIV/AIDS surveillance report. *MMWR Morb Mortal Wkly* 2001; **13**: 1–48.

2. Palella FJ, Delaney KM, Moorman AC, *et al.* Declining morbidity and mortality among patients with advanced human immunodeficiency virus infection: the HIV Outpatient Study Investigators. *N Engl J Med* 1998; **338**: 853–60.

3. Valdez H, Chowdhry TK, Asaad R, *et al.* Changing spectrum of mortality due to human immunodeficiency virus: analysis of 260 deaths during 1995–1999. *Clin Infect Dis* 2001; **32**: 1487–93.

4. Murphy EL, Collier AC, Kalisch LA, *et al.* Highly active antiretroviral therapy decreases mortality and morbidity in patients with advanced HIV disease. *Ann Intern Med* 2001; **135**: 17–26.

5. Narasimhan M, Posner AJ, DePalo VA, *et al.* Intensive care in patients with HIV infection in the era of highly active anti retroviral therapy. *Chest* 2004; **125**: 1800–4.

6. Nagachinta T, Gold CR, Cheng F, *et al.* Unrecognized HIV-1 infection in inner-city hospital emergency department patients. *Infect Control Hosp Epidemiol* 1996; **17**: 174–7.

7. Kelen GD, Fritz S, Qaqish B, *et al.* Unrecognized human immunodeficiency virus infection in emergency department patients. *N Engl J Med.* 1988; **318**: 1645–50.

8. Unrecognized HIV infection, risk behaviors, and perceptions of risk among young black men who have sex with men – six US cities, 1994–1998. *MMWR Morb Mortal Wkly Rep* 2002; **51**: 733–6.

9. Curtis JR, Bennett CL, Horner RD, *et al.* Variations in intensive care unit utilization for patients with HIV related PCP pneumonia. Importance of hospital characteristics and geographic location. *Crit Care Med* 1998; **26**: 668–75.

10. Afessa B, Green B. Clinical course prognostic factors and outcome prediction for HIV patients in the ICU. The PIP (Pulmonary complications, ICU support, and prognostic factors in hospitalized patients with HIV) Study. *Chest* 2000; **118**: 138–45.

11. Cheeseman SH, Rosen MJ. Infectious disease problems in the intensive care unit. In: Irwin RS, *et al.*, eds. *Irwin and Rippe's Intensive Care Medicine.* Philadelphia: Lippincott Williams & Willkins, 2003: 1958.

12. Maxfield RA, Sorkin B, Fazzini ET, *et al.* Respiratory failure in patients with acquired immunodeficiency syndrome and *Pneumocystis carinii* pneumonia. *Crit Care Med* 1986; **14**: 443–9.

13. Karpel JP, Prezant D, Appel D, *et al.* Endotracheal lavage for the diagnosis of PCP pneumonia in intubated patients with acquired immune deficiency syndrome. *Crit Care Med* 1986; **14**: 741.

14. Golden JA, Hollander H, Stulbarg MS, *et al.* Bronchoalveolar lavage as the exclusive diagnostic modality for Pneumocystis carinii pneumonia. A prospective study among patients with acquired immunodeficiency syndrome. *Chest* 1986; **90**: 18–22.

15. Levine SJ, Masur H, Gill VJ, *et al.* Effect of aerosolized pentamidine prophylaxis on the diagnosis of Pneumocystis carinii pneumonia by induced sputum examination in patients infected with the human immunodeficiency virus. *Am Rev Respir Dis* 1991; **144**: 760–4.

16. Gagnon S, Boota AM, Fischl MA, *et al.* Corticosteroids as adjunctive therapy for severe *Pneumocystis carinii* pneumonia in the acquired immunodeficiency syndrome. A double blind, placebo-controlled trial. *N Engl J Med* 1990; **323**: 1444–50.

17. Bozzette SA, Sattle FR, Chiu J, *et al.* A controlled trial of early adjunctive treatment with corticosteroids for Pneumocystis carinii pneumonia in the acquired immunodeficiency syndrome. California Collaborative Treatment Group. *N Engl J Med* 1990; **323**: 1451–7.

18. Wolff AJ, O'Donnell AE. Pulmonary manifestations of HIV infection in the era of highly active antiretroviral therapy. *Chest* 2001; **120**: 1888–93.

19. Confalonieri M, Calderini E, Terraciano S, *et al.* Noninvasive ventilation for treating acute respiratory failure in AIDS patients with *Pneumocystis carinii* pneumonia. *Intensive Care Med* 2002; **9**: 1233–8.

20. Hirschtick RE, Glassroth J, Jordan MC, *et al.* Bacterial pneumonias in patients infected with HIV, pulmonary complications study group. *N Engl J Med* 1995; **333**: 845–51.

21. Afessa B, Green B. Bacterial pneumonia in hospitalized patients with HIV infection. *Chest* 2000; **117**: 1017–22.

22. Baron AD, Hollander H. Pseudomonas aeruginosa bronchopulmonary infection in late HIV infection. *Am Rev Respir Dis* 1993; **148**: 992–6.

23. Rimland D, Navin TR, Lennox JL, *et al.* Prospective study of etiologic agents of community acquired pneumonia in patients with HIV infection. *AIDS* 2002; **16**: 85–95.

24. Maynaud C, Parrot A, Cadranel J. Pyogenic bacterial lower respiratory tract infections in HIV infected patients. *Eur Respir J* 2002; **20**(Suppl 36): 28s–39s.

25. Gil Suay V, Cordero PJ, Martinez E, *et al.* Para pneumonic effusions secondary to community-acquired bacterial pneumonia in human immunodeficiency virus-infected patients. *Eur Respir J* 1995; **8**: 1934–9.

26. Cordero E, Pachnon J, Rivero A, *et al.* Usefulness of sputum culture for diagnosis of bacterial pneumonia in HIV infected patients. *Eur J Clin Microbiol Infect Dis* 2002; **36**: 28.

27. Friedland IR, McCracken GH. Management of infections caused by antibiotic resistant *Streptococcus* pneumonia. *N Engl J Med* 1994; **331**: 377–82.

28. Markowitz N, Hansen NI, Hopewell PC, *et al.* Incidence of tuberculosis in the United States among HIV infected persons. *Ann Intern Med* 1997; **126**: 123–32.

29. Frye MD, Pozsik CJ, Sahn SA, *et al.* Tuberculous pleurisy is more common in AIDS than in non AIDS patients with tuberculosis. *Chest* 1997; **112**: 393–7.

30. Perlman DC, El-Sadr WM, Nelson ET, *et al.* Variation of chest radiographic patterns in pulmonary tuberculosis by degree of HIV related immunosuppression: at the Terry Berin community programs for clinical research on AIDS. *Clin Infect Dis* 1997; **25**: 242–6.

31. Gold JA, Rom WN, Harkin TJ. Significance of abnormal chest radiograph findings in patients with HIV-1 infection without respiratory symptoms. *Chest* 2002; **121**: 1472–7.

◆ 32. Barnes PF, Bloch AB, Davidson PT Jr. Tuberculosis in patients with human immunodeficiency virus infection. *N Engl J Med* 1991; **324**: 1644–50.

33. Garay SM. Tuberculosis and HIV infection. *Semin Respir Crit Care Med* 1995; **16**: 187.

34. Halvir D, Barnes P. Tuberculosis in patients with HIV Infection. *N Engl J Med* 1999; **340**: 367–73.

35. Centers for Disease Control and Prevention. Treatment of tuberculosis, American Thoracic Society, CDC and Infectious Diseases Society of America. *MMWR* 2003; **52**: 1–77.

36. Shneerson JM. Respiratory failure in tuberculosis: a modern perspective. *Clin Med* 2004; **4**: 72–6.

37. Penner C, Roberts, D Kunnimotto D, *et al.* Tuberculosis as a primary cause of respiratory failure requiring mechanical ventilation. *Am J Respir Crit Care Med* 1995; **151**: 867–72.

38. Mann M, Shelhamer J, Masur H, *et al.* Lack of clinical utility of bronchoalveolar lavage cultures for Cytomegalovirus in HIV infection. *Am J Respir Crit Care Med* 1997; **155**: 1723–8.

39. Miles P, Baughman R, Linnemann C. Cytomegalovirus in the bronchoalveolar lavage fluid of patients with AIDS. *Chest* 1990; **97**: 1072–6.

40. Huang L, Stansell JD. Respiratory manifestations of extra pulmonary disorders. In: Murray JE, Nadel JA, eds. *Textbook of Respiratory Medicine*. Philadelphia: WB Saunders, 2000.

41. Tamm M, Traenkle P, Grilli B, *et al.* Pulmonary cytomegalovirus infection in immunocompromised patients. *Chest* 2001; **119**: 838–43.

42. Hopewell PC, Luce JM. Pulmonary involvement in patients with acquired immune deficiency syndrome. *Chest* 1985; **87**: 104–12.

43. Cameron ML, Bartlett JA, Gallis HA, Waskin HA. Manifestations of pulmonary cryptococcosis in patients with AIDS. *Rev Infect Dis* 1991; **13**: 64–7.

44. Wassar L, Talvera W. Pulmonary cryptococcosis in AIDS. *Chest* 1987; **92**: 692–5.

45. Baughman RP, Rhodes JC, Dohn MN, *et al.* Detection of cryptococcal antigen in bronchoalveolar lavage fluid: a prospective study of diagnostic utility. *Am Rev Respir Dis* 1992; **145**: 1226–9.

46. Kerkering TM, Duma RJ, Shadomy S. The evolution of pulmonary cryptococcosis: clinical implications from a study of 41 patients with and without compromising host factors. *Ann Intern Med* 1981; **94**: 611–16.

47. Visnegarwala F, Graviss EA, Lacke E, *et al.* Acute respiratory failure associated with cryptococcosis in patients with AIDS analysis of predictive factors. *Clin Infect Dis* 1998; **27**: 1231–7.

48. Mylonikis E, Barlam TF, Flanigan T, Rich JD, *et al.* Pulmonary aspergillosis and invasive disease in AIDS. *Chest* 1998; **114**: 251–62.

49. Miller WT Jr, Sais GJ, Frank I, *et al.* Pulmonary aspergillosis in patients with AIDS. Clinical and radiographic correlations. *Chest* 1994; **105**: 37.

50. Denning DW. Unusual manifestations of aspergillosis. *Thorax* 1995; **50**: 812.

51. Kemper CA, Hostetler JS, Follansbee SE, *et al.* Ulcerative and plaque-like tracheobronchitis due to infection with aspergillus in patients with AIDS. *Clin Infect Dis* 1993; **17**: 344.

52. Pervez NK, Kleinerman J, Kattan, M, Freed JA. Pseudomembraneous necrotizing bronchial aspergillosis. A variant of invasive aspergillosis in a patient with hemophilia and acquired immune deficiency syndrome. *Am Rev Respir Dis* 1985; **131**: 961.

53. Pisani RJ, Wright AJ. Clinical utility of bronchoalveolar lavage in immunocompromised host. *Mayo Clin Proc* 1992; **67**: 221–7.

54. Fouret PJ, Touboul JL, Maynaud CM, *et al.* Pulmonary Kaposi's sarcoma in patients with acquired immunodeficiency syndrome: a clinicopathological study. *Thorax* 1987; **42**: 262–8.

55. Garay SM, Belenko M, Fazzini E, *et al.* Pulmonary manifestations of Kaposi's sarcoma. *Chest* 1987; **91**: 39–43.

56. Stover DE, White DA, Romano PA, *et al.* Spectrum of pulmonary diseases associated with acquired immune deficiency syndrome. *Am J Med* 1985; **78**: 429–43.

57. Lemlich G, Schwam L, Lebwhol M. Kaposi's sarcoma in acquired immunodeficiency syndrome: postmortem findings in twenty-four cases. *J Am Acad Dermatol* 1987; **16**: 319–25.

◆ 58. Aboulafia MD. The epidemiologic, pathologic, and clinical features of AIDS-associated pulmonary Kaposi's sarcoma, *Chest.* 2000; **117**: 1128–45.

59. McGuinness G. Changing trends in the pulmonary manifestation of AIDS. *Radiol Clin North Am* 1997; **35**: 1029–82.

60. Denton AS, Miller RF, Spittle MF. Management of pulmonary Kaposi's sarcoma: new perspectives. *Br J Hosp Med* 1995; **53**: 344–50.

61. Sivit CJ, Schwartz AM, Rockoff SD. Kaposi's sarcoma of the lung in AIDS: radiologic-pathologic analyses. *AJR Am J Roentgenol* 1987; **145**: 25–8.

62. Hamm PG, Judson MA, Aranda CP. Diagnosis of pulmonary Kaposi's sarcoma with fiberoptic bronchoscopy and endobronchial biopsy: a report of five cases. *Cancer* 1987; **59**: 807–10.

63. Meduri GU, Stover DE, Lee M, *et al.* Pulmonary Kaposi's sarcoma in the acquired immune deficiency syndrome: clinical, radiographic, and pathologic manifestations. *Am J Med* 1986; **81**: 11–18.

64. Beral V, Peterman T, Berkelman R, Jafffe H. AIDS-associated non Hodgkin's lymphoma. *Lancet* 1991; **337**: 805–9.

65. Polish LB, Cohn DL, Ryder JW, *et al.* Pulmonary non-Hodgkin's lymphoma in AIDS. *Chest* 1989; **96**: 1321.

66. Braun MA, Killam DA, Remick SC, *et al.* Lung cancer in patients seropositive for human immunodeficiency virus. *Radiology* 1990; **175**: 341–3.

67. Parker MS, Leveno DM, Campbell TJ, *et al.* AIDS-related bronchogenic carcinoma. Fact or fiction? *Chest* 1998; **113**: 154–61.

68. Sridhar KS, Flores MR, Raub WA, *et al.* Lung cancer in patients with human immunodeficiency virus

infection compared with historic control subjects. *Chest* 1992; **102**: 1704–8.

69. Vyzula R, Remick SC. Lung cancer in patients with HIV-infection. *Lung Cancer* 1996; **15**: 325–39.

70. Swigris JJ, Berry GJ, Raffin TA, Kuschner WG. Lymphoid interstitial pneumonia: a narrative review. *Chest* 2002; **122**: 2150–64.

71. Prosper M, Omene JA, Ledlie, Odita JC. Clinical significance of resolution of chest X-ray findings in HIV-infected children with lymphocytic interstitial pneumonitis (LIP). *Pediatr Radiol* 1995; **25**: 243–6.

72. Teirstein AS, Rosen MJ. Lymphocytic interstitial pneumonia. *Clin Chest Med* 1988; **9**: 467–71.

73. Speich R, Jenni R, Opravil M, *et al.* Primary pulmonary hypertension and HIV infection. *Chest* 1991; **100**: 1268–71.

74. Seoane L, Shellito J, Welsh D, de Boisblanc BP. Pulmonary hypertension associated with HIV infection. *South Med J* 2000; **94**: 635–9.

75. Mette, SA, Palevsky, HI, Pietra, GG, *et al.* Primary pulmonary hypertension in association with human immunodeficiency virus infection: a possible viral etiology for some forms of hypertensive pulmonary arteriopathy. *Am Rev Respir Dis* 1992; **145**: 1196–200.

76. Mehta NJ, Khan IA, Mehta RN, Sepkowitz DA. HIV-related pulmonary hypertension: analytic review of 131 cases. *Chest* 2000; **118**: 1133–41.

77. Opravil M, Pechere M, Speich R, *et al.* HIV-associated primary pulmonary hypertension. A case control study. Swiss HIV Cohort Study. *Am J Respir Crit Care Med* 1997; **155**: 990–5.

78. Afessa B. Pleural effusion and pneumothorax in hospitalized patients with HIV infection. *Chest* 2000; 117: 1031–7.

79. Joseph J, Strange C, Sahn SA. Pleural effusions in hospitalized patients with AIDS. *Ann Intern Med* 1993; **118**: 856–9.

◆ 80. Light RW, Hamm H. Pleural disease and AIDS. *Eur Respir J* 1997; **10**: 2638–43.

81. Katz AS, Nisenbaum L, Mass B. Pleural effusion as the initial manifestation of disseminated cryptococcosis in AIDS. *Chest* 1989; **96**: 440–1.

82. O'Brien RF, Cohn DL. Serosanguinous pleural effusions in AIDS associated KS. *Chest* 1989; **96**: 460–6.

83. Nador RG; Cesarman E, Chadburn A, *et al.* Primary effusion lymphoma: a distinct clinicopathologic entity associated with Kaposi sarcoma associated herpes virus. *Blood* 1996; **88**: 645–56.

84. Sepkowitz KA, Telzak EE, Gold JW *et al.* Pneumothorax in AIDS. *Ann Intern Med* 1991; **114**: 455–9.

85. McClellan MD, Miller SB, Parsons PE, *et al.* Pneumothorax with PCP in AIDS: incidence and clinical characteristics. *Chest* 1991; **100**: 1224–8.

86. Metersky ML, Colt HG, Olson LK, Shanks TG. AIDS related spontaneous pneumothorax: risk factors and treatment. *Chest* 1995; **108**: 946–51.

87. Tumberello M, Tacconelli E, Pirronti T, *et al.* Pneumothorax in HIV infected patients, role of PCP and tuberculosis. *Eur Respir J* 1997; **10**: 1332–5.

88. Cheng VC, Yuen KY, Chan WM, *et al.* Immunorestitution disease involving the innate and adaptive response. *Clin Infect Dis* 2000; **30**: 882–92.

89. Hirsch HH, Kaufmann G, Sendi P, Battegay M. Immune reconstitution in HIV infected patients. *Clin Infec Dis* 2004; **38**: 1159–66.

90. Cooney EL. Clinical indicators of immune restoration following highly active antiretroviral therapy. *Clin Infect Dis* 2002; **34**: 224–33.

91. French MA, Lenzo N, John M, *et al.* Immune restoration disease after the treatment of immunodeficient HIV infected patients with highly active antiretroviral therapy. *HIV Med* 2000; **1**: 107–15.

92. Davaro RE, Himlan PH. Immune restoration disorders following HAART. *AIDS Read* 1999; **9**: 167–9.

93. Arenas-Pinto A, Grant AD, Dwards S, Weller D. IV Lactic acidosis in HIV infected patients: A systematic review of published cases. *Sex Transm Infect* 2003; **79**: 340–4.

94. Falcó V, Rodríguez D, Ribera E, *et al.* Severe nucleoside-associated lactic acidosis in human immunodeficiency virus-infected patients: report of 12 cases and review of the literature. *Clin Infect Dis* 2002; **34**: 838–46.

95. Stenzel MS, Carpenter CCJ. The management of the complications of antiretroviral therapy. *Infect Dis Clin North Am* 2000; **14**: 851–78.

96. De Palo VA, Millstein BH, Mayo PH, *et al.* Outcome of intensive care in patients with HIV infection. *Chest* 1995; **107**: 506–10.

97. Rosen MJ, Clayton K, Schneider RF, *et al.* Intensive care of patients with HIV infection: utilization, critical illness, and outcome. *Am J Respir Crit Care Med* 1997; **155**: 67–71.

98. Lazard T, Retel O, Guidet B, *et al.* AIDS in a medical intensive care unit: immediate prognosis and long-term survival. *JAMA* 1996; **276**: 1240–5.

99. Casalino E, Mendoza-Sassi G, Wolff M, *et al.* Predictors of short- and long-term survival in HIV-infected patients admitted to the ICU. *Chest* 1998; 113: 421–9.

100. Torres A, El-Ebiary M, Marrades R, *et al.* Etiology and prognostic factors of patients with AIDS presenting life-threatening acute respiratory failure. *Eur Respir J* 1995; 8: 1922–8.

18

Respiratory illnesses related to the intentional release of chemical and biological agents of terror

LISA K MOORES, JAMES A GEILING, ASHA DEVEREAUX, BRIAN M CUNEO

INTRODUCTION

The intentional release of chemical and biologic agents on both the modern battlefield and in civilian terrorist acts has become a realistic threat. The events of September 11, 2001 have reinforced the need for all clinicians to study the medical effects of disasters, particularly those associated with weapons of mass destruction. Although not as common or easy to produce as explosive devices, biologic or chemical weapons nevertheless remain attractive weapons for terrorists' armamentarium for a variety of reasons:[1]

- They are available in stores everywhere.
- They come at a relatively low discount price.
- They have no roaming charges (i.e. a program can be started with a small amount of initial product).
- They are typically odorless, colorless, and tasteless.
- They do not destroy infrastructure.
- They possess a latency period.
- They have previously been used by government institutions (e.g. programs in the former Soviet Union).
- They are poorly detected.
- Many physicians who act as terrorists are knowledgeable about biologic or chemical agents of terror.
- They produce mass media response.

Pulmonary and critical care physicians will treat patients who present to a hospital emergency department or intensive care unit (ICU) following the release of a chemical or biologic agent much as they would for any hazardous material release. Nevertheless, much work lies ahead for these physicians and their institutions, for at least in the United States >70 percent of hospitals may not be prepared to handle such incidents,[2] and recently it was reported that only 20 percent have any plans for managing biologic or chemical agents.[3] This chapter details the recognition and management of patients exposed to chemical or biologic agents of terror, concentrating on those agents likely to be transmitted via the inhalational route or those whose acute presentation is respiratory, regardless of the route of transmission.

DEFINITIONS

Agents likely to be used

Chemical agents of warfare are gaseous, liquid, or solid substances that may be used because of their direct toxic effects. Although any chemical substance can be used, a certain number have been designed as weapons because they are easy to produce, easy to assemble, disperse relatively quickly, have the potential to produce a large number of casualties, and are difficult to treat.[4] Chemical agents are classified according to their physiologic effects.

Nerve agents are irreversible inhibitors of cholinesterase enzymes and lead to neuropathies and respiratory failure. Blistering agents cause chemical burns and when inhaled or ingested can cause respiratory failure, pancytopenia, and cancer. Choking agents often lead to pulmonary edema and can cause permanent lung damage in survivors. Blood agents (cyanide) inhibit cellular respiration, leading to hypoxia and respiratory arrest.[4]

Biologic agents of warfare are defined as living organisms, or material derived from them, intended to cause death. Similar to the chemical agents, those most likely chosen for use in a terrorist attack are those that are easy to produce, require a low dose to cause disease, rapidly lead to death or incapacitance, and are difficult to treat. They are subclassified according to the nature of the agent into viruses (viral hemorrhagic fevers, viral encephalitides, smallpox), rickettsiae (Q fever and Rocky Mountain Spotted Fever), bacteria (anthrax, plague, tularemia), and fungi and protozoa (although these are difficult to weaponize and not likely to be used).[4] The most likely form of release of any of these agents will be the airborne release of an aerosolized or powder preparation. This is because this route is not easy to detect and leads to a rapid dispersal over a large area. It also will lead to a high degree of absorption because of the large surface area of the alveolar bed.

The Centers for Disease Control and Prevention (CDC) classifies bacterial pathogens or their byproducts into three categories based on their infectiousness, ease of dissemination, predicted mortality, availability, and ease of dissemination or weaponization.[5] Anthrax, botulism, plague, smallpox, tularemia, and viral hemorrhagic fevers are considered top priority, or category A agents. This chapter will concentrate on inhalational anthrax, plague pneumonia, and tularemic pneumonia, as these are the agents most likely to lead to a respiratory emergency.

CLINICAL PRESENTATION

Initial approach to victims of chemical or biologic agents

As timely recognition and management is extremely important to the outcome of each individual patient and to containment of further spread of casualties, the initial approach will likely be somewhat empiric. Cieslak[6] has proposed that a simplified, expedient algorithm may aid first-response healthcare providers until more definitive diagnoses can be made. All medical diagnoses depend upon the clinician's initial suspicion that a particular disorder is present. In the case of potential chemical or biologic warfare and terrorism, this is of paramount import, as the incubation period for these agents will lead to an initial delay in the appearance of clinical symptoms. This incubation period can vary from a few hours to a few weeks, but in all cases is longer

for biologic agents than for chemical weapons. Chemical casualties might present within a few minutes to hours, whereas biologic casualties would present over a longer period of time, and generally after a several-day incubation period. As all of these weapons are most effectively disseminated in the aerosol form, the respiratory care provider will likely be involved in the initial decision making concerning the potential agents that may have been used. Use of the epidemiologic distinctions noted above can help formulate the approach.

Another important distinction is that, in a simplified categorization, chemical and biologic agents can also be divided into those that present primarily with respiratory symptoms and those that present with neurologic symptoms. It should be noted that this simplified approach does not allow for the categorization of all potential agents that might be employed in a terrorist or battlefield attack. Nerve agents and botulinum toxin can present with both respiratory and neurologic symptoms. Smallpox is distinguishable by its exanthem, mustard exposure by its skin lesions, and viral hemorrhagic fevers by their bleeding diatheses. In addition, many of the agents that are likely to be used, such as anthrax, plague, and tularemia, may present as a nonspecific febrile illness during their prodromal period. Nonetheless, using the time of onset and whether the symptoms are primarily respiratory or neurologic, Cieslak et al.[6] have proposed a simplified two-by-two matrix for categorization of chemical and biologic casualties. In the initial response, the respiratory care provider will naturally be most concerned about differentiating those conditions that require immediate definitive care from those that require only supportive care. With this in mind, the initial approach can be simplified to include only those agents shown in Table 18.1.

The fact that nerve agents and cyanide can present as both rapid respiratory or neurologic casualties is not of clinical import, as both can be treated in the initial empiric phase. As mentioned earlier, this grouping does omit those diseases presenting with undifferentiated febrile illnesses. However,

Table 18.1 *Classification of agents likely to be used in a terrorist attack*

Rapid-onset respiratory casualties	Delayed-onset respiratory casualties
Nerve agents Cyanide	Inhalational anthrax Pneumonic plague Pneumonic tularemia
Rapid-onset neurologic agents	**Delayed-onset neurologic casualties**
Nerve agents Cyanide	Botulism

Modified from Cieslak et al.[6]

the life-threatening diseases in this category are, for the most part, those that progress to the delayed-onset respiratory syndromes. Therefore, initial empiric therapy would be similar[6]. Using this simplified categorization, initial therapy can be proposed as shown in Table 18.2.

The challenge facing emergency room physicians and respiratory care providers will be to differentiate between diseases that have similar features, or to separate diseases due to exposure to biologic agents from other conditions that occur commonly in the community. Using a syndromic or radiographic approach may help in this regard. Although each disease will be discussed in detail later in the chapter, an initial differential diagnosis based upon the clinical syndrome or radiographic appearance is introduced here.

Table 18.2 *Recommended empiric treatment of casualties in a potential terrorist attack*

Rapid-onset respiratory casualties	Delayed-onset respiratory casualties
Nerve agent antidote and diazepam 10 mg intramuscularly Cyanide antidote if no response to nerve agent antidote	Ciprofloxacin 400 mg intravenously BID or 500 mg orally BID; or doxycycline 100 mg intravenously or orally BID
Rapid-onset neurologic casualties	**Delayed-onset neurologic casualties**
NAAK and diazepam Cyanide antidote kit (if no response to nerve agent kit)	Botulinum antitoxin

Modified from Cieslak et al.[6]

NAAK, Nerve agent antidote kit; BID, twice daily.

Syndromic approach

BIOLOGIC AGENTS

Pulmonary syndromes associated with biologic agents include acute pneumonitis and hemorrhagic mediastinitis. Primary pneumonic plague, which can be distinguished from naturally occurring secondary pneumonic plague by the absence of buboes, presents as an acute febrile illness with pneumonitis. In addition to the fever, patients complain of chest pain, dyspnea, and cough productive of bloody sputum. In the absence of immediate antimicrobial treatment, the disease rapidly progresses to extensive pulmonary consolidation, respiratory failure, sepsis, multiple organ system failure, and death. Unfortunately, there are no radiographic features pathognomonic for plague. Gram stain of sputum, however, should reveal the typical bipolar or 'safety pin' staining pattern of the Gram-negative bacillus.[5]

Inhalational tularemia will also present as an acute pneumonitis. Onset of symptoms is typically abrupt and includes high fevers with chills, rigors, headache, myalgias, sore throat, anorexia, and chest tightness with an associated nonproductive cough. The respiratory symptoms, however, may not be prominent in the early course of the disease. Early radiographs may reveal only peribronchial cuffing, but as the disease progresses there is often consolidation that involves one or more lobes. Pleural effusions and hilar adenopathy may also be present. Diagnosis can be made by fluorescent antibody of sputum or gastric washings; blood cultures are not sensitive.[5]

Inhalational anthrax should be the prime consideration in patients who present with a hemorrhagic mediastinitis. The illness is generally described as biphasic. Initially there is a nonspecific febrile prodrome characterized by fever, chills, malaise, myalgias, and gastrointestinal distress. The pulmonary symptoms will include dyspnea, nonproductive cough, and chest discomfort. Patients may then experience transient improvement, but without treatment they will progress to fulminant septic shock and death. The most sensitive, early sign of anthrax infection is a widened mediastinum with pleural effusions on chest radiography. Computed tomography (CT) scanning is more sensitive and should be performed in those suspected of having inhalational anthrax whose initial plain chest film is unremarkable.[7] Blood cultures, if obtained early, are also usually positive.[5]

CHEMICAL AGENTS

Pulmonary syndromes associated with chemical agents include autonomic dysfunction, irritant or inflammatory effects on the airways, and asphyxiants. Autonomic dysfunction suggests exposure to the organophosphate-based nerve agents. The characteristic 'SLUDGE' toxidrome describes the symptoms seen during the acute phase of nerve agent exposure: salivation, lacrimation, urination, defecation, gastrointestinal distress, and emesis. The pulmonary symptoms seen include chest tightness, wheezing, cough, and bronchorrhea. Death during the acute phase is typically due to respiratory failure. The rapidity and severity of the symptoms will depend upon the method of exposure, as well as the quantity and duration of exposure. High concentration vapor exposure will lead to onset of symptoms within seconds and will progress rapidly to fulminant systemic symptoms, to include unconsciousness, seizures, apnea, and death. With severe dermal exposure, there may be an asymptomatic period of up to 30 minutes, followed by the precipitous onset of the aforementioned systemic symptoms.[5]

Although the nonpulmonary effects of blister agents are myriad, the inflammatory airway symptoms are an early clue to potential exposure to these agents. The clinical effects of the vesicants are similar; the timing of symptom onset often distinguishes lewisite and phosgene oxime, which present within minutes, from mustard, which has a delayed onset of action after 4–8 hours. All agents cause damage to the respiratory tree, beginning with the upper airways. Mild exposures are manifest by ocular symptoms, pharyngeal swelling, pain, and edema, and airway symptoms of dry cough, hoarseness, and wheezing. More severe exposures may result in lower airway inflammation, pseudomembrane formation, or hemorrhagic bronchitis. Exposure to these vesicants can be confused with lung (choke) agents, such as chlorine and phosgene, which will also cause irritation to the tracheobronchial tree. These agents will also cause initial hoarseness, cough, and chest tightness. However, because these agents also cause increases in vascular permeability, they can often be distinguished by the early development of pulmonary edema following the airway symptoms.[5]

The final pulmonary syndrome that may be seen after chemical exposure is that of progressive tissue hypoxia and death. Early signs may include hyperventilation, hypertension, tachycardia, and dyspnea. Later symptoms include central nervous system (CNS) depression progressing to coma, apnea, and death. Recognition of this syndrome should alert the provider to the potential exposure to a blood agent, such as hydrogen cyanide or cyanogen chloride.

Radiographic approach

Being aware of the typical radiographic presentations of the most likely agents is also useful in distinguishing an outbreak. Useful radiographic features are summarized in the Table 18.3. Imaging findings of inhalational anthrax are hilar prominence and mediastinal widening (Fig 18.1). Pleural effusions are also usually present (Fig. 18.2). In contrast, the radiographic manifestation of primary pneumonic plague is a multilobar pneumonia without the presence of hilar or mediastinal adenopathy (Fig.18.3). The radiographic appearance of inhalational tularemia is less specific, and is described as multifocal segmental or lobar infiltrates. Although mediastinal adenopathy is not characteristic, some patients will develop enlarged hilar nodes. Patients with naturally occurring tularemia will often have a bronchopneumonia that is usually bilateral and may cavitate; lymphadenopathy and pleural effusions develop in approximately a third of these patients.[8] The rapid onset of diffuse pulmonary edema should suggest a chemical agent exposure.

Suspecting biologic agents

Finally, the astute physician must keep in mind diseases that occur commonly in the community and may mimic many of the illness caused by the intentional release of biologic agents. Early recognition of disease patterns that are not typical for normal, local occurrence patterns is a key factor in 'syndromic surveillance' for the intentional release of

Table 18.3 *Radiographic patterns in illness resulting from release of biologic agents*

Disease	Interstitial edema	Hilar or mediastinal adenopathy	Segmental or lobar consolidation	Diffuse airspace disease
Anthrax	No	Mediastinal, extensive	Uncommon	No
Plague	No	No	Common	Sometimes
Tularemia	No	Hilar, sometimes	Common	No

Modifed from Ketai *et al.*[8]

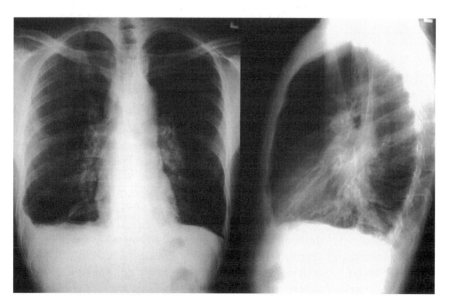

Figure 18.1 *Anteroposterior and lateral chest films of a patient with inhalational anthrax, demonstrating a widened mediastinum and hilar enlargement. (Downloaded, with permission from the Department of Radiographic Pathology, Armed Forces Institute of Pathology.)*

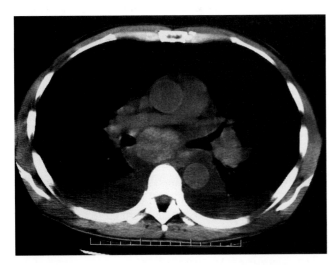

Figure 18.2 *Chest computed tomography scan (enhanced) obtained 4 days after the chest radiograph reveals massive enlargement of subcarinal (arrow) and left hilar lymph nodes (arrowhead), and large bilateral pleural effusions. (Downloaded, with permission from the Department of Radiographic Pathology, Armed Forces Institute of Pathology.)*

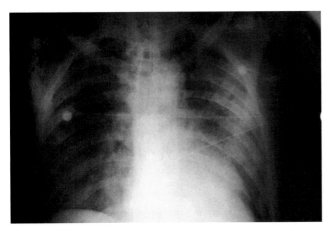

Figure 18.3 *Chest radiograph from a patient with pneumonic plague. (Copied from the Centers for Disease Control and Prevention Pubic Health Information Library.)*

biologic weapons. When first identified, it may not be clear whether an index case is a result of naturally occurring disease or hostile actions. Certain factors, however, make a terrorist attack more likely. Cunha[9] has created a useful comparison of the clinical syndromes of potential bioterrorist agents and their naturally occurring mimics:

- community-acquired pneumonia with hemoptysis – plague or tularemic pneumonia versus cavitary pneumonia, pulmonary embolism, or infarction
- community-acquired pneumonia with nausea, vomiting, diarrhea, and abdominal pain (atypical pneumonia) –

plague or tularemic pneumonia versus *Legionella* or *Mycoplasma pneumoniae*
- pneumonia with chest pain/shock – inhalational anthrax versus acute aortic dissection or myocardial infarction.

Suspecting chemical agents

The most important tool in detecting the use of chemical agents is intelligence information that prompts the use of detection equipment. Unfortunately the first warning of the use of these agents will likely be victims who succumb to their effects. Equipment that senses the presence of chemical agents predominantly consists of point-source detectors, that is they detect the presence of agents from a fixed source close to the agent. The chemical agent monitor or varieties of this technology use ion mobility spectrometry to detect mustard or nerve agents. Chemical agent detector paper and other chemical agent detector kits can sense nerve, blister, and cyanide, though their technologies continue to improve. Standoff detection capability exists to sense agents at a distance, although could clearly be inhibited by meteorologic or geographic constraints. For example, the US Military's Remote Sensing Chemical Agent Alarm (RSCAAL) can sense nerve and blister agents at a distance of 1.5 km. Finally, specialty vehicles such as the Fox NBC Mobile Detector or Recon Vehicle can enter a suspected dangerous area and determine the presence of most chemical as well as biologic agents.

In addition to actively seeking to detect the presence of chemical or biologic agents, a variety of clues may assist medical personnel or others in determining the presence of a chemical or biologic terrorist attack. These include:

- large number of ill persons with a similar syndrome
- large number of cases of unexplained diseases or deaths
- unusual illnesses in a population
- higher morbidity or mortality in a common disease or syndrome
- single case of a disease caused by an uncommon agent
- several unusual or unexplained diseases occurring in the same patient
- disease with an unusual geographic or seasonal distribution
- a lower attack rate in people who were indoors than in those who were outdoors
- illness that is unusual for a given population or age group
- unusual disease presentation
- similar genetic type among agents isolated from distinct sources at different times or locations
- unusual, atypical, genetically engineered, or antiquated agent strain
- stable endemic disease with an unexplained increase in incidence
- simultaneous clusters of a similar illness in noncontiguous areas

- atypical disease transmission through aerosols, food, or water
- point source of disease outbreak with a compressed epidemic curve
- patterns of illness related to ventilation systems
- unusual animal deaths or illnesses preceding or accompanying human disease.

OVERVIEW OF CHEMICAL AGENTS

Decontamination issues regarding management of chemical agent exposures

To adequately care for respiratory emergencies due to a disaster, physicians, staff, and facilities need to maintain a state of readiness and perform regular simulations as currently is standard for a cardiac arrest. In a mass casualty situation, physicians can expect not only the possibility of being the first-responder but also becoming a victim of a chemical event. Patients commonly arrive at a hospital after bypassing any established 'hot zones' put in place by area first-responders or hazardous materials (HAZMAT) personnel.[10,11] Unlike military personnel, for whom personal protective equipment (PPE) is mandated based on intelligence information regarding potential threats, civilians are relatively unprotected. Based on the military experience, mortality approaches 5 percent, but a majority of patients exposed to a chemical agent experience long-term medical issues.[12] Minimizing exposure and maximizing decontamination are the key steps in limiting toxicity following an attack. Effective decontamination decreases further injury to the patient and contamination of medical personnel. Due to the complex nature of the presenting injuries, critical care physicians will be called upon in the management of these victims and therefore can be expected to take a leading role in establishing the policies and protocols for decontamination. Therefore, the initial hospital response to massive decontamination is reviewed prior to presenting details about management of specific chemical agent exposures.

Equipment and supplies needed for mass decontamination

Hospitals must be prepared for ambulatory and nonambulatory decontamination. Most patients arriving without prior decontamination at the site will initially be ambulatory, but preparation for clinical deterioration of these patients should be paramount as they will likely succumb to the effect of any agents on their clothing.[13] The decontamination site should be near the medical treatment facility and away from the ventilatory source. Supplies and equipment recommended for this area are listed in Boxes

18.1 and 18.2. Personnel performing decontamination should wear appropriate PPE. Addressing the ABCs of emergency medical care may supersede decontamination, but can be done safely to protect medical personnel.[14]

Federal regulations and OSHA (Occupational Safety and Health Administration) require that employees be trained to perform their jobs without endangering themselves or others. Of the 1364 emergency personnel responding to the Tokyo sarin gas incident in 1995, 135 (9.9 percent) became symptomatic from the nerve gas and required medical attention. None wore any respiratory protection and exposure was felt to be from the victims' clothing.[16] In addition, 23 percent of staff at the receiving hospital also

---

Box 18.1 Recommended hospital decontamination supply list

- Source of warm water and at least two spray hoses
- Garden hoses
- Spray nozzles
- 600 red bags
- Trauma scissors
- Seat-belt rippers
- 8–10 decontamination litters
- 8–10 38 L (10 gallon) buckets
- Concentrated soap detergent
- Soft brushes
- Sponges
- 300 towels
- 300 patient gowns
- Hazardous material drums
- Barricade tape and portable poles/stands to form barrier
- Privacy screens
- Soap dispensers
- Decontamination powders/solutions
- Tags/bands to match patients to belongings
- Duct tape
- Source for electricity and light[15]

Box 18.2 Medical equipment for the decontamination area

- Endotracheal intubation equipment (laryngeal mask airways may not be effective due to volume of secretions and central nervous system alteration)
- Suction devices
- Ambu Mk 3 bag with self-inflating bag and NATO filtration canister
- Portable ventilator units
- Specific antidotes: atropine, oximes, diazepam, and bronchodilators

experienced symptoms.[16] Since every healthcare facility can expect to receive contaminated patients, there must be written plans and teams trained to decontaminate patients wearing appropriate PPE.[17]

Personnel protective equipment is characteristically divided into four levels of chemical protection from the highest level A (self-contained breathing apparatus [SCBA] with full-body suits) to level D, a simple work uniform.

Level A: Highest level of total body protection. This is a fully encapsulated, chemical-resistant suit and SCBA.

Level B: Highest level of respiratory protection but lesser degree of skin and eye protection; SCBA plus overalls, long sleeves, jacket.

Level C: Used when known substance exposure with unlikely skin and ocular exposure risks. This includes a full facemask with an air-purifying canister respirator and chemical-resistant clothing.

Level D: Work uniform or scrubs. Surgical masks do not protect from toxic gases, vapors, or fumes.

Depending on the agent and level of decontamination performed outside of the facility, most healthcare workers within the ICU or hospital will be working in Level C or D protective gear *as long as decontamination has been performed*.[10] When in doubt, respiratory protection should be used.[14]

Liquid evaporation of chemical agents may take hours depending on their composition, persistence and volatility; therefore, clothing should be carefully removed with attention to avoiding contact with medical personnel's unexposed skin surfaces. Chemicals in contact with a patient's skin should be considered analogous to unextinguished flames as long as the chemical remains in contact with the patient.[18] Dispose of the contaminated garments in impermeable bags or containers with bleaching/decontamination powders. Simple laundering of the clothes exposed to nerve agents should not be considered adequate as toxic levels of residual pesticides have been shown to persist despite laundry with the laundry detergent Cheer®.[19] Removal of contaminated clothing can eliminate 85–90 percent of trapped chemical substances.[20]

Since September 11, 2001, there has been a great deal of research and development of effective decontamination agents. Biocatalytic enzymes that hydrolyze nerve and chemical agents as well as biotoxins are being continually explored for use on skin and equipment. Storage, cost, degradation, and specificity of use are some of the limitations encountered.[21] A relatively new product by Sandia National Laboratories called EasyDECON has a 99.9 percent kill rate for: sarin, soman, tabun, VX, mustard, diphenyl chlorophosphate, *O*-ethyl *S*-ethyl phenyl-phosphonothioate, malathion, 2-chloroethyl ethyl sulfide (half mustard), and 2-chloroethyl phenyl sulfide. It works quickly and deploys as a foam, liquid, aerosol, or a gas leaving

minimal toxicity.[22] Unfortunately, this agent offers no personal protection or passive decontamination. Future investigations continue in the development of a passive means of personal and equipment protection with self-decontaminating materials and fibers.[21]

For ocular emergencies, experience with the decontaminate Diphoterine® in Europe following accidental chemical splashes with 30 percent sodium hydroxide, nitric acid, sulfuric acid, and phosphoric acid show superiority over water or saline irrigation. There is a notable reduction in conjunctival edema and pain relief with initial Diphoterine® use. This agent has been shown *in vitro* to neutralize approximately 600 chemical compounds including sulfur mustard and radionuclides.[23]

In the event of a nonaccidental release of chemicals, as in a terrorist event, people in the vicinity of an explosion are likely to sustain traumatic injuries. Management of these patients can be complicated by the need for stabilization of hemorrhage, drug–chemical agent interactions resulting in challenging anesthesia requirements, and concomitant decontamination issues.[24] Although there are no prospective trials in this area, general consensus remains that the wound should be rinsed with a neutral solution such as saline. Previous military literature cites the use of sodium hypochlorite (0.5 percent and 2.5 percent solutions) to decontaminate patients exposed to chemical and nerve agents. Based on some animal studies, it is believed that this practice would likely potentiate further skin damage.[25] Therefore, sodium bicarbonate or saline solutions are currently recommended for wound irrigation. Cloth fragments or plugs may be embedded in the wound and are not likely to be a threat to medical personnel if the patient arrives with a dressing in place and requires further critical care stabilization. However, thorough excision and debridement of the wound with irrigation should be the goal. During debridement, periodic evaluation of the wound by a chemical detector (CAM, chemical agent monitor) may be helpful to locate unidentified contaminated cloth fibers. However, 'when in doubt, irrigate'.[26] Moreover, during a mass casualty, some aspects of the physical exam may have been overlooked during the initial survey. Ear canals, the axillae, groin, and creases of the buttocks are potential sites of systemic absorption of chemical agents and need to be thoroughly cleansed.[27] Algorithmic steps for treating conventional trauma patients with chemical injuries include:[28]

- airway management – if not intubated, lay patient in lateral decubitus position to manage secretions and vomiting
- securing breathing
- hemorrhage/circulation control
- antidote administration
- decontamination
- dressing of the wound
- rapid evacuation to a noncontaminated site

The hospital as the victim of disaster

Physicians today must not depend on their current work environment as the setting in which they may be required to deliver care in the event of a disaster. Back-up facilities such as schools, community centers, and field hospitals may serve as the hospital. Anticipating lack of communication, power issues, and failure of back-up generators should be included in any practice drill. Following the Northridge earthquake in California in 1994, area hospitals needed to evacuate patients (due to resultant or anticipated structural damage of their facilities) using flashlights, and personnel had to manually ventilate intubated ICU patients for up to 2 hours until they could be managed with portable generators and ventilator units on a nearby lawn.[29] Performing any of these activities in PPE adds a significant challenge to performance of clinical tasks and interpersonal communication, and can cause an increase in heat-related stress and injuries.[30] Tasks such as endotracheal intubation can be prolonged by as much as 46 percent when compared with performance without PPE. In one report tube fixation and manual dexterity were the most common problems cited for the delay.[31] Each hospital now must be prepared to anticipate their 'surge capacity' in the event of a disaster and coordinate evacuation of existing patients to facilitate management of disaster victims.

When any mass casualty occurs, everyone is caught by surprise and frequently a chaotic atmosphere dominates. Actions taken during first aid and decontamination will determine the extent of morbidity and mortality for casualties of chemical victims. It is important to also establish a chain of command for reporting and a method to systematically gather information and data on each patient. Although these 'rules of thumb' were known, it was very difficult to implement during the World Trade Center bombing in New York City on September 11, 2001. Heightened awareness and disaster preparedness will be the cornerstone of management of chemical agent victims and physicians must be aware of the resources available to them.

Agent characteristics

Chemical agents are divided into broad categories based upon their physiologic effects and mechanisms of action. The most common categories include: pulmonary agents; cyanide; vesicants; incapacitating agents; riot control agents; and nerve agents.

PULMONARY AGENTS

The pulmonary agents include chlorine, phosgene (carbonyl chloride [CG]) and diphosgene (trichloromethyl chloroformate [DP]). These agents are denser than air and tend to accumulate in low-lying areas. When exposed to water, they produce hydrochloric acid; in addition, phosgene acylates amino, hydroxyl, and sulfhydryl groups in tissue that results in oxidative injury. The clinical effects are most common in hydrated, mucous membranes such as the conjunctiva and bronchoalveolar spaces.[32]

Clinically, chlorine tends to react in the upper airway, resulting in rhinorrhea, hypersalivation with laryngeal edema as well as some lower airway findings such as cough, wheezing, and rales. Phosgene and diphosgene tend to bypass the upper respiratory tract and become slowly absorbed in the lower tract, resulting in more diffuse bronchoalveolar injury, dyspnea, bronchospasm, and pulmonary leak. The clinical effects have a dose–time response variability. Low dose, short exposure tends to produce minor symptoms, whereas higher doses can result in laryngospasm, pneumonitis, and acute lung injury. Classically the acute respiratory distress syndrome (ARDS) can be delayed for up to 48 hours after exposure.[32] Most chemical agent detection devices can identify these compounds, although some military detection kits and papers cannot. The gases tend to have the odor of newly mown hay or freshly cut grass or corn. Decontamination consists simply of fresh air and copious water irrigation for liquid exposure.

Management of these patients includes enforced rest as exertion can exacerbate symptoms or the appearance of ARDS. Other supportive care includes oxygen and bronchodilators. Corticosteroids have been tried during the latency period following phosgene exposure in an attempt to prevent the appearance of pulmonary edema, although they clearly play no role in the management of the edema once it appears. In addition, animal studies have demonstrated the possible effectiveness of large doses of ibuprofen and acetylcysteine aerosol, but these therapies remain unproved in humans.[33]

CYANIDE

Cyanide is a chemical asphyxiant that in the past has been termed a 'blood agent.' The most common forms include hydrogen cyanide (AC) and cyanogen chloride (CK). The gases are ubiquitous in nature but become poisonous in high concentrations. They are highly volatile gases or colorless liquids; because of their volatility, they are the least toxic of the lethal chemical agents. Absorption tends to occur through inhalation, whereupon they become widely distributed through the blood. They act primarily upon metal-containing enzymes such as cytochrome oxidase in the mitochondria, thereby inhibiting cellular respiration and forcing cells to use anaerobic metabolism.[34]

Symptoms following exposure tend to be few unless victims are exposed to high concentrations. Once cellular respiration becomes impaired, metabolic acidosis develops and the patient becomes restless with tachycardia and tachypnea. Later, these compensatory mechanisms become overwhelmed and patients develop vomiting, respiratory arrest, seizures, and eventually cardiac arrest. Symptoms can appear within 15 seconds following the inhalation of extremely high concentrations and progress to cardiac arrest by 6–8 minutes.[35]

Chemical agent monitors except some detection papers can sense the presence of cyanogens. Decontamination consists simply of removing the victim from the area of exposure as the agents evaporate quickly. Management of cyanide poisoning focuses on increasing the body's detoxification and excretion capabilities. Sodium thiosulfate as a 12.5 g intravenous injection creates thiocyanate from the conversion of cyanide and sodium thiosulfate by the enzyme rhodanese. In addition, patients receive sodium nitrite as 300 mg in 10 mL diluent administered intravenously over 2–4 minutes. Sodium nitrite assists in the formation of methemoglobin that competitively binds the cyanide ions with greater affinity than cytochrome oxidase.[36] Other supportive care includes oxygen and management of the metabolic acidosis that usually appears.

VESICANTS

Vesicants derive their name from the vesicles the agents produce. Two agents comprise this group, mustard (bis-2-chloroethyl sulfide [HD]) and lewisite (2-chlorovinyl dichloroarsine [L]). They have also been combined into mustard-lewisite (HL) mixture. These agents cause a variety of irritant signs and symptoms including ocular irritation, conjunctivitis, and corneal opacity. Inhalation results range from mild upper respiratory complaints to marked airway damage including asthma, chronic bronchitis, bronchiectasis, pulmonary fibrosis, and bronchiolitis obliterans.[37,38] Skin exposure results in erythema at low doses and eventual vesicle formation at higher doses. The principal difference in the agents is the latency of mustard, an asymptomatic period of hours that varies somewhat with the strength of the exposure. Mustard also can cause gastrointestinal effects as well as bone marrow suppression as seen in its use as a chemotherapeutic agent. These agents can be detected by a variety of devices, papers, and alarms.

The recommended decontamination solution is hypochlorite in large amounts, though large quantities of soap and water are more practically employed. Early treatment with nonsteroidal anti-inflammatory drugs has been shown to be beneficial against the cutaneous injury caused by mustard.[20] Skin lesions can also be treated as burns through cooling the skin to approximately 15°C; applying zinc chloride and desferrioxamine to skin lesions may also be effective.[39,40] Respiratory management is mostly symptomatic although patients may benefit from bronchoscopy, including bougienage and laser photoresection if their findings progress.[41] Lewisite has a specific antidote known as British anti-lewisite that may decrease some of the systemic effects.[36]

INCAPACITATING AGENTS

Incapacitating agents serve as tools to suppress a person's defense mechanisms. The classic agent in this group is known as BZ (3-quinuclidinyl benzilate [QNB]). Its actions and effects are anticholinergic, resulting in mydriasis, dry mouth, dry skin, increased deep tendon reflexes, decreased ability to concentrate, disturbed perception and interpretation (illusions and/or hallucinations), denial of illness, short attention span, and finally impaired memory. Not identified by most field detectors, its use must be suspected based upon its toxidrome. Decontamination should be effective with soap and water. Therapy is mostly supportive, though physostigmine can be used for significantly affected individuals.[36]

A variety of other agents can be used to incapacitate patients. Although not normally considered important in discussions on chemical agents, an assortment of nonchemical 'incapacitating agents' needs to be considered when patients present with a variety of symptom complexes. If not directly caused by these 'agents', they can clearly aggravate or mimic the clinical effects of chemical agents. Such products include noise, microwave, high-intensity photostimulation, olfactory assault, staphylococcal enterotoxin B (SEB), riot control agents, nausea-producing agents (DM/adamsite), or psychochemical agents such as stimulants, depressants, barbiturates, opioids, and psychedelics (including LSD, MDMA/ecstasy, PCP). For example, the agent used by Russian authorities to release the 800 hostages in Moscow's Dubrovka Theater in 2002 included the 'calmative' agent carfentanil and possibly halothane.[42]

RIOT CONTROL AGENTS

Other incapacitating agents that have been used include the riot control agents or tear gases, which typically have been placed into their own classification. There are two major versions of these irritants, 2-chloro-1-phenylethanone (CN or MACE™, Mace Security International, Inc., Bennington, VT) and 2-chlorobenzalmalononitrile. More recently a third agent, capsaicin or pepper spray, has been added to this category. These agents cause irritation to exposed mucous membranes and skin, resulting in eye pain and tearing, nasal burning, respiratory discomfort, and tingling of exposed skin. No easily available detector exists, so first indications of its use will be the presentation of casualties. Because these agents are solids, which are dispersed as powders, decontamination consists of fresh air, shaking of clothes, and irrigation of mucous membranes with water. The clinical conditions tend to be mild and effects are self-limiting.[43]

However, more serious complications of these agents have been described, particularly with high-dose exposure. Eye symptoms can progress to a transient conjunctivitis and blepharospasm. Skin findings may eventually include late-onset erythema with vesicle formation, perhaps confusing symptoms with possible mustard exposure. High dose, close proximity exposure to CS has been described to cause profound hypoxia with exercise after exposure, and associated interstitial pneumonitis has been seen on CT scan. Death has also been associated with the use of pepper spray.

Irritation of airways with the spray resulting in laryngospasm, bronchospasm, and eventually respiratory arrest has also been described.[43]

OVERVIEW OF NERVE AGENTS

The nerve agents are the most notorious and feared chemical agents, principally because they are the most toxic. The commonly known agents include:

- GA (tabun): Ethyl N,N-dimethylphosphoramidocyanidate
- GB (sarin): Isopropyl methyl phosphonofluoridate
- GD (soman): Pinacolyl methyl phosphonofluoridate
- GF: O-cyclohexyl-methylphosphonofluoridate
- VX: O-ethyl S-(2-(diisopropylaminoethyl) methyl phosphonothiolate.[44]

These agents can be dispersed from missiles, rockets, bombs, artillery shells, spray tanks, land mines, and a variety of other munitions.

They act through their inhibition of organophosphorus cholinesterases, specifically plasma butyrylcholinesterase, red blood cell (RBC) acetylcholinesterase, and acetylcholinesterase (AChE) at tissue cholinergic receptor sites. Following an acute exposure, the RBC enzyme activity best reflects the tissue AChE activity during recovery. Nerve agents irreversibly bind to AChE and thereby prevent the hydrolysis of the neurotransmitter acetylcholine (ACh); the resultant excess ACh produces the clinical effects of nerve agent toxicity. Because the binding of agent to enzyme is permanent, its activity returns only with new enzyme synthesis or RBC turnover (1 percent/day).[35] Excess ACh affects both muscarinic and nicotinic sites. Affected muscarinic sites include postganglionic parasympathetic fibers, glands, pulmonary and gastrointestinal smooth muscles, and organs targeted by CNS efferent nerves, such as the heart via the vagus nerve. Nicotinic sites include autonomic ganglia and skeletal muscle.

Nerve agents produce a similar clinical syndrome to that of organophosphate insecticide poisoning. The symptom complex has been previously described by the 'SLUDGE' toxidrome: increased salivation, lacrimation, urination, defecation, gastric distress, and emesis.[45] In contrast with insecticides or other cholinesterase inhibitors, nerve agents are more toxic. For example, in vitro sarin has a 1000-fold greater inhibitory action on human blood, brain, and muscle cholinesterase than the insecticide parathion.[46] The agents are most commonly liquids at standard temperatures, with 'G' agents being the most volatile; of the common agents, sarin is the most volatile and VX the least. Vapor or aerosol exposure that, when exposed to a population results in 50 percent of the victims dying, is known as LCt_{50}. Estimated human LCt_{50} for the common nerve agents are:

- tabun vapor – 400 mg min/m^3
- sarin vapor – 100 mg min/m^3
- soman vapor – 50 mg min/m^3
- VX vapor – 30 mg min/m^3.

In contrast with vapor exposure, the cutaneous absorption or LD_{50} for the four agents are:[46]

- tabun – 1000 mg
- sarin – 700 mg
- soman – 350 mg
- VX – 6–10 mg.

Clinical effects

The principal effect on the eyes is miosis, which occurs as a consequence of direct contact with vapor. Rarely does this effect appear in the setting of dermal absorption of an agent unless present in high dose. The symptoms appear shortly after exposure, often within seconds. The pupillary constriction is often associated with an intense sharp or dull pain (which may consequently induce nausea and vomiting). Miosis results in dim or blurred vision and the conjunctive often become injected. Significant lacrimation also usually appears. Rhinorrhea may be the first sign of nerve agent exposure, its significance being dose dependent. Associated bronchorrhea with bronchoconstriction may appear, again depending upon the severity of exposure. Further respiratory compromise develops with diaphragm and other muscle weakness. High-dose exposure may result in CNS-mediated apnea. Usually, a vagally mediated bradycardia may be expected with these agents. However, typically these patients have a 'fight or flight'-induced tachycardia, which in addition to adrenergic surge, may also occur because of hypoxia. Blood pressure remains normal until terminal decline. A variety of dysrhythmias develop, including torsades de pointes. In concert with torsades, QTc prolongation may develop on the electrocardiogram, which, if it appears, may portend a poor prognosis.[47,48]

Exposure results in increased salivary gland secretion as well as other gastrointestinal glandular secretion. Victims may present with significant nausea, vomiting, and diarrhea. Localized sweating may occur at the site of exposure to nerve agent droplets. Generalized sweating typically appears only with a large vapor or skin exposure. Skeletal muscles initially develop fasciculations and twitching, but they become weak, fatigued, and eventually flaccid.

Small exposure to nerve agents produce variable and nonspecific CNS findings, including an inability to concentrate, insomnia, bad dreams, irritability, impaired judgment, and depression. Larger exposure may result in loss of consciousness, seizure activity, and apnea. Psychological and behavioral changes are comprised of anxiety, tenseness, fatigue, forgetfulness, irritability, impaired judgment, and mild confusion. Complete disorientation and hallucinations do not occur. A chronic decline in memory function was seen in rescue teams and police officers at the Tokyo sarin gas release.[49]

Initial effects from nerve agent exposure can be seen within seconds to minutes; the rapidity and severity of symptoms again depend upon the dose. High-dose vapor exposure may present as seizures or loss of consciousness in less than 1 minute, whereas low-dose skin contact may not present as long as 18 hours later when the victim appears with gastrointestinal complaints. The differential diagnosis of patients presenting after nerve agent exposure is limited, though low-dose sporadic cases may be initially diagnosed as upper respiratory tract infections, allergic rhinitis, or gastroenteritis.

Documentation of exposure to nerve agents has both medical and legal implications. Measurement of red cell ChE inhibition is more sensitive than measurement of plasma ChE activity in the setting of nerve agent exposure. However, although helpful in confirming exposure to a nerve agent, the level of enzyme activity inhibition does not correlate with symptom activity. Other laboratory findings that appear include hypoxemia and respiratory acidosis as a consequence of the previously described respiratory signs.[50]

Medical management

Decontamination remains the key element in mitigating the effects of nerve agent poisoning on patients, equipment, and healthcare workers. Following removal of agent, airway and breathing management become paramount. Because of the associated nausea and vomiting seen in these patients, they should be considered to have a full stomach and therefore should undergo cricoid pressure during intubation. Ventilatory support may be problematic because of the increased airway resistance (50–70 cm H_2O). This elevated airway resistance in combination with increased airway secretions makes the laryngeal airway mask less desirable than the esophageal-tracheal CombiTube® if a cuffed endotracheal cannot be placed.[30] Even if adequately treated, assisted ventilation may be required for 30 minutes to 3 hours in severe cases.

In addition to standard supportive care, management of nerve agent casualties hinges on the administration of antidotes. Atropine serves as the principal medication in the treatment of victims of nerve agent exposure. It functions primarily as a cholinergic blocking agent (i.e. it is anticholinergic) and works most effectively at muscarinic sites. The standard 2 mg dose when administered to a nonexposed person will result in mydriasis, decreased secretions and sweating, mild sedation, decreased gastrointestinal motility, and tachycardia. For the treatment of nerve-agent casualties, the recommended atropine dosage is 2 mg every 3–5 minutes, titrated to secretions.[46] Atropine should not be dosed to miosis or eye symptoms, which in the past were treated with topical atropine or homatropine, but currently appear to benefit from the use of tropicamide.[51]

Atropine will usually not be effective in terminating seizures, though other anticholinergics may be successful if given early; these agents include benactyzine, procyclidine, and aprophen.[52]

An additional agent that may be a helpful antidote for nerve agent poisoning is pralidoxime chloride (2-PAMCl), an oxime that attaches to the agent and breaks the agent–enzyme bond. It is effective only at nicotinic sites but thus may help improve muscle strength. It is ineffective in decreasing secretions. Additionally, 'aging' decreases effectiveness, that is the longer nerve agent has been present to bond with AChE, the less likely it will be able to break that agent–enzyme bond. Aging occurs within 2 minutes for soman but within 3–4 hours for sarin. Dosing is 15–25 mg/kg or 1 g intravenously piggyback over 20–30 minutes. Other oximes including obidoxime and the H oximes, HI-6, Hlö-7 and methoxime may eventually provide additional options to reactivate ChE.[53]

Atropine and 2-PAMCl are often combined into an injector kit or system. The MARK I kit (Meridian Medical Technologies, Inc.; Columbia, MD) used by the US military is increasingly becoming available on the civilian market. The AtroPen® Auto-Injector (Meridian Medical Technologies, Inc.) contains 2 mg of atropine and a ComboPen® Auto-Injector (Meridian Medical Technologies, Inc.) contains 600 mg of 2-PAMCl (8.9 mg/kg in a 70 kg person). In the US Army, each soldier is usually issued three kits. Military doctrine recommends that individuals exposed to nerve agent self-administer one MARK I kit if they are experiencing the effects of a nerve agent. If they remain symptomatic, they are instructed to seek 'buddy aid' to determine if additional injections are necessary.

Diazepam remains the anticonvulsant of choice, based primarily on its historical use and demonstrated effectiveness. In settings of high threat of the use of chemical agents, the US military issues a 10 mg auto-injector, which soldiers are trained to administer to their buddy after three MARK Is are given. Medical personnel carry additional diazepam. The centrally acting anticholinergic agent scopolamine may also be effective in the initial phases of seizures.[54] Ketamine has also been shown to have a role as an anticonvulsant because of its a neuroprotective and antiepileptic activities.[55]

Other modalities that have been shown to be effective in nerve agent poisoning include the use of nebulized ipratropium bromide, which may help manage agent-induced bronchospasm. More aggressive therapy may include the use of hemodiafiltration (for 4 hours) followed by hemoperfusion, which was successfully employed in the management of one victim of the Tokyo sarin attack.[35] Future therapies may include bacterial detoxification, the use of nerve agent scavengers such as organophosphorus acid anhydride hydrolase (OPAH), benzodiazepine receptor partial agonists (e.g. bretazenil) in the prophylactic treatment of nerve agent poisoning, or peroxidases that enzymatically break down nerve agent.[56–59]

In scenarios where the use of nerve agents against military personnel or the civilian population is likely, pretreatment with pyridostigmine bromide provides an additional layer of protection. Administered as a 30 mg tablet every 8 hours, pyridostigmine bromide increases the LD_{50} severalfold for soman. It functions by binding to ChE (carbamylation), thereby blocking nerve agent from attaching to ChE. Decarbamylation then occurs after 4 hours whereupon ChE becomes fully functional.[60] These agents are not without their side effects. When used in Desert Storm, approximately half of military personnel complained of mild gastrointestinal symptoms, including abdominal cramping, soft stools, and increased flatus. However, only 0.07 percent of soldiers required to take this medication discontinued it because of the gastrointestinal problems, asthma exacerbations, hypertension, or non-specific allergic reactions.[60]

In managing victims of nerve agent poisoning, several treatment caveats have developed over time. Antidote administration with atropine should be titrated to treat secretions, dyspnea, or retching and vomiting. Again, miosis does not typically respond to atropine. Victims with eye pain and headache should be treated with topical tropicamide. Of note, fasciculations can persist after restoration of consciousness, spontaneous ventilation, and even ambulation.

As with other chemical agents, all suspected nerve agent casualties should be decontaminated prior to evaluation inside a medical facility. Asymptomatic 'casualties' who present more than seconds to minutes after an event are unlikely to have sustained a significant vapor exposure. If exposed to liquid agent, even asymptomatic victims should be observed for 18 hours. Red blood cell ChE activity should be assessed if available; even if that capability does not exist locally, obtaining a sample for later medicolegal or forensic analysis may be beneficial. When triaging multiple casualties, patients recovering from exposure and treatment in the field can usually be placed into a 'delayed' category. Ambulatory patients and those with normal vital signs can be categorized as 'minimal'. 'Immediate' patients are those with unstable vital signs or seizure activity. Patients who are apneic, pulseless, or without a blood pressure will most likely be declared 'expectant.' Determining which patients should return to work depends in large part on the extent of symptoms. The presence of disability, and the number of victims affected by the incident, will play a large role in that decision. For occupational exposure, return to a normal functioning level can be expected when the RBC ChE activity returns to about 75 percent of baseline (approximately 45 days). All but the mildest of exposures should be observed for about a week.[36]

Many long-term effects of nerve agent exposure have been described. Neuropsychiatric symptoms include memory and sleep disturbances, depression, anxiety, and irritability. In addition, an 'intermediate syndrome' has been described in organophosphorus insecticide poisoning; symptoms include limb proximal muscle weakness, cranial nerve muscle weakness, and areflexia.[46]

OVERVIEW OF SPECIFIC BIOLOGIC AGENTS

Anthrax

Bacillus anthracis is a bacterium which occurs in spore form and a vegetative form. The spore form is a hibernating form, which predominates when nutrients are lacking. Anthrax spores have been reported to survive in the environment for 40 years. The spore is small enough (1×1.5 μm) to be easily aerosolized and inhaled and deposited in the lungs at the alveolar level. Alveolar macrophages ingest the spores and travel via the pulmonary lymphatic system to the mediastinal lymph nodes. The germination of the spores may occur within a few days or be delayed for up to 2 months. Once the spore reaches an area with adequate nutrients, it germinates to form the vegetative cell, which feeds and reproduces. The vegetative cell is a Gram-positive aerobic rod or bacillus that occurs as single cells or short chains (Fig. 18.4). It cannot survive for long outside an animal host (or in appropriate media), but in the animal host it is extremely virulent. The vegetative cells produce and release a lethal factor, which causes cell damage and immunosuppression, and an edema factor, which causes edema and further immunosuppression. Both of these toxins contain a protein component called protective factor or antigen. The vegetative cells reproduce rapidly and the patient becomes massively bacteremic.[61]

The bacterial proliferation and toxin production leads to a clinical syndrome of hemorrhagic lymphadenitis and mediastinitis. Although imaging studies will show infiltrates, this is not a true pneumonia because there is no infection of the alveolar spaces. Autopsy examination may show focal hemorrhagic pulmonary parenchymal lesions, but not the

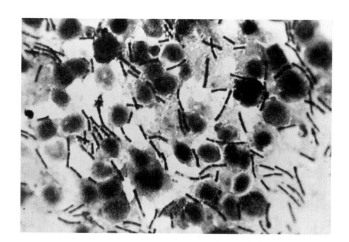

Figure 18.4 *Photomicrograph of* Bacillus anthracis. *(Copied from the Centers for Disease Control and Prevention Pubic Health Information Library.)*

usual inflammatory cells and bacteria associated with pneumonia. For this reason, the term inhalational anthrax is used, as opposed to anthrax pneumonia. Although naturally occurring anthrax infection can occur in the cutaneous and gastrointestinal forms, when used as an agent of terror, it will be dispersed as an aerosol, leading to the inhalational form of disease. Historically, mortality for advanced anthrax with respiratory failure has been close to 100 percent. However, the most recent outbreak had an overall mortality of 45 percent. This improved survival may indicate that with aggressive modern critical care many patients might survive.[62]

CLINICAL FEATURES

Unfortunately, the initial symptoms of inhalational anthrax are nonspecific and difficult to differentiate from the common and benign respiratory illnesses that occur in patients presenting to pulmonary and emergency medicine physicians. The incubation period from exposure to onset of illness may vary from 4 to 60 days. Since the initial symptoms are nonspecific, one of the most important clues to an early diagnosis is an exposure history to a credible potential source. This means that in a new outbreak the index case may be impossible to diagnose until the more classic or defining features of the disease are apparent.

The initial signs and symptoms of inhalational anthrax are nonspecific and difficult to differentiate from other febrile illnesses. In the October to November 2001 US Postal Service anthrax outbreak, all patients presented with fever, fatigue and malaise. Cough and nausea and vomiting occurred in the majority. Other common symptoms included dyspnea, chest pain, myalgias, headache, confusion, and abdominal pain.[62] Some symptoms are helpful in differentiating inhalational anthrax from other common respiratory illnesses. In the influenzalike viral syndromes, the significant shortness of breath, nausea, and vomiting seen in inhalational anthrax are *not* common. On the other hand, nasal congestion and rhinorrhea are common in the influenzalike illnesses but distinctly unusual in anthrax.[63] Fever and tachycardia are common initial signs. Later presentations are significant for hypotension, pulmonary consolidation, and confusion.[62] Elevated liver associated enzymes are common. There may be a mild leukocytosis with a predominance of immature neutrophils. Most patients will be hypoxic.[62]

Chest radiographs often show abnormal findings with a predominance of mediastinal widening (see Fig. 18.1); pleural effusions may also be present.[62] Chest CT may show hemorrhagic mediastinal adenopathy with mediastinal edema and hemorrhagic pleural and pericardial effusions (see Fig. 18.2). Central infiltrates may be present. One report noted that on the initial CT with intravenous contrast the appearance of the lymph nodes was nonspecific, but delayed images obtained 20 minutes later showed peripheral enhancement with central hypodensity in the nodes. This finding is consistent with hemorrhagic mediastinal adenopathy and is more specific for anthrax. Therefore, if anthrax is suspected it may be helpful to obtain 20-minute post-contrast delayed images.[7] In addition, a chest CT, due to the greater sensitivity of CT compared with plain films, should be obtained even if the chest radiograph is normal in any case of suspected inhalational anthrax.

DIAGNOSIS

Blood cultures should be positive within the first 24 hours in the untreated patient. However, after only one to two doses of antibiotics, the blood cultures may be sterile. Due to the high bacterial load, a Gram stain of the blood may be positive. Sputum Gram stain and culture usually do not contain organisms. Cerebrospinal fluid Gram stain and culture may be positive in patients with inhalational anthrax complicated by meningitis.[64] Nasal swabs for anthrax have been used to screen populations at risk after the 2001 incident, but the accuracy of this test is uncertain. A fatal human case of anthrax, which had a negative nasal swab, suggests that the sensitivity may not be ideal. A positive swab, however, is evidence of exposure and is an indication for prophylactic therapy. In general, nasal swabs for anthrax should not be used for individual patient management, but may be useful for epidemiologic study.[65]

Preliminary study indicates that a fluorescent antibody assay against *B. anthracis* cell wall and capsular antigens may be sensitive and specific. Although this has been tested on human specimens, it is still considered experimental. A polymerase chain reaction (PCR) assay of sterile fluids such as blood, pleural, and pericardial fluid is available as well, and may be helpful in making a rapid diagnosis.[66] Data based on clinical human isolates, animal samples, and laboratory studies indicate that the three-target PCR assay approaches a sensitivity and specificity of 100 percent.[67] Serologic studies that measure antibody response against *B. anthracis* are not helpful given that the diagnosis requires comparison of acute and convalescent titers obtained 6 weeks apart. This may be helpful in defining the epidemiology of an outbreak, but is not useful for individual patient management.

TREATMENT

Early antibiotic administration is of primary importance. Both the CDC and the Working Group on Civilian Biodefense have recently made treatment recommendations. For inhalational anthrax, ciprofloxacin should be given intravenously at a dose of 400 mg every 12 hours. Alternatively, doxycycline can be given intravenously at a dose of 100 mg every 12 hours. For moderate or severely ill patients, a second or third antibiotic should accompany either medication. Other agents include: rifampin, vancomycin, penicillin, ampicillin, chloramphenicol, imipenem, clindamycin, or clarithromycin. Clindamycin, at least theoretically, may be a good choice due to its ability to suppress the bacteria's toxin production.[68]

Genetically engineered strains of anthrax exist that carry resistance to tetracyclines and fluoroquinolones. The anthrax strain in the 2001 outbreak contained an inducible β-lactamase, and therefore monotherapy with a penicillin or an ampicillin derivative is not recommended. Multidrug resistance must be assumed until sensitivities are available. Duration of antibiotic therapy is prolonged due to the possible sequestration of anthrax spores in lymph nodes and other tissue. The recommended total duration of oral and intravenous therapy is 60 days.[68]

In the case of confirmed or suspected anthrax meningitis, high-dose penicillin therapy is recommended due to its proved efficacy and ability to cross the blood–brain barrier. In addition, dexamethasone (10 mg intravenously every 6 hours for the first 4 days) should be considered. This regimen has been shown to decrease mortality and rate of neurologic complications in adults with bacterial meningitis (although no patients in this study had anthrax).[69] Other indications for steroid therapy may include patients with severe mediastinal edema (which can compress and compromise airways and vascular structures) and severe edema affecting the intrathoracic or extrathoracic airways.[70] In addition, patients with relative adrenal insufficiency in the setting of septic shock (defined as a baseline cortisol of less than 248.3 mmol/L [9 µg/dL] or a baseline cortisol of between 413.8 mmol/L [15 µg/dL] and 938.1 mmol/L [34 µg/dL] with an inappropriately low increase in cortisol at 30–60 minutes of less than 9 µg/dL) may have a survival benefit with the addition of 50 mg of hydrocortisone every 6 hours for 7 days. The adjunctive use of fludrocortisone 50 µg per day may also be considered.[71,72]

In the case of large pleural effusions, chest tube thoracostomy will likely be necessary to allow for adequate ventilation and to remove infected material. Other standard therapies for shock, such as mechanical ventilation, volume resuscitation, and vasopressors, should be used as indicated.

POSTEXPOSURE PROPHYLAXIS

If a history of exposure to aerosolized anthrax spores is probable, then prophylactic antibiotics are indicated. The recommended regimen is ciprofloxacin 500 mg orally every 12 hours for 60 days. Alternative therapies include doxycycline 100 mg orally every 12 hours or amoxicillin 500 mg orally every 8 hours. For children and pregnant or lactating women, the doxycycline alternative is not offered due to possible adverse effects on developing bones and teeth.[65,66,70]

INFECTION CONTROL

Although there have been rare cases of cutaneous anthrax spread from person to person, inhalational anthrax is not spread in this manner. However, any patient who presents with anthrax exposure may have anthrax spores contaminating their clothing and hair. Clothing should be bagged and disposed off, and the hair should be washed.

In any case of suspected or confirmed anthrax, the microbiology lab with biosafety level 2 precautions should handle most patient specimens. This means that the microbiology lab needs to be alerted prior to the arrival of the specimen that anthrax is a possibility. Specimens that are easily aerosolized, such as a powder, need to be handled with much more stringent precautions, but are unlikely to be isolated in a patient care setting.[64]

ANTHRAX VACCINE

The only anthrax vaccine (anthrax vaccine adsorbed [AVA]) licensed in the United States was developed in the 1950s and consists of a cell-free filtrate derived from a nonencapsulated attenuated strain of B. anthracis containing no whole or live bacteria.[73] The vaccine is administered subcutaneously in 6 doses over 18 months, at weeks 0, 2, and 4, and months 6, 12, and 18. Yearly boosters are recommended. Anthrax vaccination is currently recommended for individuals at risk such as military and civilians being deployed to areas with a biowarfare threat, those exposed to animal products, and laboratory workers. The vaccine is contraindicated in patients allergic to any of the components and patients who are pregnant. In human studies, 95 percent of vaccinees show a fourfold increase in antibodies to the protective antigen (anti-PA); after three doses, however, the correlation between antibody levels and protection from disease is not defined. The only trial documenting efficacy in humans was performed in mill workers in 1962. This trial showed a 92 percent efficacy against cutaneous and inhalational anthrax based on occupational exposure.[74] Efficacy and safety in children, adults over 65, and pregnant women have not been established.

Typically the anthrax vaccine is recommended for pre-exposure use. During the 2001 US Postal Service anthrax attacks, the question of using the vaccine for postexposure prophylaxis was raised to protect against germination of residual spores that could later result in active infection.[65] Based on a prior animal study,[75] postal employees exposed during the outbreak were offered either antibiotic therapy alone for 100 days or 60 days of antibiotic treatment with three doses of anthrax vaccine on days 0, 14, and 28. Although these data should be used cautiously, to date there have been no cases of anthrax in either group.[65]

The anthrax vaccine has been shown overall to be relatively safe. Post licensure surveillance, through the Vaccine Adverse Event Reporting System (VAERS) including the DoD data from 1998–2000 and civilian data, revealed a 5 percent serious adverse event rate after 1 859 00 doses of vaccine. The reactions ranged from injection site hypersensitivity, pain, edema, and headache to Guillain–Barré syndrome, multiple sclerosis, anaphylaxis, and death. The only reactions confirmed to be vaccine related were the injection site reactions.[76] The biggest concern about the safety of AVA stems from allegations that the vaccine was the cause of the Gulf War syndrome.

However, after extensive review, the CDC concluded that there is no association between AVA and Gulf War syndrome.[76]

Plague

Plague is a zoonotic infection caused by the Gram-negative rod *Yersinia pestis*, a nonspore-forming, bipolar-staining bacillus of the family Enterobacteriaceae. The plague bacillus produces virulence factors encoded on chromosomes and plasmids that help play a role in adapting the organism to survival intracellularly. One of the plasmids, encoded for a plasminogen activator protease, is required for the systemic spread of infection. Other important virulence factors include the production of a lipopolysaccharide endotoxin and a capsular envelope containing the antiphagocytic principal factor I antigen.[77–83]

Plague primarily is an infection seen in rodents and rabbits. However, humans may become an accidental host. Although the incidence of naturally occurring plague in humans is small, it is felt that aerosolized droplets of *Y. pestis* could be used as a biological warfare agent.[68,84,85] The aerosolized form would result in the highly contagious and fatal pneumonic form of plague. In nonhuman primates, inhalation of as few as 100–20 000 organisms has been shown to cause infection.[86] The World Health Organization (WHO) estimates that dissemination of 50 kg of aerosolized *Y. pestis* over a population of 5 million would cause 150 000 infections and 36 000 deaths. Any cases of plague pneumonia in a nonendemic area or those that are not a complication of an ongoing bubonic epidemic should be considered a result of bioterrorism.

CLINICAL PRESENTATION

The incubation period and clinical manifestations of plague depend on the mode of transmission. If plague is used as a weapon of mass destruction, it will most likely be aerosolized, leading to the pneumonic form. However, the bubonic or septicemic forms may be seen if infected fleas are used.[84,85,87] Patients with primary pneumonic plague usually present with severe, rapidly progressive pneumonia with septicemic features which can become rapidly fatal. One should consider plague when a large number of previously healthy people present with acute fulminant pneumonia. Plague is highly contagious by the airborne route. The incubation period is 1–6 days in most epidemics. Clinical signs and symptoms of infection include rapid onset of fever, dyspnea, chest pain, and cough that may produce bloody, watery, or purulent sputum. Tachycardia, dyspnea, and cyanosis are also noted. There are often accompanying gastrointestinal symptoms of nausea, vomiting, diarrhea, and abdominal pain. The classic buboes (tender, enlarged lymph nodes with surrounding erythema) associated with other types of plague are nearly always absent (with the rare exception of cervical buboes). The clinical presentation of plague in children is similar to that of adults.[88] The clinical data regarding manifestations of plague in pregnant women are limited.[89]

As with other Gram-negative organisms, *Y. pestis* produces endotoxin that leads to shock, multiorgan failure, and disseminated intravascular coagulation. Acute respiratory failure requiring mechanical ventilation may occur. Extreme caution regarding respiratory isolation must be taken as pneumonic plague can result in human spread.[84,90–93] Mortality in pneumonic plague is very high. The disease is uniformly fatal if appropriate antibiotics are not instituted within 24 hours.

LABORATORY FINDINGS

In all forms of plague, laboratory testing often reveals a mild to moderate leukocytosis (white blood cell count 10 000–20 000/μL) with a neutrophil predominance and toxic granulations. Elevated liver enzyme levels, azotemia, and coagulopathy are common. Evidence of disseminated intravascular coagulation is seen in severe cases. Chest radiographs often show bilateral infiltrates, lobar consolidations, and pleural effusions. Cavities can be seen, but are much less common. Mediastinal adenopathy is rare, and distinguishes plague from anthrax in uncertain exposures (see Fig. 18.3).[94] The sputum is usually purulent, often blood tinged, and contains plague bacilli.

DIAGNOSIS

A high index of clinical suspicion is critical for timely diagnosis of plague. Early pneumonic plague can mimic inhalational anthrax. However, the initial radiographic finding of anthrax is a predominance of mediastinal widening from hilar and mediastinal lymphadenopathy, whereas pneumonic plague is primarily an airspace disease.

Gram staining of blood, sputum, or bubo aspirates reveal the characteristic Gram-negative rod with bipolar staining (often referred to as a 'safety-pin') (Fig. 18.5). Staining with Wright, Giemsa, or Wayson stains can also demonstrate the organism. Cultures of blood, sputum or aspirates are often positive within 24–48 hours. The laboratory should be notified regarding the clinical suspicion of plague because cases of laboratory-acquired plague have occurred.[93] In the United States, rapid diagnostic tests such as IgM immunoassay, direct fluorescent antibody testing and PCR are available in certain laboratories (the CDC plague laboratory, a few state departments of health, and military laboratories). Direct fluorescent antibody staining for *Y. pestis* and dipstick antigen detection tests, which are highly specific for plague, are also available at some centers.[95–97] A rapid diagnostic test using monoclonal antibodies to the F-1 antigen was recently field tested in Madagascar and shown to be comparable in specificity and sensitivity to bacteriology and detection by ELISA in bubonic and pneumonic plague.

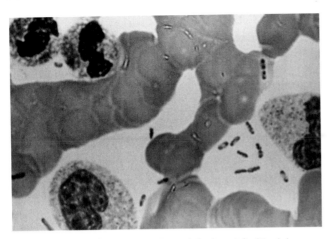

Figure 18.5 *Dark stained bipolar ends (safety pin) of* Yersinia pestis *can clearly be seen in this Wright stain of blood from a plague victim. (Copied from the Centers for Disease Control and Prevention Pubic Health Information Library).*

This rapid diagnostic test shows promise for early and rapid diagnosis of plague.[98]

TREATMENT

The mainstay of therapy for *Y. pestis* has traditionally included antibiotic therapy with streptomycin or gentamicin. Other acceptable alternatives include ciprofloxacin, tetracycline, doxycycline, and chloramphenicol.[84,99–102] In 1995, a multidrug-resistant *Y. pestis* was isolated in a patient with bubonic plague in Madagascar.[103] Other than this case, there have been no additional reports of resistance and many episodic cases and outbreaks of plague have responded to currently recommended antibiotics. Most patients generally respond quite rapidly and are afebrile in about 3 days. A 10-day course of therapy is recommended to prevent relapses.

The management of plague in a mass casualty situation such as can occur with bioterrorism will pose major threats to the availability of medical resources. Failure to institute antibiotics within 24 hours of onset of pneumonic plague will likely result in the death of the patient. The ability to give intravenous or intramuscular streptomycin or gentamicin may not be feasible. The Working Group on Civilian Biodefense recommends oral treatment in this setting; either doxycycline 100 mg twice daily, ciprofloxacin 500 mg twice daily, or chloramphenicol 25 mg/kg four times a day.[65] All patients suspected of having plague should be put in respiratory isolation and therapy should be instituted promptly. Universal precautions and special handling of blood and discharge from the bubo must be taken.[104] In cases of pneumonic plague, strictly enforced respiratory isolation in addition to the use of gloves, gowns, and eye protection must be undertaken and such measures should be continued for the first few days of antibiotic therapy. The patients may be taken off isolation after 4 days of antibiotics for the pneumonic form.

POSTEXPOSURE PROPHYLAXIS

Prophylaxis with tetracycline or doxycycline has been used for people who have been in close contact (within 60–150 cm [2–5 feet]) with an infected person. Ciprofloxacin has proved effective in animal models of *Y. pestis* pneumonia, but quinolones have not been used in human trials.[77,105] Pregnant women and children under 8 years of age should receive trimethoprim-sulfamethoxazole in two divided doses for 6 days.

PLAGUE VACCINE

The licensed plague vaccine is a killed, whole cell vaccine originally developed prior to World War II.[106] The vaccine is administered first at a high dose then one fifth of the dose at 1–3 months and 5–6 months followed by similar dose boosters every 6 months for 1.5 years, then yearly.[106] The vaccine is recommended for laboratory workers, military troops, and people living in endemic areas. It is contraindicated in patients allergic to any of its components. Although it has been shown to be effective against bubonic plague, it is unknown if protection is provided against pneumonic plague. The vaccine has not been studied in children and is contraindicated during pregnancy. Vaccine side effects include local tenderness, erythema, and pain in 11 percent of vaccinees with the incidence of large local reactions increasing with successive doses. Hence, the dose of the second and third inoculations is reduced. Headache, malaise, and myalgias are seen in 4 percent of vaccinees. Rarely, sterile abscesses, anaphylaxis, or necrotic lesions develop.[106]

Unfortunately, the manufacturer discontinued the vaccine in 1999 because of production problems. It is unclear if production will resume as the threat of biological warfare increases. To provide protection against pneumonic plague, studies are ongoing to develop an effective vaccine against all forms of the disease. The most promising research has been the development of a recombinant vaccine combining the F1 and V antigens. It was effective in preventing inhalational disease in laboratory animals but has not been studied in humans. Passive immunization with V-antigen polyclonal antiserum or monoclonal anti-V antibody in mice protected them against lethal challenge with *Yersinia*. Treatments targeting other virulence factors are also under investigation.[107]

Tularemia

Tularemia is a bacterial zoonosis caused by *Francisella tularensis*, a Gram-negative coccobacillus (Fig. 18.6) which can be found in contaminated water and soil as well as infected ticks and animals. Infected arthropods (notably the dog tick (*Dermacentor variabilis*), the wood tick (*Dermacentor andersoni*), and the Lone Star tick (*Amblyomma americanum*)) and flies are the most important

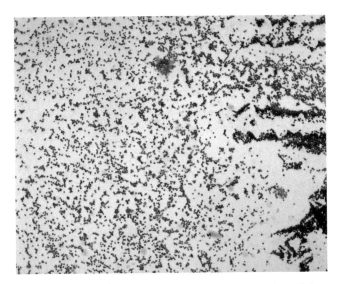

Figure 18.6 Francisella tularensis *is Gram-negative in its staining morphology. (Copied from the Centers for Disease Control and Prevention Pubic Health Information Library.)*

vectors in the United States. Contact with infected animals is another mode of contracting tularemia, and skinning, dressing, and eating animals such as rabbits have resulted in infection.[108] Recently, an outbreak of tularemia in 15 patients (including 11 with primary pneumonic tularemia) was reported on Martha's Vineyard, Massachussets, and was associated with lawn mowing and brush cutting.[109] Although tularemia could be used as a weapon in a variety of way, an aerosol release would likely have the greatest impact on the public health system. In 1969, a WHO committee estimated that aerosol dispersal of 50 kg of *F. tularensis* over a metropolitan area of 5 million inhabitants could lead to 250 000 incapacitating casualties and 19 000 deaths.[110]

CLINICAL PRESENTATION

In a terrorist attack, pneumonic tularemia would result from direct inhalation of the organism. Once inhaled, the bacilli multiply, spread to regional lymph nodes and further multiply, and can then disseminate throughout the body. Bacteremia is common in the early phase of the infection. Inhalational illness commonly results in an initial systemic illness without prominent pulmonary symptoms.[110] The onset of symptoms is abrupt and characterized by high fever, severe headache, chills, myalgias, and sore throat. Patients may have a dry or slightly productive cough. Some inhalational exposures will lead to hemorrhagic inflammation of the airways and more rapid progression to pneumonia. In untreated disease, symptoms can persist for weeks or months with progressive disability. Even after the institution of antibiotics, symptoms can be incapacitating for several days.

The earliest abnormality on chest radiography may be only mild peribronchial cuffing or several small, discrete

infiltrates.[110] Other descriptions include subsegmental or lobar infiltrates, hilar adenopathy, pleural effusion (up to 25 percent in one report[111]), and apical or miliary infiltrates, with less common changes including cavitation and bronchopleural fistulas.[112–114]

DIAGNOSIS

Tularemia can be difficult to diagnose, especially without epidemiological evidence to suggest exposure to the organism. Although *F. tularensis* can be grown in culture, it requires special media and its propagation in the routine diagnostic laboratory represents a potential danger to laboratory personnel (tularemia has been ranked as the third most common cause of accidental infection among laboratory workers[115]). For these reasons, in isolated, naturally occurring cases of tularemia, serologic testing is the suggested method of diagnosis. Antibodies usually become detectable by the end of the second week of infection, and a firm diagnosis can be made by demonstrating a fourfold or greater increase in titer. As this is not helpful in identifying the index cases of a potential mass exposure, one should collect sputum and blood specimens and notify the laboratory personnel that tularemia is suspected, allowing for adequate safety precautions. Designated reference laboratories can perform rapid testing for *F. tularensis* using antigen detection assays, PCR, enzyme-linked immunoassays, immunoblotting and other specialized techniques, allowing for identification of the organisms within several hours.[110]

TREATMENT

Streptomycin is the drug of choice for tularemia, and a clinical response is usually seen with 48 hours of administration. Alternative agents include gentamicin and doxycycline, although doxycycline has been associated with relapses.[116] Notably, although ceftriaxone has shown *in vitro* activity against *F. tularensis*, clinical reports demonstrate failure with ceftriaxone treatment.[117] A pneumonia that fails to respond to a β-lactam antibiotic has been suggested as a potential clue to the diagnosis of tularemia.[118] In a mass casualty setting, either doxycycline 100 mg orally twice daily or ciprofloxacin, 500 mg orally twice daily, is the recommended treatement.[110]

TULAREMIA VACCINE

The United States does not have a licensed tularemia vaccine for general usage. A live investigational product, known as the live vaccine strain (LVS) is available through the US Army Material Research Command at Fort Detrick, Maryland.[110,119] Evaluations have demonstrated that the LVS vaccine protected human volunteers against an aerosol challenge with virulent *F. tularensis*, although it was not always complete.[120] Several limitations of the current LVS vaccine indicate a need for a new one. These include the method of administration, which requires scarification similar to the vaccina vaccine, making standardization difficult. In addition, there is a lack of understanding of the factors responsible for conferring virulence as well as genetic instability of the organism. Finally, antigens serving as targets for generating cell-mediated immunity are not well understood.[121] After the September 11, 2001 attacks, the US is again attempting to develop, manufacture, test, and license a LVS vaccine from the current strain. Internationally, several efforts are under way to develop new tularemia vaccines. In particular, Sweden is attempting to develop a subunit vaccine against aerosolized forms of *F. tularensis*.[121]

SUMMARY

Healthcare providers will play a critical role in recognizing and responding to illnesses caused by the intentional release of chemical or biologic agents. The syndrome descriptions, radiographic presentations, and characteristics of the most likely agents presented in this chapter are intended to introduce the respiratory care provider to this vital role. These agents will remain a favorite weapon for terrorists to employ and will result in casualties that stress current medical infrastructure. Further study and training in the care of victims of these agents must occur on a recurring basis in order to maximize medical effectiveness when a terrorist event that employs these agents takes place. The following 10 steps summarize the approach to and the management of chemical and biologic agent casualties:

1. maintain an index of suspicion
2. protect yourself
3. assess the patient
4. decontaminate as appropriate
5. establish a diagnosis
6. render prompt treatment
7. practice good hazmat protection
8. alert the proper authorities
9. assist in the epidemiologic/criminal investigation
10. maintain proficiency and continue to educate and train healthcare providers on these agents and their effects.

Key learning points

- The intentional release of chemical or biologic agents of terror is a realistic threat.

- All medical providers are essential to community and hospital preparedness.

- The use of chemical agents will necessitate that hospitals design and develop appropriate decontamination areas and procedures.

- Chemical agents will present as autonomic dysfunction, airway inflammation, pulmonary edema, or tissue hypoxia.

- Biologic agents will present as acute pneumonitis or hemorrhagic mediastinitis.

- Inhalational anthrax, pneumonic plague, and pneumonic tularemia are the most likely biologic agents that the respiratory care provider will encounter.

- An empiric approach to treatment that assesses the rapidity of onset and whether the symptoms are primarily respiratory or neurologic is essential until specific causative agents can be confirmed.

COMPETING INTERESTS

This chapter portrays the views of the authors and does not reflect those of the Department of Defense, the Department of Veterans Affairs, or Dartmouth Medical School.

ACKNOWLEDGMENT

Dr Geiling would like to acknowledge the assistance of the Chemical Casualty Care Division, US Army Medical Research Institute of Chemical Defense.

APPENDIX: REFERENCE WEBSITES

- Background on chemical warfare: http://www.mitretek.org/HomelandSecurityAndCounter terrorism.htm (accessed April 2006)
- BioMed Training: http://www.biomedtraining.org (accessed February 2003)
- Terrorism: http://www.csis-scrs.gc.ca/en/publications/publications_proliferation.asp (accessed April 2006)
- Domestic Preparedness: http://hld.sbccom.army.mil/ (accessed March 2004)
- Medical NBC Online: http://www.nbc-med.org/ (accessed April 2006)
- National Disaster Medical System: http://ndms.dhhs.gov/index.html
- NBC Links: www.nbc-links.com/
- OSHA: www.osha.gov/
- US Army Medical Research Institute of Chemical Defense: http://ccc.apgea.army.mil/ (accessed April 2006)
- US Army Medical Research Institute of Infectious Diseases: www.usamriid.army.mil/

- Virtual Hospital War Health Topics for Providers: www.vh.org/adult/provider/emergencymedicine/wartopics
- WMD First Responders: http://wmdfirstresponders.com

REFERENCES

1. Cieslak TJ. *Biological Warfare and Terrorism*. USA: US Army Medical Research Institute of Infectious Diseases, 2000.

2. Treat KN, Williams JM, Furbee PM, *et al.* Hospital preparedness for weapons of mass destruction incidents: an initial assessment. *Ann Emerg Med* 2001; **38**: 562–5.

3. Wetter DC, Daniell WE, Treser CD. Hospital preparedness for victims of chemical or biological terrorism. *Am J Public Health* 2001; **91**: 710–16.

4. White SM. Chemical and biological weapons. Implications for anaesthesia and intensive care. *Br J Anaesth* 2002; **89**: 306–24.

5. Bogucki S, Weir S. Pulmonary manifestations of intentionally released chemical and biological agents. *Clin Chest Med* 2002; **23**: 777–94.

6. Cieslak TJ, Rowe JR, Kortepeter MG, *et al.* A field-expedient algorithmic approach to the clinical management of chemical and biological casualties. *Mil Med* 2000; **165**: 659–62.

7. Krol CM, Uszynski M, Dillon EH, *et al.* Dynamic CT features of inhalational anthrax infection. *AJR Am J Roentgenol* 2002; **178**: 1063–6.

8. Ketai L, Alrahji AA, Hart B, Enria D, Mettler F, Jr. Radiologic manifestations of potential bioterrorist agents of infection. *AJR Am J Roentgenol* 2003; **180**: 565–75.

9. Cunha BA. Anthrax, tularemia, plague, Ebola or smallpox as agents of bioterrorism: recognition in the emergency room. *Clin Microbiol Infect* 2002; **8**: 489–503.

10. Bradley R. Health care facility preparation for weapons of mass destruction. *Prehospital Emergency Care* 2000; **4**: 261–9.

11. Okumura T, Suzuki K, Fukuda A, *et al.* The Tokyo subway attack: disaster management, part 1: community emergency response. *Acad Emerg Med* 1998; **5**: 613–17.

12. Betts-Symonds G. Major disaster management in chemical warfare. *Accid Emerg Nurs* 1994; **2**: 122–9.

13. Burgess J, Blackmon GM, Brodkin CA, Robertson WO. Hospital preparedness for hazardous materials incidents and treatment of contaminated patients. *West J Med* 1997; **167**: 387–91.

14. Schulz M, Cisek J, Wabeke R. Simulated exposure of hospital emergency personnel to solvent vapors and respirable dust during decontamination of chemically exposed patients. *Ann Emerg Med* 1995; **26**: 324–9.

15. Hudson T, Reilly K, Dulaigh J. Considerations for chemical decontamination shelters. *Disaster Management and Response* 2003; **1**: 110–13.

16. Okumura T, Suzuki K, Fukuda A, *et al.* The Tokyo subway sarin attack: disaster management, part 2: hospital response. *Acad Emerg Med* 1998; **5**: 618–24.

17. Horton D, Berkowitz Z, Kaye, WE. Secondary contamination of ED personnel from hazardous materials events, 1995–2001. *Am J Emerg Med* 2003; **21**: 199–204.

18. Kirk M, Cisek J, Rose SR. Emergency department response to hazardous materials incidents. *Concepts and Controversies in Toxicology* 1994; **12**: 461–81.

19. Nelson C, Laughlin J, Kim C, *et al.* Laundering as decontamination of apparel fabrics: residues of pesticides from six chemical cases. *Archives of Environmental Contamination and Toxicology* 1992: 85–90.

20. Kales SN, Christiani DC. Acute chemical emergencies. *N Engl J Med* 2004; **350**: 800–8.

21. Russell A, Berberich JA, Drevon GF, Koepsel RR. Biomaterials for mediation of chemical and biological warfare agents. *Annu Rev Biomed Eng* 2003; **5**: 1–27.

22. Lindsey J. Amazing terrorism tool: new foam could revolutionize decon. *JEMS* 2003:84–6.

23. Hall A, Blomet J, Mathieu, L. Diphoterine for emergent eye/skin chemical splash decontamination: a review. *Vet Hum Toxicol* 2002; **44**: 228–31.

24. Shapira I, Abraham RB, Weinbroum AA. Anesthesia for victims of nerve agents undergoing surgery: establishment of a management protocol. *J Med* 2000; **31**: 143–8.

25. Gold M, Bongiovanni R, Scharf BA, *et al.* Hypochlorite solution as a decontaminant in sulfur mustard contaminated skin defects in the euthymic hairless guinea pig. *Drug Chemical Toxicol* 1994; **17**: 499–527.

26. Cooper G, Ryan J, Galbraith, K. The surgical management in war of penetrating wounds contaminated with chemical warfare agents. *J R Army Med Corps* 1994; **140**: 113–18.

27. Leonard R. Hazardous materials accidents: initial scene assessment and patient care. *Aviat Space Environ Med* 1993: 546–50.

28. Berkenstadt H, Marganitt B, Atsmon J. Combined chemical and conventional injuries-pathophysiological, diagnostic, and therapeutic aspects. *Israel J Med Sci* 1991; **27**: 623–6.

29. Schultz C, Koenig KL, Lewis RJ. Implications of hospital evacuation after the Northridge, California, earthquake. *N Engl J Med* 2003; **348**: 1349–55.

30. de Jong RH. Nerve gas terrorism: a grim challenge to anesthesiologists. *Anesth Analg* 2003; **96**: 819–25.

31. Hendler I, Nahtomi O, Segal E, *et al.* The effect of full protective gear on intubation performance by hospital medical personnel. *Military Med* 2000; **165**: 272–4.

32. Prevention and treatment of injury from chemical warfare agents. *Med Lett Drugs Ther* 2002; **44**: 1–4.

33. Smith D. Inhalational injuries. CHEST, the Annual Conference of the American College of Chest Physicians, Orlando, FL, October 25–30, 2003.

34. Chemical agents and syndromes. In: Farmer C, ed. *Fundamentals of Disaster Medicine*. Des Plaines: Society of Critical Care Medicine, 2003.

◆ 35. Leikin JB, Thomas RG, Walter FG, *et al.* A review of nerve agent exposure for the critical care physician. *Crit Care Med* 2002; **30**: 2346–54.

36. *Medical Management of Chemical Casualties Handbook*. Aberdeen Proving Ground: US Army Medical Research Institute of Chemical Defense (USAMRICD), 2000.

37. Emad A, Rezaian GR. The diversity of the effects of sulfur mustard gas inhalation on respiratory system 10 years after a single, heavy exposure: analysis of 197 cases. *Chest* 1997; **112**: 734–8.

38. Thomason JW, Rice TW, Milstone AP. Bronchiolitis obliterans in a survivor of a chemical weapons attack. *JAMA* 2003; **290**: 598–9.

39. Karayilanoglu T, Gunhan O, Kenar L, Kurt B. The protective and therapeutic effects of zinc chloride and desferrioxamine on skin exposed to nitrogen mustard. *Mil Med* 2003; **168**: 614–17.

40. Sawyer TW, Nelson P, Hill I, *et al.* Therapeutic effects of cooling swine skin exposed to sulfur mustard. *Mil Med* 2002; **167**: 939–43.

41. Freitag L, Firusian N, Stamatis G, Greschuchna D. The role of bronchoscopy in pulmonary complications due to mustard gas inhalation. *Chest* 1991; **100**: 1436–41.

42. Wax PM, Becker CE, Curry SC. Unexpected 'gas' casualties in Moscow: a medical toxicology perspective. *Ann Emerg Med* 2003; **41**: 700–5.

43. Thomas R, Smith P. Riot control agents. In: Roy M, ed. *Physician's Guide to a Terrorist Attack*. Totowa, NJ: Human Press, Inc, 2004: 325–36.

44. Information Paper. The Fox NBC Reconnaissance Vehicle. 2004 vol. Available at: www.gulflink.osd.mil/foxnbc/ (accessed April 19, 2006).

45. Heck J, Geiling J, Bennet B. Chemical weapons: history, identification, and management. *Crit Decis Emerg Med* 1999; **13**: 1–8.

46. Sidell F. Nerve agents. In: Zajtchuck R, Bellamy R, eds. *Textbook of Military Med: Medical Aspects of Chemical and Biological Warfare*. Washington, DC: Office of the Surgeon General, Department of the Army; **1997**: 129–79.

47. Abraham S, Oz N, Sahar R, Kadar T. QTc prolongation and cardiac lesions following acute organophosphate poisoning in rats. *Proc West Pharmacol Soc* 2001; **44**: 185–6.

48. Chuang FR, Jang SW, Lin JL, *et al.* QTc prolongation indicates a poor prognosis in patients with organophosphate poisoning. *Am J Emerg Med* 1996; **14**: 451–3.

49. Nishiwaki Y, Maekawa K, Ogawa Y, *et al.* Effects of sarin on the nervous system in rescue team staff members and police officers 3 years after the Tokyo subway sarin attack. *Environ Health Perspect* 2001; **109**: 1169–73.

50. Ben Abraham R, Weinbroum AA. Resuscitative challenges in nerve agent poisoning. *Eur J Emerg Med* 2003; **10**: 169–75.

51. Lee EC. Clinical manifestations of sarin nerve gas exposure. *JAMA* 2003; **290**: 659–62.

52. McDonough JH, Jr, Zoeffel LD, McMonagle J, *et al.* Anticonvulsant treatment of nerve agent seizures: anticholinergics versus diazepam in soman-intoxicated guinea pigs. *Epilepsy Res* 2000; **38**: 1–14.

53. Kassa J. Review of oximes in the antidotal treatment of poisoning by organophosphorus nerve agents. *J Toxicol Clin Toxicol* 2002; **40**: 803–16.

54. Krivoy A, Layish I, Rotman E, Yehezkelli Y. Treatment of sarin exposure. *JAMA* 2004; **291**: 181; author reply 182–3.

55. Mion G, Tourtier JP, Petitjeans F, *et al.* Neuroprotective and antiepileptic activities of ketamine in nerve agent poisoning. *Anesthesiology* 2003; **98**: 1517; author reply 1517–18.

56. Raushel FM. Bacterial detoxification of organophosphate nerve agents. *Curr Opin Microbiol* 2002; **5**: 288–95.

57. Tashma Z, Raveh L, Liani H, *et al*. Bretazenil, a benzodiazepine receptor partial agonist, as an adjunct in the prophylactic treatment of OP poisoning. *J Appl Toxicol* 2001; **21**(Suppl 1): S115–19.

58. Rincon P. Push for anti-nerve agent drug. BBC News, 2004. Available at: newsvote.bbc.co.uk/mpapps/pagetools/print/news.bbc.co.uk/2/hi/science/nature/3671827.stm (accessed April 2, 2006).

59. Broomfield CA, Kirby SD. Progress on the road to new nerve agent treatments. *J Appl Toxicol* 2001; **21**(Suppl 1): S43–6.

60. Keeler JR, Hurst CG, Dunn MA. Pyridostigmine used as a nerve agent pretreatment under wartime conditions. *JAMA* 1991; **266**: 693–5.

◆ 61. Swartz MN. Recognition and management of anthrax – an update. *N Engl J Med* 2001; **345**: 1621–6.

● 62. Jernigan JA, Stephens DS, Ashford DA, *et al*. Bioterrorism-related inhalational anthrax: the first 10 cases reported in the United States. *Emerg Infect Dis* 2001; **7**: 933–44.

63. Considerations for distinguishing influenza-like illness from inhalational anthrax. *MMWR Morb Mortal Wkly Rep* 2001; **50**: 984–6.

64. Anthrax medical summary. In: America IDSo, ed. 2003 vol. Available at: www.cidrap.umn.edu/idsa/bt/anthrax/biofacts/anthraxfactsheet.html (accessed April 19, 2006).

◆ 65. Inglesby TV, O'Toole T, Henderson DA, *et al*. Anthrax as a biological weapon, 2002: updated recommendations for management. *JAMA* 2002; **287**: 2236–52.

66. Bell DM, Kozarsky PE, Stephens DS. Clinical issues in the prophylaxis, diagnosis, and treatment of anthrax. *Emerg Infect Dis* 2002; **8**: 222–5.

67. Hoffmaster AR, Meyer RF, Bowen MD, *et al*. Evaluation and validation of a real-time polymerase chain reaction assay for rapid identification of Bacillus anthracis. *Emerg Infect Dis* 2002; **8**: 1178–82.

◆ 68. Darling RG, Catlett CL, Huebner KD, Jarrett DG. Threats in bioterrorism. I: CDC category A agents. *Emerg Med Clin North Am* 2002; **20**: 273–309.

69. de Gans J, van de Beek D. Dexamethasone in adults with bacterial meningitis. *N Engl J Med* 2002; **347**: 1549–56.

70. Bartlett JG, Inglesby TV, Jr, Borio L. Management of anthrax. *Clin Infect Dis* 2002; **35**: 851–8.

71. Annane D, Sebille V, Charpentier C, *et al*. Effect of treatment with low doses of hydrocortisone and fludrocortisone on mortality in patients with septic shock. *JAMA* 2002; **288**: 862–71.

72. Cooper MS, Stewart PM. Corticosteroid insufficiency in acutely ill patients. *N Engl J Med* 2003; **348**: 727–34.

73. Nass M. Model of a response to the biological warfare threat. *Infect Dis Clin North Am* 1999; **13**: 187–210.

74. Brachman P, Gold S, Plotkin R. Field evaluation of a human anthrax vaccine. *Am J Public Health* 1962; **52**: 356–63.

75. Friedlander AM, Welkos SL, Pitt ML, *et al*. Postexposure prophylaxis against experimental inhalation anthrax. *J Infect Dis* 1993; **167**: 1239–43.

76. Use of anthrax vaccine in the United States – recommendations of the Advisory Committee on Immunization Practices: Advisory Committee on Immunization Practices, Recommendations, and Reports; 2000: 1–20.

77. Smego RA, Frean J, Koornhof HJ. Yersiniosis I: microbiological and clinicoepidemiological aspects of plague and non-plague Yersinia infections. *Eur J Clin Microbiol Infect Dis* 1999; **18**: 1–15.

78. Straley SC. The plasmid-encoded outer-membrane proteins of *Yersinia pestis*. *Rev Infect Dis* 1988; **10**(Suppl 2): S323–6.

79. Sodeinde OA, Subrahmanyam YV, Stark K, *et al*. A surface protease and the invasive character of plague. *Science* 1992; **258**: 1004–7.

80. Straley SC, Skrzypek E, Plano GV, Bliska JB. Yops of *Yersinia* spp. pathogenic for humans. *Infect Immun* 1993; **61**: 3105–10.

81. Oyston P. Plague virulence. *J Med Microbiol* 2001; **50**: 1015–17.

82. Lindler LE, Klempner MS, Straley SC. *Yersinia pestis* pH 6 antigen: genetic, biochemical, and virulence characterization of a protein involved in the pathogenesis of bubonic plague. *Infect Immun* 1990; **58**: 2569–77.

83. Guan KL, Dixon JE. Protein tyrosine phosphatase activity of an essential virulence determinant in *Yersinia*. *Science* 1990; **249**: 553–6.

◆ 84. Inglesby TV, Dennis DT, Henderson DA, *et al*. Plague as a biological weapon: medical and public health management. Working Group on Civilian Biodefense. *JAMA* 2000; **283**: 2281–90.

85. Recognition of illness associated with the intentional release of a biologic agent. *MMWR Morb Mortal Wkly Rep* 2001; **50**: 893–7.

86. Speck RS, Wolochow H. Studies on the experimental epidemiology of respiratory infections. VIII. Experimental pneumonic plague in *Macacus rhesus. J Infect Dis* 1957; **100**: 58–69.

87. Poland J, Dennis D. Plague. In: Evans A, Brachman P, eds. *Bacterial Infections of Humans: Epidemiology and Control.* New York: Plenum Medical Book Company, 1998: 545–58.

88. Burkle FM, Jr. Plague as seen in South Vietnamese children. A chronicle of observations and treatment under adverse conditions. *Clin Pediatr (Phila)* 1973; **12**: 291–8.

89. Wong TW. Plague in a pregnant patient. *Trop Doct* 1986; **16**: 187–9.

90. Pneumonic plague – Arizona, 1992. *MMWR Morb Mortal Wkly Rep* 1992; **41**: 737–9.

91. Ratsitorahina M, Chanteau S, Rahalison L, *et al.* Epidemiological and diagnostic aspects of the outbreak of pneumonic plague in Madagascar. *Lancet* 2000; **355**: 111–13.

92. Davis KJ, Fritz DL, Pitt ML, *et al.* Pathology of experimental pneumonic plague produced by fraction 1-positive and fraction 1-negative *Yersinia pestis* in African green monkeys (*Cercopithecus aethiops*). *Arch Pathol Lab Med* 1996; **120**: 156–63.

93. Burmeister RW, Tigertt WD, Overholt EL. Laboratory-acquired pneumonic plague. Report of a case and review of previous cases. *Ann Intern Med* 1962; **56**: 789–800.

94. Alsofrom DJ, Mettler FA, Jr, Mann JM. Radiographic manifestations of plaque in New Mexico, 1975–1980. A review of 42 proved cases. *Radiology* 1981; **139**: 561–5.

95. Rahalison L, Vololonirina E, Ratsitorahina M, Chanteau S. Diagnosis of bubonic plague by PCR in Madagascar under field conditions. *J Clin Microbiol* 2000; **38**: 260–3.

96. Williams JE, Gentry MK, Braden CA, *et al.* Use of an enzyme-linked immunosorbent assay to measure antigenaemia during acute plague. *Bull World Health Organ* 1984; **62**: 463–6.

97. Hinnebusch J, Schwan TG. New method for plague surveillance using polymerase chain reaction to detect Yersinia pestis in fleas. *J Clin Microbiol* 1993; **31**: 1511–14.

● 98. Chanteau S, Rahalison L, Ralafiarisoa L, *et al.*

Development and testing of a rapid diagnostic test for bubonic and pneumonic plague. *Lancet* 2003; **361**: 211–16.

99. Bonacorsi SP, Scavizzi MR, Guiyoule A, *et al.* Assessment of a fluoroquinolone, three beta-lactams, two aminoglycosides, and a cycline in treatment of murine *Yersinia pestis* infection. *Antimicrob Agents Chemother* 1994; **38**: 481–6.

100. Russell P, Eley SM, Green M, *et al.* Efficacy of doxycycline and ciprofloxacin against experimental Yersinia pestis infection. *J Antimicrob Chemother* 1998; **41**: 301–5.

101. Rasoamanana B, Coulanges P, Michel P, Rasolofonirina N. [Sensitivity of *Yersinia pestis* to antibiotics: 277 strains isolated in Madagascar between 1926 and 1989]. *Arch Inst Pasteur Madagascar* 1989; **56**: 37–53.

102. Smith MD, Vinh DX, Nguyen TT, *et al.* In vitro antimicrobial susceptibilities of strains of *Yersinia pestis. Antimicrob Agents Chemother* 1995; **39**: 2153–4.

103. Galimand M, Guiyoule A, Gerbaud G, *et al.* Multidrug resistance in Yersinia pestis mediated by a transferable plasmid. *N Engl J Med* 1997; **337**: 677–80.

104. Garner JS. Guideline for isolation precautions in hospitals. The Hospital Infection Control Practices Advisory Committee. *Infect Control Hosp Epidemiol* 1996; **17**: 53–80.

105. Butler T. *Yersinia* infections: centennial of the discovery of the plague bacillus. *Clin Infect Dis* 1994; **19**: 655–61; quiz 662–3.

106. Plague Vaccine. *Mosby's Drug Consult,* 12th Edition. 2003 vol, 2002. Available at: http://home.mdconsult.com/das/drug/view/2670136 6/1/2050/top?sid=165273780 (accessed April 19, 2006).

107. Fauci A. NIAID biodefense research agenda for CDC category A agents. 2002 vol, www.niaid.nih.gov/biodefense/research/biotresearch agenda.pdf (accessed April 19, 2006).

108. Langley R, Campbell R. Tularemia in North Carolina, 1965–1990. *N C Med J* 1995; **56**: 314–17.

109. Feldman KA, Enscore RE, Lathrop SL, *et al.* An outbreak of primary pneumonic tularemia on Martha's Vineyard. *N Engl J Med* 2001; **345**: 1601–6.

◆ 110. Dennis DT, Inglesby TV, Henderson DA, *et al.* Tularemia as a biological weapon: medical and public health management. *JAMA* 2001; **285**: 2763–73.

111. Scofield RH, Lopez EJ, McNabb SJ. Tularemia pneumonia in Oklahoma, 1982–1987. *J Okla State Med Assoc* 1992; **85**: 165–70.

112. Overholt EL, Tigertt WD. Roentgenographic manifestations of pulmonary tularemia. *Radiology* 1960; **74**: 758–65.

113. Archer V, Blackford S, JE. Pleuropulmonary manifestations in tularemia: A roentgenogrpahic study base on thirty-four unselected cases. *JAMA* 1935; **104**: 897–8.

114. Rubin SA. Radiographic spectrum of pleuropulmonary tularemia. *AJR Am J Roentgenol* 1978; **131**: 277–81.

115. Overholt EL, Tigertt WD, Kadull PJ, *et al.* An analysis of forty-two cases of laboratory-acquired tularemia. Treatment with broad spectrum antibiotics. *Am J Med* 1961; **30**: 785–806.

116. Enderlin G, Morales L, Jacobs RF, Cross JT. Streptomycin and alternative agents for the treatment of tularemia: review of the literature. *Clin Infect Dis* 1994; **19**: 42–7.

117. Cross JT, Jacobs RF. Tularemia: treatment failures with outpatient use of ceftriaxone. *Clin Infect Dis* 1993; **17**: 976–80.

118. Fredricks DN, Remington JS. Tularemia presenting as community-acquired pneumonia. Implications in the era of managed care. *Arch Intern Med* 1996; **156**: 2137–40.

119. Evans M, Freidlander A. Tularemia. In: Zajtchuck R, Bellamy R, eds. *The Textbook of Military Med: Medical Aspects of Chemical and Biological Warfare.* Washington, DC: The Office of the Surgeon General, Department of the Army, 1997: 503–12.

120. Foshay L, Hesselbrock W, Wittenberg M. Vaccine prophylaxis against tularemia in man. *Am J Public Health* 1942; **32**: 1131–45.

121. Ales NC, Katial RK. Vaccines against biologic agents: uses and developments. *Respir Care Clin North Am* 2004; **10**: 123–46.

122. Brennan RJ Waeckerle J, Sharp TW, Lillibridge, SR. Chemical warfare agents: emergency medical and emergency public health issues. *Ann Emerg Med* 1999; **34**: 191–204.

123. Baker D. Management of respiratory failure in toxic disasters. *Resuscitation* 1999; **42**: 125–31.

19

Pediatric respiratory emergencies

ALI M NADROO, NITIN P RON, PRAMOD NARULA

INTRODUCTION

Respiratory emergencies are common in infancy and childhood. They are also a common cause of cardiac arrest in this age group.[1] Although the survival rate of out-of-hospital cardiopulmonary arrest is only 3–17 percent in many studies, and this is accompanied by significant neurologic damage, the survival for respiratory arrest alone, in children, is greater than 50 percent where resuscitation is provided.

The pediatric airway differs from the adult airway as it is shorter and narrower, and the epiglottis is long and floppy. Therefore, a relatively small airway obstruction can cause significant reduction in airway diameter with increased airflow resistance and work of breathing. Over the past few years, there have been significant advances in the etiopathology and management of respiratory diseases. Interleukins, aquaporins, cytokines, and other molecules as well as free radicals, have been described to mediate inflammation and repair.

Pharmacologic therapy for many diseases, including bronchopulmonary dysplasia (BPD) and pediatric asthma focuses on use of 'free radical sinks' and cytokine inhibitors. Recent ventilatory strategies have moved away from mimicking the volumes and pressures of physiologic ventilation toward using low-pressure and low-volume strategies as well as ventilation in prone position.[1–6] High-frequency oscillatory ventilation (HFOV) in the pediatric and more so in the neonatal age group has improved alveolar recruitment and reduced barotrauma and volutrauma.[7] Adjunctive therapies such as the use of pulmonary surfactant have improved the short-term response of the lungs in neonates to ventilation and reduced the incidence of patent ductus arteriosus, intraventricular hemorrhage, and pneumothorax.[8–10] Surfactant has also been used in children for respiratory distress syndrome (RDS), although the results have been mixed. A randomized controlled trial found no benefit of nebulized surfactant in adult patients with sepsis-induced adult respiratory syndrome.[11] However, another trial involving use of bovine surfactant in acute RDS patients of different age groups showed superior air exchange and improved lung physiology in the surfactant-treated child patients without a change in the outcome.[12]

Inhaled nitric oxide (iNO) is now routinely being used in the treatment of persistent pulmonary hypertension of the new born (PPHN). However, trials of iNO after the newborn period and in adults for ARDS have shown only transient improvement in lung function and oxygenation.[13–16] Extracorporeal membrane oxygenation (ECMO) is now being used to manage neonates with PPHN not responding to conventional therapy and iNO. However, outcomes of pediatric ECMO are not as good as for neonates, with an overall survival rate of 40–50 percent.[17–19] Newer therapeutic modes such as liquid ventilation are limited to animal experiments and a few human studies. A study of the efficacy of liquid ventilation in adults with ARDS failed to demonstrate any benefit among the treatment group.[20]

CROUP

Croup refers to a clinical syndrome characterized by barking cough, inspiratory stridor, and hoarseness of the voice. It is also referred to as laryngotracheobronchitis. Croup is a common cause of upper airway obstruction in children, and about 6 percent of children require hospitalization. Most cases of croup are viral in etiology, the most common causative agent being parainfluenza virus (75 percent of viral cases). Other viruses that can cause croup are adenovirus, respiratory syncytial virus (RSV), and measles virus. Viral croup shows a biannual peak in incidence.

Clinical features

There may be a short history suggestive of a viral upper respiratory infection, such as cough, cold, and fever. Subsequently the child develops a hoarse voice, brassy cough, and stridor, which is usually inspiratory, though it can be both inspiratory and expiratory. The illness usually lasts for several days but may last for several weeks. Agitation and crying can worsen the symptoms. If croup progresses in severity, the child may appear cyanotic and pale due to hypoxemia, and the disease may lead to respiratory failure.

Investigations

Radiography of the upper airways shows subglottic narrowing, referred to as the 'steeple sign'.

Management

MILD CROUP (NO STRIDOR AT REST)

The child should be disturbed as little as possible. They can generally be managed at home. The use of steam from a shower or bath, historically, is known to terminate acute spasm. However, as this could inadvertently cause complications such as burns and scalds, cold mist from a humidifier by the bedside may be more helpful. Treatment of fever, if present, with antipyretics, is also indicated.

MODERATE TO SEVERE CROUP (STRIDOR AT REST)

Mist therapy

Misting through a tent or humidifier has been one of the mainstays of the treatment of croup that relieves the symptoms by soothing the inflamed upper airway mucosa. However, placing the child in an unfamiliar atmosphere of a croup tent may further agitate the child and therefore worsen the spasm. It may also make the evaluation of progressive respiratory distress more difficult. Randomized controlled trials have failed to demonstrate the efficacy of this technique.[21]

Corticosteroids

Corticosteroids may act by reduction of inflammation and swelling of the respiratory mucosa. Dexamethasone in a dose of 0.15–0.6 mg/kg orally or intramuscularly is recommended. Budesonide in a dose of 2 mg by nebulizer can also be used. A few trials have found dexamethasone superior to budesonide. Both dexamethasone and budesonide have been found to reduce stay in the emergency room and in inpatient settings.[22,23]

Epinephrine

Racemic epinephrine, in a dose of 0.05 mL/kg, to a maximum of 0.5 mL/dose diluted in normal saline, given by nebulization, reduces secretions and inflammation of the respiratory mucosa. Racemic epinephrine can be given every 2 hours, and children needing more frequent administration should be considered for admission to the pediatric intensive care unit. The child who has been administered racemic epinephrine should be observed for at least 2 hours subsequently for rebound symptoms.[24,25] However, rebound of symptoms is uncommon if racemic epinephrine is administered along with corticosteroids.

Intubation

If the child with croup shows evidence of impending or imminent respiratory failure, intubation and mechanical ventilation should be considered.

EPIGLOTTITIS

Epiglottitis is the inflammation of the epiglottis and the supraglottic portion of the airway. This disease has become much less common after the introduction of the influenza (HiB) vaccine. It affects children between 2 and 6 years of age, the peak incidence being at about 3 years. The commonest causative organism is *Haemophilus influenzae*, but other bacteria and viruses can cause epiglottitis.

Clinical features

The child with epiglottitis may present with a history of high fever. The child may have a 'toxic' and anxious look, with drooling, and may adopt a 'tripod position' sitting with both arms extended and face in the sniffing position, in order to maintain patency of the airway. If epiglottitis is suspected, the pharynx should be examined in the operating room with trained personnel ready to intubate. The epiglottis will be seen to be inflamed and 'cherry red' in color.

Investigations

Radiographs should never be done when moderate to severe airway obstruction is suspected. In case of mild airway obstruction, radiographs may show an enlarged epiglottis. The aryepiglottic folds may be markedly thickened, separating the tracheal and esophageal air columns in the hypopharyngeal area.

Management

The child with suspected epiglottitis should not be agitated or disturbed, as this could increase the laryngospasm and worsen respiratory distress. Humidified oxygen by mask should be administered if this does not upset the child. An airway team should be called to the emergency room and should accompany the child to the operating room. The epiglottis should be visualized to confirm the diagnosis. Swabs should be taken from the pharyngeal and epiglottic surface, and the child should be intubated under anesthesia and put on mechanical ventilation.[26,27] If the vocal cord edema is severe, tracheostomy may be indicated. Antibiotics such as ceftriaxone should be started. Antibiotics should be continued for 7–10 days, and the child should be gradually weaned off mechanical ventilation.

BRONCHIAL FOREIGN BODY ASPIRATION

Foreign body aspiration is not unusual in children. They can either be extruded by the child's cough reflex or lodge themselves in the larynx, trachea, or bronchi. A common site for lodgment is the right main stem bronchus, as it is shorter, straighter and wider than the left main stem bronchus.[28]

Pathophysiology

A foreign body lodged in the right main stem bronchus may cause either partial or complete obstruction. If it causes partial obstruction, it can act as a ball valve or check valve. Air can, therefore, enter the bronchus on inspiration, but is unable to leave the bronchus on expiration, as the airflow is blocked by the foreign body. This results in overinflation and emphysema of the segment distal to the obstruction, with poor air exchange. If the obstruction is complete, the air in the segment distal to the bronchus eventually gets absorbed and this causes atelectasis. Both situations can lead to secondary infection and abscess formation.

Clinical features

Immediately after the foreign body is aspirated, there may be paroxysmal coughing. If the foreign body irritates the mucosa and causes total obstruction, there may be wheezing. The coughing and wheezing may last for an indefinite period. Dullness to percussion and reduced air entry on the affected side may be perceived on examination.

If it is a nonirritating foreign body and the obstruction is partial, then the child may be relatively asymptomatic after the initial symptoms. If postobstruction emphysema develops, there may be respiratory distress and there may be reduced air entry on examination and hyperresonance on percussion. In either case, fever and respiratory distress may develop in case of superadded infection.

Investigations

In case of complete foreign body obstruction, the chest radiograph may show atelectasis and mediastinal shift to the same side. A radioopaque foreign body may be visualized. Both expiratory and inspiratory films should be taken. In case of check valve obstruction with emphysema, expiratory films may show mediastinal shift to the side opposite to the obstruction. This may be better visualized on fluoroscopy. However, the chest radiograph can show normal findings in the case of foreign body aspiration, and rigid bronchoscopy should be done for both diagnosis and management, if aspiration is strongly suspected.

Treatment

The child should be administered oxygen if in respiratory distress, and appropriate respiratory support should be provided. Bronchodilators can be administered by nebulization if the child is wheezing. Children who are symptomatic with strong suspicion of foreign body aspiration should be admitted to the hospital. Rigid bronchoscopy should be performed, and the foreign body removed, if visualized. Treatment with antibiotics should be instituted if superadded infection is suspected.

STATUS ASTHMATICUS

Asthma is characterized by diffuse, reversible lower airway obstruction with evidence of lower airway inflammation and edema, bronchial smooth muscle spasm and mucus plugging. Worsening acute severe asthma, when not responsive to conventional bronchodilator treatment, can lead to status asthmaticus. There is no consensus in the literature about the exact definition of the condition – a patient who is not responsive to initial doses of nebulized bronchodilators should be considered to be in status asthmaticus. Some authors characterize a patient with severe asthma as being in status asthmaticus if they fail to respond to at least three doses of nebulizers or bronchodilators.[29]

Epidemiology

The prevalence of asthma is on the rise worldwide. In the United States it is about 10 percent.[30] The morbidity and mortality related to asthma is also on the rise both in the United States and worldwide. The risk factors for potentially fatal asthma include medical factors such as a history of previous asthma attack with seizure; loss of consciousness or respiratory failure; psychosocial factors such as noncompliance or depression; and ethnic factors, with nonwhite children being more at risk than white children.

Clinical features

The child with status asthmaticus usually presents with cough and wheezing, and increased work of breathing. Bilateral wheezing may be heard on auscultation, with reduced air entry. However, if air entry is significantly reduced, wheezing may not be heard, and a 'silent chest' may be an ominous sign.[31] Children may also present in respiratory failure or cardiopulmonary arrest. They may have low oxygen saturation on pulse oximetry and may demonstrate pulsus paradoxus.[32–34]

Investigations

The diagnosis of status asthmaticus is mainly clinical. Arterial blood gas may show evidence of respiratory and metabolic acidosis.

Management

GENERAL

The cardiopulmonary status of the child in status asthmaticus should be continuously monitored, along with blood pressure measurement.

OXYGEN

Adequate humidified oxygen should be provided to keep saturations above 95 percent via non-rebreather mask.

NEBULIZED BRONCHODILATORS

Albuterol should be administered, either by frequent nebulization or as continuous nebulization. Most studies have used low doses (4–10 mg/h) of continually nebulized albuterol, but recent studies recommend much higher doses (up to 150 mg/h at 10–12 L/min flow).[35] It must be noted that very small quantities of nebulized medications may reach the targeted bronchioles in the presence of severe bronchospasm.[36]

CORTICOSTEROIDS

Intravenous methylprednisolone, 0.5–1 mg/kg every 4–6 hours, or hydrocortisone, 2–4 mg/kg every 4–6 hours, should be administered. Intravenous steroids may take over 4 hours to start having effect.

ANTICHOLINERGICS

Ipratropium can be used by nebulization in a dose of 250–500 µg every 6 hours, in addition to albuterol administration.[37]

INTRAVENOUS BRONCHODILATORS

Intravenous terbutaline in a dose of 0.1–10 µg/kg per minute should be considered in children unresponsive to continuous nebulization. Some trials have suggested using intravenous aminophylline, but this remains controversial.[38] Other authors suggest using this in critically ill children when standard treatment for status asthmaticus has been unsuccessful.[38]

MAGNESIUM SULFATE

Intravenous magnesium sulfate has been recommended for the treatment of severe asthma, in a dose of 75 mg/kg over 20 minutes.[39,40] The efficacy of magnesium sulfate in children with bronchospasm is, however, doubtful.

HELIOX

Helium-oxygen mixture with a concentration of helium between 60 percent and 80 percent can be used to reduce the density of the mixture as compared with nitrogen-oxygen mixture and therefore increase oxygen delivery to the distal bronchioles.[41,42] However, this cannot be used in children with a relatively high oxygen requirement due to the relatively lower concentration of oxygen in the mixture.[43]

VENTILATION

Mechanical ventilation should be avoided, if possible, in patients with severe asthma, as it increases the incidence of complications such as barotrauma and air trapping.[44–46] The indications for ventilation include deterioration in the child's mental state, cardiac and respiratory arrest and evidence of severe hypoxia. If the child needs to be ventilated, a long expiratory time and low rate strategy should be employed, with appropriate pressure support as the child improves.[47]

KETAMINE

Ketamine is an anesthetic and analgesic agent, which also mediates bronchodilatation. Therefore it has been used in children with severe asthma on mechanical ventilation (2 mg/kg bolus followed by a continuous infusion of 0.5 mg/kg per hour).[48] However, it should be used with caution in patients with hypercarbia as it may cause increased intracranial tension due to its ability to cause cerebral vasodilatation.[49]

SMOKE INHALATION

Smoke inhalation is associated with over half of burn deaths in the United States. Advances in technology have been contributing to reducing the mortality due to surface burns. However, this has led to an increase in the morbidity and mortality due to pulmonary injury as a result of concomitant smoke inhalation.

Pathophysiology and clinical features

Injury due to smoke inhalation may be due to injury at a cellular level, or due to local or systemic effects. Injury immediately after exposure may be due to the effects of hypoxia or carbon monoxide. Carbon monoxide causes poor release of oxygen to the tissues, and it also may have a myocardial depressant effect leading to ventricular arrhythmias.[50] At the cytochrome oxidase level it may cause neurologic manifestations. Combustion of plastic may cause cyanide toxicity, and other toxic gases may contribute to morbidity as well.

The mechanism and effects of smoke inhalation injury may be divided into five phases:[51]

1. Immediate heat transfer may result in severe mucosal injury, and may cause acute respiratory distress due to bronchospasm and laryngeal edema. This may go on for 6–12 hours, and the bronchospasm may not be reversed by administering β-agonists.
2. At 6–72 hours pulmonary edema may occur, initially due to increased capillary permeability and subsequently worsened by surfactant deficiency.
3. At 2–4 days respiratory distress may occur or be worsened by the presence of a cervical eschar.
4. After 2–4 days, pneumonia may develop as a result of either restrictive disease or decreased ability of the mucociliary apparatus to clear the airways of bacteria.
5. Late effects of smoke inhalation may be manifested by increased predisposition to airway hyperactivity.

Investigations

Studies have shown that in 92 percent of patients with inhalation injury the radiograph revealed normal findings if it was taken early.[52] Therefore in the absence of respiratory signs, early chest films may not be useful in the diagnosis of inhalation injury. Bronchoscopy is a useful investigation in evaluating inhalation injury and studies have shown up to 86 percent diagnostic accuracy.[53] It has also been used for therapeutic purposes in the presence of atelectasis.[53] Pulmonary function tests, when performed, may be abnormal, but they are more useful as a follow-up tool rather than for diagnosis. Radionuclide xenon scanning has not been shown to be of practical value.

Management

Prehospital emergency personnel should follow a trauma management protocol, including spinal immobilization if a fall or spinal trauma is suspected. Airway, breathing, and circulation should be assessed and appropriately managed; 100 percent oxygen should be provided through a non-rebreather. Carboxyhemoglobin levels, total and differential white blood cell (WBC) count, electrolytes, blood urea nitrogen (BUN), and glucose should be measured. Blood should be cross-matched and kept ready if need for transfusion arises. Burns, if present, should be assessed and managed, and appropriate intravenous fluids administered. Asymptomatic low-risk children should be observed for 4–12 hours. Severe respiratory distress should be managed with endotracheal intubation and oxygenation. Bronchospasm, if present, can be treated with bronchodilators.

The role of corticosteroids is controversial. Although steroids have been used to treat upper airway burns and edema, their use has been reported to be associated with increased rate of pulmonary infection.[54] If cyanide toxicity is suspected, antidotes in the form of sodium nitrate and sodium thiosulfate should be used. The use of prophylactic antibiotics is controversial as well, and is not generally recommended. Parenteral coverage of antibiotics should be provided when infection is suspected. Hyperbaric oxygen has been tried for management of carbon monoxide poisoning. However, in a gravely ill patient, it may be advisable to provide high-flow 100 percent oxygen, as it may be difficult to treat such a child if enclosed in a hyperbaric chamber.

DROWNING AND NEAR-DROWNING

Epidemiology and definition

Drowning is responsible for about 500 000 deaths around the world every year, and is the third most common cause of death by unintentional injury for people between 5 and 44 years of age.[55] Drowning is defined as death resulting from suffocation within 24 hours of submersion in a liquid medium, and near-drowning as survival at least 24 hours after an episode of suffocation caused by submersion in a liquid medium. The immersion syndrome is defined as syncope provoked by bradycardia, tachycardia, or arrhythmia precipitated by sudden contact with water at a temperature of at least 5° less than the body temperature.

Pathophysiology

The pathophysiology of drowning and near-drowning involves hypoxia and metabolic acidosis, and hypercarbia leading to respiratory acidosis.[56] Although experimental models demonstrate a difference in the pathophysiologic mechanisms and effects in freshwater and saltwater drowning, this is often of little practical significance. There is initial laryngospasm or breath-holding, followed by aspiration of water. This leads to pulmonary surfactant depletion, alveolar damage, pulmonary edema, intrapulmonary shunting, and hypoxia. Ventricular fibrillation may occur due to hypoxia and acidosis, and there may be severe peripheral vasoconstriction due to hypoxia, catecholamine release, and hypothermia.

Management

It is important to remember that artificial or assisted breaths must be started at the site of rescue of the drowning victim if possible, and should not be deferred. Time should not be wasted in trying to extrude the water from the lungs before cardiopulmonary resuscitation is started. This is because the water quickly dissipates into the vascular compartment in case of freshwater immersion, and will continue to cause fluid to be poured into the lungs due to pulmonary edema in case of saltwater drowning. Suctioning fluid from the airways may be necessary in case of saltwater drowning, due to pulmonary edema. Cardiopulmonary resuscitation should be continued as long as needed until the victim arrives at an emergency care facility.

Admission to a hospital for a minimum of 24 hours is indicated for any drowning victim who was submerged for at least 1 minute, was apneic or cyanotic, or required pulmonary resuscitation. Fulminant pulmonary edema despite normal chest radiograph findings has been reported to develop as long as 12 hours after the episode. Monitoring should be done by serial measurement of blood gases, electrolytes, BUN, creatinine, and hemoglobin.

Adequate respiratory support should be provided in the form of high-flow oxygen, continuous positive airway pressure (CPAP) or mechanical ventilation, if indicated. Cardiac dysfunction, if present, should be treated with pressors such as dobutamine. Administration of diuretics such as furosemide may lead to volume depletion. Cerebral anoxia and edema should be appropriately monitored and treated, if present. Hyperpyrexia due to failure of the hypothalamic thermostat has been treated with body cooling, and dexamethasone can be used for management of cerebral edema. Any drowning victim should be examined for the presence of cranial and spinal trauma. Recent studies have explored the administration of surfactant, instituting ECMO, nitric oxide, and liquid ventilation, but these are still in the experimental stage.

Prevention

The key to minimize injury or death due to drowning is prevention. Pediatricians, in consonance with parents, children, caregivers, and the community must be proactive in implementing the American Academy of Pediatrics (AAP) recommendations for the prevention of drowning.[57]

BRONCHIOLITIS

Epidemiology and etiology

Bronchiolitis is a common viral respiratory infection in children. In the United States, the rate of admission for bronchiolitis among children under 1 year of age has increased from 12.9 per 1000 children in 1980 to 31.2 per 1000 children in 1996, possibly partly due to an increase in the number of premature children and partly as a result of changes in admission criteria.[58] The respiratory syncytial virus (RSV) is responsible for bronchiolitis in over 50 percent of cases, other agents being parainfluenza virus, adenovirus, mycoplasma, etc. Bronchiolitis is more common in boys, and peaks during winter and early spring.

Pathophysiology

Pathophysiologic processes occur both at the cellular and molecular levels. Infection by the virus leads to edema and accumulation of cellular debris, thus causing airway obstruction, air trapping, and atelectasis.[59] At a molecular level, cytokines, interleukins, and IgE are involved.[60]

Clinical features

Clinical features are often more severe in the younger age groups, especially babies under 1 year of age. There may be evidence of a mild upper respiratory tract infection with sneezing and rhinorrhea, with or without fever. This is followed by respiratory distress and wheezing. Very young babies may have apnea. Examination may therefore reveal respiratory distress in the form of nasal flaring, retractions, and crackles or wheezing on auscultation. Pulse oximetry may show evidence of hypoxia, and there may not always be a correlation between the degree of respiratory distress and hypoxemia.

Differential diagnosis

In a younger child, the diagnosis of asthma rather than bronchiolitis may be entertained if there are repeated episodes of wheezing, absence of a viral prodrome, and presence of a family history of atopy or asthma. In babies and children presenting with wheezing or stridor, tracheomalacia or bronchomalacia and vascular rings and slings should be ruled out. Pertussis should be considered as a differential diagnosis in babies with persistent and continuous coughing.

Investigations

The chest radiograph may show evidence of hyperinflation or atelectasis. The WBC and differential counts may be normal or affected. Viral testing can be done by rapid immunofluorescence, and this may often avoid the need for sepsis evaluation in an infant.

Management

The management of bronchiolitis is mainly supportive. Babies with significant respiratory distress should be hospitalized, and so should very young infants because of the risk of apnea.[61–63] Cool humidified oxygen should be provided. The baby should not be fed orally and parenteral fluids should be provided if there is risk of aspiration.

Bronchodilators may provide some short-term improvement, although there are few data to support administering bronchodilators to all patients. A Cochrane metaanalysis suggested improved clinical scores for hospitalized patients and outpatients receiving bronchodilator therapy, but the authors mention possible bias in data.[64] Therefore it may be reasonable to offer an initial treatment with a bronchodilator, with further treatment depending on the response. Nebulized epinephrine has also been tried as a therapeutic modality, although trials have not shown this to be efficacious.[65–67]

Corticosteroids have been widely used by the oral, inhaled, or intravenous route. However, there is little evidence to show that corticosteroids are beneficial, except in cases of recurrent wheezing where reactive airway disease may figure as a differential diagnosis.[68] Ribavirin, an antiviral agent, has been administered by aerosol to infants with chronic lung disease or congenital cardiac disease, but there is no convincing evidence of its efficacy.[69] Respiratory syncytial virus immune globulin has no role in acute bronchiolitis, and antibiotics are indicated only in the presence of bacterial pneumonia.[70]

There has been a recent interest in the administration of heliox for moderate to severe bronchiolitis. Some trials have been conducted using heliox. They have shown some improvement in clinical scores and length of stay, but all had limitations such as only short-term use of heliox, lack of standardization or absence of randomization and blinding.[71,72]

Prevention

Palivizumab, a monoclonal antibody to the RSV F protein, has been effective in reducing the risk of RSV infection before and during the RSV season. The latest AAP recommendations for administration of palivizumab should be followed (monthly intramuscular injections for high-risk groups).[73] Pooled RSV immunoglobulin has also been used, although this involves intravenous administration. Thorough handwashing is an extremely effective method to prevent nosocomial transmission of RSV.

RESPIRATORY EMERGENCIES IN THE NEONATE

After birth a normal neonate establishes the lungs as the site of gas exchange. This involves absorption of the lung fluid and a change from fetal to neonatal circulation – a transition from blood being shunted away from the lungs to now fully perfused pulmonary vasculature. The lung fluid is absorbed into the interstitium by active transport and drainage through pulmonary circulation. This process starts before the labor and is influenced by the increasing levels of catecholamines. The fluid absorption is accelerated by the onset of labor and after birth. The first few breaths facilitate the drainage of lung fluid and establish functional residual capacity (FRC). To maintain the FRC the alveoli must stay patent at the end of expiration. This process is facilitated by the presence of endogenous surfactant. Thus any condition that leads to surfactant deficiency (such as prematurity) or its inactivation (meconium stained amniotic fluid, hypoxia, and pulmonary hemorrhage) can lead to loss of FRC and inadequate gas exchange.

The transition from fetal to neonatal circulation involves decrease in pulmonary resistance as a result of expansion of lungs, fall in arterial carbon dioxide, rise in pH and oxygen, an increase in systemic blood pressure, and closure of the ductus arteriosus.[74–76] Thus respiratory distress in a neonate may be the result of several factors that operate individually or in combination with each other. These causes include surfactant deficiency, delayed absorption of lung fluid, aspiration of meconium into the lungs, and failure of decrease in pulmonary resistance leading to persistence of the fetal circulatory pattern. Neonatal sepsis especially group B streptococcal infection also remains a leading cause of neonatal respiratory distress.[77–80] Furthermore any anatomic abnormality in the respiratory tract or related structures may also lead to respiratory difficulty.[81]

During evaluation of a neonate with respiratory distress these etiological factors should be kept in mind and the management planned accordingly.[79] Significant advances in the understanding of the physiology of the premature neonate and in technology have markedly improved the survival of these babies. Some of the newer modes of treatment include use of iNO to lower the pulmonary resistance, HFOV, and ECMO. However, optimal antenatal care, prevention of preterm delivery, and proper handling of the newborn baby at birth remain key factors in the management of these patients.[80–82]

Developmental aspects of neonatal lung disease

The maturational changes that take place before the onset of normal respiratory function in the newborn include structural development of the lung to ensure adequate sites for gas exchange, maturation of the surfactant system, and maturation of the neuromuscular control of respiration. Lung development can be divided into five phases: embryonic, pseudoglandular, canalicular, saccular, and alveolar.[83–85]

EMBRYONIC PHASE

The primordial lung bud appears on day 26 of gestation as a ventral epithelial outgrowth from the foregut and forms the two primary bronchial buds. During the fifth week these primary bronchi divide to form the lobar bronchi and the lung buds grow laterally into the walls of the pericardioperitoneal canals. Segmental bronchi form establishing the bronchopulmonary segments in the sixth week.

PSEUDOGLANDULAR PERIOD

Dichotomous branching of the bronchial buds during the subsequent 10-week period forms all the conducting airways, after which they only grow in size. The pleural membranes and pulmonary lymphatics also develop between 8 and 10 weeks. The malformation arising during this period is pulmonary sequestration, which is thought to originate as accessory or ectopic bronchial buds or branches. Separation of the pleuroperitoneal canals into the thoracic cavity and the peritoneal cavity is completed before the seventh week of gestation by formation of the diaphragm from the pleuroperitoneal membranes. Failure of closure of this canal, before the tenth week of gestation when the developing intestine return to the abdominal cavity, may lead to diaphragmatic hernia.

CANALICULAR PERIOD

In the 17–28 weeks of gestation the basic structure of the gas-exchanging portion of the lung is formed and vascularized. The epithelial growth predominates over the mesenchymal growth. The main features of this phase are appearance of acini, epithelial differentiation with the development of the potential air–blood barrier, and the expression of antigenic markers that lead to differentiation into type I or type II (surfactant-producing pneumocytes). At 17 weeks the first intraacinar respiratory bronchioles develop. From 18 weeks multiple saccules arise from the last generation of respiratory bronchioles. Glycogen-rich type II pneumocytes are usually distinguished at 20 weeks by the appearance of lamellar inclusions, but lamellar bodies are not seen until a later date. The abnormalities that occur during this period of acinar development may lead to pulmonary hypoplasia, with deficient gas exchange tissue. Failure of fusion of the double capillary membrane results in alveolar capillary dysplasia leading to severe hypoxia.

SACCULAR PERIOD

The saccular period begins at about 25–28 weeks of gestation and is associated with continued widening of terminal airways and formation of cylindrical structures called saccules.

ALVEOLAR PERIOD

The alveolar phase continues from 36 weeks of gestation to 3 years of postnatal life. At term gestation about 50–150 million alveoli are present. There is a rapid increase in their number during the first years of life, reaching the adult number of approximately 300 million by 3 years of age. Vitamin A and thyroxine (T_4) stimulate alveolarization, whereas mechanical ventilation, glucocorticoids, pro-inflammatory cytokines, and poor nutrition adversely affect it.[86]

Pulmonary fluid

Approximately 30 mL/kg of fluid fills the potential air spaces of the fetal lung. It contains large amount of chloride, small amounts of bicarbonate and almost no protein. Its potassium concentration is similar to that of the plasma until near term. Fetal lung fluid is secreted at 4–5 mL/kg per hour as a result of active secretion of chloride ions into the pulmonary fluid. The pressure in the trachea exceeds that in the amniotic fluid by about 2 mm Hg. Thus amniotic fluid rarely enters the developing lung, except in circumstances of fetal distress. The lung must clear this liquid soon after birth for the fetus to complete the transition from intrauterine to extrauterine life. The process of clearing begins 2–3 days before birth with a decrease in the rate of secretion of fetal lung liquid. During active labor and delivery the fetal lung fluid decreases to about 35 percent of the earlier volume. This amount must be absorbed after the birth. When the lungs expand water moves rapidly from the air spaces into the interstitium and is subsequently absorbed by the lymphatics and pulmonary blood vessels. Delayed absorption of the pulmonary fluid leads to transient tachypnea of the newborn and is more common among babies born by a cesarean section to mothers who did not go into active labor.[87,88]

Clinical signs of respiratory distress in a neonate

The clinical signs commonly used to assess the pulmonary function in a neonate are: respiratory rate, retractions, nasal flaring, grunting, and cyanosis.[89]

RESPIRATORY RATE

Neonates with abnormal elastic and resistive components of the work of breathing tend to adjust their respiratory rate to minimize the work. Thus, in neonates with decreased lung compliance such as in those with RDS, respiratory rate is rapid and shallow, whereas those with increased airway resistance (such as caused by subglottic stenosis) may exhibit respiration that is slower and deeper.

RETRACTIONS

The negative intrapleural pressure generated during inspiration is determined by balance between the force of the diaphragm and the compliance of the lung and the chest wall. The neonatal chest being very compliant, substernal, subcostal, and intercostal retractions are readily seen with relatively small changes in lung mechanics. In neonates with respiratory distress, retractions become more apparent as the lungs compliance decreases. Severe retractions may also indicate complications of respiratory disease such as airway obstruction, misplacement of an endotracheal tube, pneumothorax, or atelectasis. In smaller infants the retractions may even precede blood gases changes.

NASAL FLARING

The enlargement of the effective air passage produced by activation of alae nasi results in the reduction of the resistance. Because newborns are obligatory nose breathers, nasal resistance contributes significantly to the total lung resistance. Nasal flaring decreases work of breathing by decreasing the resistance. It is commonly observed in infants with respiratory distress.

GRUNTING

During normal respiration the vocal cords abduct during inspiration and adduct during expiration without producing any sound. In the presence of increased work of breathing, neonates attempt to compensate by closing their vocal cords during expiration thereby increasing lung volume, which leads to an improved ventilation/perfusion ratio. Expiration through partially closed vocal cords produces the grunting sound. Grunting may be intermittent or continuous depending on the severity of the lung disease.

CYANOSIS

Cyanosis reflects the presence of a minimum of 50 g/L of reduced hemoglobin in systemic capillaries. Peripheral cyanosis is often a manifestation of peripheral vascular constriction in response to low environmental temperature. It may also reflect a low cardiac output state leading to slow capillary circulation and decrease in oxygenated hemoglobin. In contrast, central cyanosis is always pathologic and a manifestation of significant hypoxia. Fetal hemoglobin has a higher affinity for oxygen. Therefore presence of cyanosis in a neonate signifies relatively higher degree of hypoxia than in older children or adults.

Persistent pulmonary hypertension of the newborn

As a result of the high pulmonary vascular resistance prior to birth, blood is diverted away from the lungs through the foramen ovale and the patent ductus arteriosus into the low resistance systemic and placental circulation. With the loss of the placenta at the time of birth, systemic vascular resistance increases concomitantly with a significant drop in pulmonary vascular resistance. That results in increased blood flow to lungs and cessation of right to left shunt across the ductus arteriosus and foramen ovale thus completing the cardiopulmonary adaptation at birth. Failure of the decrease in pulmonary resistance can lead to persistence of the fetal circulatory pattern.[90]

TRANSITION AT BIRTH

Abolition of placental circulation leads to increase in systemic vascular resistance, increase in the left ventricular and left atrial pressure that in turn results in functional closure of the foramen ovale. Onset of ventilation and expansion of the lungs straightens out mechanically compressed vessels and results in increase in oxygen tension in the alveolus and in arterial blood. That leads to pulmonary vascular relaxation and constriction of ductus arteriosus. Both these changes together result in the closure of the fetal conduits that diverted blood away from the lungs. With increased systemic vascular resistance more blood flows into the low-resistance pulmonary bed. The ductus arteriosus remains anatomically patent for several weeks after birth, but because the neonate is so much better oxygenated than the fetus the ductus becomes functionally closed in the full-term infant by 24–36 hours after birth.

DEFINITION

Persistent pulmonary hypertension of the newborn is the result of elevated pulmonary vascular resistance to the point that venous blood is diverted through the ductus arteriosus and foramen ovale away from the lungs into the systemic circulation resulting in systemic arterial hypoxemia. It can be classified into three forms:

- No evidence of parenchymal disease with radiographically normal lungs –primary pulmonary hypertension.
- PPHN associated with pulmonary parenchymal disease, such as hyaline membrane disease, meconium aspiration, or pneumonia or other diseases leading to alveolar hypoxia – secondary PPHN.
- PPHN associated with hypoplasia of the lungs – most often in the form of diaphragmatic hernia associated with an anatomic reduction in capillary number.

It is essential to rule out cyanotic heart disease which can clinically mimic PPHN.

PATHOPHYSIOLOGY

Failure of pulmonary vascular resistance to decrease after birth (despite improved alveolar oxygenation, lung expansion, and increased systemic resistance) results in continuing blood flow through the foramen ovale and ductus arteriosus from right to left. With inability to increase pulmonary blood flow the arterial oxygen tension falls to very low levels. To pump blood to either vascular bed, the right heart is subjected to a large mechanical load in the presence of high pulmonary (supra-systemic) and systemic resistance. Persistence of high vascular resistance and hypoxemia may lead to poor myocardial performance resulting in right heart dilation, tricuspid insufficiency, and right heart failure. Several mechanisms have been proposed that may lead to persistent pulmonary hypertension:

1. High dose intake of aspirin by mothers near term may lead to repeated intrauterine closure of the ductus with redirection of blood flow into the high-resistance fetal pulmonary vasculature.

2. There is pathologic evidence that babies with PPHN have greater thickness of medial muscle in pulmonary arteries than in normal full-term infants. This has been attributed to repeated intrauterine hypoxia that stimulates the hypertrophy of medial smooth muscle surrounding the pulmonary arterioles, resulting in constriction of vessels to an extreme degree for long periods of time. This may lead to abnormal responsiveness of the pulmonary vasculature to hypoxia with an inability to relax after the stimulus for vasoconstriction is removed, i.e. birth asphyxia.

3. Poor regional ventilation and alveolar hypoxia may lead to localized vasoconstriction, even though other parts of the lung are ventilating normally.

4. Congenital diaphragmatic hernia or other causes of pulmonary hypoplasia are frequently accompanied by undergrowth of the pulmonary vascular tree and increased vascular resistance.

5. Nitric oxide, eicosanoids, and endothelin are among some of the vasoactive mediators that play a role in transitional circulation. Other mediators such as leukotrienes, tumor necrosis factor, and platelet activating factor may participate in active pulmonary vasoconstriction. Alteration in the level of these substances may lead to pulmonary vasoconstriction.

6. Pathologic evidence of platelet-fibrin microthromboembolism has been reported in infants who succumb to PPHN. The mechanical obstruction caused by these microthrombi and vasoconstriction, which is caused by the accompanying release of vasoactive mediators, may induce pulmonary hypertension. PPHN is most often associated with perinatal asphyxia and less frequently associated with other disorders such as hypoglycemia, hypocalcemia, hyperviscosity syndrome, and sepsis.[90]

CLINICAL DIAGNOSIS

Primary PPHN presents in the early postnatal period as cyanosis and tachypnea that closely mimic the presentation of cyanotic congenital heart disease. There may be differential cyanosis between upper and lower body. The lung fields are usually clear on a radiograph. The degree of hypoxia is variable and the Pa_{CO_2} is normal or low. Secondary PPHN presents primarily as respiratory distress due to underlying lung disease. As the lung disease deteriorates and the patient needs increasing respiratory support, PPHN becomes apparent. Chest radiograph findings are consistent with the underlying disease. In both types clinical evidence of tricuspid incompetence may be present.

Echocardiography should be performed to exclude congenital heart disease; determine the pulmonary artery pressure; the presence, degree, and direction of shunt through the duct and foramen ovale; and right or left ventricular function and output.[91–94]

MANAGEMENT

The treatment is aimed at maintenance of normal arterial levels of oxygen and its delivery to the organs of the body, and minimizing pulmonary vasoconstriction. The most potent natural pulmonary vasodilators are oxygen and optimal lung inflation.

Oxygen

Improving alveolar oxygenation with supplemental oxygen early on, in the presence of pulmonary parenchymal disease is particularly useful as it often results in relaxation of the pulmonary arteries and improved pulmonary blood flow. Animal data suggest that optimal pulmonary vasodilatation occurs with a Pa_{CO_2} of 100–120 mm Hg. The Pa_{CO_2} should be maintained between 80 mm Hg and 100 mm Hg. Higher levels of inspired oxygen offer no benefit but may instead contribute to secondary lung injury.

Conventional ventilation

This is the mainstay of respiratory support. The ventilatory strategy should be based according to the underlying pulmonary disease if any. Patients should be well sedated and term and near-term babies even paralyzed to ensure optimal ventilator efficiency. It is often necessary to ventilate with high minute volumes (>300 mL/kg) to achieve normal blood gases. Small reductions in minute volume that may occur with retained secretions or minor painful procedures may lead to significant changes in oxygenation.

Sedation

Because catecholamines stimulate α-adrenergic receptor release and thereby increase pulmonary vascular resistance, use of a strong narcotic analgesic like fentanyl at a dose of 3–8 µg/kg per hour can prevent pulmonary vasospasm due to minor variability in oxygenation. Alternatively continuous infusion of morphine sulfate starting at 10 µg/kg per hour and/or bolus or continuous infusion of lorazepam may be used. Paralysis is usually achieved with pancuronium bromide administered every 1–3 hours intravenously at 0.1–0.2 mg/kg per dose. Pa_{CO_2} should be maintained between 35 mm Hg and 40 mm Hg and lower levels than this may cause cerebral vasoconstriction.[95,96]

High frequency oscillatory ventilation

The best effect of HFOV is seen in babies with underlying severe lung disease. It probably works by allowing better lung inflation and alveolar recruitment.[96–98]

Inotropes

Low-ventricular outputs are common in babies with PPHN. The low output may reflect the inability of right ventricle to pump blood through the lungs against high resistance, which in turn causes a low left ventricular output. In animal studies, dopamine has similar vasoconstrictor activity on the pulmonary and systemic vasculature, so at an empiric level, dobutamine is the preferred inotrope starting at 10 µg/kg per minute. Significant increase in ventricular outputs with nitric oxide in term babies has been reported and this may be a more rational approach to circulatory support than inotropes.[90]

Vasodilators

Vasodilators that have been used to treat pulmonary hypertension include tolazoline, prostacyclin, magnesium sulfate, and nitric oxide. Tolazoline and prostacyclin have been widely used and both drugs have similar vasodilator effects on the systemic and the pulmonary circulations and may cause systemic hypotension. Prostaglandin I_2 (prostacyclin), one of the major endogenous pulmonary vasodilators, is normally produced by the lung when lung vessels are in a constricted state. Whether PPHN is the result of faulty PGI_2 production is not known. Administration of pharmacologic doses of PGI_2 to babies with persistent pulmonary hypertension has proved successful even when tolazoline failed.

Inhaled nitric oxide is a more specific pulmonary vasodilator and has become the therapy of choice in term infants with PPHN. Randomized trials in infants with primary and secondary PPHN have shown that nitric oxide significantly improves oxygenation and reduces the need for ECMO. Response to nitric oxide depends on the underlying pathophysiology. Marked improvement is seen with nitric oxide alone in babies with primary PPHN. In babies with secondary PPHN, the effects of nitric oxide are augmented by HFOV.

Inhaled nitric oxide directly activates soluble guanylate cyclase resulting in increased levels of cyclic guanosine monophosphate (GMP) in vascular smooth muscle cells. This results in vascular relaxation by prohibition of myosin protein cross-bridge formation in smooth muscle. A controlled trial of iNO in infants with congenital diaphragmatic hernia demonstrated no efficacy. The US Food and Drug Administration approved nitric oxide in 1999 for use in term and near-term infants with hypoxic respiratory failure requiring ventilatory support with clinical and/or echo-cardiographic evidence of pulmonary hypertension.[99–101]

In critical situations where there is no time to set up the NO circuit or it is not available, a slow intravenous bolus of tolazoline (0.5–1 mg/kg) can be life saving. However, patients should be closely monitored for hypotension. Extracorporeal membrane oxygenation should be considered only in babies who fail to respond to HFOV and nitric oxide. Since the introduction of nitric oxide and HFOV, the need for ECMO has declined.[102–103]

Apnea

Apnea in a neonate is the cessation of inspiratory gas flow for 20 seconds or for a shorter duration if accompanied by bradycardia (heart rate less than 100 beats per minute), cyanosis, or pallor or desaturation as observed on pulse oximeter. Apnea is the most common respiratory problem in the premature infant frequently prolonging hospitalization and the need for monitoring.

TYPES OF APNEA

Obstructive and central apnea

Obstructive apnea is characterized by the presence of inspiratory muscle activity without inspiratory airflow whereas central apnea is defined as absence of inspiratory muscle activity. Obstructive apnea may be followed by central apnea, thus both types occur during the same episode; this is termed as mixed apnea.

Apnea of prematurity

Incidence and severity of apnea in premature infants are both inversely related to gestational age. Approximately 50 percent of infants less than 1500 g birth weight require either pharmacologic intervention or ventilatory support for recurrent prolonged apneic episodes. The peak incidence occurs between 5 and 7 days postnatal age. It is unlikely to occur beyond the first 7 days of life. It usually resolves between 34 and 36 weeks postconceptual age. However, apnea of prematurity has been reported to occur up to 41 weeks of postconceptaual age in extreme low birth weight infants.[104–105]

Epileptic apnea

Neonates can develop apnea during seizures and it may be difficult to distinguish this type of apnea from the one due to the other causes mentioned above. Epileptic apnea rarely lasts for longer than 10–20 seconds and is usually accompanied by initial tachycardia followed by later bradycardia if seizures are prolonged. In contrast, nonepileptic apnea is frequently accompanied by early bradycardia. Continuous electro-encephalographic monitoring can also be useful in distinguishing the two types.

ETIOLOGY

Apnea of prematurity is the most common cause of apnea in the neonatal intensive care unit (NICU). It is a specific diagnosis and also one of exclusion. Other causes of apnea should be looked for if the apnea progresses in severity, fails to respond to appropriate therapy, severe episodes occur on the first day of life, or it appears at a gestational age when it should not occur. Apnea in a term or near-term baby in the absence of maternal sedation or hypoxia at birth should raise suspicion of serious underlying cause. Factors that can lead to apnea include:

- impairment of oxygenation secondary to cardiac (congestive heart failure, and pulmonary edema due to patent ductus arteriosus, coarctation of aorta, or from shunting due to cyanotic heart disease) and lung disease (surfactant deficiency, pneumonia, air leaks, atelectasis)
- sepsis
- neurologic disorders such as intracranial hemorrhage of various types, neonatal seizures, hypoxic ischemic encephalopathy, or other disorders that lead to increased intracranial pressure

- exposure to various drugs (narcotics, β-blockers) during the prenatal period due to maternal use or postnatal exposure to sedatives, hypnotics or narcotics in the neonatal unit
- metabolic causes – hypoglycemia, hyponatremia, hypocalcemia, hypercalcemia or acidosis
- hypothermia or hyperthermia
- hematological causes – severe anemia
- gastrointestinal causes – necrotizing enterocolitis or gastroesophageal reflux.

PATHOPHYSIOLOGY OF APNEA

Developmental immaturity

More frequent occurrence of apneic episodes in immature infants and decrease in their frequency during the period in which brainstem conduction time of the auditory evoked response shortens with advancing gestational age suggests that immaturity of brainstem control of central respiratory drive may be a contributory factor for apnea of prematurity.[106]

Sleep state

Rapid eye movement (REM) sleep is marked by irregularity of frequency as well as depth of breathing. Since REM sleep predominates in the preterm infants they are prone more frequently to apneic episodes.[107,108]

Immature response to peripheral vagal stimulation

Stimulation of laryngeal receptors in the adult results in coughing whereas stimulation of the same receptors in the premature infant results in apnea. Gavage feeding, aggressive pharyngeal suctioning, and gastroesophageal reflux may also induce this reflex apnea.

Chemoreceptor response

Increased breathing effort and ventilation in response to elevated carbon dioxide level reflects predominantly central medullary chemoreceptor response and to a lesser extent carotid body chemoreceptor activity. The ventilatory response to increased carbon dioxide is decreased in preterm babies with apnea compared to those without apnea, which suggests that abnormal respiratory control may contribute to the causation of apnea.

Adults respond to decreased inspiratory oxygen by a sustained increase in ventilation. In contrast, preterm neonates respond to decreased inspiratory oxygen by an initial increase in ventilation followed by a sustained depression of ventilation or even apnea. This biphasic response may represent initial peripheral chemoreceptor stimulation followed by overriding depression of the respiratory center as a result of hypoxia. Progressive decrease in inspiratory oxygen also causes a significant flattening of carbon dioxide response in preterm infants.[109]

Obstructive apnea

A pause in alveolar ventilation due to obstruction of airflow within the upper airway, particularly at the level of the pharynx, causes obstructive apnea. Because the muscles (genioglossus and geniohyoid) that are responsible for keeping the airway open are too weak in the premature infant, the pharynx tends to collapse from negative pressure generated during inspiration. Mucosal adhesive forces tend to prevent the reopening of the collapsed airway during expiration. Neck flexion may worsen this form of apnea.[110,111]

Mixed apnea

A combination of both types of apnea represents as much as 50 percent of all episodes.[112]

MONITORING

All neonates under 34 weeks' gestational age should be monitored for both apnea and bradycardia. An alarm should sound if respiration ceases for more than 20 seconds or if the heart rate drops below 100 beats per minute. Impedance monitors routinely used in NICUs cannot detect an obstructive type of apnea because chest movement is present with no airflow. Such apneic episodes may only be detected when the monitor displays bradycardia. Also reflex apnea can lead to bradycardia within seconds of onset thus setting off the cardiac alarm 10–15 seconds ahead of the apnea alarm.

MANAGEMENT

When the monitor alarm sounds the baby should be observed for signs of breathing and skin color. If the baby is apneic, pale, cyanotic, or bradycardic, tactile stimulation should be provided. If the baby does not respond, bag and mask ventilation along with suctioning should be applied. Oxygen saturation should be maintained between 88 percent and 92 percent with supplemental oxygen if needed.

Nasal CPAP of 3–4 cm H_2O may be needed in babies who have recurrent apnea. The CPAP splints the upper airway with positive pressure during both inspiration and expiration, thereby preventing pharyngeal collapse. Its use can reduce the frequency of both obstructive and mixed types of apnea. Other mechanisms proposed include alteration of the Hering–Breuer reflex, stabilization of the chest wall musculature, and elimination of the intercostal inspiratory inhibitory reflex. Extreme degrees of flexion and extension of the neck should be avoided. Suctioning of the pharynx should be performed cautiously since suctioning itself may stimulate reflexes that lead to apnea. The baby should be evaluated for any underlying cause, so that therapy can be directed accordingly.

Pharmacological therapy

The most common drugs used to treat apnea of prematurity are the methylxanthines (caffeine and theophylline). Aminophylline is theophylline combined with ethylenediamine to increase water solubility. Mechanism of action of methylxanthines is as follows. Adenosine is a neurotransmitter that inhibits the respiratory drive and can cause respiratory depression, Methylxanthines antagonize adenosine, thus blocking inhibition. Stimulation of respiratory neurons results in an enhancement of minute ventilation, chemoreceptor sensitivity to carbon dioxide, and cardiac output. Other mechanisms by which methylxanthines may reduce apnea are improvement of diaphragmatic activity and stimulation of the respiratory center.

Aminophylline is administered as a loading dose of 5–6 mg/kg orally or as an intravenous infusion over 30 minutes followed by a maintenance dose of 1.5–2 mg/kg per dose intravenously or orally given every 8–12 hours started 8–12 hours after loading dose to achieve the therapeutic level of 6–13 µg/mL. Plasma half-life of aminophylline is 20–30 hours. Trough level should be obtained at 48–72 hours after loading dose. Levels >20 µg/mL are considered toxic. Aminophylline has a narrower difference between the toxic and therapeutic range than caffeine.

Caffeine citrate is administered as a loading dose of 20 mg/kg orally or intravenously as a single dose or divided in two doses of 10 mg/kg each followed by a maintenance dose of 2.5–5 mg/kg per dose orally or intravenously every 24 hours, started 24 hours after the loading dose. The therapeutic level of caffeine is 5–25 µg/mL. Trough level may be obtained on day 5 or 6 after loading dose.

Toxic level is greater than 40–50 µg/mL. Since there is a greater margin of safety, routine monitoring of blood levels may not be needed. Caffeine citrate has a longer plasma half-life of 40–230 hours and has fewer side effects. Methylxanthine therapy is usually continued until the baby has reached 32–37 weeks' postconceptual age and apneic episodes have ceased. The baby should be monitored for any recurrence of apnea for at least 5 days after the medication has been discontinued. Major side effects of methylxanthines are tachycardia, vomiting, feeding intolerance, jitteriness, and seizures. Generally, the dose is held if heart rate exceeds 180/minute.[113]

Intermittent mandatory ventilation

Intermittent mandatory ventilation may be needed if significant apnea persists despite using both pharmacotherapy and CPAP. It has been recently suggested that nasal intermittent positive pressure is more beneficial than CPAP alone in reducing frequency of apnea of prematurity.[114]

SUDDEN INFANT DEATH SYNDROME AND APNEA OF PREMATURITY

There is no evidence that apnea of prematurity is an independent risk factor for sudden infant death syndrome (SIDS). Although preterm babies constitute about 18 percent of all babies that die of SIDS, only 2–4 percent of SIDS cases had a hospital record of apnea of prematurity. Because of increased parental concern for apnea in such babies a SIDS-prevention strategy should be discussed with the parents. Factors that reduce the risk of SIDS include sleeping on the back, encouraging breast feeding, and avoiding exposure to smoking and overheating.[115]

Meconium aspiration syndrome

Meconium aspiration syndrome is defined as respiratory distress in an infant born through meconium-stained amniotic fluid (MSAF) whose symptoms cannot be otherwise explained. It is caused by aspiration of meconium that may occur in utero or after delivery with the first few breaths. About 13 percent of all live births are associated by MSAF whereas only 5 percent of those born through MSAF develop meconium aspiration syndrome. Meconium aspiration syndrome accounts for about 1000 deaths annually in the United States.[116,117]

PATHOGENESIS

Passage of meconium by the fetus into the amnion fluid does not necessarily indicate fetal distress. It may represent an adaptation reflux developed by a mature fetus with age-appropriate levels of motilin in the gastrointestinal tract. Cord or head compression also may lead to passage of meconium through vagal stimulation in the absence of fetal distress. Passage of meconium may also be secondary to an in utero stress as a result of fetal hypoxia and acidosis producing relaxation of the anal sphincter. Term and post-mature fetuses are more likely to pass meconium in response to such a stress than are preterm. Perinatal conditions that increase the risk of meconium aspiration syndrome include maternal hypertension, diabetes mellitus, heavy cigarette smoking, pre-eclampsia, eclampsia, intrauterine growth retardation, oligohydramnios, and intrauterine hypoxia due to any other cause.

It is not clear why only 5 percent of babies born through MSAF develop meconium aspiration syndrome whereas others do not. Chronic fetal hypoxia and acidosis may lead to fetal gasping, further leading to in utero aspiration of meconium. Recently it has been suggested that a chronic in utero insult may be responsible for most cases of severe meconium aspiration syndrome as compared with an acute peripartum hypoxia. A vigorous baby who aspirates meconium-stained fluid from the nasopharynx at birth usually develops a milder form of the disease compared with the severe cases caused by chronic fetal hypoxia.[118]

MECHANISMS OF INJURY

Aspiration of meconium can adversely affect the lung function in several ways including mechanical obstruction of airways, inactivation of surfactant, vasoconstriction of pulmonary vessels, and chemical pneumonitis.[119] Thick and viscous meconium when aspirated may cause partial or complete airway obstruction. Partial obstruction produces a 'ball-valve' effect in which air can enter the alveoli but is unable to escape. This causes air trapping in the alveoli with ventilation/perfusion mismatch. It may lead to hyperexpansion and various types of air leak syndromes whereas complete obstruction of the small airways leads to atelectasis and areas of unventilated lung with further ventilation/perfusion mismatch and hypoxemia. The risk of pneumothorax is estimated to range from 15 percent to 33 percent.

A full-term baby with meconium aspiration syndrome can develop secondary surfactant deficiency due to inactivation that leads to increased surface tension with atelectasis, diminished lung compliance, decreased lung volumes, and resultant poor oxygenation. Meconium has a direct inhibitory effect on the function of surfactant and displaces surfactant from the alveolar surface.[120–123] It causes chemical pneumonitis associated with release of cytokines such as tumor necrosis factor-α, interleukin-1β, and interleukin-8, and it may directly injure lung parenchyma or lead to vascular leakage (which causes a toxic pneumonitis with hemorrhagic pulmonary edema). Vasoconstriction caused by several underlying factors such as hypoxia acidosis, release of vasoactive mediators, e.g. eicosanoids, endothelin-1, and PGE_2, may lead to persistent pulmonary hypertension.[120]

DIAGNOSIS

Meconium aspiration syndrome should be considered in any baby born through MSAF who develops respiratory distress. The radiographic findings include diffuse, asymmetric patchy infiltrates, consolidation or atelectasis, over-aeration leading to air leak syndromes such as pneumothorax or pneumomediastinum, or pulmonary interstitial emphysema.[124] These classic radiographic findings of meconium aspiration syndrome may take a period of days or weeks to clear. A two-dimensional echocardiogram to evaluate for pulmonary hypertension may be useful early in a neonate's course.

PERINATAL MANAGEMENT

One should consider MSAF as a possible warning sign of fetal distress. It is recommended that obstetricians should monitor the fetal heart rate tracing and have a low threshold for performing additional testing, such as fetal scalp pH. Amnioinfusion is the infusion of a sterile isotonic solution into the amniotic cavity in order to dilute the meconium. It also increases the volume of amniotic fluid and thus may decrease the risk of cord compression, which could be a cause for fetal hypoxia and fetal gasping. A recent metaanalysis found a 76 percent reduction in meconium aspiration syndrome with amnioinfusion. However, benefits of prophylactic amnioinfusion for MSAF when the fetus otherwise seems well are not clear.[125–127]

Intrapartum suctioning

The aim is to clear as much meconium as possible from the oropharynx, before the baby is able to take a breath, in order to prevent its aspiration. The mouth, pharynx, and nose should be suctioned with either a large-bore suction catheter (12–14 Fr) or a bulb syringe as soon as the head is delivered and before the shoulders are delivered in a cephalic presentation or immediately after the head is delivered with a breech presentation. Although intrapartum suctioning has been considered standard procedure for more than two decades based on the work of Carson et al.,[128] a multicenter, randomized controlled trial has demonstrated that routine intrapartum oropharyngeal and nasopharyngeal suctioning of term-gestation babies born through MSAF does not prevent meconium aspiration syndrome.[129–131]

Neonatal management

A skilled resuscitation team should be present at all deliveries that involve MSAF. The nature of pediatric intervention in babies born through MSAF depends on whether the baby is depressed or vigorous. A baby with a strong respiratory effort, good muscle tone, and a heart rate more than 100 beats/min is defined as vigorous. In such babies intubation is not indicated.[132] When a neonate is depressed (i.e. poor respiratory effort, limp, heart rate <100 beats/min) the airway should be cleared as soon as possible from the hypopharynx and upper airways to minimize the amount of meconium aspiration. The neonate is placed under a radiant heater and drying and stimulating is delayed. Direct laryngoscopy should be performed, and the mouth and hypopharynx suctioned under direct vision with a 12 Fr or 14 Fr suction catheter, followed by intubation. A negative suction (approximately 100 mm Hg) is directly applied to the endotracheal tube as it is slowly withdrawn. The process may be repeated until no additional meconium is recovered. The baby's heart rate is closely monitored, if it drops the resuscitation must proceed without delay and positive pressure ventilation should be applied.[129–132]

Most babies born through MSAF do not require any intervention and can stay with their mother. Since meconium aspiration syndrome does not always present immediately, these babies should be closely monitored for signs of respiratory distress. They may exhibit features of postmaturity, such as peeling and yellow staining of skin, long fingernails, and stained umbilical cord. Besides the other signs of respiratory distress, the chest may appear barrel shaped as a result of overinflation. Rales and rhonchi may be heard on auscultation. Most babies who develop symptoms do so in the first few hours of life. Babies at risk for meconium aspiration syndrome who show signs of respiratory distress must be transferred to the NICU. Since babies with meconium aspiration syndrome are highly prone to air leak syndromes, therapy is aimed at increasing oxygenation while minimizing the barotraumas. The type of respiratory support depends upon the severity of respiratory distress. It varies from a simple oxygen hood to mechanical ventilation, iNO and even ECMO. In severe cases there is a vicious cycle of hypoxemia that further leads to acidosis, and which together cause pulmonary vasoconstriction and may lead to PPHN, the management of which has been described earlier in this chapter. Hyperventilation with resultant alkalinization has been used earlier to decrease pulmonary vascular resistance, but adverse affects of hypocarbia on the already vulnerable brain have raised concerns about its use. Use of HFOV may minimize barotrauma through the use of subnormal tidal volumes at supraphysiologic rates. It allows use of high mean airway pressures without the concurrent use of high peak pressures.[133]

Surfactant

Use of surfactant in severe cases of meconium aspiration syndrome has been shown to decrease the need for ECMO and possibly to reduce the risk of pneumothorax.[123,133] There was, however, no difference in mortality. There seems to be a differential resistance between types of surfactant to the surfactant inhibitors seen in meconium aspiration syndrome.[134] The search is ongoing for new synthetic surfactant preparations that may be more resistant to inactivation by meconium. The dose of surfactant used in meconium aspiration syndrome has not been clearly defined. An animal study has recently demonstrated that two doses of surfactant (100 and 200 mg/kg) used in experimentally induced meconium aspiration syndrome in newborn rabbits were equally effective.[135]

Surfactant lavage

It has been suggested that the use of large-volume lung lavage with dilute surfactant may be effective in removing particulate meconium from the lung, minimize obstruction, and simultaneously offset the inactivation of surfactant by meconium. Its use in the neonate with severe meconium aspiration syndrome may carry substantial risks. Use of large-volume lung lavage might exacerbate hemodynamic instability, and pulmonary hypertension that commonly occur in association with meconium aspiration syndrome, and lead to acute deterioration. Evidence for the efficacy of surfactant lavage awaits the conclusion of the multicenter, randomized trial of KL4-surfactant that is currently underway.[134–139]

Inhaled nitric oxide (see also section on PPHN)

Since iNO is effective as a local vasodilator, its adequate delivery to the alveoli should be ensured. Pretreatment with surfactant may enhance the delivery of iNO to the alveoli, with a resultant increase in oxygenation. A large, randomized multicenter trial has demonstrated that infants with meconium aspiration syndrome responded better to the combination of iNO and HFOV, possibly because of improved lung inflation and better delivery of nitric oxide to alveoli .[96,139–141]

Extracorporeal membrane oxygenation

Since the introduction of iNO for the treatment of PPHN, the need for ECMO has significantly decreased. However, babies with meconium aspiration syndrome still make up approximately 35 percent of those neonates who require ECMO.

RESPIRATORY DISTRESS SYNDROME

Respiratory distress syndrome, also called hyaline membrane disease, is the most common cause of respiratory morbidity in neonates. It occurs in up to 50 percent of babies born at 28–32 weeks and the incidence approaches nearly 100 percent at 24 weeks. In the United States, 40 000 infants develop RDS each year.[142–144]

Surfactant system

Surfactant is the substance that lowers the surface tension and is produced by the alveolar type II cells. It is composed of two main fractions: lipids and surfactant-specific proteins. Lipids account for 90 percent and phospholipids form the bulk of the lipids. Other lipids that are found are cholesterol, triacylglycerol, and free fatty acids. Phosphatidylcholine (PC) forms 70–80 percent of the total amount of lipid. Approximately 50–70 percent of PC is saturated, especially the dipalmitoyl form (DPPC). The anionic PG accounts for approximately 8 percent. Other lipids are phosphatidylethanolamine (PE, ± 5 percent), phosphatidylinositol (PI, ± 3 percent); and phosphatidylserine (PS), lysophosphatidylcholine, and sphingomyelin in small quantities (less than 2 percent).

About 10 percent of surfactant consists of four surfactant-associated proteins: SP-A and SP-D are hydrophilic, and SP-B and SP-C hydrophobic. SP-A does not have direct surface tension lowering properties but may contribute in formation of tubular myelin, regulation of phospholipid insertion into the monolayer, modulation of uptake and secretion of phospholipids by type II cells, activation of alveolar macrophages and binding and clearance of bacteria and viruses. Most putative functions of SP-D described so far include activation of alveolar macrophages, agglutination of bacteria, protection against nonbacterial microorganisms and viruses, and in phosphatidylinositol metabolism. SP-B enhances the formation of a stable surface film by inducing the insertion of phospholipids into the monolayer at the air liquid interface. Together with SP-A it helps in the formation of tubular myelin. It also reduces the inactivation of surfactant by serum proteins. Absence of SP-B results in phenotypic expression of a lethal form of RDS in term infants.

Surfactant is stored and exported to the alveolar surface as lamellar bodies. After secretion, surfactant is transformed into specific structures, called tubular myelin, from which phospholipids are inserted into an air–liquid interface thus reducing the surface tension during expiration. During the next inhalation, surfactant components are lost from the interface and taken back into the type II cell for recycling.[145–149]

Etiology/pathophysiology

Avery and Mead established surfactant deficiency as the cause of RDS in 1959.[150] Earlier than that, Rogers and

Gruenwald had proposed that high surface tension might cause the atelectasis in hyaline membrane disease.[151] Fujiwara and Adams in 1980 were the first to demonstrate the therapeutic role of surfactant in human neonates.[152] Subsequently synthetic and natural surfactant preparations were used in a series of multicenter trials. Respiratory distress syndrome is the result of primary absence or deficiency of surfactant. Surfactant lowers the surface tension of the alveolar membrane. Without surfactant the alveoli collapse at the end of expiration. Preterm neonates have both structural immaturity of the lung as well as surfactant deficiency.[153–157] Surfactant replacement therapy is the standard of care for preterms with RDS and has significantly decreased the mortality.

Clinical features

Surfactant deficiency leads to progressive atelectasis, loss of functional residual capacity, resulting in hypoventilation and ventilation/perfusion mismatch. This in turn leads to hypoxia, hypercarbia, metabolic acidosis, and respiratory failure. Respiratory distress syndrome is further complicated in premature babies by weak respiratory muscles and compliant chest wall, which impair alveolar ventilation. The neonate presents at birth or within several hours after birth with signs of respiratory distress that include tachypnea, expiratory grunting (caused by partially closed glottis), retractions (secondary to decreased lung compliance and increased rib cage compliance), nasal flaring, cyanosis, and increasing oxygen requirement. Other clinical features include pallor, cardiovascular instability, and extremity edema that develops after several hours due to altered capillary permeability.

Investigations

Chest radiographs are characterized by diffuse reticulogranular pattern caused by alveolar microatelectasis, giving the classic ground glass appearance. Aerated bronchioles superimposed on collapsed alveolar give rise to widely distributed airbronchogram. In more severe cases complete white-out of the lungs with loss of cardiac borders may be seen. However, radiographic appearances in RDS are variable and may not reflect the degree of respiratory compromise. Neonatal pneumonia, especially that caused by group B streptococci, may present with radiographic features similar to RDS.

Clinical features

The clinical course depends upon the severity of RDS, the gestation age, and birth weight. The uncomplicated clinical course is characterized by progressive worsening of symptoms with a peak severity by 2–3 days following which

recovery begins. However, surfactant therapy may shorten this course. When the disease process is severe enough to require assisted ventilation, recovery may take several days or even weeks.

Clinical management

The basic management of RDS includes supportive therapy. Adequate oxygenation, ventilation, temperature, and circulation must be assured before the baby is transferred from the delivery room. Oxygen therapy by means of CPAP or positive pressure ventilation is often initiated in the delivery room for smaller babies and continued in NICU. The baby is placed in a thermoneutral environment to reduce oxygen consumption. Close monitoring of vital signs, oxygen saturation, and blood gases by noninvasive monitoring is required, and an umbilical arterial line for frequent sampling and accurate blood pressure is often necessary.

Mild or moderate RDS is often managed by CPAP. Usually, 3–6 cm of water pressure applied to baby's airways helps to open up the alveoli and prevent atelectasis. Adequacy of ventilation and oxygenation must be closely monitored and mandatory ventilation instituted well in advance of respiratory failure to avoid hypoxemia, respiratory acidosis, and secondary pulmonary vasoconstriction. Pressure-cycled ventilators are most frequently used in the NICU and are controlled by setting positive inspiratory pressure, positive end-expiratory pressure (PEEP), rate, inspiratory pressure, and FiO_2. PaO_2, $PaCO_2$, pH, and oxygen saturation should be maintained within acceptable limits with minimal ventilator parameters to avoid barotrauma and oxygen toxicity to the immature lung. Frequent adjustments are needed in the face of rapidly changing compliance of the lungs after surfactant therapy or during the recovery phase. Hyperoxia is associated with retinopathy of prematurity, a leading cause of blindness among premature babies. PO_2 is generally maintained between 50 mm Hg and 80 mm Hg. Hypocarbia of less than 30 mm Hg has been associated with higher incidence of periventricular leukomalacia. In severe forms of RDS nonresponsive to conventional ventilation and surfactant therapy, use of other modes of ventilation such as HFOV or jet ventilators may be necessary.[158–161]

SURFACTANT THERAPY

Several forms of natural as well as synthetic surfactant have been used in various regimens. Surfactant therapy appears to decrease the incidence of air leaks, improve oxygenation, and reduce the mortality from RDS among preterm ventilated neonates. The incidence of BPD, intraventricular hemorrhage, sepsis, and symptomatic patent ductus arteriosus seems to be unaltered. Surfactant is administered through the endotracheal tube either through a sidehole adapter connected to an endotracheal tube or a catheter. Dramatic improvement in oxygenation after surfactant therapy correlates well with improvement in lung volume and stabilization of FRC. If ventilator pressures are promptly lowered a significant improvement in compliance is seen. The dose is repeated if the oxygen requirement stays more than 30 percent after 8–12 hours. It is unclear whether a prophylactic dose of surfactant administered intratracheally within the first minutes of birth has any advantage over its use as a rescue therapy after the symptoms have developed. Although earlier therapy has been shown to reduce the need for subsequent treatment, supplemental oxygenation, and mechanical ventilation, it should be reserved for babies who need endotracheal intubation and are likely to develop more severe lung disease.

The currently available surfactant preparations are not ideal and require further refinement. As the role of surfactant proteins in the surface tension lowering function of lipids has been defined, recombinant DNA technology may aid in production of protein-containing surfactant preparations.[150–161]

Prevention of respiratory distress syndrome

Although the incidence of premature birth has remained unchanged in United States, the incidence of RDS has shown a significant decrease at each gestational age. Antenatal steroids, administered to mother at least 24–48 hours before the birth, seem to decrease both the incidence and severity of RDS and also appear to reduce the incidence of intraventricular hemorrhage in premature babies. Its effectiveness is enhanced if used prior to gestation of 34 weeks. However, use of multiple courses of antenatal steroids has been reported to be associated with poorer neurodevelopmental outcome and decreased fetal growth. The physiologic role of thyroid hormone in lung development and surfactant maturation has been demonstrated in lung cell culture of humans and other animals as well as in initial clinical trials.[162,163] But subsequent multicenter studies performed in the United States and Australia did not show any significant synergistic effect of combined steroid and thyrotropin-releasing hormone (TRH) therapy as compared with steroids alone.[164,165]

SURGICAL PROBLEMS PRESENTING AS RESPIRATORY DISTRESS IN A NEONATE

Two to three percent of neonates are born with a congenital anomaly that may require intervention soon after birth. Disorders such as diaphragmatic hernia, bilateral choanal atresia, or hydrops fetalis with pericardial and pleural effusion can be life threatening, whereas other problems such as esophageal atresia with tracheoesophageal fistula may present later with aspiration pneumonia. A quick and thorough screening exam for congenital anomalies should be part of routine management in the delivery room.[166]

Choanal atresia

Choanal atresia is the congenital absence of the posterior nasal aperture (the choanae). It results from bony fusion or persistence of the buccopharyngeal membrane or mixture of both – thus classified into three types: bony, membranous, or mixed.[167] It could be unilateral or bilateral.

Bilateral choanal atresia presents at birth. As neonates are obligatory nasal breathers for 4–6 weeks after birth, bilateral choanal atresia can present as upper airway obstruction leading to respiratory distress and hypoxia. The baby becomes cyanotic and struggles for air when quiet and becomes pink while crying.[167,168] Bilateral choanal atresia is the most common cause of complete upper airway obstruction at birth with an incidence of 1 in 7000 live births. Twenty to 50 percent of patients with bilateral choanal atresia have associated anomalies that include various syndromes such as the CHARGE association, Treacher Collins, Apert, Lenz–Majewski hyperostosis, Antley–Bixler–Downs, and Crouzon syndromes.[166–168]

Unilateral choanal atresia may not be symptomatic. Infants may initially present with foul-smelling secretions on the effected side or with respiratory distress associated with upper respiratory obstruction. It is twice as frequent in girls as in boys and occurs twice as often on the right side as the left. Inability to pass a 6 Fr catheter through the nares into the pharynx suggests the diagnosis.

Management at birth depends upon the severity of symptoms and if it is bilateral or unilateral. An appropriate oral airway (size 0 or 00) should be placed and properly secured to prevent dislodging. A thorough evaluation for other congenital anomalies should be performed including echocardiogram (70 percent have associated heart defects).[169,170] A computed tomography scan should be performed to differentiate between the bony, membranous, and mixed type of choanal atresia.[171] If the baby tolerates an oral airway surgical correction may be deferred until 4–6 weeks of age. Immediate repair is recommended if the patients need endotracheal intubation. Transnasal endoscopic repair has been used with better results.[172] Some babies may need repeated dilatation in the postoperative period. Use of topical mitomycin as an adjunct to surgical repair has been proposed to reduce the need for repeated surgery by decreasing the granulation tissue and cicatrix.[173,174]

Esophageal atresia

In esophageal atresia, the proximal and distal portions of the esophagus do not communicate. The upper segment of the esophagus is a dilated blind-ending pouch with hypertrophied muscular and the distal esophageal portion is an atretic pouch with a small diameter and a thin muscular wall. An abnormal communication between the trachea and esophagus may exist and occurs most commonly between the distal esophageal segment and the trachea just above the carina. Five types of esophageal atresia and tracheoesophageal fistula (TEF) have been described. The most common abnormality is esophageal atresia with a distal TEF (84 percent). Other types are isolated atresia with no fistula (8 percent), TEF with no atresia or H-type (4 percent), esophageal atresia with proximal and distal fistulas (3 percent), and esophageal atresia with a proximal fistula (1 percent). An H-type TEF represents a TEF without esophageal atresia. It can occur at any level from the cricoid cartilage to the carina. It occurs with a frequency of 1 in 3000 live births with a male-to-female ratio of 1.26. Esophageal atresia and tracheoesophageal atresia are congenital malformations that are typically diagnosed in neonates within the first few hours of life.[175–179]

INITIAL STABILIZATION

Once tracheoesophageal fistula is suspected the baby should be stabilized to prevent aspiration pneumonia. A 10 Fr Replogle catheter should be placed in the upper pouch and connected to an intermittent suction (or aspirate every 5 minutes with a syringe). The pouch fills with secretions, which can overflow into the lungs if not continuously emptied. The baby should be placed at a 30° angle, head up position in an incubator for temperature maintenance and close observation. Sedation may be used to prevent the baby from crying as this causes air to be forced into the stomach through the fistula, causing distension that can result in reflux of air carrying gastric contents into the lung. The baby should be examined for other congenital anomalies that may have an effect on surgical intervention.

CLINICAL SIGNS

The inability to swallow and absorb amniotic fluid through the gut leads to polyhydramnios and increased pressure due to the accumulation of amniotic fluid results in a greater number of premature births. Polyhydramnios is seen in 95 percent of babies with esophageal atresia and no fistula and in 35 percent of those who have esophageal atresia with a distal fistula.[180–184]

Diagnosis can be made by the inability to pass a large radioopaque (10 Fr) catheter into the stomach. The catheter gets coiled up in the upper pouch and can be seen in posteroanterior and lateral chest radiographs. Injection of 10 mL of air into the catheter while simultaneously taking a radiograph of the chest and abdomen may outline the pouch. Injection of barium and other contrast materials are not necessary and may pose a risk of aspiration through the fistula. The chest films may also show radiographic signs of right-sided aortic arch, vertebral anomalies, aspiration pneumonia, and patchy atelectasis.[185–188]

PATHOPHYSIOLOGY OF RESPIRATORY SYMPTOMS

The inability of babies with esophageal atresia to clear their secretions leads to persistent regurgitation, frothy bubbles in the mouth and sometimes nose, drooling, and aspiration of secretions. Any attempts at feeding result in choking, coughing, cyanotic episodes, and regurgitation of feeds. In addition, when these babies strain, cough, or cry, air enters the stomach through the fistula leading to dilatation of the stomach and small intestine and elevation of the diaphragm, which makes respiration more difficult. The reflux of gastric secretions may also occur through the fistula into the tracheobronchial tree and contributes to pneumonia and atelectasis.[176–183]

With atresia alone, the abdomen appears scaphoid. In 50–70 percent of babies with esophageal atresia there may be other anomalies including vertebral, anorectal, cardiac, tracheal, renal, and limb (VACTERL association). Cardiac abnormalities are the most common, especially ventricular septal defects and tetralogy of Fallot.

COMPLICATIONS

Preoperatively, the greatest risk to the child with esophageal atresia and/or TEF is aspiration. Gastric rupture has been reported in babies with TEF who were receiving ventilatory support. Air is forced through the fistula into the distal esophagus and then into the stomach.

The severity of complications after esophageal atresia repair is often dictated by the extent of the repair required. Primary anastomosis and fistula closure has fewer complications than esophageal replacement. The most common complications include anastomotic leak, recurrent fistula, stricture, and gastroesophageal reflux. Anastomotic leakage into the mediastinum occurs in 14–21 percent of babies. Most leaks are small, occur usually after the first 48 hours after surgery, and require only conservative management with cessation of oral intake and antibiotic therapy. Spontaneous healing occurs in 95 percent of leaks when a mediastinal drain is present. Major anastomotic disruptions occur in only 3–5 percent of leaks, but large leaks can be fatal and require surgical repair. Mediastinal leaks can lead to TEF recurrence; therefore, they should be monitored carefully.

An anastomotic leak can present with choking episodes during feeding and/or recurrent pneumonia. The best methods of diagnosis are bronchoscopy and esophagography. Tracheomalacia is seen postoperatively in almost all cases of TEF.[188–192]

Congenital lobar emphysema

Congenital lobar emphysema is the result of a group of heterogeneous disorders that lead to overdistension and air trapping within the alveoli involving a part or whole lobe of a lung. The left upper lobe is most commonly involved (50 percent), followed by the right middle lobe (24 percent) and the right upper lobe (18 percent). Partial bronchial obstruction has been attributed to defective or overtly compliant cartilage, valvelike obstruction created by mucosal folds, bronchial stenosis, and external compression by aberrant blood vessels, mediastinal, or intrapulmonary masses. Familial form has also been reported. Boys are affected more often than girls (1.8:1). About 30 percent of cases have associated heart anomalies such as tetralogy of Fallot, ventricular septal defect, or anomalous pulmonary venous return.[193–196]

Pathophysiology

The obstruction is ball valve type and leads to progressive distension of the alveoli that compress the surrounding normal lung tissue and in some cases the contralateral lung by crossing over the mediastinum. The alveoli may be distended up to 3–10 times the normal size.

Clinical presentation

Patients usually present at 1–2 months of age but many neonates may exhibit symptoms soon after birth or within the first 6 months of life. Rarely, a child remains undiagnosed up to school age. Severity of symptoms depends upon size of the overinflated lobe and the resultant compression, as well as the mediastinal shift. Some children may remain asymptomatic whereas others present with variable degrees of respiratory distress. Physical findings include a hyper-resonant note on percussion, decreased breath sounds over the affected lobe, and signs of mediastinal shiftlike displacement of apical heart beat.[197,198]

Diagnosis

Chest radiograph shows a unilateral hyperinflated lobe, bronchovascular markings to the periphery of the involved lobe, and possibly a mediastinal shift and/or atelectasis or collapse of the adjacent lobe.[199]

Management

For infants with severe respiratory symptoms, segmentectomy or lobectomy is the treatment of choice. The incidence of complications is low. Asymptomatic children may not require any definitive treatment. Most respiratory symptoms do not progress and resolve within a year of age. Lobectomy has been successfully avoided in occasional cases by the use of selective endotracheal intubation on the unaffected side or HFOV.[199,200]

Diaphragmatic hernia

PATHOPHYSIOLOGY

Congenital diaphragmatic hernia (CDH) is characterized by a defect in the diaphragm that occurs due to failure of closure of the pleuroperitoneal canal during the sixth to eighth week of gestation. In approximately 85–90 percent, the hernia occurs through the posterolateral lumbocostal triangle called Bochdalek hernia, whereas 10–15 percent are right-sided hernias, also called Morgagni hernia. Bilateral hernias occur in less than 1 percent and are usually fatal. A left-sided hernia allows herniation of both small and large bowel as well as intraabdominal solid organs into the thoracic cavity. In right-sided hernias, only the liver and a portion of the large bowel tend to herniate. The severity and size of defect and the timing of herniation of bowel into the thoracic cavity result in varying degrees of pulmonary hypoplasia associated with a decrease in cross-sectional area of the pulmonary vasculature and dysfunction of the surfactant system. In addition to parenchymal disease, the intraacinar pulmonary arteries appear to have increased musculature.

Pulmonary capillary blood flow is decreased because of the small cross-sectional area of the pulmonary vascular bed, and flow may be further decreased by abnormal pulmonary vasoconstriction. Right-sided hernias may not be symptomatic early because the liver may seal the defect.[201–206]

EPIDEMIOLOGY

Congenital diaphragmatic hernia occurs in 1 in 2000–4000 live births. Isolated posterolateral CDH is 1.5 times more frequent in boys than girls. The risk of recurrence of isolated CDH for future siblings is approximately 2 percent. Familial CDH has been reported and may be multifactorial or due to an autosomal recessive pattern. Although CDH is most commonly a disorder of the neonatal period, as many as 10 percent of patients may present after the neonatal period and even during adulthood. Outcome in patients with late presentation of CDH is extremely good, with low or no mortality.[201,202]

ETIOLOGY

No single gene mutation has been identified as producing or contributing to this anomaly. A variety of chromosomal anomalies including trisomy 13, trisomy 18, and tetrasomy 12p mosaicism have been reported in 4 percent of infants with CDH. Congenital diaphragmatic hernia may be associated with nonchromosomal disorders such as the de Lange syndrome.[202]

CLINICAL FEATURES

In most patients the diagnosis is established by an antenatal sonogram. Infants most commonly present with a history of cyanosis and respiratory distress in the first minutes or hours of life, although a later presentation is possible. They frequently exhibit a scaphoid abdomen, respiratory distress, and cyanosis. In left-sided hernia, auscultation of the lungs reveals poor air entry on the left, with a shift of cardiac sounds over the right chest. Posterolateral hernia may occur as an isolated defect or in association with other congenital anomalies. Congenital diaphragmatic hernia can occur as part of a multiple malformation syndrome in up to 40 percent of infants, principally with cardiovascular, genitourinary, and gastrointestinal malformations. Lethal anomalies are present in up to 16 percent.[202–204]

PERINATAL MANAGEMENT

Bag-and-mask ventilation should be avoided in the delivery room because the stomach and intestines become distended with air and further compromise pulmonary function. Neonates with prenatal diagnosis or with symptoms should immediately undergo endotracheal intubation and mechanical ventilation. Placement of an orogastric tube may prevent further compression of the lung secondary to bowel distension. It also helps to determine the position of the stomach. The resuscitation team should consider the possibility of early pneumothorax if the baby does not stabilize.[205–208]

NICU MANAGEMENT

All neonates with severe CDH who present in the first few hours of life require endotracheal intubation and mechanical ventilation. High-frequency oscillatory ventilation should be considered if high peak inspiratory pressures are needed. Surfactant administration may be helpful because of associated lung immaturity and surfactant deficiency. Inhaled nitric oxide may be used to lower the pulmonary vascular resistance. However, its use has not been shown to reduce mortality or the need for ECMO in infants with CDH. Arterial blood gases should be monitored frequently because of persistent pulmonary hypertension. Placement of venous and arterial lines is essential because many infants may require use of inotropic agents, multiple infusions, and frequent blood sampling. Associated PPHN should be managed as described earlier in the section on persistent pulmonary hypertension. Patients should be adequately sedated or paralyzed to achieve optimal oxygenation. Pulse oximeter probes at preductal (right-hand) and postductal (either foot) sites may help in assessing a right-to-left shunt at the level of the ductus arteriosus.[209–212] If optimal oxygenation and perfusion is not achieved by ventilation and medical therapy ECMO is indicated.

CHEST RADIOGRAPHY

Typical findings in left-sided posterolateral CDH include air- or fluid-filled loops of the bowel in the left hemithorax and shift of the cardiac silhouette to the right. Due to underlying lung hypoplasia these patients are prone to development of pneumothorax. Placement of an orogastric tube prior to the study helps determine the position of the stomach.

ECHOCARDIOGRAM

An echocardiogram should be performed to rule out PPHN and associated cardiac anomalies. If the infant is being considered for ECMO it is essential to perform cranial ultrasonographic examination to evaluate for intracranial bleeding and anomalies. Patients should also have a renal sonogram. Consultation with a geneticist and chromosome studies may be helpful, especially in the presence of dysmorphic features.[202,207]

SURGICAL CARE

Preoperative stabilization significantly decreases morbidity and mortality. The ideal time to repair a CDH is not known.

Many surgeons prefer to operate when echocardiographic evidence for normal pulmonary artery pressures is maintained for at least 24–48 hours. Delays of up to 7–10 days are often well tolerated. A single lung transplant has been successfully performed. It allows the remaining hypoplastic lung to increase in size and recover from injury while allowing for optimal ventilation and oxygenation.[209,212,213]

Key learning points

- In children a relatively small airway obstruction can cause significant reduction in airway diameter with increased airflow resistance and work of breathing.

- Croup is a common cause of upper airway obstruction in children, and about 6 percent of children require hospitalization.

- If epiglottitis is suspected, the pharynx should be examined in the operating room with trained personnel ready to intubate. Radiographs should never be done when moderate to severe airway obstruction is suspected. The child with suspected epiglottitis should not be agitated or disturbed, as this could increase the laryngospasm and worsen respiratory distress.

- A common site for foreign body lodgment is the right main stem bronchus, as it is shorter, straighter and wider than the left main stem bronchus.

- A child with asthma who is not responsive to initial doses of nebulized bronchodilators should be considered to be in status asthmaticus. If air entry is significantly reduced, wheezing may not be heard, and a 'silent chest' may be an ominous sign. The cardiopulmonary status of the child in status asthmaticus should be continuously monitored.

- Mechanical ventilation should be avoided, if possible, in patients with severe asthma, as it increases the incidence of complications such as barotrauma and air trapping.

- In the absence of respiratory signs, early chest films may not be useful in the diagnosis of inhalation injury.

- Pediatricians, in consonance with parents, children, caregivers, and the community must be proactive in implementing the AAP recommendations for the prevention of drowning.

- In the RSV season, the latest AAP recommendations for administration of palivizumab should be followed (monthly intramuscular injections for high-risk groups) for prevention.

- Respiratory distress in a neonate may be result of several factors that operate individually or in combination with each other. These causes include surfactant deficiency, delayed absorption of lung fluid, aspiration of meconium into the lungs, and failure of decrease in pulmonary resistance leading to persistence of the fetal circulatory pattern.

- Optimal antenatal care, prevention of preterm delivery, and proper handling of the newborn baby at birth remain key factors in the management of these patients.

- The clinical signs commonly used to assess the pulmonary function in a neonate are: respiratory rate, retractions, nasal flaring, grunting, and cyanosis.

- Presence of cyanosis in a neonate signifies relatively higher degree of hypoxia than in older children or adults.

- Apnea is the most common respiratory problem in the premature infant frequently prolonging hospitalization and the need for monitoring.

- Apnea in a term or near-term baby in absence of maternal sedation or hypoxia at birth should raise suspicion of serious underlying cause.

- Adults respond to decreased inspiratory oxygen by a sustained increase in ventilation. In contrast, preterm neonates respond to decrease inspiratory oxygen by initial increase in ventilation followed by a sustained depression of ventilation or even apnea.

- There is no evidence that apnea of prematurity is an independent risk factor for SIDS.

- A skilled resuscitation team should be present at all deliveries that involve MSAF. The nature of pediatric intervention in babies born through MSAF depends on whether the baby is depressed or vigorous.

- Since the introduction of iNO for the treatment of PPHN, the need for ECMO has significantly decreased.

- Surfactant replacement therapy is the standard of care for preterms with RDS and has significantly decreased the mortality.

- Disorders such as diaphragmatic hernia, bilateral choanal atresia, or hydrops fetalis with pericardial and pleural effusion can be life threatening, whereas other problems such as esophageal atresia with tracheoesophageal fistula may present later with aspiration pneumonia.

REFERENCES

1. Fingerhut LA, Cox CS, Warner M. International comparative analysis of injury mortality: findings from the ICE on injury statistics. *Adv Data* 1998; **7**: 1–20.

2. Brochard L, Roudot-Thorawal F, Roupie E, *et al.* Tidal volume reduction for prevention of ventilator-induced lung injury in acute respiratory distress syndrome. The Multicenter Trial Group on Tidal reduction in ARDS. *Am J Respir Crit Care Med* 1998; **158**: 1831–8.

3. Brower RG, Shanholtz CB, Fessler HE, *et al.* Prospective, randomized, controlled clinical trial comparing traditional versus reduced tidal volume ventilation in acute respiratory distress syndrome patients. *Crit Care Med* 1999; **27**: 1492–8.

4. Stewart TE, Mead MO, Cook DJ, *et al.* Evaluation of a ventilation strategy to prevent barotrauma in patients at high risk for acute respiratory distress syndrome. Pressure- and Volume-limited Ventilation Strategy Group. *N Engl J Med* 1998; **338**: 355–61.

5. Curley MA, Thompson JE, Arnold JH. The effects of early and repeated prone positioning in pediatric patients with acute lung injury. *Chest* 2000; **118**: 156–63.

6. Kornecki A, Frndova H, Coates AL, Shemie SD. A randomized trial of prolonged prone positioning in children with acute respiratory failure. *Chest* 2001; **119**: 211–18.

7. Arnold JH, Hanson JH, Toro-Figuero LO, *et al.* Prospective, randomized comparison of high-frequency oscillatory ventilation and conventional mechanical ventilation in pediatric respiratory failure. *Crit Care Med* 1994; **22**: 1530–9.

8. HIFI Study Group: High-frequency oscillatory ventilation compared with conventional mechanical ventilation in the treatment of respiratory failure in preterm infants. *N Engl J Med* 1989; **320**: 88–93.

9. Jobe AH. Pulmonary surfactant therapy. *N Engl J Med* 1993; **328**: 861–8.

10. Lopez-Herce J, de Lucas N, Carrillo A, *et al.* Surfactant treatment for acute respiratory distress syndrome. *Arch Dis Child* 1999; **80**: 248–52.

11. Anzueto A, Baughman RP, Guntupalli KK, *et al.* Aerosolized surfactant in adults with sepsis-induced acute respiratory distress syndrome. Exosurf Acute Respiratory Distress Syndrome Sepsis Study Group. *N Engl J Med* 1996; **334**: 1417–21.

12. Gregory TJ, Steinberg KP, Spragg R, *et al.* Bovine surfactant therapy for patients with acute respiratory distress syndrome. *Am J Respir Crit Care Med* 1997; **155**: 1309–15.

13. Dellinger RP. Inhaled nitric oxide in acute lung injury and acute respiratory distress syndrome. Inability to translate physiologic benefit to clinical outcome benefit in adult clinical trials. *Intensive Care Med* 1999; **25**: 881–3.

14. Day RW, Allen EM, Witte MK. A randomized, controlled study of the 1-hour and 24-hour effects of inhaled nitric oxide therapy in children with acute hypoxemic respiratory failure. *Chest* 1997; **112**: 1324–31.

15. Dobyns EL, Cornfield DN, Anas NG, *et al.* Multicenter randomized controlled trial of the effects of inhaled nitric oxide therapy on gas exchange in children with acute hypoxemic respiratory failure. *J Pediatr* 1999; **134**: 406–12.

16. Lundin S, Mang H, Smithies M, *et al.* Inhalation of nitric oxide in acute lung injury: results of a European multicenter study. The European Study Group of Inhaled Nitric Oxide. *Intensive Care Med* 1999; **25**: 911–19.

17. Moler FW, Custer JR, Bartlett RH, *et al.* Extracorporeal life support for severe pediatric respiratory failure: an updated experience 1991–1993. *Pediatr* 1994; **124**: 875–80.

18. Swaniker F, Kolla S, Moler F, *et al.* Extracorporeal life support outcome for 128 pediatric patients with respiratory failure. *J Pediatr Surg* 2000; **35**: 197–202.

19. Vats A, Pettignano R, Culler S, Wright J. Cost of extracorporeal life support in pediatric patients with acute respiratory failure. *Crit Care Med* 1998; **26**: 1587–92.

20. Hirschl RB, Conrad S, Kaiser R, *et al.* Partial liquid ventilation in adult patients with ARDS: a multicenter phase I-II trial. Adult PLV Study Group. *Ann Surg* 1998; **228**: 692–700.

21. Bourchier D, Dawson KP, Fergusson DM. Humidification in viral croup: A controlled trial. *Aust Paediatr J* 1984; **20**: 289–91.

22. Super DM, Cartelli NA, Brooks LJ, *et al.* A prospective randomized double-blind study to evaluate the effect of dexamethasone in acute laryngotracheitis. *J Pediatr* 1989; **115**: 323–9.

23. Klassen TP, Feldman ME, Watters LK, *et al.* Nebulized budesonide for children with mild-to-moderate croup. *N Engl J Med* 1994; **331**: 285–9.

24. Kelley PB, Simon JE. Racemic epinephrine use in croup and disposition. *Am J Emerg Med* 1992; **10**: 181–3.

25. Prendergast M, Jones JS, Hartman D. Racemic epinephrine in the treatment of laryngotracheitis: can we identify children for outpatient therapy? *Am J Emerg Med* 1994; **12**: 613–16.

26. Schuller DE, Birck HG. The safety of intubation in croup and epiglottitis: an eight-year follow-up. *Laryngoscope* 1975; **85**: 33–46.

27. Zulliger JJ, Schuller DE, Beach TP, *et al.* Assessment of intubation in croup and epiglottitis. *Ann Otol Rhinol Laryngol* 1982; **91**: 403–6.

28. Black R, Johnson D. Bronchoscopic removal of aspirated foreign bodies in children. *J Pediatr Surg* 1994; **29**: 682–4.

29. Halfaer MA, Nichols DG, Rogers MC. Lower airway disease: bronchiolitis and asthma. In: Rogers M, Nichols D eds. *Textbook of Pediatric Intensive Care*, 3rd ed. Baltimore MD: Williams and Wilkins, 1996; 127–64.

30. Gergen PJ, Mullally DI, Evans R. National survey of prevalence of asthma among children in the United States, 1976–1980. *Pediatrics* 1988; **81**: 1–7.

31. McFadden ER Jr, Kiser R, DeGroot WJ. Acute bronchial asthma. Relations between clinical and physiologic manifestations. *N Engl J Med* 1973; **288**: 221–5.

32. Rebuck AS, Pengelly LD. Development of pulsus paradoxus in the presence of airways obstruction. *N Engl J Med* 1973; **288**: 66–9.

33. Pierson RN Jr, Grieco MH. Pulmonary blood volume in asthma. *J Appl Physiol* 1972; **32**: 391–6.

34. Wright RO, Steele DW, Santucci KA, *et al.* Continuous, noninvasive measurement of pulsus paradoxus in patients with acute asthma. *Arch Pediatr Adolesc Med* 1996; **150**: 914–18.

35. Ibsen LM, Bratton SL. Current therapies for severe asthma exacerbations in children. *New Horiz* 1999; **7**: 312–15.

36. Bisgaard H. Delivery of inhaled medication to children. *J Asthma* 1997; **34**: 443–67.

37. Rebuck AS, Chapman KR, Abboud R, *et al.* Nebulized anticholinergic and sympathomimetic treatment of asthma and chronic obstructive airways disease in the emergency room. *Am J Med* 1987; **82**: 59–64.

38. Yung M, South M. Randomized controlled trial of aminophylline for severe acute asthma. *Arch Dis Child* 1998; **79**: 405–10.

39. Ciarallo L, Sauer AH, Shannon MW. Intravenous magnesium therapy for moderate to severe pediatric asthma: results of a randomized, placebo-controlled trial. *J Pediatr* 1996; **129**: 809–14.

40. Monem GF, Kissoon N, DeNicola L. Use of magnesium sulfate in asthma in childhood. *Pediatric Ann* 1996; **136**: 139–44.

41. Curtis JL, Mahlmeister M, Fink JB, *et al.* Helium-oxygen gas therapy. Use and availability for the

emergency treatment of inoperable airway obstruction. *Chest* 1986; **90**: 455–7.

42. Rodeberg DA, Easter AJ, Washam MA, *et al.* Use of a helium-oxygen mixture in the treatment of postextubation stridor in pediatric patients with burns. *J Burn Care Rehabil* 1995; **16**: 476–80.

43. Madison JM, Irwin RS. Heliox for asthma. A trial balloon. *Chest* 1995; **107**: 597–8.

44. O'Rourke PP, Crone RK. Halothane in status asthmaticus. *Crit Care Med* 1982; **10**: 341–3.

45. Williams TJ, Tuxen DV, Scheinkestel CD, *et al.* Risk factors for morbidity in mechanically ventilated patients with acute severe asthma. *Am Rev Respir Dis* 1992; **146**: 607–15.

46. Tuxen DV, Lane S. The effects of ventilatory pattern on hyperinflation, airway pressures, and circulation in mechanical ventilation of patients with severe airflow obstruction. *Am Rev Respir Dis* 1987; **136**: 872–9.

47. Wetzel RC. Pressure-support ventilation in children with severe asthma. *Crit Care Med* 1996; **24**: 1603–5.

48. Rock MJ, Reyes de la Rocha S, L'Hommedieu CS, Truemper E. Use of ketamine in asthmatic children to treat respiratory failure refractory to conventional therapy. *Crit Care Med* 1986; **14**: 514–16.

49. Oren RE, Rasool NA, Rubinstein EH. Effect of ketamine on cerebral cortical blood flow and metabolism in rabbits. *Stroke* 1987; **18**: 441–4.

50. Ginsberg MD, Myers RE, McDonagh BF. Experimental carbon monoxide encephalopathy in the primate. II. Clinical aspects, neuropathology, and physiologic correlation. *Arch Neurol* 1974; **30**: 209–16.

51. Stone HH. Pulmonary burns in children. *J Pediatr Surg* 1979; **14**: 48–52.

52. Clark WR, Bonaventura M, Myers W. Smoke inhalation and airway management at a regional burn unit: 1974–1983. Part I: Diagnosis and consequences of smoke inhalation. *J Burn Care Rehabil* 1989; **10**: 52–62.

53. Pruitt BA Jr, Cioffi WG, Shimazu T, *et al.* Evaluation and management of patients with inhalation injury. *J Trauma* 1990; **30**: S63–8.

54. Haponik EF, Crapo RO, Herndon DN, *et al.* Smoke inhalation. *Am Rev Respir Dis* 1988; **138**: 1060–3.

55. Leads from the MMWR. Progress toward achieving the national objectives for injury prevention and control. *JAMA* 1988; **259**: 2069, 2073, 2076–7.

56. Guidelines for cardiopulmonary resuscitation and emergency cardiac care. Emergency Cardiac Care Committee and Subcommittees, American Heart Association. Part IV. Special resuscitation situations. *JAMA* 1992; **268**: 2242–50.

57. American Academy of Pediatrics Committee on Injury, Violence, and Poison Prevention. Prevention of drowning in infants, children, and adolescents. *Pediatrics* 2003; **112**: 437–9.

58. Denny FW, Collier AM, Henderson FW, Clyde WA Jr. The epidemiology of bronchiolitis. *Pediatr Res* 1977; **11**: 234–6.

59. Sigurs N. Epidemiologic and clinical evidence of a respiratory syncytial virus-reactive airway disease link. *Am J Respir Crit Care Med* 2001; **163**: S2–6.

60. Welliver RC. Immunology of respiratory syncytial virus infection: eosinophils, cytokines, chemokines and asthma. *Pediatr Infect Dis J* 2000; **19**: 780–3.

61. Kneyber MCJ, Steyerberg EW, de Groot R, Moll HA. Long-term effects of respiratory syncytial virus (RSV) bronchiolitis in infants and young children: a quantitative review. *Acta Paediatr* 2000; **89**: 654–60.

62. Bruhn FW, Mokrohisky ST, McIntosh K. Apnea associated with respiratory syncytial virus infection in young infants. *J Pediatr* 1977; **90**: 382–6.

63. Anas N, Boettrich C, Hall CB, Brooks JG. The association of apnea and respiratory syncytial virus infection in infants. *J Pediatr* 1982; **101**: 65–8.

64. Kellner JD, Ohlsson A, Gadomski AM, *et al.* Bronchodilators for bronchiolitis. *The Cochrane Database Syst Rev* 2000; (**2**): CD001266.

65. Abul-Ainine A, Luyt D. Short term effects of adrenaline in bronchiolitis: a randomised controlled trial. *Arch Dis Child* 2002; **86**: 276–9.

66. Kristjansson S, Lodrup Carlsen KC, Wennergren G, *et al.* Nebulised racemic adrenaline in the treatment of acute bronchiolitis in infants and toddlers. *Arch Dis Child* 1993; **69**: 650–4.

67. Hariprakash S, Alexander J, Carroll W, *et al.* Randomized controlled trial of nebulized adrenaline in acute bronchiolitis. *Pediatr Allergy Immunol* 2003; **14**: 134–9.

68. Garrison MM, Christakis DA, Harvey E, *et al.* Systemic corticosteroids in infant bronchiolitis: A meta-analysis. *Pediatrics* 2000; **105**: E44.

69. Law BJ, Wang EE, MacDonald N, *et al.* Does ribavirin impact on the hospital course of children with respiratory syncytial virus (RSV) infection? An analysis using the pediatric investigators

collaborative network on infections in Canada (PICNIC) RSV database. *Pediatrics* 1997; **99**: E7.

70. Rodriguez WJ, Gruber WC, Groothuis JR, *et al.* Respiratory syncytial virus immune globulin treatment of RSV lower respiratory tract infection in previously healthy children. *Pediatrics* 1997; **100**: 937–42.

71. Hollman G, Shen G, Zeng L, *et al.* Helium-oxygen improves Clinical Asthma Scores in children with acute bronchiolitis. *Crit Care Med* 1998; **26**: 1731–6.

72. Martinon-Torres F, Rodriguez-Nunez A, Martinon-Sanchez JM. Heliox therapy in infants with acute bronchiolitis. *Pediatrics* 2002; **109**: 68–73.

73. The Impact-RSV Study Group. Palivizumab, a humanized respiratory syncytial virus monoclonal antibody, reduces hospitalization from respiratory syncytial virus infection in high-risk infants. *Pediatrics* 1998; **102**: 531–7.

74. Venkatesh VC, Katzberg HD. Glucocorticoid regulation of epithelial sodium channel genes in human fetal lung. *Am J Physiol* 1997; **273**: L227–33.

75. Saunders RA, Milner AD. Pulmonary pressure/volume relationships during the last phase of delivery and the first postnatal breaths in human subjects. *J Pediatr* 1978; **93**: 667–73.

76. Clark RH. Gibbs RS, Schrag S, Schuchat A. Perinatal infections due to group B streptococci. *Obstet Gynecol* 2004; **104**: 1062–76.

77. Meadow W, Lee G, Lin K, Lantos J. Changes in mortality for extremely low birth weight infants in the 1990s: implications for treatment decisions and resource use. *Pediatrics* 2004; **113**: 1223–9.

78. Lukacs SL, Schoendorf KC, Schuchat A. Trends in sepsis-related neonatal mortality in the United States, 1985–1998. *Pediatr Infect Dis J* 2004; **23**: 599–603.

79. Fraser J, Walls M, McGuire W. Respiratory complications of preterm birth. *BMJ* 2004; **329**: 962–5.

80. Dinwiddie R. Congenital upper airway obstruction. *Paediatr Respir Rev* 2004; **5**: 17–24.

81. Flamant C, Nolent P, Hallalel F, *et al.* Evolution of extracorporeal membrane oxygenation (ECMO) in neonatal acute respiratory failure, fifteen years of experience. *Arch Pediatr* 2004; **11**: 308–14.

82. Carlo WA, Prince LS, St John EB, Ambalavanan N. Care of very low birth weight infants with respiratory distress syndrome: an evidence-based review. *Minerva Pediatr* 2004; **56**: 373–80.

83. deMello DE. Pulmonary pathology. *Semin Neonatol* 2004; **9**: 311–29.

84. Langston C. Langston C. New concepts in the pathology of congenital lung malformations. *Semin Pediatr Surg* 2003; **12**: 17–37.

85. Sadler TW. Respiratory system. In: *Longman's Medical Embryology*. Baltimore: Williams and Wilkins, 1990: 228–37.

86. Jobe AH, Ikegami M. Mechanisms initiating lung injury in the preterm. *Early Hum Dev* 1998; **53**: 81–94.

87. Olver RE, Walters DV, Wilson S. Developmental regulation of lung liquid transport. *Annu Rev Physiol* 2004; **66**: 77–101.

88. Pitkanen O. Lung epithelial ion transport in neonatal lung disease. *Biol Neonate* 2001; **80**(Suppl 1): 14–17.

89. Carlo WA, Martin RJ, Bruce EN, *et al.* Alae nasi activation (nasal flaring) decreases nasal resistance in preterm infants. *Pediatrics* 1983; **72**: 338–43.

90. Kinsella JP, Abman SH. Recent developments in the pathophysiology and treatment of persistent pulmonary hypertension of the newborn. *J Pediatr* 1995; **126**: 853–64.

91. Evans N, Kluckow M, Currie A. Range of echocardiographic findings in term and near term babies with high oxygen requirements. *Arch Dis Child Fetal Neonatal Ed* 1998; **78**: F105–11.

92. Fox WW, Duara S. Persistent pulmonary hypertension in the neonate: diagnosis and management. *J Pediatr* 1983; **103**: 505–14.

93. Evans N, Kluckow M. Early determinants of right and left ventricular output in ventilated preterm infants. *Arch Dis Child Fetal Neonatal Ed* 1996; **74**: F88–94.

94. Su BH, Peng CT, Tsai CH. Persistent pulmonary hypertension of the newborn: echocardiographic assessment. *Acta Paediatr Taiwan* 2001; **42**: 218–23.

95. Skinner JR, Hunter S, Hey E. Haemodynamic features at presentation in persistent pulmonary hypertension of the newborn and outcome. *Arch Dis Child Fetal Neonatal Ed* 1996; **74**: F26–32.

96. Kinsella JP, Truog WE, Walsh WF, *et al.* Randomized, multicenter trial of inhaled nitric oxide and high-frequency oscillatory ventilation in severe, persistent pulmonary hypertension of the newborn. *J Pediatr* 1997; **131**: 55–62.

97. Clark RH, Yoder BA, Sell MS. Prospective, randomized comparison of high-frequency oscillation and conventional ventilation in candidates for extracorporeal membrane oxygenation. *J Pediatr* 1994; **124**: 447–54.

98. Finer NN. Inhaled nitric oxide in neonates. *Arch Dis Child Fetal Neonatal Ed*. 1997; **77**: F81–4.

99. Roberts JD, Jr, Fineman JR, Morin FC, 3rd, *et al.* Inhaled nitric oxide and persistent pulmonary hypertension of the newborn. The Inhaled Nitric Oxide Study Group. *N Engl J Med* 1997; **336**: 605–10.

100. Clark RH, Kueser TJ, Walker MW. Low-dose nitric oxide therapy for persistent pulmonary hypertension of the newborn. Clinical Inhaled Nitric Oxide Research Group. *N Engl J Med* 2000; **342**: 469–74.

101. The Neonatal Inhaled Nitric Oxide Study Group. Inhaled nitric oxide in full-term and nearly full-term infants with hypoxic respiratory failure. *N Engl J Med* 1997; **336**: 597–604.

102. UK collaborative randomized trial of neonatal extracorporeal membrane oxygenation. UK Collaborative ECMO Trail Group. *Lancet* 1996; **348**: 75–82.

103. Kim ES, Stolar CJ. ECMO in the newborn. *Am J Perinatol* 2000; **17**: 345–56.

104. Eichenwald EC, Aina A, Stark AR. Apnea frequently persists beyond term gestation in infants delivered at 24–28 weeks. *Pediatrics* 1997; **100**: 354–9.

105. Cote A, Hum C, Brouillette RT, Themens M. Frequency and timing of recurrent events in infants using home cardio respiratory monitors. *J Pediatr* 1998; **132**: 783–9.

106. Gerhardt T, Bancalari E. Apnea of prematurity: I. Lung function and regulation of breathing. *Pediatrics* 1984; **74**: 58–62.

107. Holditch-Davis D, Edwards LJ, Wigger MC. Pathologic apnea and brief respiratory pauses in preterm infants: relation to sleep state. *Nurs Res* 1994; **43**: 293–300.

108. Lehtonen L, Martin RJ. Ontogeny of sleep and awake states in relation to breathing in preterm infants. *Semin Neonatol* 2004; **9**: 229–38.

109. Theobald K, Botwinski C, Albanna S, McWilliam P. Apnea of prematurity: diagnosis, implications for care, and pharmacologic management. *Neonatal Netw* 2000; **19**: 17–24.

110. Thach BT, Stark AR. Spontaneous neck flexion and airway obstruction during apneic spells in preterm infants. *J Pediatr* 1979; **94**: 275–81.

111. Abu-Osba YK, Brouillette RT, Wilson SL, Thach BT. Breathing pattern and transcutaneous oxygen tension during motor activity in preterm infants. *Am Rev Respir Dis* 1982; **125**: 382–7.

112. Miller MJ, Martin RJ. Apnea of prematurity. *Clin Perinatol* 1992; **19**: 789–8.

113. Bhatt-Mehta V, Schumacher RE. Treatment of apnea of prematurity. *Paediatr Drugs* 2003; **5**: 195–210.

114. Lemyre B, Davis PG, de Paoli AG. Nasal intermittent positive pressure ventilation (NIPPV) versus nasal continuous positive airway pressure (NCPAP) for apnea of prematurity. *Cochrane Database Syst Rev* 2002; **1**: CD002272.

115. Baird TM. Clinical correlates, natural history and outcome of neonatal apnea. *Semin Neonatol* 2004; **9**: 205–11.

116. Wiswell TE. Advances in the treatment of the meconium aspiration syndrome. *Acta Paediatr Suppl* 2001; **90**: 28–30.

117. Yoder BA, Kirsch EA, Barth WH, Gordon MC. Changing obstetric practices associated with decreasing incidence of meconium aspiration syndrome. *Obstet Gynecol* 2002; **99**: 731–9.

118. Ghidini A, Spong CY. Severe meconium aspiration syndrome is not caused by aspiration of meconium. *Am J Obstet Gynecol* 2001; **185**: 931–8.

119. Hageman JR, Caplan MS. An introduction to the structure and function of inflammatory mediators for clinicians. *Clin Perinatol* 1995; **22**: 251–61.

120. Moses D, Holm BA, Spitale P, *et al.* Inhibition of pulmonary surfactant function by meconium. *Am J Obstet Gynecol* 1991; **164**: 477–81.

121. Cleary GM, Antunes MJ, Ciesielka DA, *et al.* Exudative lung injury is associated with decreased levels of surfactant proteins in a rat model of meconium aspiration. *Pediatrics* 1997; **100**: 998–1003.

122. Dargaville PA, South M, McDougall PN. Surfactant and surfactant inhibitors in meconium aspiration syndrome. *J Pediatr* 2001; **138**: 113–15.

123. Findlay RD, Taeusch HW, Walther FJ. Surfactant replacement therapy for meconium aspiration syndrome. *Pediatrics* 1996; **97**: 48–52.

124. Yeh TF, Harris V, Srinivasan G, Lilien L *et al.* Roentgenographic findings in infants with meconium aspiration syndrome. *JAMA* 1979; **242**: 60–3.

125. Hofmeyr GJ. Amnioinfusion for meconium-stained liquor in labor (Cochrane review). *Cochrane Database Syst Rev* 2002; **1**: CD000014.

126. Cialone PR, Sherer DM, Ryan RM, *et al.* Amnioinfusion during labor complicated by particulate meconium stained amniotic fluid

decreases neonatal morbidity. *Am J Obstet Gynecol* 1994; **170**: 842–9.

127. Macri CJ, Schrimmer DB, Leung A, *et al.* Prophylactic amnioinfusion improves outcome of pregnancy complicated by thick meconium and oligohydramnios. *Am J Obstet Gynecol* 1992; **167**: 117–21.

128. Carson BS, Losey RW, Bowes Jr WA, Simmons MA. Combined obstetric and pediatric approach to prevent meconium aspiration syndrome. *Am J Obstet Gynecol* 1976; **126**: 712–15.

129. Wiswell TE, Gannon CM, Jacob J, *et al.* Delivery room management of the apparently vigorous meconium-stained neonate: results of the multicenter, international collaborative trial. *Pediatrics* 2000; **105**: 1–7.

130. Vain NE, Szyld EG, Prudent LM, *et al.* Oropharyngeal and nasopharyngeal suctioning of meconium-stained neonates before delivery of their shoulders: multicenter, randomized controlled trial. *Lancet* 2004; **364**: 597–602.

131. Locus P, Yeomans E, Crosby U. Efficacy of bulb versus DeLee suction at deliveries complicated by meconium stained amniotic fluid. *Am J Perinatol* 1990; **7**: 87–91.

132. Halliday HL. Endotracheal intubation at birth for preventing morbidity and mortality in vigorous, meconium-stained infants born at term. *Cochrane Database Syst Rev* 2001; **1**: CD000500.

133. Hachey WE, Eyal FG, Curtet-Eyal NL, Kellum FE. High-frequency oscillatory ventilation versus conventional ventilation in a piglet model of early meconium aspiration. *Crit Care Med* 1998; **26**: 556–61.

134. Lotze A, Mitchell BR, Bulas DI, *et al.* Multicenter study of surfactant use in the treatment of term infants with severe respiratory failure. *J Pediatr* 1998; **132**: 40–7.

135. Lyra JC, Mascaretti RS, Precioso AR, *et al.* Different doses of exogenous surfactant for treatment of meconium aspiration syndrome in newborn rabbits. *Rev Hosp Clin Fac Med Sao Paulo* 2004; **59**: 104–12.

136. Herting E, Rauprich P, Stichtenoth G, *et al.* Resistance of different surfactant preparations to inactivation by meconium. *Pediatr Res* 2001; **50**: 44–9.

137. Lam BCC, Yeung CY. Surfactant lavage for meconium aspiration syndrome: a pilot study. *Pediatrics* 1999; **103**: 1014–18.

138. Wiswell TE, Knight GR, Finer NN, *et al.* A multicenter, randomized, controlled trial comparing Surfaxin (lucinactant) lavage with standard care for treatment of meconium aspiration syndrome. *Pediatrics* 2002; **109**: 1081–7.

139. Kinsella JP. Meconium aspiration syndrome: is surfactant lavage the answer? *Am J Respir Crit Care Med* 2003; **168**: 413–14.

140. Rais-Bahrami KRO, Seale WR, Short BL. Effect of nitric oxide in meconium aspiration syndrome after treatment with surfactant. *Crit Care Med* 1997; **25**: 1744–7.

141. Kinsella JP, Neish SR, Shaffer E, Abman SH. Low-dose inhalation nitric oxide in persistent pulmonary hypertension of the newborn. *Lancet* 1992; **340**: 819–20.

142. Perelman RH, Farrell PM. Analysis of causes of neonatal death in the United States with specific emphasis on fatal hyaline membrane disease. *Pediatrics* 1982; **70**: 570–5.

143. Malloy MH, Hartford RB, Kleinman JC. Trends in mortality caused by respiratory distress syndrome in the United States, 1969–83. *Am J Public Health* 1987; **77**: 1511–14.

144. Farrell PM, Wood R. Epidemiology of hyaline membrane disease in the United States: analysis of national mortality statistics. *Pediatrics* 1976; **58**: 167–76.

145. Van Golde LM, Batenburg JJ, Robertson B. The pulmonary surfactant system: biochemical aspects and functional significance. *Physiol Rev* 1988; **68**: 374–455.

146. Creuwels LA, van Golde LM, Haagsman HP. The pulmonary surfactant system: biochemical and clinical aspects. *Lung* 1997; **175**: 1–39.

147. Jobe AH, Ikegami M. Biology of surfactant. *Clin Perinatol* 2001; **28**: 655–69.

148. Ikegami M, Jobe AH. Surfactant protein metabolism in vivo. *Biochim Biophys Acta* 1998; **1408**: 218–25.

149. Veldhuizen R, Possmayer F. Phospholipid metabolism in lung surfactant. *Subcell Biochem* 2004; **37**: 359–88.

150. Avery ME, Mead J. Surface properties in relation to atelectasis and hyaline membrane disease. *Am J Dis Child* 1959; **97**: 517–23.

151. Rogers WS, Gruenwald P. Hyaline membranes in the lungs of premature infants. *Am J Obstet Gynecol* 1956; **71**: 9–15.

152. Fujiwara T, Adams FH. Surfactant for hyaline membrane disease. *Pediatrics* 1980; **66**: 795–8.

153. Corbet AJ, Long WA, Murphy DJ, *et al.* Reduced mortality in small premature infants treated at birth with a single dose of synthetic surfactant. *J Paediatr Child Health* 1991; **27**: 245–9.

154. Bose C, Corbet A, Bose G, *et al.* Improved outcome at 28 days of age for very low birth weight infants treated with a single dose of a synthetic surfactant. *J Pediatr* 1990; **117**: 947–53.

155. Long W, Corbet A, Cotton R, *et al.* A controlled trial of synthetic surfactant in infants weighing 1250 g or more with respiratory distress syndrome. The American Exosurf Neonatal Study Group I, and the Canadian Exosurf Neonatal Study Group. *N Engl J Med* 1991; **325**: 1696–703.

156. Goldsmith LS, Greenspan JS, Rubenstein SD, *et al.* Immediate improvement in lung volume after exogenous surfactant: alveolar recruitment versus increased distention. *J Pediatr* 1991; **119**: 424–8.

157. Kelly E, Bryan H, Possmayer F, *et al.* Compliance of the respiratory system in newborn infants pre- and post surfactant replacement therapy. *Pediatr Pulmonol* 1993; **15**: 225–30.

158. Rodriguez RJ. Management of respiratory distress syndrome: an update. *Respir Care* 2003; **48**: 279–86.

159. Dunn MS, Reilly MC. Approaches to the initial respiratory management of preterm neonates. *Paediatr Respir Rev* 2003; **4**: 2–8.

160. Egberts J, de Winter JP, Sedin G, *et al.* Comparison of prophylaxis and rescue treatment with Curosurf in neonates less than 30 weeks' gestation: a randomized trial. *Pediatrics* 1993; **92**: 768–74.

161. American Academy of Pediatrics. Committee on Fetus and Newborn. Surfactant replacement therapy for respiratory distress syndrome. *Pediatrics* 1999; **103**: 684–5.

162. Knight DB, Liggins GC, Wealthall SR. A randomised, controlled trial of ante partum thyrotropin-releasing hormone and betamethasone in the prevention of respiratory disease in preterm infants. *Am J Obstet Gynecol* 1994; **1**: 11–16.

163. Moraga FA, Riquelme RA, Lopez AA, *et al.* Maternal administration of glucocorticoid and thyrotropin-releasing hormone enhances fetal lung maturation in undisturbed preterm lambs. *Am J Obstet Gynecol* 1994; **3**: 729–34.

164. Jobe AH, Mitchell BR, Gunkel JH. Beneficial effects of the combined use of prenatal corticosteroids and postnatal surfactant on preterm infants. *Am J Obstet Gynecol* 1993; **168**: 508–13.

165. Maher J, Goldenberg RL. Outcomes of very-low-birth-weight infants after maternal corticosteroid therapy before 28 weeks' gestation. *Am J Obstet Gynecol* 1993; **169**: 1363–4.

166. Weintraub AS, Holzman IR. Neonatal care of infants with head and neck anomalies. *Otolaryngol Clin North Am* 2000; **33**: 1171–89.

167. Brown OE, Pownell P, Manning SC. Choanal atresia: a new anatomic classification and clinical management applications. *Laryngoscope* 1996; **106**: 97–101.

168. Leraillez J. Neonatal nasal obstruction. *Arch Pediatr* 2001; **8**: 214–20.

169. Keller JL, Kacker A. Choanal atresia, CHARGE association, and congenital nasal stenosis. *Otolaryngol Clin North Am* 2000; **33**: 1343–51.

170. Nanni L, Ming JE, Du Y, *et al.* SHH mutation is associated with solitary median maxillary central incisor: a study of 13 patients and review of the literature. *Am J Med Genet* 2001; **102**: 1–10.

171. Faust RA, Phillips CD. Assessment of congenital bony nasal obstruction by 3-dimensional CT volume rendering. *Int J Pediatr Otorhinolaryngol* 2001; **61**: 71–5.

172. Deutsch E, Kaufman M, Eilon A. Transnasal endoscopic management of choanal atresia. *Int J Pediatr Otorhinolaryngol* 1997; **40**: 19–26.

173. Friedman NR, Mitchell RB, Bailey CM, *et al.* Management and outcome of choanal atresia correction. *Int J Pediatr Otorhinolaryngol* 2000; **52**: 45–51.

174. Prasad M, Ward RF, April MM, *et al.* Topical Mitomycin as an adjunct to choanal atresia repair. *Arch Otolaryngol Head Neck Surg* 2002; **128**: 398–400.

175. Spitz L. Esophageal atresia: past, present, and future. *J Pediatr Surg* 1996; **31**: 19–25.

176. Engum SA, Grosfeld JL, West KW, *et al.* Analysis of morbidity and mortality in 227 cases of esophageal atresia and/or tracheoesophageal fistula over two decades. *Arch Surg* 1995; **130**: 502–8.

177. Moore KL. The respiratory system. In: Moore KL, ed. *The Developing Human: Clinically Oriented Embryology*, 4th ed. Philadelphia: Saunders, 1988:207–10.

178. Diez-Pardo JA, Baoquan Q, Navarro C, Tovar JA. A new rodent experimental model of esophageal atresia and tracheoesophageal fistula: preliminary report. *J Pediatr Surg* 1996; **31**: 498–502.

179. Felix JF, Keijzer R, van Dooren MF, *et al.* Genetics and developmental biology of oesophageal atresia and tracheo-oesophageal fistula: lessons from mice

relevant for paediatric surgeons. *Pediatr Surg Int* 2004; **20**: 731–6.

180. German JC, Mahour GH, Woolley MM. Esophageal atresia and associated anomalies. *J Pediatr Surg* 1976; **11**: 299–306.

181. Poenaru D, Laberge JM, Neilson IR, Guttman FM. A new prognostic classification for esophageal atresia. *Surgery* 1993; **113**: 426–32.

182. Chittmittrapap S, Spitz L, Kiely EM, Brereton RJ. Oesophageal atresia and associated anomalies. *Arch Dis Child* 1989; **64**: 364–8.

183. Rokitansky A, Kolankaya A, Bichler B, *et al.* Analysis of 309 cases of esophageal atresia for associated congenital malformations. *Am J Perinatol* 1994; **11**: 123–8.

184. Kallen K, Mastroiacovo P, Castilla EE, *et al.* VATER non-random association of congenital malformations: study based on data from four malformation registers. *Am J Med Genet* 2001; **101**: 26–32.

185. Karnak I, Senocak ME, Hicsonmez A. The diagnosis and treatment of H-type tracheoesophageal fistula. *J Pediatr Surg* 1997; **2**: 1670–4.

186. Vijayaraghavan SB. Antenatal diagnosis of esophageal atresia with tracheoesophageal fistula. *J Ultrasound Med* 1996; **15**: 417–19.

187. Ratan SK, Varshney A, Mullick S, *et al.* Evaluation of neonates with esophageal atresia using chest CT scan. *Pediatr Surg Int* 2004; **27**: 757–61.

188. Dutta HK, Rajani M, Bhatnagar V. Cineradiographic evaluation of postoperative patients with esophageal atresia and tracheoesophageal fistula. *Pediatr Surg Int* 2000; **16**: 322–5.

189. Sillen U, Hagberg S, Rubenson A, Werkmaster K. Management of esophageal atresia: review of 16 years' experience. *J Pediatr Surg* 1988; **23**: 805–9.

190. Erdogan E, Emir H, Eroglu E, *et al.* Esophageal replacement using the colon: a 15-year review. *Pediatr Surg Int* 2000; **16**: 546–9.

191. Kovesi T, Rubin S. Long-term complications of congenital esophageal atresia and/or tracheoesophageal fistula. *Chest* 2004; **126**: 915–25.

192. Michaud L, Guimber D, Sfeir R, *et al.* Anastomotic stenosis after surgical treatment of esophageal atresia: frequency, risk factors and effectiveness of esophageal dilatations. *Arch Pediatr* 2001; **8**: 268–74.

193. Mani H, Suarez E, Stocker JY. The morphologic spectrum of infantile lobar emphysema: a study of 33 cases. *Paediatr Respir Rev* 2004; **5**(Suppl A): S313–20.

194. Tander B, Yalcin M, Yilmaz B, *et al.* Congenital lobar emphysema: a clinicopathologic evaluation of 14 cases. *Eur J Pediatr Surg* 2003; **13**: 108–11.

195. Hishitani T, Ogawa K, Hoshino K, *et al.* Lobar emphysema due to ductus arteriosus compressing right upper bronchus in an infant with congenital heart disease. *Ann Thorac Surg* 2003; **75**: 1308–10.

196. Aslan AT, Yalcin E, Ozcelik U, *et al.* Foreign-body aspiration mimicking congenital lobar emphysema in a forty-eight-day-old girl. *Pediatr Pulmonol* 2005; **39**: 189–91.

197. Ankermann T, Oppermann HC, Engler S, *et al.* Congenital masses of the lung, cystic adenomatoid malformation versus congenital lobar emphysema: prenatal diagnosis and implications for postnatal treatment. *J Ultrasound Med* 2004; **23**: 1379–84.

198. Schwartz MZ, Ramachandran P. Congenital malformations of the lung and mediastinum – a quarter century of experience from a single institution. *J Pediatr Surg* 1997; **32**: 44–7.

199. Ozcelik U, Gocmen A, Kiper N, *et al.* Congenital lobar emphysema: evaluation and long-term follow-up of thirty cases at a single center. *Pediatr Pulmonol* 2003; **35**: 384–91.

200. Ayed AK, Owayed A. Pulmonary resection in infants for congenital pulmonary malformation. *Chest* 2003; **124**: 98–101.

201. Langham MR Jr, Kays DW, Ledbetter DJ. Congenital diaphragmatic hernia. Epidemiology and outcome. *Clin Perinatol* 1996; **23**: 671–88.

202. Enns GM, Cox VA, Goldstein RB, *et al.* Congenital diaphragmatic defects and associated syndromes, malformations, and chromosome anomalies: a retrospective study of 60 patients and literature review. *Am J Med Genet* 1998; **79**: 215–25.

203. Nobuhara KK, Wilson JM. Pathophysiology of congenital diaphragmatic hernia. *Semin Pediatr Surg* 1996; **5**: 234–42.

204. O'Toole SJ, Irish MS, Holm BA. Pulmonary vascular abnormalities in congenital diaphragmatic hernia. *Clin Perinatol* 1996; **23**: 781–94.

205. Wilcox DT, Irish MS, Holm BA, Glick PL. Prenatal diagnosis of congenital diaphragmatic hernia with predictors of mortality. *Clin Perinatol* 1996; **23**: 701–9.

206. Nadroo AM, Levshina R, Tugertimur A, *et al.* Congenital diaphragmatic hernia: atypical presentation *J Perinat Med* 1999; **27**: 276–8.

207. Witters I, Legius E, Moerman P, *et al.* Associated malformations and chromosomal anomalies in 42 cases of prenatally diagnosed diaphragmatic hernia. *Am J Med Genet* 2001; **103**: 278–82.

208. Steinhorn RH, Kriesmer PJ, Green TP. Congenital diaphragmatic hernia in Minnesota. Impact of antenatal diagnosis on survival. *Arch Pediatr Adolesc Med* 1994; **148**: 626–31.

209. Doyle NM, Lally KP. The CDH Study Group and advances in the clinical care of the patient with congenital diaphragmatic hernia. *Semin Perinatol* 2004; **28**: 174–84.

210. Clark RH, Hardin WD Jr, Hirschl RB. Current surgical management of congenital diaphragmatic hernia: a report from the Congenital Diaphragmatic Hernia Study Group. *J Pediatr Surg* 1998; **33**: 1004–9.

211. NINOS. Inhaled nitric oxide and hypoxic respiratory failure in infants with congenital diaphragmatic hernia. The Neonatal Inhaled Nitric Oxide Study Group (NINOS). *Pediatrics* 1997; **99**: 838–45.

212. Nobuhara KK, Lund DP, Mitchell J. Long-term outlook for survivors of congenital diaphragmatic hernia. *Clin Perinatol* 1996; **23**: 873–87.

213. Sydorak RM, Harrison MR. Congenital diaphragmatic hernia: advances in prenatal therapy. *Clin Perinatol* 2003; **30**: 465–79.

Index

Note: abbreviations used in the index are explained on pp. xiii–xiv; page numbers in **bold** refer to figures.